MAXILLOFACIAL TRAUMA

& ESTHETIC FACIAL RECONSTRUCTION

MAXILLOFACIAL TRAUMA & ESTHETIC FACIAL RECONSTRUCTION

PETER WARD BOOTH, FDS, FRCS

Consultant Maxillofacial Surgeon
Department of Maxillofacial Surgery
The Queen Victoria Hospital
East Grinstead, West Sussex, United Kingdom

BARRY L. EPPLEY, MD, DMD

Plastic and Maxillofacial Surgeon
Indiana University Health North and West Hospitals
Indianapolis, Indiana, United States of America

RAINER SCHMELZEISEN, MD, DDS

Professor and Chairman
Department of Oral and Maxillofacial Surgery
Albert Ludwigs University and Hospital
Freiburg, Germany

EDITION 2

ELSEVIER

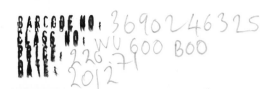
MAXILLOFACIAL TRAUMA AND ESTHETIC FACIAL RECONSTRUCTION   ISBN: 978-1-4377-2420-2
Copyright © 2012, 2003 by Saunders, an imprint of Elsevier Inc.

Notices

Knowledge and best practice in this field are constantly changing. As new research and experience broaden our understanding, changes in research methods, professional practices, or medical treatment may become necessary.

Practitioners and researchers must always rely on their own experience and knowledge in evaluating and using any information, methods, compounds, or experiments described herein. In using such information or methods they should be mindful of their own safety and the safety of others, including parties for whom they have a professional responsibility.

With respect to any drug or pharmaceutical products identified, readers are advised to check the most current information provided (i) on procedures featured or (ii) by the manufacturer of each product to be administered, to verify the recommended dose or formula, the method and duration of administration, and contraindications. It is the responsibility of practitioners, relying on their own experience and knowledge of their patients, to make diagnoses, to determine dosages and the best treatment for each individual patient, and to take all appropriate safety precautions.

To the fullest extent of the law, neither the Publisher nor the authors, contributors, or editors, assume any liability for any injury and/or damage to persons or property as a matter of products liability, negligence or otherwise, or from any use or operation of any methods, products, instructions, or ideas contained in the material herein.

Previous editions copyrighted

Library of Congress Cataloging-in-Publication Data
Maxillofacial trauma and esthetic facial reconstruction / [edited by] Peter Ward Booth, Barry L. Eppley, Rainer Schmelzeisen.—2nd ed.
    p. ; cm.
    Includes bibliographical references and index.
    ISBN 978-1-4377-2420-2 (hardcover : alk. paper)
    I. Ward Booth, Peter.   II. Eppley, Barry L.   III. Schmelzeisen, R. (Rainer)
    [DNLM: 1. Maxillofacial Injuries—surgery. 2. Esthetics. 3. Reconstructive Surgical Procedures—methods.   WU 610]
    LC classification not assigned
    617.9′52—dc23
                                                                    2011031518

Vice President and Publishing Director: Linda Duncan
Acquisitions Editor: John J. Dolan
Developmental Editor: Brian S. Loehr
Publishing Services Manager: Catherine Jackson
Project Manager: Sara Alsup
Design Direction: Teresa McBryan

Printed in China

Last digit is the print number: 9 8 7 6 5 4 3 2 1

Contributors

Khalid Abdel-Galil, BDS (hons), MBBS (Lon), DIC MSc (Lon), FDSRCS (Lon), FRCS (Eng), OMFS
Specialist Registrar
Department of Oral & Maxillofacial Surgery
Leeds Teaching Hospital NHS Trust
Leeds, United Kingdom

Peter Ayliffe, FDS, RCS (Eng), FRCS, OMFS
Department of Maxillofacial Surgery
Great Ormond Street Hospital
London, United Kingdom

Nicholas J. Baker, FDSRCS, FRCS, FRCS (Maxfac)
Consultant Oral and Maxillofacial Surgeon
Department of Oral and Maxillofacial Surgery
Southampton University Hospital NHS Trust
Southampton, United Kingdom

Mark S. Ballard, MBBS, BSc, RAMC
Radiologist Specialist Registrar
Department of Imaging
Brighton and Sussex University Hospitals NHS Trust
Queen Victoria NHS Foundation Trust
Brighton, United Kingdom

Stephen E. Bond, MB, MS, FDSRCS (Eng), FRCS (Ed), FRCS (Ed) (OMFS)
Specialist Registrar
Department of Oral and Maxillofacial Surgery
John Radcliffe Hospital
Oxford, UK

Rudolf R.M. Bos, DMD, PhD
Professor
Department of Oral and Maxillofacial Surgery
University Medical Center Groningen
University of Groningen
Groningen, The Netherlands

Henk J. Busscher
Professor
Department of BioMedical Engineering
University Medical Center Groningen
University of Groningen
Groningen, The Netherlands

Malcolm Cameron, MBBS, BDS, FRCS (Eng), FDSRCS (Eng), FRCS (OMFS)
Department of Oral and Maxillofacial Surgery
Addenbrooke's Hospital
Cambridge University Hospitals NHS Trust
Cambridge, United Kingdom

Alexandra Clarke, DPsych, MSc, BSc (hons), AFBPsS
Professor (Visiting)
Faculty of Applied Science
University of the West of England
Bristol, United Kingdom

Consultant Psychologist
Plastic and Reconstructive Surgery
Royal Free Hospital
London, United Kingdom

Jeremy Collyer, FRCS (Maxfac), FDS
Consultant Oral and Maxillofacial Surgeon
Department of Maxillofacial Surgery
Queen Victoria Hospital
East Grinstead, United Kingdom

John E. Crossman, BSc, MBBS, MD, FRCS (SN)
Consultatnt Neurosurgeon
Department of Neurosurgery
Royal Victoria Infirmary
Newcastle upon Tyne NHS Trust
Newcastle upon Tyne, United Kingdom

Bernard Devauchelle, PhD, MD FRCS (Eng),
    FDSRCS (Eng)
Department of Maxillofacial Surgery
Amiens University Hospital
Amiens, France

Mark F. Devlin, FRCD (Ed) (OMFS), FRCS (Ed), MBChB,
    FDSRCPS
Honourary Clinical Senior Lecturer
Department of Oral and Maxillofacial Surgery
University of Glasgow
Glasgow, Scotland, United Kingdom

M. Stephen Dover, FDSRCS, FRCS
Consultant
Maxillofacial Unit
University Hospital Birmingham
Birmingham, United Kingdom

Consultant and Clinical Lead
Craniofacial Unit
Birmingham Children's Hospital
Birmingham, United Kingdom

Georg Eggers, MD, DDS, FEBOUFS
Professor
Department of Oral and Maxillofacial Surgery
Heidelberg University
Heidelberg, Germany

Head
Department of Oral and Maxillofacial Surgery
Weinheim Head Center
Weinheim, Germany

Barry L. Eppley, MD, DMD
Associate Professor of Plastic Surgery
Division of Plastic Surgery
Indiana University School of Medicine
Indianapolis, Indiana, United States of America

Barrie T. Evans, FRCS (Eng & Edin), FDSRCS (Eng),
    FFDRCS (Ire)
Consultant Surgeon
Department of Oral and Maxillofacial Surgery
Southampton University Hospitals NHS Trust
Hampshire, United Kingdom

Honorary Consultant Oral & Maxillofacial Surgeon to the
    Royal Navy
Ministry of Defense
London, United Kingdom

Honorary Senior Clinical Lecturer
Southampton University Medical School
Hampshire, United Kingdom

Miriam A. Farley, LLB (Hons)
Senior Solicitor
Hempsons London
London, United Kingdom

Ian Francis, MA, FRCR, FRCS, BDS (Hons)
Consultant Radiologist
Department of Radiology
Brighton and Sussex University Hospitals NHS Trust
Queen Victoria NHS Foundation Trust
Brighton, United Kingdom

Nils-Claudius Gellrich, MD, DDS, PhD
Professor
Department of Oral and Maxillofacial Surgery
Hannover Medical School
Hannover, Germany

Stefan Hassfeld, MD, DMD, PhD
Professor and Chairman
Maxillofacial and Craniofacial Surgery
University of Witten/Herdecke
Dortmund General Hospital
Dortmund, Germany

Jarg-Erich Hausamen, MD, DDS, PhD
Former Professor and Chairman
Department of Oral and Maxillofacial Surgery
Hannover Medical School
Hannover, Germany

C. Michael Hill, FDSRCS (Ed), MSc, BDS, MDSc,
    FDSRCS (Eng)
Honorary Senior Lecturer
Department of Oral and Maxillofacial Surgery
Cardiff University
Cardiff, Wales, United Kingdom

Consultant Oral and Maxillofacial Surgeon
Department of Oral and Maxillofacial Surgery
Cardiff University
Cardiff, Wales, United Kingdom

Ian S. Holland, FDS, FRCS
Consultant Oral and Maxillofacial Surgeon
Department of Oral and Maxillofacial Surgery
Regional Maxillofacial Unit
Southern General Hospital
Glasgow, Scotland, United Kingdom

Alistair Jenkins, MD, FRCS (Ed)
Consultant Neurosurgeon
Department of Neurosurgery
Newcastle General Hospital
Newcastle upon Tyne, United Kingdom

D. Carl Jones, FRCS, FDCRCS
Consultant Maxillofacial Surgeon
Department of Maxillofacial Surgery
Wirral University Teaching Hospital
Wirral, United Kingdom

Risto Kontio, MD, DDS, PhD
Maxillofacial Surgeon
Department of Oral and Maxillofacial Surgery
Helsinki University Hospital
Helsinki, Finland

David Andrew Koppel, MBBS, BDS, FDS, FDSRCPS,
    FRCS (Eng, Glasg)
Honorary Senior Clinical Lecturer
Faculty of Medicine
University of Glasgow
Glasgow, Scotland, United Kingdom

Consultant Cranofacial / Oral and Maxillofacial Surgeon
Lead Clinician
Department of Oral and Maxillofacial Surgery
Regional Maxillofacial Unit
Southern General Hospital
Glasgow, Scotland, United Kingdom

Alexander C. Kübler, MD, DMS, PhD
Department of Oral and Maxillofacial Surgery
Julius-Maximilians University at Würzburg
Würzburg, Germany

Dorothy A. Lang, FRCS (Glasg), FRCS (Lond)
Consultant Neurosurgeon
Wessex Neurological Centre
Southampton University Hospitals
Southampton, United Kingdom

Richard A. Loukota, FDSRCS, FRCS
Professor and Consultant Oral and Maxillofacial Surgeon
Department of Oral and Maxillofacial Surgery
Leeds Teaching Hospital NHS Trust
Leeds, United Kingdom

David W. MacPherson, MBBS, FDSRCS, FRCS
Consultant Maxillofacial Surgeon
The Maxillofacial Unit
St. Richard's Hospital, Chichester and Worthing Hospitals
Chichester, United Kingdom

Jeremy D. McMahon, MBChB, FRACDS, FRCS
Maxillofacial Head and Neck Surgeon
Royal Hallamshire Hospital
Sheffield Teaching Hospitals NHS Trust
Sheffield, United Kingdom

Marc C. Metzger, MD, DMD
Professor
Department of Craniomaxillofacial Surgery
Freiburg University Hospital
Freiburg, Germany

Andrew M. Monaghan, BDS, FDSRCS, MB, BS, FRCS
Consultant Oral and Maxillofacial Surgeon
Department of Maxillofacial Surgery
University Hospital Birmingham
Birmingham, United Kingdom

Khursheed F. Moos, MBBS, BDS, FRCS (Ed), FDSCRCS
    (Eng & Edin), FRCPS (Glasg)
Professor Emeritus & Honorary Senior Research Fellow
Department of Oral and Maxillofacial Surgery
Glasgow Dental Hospital and School
Glasgow, Scotland, United Kingdom

Joachim Mühling, MD, DMD, PhD[†]
Former Head of Maxillofacial and Craniofacial Surgery
Heidelberg University Clinic
Heidelberg, Germany

Justin Nissen, FRCS
Consultant Neurosurgeon
Department of Neurosurgery
Newcastle General Hospital
Newcastle upon Tyne, United Kingdom

Chi Wang Peter Pang, MBChB, FRCS (Edin), FHKAM
    (Surgery)
Honorary Clinical Assistant Professor
Department of Surgery
The Chinese University of Hong Kong
Hong Kong, SAR

Director
Plastic and Aesthetic Centre
The Union Hospital
Hong Kong, SAR

Mike Perry, FRCS, FDS, BSc
Consultant Oral and Maxillofacial Surgeon
Lead Clinician – Craniomaxillofacial Trauma
Regional Maxillofacial Unit
Ulster Hospital
Dundonald, Northern Ireland, United Kingdom

David Richardson, FRCS, FDSRCS
Consultant Maxillofacial Surgeon
Maxillofacial Unit
Aintree University Hospital
Liverpool, United Kingdom

Henning Schliephake, MD, DDS, PhD
Professor and Chair
Department of Oral and Maxillofacial Surgery
University of Goettingen
Goettingen, Germany

† Deceased

Rainer Schmelzeisen, MD, DDS
Professor and Chairman
Department of Oral and Maxillofacial Surgery
Albert Ludwigs University and Hospital
Freiburg, Germany

Ralf Schön, MD, DDS, PhD
Professor
Department of Oral and Maxillofacial Surgery
Heinrich-Heine-Universität
Duesseldorf, Germany

Department of Oral and Maxillofacial Surgery
St. Joseph Hospital
Krefeld, Germany

Alexander Schramm, MD, DDS, PhD
Professor & Chairman
Department of Maxillofacial Surgery
Ulm Military Hospital
Academic Hospital of the University of Ulm
Ulm, Germany

Kenneth J. Sneddon, BDS, MBBS, FDSRCS, FRCS
Consultant Oral and Maxillofacial Surgeon
Department of Oral and Maxillofacial Surgery
The Queen Victoria Hospital
East Grinstead, West Sussex, United Kingdom

Leo F. A. Stassen, MB, MCH, BAO, B.Dent.Sc, FRCS
(Ed), FDSRCS, MA, FTCD, FFSEM (UK)m, FFDRCSI
Professor
Department of Oral and Maxillofacial Surgery
Oral and Maxillofacial Unit
Dublin University—Trinity College
Dublin, Republic of Ireland

Professor
Department of Oral and Maxillofacial Surgery
National Maxillofacial Unit
St. James's Hospital
Dublin, Republic of Ireland

David W. Thomas, PhD, FDSRCS (Ed), FDSRCS (Eng)
Professor of Oral Surgery
Department of Oral and Maxillofacial Surgery
School of Dentistry
University of Cardiff
Cardiff, Wales, United Kingdom

Edward Wai-Hei To, BDS (Lon), MBChB (Eng), FRCS
(Eng), FFDRCS, FRACDS, FCDSHK (Max-Fac),
FCSHK, FHKAM
Honorary Clinical Associate Professor
Department of Surgery
Li Ka Shing Medical School
University of Hong Kong
Hong Kong, China

Man Kwong Tung, MBBS (HKU), FRCS (Ed), FRCS
(Glas), FCSHK, FHKAM (Surgery)
Honorary Consultant and Associate Director
Plastic and Reconstructive Surgery Center
Hong Kong Sanatorium and Hospital
Hong Kong, China

Anthony G. Tyers, FRCS, FRCS (Ed), FRCOphth
Department of Ophthalmology
Salisbury District Hospital
Salisbury, United Kingdom

Pit J. Voss, MD, DMD
Department of Oral and Maxillofacial Surgery
University Hospital of Freiburg
Freiburg, Germany

Peter Ward Booth, FDS, FRCS
Consultant Maxillofacial Surgeon
Department of Maxillofacial Surgery
The Queen Victoria Hospital
East Grinstead, West Sussex, United Kingdom

Roger M. Webb, FDSRCS (Eng), MRCS (Eng), FRCS
(OMFS)
Consultant Oral and Maxillofacial Surgeon
Department of Oral and Maxillofacial Surgery
King's College Hospital
London, United Kingdom

Richard R. Welbury, MBBS, BDS, PhD, FDSRCS,
FDSRCPS, FRCPCH
Professor
Department of Pediatric Dentistry
University of Glasgow Dental School
University of Glasgow
Glasgow, Scotland, United Kingdom

Joachim E. Zöller, MD, DMD, PhD
Professor
Department of Craniomaxillofacial and Plastic Surgery
University of Cologne
Cologne, Germany

Preface

It gives me great pleasure to pen the Preface to this Second edition, but in the same measure I want to express my sincere gratitude to the contributors who make the whole thing possible. The contribution of the joint editors, Barry Eppley and Rainer Schmelzeisen has been outstanding not only from their contributions, but the planning and the all important "encouragement" to the contributors.

There is no "correct" answer to the dilemma between the benefits of a single author book and that produced by multiple authors. My view is clear; no one person has a monopoly of wisdom in every aspect of facial trauma, so we as a team aim to harness individual's expertise. So you may read conflicting advice within the book. I have every confidence however, our sophisticated readership will, in the light of the evidence we present, form their own views.

As I said in the Preface for the first edition, the etiology of facial trauma has changed, and certainly in the UK, it remains a "disease" of the young male, predominately as the result of excessive alcohol consumption. Just as the society and the car industry modified designs and introduced innovations to curb the hazards of driving vehicles, so we are now seeing the first glimmers of change in society towards alcohol consumption, if not yet the drinks industry. At least the problem is in the public domain and the unnecessary toll on otherwise fit healthy males is being recognized. It is to be hoped society continues to introduce preventative measures, and recognizes other emerging factors like drug and solvent misuse.

As in the first edition we have sought the wisdom of world experts, who have reviewed and updated their contributions. This has introduced new concepts as the result of looking at "outcomes". It has indeed introduced totally new approaches, like face transplants.

We hope this second edition, reflects the latest trends, concepts and innovations in the care of patients with facial trauma. As always, only by careful disinterested audit can the long-term value of these innovations be evaluated. I am sure the UK is a barometer of the industrialized world, and we are seeing much greater economic pressure on health care services. As surgeons we must respect these changes and seek greater efficiencies, but equally we must resist lowering of standards of care. It is equally exciting to see the new economic tigers like China, Brazil, and India contributing so much more innovation and audit in all aspects of health care and facial trauma management in particular.

Finally I would like to thank Elsevier, and Brian Loehr and Sara Alsup in particular, for their continued support, patience and skill in bringing this edition to print.

Peter Ward Booth

Table of Contents

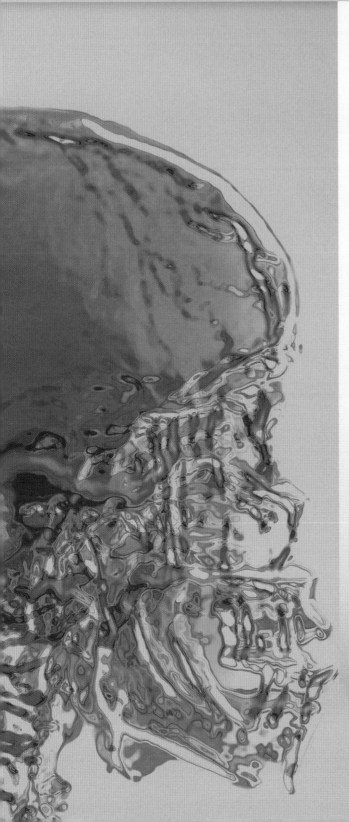

CHAPTER 1

Etiology and Prevention of Craniomaxillofacial Trauma

C. Michael Hill, Barry L. Eppley, David W. Thomas, Stephen E. Bond, Andrew M. Monaghan, M. Stephen Dover

Injuries to the face, head, and neck are relatively common, but in the overall trauma literature, the etiology of maxillofacial injuries has received relatively little attention. Almost all injuries result from some form of trauma, which may be defined as a physical force resulting in injury. Injuries may also be the result of chemical, thermal, or even radiation trauma, but these occur far less commonly than physical trauma.

Despite the high incidence of facial injuries, there has been relatively little research until recently into their etiology, treatment, and prognosis. Nevertheless, such injuries are clinically important for several reasons:

- The soft tissues and bones of the face give anterior protection to the cranium.
- Facial appearance is a major factor, if not the most significant factor, in appearance and perception of self.
- The whole anatomic region is associated with several important functions of daily life, including sight, smell, eating, breathing, and talking. Significant impairment in any of these functions has potentially serious effects on the patient's lifestyle and quality of life.

Trauma has traditionally been classified according to anatomic site. Although this is a logical approach on which to base treatment, in terms of developing strategies to prevent injury it is more informative to consider the etiology and the applied forces that produce injuries of differing types. Patterns of injury can be described that relate to certain types of accidents, and it is important to understand these patterns in relation to forensic evidence. In addition, strategies to reduce the incidence of maxillofacial injuries need to be developed, because the cost of treatment of these injuries can be high.

The reaction of the body to trauma depends on the nature of the assault and the response of the victim. The applied force and the extent of injury after trauma are affected by several factors. The kinetic energy (or potential to inflict damage) is calculated as one half of the mass of the object striking the face or head multiplied by the velocity squared; this is usually represented by the formula, $K = \frac{1}{2} MV^2$. Sometimes the situation is the opposite, and the momentum is generated by movement of the head striking a static object (e.g., in a fall). In all cases, it is the velocity rather than the mass of an object that has the greater proportional effect because of the kinetic energy generated. This is clearly demonstrable in road traffic accidents (RTAs): The severity of injuries associated with collisions at speeds greater than 20 mph (32 kph) is disproportionately increased compared with injuries sustained at lower speeds, and the risk of serious or fatal injury is much greater. The same principle applies to ballistic injuries: Although rifle or gunshot injuries may appear to be more damaging, they are seldom as severe as injuries caused by high-velocity bullets.

In most cases, the applied force is predetermined, but there are four other variables that affect the type and severity of injury sustained:

- The position of impact—the anatomic region to which the force is applied
- The area of impact—the wider the area, the greater the dissipation of force (given that pressure equals force per unit area)
- The resistance—whether there is any movement of the head or the soft tissues, or whether there is contact with bone; any restriction of movement potentially increases the severity of injury
- The angulation of the strike—a glancing blow causes a less serious injury

The strength of the soft tissues and underlying bone also plays a part in the extent of any injury, but there has been little work to assess susceptibility to injury in those terms.

CLASSIFICATION OF FACIAL TRAUMA

The classification of maxillofacial trauma should be related to outcome (i.e., type of injury sustained) to be valuable in audit of outcomes. It can also be considered with respect to etiology under a variety of headings, including assaults, falls, industrial injuries, RTAs, animal bites, sports injuries, burns, and war injuries. Other categories could also be included, such as iatrogenic and self-inflicted injuries. In all published studies, industrial injuries have represented only a small percentage of the overall total, although such injuries may be underreported. Many of these injuries are the result of falls at work, but equipment breakages and malfunctions also account for a significant proportion.

Several difficulties exist in comparing published reports because of variations in data collection and classification of injuries.[1] Soft tissue injuries, nasal bone fractures, dental injuries, and dentoalveolar fractures are presented in different ways by different centers, and in some studies, they are completely omitted. True comparison of published studies is also made difficult by the use of different selection criteria and the frequent reporting of retrospective, poorly collected data (which are commonly restricted to either causes or types of injury). Even so, the existing data have been useful in helping to promote changes in legislation and practice aimed at reducing the number and extent of maxillofacial injuries.

Attempts to standardize the recording of injury pattern and severity have been made.[1] With respect to assessing the injury severity associated with maxillofacial trauma, a number of scales have been described. These have three important uses:

- They promote targeted care (e.g., the Glasgow Coma Scale[2]).
- They help to predict the likely outcome (e.g., the Abbreviated Injury Scale [AIS][3] and the Injury Severity Score [ISS][4]).
- They encourage the accurate assessment and outcome of critically injured patients (e.g., Acute Physiology and Chronic Health Evaluation [APACHE II] Disease Classification System[5]).

It is well recognized that scoring systems are useful for determining the extent of maxillofacial trauma, but they do have a number of drawbacks. For example, whereas the International Classification of Diseases (ICD) describes diagnostic codes for most injuries,[6] in practice the coding for patients with multiple craniofacial injuries may be complex,[7] and data recovery almost certainly introduces bias in retrospective studies. There can be little doubt, therefore, that the prospective, systematic collection of data is always to be preferred in considering the etiology of facial injuries.

ASSAULT

From a forensic viewpoint, *assault* can be defined as the perceived threat of an imminent attack. Any act of physical violence is legally referred to as *battery*. In medical parlance, the word *assault* has become synonymous with the act of violence itself.

The comparative study of the prevalence of maxillofacial trauma as a result of assault (battery) is not easy. This is again due to the fact that relatively few studies have considered consecutive, nonselective data in estimating the pattern of injuries sustained, the actual treatment delivered, or the resulting demand for services.

It is well accepted that there is an increasing incidence of maxillofacial trauma associated with the rise in interpersonal violence in much of Western society (Fig. 1-1). In the developed world, there has been a pattern of increasing violence in urbanized settings since World War II, but in the developing nations, this pattern is less evident. With the increase in interpersonal violence in the developed world (coupled with improvements in road safety and car design), assaults are replacing RTAs as the most common etiologic factor in maxillofacial trauma[8,9] (Table 1-1); in the Third World, this is not yet the case. This trend has been observed in many countries, including the United States, United Kingdom, Scandinavia, Australia, and New Zealand.[10-14] The pattern in many other societies is different, with RTAs often remaining the most common cause of maxillofacial trauma.[15-19] In the Netherlands, RTAs still predominate because of the number of bicycle accidents that occur.

When considering interpersonal violence, the frequency with which the face is involved in assaults was shown in one study to approach 50% of all reported cases. Approximately 40% of individuals who presented at emergency departments because of assault had facial injuries, and almost 30% of assault victims had fractures, 83% of which affected the facial

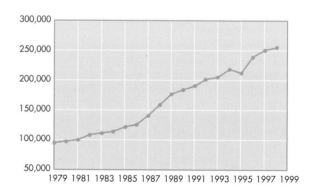

FIGURE 1-1   The increasing incidence of violence in the United Kingdom as demonstrated by government statistics.

TABLE 1-1	Etiology of Facial Injuries in Studies from Around the World								
	Australia[7]	New Zealand[12]	Japan[16]	Norway[23]	United Kingdom[14]	USA[19]	India[16]	Nigeria[39]	Tanzania[13]
Assaults	52	32	15.5	49	52	49	25	43	14.5
RTAs	19	30	38.5	14	16	43	40	27	81
Sports	16	20	16.5	8	19	4	4	9	<2
Falls	10	9	28.5	15	11	3.5	24	18	<2
Industrial	1.5	—	0.3	9	2	0.5	1.3	3	1
Other	1.5	9	0.7	4	—	—	1.2	—	—

RTAs, road traffic accidents.

skeleton.[18] The rise in interpersonal violence has directly increased the trauma workload, particularly for oral and maxillofacial surgeons, and especially with regard to the more serious facial injuries.[20]

With the exception of the sex of the assailant, which is usually male, the single most important etiologic factor in assault cases appears to be alcohol consumption (by both the assailant and the victim). Almost 50% of assault victims are found to have an increased blood alcohol concentration (>100 mg/dL), and alcohol abuse has been described as a contributing factor to assault in almost all independent studies.[21,22] It is difficult to obtain accurate figures on the numbers of assailants who have consumed alcohol because so many escape. However, this information is widely reported, and the fact that so many assaults take place in or near locations where alcoholic beverages are supplied gives further confirmation to this hypothesis that alcohol consumption is an important factor in assault. In the British Association of Oral and Maxillofacial Surgeons' survey of facial injuries (an intensive multicenter study), 55% of assaults were related to alcohol consumption, and 24% of the facial injuries recorded were caused by assaults. However, this study is still incomplete, and formal testing of all those involved was not possible.

The victims of trauma from assaults are most frequently young adult men in the 18- to 25-year-old age group, and they are most commonly assaulted by an unknown assailant.[8] Those affected tend to be employed in manual labor, suggesting a possible causal link between social deprivation and aggression, but this has not been confirmed in other studies.[23] Assaults leading to facial injuries typically occur in a bar or a public place near a bar and frequently late at night[18,24]; the effects of cumulative alcohol consumption compounded by tiredness have not been independently studied but may offer a simple explanation for this fact. The relationship between alcohol and assault was even clearer in a U.K. study which showed that, among those older than 15 years of age, alcohol consumption was associated with 90% of facial injuries occurring in bars, 45% of those occurring in the street, and 25% of those occurring in the home situation. Almost one quarter of all facial injuries in all age groups were related to consumption of alcohol within 4 hours of the injury.

Studies in large cities have shown that assaults often occur within a relatively limited geographic area and that they tend to be focused in areas adjacent to licensed premises.[25] Assaults make up a slightly larger proportion of facial injuries seen in emergency departments in cities (26%) than in county towns (21%).

Whereas males are more commonly assaulted by unknown assailants, the converse is true of female victims. Typically, women are assaulted by a partner or ex-partner, and the assault occurs in or around the home. Moreover, a greater percentage of women are assaulted at home in county towns (52%) compared with cities (38%), and fewer females are assaulted in public bars in all environments.

The number of injuries caused by female assailants is small, but there is some evidence that it is growing. Again, alcohol appears to be the main factor in the etiology of such attacks.

The pattern of injury sustained depends largely on the implement used. Whereas studies of maxillofacial trauma have often considered bony injury in isolation, soft tissue lacerations are the most common maxillofacial injuries sustained.[26,27] Despite their frequency, soft tissue injuries are often overlooked in trauma epidemiology. More than two thirds of the injuries sustained in assaults are lacerations; almost 40% of all assault victims[18] and 95% of victims of domestic violence[28] have facial lacerations. Soft tissue injuries are most frequently inflicted by direct, blunt trauma. Stab injuries to the face are uncommon,[29] but the use of broken glass or blades was responsible for 11% of facial injuries in one study.[18]

A number of studies have considered hard tissue injuries in isolation. Assault-related fractures most frequently involve (in order of descending frequency) the nasal bones, the mandible, the zygoma, and the midface. This contrasts with the pattern observed in RTAs, which cause injury principally to the midface (see later discussion).

The pattern of injury is affected greatly by the weapon selected. In the past, fists, feet, blunt instruments, and broken glass were commonly used. More recently, baseball bats and automatic and semiautomatic weapons have been more frequently used in premeditated assaults, principally in the United States, and this has had a considerable impact on the extent and pattern of injuries in some studies.[30-32] Despite attempts to reduce the incidence of injuries due to assault[33] (including education about alcohol consumption, introduction of drinking glasses made of toughened safety glass in licensed premises, increased policing, and improved street lighting), the available data suggest that maxillofacial trauma due to assaults and interpersonal violence will continue to increase for some time yet.

MEDICOLEGAL DESCRIPTION OF INJURIES

BRUISES OR CONTUSIONS

A *bruise* is the result of subcutaneous bleeding that occurs after an impact from a blunt object. Bruises may be seen adjacent to lacerations or abrasions, but they also frequently occur without rupture of the skin. The extent of any bruising is related to the severity of the impact, the laxity of the tissues, the individual's propensity to bruising, and age (older people and children being most susceptible). Particular care needs to be taken in trying to correlate the severity of a blow with the extent of bruising, particularly in older patients and in those taking anticoagulants, who may have disproportionately excessive bruising.

ABRASIONS

An *abrasion* is a superficial wound that does not fully penetrate the dermis. The point at which an abrasion may be termed a *laceration* is not always easy to determine, because deeper abrasions frequently bleed (sometimes excessively) and therefore must have penetrated the dermis. This is especially apparent after an RTA in which the victim's head skidded over a gravel surface.

Careful examination of abrasions often reveals a "heaping" of skin at the distal end of the impact area. This raised skin or small skin tags can indicate the direction of impact and therefore can be useful in helping to establish possible causes.

Deeper wounds are often accompanied by foreign bodies—wood splinters, road dirt, paint specks, and the like—all of which can be used to provide forensic evidence. It is clearly good medical practice to clean wounds before repair or dressing, but few practitioners collect any debris removed from a wound, although this practice could be of considerable legal benefit.

LACERATIONS

A *laceration* is a full-thickness wound of the skin that is caused by compression of the skin against the bone with a blunt object. A blunt weapon such as a fist or a bat may have been used, or the head or other body part may have struck a blunt object (e.g., in a fall). There is no way of distinguishing the cause with certainty unless the wound contains foreign matter.

On occasion, it can be difficult to distinguish a laceration from an incision, although the former usually shows mild inversion of the wound edges on close examination—a feature not seen in wounds caused by sharp objects. Lacerations may bleed profusely, but they frequently do not because of retraction of the blood vessels that were compressed during the creation of the injury.

INCISIONS

An *incision* is a full-thickness skin wound that is caused by a sharp instrument. If the length of the wound exceeds its depth, it is referred to as a *slash wound*; if the converse is true, it is a *stab wound*.

The clinical appearance of a slash wound is affected by the muscular pull and the crease lines of the skin. Such wounds may bleed profusely, and it is not always easy to identify and occlude vessels that have been cut. From a forensic point of view, it is not easy to glean much information from a slash wound, although the deeper end of the incision tends to be the origin. Ragged edges may suggest a blunter implement, but the actual type of implement used cannot be categorized with any certainty.

Although stab wounds to the face are less common than stab wounds to other sites, they yield more forensic information, and good close-up photographs of such wounds should be taken before suturing. Multiple stab wounds in the region of the neck should lead the clinician to consider a possible diagnosis of attempted suicide, although stabbing of other areas of the body (e.g., chest, wrists) is more common in such cases. The unpredictable direction of the stab may cause unpredictable severity to the wound.

ROAD TRAFFIC ACCIDENTS

MOTOR VEHICLE ACCIDENTS

RTAs are a major health problem. In the United States alone, they account for an estimated 50,000 deaths and more than 3 million injuries annually. Although RTAs are frequently associated with severe maxillofacial injuries, most of these injuries are facial lacerations. In Western countries, the highest rate of maxillofacial trauma in many studies occurred during the 15 years following World War II (see Table 1-1).[34]

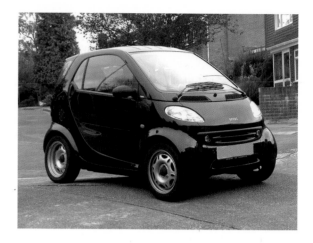

FIGURE 1-2 The Smart microcar—small in size but big in safety features.

In the developing world, RTAs still account for the majority of maxillofacial trauma,[35-38] but the introduction of seat-belt and drunk-driving legislation and improvements in car design (discussed later) have greatly decreased the incidence of fatalities and RTA-associated maxillofacial trauma.[39,40] This serves to illustrate not only the progress of car design but also the benefits of the detailed study of facial trauma. The most important factor in determining the extent of injuries sustained in RTAs is the direction of the collision; for example, drivers involved in head-on collisions are 18% more likely to survive.

In the past 30 years, modern car designers have developed an impressive array of safety features to reduce the risk of serious injury in RTAs (Fig. 1-2). Some of these are principally improvements in the design features of the car, such as crumple zones, collapsing steering wheels, and side-impact bars. Others have involved the development of new technologies (often adopted from the aviation industry), including improved seat restraints, laminated windshields, air bags, computerized warning systems, and antilock and assisted braking systems.[41] Improvements have also been made to the environment, such as enhanced road design, better signposting and lighting, rumble strips, and bright "cats' eyes." Recent innovations have included car designs that minimize injuries to pedestrians or cyclists struck by vehicles.

External Support Devices

Supportive and protective devices play a major role in preventing facial injuries and significantly reducing the magnitude of the facial damage. They can be divided into protective devices that are installed as part of a vehicle or sporting equipment and those devices that are carried or worn by the individual.

The decrease in maxillofacial trauma associated with RTAs has been dramatic. In the United Kingdom, car ownership has increased rapidly in the past 20 years, but the total incidence of facial fractures associated with RTAs has decreased by one third.[42] Most encouragingly, the percentage of all facial fractures associated with RTAs has decreased from 46.8% in 1948 to 18.6% over the same period.[34] The severity of injuries has also decreased: 54% of RTA-associated midfacial injuries were at Le Fort II or III levels in 1948-1955, compared with 8.6% in 1987-1993.[34] These dramatic improvements occurred after the introduction of drunk-driving legislation in the 1970s and compulsory seat-belt wearing in 1983: The incidence of facial injuries in patients involved in RTAs was reduced from 21% to 6% in less than 2 years.[43]

Similar findings have been noted in several other countries. However, Tanaka and colleagues[15] reported that seat-belt legislation in Japan did not make a great difference in the pattern of facial injuries, whereas Imai and co-workers[44] concluded that the number of midfacial fractures was significantly reduced. It is difficult to postulate why these findings differed and whether the perceived lack of improvement may have been related to poor compliance or to an already low incidence of such injuries.

Compliance with seat-belt legislation is another area in which there is considerable national variation. Despite the proven benefits of seat belts, almost 70% of individuals involved in RTAs were not using any form of restraint. Particularly alarming was a study of pediatric RTA-related facial trauma in the United States, which demonstrated that only 138 of 412 children with facial trauma were restrained at the time of impact.

Seat Belts and Lap Belts

Seat belts work in three different ways. Perhaps most obvious is the restraint of the person within the vehicle, which prevents their expulsion through the windshield. Seat belts also spread the area over which the energy of impact is dissipated. Finally, seat belts are made of a fabric that has a slight degree of elasticity; this increases the time during which the energy of impact is dissipated.

The current three-point combination lap and diagonal belt positioned across the pelvis and the rib cage was developed by a Swedish aircraft engineer and was introduced in 1959. It provides a strong three-point harness with a simple pendulum and ratchet mechanism that locks the belt in sudden-stop situations. The lap belt spreads crash forces across the strong pelvic bone and keeps the passenger from being tossed around inside the car, whereas the shoulder harness spreads forces across the rib cage and prevents the upper body from jack-knifing forward. In the United States, this three-point system has been mandatory in automobiles since 1974 and saves thousands of lives each year.[45]

It is universally accepted that the use of seat belts and lap belts is associated with a lower risk of serious injury, particularly to the head and face (Fig. 1-3). The difference in injury

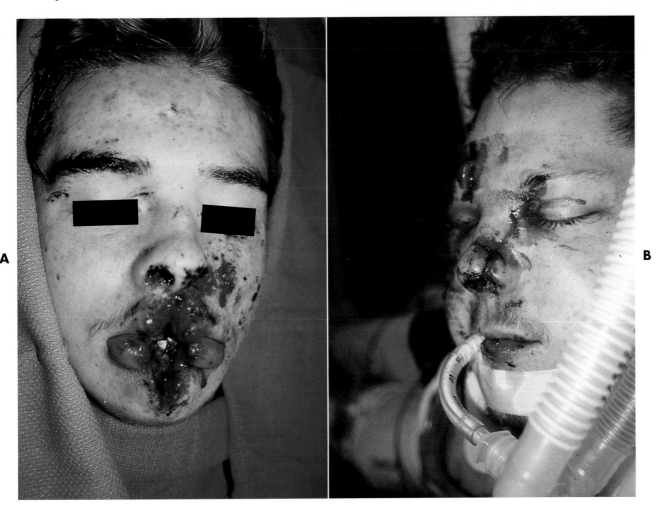

FIGURE 1-3 The combination of seat belt and lap belt prevents the driver's face from striking the steering wheel as well as direct impact of passengers' faces onto the dashboard or the back of the seat. **A,** Unrestrained driver in motor vehicle accident. **B,** Unrestrained passenger in motor vehicle accident.

rate is so significant that the use of these devices is mandated by law in all parts of the United States and the United Kingdom, and violations are punishable by monetary fines. Despite these recognized safety facts, seat belts and lap belts frequently are not used (e.g., by up to 33% of front seat occupants), and the results are manifested in trauma registry records.

For children, the rate of restraint use is better (78%), according to the latest National Pediatric Trauma Registry information from 92 centers reporting throughout the United States. This probably reflects the effects of pediatric education campaigns and the legal requirement for use of restraints in children up to the age of 4 years or 40 lb in weight (Fig. 1-4).[46]

Despite the craniofacial protection provided by seat belts and lap belts, severe systemic injuries still do occur in belted individuals.[47,48] Certain specific injuries occur with belt use, including cervical, lumbar, and intra-abdominal injuries; this has been referred to as *seat-belt syndrome*. However, critical

analysis suggests that, with the exception of sternal fractures, injuries previously associated with seat-belt syndrome occur in similar proportions in belted and unbelted patients.

Air Bags

Like seat belts and lap belts, the air bag has proved to be effective in reducing injuries and fatalities in motor vehicle accidents.[49,50] They work best for belted drivers, reducing fatalities by more than 50%. With unbelted drivers, fatalities are reduced by up to one third, and facial injuries are decreased due to the prevention of direct facial impact onto the steering wheel, dashboard, or seat (Fig. 1-5). Of all automotive safety devices, air bags probably provide the single best protection for the driver, preventing lacerations and facial fractures. Among passengers, air bags have been reported to reduce the incidence of facial lacerations but not that of fractures.[47]

The air bag is a round, inflatable nylon bag that is slightly larger than the steering wheel and less than 1 foot in thickness at its central section when fully inflated. It is deployed when sudden longitudinal deceleration occurs by means of sensors located within the forward portion of the vehicle. The deployment is almost instantaneous, with the bag becoming fully inflated in about 0.01 second and coming out of the dashboard at up to 200 mph. This provides a temporary cushion that is subsequently deflated over several seconds by the release of hot gases through exhaust ports on the back of the air bag. The United States Congress has mandated the installation of dual air bags in all new passenger cars since 1997 and in all vans, trucks, and utility vehicles since 1998.

Although severe facial trauma is clearly reduced by the use of air bags, some facial injuries still occur. The rapid deployment of the air bag is caused by a combustion process that releases a significant amount of heat, which can burn a patient's face, although the exhaust ports are positioned to blow away from the driver. Most commonly, burns attributed to air bags are minor and are frictional in nature, resulting from the high-velocity impact of the fabric to the face, chin, and neck (Fig. 1-6). More serious is the potential for alkali burns to the eye caused by the fine aerosol byproducts of

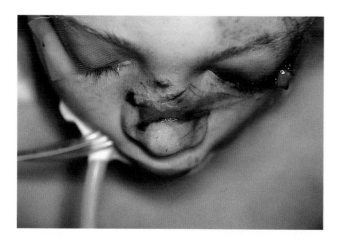

FIGURE 1-4   Four-year-old girl with nasal and orbital fractures who was not restrained in a car seat at the time of a motor vehicle accident.

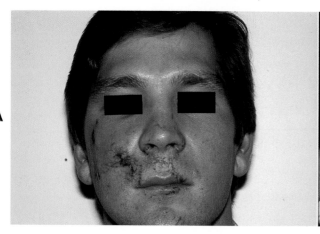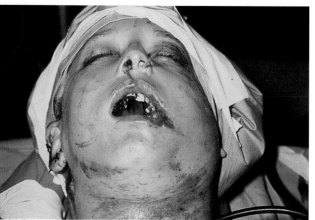

A   **B**

FIGURE 1-5   The deployment of air bags significantly reduces the magnitude of facial injuries from motor vehicle accidents. **A,** Minimal facial injuries (abrasions, small lacerations) with the use of an air bag in a restrained driver. **B,** Significant facial injuries (Le Fort fractures) affecting an unrestrained driver with no air bag.

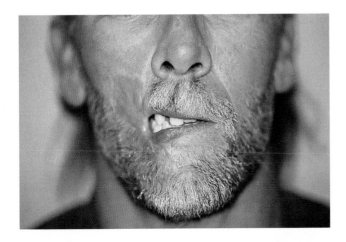

FIGURE 1-6 Air bags can cause some minor injuries, particularly friction burns. This 35-year-old man suffered significant burns from an air bag, sustaining full-thickness injury to the right commissure and cheek with resultant severe contracture.

combustion, which include sodium hydroxide, sodium carbonate, and other metallic oxides.[51] This risk and that of frictional burns can be decreased by positioning the driver's seat as far back as possible when driving, to decrease the force of the air-bag deployment onto the face.

In addition, the risk of injury to children can be reduced by never having an infant in the front seat of a vehicle with an air bag (or by immobilizing the air bag) and by properly restraining children younger than 12 years of age in a child safety seat or with a safety belt in the back seat of the car.

Side-impact air bags have also been developed and are available on more expensive vehicle models.

Some controversy remains regarding the influence of air bags on the pattern of injury sustained in RTAs. However, a 2000 study conclusively showed that deployment of a driver's air bag in a collision significantly prevents facial fractures, although the protective benefit against facial lacerations was unproven.[50] Another U.S. study reported AIS scores of 1.13 for subjects using an air bag together with a seat belt, 1.29 for those using a seat belt only, and 1.46 for unrestrained subjects.

Other Safety Features
Among other safety features that have been introduced, the use of laminated safety glass for windshields has virtually eliminated the multiple penetrating facial and frontal injuries that previously were often seen in emergency departments after RTAs.

Summary
Injuries resulting from RTAs typically affect men aged 18 to 25 years.[7] The fractures incurred in these accidents are caused by rapid deceleration and direct impact of the head with an object, usually with the steering wheel, the frame of the car, or the dashboard. Numerous studies have shown that these injuries are typically midfacial, principally affecting the nasal bones, zygoma, and maxilla. The incidence and severity of maxillofacial injuries vary greatly in different parts of the world, and in some countries RTAs are still the most common cause of maxillofacial fractures.[15,35-38,45]

MOTORCYCLE ACCIDENTS

Motorcycle accidents account for about 50% of all traffic-related injuries. Studies have shown that most of the remaining injuries involve motor and pedal cycles with relatively few pedestrian accidents. The incidence and severity of head injuries associated with motorcycle accidents has decreased drastically since the mandatory introduction of crash helmets and drunk-driving legislation.[47] The risk of death is reduced by almost 30% with the use of a crash helmet. Consequently, crash helmets are compulsory even for pedal cyclists in parts of Australia.[7] In some countries, however, they are not obligatory even for motorcycle riders, and in regions of China (where helmet wearing is rare) almost 60% of head injuries are associated with motorcycle accidents.

The incidence of facial injuries in motorcycle and bicycle accidents is predictably significant. On average, between one third and one half of all such accidents result in facial trauma, depending on the hospital setting, the study population, and the case identification methods. The magnitude of the facial trauma is understandably higher in accidents involving motorcycles as opposed to pedal cycles due to the higher speeds involved and the open traffic conditions in which such accidents occur.

Helmets
The scientific evidence that helmets protect against head, brain, and facial injuries in motorcycle and bicycle accidents has been well established by multiple, well-designed, case-control studies.[52,53] Helmet use by motorcycle riders not only decreases the risk of facial injuries by more than 50% but also is associated with fewer fractures and a decreased number of moderate and severe systemic injuries (Fig. 1-7). Studies have also shown a lower incidence of facial injuries among those riders who use a full-face helmet compared with an open-face or jet helmet.

Facial injuries to pedal cyclists occur at a rate comparable to that of head injuries. Helmets are protective against trauma to the upper and midfacial regions, reducing injuries by two thirds. Although a well-fitting helmet covers only the forehead, the midface gets some protection, probably through a shadow effect. Historically, the use of protective headgear by cyclists was quite low throughout the world. Helmet use has now risen dramatically in many areas due to community-wide helmet campaigns and legislative efforts. Because cycle speed is an independent risk factor for injury, helmet wearing should be compulsory for both recreational riders and serious competitors.

Despite the incontrovertible evidence, a large number of car occupants and motorcyclists involved in RTAs were wearing neither safety belts nor crash helmets at the time of the accident. These may be partially explained by the association of injuries with the use of alcohol[56] or drugs.[52] The other factor that significantly affects the severity of injury is the speed at which an accident occurs. Because of the dynamics of applied force or kinetic energy ($K = \frac{1}{2}MV^2$), even small increases in speed result in disproportionate intensification of injury. The converse is also true: Small reductions in speed reduce the seriousness of the injuries sustained.

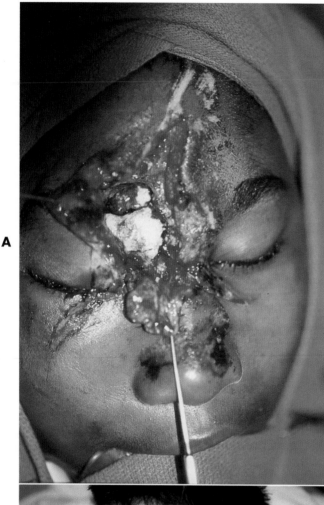

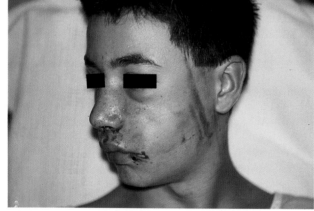

FIGURE 1-7   The lack of any safety gear in low-velocity motorized vehicle accidents is a frequent source of facial injuries in young patients. **A,** An 8-year-old girl with open frontal sinus fractures resulting from a head-on collision with a pole while driving a moped. **B,** A 14-year-old boy with zygomaticomaxillary fractures sustained while driving a motorbike.

OTHER CYCLING INJURIES

Cycling has seen a rise in popularity in recent years, and much attention has been given to the prevention of head injury in cyclists.

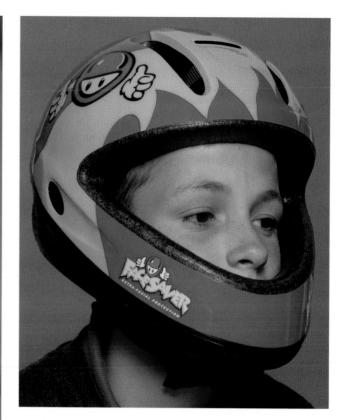

FIGURE 1-8   A child's full-face cycling helmet designed for comfort and better facial protection.

In the United Kingdom, as in the United States, there is at present no legal requirement for cyclists to wear protective helmets. A 2-year case-control trial in the United States reported that 20.7% of patients presenting to emergency departments after cycling accidents had serious facial injuries.[56,57] After adjustments for age, sex, speed, and road surface, it was concluded that helmets reduced the risk of lacerations and fractures to the upper and middle face by 65% but had no effect in preventing serious injury to the lower face.

One recommendation is that consideration be given to the fitting of chin protection, which may decrease the risk to the lower face. A prototype helmet of this kind has been developed (Fig. 1-8). Its acceptance will depend on the creation of an ethos among younger people that encourages use of helmets rather than resentment of them, as is largely the case at present.

The epidemiology of maxillofacial injuries observed in pedestrians contrasts markedly with that of drivers, with more severe cranial fractures and increased AIS scores. Injuries to pedestrians more frequently affect children, and complex craniomaxillofacial trauma is an important cause of mortality and morbidity in the community.[53]

Mountain bike–related accidents show a different profile of facial injuries, probably reflecting the terrain in which they are ridden (Fig. 1-9). Mountain bike accidents result in a higher percentage of facial fractures, especially severe midfacial fractures, and more associated systemic injuries. This strongly suggests that the addition of faceguards to helmets, particularly in this specialty riding group, should be considered.

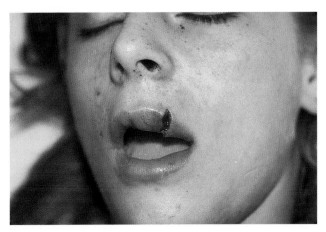

FIGURE 1-10   Facial laceration sustained when the patient fell from rollerblades and struck the face on a mailbox.

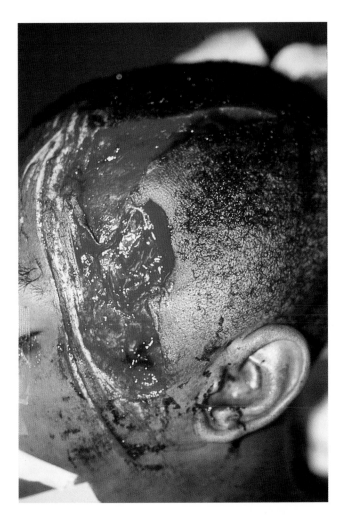

FIGURE 1-9   A teenage boy who sustained severe facial lacerations from striking a tree branch while falling from a mountain bike.

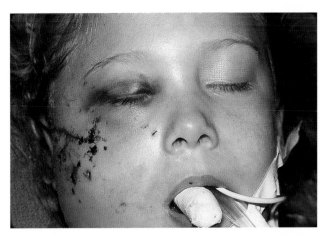

FIGURE 1-11   Facial lacerations sustained when the patient fell from a skateboard and was struck by the tip of the board.

Two recent additions to recreational activities for nonathletes that pose facial injury risks are in-line skating (rollerblading) and skateboarding. Rollerblading has become popular, and it provides a good aerobic workout. However, it is not without risk, and between 1993 and 1995, almost 100,000 skaters were injured severely enough to require emergency care. Almost 20% of rollerblading injuries were to the head, face, or chin (Fig. 1-10). Of these injured skaters, almost half (46%) were wearing no safety equipment at the time of injury, and only 7% were fully outfitted including a helmet.[54]

In contrast, the traditional form of skateboarding, in which jumping and aerobatic maneuvers are done, has always been associated with the wearing of safety gear due to the more obvious risk exposure (Fig. 1-11). A recent variation of this activity is the so-called scooter form of skateboarding, in which an upright handle is added to the front of the board (sometimes known as a razor scooter). This enables very young and inexperienced riders to enjoy this form of skateboarding. Injury risk is significant because the front wheel beneath the handle is small and can easily get caught in small depressions and flip the rider. The presence of the upright handlebar puts the face at greater risk than in traditional skateboarding, and safety equipment should always be used.

GUN AND WAR INJURIES

War was a feature in some part of the world for almost the whole of the 20th century. In addition to conventional war, the rise of terrorism has added another dimension to the potential for battle-type injuries. Ballistic injuries—from bullets, shells, or bombs—produce unpredictable and complex tissue damage because of the high-velocity impact, which imparts high levels of kinetic energy to the tissues. In addition, wound contamination is common. Where such conflict is prevalent, it is an important cause of facial injuries.

Previous studies showed that 16% of all gun- and war-related injuries were to the head and neck. However, more recent analysis of casualty numbers from Iraq and Afghanistan showed a much higher proportion of maxillofacial injuries, approaching 30%.[58] This has been explained by the improvements in torso protection afforded by the use of body armor: Patients are surviving wounds that previously would have been fatal. Studies of U.S. servicemen have shown that the principal cause of injury at all sites in wartime is shrapnel from exploding armaments; some 60% of injuries occurring during World War II and 75% of those sustained in the Vietnam conflict were from this cause.[59,60] In Iraq and Afghanistan, improvised explosive devices and other forms of explosives have been more common than in previous conflicts and account for more than 80% of injuries.[59] It is postulated that these devices are more likely than other weapons to produce facial injury, offering a further explanation for the change in incidence.[62]

The pattern and extent of war injuries have changed with the development of armaments technology and the use of antipersonnel devices. Correspondingly, the role of the maxillofacial surgeon in the treatment of these injuries has developed from providing a small amount of technical assistance to being pivotal in the management of injured personnel.

Injuries sustained as a result of high-velocity bullets impacting the head and neck are frequently fatal because of the dispersal of energy distant to the entry site. Whereas in past wars, young adult men were those principally affected, recent conflicts have produced a dramatic rise in the number of women and children who are wounded.[63]

Although the incidence of war injuries obviously varies throughout the world, in Western societies gunshot wounds are becoming more common and are most likely to result from violent crime or attempted suicide rather than war or terrorism.[7]

Modern warfare has considerably changed the pattern of facial injuries, and this can be seen in the evolution of the literature on maxillofacial injuries from this cause. In the United States, however, shotgun injuries are more commonly sustained because of assault or attempted suicide.[64] Despite figures showing that the United States has an eightfold higher incidence of gun fatalities than all its economic counterparts combined, the American gun lobby remains a powerful and vocal body, presenting gun ownership as a human rights issue. It is salutary to realize that more than 30,000 people die annually in the United States alone as a result of gunshot wounds; of these, approximately half are suicides.

SPORTS INJURIES

Participation in sports has become increasingly popular, and this has focused attention on the epidemiology of sports injuries. A limited number of studies have investigated the causes and types of maxillofacial injuries associated with sports.[65] Workers have investigated both the overall distribution and severity of sports trauma and that associated with individual sports.[66-69] It must be remembered, however, that the treatment of such injuries relates not only to the repair of maxillofacial and dentoalveolar fractures but also to the treatment of soft-tissue injuries.

There are several ways of classifying generalized sports injuries, but they have commonly been described as acute or repetitive. However, most injuries in published surveys of maxillofacial trauma are acute. The etiology of sports-related trauma varies according to the type of sport played. Consequently, the reporting of sports injuries varies considerably among studies from different countries as well as among studies of specific sports.[65,67,68] Whereas the face is the most frequently affected area of the body in some studies, in others the limbs are more commonly affected.[67] A prospective U.K. study demonstrated that almost 80% of injuries affect solely the soft tissues, confirming that investigation of only facial fractures or dentoalveolar injuries associated with sports does not accurately indicate maxillofacial service demand.

Again, the majority of sports-related injuries occur in men aged 18 to 25 years. Moreover, in almost all sports played by both genders, there is a positive male/female ratio which has varied in different studies from 1.2 : 1 to 3 : 1.

There is seasonal variation in the presentation of patients with sports injuries in the United Kingdom. The incidence of these injuries is highest at the beginning of the main sporting season (i.e., late August through September). This presumably results from the low level of general fitness and lack of timing that follow a long period of rest. There is a decreased incidence of sports injuries among fit, professional athletes. When the type of sport is considered, rugby is the sport most commonly associated with facial injuries in the United Kingdom. This has been a finding in studies of facial fractures in both the United Kingdom and Japan, where rugby is increasing in popularity.[63-67]

Studies in both the United Kingdom and the United States have shown that prevention has decreased the number of sports-related dental and dentoalveolar injuries.[68] The reason for the reduction may be the increased use of mouthguards and protective headgear, but it may also be due to better safety awareness in general.[70] The relatively low incidence of facial injuries in contact sports may reflect the wearing of mouthguards and protective headgear, but it may also be a result of underreporting.

Several other factors can be identified in relation to risk, including a dental overjet of greater than 5 mm, left-handedness, and parental attitude. Another obvious factor is the relative prevalence of any particular sport. For example, although skiing injuries are unknown in countries without snow, where skiing is a national pastime, injuries related skiing or ice sports may represent a significant proportion of the overall workload of the oral and maxillofacial surgeon. The occasional skier is particularly at risk due to a combination of lack of fitness and lack of skill.

FALLS

Injuries sustained as a result of falls are somewhat different from other facial injuries because they usually are caused by impact onto a static object of variable size and density. Whereas maxillofacial trauma associated with assaults, RTAs, and sports is found predominantly in the 17- to 26-year-old age group, a bimodal age distribution can be identified in the pattern of fall injuries. The initial peak occurs during the first 10 years of life, and the second peak occurs (as frailty increases) in patients older than 65 years of age.[71,72] In the younger age group, boys are predominantly affected, whereas women have a somewhat higher incidence of fractures in the older age group. The reasons for this distinction are not entirely clear but probably relate to changes in bone density, with osteoporosis affecting women earlier in life.

The distribution and severity of maxillofacial injuries after a fall depend on the terminal velocity and mass of the victim and the density, mobility, and area of contact of the object that was struck. There are two distinct patterns of fall injuries: tripping while walking or running and falling from a height. The latter is more common in the developing world, where lack of safety measures and design inadequacies frequently contribute to accidents, particularly among children. In most published series from the developing world, falls are the second most frequent cause of maxillofacial injuries, accounting for up to 40% of such injuries in some studies but 15% to 20% more commonly.

The actual injury pattern in this type of accident is affected by the ability (or inability) of the victim to cushion the fall with outstretched arms and to involuntarily rotate the head as it approaches its target. In high-speed falls, the central section of the face is more vulnerable, and there is a tendency to sustain dentoalveolar injuries, avulsed teeth, fractured nasal bones, and abrasions. If the arms are pushed forward, there is usually rotation of the body and head so that the injury pattern is more often unilateral, with the zygoma and mandible more frequently involved. For some reason, the left side of the face is slightly more commonly affected than the right side. Younger patients tend to have higher rates of distal-extremity injuries from falls, whereas the elderly tend to have a more central type of injury involving the face and scalp, possibly because of diminished protective reflexes. Repeated falls in the elderly should be thoroughly investigated to determine whether there is a treatable medical or social cause for the falls.[72]

Although falls cannot be completely eliminated, many can be prevented. In the developing world, working and living on mountainous terrain, inadequate or absent railings, and open-plan windows all increase the risk of falls. All of these situations are readily amenable to safety improvements (at a comparatively low cost). They are relatively rarely implicated as causes of injury in developed countries, where legislation and fear of litigation often dictate safety design features.

PREVENTION OF CRANIOMAXILLOFACIAL TRAUMA

MEDICAL PREVENTION

The primary arena for medical prevention of craniomaxillofacial trauma is in the use of medications to treat various abnormal physiologic conditions that may result in trauma due to falling. Such conditions include circulatory disturbances and vasovagal reactions, transient ischemic attacks due to intracranial or carotid vessel arteriosclerosis, and inadequate insulin replacement in severe diabetes. This pharmacologic approach is aimed at preventing loss of consciousness and subsequent falls.

One of the most common traumatic effects from facial accidents is dental injury. Tooth fracture, luxation, and avulsion can be partially prevented in some patients by proper and regular dental care and maintenance. The preservation of alveolar bone height through long-term tooth retention and periodontal care can prevent complete tooth avulsion in some cases and may make it more likely that splinting of loose teeth will be successful. In addition, some facial injuries are avoided by better maxillomandibular bone stock preservation, because more force can be absorbed and transferred without fracture (Fig. 1-12).

Orthodontic or orthognathic correction of severe malocclusions, particularly those in which the anterior teeth are in a proclined position, can help decrease the number of

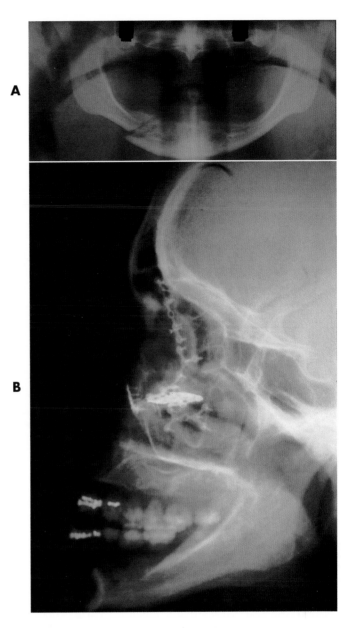

A

B

FIGURE 1-12 Significant loss of alveolar bone (edentulous state) weakens the jawbones and predisposes them to fracture. **A,** Fracture of mandibular body. **B,** Repair of severe zygomaticomaxillary fracture in edentulous maxilla.

traumatized teeth. Early removal of impacted third molars and subsequent replacement by bone decreases the risk of mandibular angle fracture later in life, although this is not an indication for prophylactic removal of wisdom teeth.

PREVENTION THROUGH EXTERNAL SUPPORT DEVICES

Mouthguards and Protectors

With the increased participation and competitiveness of athletics around the world, sports-related injuries are occurring more frequently. In particular, orofacial trauma to the teeth, gums, and lips is more prevalent. Fractured, partially avulsed, and completely knocked-out teeth are common, with

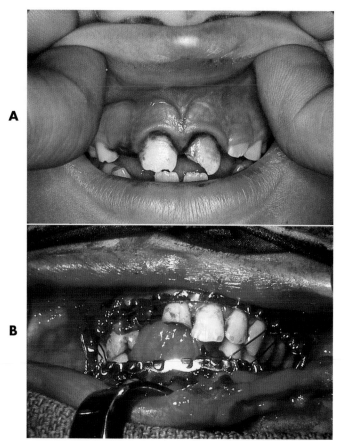
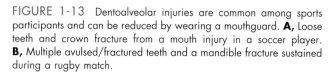

FIGURE 1-13 Dentoalveolar injuries are common among sports participants and can be reduced by wearing a mouthguard. **A,** Loose teeth and crown fracture from a mouth injury in a soccer player. **B,** Multiple avulsed/fractured teeth and a mandible fracture sustained during a rugby match.

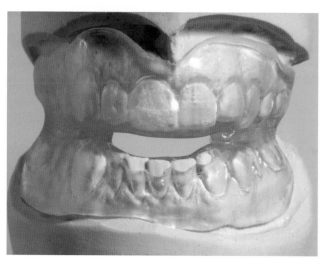

FIGURE 1-14 A bimaxillary mouthguard protects the teeth and possibly the jaws. *(Design and photograph courtesy Mr. P. Millward, Cardiff, UK.)*

associated lacerations to the gums, tongue, and lips (Fig. 1-13). In the United States, the National Youth Sports Foundation estimated that more than 5 million teeth are knocked out and more than 200,000 other oral injuries occur during sporting activities each year. Many orofacial injuries can be prevented through the use of a mouthguard.[71]

Although mouthguards have been used in boxing for almost a century and have been advocated by the American Dental Association in football and hockey for several decades, many participants in other sports (e.g., basketball, soccer, baseball, rugby) have been reluctant to wear them. The benefits of wearing a sports mouthguard have been well documented. In (American) football, where mouthguards are mandatory, fewer than 1% of all injuries involve the teeth and mouth. Conversely, in basketball, where mouthguards are not routinely worn, more than one quarter of all player injuries involve the teeth, tongue, and lips.[69,70]

Mouthguards provide a number of advantages to both amateur and professional athletes. Most obvious is the protection of the teeth, which is achieved by the use of a plastic interface to separate the dental arches. Mouthguards protect against oral lacerations and contusions by holding the lips and cheek tissues away from the teeth. In addition, they absorb and distribute the force of the impact, decreasing the risk of mandibular angle and condylar fractures. When properly fitted, mouthguards are comfortable to wear, rarely cause gagging, and provide no obstruction to breathing.

Mouthguards come in two basic types: stock ("boil and bite") guards, which are typically available in retail stores, and custom-fabricated guards, which are made by a dentist. Stock mouthguards do not fit as accurately as custom guards, are often uncomfortable, and frequently interfere with breathing and speaking. In addition, stock guards provide a false sense of protection from the dramatic decrease in interocclusal thickness that occurs when one bites it into place in the softened state. Given that the total replacement cost for a single knocked-out tooth is more than 20 times the cost of a custom-fabricated mouthguard, it makes sense that every person should wear one if the sport involves contact or the possibility of falling. This is especially true in sports such as football, hockey, basketball, boxing, rugby, lacrosse, martial arts, soccer, skating, and cycling, in which traumatic contact can be expected.

Although the overall severity of maxillofacial sports injuries tends to be less serious than for injuries sustained in assaults or RTAs, facial bone fractures remain common.[64] Research has shown that the number and severity of these injuries can be reduced with appropriate rule changes and improved protective clothing where necessary. Vacuum-formed mouthguards are particularly effective at preventing dental injuries, and the newer, bimaxillary mouthguards (Fig. 1-14) provide added support to the mandible. Whether these devices decrease the risk of injury to the mandible or maxilla is uncertain, but they are popular with players once they have gotten used to them.

Overall, however, attitudes to mouthguards remain problematic, with evidence that both players and coaches sometimes do not support their use. Despite all the published studies supporting the effectiveness of mouthguards, large numbers of players are still not convinced of their effectiveness and personal desirability. It is difficult to know how far sports' governing bodies should be encouraged to enforce protective measures, but the medical profession could clearly do more to promote the message of effectiveness of such measures in preventing injury.

The cost to society as a whole of failing to reduce the rates of sports-related injuries is considerable, and the balancing of individual freedom against corporate responsibility is not easy. What is certain is that good protective measures are effective (see, for example, Castaldi's paper[70] about the effect of protective measures in hockey) and can be promoted wholeheartedly to try and induce societal change.

Eye Protection

Sports injuries are a common mechanism of ocular trauma and typically occur in ball-related activities. The curved surface of a small-sized ball is capable of bypassing the surrounding protruding orbital rims and making direct contact with the globe. It is estimated that more than 100,000 sports-related eye and orbital wall injuries requiring physician evaluation or treatment occur annually in the United States. Baseball players are particularly at risk: Roughly 10% to 20% of all injuries in the sport occur to the face, accounting for almost one third of all sports-related eye injuries. Other ball sports with significant ocular trauma risk are handball, squash, racquetball, and basketball.

Virtually all ocular injuries should be preventable with the appropriate protection. Protective eyewear such as goggles should be composed of shatter-resistant plastics that wrap around the lateral rim of the orbit for maximal globe protection (Fig. 1-15). Failure to use safety gear is largely due to comfort considerations and lack of perceived risk by the participant.

Eye protection can significantly influence the outcome of explosive injuries in martial conflicts.[73] Their use by troops is variable.

PROTECTION THROUGH EDUCATION

Education in all aspects of life in which the face is exposed to trauma is important, including motorized and pedaled transportation and other outdoor activities. In most of these exposures, the face is known to be at risk and protective devices are recommended and commonly used.[69] In examining different sports, the incidence of facial injury compared with injury to other body locations varies from 26% in ice hockey to 36% in wrestling, 11% in basketball, 7% in baseball, 7% in handball, and 4% in skiing.

Numerous other risk exposures are not as easily recognized. One that deserves special mention because it is often a source of severe facial disfigurement and scarring is that of dog bites, for which education is the only means of prevention. Dog bites commonly occur in small children and teenagers, in whom the evidence of the repaired facial injuries will remain for the rest of their lives. In the United States, several million people are bitten each year, one every 40 seconds. More than 300,000 of these dog-bite injuries require emergency treatment, leading to more than 6000 reconstructive surgeries and hospitalizations and almost 20 deaths per year. Total medical costs related to dog bites exceed $250 million per year, and the cost of the associated human suffering is incalculable.[74]

More than 60% of dog-bite victims are children, with the highest incidence occurring among those younger than 15

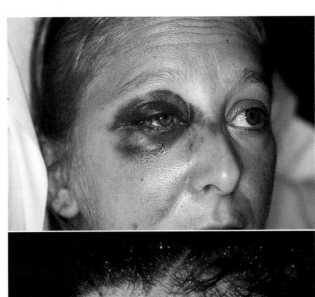

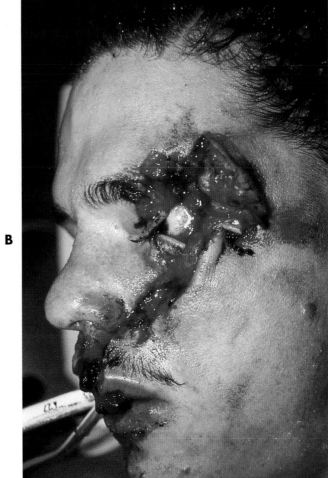

FIGURE 1-15 The potential injuries from orbital trauma can be reduced by use of proper safety eyewear. **A,** A 27-year-old woman with an orbital floor blowout fracture after being struck in the eye with a softball. She was not wearing protective eyewear. **B,** A 25-year-old man with severe facial lacerations and orbital fractures from being struck by the loose cable of a chainsaw. He was not wearing protective gear.

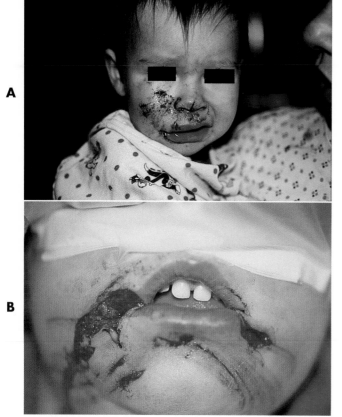

FIGURE 1-16   Dog bites are common sources of facial injuries in young children. **A,** Multiple puncture marks in a 2-year-old boy which occurred while he was playing (unsupervised) with a neighbor's dog. **B,** Severe facial lacerations in a 3-year-old who tried to kiss an unknown dog.

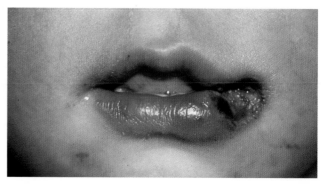

FIGURE 1-17   Typical commissure burn in an 18-month-old boy who chewed on an electrical cord.

years of age, who frequently are bitten in the face, neck, and head (Fig. 1-16). A 10-year retrospective internal review of all dog bites from the trauma registry (143 cases) at the Riley Hospital for Children in Indianapolis, Indiana, revealed several interesting and underappreciated findings. In 84% of cases, the dog was either a family pet or well known to the victim (i.e., belonging to a neighbor or a relative). Most dog bites occurred when the dog was on the owner's property (89%). Seventy-two percent of the dog-bite patients were infants and children younger than 5 years of age. The three breeds most commonly identified as biting were pit bull terriers, chows, and rottweilers, which together made up 64% of the identified dogs.

Although dogs provide a wonderful source of companionship and pleasure, one must be aware that dogs are not human and may not always respond to certain situations in a completely predictable manner. This is particularly true when dogs are around children, who often do not appreciate that their behavior may be unsettling to the dog. Education can be helpful in reducing the risk of dog-bite injuries. The American Society of Plastic Surgeons endorses the following messages:

- Never approach an unfamiliar dog.
- Never run from or scream at a dog.

- Do not disturb a dog while it is eating, drinking, sleeping, or caring for puppies.
- If a dog knocks you over, roll into a ball and stay still.
- Never allow a child to play with a dog unless supervised by an adult.
- Do not stare a dog directly in the eyes.
- Do not touch a dog without allowing it to see you and sniff you first.

Another preventable facial injury that is unique to pediatric patients is the electrical commissure burn. This low-voltage electrical injury occurs when infants or children chew or suck on the live end (female end) of an electrical cord (Fig. 1-17). The combination of a violation of the plastic covering and the electrolyte-rich saliva from the mouth completes an electrical circuit as an arc burn. This can generate temperatures as high as 2500° C, causing extensive local tissue damage at the corner of the mouth with eventual sloughing, scar replacement, and subsequent contracture and microstomia. Whereas the lip injury can be initially treated with oral splints or a secondary surgical commissuroplasty, it can be completely prevented by covering electrical outlets, replacing old appliances and lights, and curbing the curiosity of toddlers who are prone to oral investigation.

The incidence of injuries to the head, neck, and face is high in cases of domestic violence, and women are the predominant victims (Fig. 1-18). Research indicates that approximately two thirds of these women suffer injuries about the face, and such injuries can be used as a diagnostic marker in the emergency department. This anatomic location of injuries is so significant that a woman presenting for evaluation of facial injuries is 7.5 times more likely to have experienced domestic violence than a woman with injuries limited to other locations.[75] This suggests that any woman who presents to the emergency department for evaluation of injuries not related to RTAs or sports accidents is at high risk for being a victim of domestic violence. Most of these injuries are caused by blunt trauma and commonly consist of facial bruising and abrasions, lip lacerations, and nasal fractures. Education and counseling remain the only preventive modalities for this cause of facial injury.

SHIFTING ETIOLOGIC FACTORS

Oral and craniomaxillofacial surgery has emerged as one of the most progressive specialties of recent years. This has led

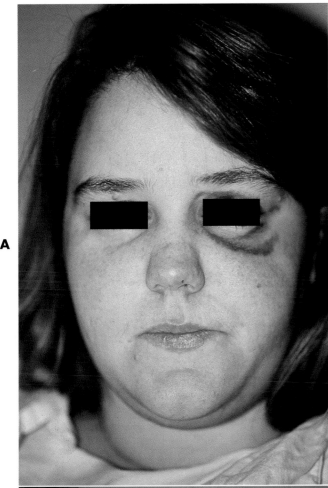

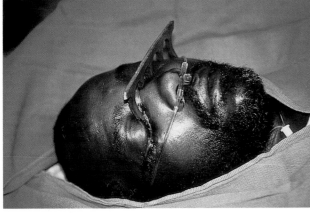

FIGURE 1-18 Domestic violence is a frequent source of facial trauma, particularly in women. **A,** A zygomaticomaxillary fracture in a young female caused by a punch thrown by a male companion. **B,** A rake was implanted in the face of a 42-year-old man while he was sleeping after a domestic argument.

to an increased awareness of the roles of dental occlusion, modern methods for repair of bony fractures, and treatment of complex orbital and soft tissue injuries, all of which have raised the profile of trauma to the face and emphasized the importance of specialist treatment.

Several factors suggest that the pattern of injuries will continue to change on a global scale, although it is difficult to predict the extent of such change. At the start of a new millennium for Western society, despite improved safety design, increased legislation, and the absence of widespread war, there are two important factors that will probably increase the need for maxillofacial trauma services in the coming decades. First is the continuing rise in interpersonal violence. Although Western society may well address the problems caused by excessive alcohol consumption (like cigarette smoking, excessive drinking is starting to become more socially unacceptable), other drug-related injuries and crimes are likely to continue increasing. The growth of legal (forensic) medicine will probably continue unabated, and clinicians will require more training in forensic techniques.

Second, the increasing age of the population will probably result in an increased prevalence of fractures in older people, and these fractures are more difficult to treat and slower to heal than in younger people. Research into aging and healing processes may offer advances in this area, but change is unlikely to be rapid.

Increasing globalization and population drift through immigration and emigration also make the future difficult to predict. With diverse cultures aspiring to move closer together, while at the same time retaining their own identity, it is conceivable that there could be some convergence of the etiologic patterns of maxillofacial trauma in the developed and developing worlds.

Although Western populations tend to oppose too much health and safety regulation, the challenges facing the developing world are to implement safety and design legislation that will minimize RTAs and falls while acting simultaneously to prevent injuries relating to violent crime and assault. Here, the changing pattern of injuries places a considerable demand on those responsible for the planning of health care. There is a need not only to plan service provision and manpower requirements but also to be aware of the continually changing incidence and nature of the injuries sustained. Prospective monitoring of the causes, severity, and treatment outcomes of maxillofacial trauma must assume a higher profile if accurate service planning is to take place. Information on these factors then needs to be shared more widely. If these things occur, it should be possible to balance the provision of health care with service demand in the most optimal way.

REFERENCES

1. Ali T, Shepherd JP: The measurement of injury severity. *Br J Oral Maxillofac Surg* 32:13-18, 1994.
2. Teasdale G, Jennet B: Assessment of coma and impaired consciousness: a practical scale. *Lancet* 1:81-84, 1974.
3. *Abbreviated injury scale*, Des Plaines, Ill, 1990, Society for the Advancement of Automotive Medicine.
4. Baker SP, O'Neill B, Haddon W et al: The Injury Severity Score: a method for describing patients with multiple injuries and evaluating emergency care. *J Trauma* 14:187-196, 1974.
5. Knaus WA, Zimmermann JE, Wagner DP et al: APACHE Acute Physiology and Chronic Health Evaluation: a physiology based classification system. *Crit Care Med* 9:591-597, 1981.
6. *Manual of the international statistical classification of diseases and related health problems*, 10th revision (ICD-10), Geneva, 1977, World Health Organization.
7. Simpson DA, McLean AJ: Epidemiology. In Simpson DA, David D, editors: *Craniomaxillofacial trauma*, London, 1995, Churchill Livingstone.
8. Brickley MR: *The circumstances and aetiology of urban violence*, MScD thesis, 1993, University of Wales.
9. Cohen LE, Felson M: Social change and crime rate trends: a routine activity approach. *Am Sociol Rev* 44:588-608, 1979.

10. Dimitroulis G, Eyre J: A 7-year review of maxillofacial trauma at a central London hospital. *Br Dent J* 170:300-302, 1991.

11. Brook I, Wood N: Aetiology and incidence of facial fractures in adult. *Int J Oral Maxillofac Surg* 12:293-298, 1983.

12. Hammond KL, Ferguson JW, Edwards JL: Fractures of the facial region in the Otago region 1979-1985. *N Z Dent J* 87:5-9, 1991.

13. Moshy J, Mosha HJ, Lema PA: Prevalence of maxillo-mandibular fractures in mainland Tanzania. *East Afr Med J* 73:172-175, 1996.

14. Telfer M, Jones GM, Shepherd JP: Trends in the aetiology of maxillofacial fractures in the UK (1977-1987). *Br J Oral Maxillofac Surg* 29:250-255, 1991.

15. Tanaka N, Tomitsuka K, Shionoya K et al: Aetiology of maxillofacial fractures. *Br J Oral Maxillofac Surg* 32:19-23, 1994.

16. Naik BK, Paul G: Incidence and aetiology of fractures of the facio-maxillary skeleton in Trivandrum: a retrospective study. *Br J Oral Maxillofac Surg* 24:40-44, 1986.

17. Thomas DW, Sageman M, Shepherd JP: Trends in the management of fractured mandibles. *Health Trends* 26:113-115, 1995.

18. Shepherd JP, Shapland M, Scully C et al: Pattern, severity and aetiology of injury in assault. *J R Soc Med* 83:75-78, 1990.

19. Scherer M, Sullivan W, Smith D et al: An Analysis of 1423 Facial Fractures in 788 Patients at an Urban Trauma Center. *J of Trauma-Injury Infection & Critical Care* 29:388-390, 1989.

20. Thomas DW, Smith AT, Walker R et al: The provision of oral and maxillofacial surgery services in England and Wales 1984-1991. *Br Dent J* 176:215-219, 1994.

21. Heather N: Relationship between delinquency and drunkenness amongst Scottish young offenders. *Br J Alcohol Alcoholism* 16:150-161,1981.

22. Torgerson S, Tornes K: Maxillofacial fractures in a Norwegian district. *Int J Oral Maxillofac Surg* 21:335-338, 1992.

23. Tarling R: Social deprivation and violence in London, *Home Office Research Bulletin*, London, 1982, HMSO.

24. McClintock FH, Wilkstrom POH: The comparative study of urban violence and criminal violence in Edinburgh and Stockholm. *Br J Criminol* 32:505-520, 1992.

25. Shepherd JP, Robinson L, Levers BGH: Roots of urban violence. *Injury* 21:139-141, 1990.

26. Hocking D: Assaults in SE London. *J R Soc Med* 82:283-284, 1989.

27. Key SJ, Thomas DW, Shepherd JP: The management of soft tissue facial wounds. *Br J Oral Maxillofac Surg* 33:76-85, 1995.

28. Ochs HA, Neuenschwander MC, Dodson TB: Are head, neck and facial injuries markers of domestic violence? *J Am Dent Assoc* 127:757-761, 1996.

29. Cascarini L, Bleetman T: Head and neck stabbing injuries. *Br J Oral Maxillofac Surg* 33:63, 1995.

30. Hussain K, Wijetunge DB, Grubnic S et al: A comprehensive analysis of craniofacial trauma. *J Trauma* 36:34-47, 1994.

31. Berlet AC, Talenti DP, Carroll SF: The baseball bat: a popular mechanism of urban injury. *J Trauma* 33:167-170, 1992.

32. Stone JL, Lichtor T, Fitzgerald LF et al: Demographics of civilian cranial gunshot wounds: devastation related to escalating semiautomatic usage. *J Trauma* 38:851-854, 1995.

33. Shepherd JP, Farrington DP: Assault as a public health problem: discussion paper. *J R Soc Med* 86:89-92, 1993.

34. Vincent-Townend JPL, Shepherd JP: The epidemiology of maxillofacial trauma. In: Williams JLL, editor: *Maxillofacial trauma*, London, 1995, Churchill Livingstone.

35. Adekeye EO: The pattern of fractures of the facial skeleton in Kaduna, Nigeria. *Oral Surg* 49:491-495, 1980.

36. Abiose BO: Maxillofacial skeleton injuries in the Western States of Nigeria. *Br J Oral Maxillofac Surg* 19:268-271, 1986.

37. Khalil AF, Shaladi OA: Fractures of the facial bones in eastern regions of Libya. *Br J Oral Maxillofac Surg* 19:300-304, 1981.

38. Adeloye A, al-Kuoka N, Semabatya-Lule GC: Pattern of acute head injuries in Kuwait. *East Afr Med J* 73:253-258, 1996.

39. Homel R, Castledene D, Kearns I: Drink-driving counter measures in Australia. *Alcohol Drugs Driving* 4:33-44, 1988.

40. Tunbridge R: The long-term effect of seat-belt legislation on road-user injury patterns. *Health Bull* 48:347-349:1990.

41. Huelke DF, Moore JL, Ostrom M: Air bag injuries and occupant protection. *J Trauma* 33:894-898, 1992.

42. Telfer M, Jones GM, Shepherd JP: Trends in the aetiology of maxillofacial fractures in the UK. *Br J Oral Maxillofac Surg* 29:250-255, 1991.

43. Perkins CS, Leyton SA: The aetiology of maxillofacial injuries and seat-belt law. *Br J Oral Maxillofac Surg* 26:353-363, 1988.

44. Imai Y, Toyohashi M, Sakamoto H et al: A clinical study of maxillo-facial fracture (1). *J Stomatol Soc (Jpn)* 40:826-829, 1991.

45. *The science of seat belts* (website): www.progressive.org. Accessed 2009.

46. Hayes JR, Groner JI: Using multiple imputation and propensity scores to test teh effect of car seats and seat belt usage on injury severity from trauma registry data. *J of Ped Surg* 43(5):924-927, 2008.

47. Porter RS, Zhao N: Patterns of injury in belted and unbelted individuals presenting to a trauma center after motor vehicle crash: seat belt syndrome revisited. *Ann Emerg Med* 32:418-424, 1998.

48. Tufts University School of Medicine: *Rehabilitation and childhood trauma*. National Pediatric Trauma Registry, phase 3, Boston, 2000, Tufts University.

49. Barry S: The effectiveness of airbags. *Accid Anal Prev* 31:781-787, 1999.

50. Murphy RX Jr, Birmingham L, Okunski WJ et al: The influence of airbag restraining devices on the patterns of facial trauma in motor vehicle collisions. *Plast Reconstr Surg* 105:516-520, 2000.

51. Baruchin AM, Jakim I, Rosenberg L et al: On burn injuries related to airbag deployment. *Burns* 25:49-52, 1999.

52. Muellman RL, Milinek EJ, Collicot PE: Motorcycle crash injuries and costs: effect of a re-enacted comprehensive helmet use law. *Ann Emerg Med* 21:266-272, 1992.

53. Evans L, Frick MC: Helmet effectiveness in preventing motorcycle driver and passenger fatalities. *Accid Anal Prev* 20:447-458, 1988.

54. Knox CL, Comstock RD, McGeehan J, Smith GA: Differences in teh reisk associated with head injury for pediatric ice skaters, roller skaters, and in-line skaters. *Pediatrics* 118(2):549-554, 2006.

55. Brown RD, Cowpe JG: Patterns of maxillofacial trauma in two different cultures: a comparison between Riyadh and Tayside. *J R Coll Surg Edinburgh* 30:299-302, 1985.

56. McDermott FT: The effectiveness of helmets in the prevention of bicyclist head injuries. *World J Surg* 16:379-383, 1992.

57. Lee MC, Chiu WT, Chang LT et al: Craniofacial injuries in un-helmeted riders of motor bikes. *Injury* 26:467-470, 1995.

58. Lew TA, Walker JA, Wenke JC et al: Characterisation of craniomaxillofacial battle injuries sustained by United States service members in the current conflicts of Iraq and Afghanistan. *J Oral Maxillofac Surg* 68:3-7, 2010.

59. Sastry MS, Sastry MC, Paul BK et al: Leading causes of facial trauma in the major trauma outcome study. *Plast Reconstr Surg* 95:196-197, 1995.

60. Dobson JE, Newell MJ, Shepherd JP: Trends in maxillofacial injuries in wartime 1914-1986. *Br J Maxillofac Surg* 27:441-450, 1989.

61. Ramasamy A, Harrison SE, Stewart MPM et al: Penetrating missile injuries in the Iraqi insurgency. *Ann R Coll Surg Engl* 91:551-558, 2009.

62. Powers D: Distribution of civilian and military maxillofacial surgical procedures performed in an air force theatre hospital: implications for training and readiness. *J R Army Med Corps* 156:117-121, 2010.

63. Taher AA: Pediatric facial injuries in Tehran: a review of 87 patients. *J Craniofac Surg* 4:21-27, 1993.

64. Haugh RH: Gunshot wounds of the face in attempted suicide patients. *Br J Maxillofac Surg* 56:933-934, 1998.

65. Hill CM, Burford K, Martin A et al: One-year review of maxillofacial sports injuries treated at an accident and emergency department. *Br J Oral Maxillofac Surg* 36:44-47, 1998.

66. Hill CM, Crosher RF, Mason DA: Dental and facial injuries following sports accidents: a study of 130 patients. *Br J Oral Maxillofac Surg* 23:268-274, 1985.

67. Schatz JP, Joho JP: A retrospective study of dento-alveolar injuries. *Endodont Dent Traumatol* 10:11-14, 1994.

68. Tanaka N, Hayashi S Suzuki K et al: Clinical study of maxillofacial fractures sustained in sports. *J Stomatolog Society (Jpn)* 59:571-577, 1992.

69. Kujala UM, Taimela S, Antti-Poika I et al: Acute injuries in soccer, ice hockey, volleyball, basketball, judo and karate: analysis of national registry data. *BMJ* 311:1465-1468, 1995.

70. Castaldi C: Sports-related oral and facial injuries in the young athlete: a new challenge for the pediatric dentist. *Pediatr Denti* 8:311-316, 1986.

71. Guven O: Fractures of the maxillofacial region in children. *J Craniomaxillofac Surg* 20:244-247, 1992.

72. Chew DJ, Edmondson HD: A study of maxillofacial injuries in the elderly resulting from falls. *J Oral Rehab* 23:505-509, 1996.

73. Ansell MJ, Breeze J, McAlister VC et al: Management of devastating ocular trauma: experience of maxillofacial surgeons deployed to a forward field hospital. *J R Army Med Corps* 156:106-109, 2010.

74. Berzon DR, DeHoff JB: Medical costs and other aspects of dog bites in Baltimore. *Public Health Rep* 89(4):377-381, 1974.

75. Wu V, Huff H, Bhandari M: Pattern of physical injury associated with intimate partner violence in women presenting to the emergency department: a systematic review and metaanalysis. *Trauma Violence Abuse* 11(2):71-82, 2010.

CHAPTER 2

Medicolegal Implications of Facial Injuries

Barry L. Eppley, Miriam A. Farley

As societies become increasingly litigious, there is a considerable likelihood that a surgeon treating patients who have sustained facial injuries will become a participant in the litigation process. The prominent visibility of the face and its importance to each individual ensures that its physical characteristics and emotional perspective are both highly valued and guarded.

Most likely, this participation will involve a civil suit in which the patient is taking action against the driver of a car, an employer, or the owner of a dog. From this perspective, the physician is providing information on the extent of the wounds, the care provided and that potentially needed, and any permanent injury (e.g., scars, dysfunction). As medical insurers become increasingly vigilant and more financially restrictive, the physician who participates in the care of the facial wound may also assist the patient's legal representative in obtaining the maximal medical benefits that are due under the guidelines of the health policy. Lastly, the specter of being a named defendant in a medical liability suit is an ever-present consideration, albeit the most unpleasant one.

When treating an individual with a facial injury, the surgeon must be aware that, as the medical record is being created, a legal record is simultaneously being formed. The recording of patient information through emergency department records, hospital charts, office notes, or operative reports establishes unchangeable evidence of what occurred and how the patient was medically treated. Being as meticulous in clinical record keeping as in the treatment of the patient will always serve the physician well.

Several aspects of the legal system are worth reviewing so that the treating physician may have some perspective on the medicolegal process. This information is useful because it relates to how these issues may directly affect the care delivered and how such events may be interpreted in the future. The first part of the chapter is written primarily from the perspective of the legal system in the United States and the second part for the United Kingdom; it is acknowledged that many countries have different medicolegal laws that are variably enforced.

TORT LAW

Tort law is the branch of the law through which an aggrieved individual seeks compensation to right a wrong that was done

to him (or her) in a civil context, usually the wrongful act of another person. However, failure to act when there is a legal duty to do so may also subject the wrongdoer to liability for his omissions. Some wrongful acts may be criminal in nature (e.g., battery) as well as being a civil tort. If the wrongdoer is prosecuted criminally, he (or she) may also be subject to civil liability without double jeopardy.

The most common tort for which a facial reconstructive surgeon may become involved in litigation is *negligence*. Although the surgeon treating facial injuries need not be overly concerned with the legal definition of negligence, its proof requires four separate elements: (1) the existence of a duty, (2) breach of the duty, (3) causation (between the breach of duty and harm suffered), and (4) damages.

Negligent operation of a motor vehicle may be the most common type of tort resulting in a facial injury. This usually occurs when an individual suffers injuries from being hit by a car operated by another driver. More rarely, an action may originate from an injured passenger against the driver of the motor vehicle in which the person was riding. Animal bites, particularly in children, are an especially obvious injurious circumstance in which litigation rates are high relative to the occurrence of injury (Figs. 2-1 through 2-3). Unsafe maintenance of premises, manufacture of defective products, and intentional torts such as battery are also commonly encountered in clinical practice.

THE TREATING PHYSICIAN AND LITIGATION

When a physician encounters a patient with a facial injury and there is some suspicion that tort litigation may result, he should be thinking of his potential role in any lawsuit.

Documentation is of the utmost importance. This means that records should be complete, accurate, and without editorial comment. The events that resulted in the facial injury should be noted in the patient's medical record. The presence of underlying medical conditions, such as acute drug or alcohol intoxication, is a very important part of the initial medical record. However, if the physician is going to document the use of illicit drugs or alcohol, he must not speculate, and there should be confirmatory medical test results to support these comments.

Documentation of a facial injury should go beyond a written chart note or dictated operative report. Exact

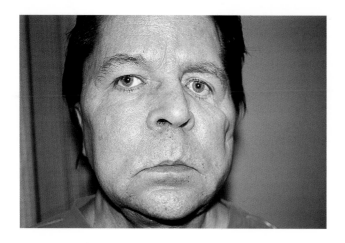

FIGURE 2-1 Facial deformity secondary to untreated zygomatico-maxillary fracture.

measurement of all lacerations should be taken and recorded, either in the emergency department note or as part of the operative report. Such wound measurements are often taken anyway, because the billing of wound closures (CPT codes) is based on the length and depth of the wound. Diagrams may be helpful, but preoperative and postoperative photographs are invaluable and should be taken whenever possible. Digital photography is the standard. Today's cell phones have such good-quality cameras that there is little reason why photographs cannot easily be taken and transferred to the patient's medical record (Fig. 2-4).

There is no aspect of medical care in which photographs are more widely helpful than the treatment of facial injuries. The establishment of visual documentation in the medical record has numerous merits in the present and potential future care of the patient. Thorough documentation of facial injuries creates a record for the patient to review in the future. This serves to educate the patient about the severity of the

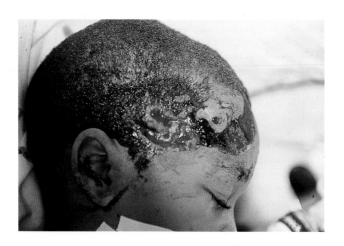

FIGURE 2-2 Forehead and facial nerve transection (frontal branch) due to dog-bite injury from a neighbor's pet.

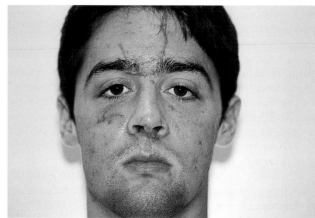

FIGURE 2-3 Scars resulting from extensive facial lacerations after the patient was hit by a drunk driver.

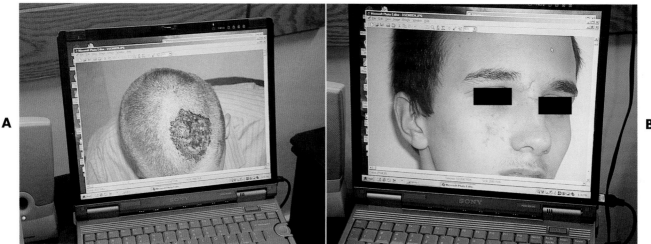

FIGURE 2-4 Facial trauma patients whose photos were taken with a digital camera and immediately downloaded to a laptop for storage, showing a partial scalp avulsion (**A**) and facial scars resulting from lacerations (**B**). Such digital images can easily be sent by e-mail or burned onto a disk.

initial injuries. This is very useful, because many facially injured patients will need reconstructive surgeries or scar revisions. An appreciation of the original problem may help the patient understand why such procedures are necessary. Furthermore, if a physician is going to become involved in any litigation, either willingly or reluctantly, good photographic documentation of the facial wounds will help both parties to understand the nature and severity of the injuries and may increase the likelihood of a settlement before trial or sometimes before a suit is filed.

The more ambiguous the nature and extent of the injuries appear in the medical record, the more room the attorneys will have for arguing a position that is favorable to their client, leaving the treating physician in the middle of a legal tug-of-war in which he is not likely to be an enthusiastic participant.

THE LITIGATION PROCESS

The treating physician may expect litigation if the patient has suffered severe, extensive, or disfiguring injuries in a setting of potential negligence. The first concrete indication of a lawsuit is a request for medical records made by the plaintiff's attorney. Each state has its own statutes governing the handling of medical records requests, and it would be prudent for the physician to become familiar with the laws in the state in which he practices. Under no circumstances should original records be provided; copies should be sent, with the original records kept in the physician's office at least as long as required by state laws. If litigation is ongoing, a patient's medical records should not be purged from the files simply because the statutory time for maintenance of medical records has expired. Additionally, a patient's confidential medical record should never be duplicated and forwarded in the absence of a properly executed release form signed by the patient or the patient's guardian.

Usually, the provision of medical records does not end the physician's involvement in the underlying legal matter. The pace of personal injury litigation is most often driven by the plaintiff's attorney; therefore, the physician's first contact is likely to be the attorney who is representing the patient. Depending on the attorney's style and practice habits, the physician may be asked to participate in an informal conference. Frequently, the plaintiff's attorney asks for a narrative statement to record in writing the content of the conference with the attorney. Typically, the physician is asked to respond to very specific questions regarding the cause of the plaintiff's injuries, history and physical examination findings, treatment, and prognosis. Some plaintiffs' attorneys choose to forego the conference, especially if there is not sufficient funding for the case, and simply ask for a narrative report.

Many physicians do not like to become involved in litigation, even if they are not a party to it. However, physicians can always be subpoenaed to testify at a deposition or trial, so this task cannot be completely avoided. In general, cases are far more likely to be settled in advance of trial if both sides have reasonable expectations and as much information as possible about liability and damages. If the response to a request for a narrative report is both clear and complete, the prospects for early settlement are better. However, there may be matters and issues beyond the physician's control, and this can cause some cases to proceed toward trial despite full cooperation in providing the medical information that is available.

DEPOSITION AND TRIAL TESTIMONY

There are two types of depositions in the litigation process: discovery (or evidentiary) depositions and trial depositions.

DISCOVERY DEPOSITIONS

The purpose of a *discovery deposition* is to learn what the deponent's testimony is likely to be at trial. Discovery depositions are usually taken by defense counsel. Because all depositions are given under oath, and under the penalties for perjury, defense counsel will seek to build a record that may be used at trial to impeach the deponent's credibility if there are inconsistencies or inaccuracies.

The attorney conducting the deposition will ask a series of questions, usually beginning by asking the deponent-physician about his medical education and training. After the preliminary questions have been asked and answered, the substance of the legal case will be explored. Unlike examination at trial, leading questions are permissible on direct examination. Objections may be made by the plaintiff's attorney, but the custom in most jurisdictions is for the deponent to go ahead and answer once the objection has been stated, unless advised otherwise. The admissibility of the objections to questions and answers at trial will be decided by the trial judge at a later date. If the plaintiff's attorney and the defense attorney disagree as to whether a particular question should be answered, they may seek to contact the trial judge for an impromptu ruling, or they may skip the question for the time being and have the deponent answer it at a later date, if that is in accordance with the trial judge's ruling.

In most jurisdictions, deposition testimony in one matter is admissible in another. If there is a significant chance of a subsequent medical malpractice action arising from the care rendered to the plaintiff, the physician would be wise to seek counsel before attending any deposition. Although medical negligence laws vary from state to state, a showing of negligent care usually must be present if the plaintiff is to prevail in a medical malpractice suit. A mere unsatisfactory medical outcome in the absence of negligence will not typically suffice. However, the requirements for filing a medical malpractice action are not as burdensome as those for sustaining the charges of negligence, so a physician may become a medical malpractice defendant even if the suit is largely without merit.

TRIAL DEPOSITIONS

The other type of deposition is a *trial deposition*. Most jurisdictions allow for some depositions to be conducted outside the courtroom and either read into evidence at trial or recorded on audiotape or, more commonly, videotape. A common setting for a trial deposition to be conducted in this fashion is when the witness is a physician whose schedule does not allow live testimony at trial. Typically, the plaintiff's attorney prefers treating physicians to give live testimony, because it holds the jury's attention better than a videotape. The plaintiff's attorney usually seeks to have the treating

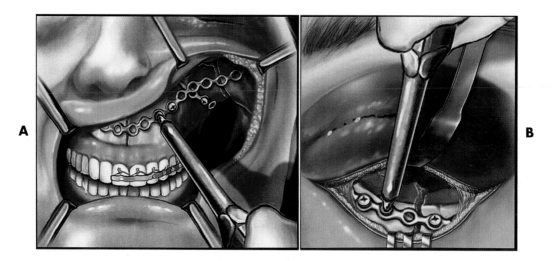

FIGURE 2-5 Artistic renderings of the intraoperative repair of a patient's facial injuries, which were used for illustration to a jury. **A,** Zygomaticomaxillary repair. **B,** Orbital repair.

physician play the role of a teacher for the laypeople on the jury, taking the medical evidence and making it easily understandable. In certain cases, especially when a medical device (e.g., metal plate and screws) has been used, the plaintiff's attorney may bring a similar device into the courtroom, have the treating physician explain its function, admit it into evidence, and perhaps pass it to the jury for inspection.

A good attorney will prepare witnesses in advance of trial testimony. The attorney wants answers that are responsive to the questions asked without going too far afield. Testimony should give the appearance of being thoughtful and complete, without seeming rehearsed or staged. In cases involving facial injuries, the plaintiff's attorney may seek the physician's guidance about the use of demonstrative aids. Photographs, diagrams, and illustrations are commonly used, especially when the damages are severe or the anatomy is complicated (Fig. 2-5). Sometimes the attorney requests several conferences with the testifying physician in advance of trial to make the presentation smooth and to anticipate the questions which are likely to arise on cross-examination by defense counsel. If liability is admitted by the defendant or is clearly apparent, the treating physician probably will be the main witness and the focus of attention for the trial.

The same caveat applies to trial testimony as to deposition testimony: Any statement made by the physician in the course of trial testimony is made under oath, under the penalties for perjury, and may be admissible as evidence in other matters. Variations or departures from the truth are to be strictly avoided.

THE PHYSICIAN AS AN EXPERT WITNESS

Most commonly, the physician caring for an individual with facial injuries will be asked to testify as a treating physician, but there are other circumstances in which testimony might be given. The term *expert witness* sometimes refers to a physician who is called to testify on the basis of specialized knowledge even when not involved in the treatment of the individual patient. However, most treating physicians are deemed to be expert witnesses as well. Jurisdictions vary as to the evidence required to designate a physician as an expert witness, but the

role of the expert is largely the same, regardless of the jurisdiction. Rule 702 of the *Federal Rules of Civil Procedure* states the following regarding expert testimony:

If scientific, technical, or other specialized knowledge will assist the trier of fact to understand the evidence or to determine a fact in issue, a witness qualified as an expert by knowledge, skill, experience, training, or education, may testify thereto in the form of an opinion or otherwise, if (1) the testimony is based upon sufficient facts or data, (2) the testimony is the product of reliable principles and methods, and (3) the witness has applied the principles and methods reliably to the facts of the case.

The role of the expert is to explain to the jury what is outside the range of knowledge of the ordinary layperson. Unlike lay witnesses, expert witnesses may give their opinions and are not restricted to a recitation of facts. Furthermore, expert witnesses may testify as to their opinion on ultimate issues, even though the trier of fact will make the final determination.

A common source of referrals for physicians to serve as expert witnesses in cases where they did not render care is from law firms that practice insurance defense law. Most jurisdictions allow for an *independent medical examination* by a physician chosen by defense counsel for this purpose. A physician who is engaged in an independent medical examination typically reviews the plaintiff's medical records, imaging studies, and any other data that are relevant to the issues of causation or damages. The rules of trial procedure in most jurisdictions require personal injury plaintiffs to submit to independent medical examinations, because the plaintiff is putting his or her medical status into the controversy. The independent medical examiner is expected to write a report of findings, including conclusions, a copy of which will be delivered to the other attorney on request.

Like the treating physician, the independent medical examiner may be subject to being deposed at a discovery deposition and perhaps at trial. Most jurisdictions allow for questioning of independent medical examiners regarding their prior testimony (in other cases) and the income derived from it. An expert who derives a substantial portion of his or her income from testifying in court, particularly if it is usually for the same side, may appear to have diminished credibility and may be perceived as a "hired gun."

MEDICAL MALPRACTICE

Almost every practicing physician has had a malpractice concern, be it real or imagined, at one time or another. Typically, concern arises in situations in which there was a less than desirable medical outcome. It is well known that the best safeguard against being named as a defendant in a medical malpractice suit is to be an effective communicator with patients and their families. Poor or suboptimal outcomes can occur even when the appropriate surgical principles and techniques are used. This is particularly true in cases of severe facial injuries, because the surgeon must deal with traumatized tissues that often will not heal in an ideal manner. Physicians who are available to speak to patients and, more importantly, to actually listen to them are less likely to be targeted in a lawsuit than those who do not communicate effectively.

Ultimately, the optimization of patient-physician rapport through the establishment of trust is the single most important factor in how patients feel about their surgical outcomes. The factors involved in obtaining a patient's trust are numerous but include a belief in the physician's honesty, effort, and concern. In short, if the patient believes that the physician cares about his problem and has made the best effort, satisfaction with the end result usually occurs.

Although most physicians believe that they know what constitutes medical negligence, they are frequently mistaken. *Medical negligence* or *medical malpractice* is a legal term, not a medical one. The elements of medical negligence are similar to those discussed earlier in the context of general negligence: duty, breach, causation, and damages. However, for a prima facie case of professional negligence, there must also be a showing of a doctor-patient relationship. As it relates to negligence that is the result of an affirmative act, the relationship may be inferred. However, if the negligence alleged is one of omission or failure to act, the doctor-patient relationship must be proved to exist for the claim to succeed.

Medical malpractice law is different from jurisdiction to jurisdiction. Although there is no one definition that will exactly fit the laws of each state, medical malpractice generally consists of rendering treatment that is "below the standard of care." *Standard of care* is an amorphous legal concept. As an example, Indiana law defines the standard of care that a physician owes to a patient as "that degree of care, skill and proficiency exercised by reasonably careful, skillful, and prudent practitioners in the same class to which he belongs, acting under the same or similar circumstances."[1] Typically, medical care need not result in a perfect outcome to avoid the attachment of liability, and physicians are not usually held liable for errors in judgment if they were made in good faith. The fact that another physician in the same specialty might have treated a given patient differently does not mean that the care rendered was negligent.

In the majority of jurisdictions, a particular physician's medical care is judged by a community standard. This means that a physician's care is not compared to a textbook standard but rather to the standard of care in his particular medical community (the "locality rule"). Many jurisdictions have supplanted this doctrine with the "modified locality rule," which allows for a physician's care to be judged by a standard in a similar community, not necessarily the same community in which he practices. Because medical negligence cases require an expert opinion, it can be difficult in smaller communities to find a plaintiff's expert to testify critically about the care given by another member of the same medical community.

Because of advances in technology and the abundance of seminars and written materials, some jurisdictions are moving toward a national standard of care. If this trend progresses, it would be detrimental to practitioners in smaller communities with less sophisticated medical resources, who currently are not held to the same standard as their counterparts in large urban centers. This is a developing area in medical negligence law, and its progress should be carefully monitored by American physicians and organized medicine.

CONTROVERSIES

Although few physicians relish participating in the medicolegal process, treating patients with facial injuries is likely to lead to multiple interactions with attorneys and the courts. This is inevitable and should not be viewed as controversial or undesirable. It is an inherent part of helping patients recover from facial injuries. It is not as glamorous nor as appealing as surgical reconstruction, but it is very important for many patients who will be scarred or deformed or suffer some lifelong orofacial dysfunction.

The acquisition of digital imaging data can be a two-edged sword. Whereas every patient has a legal right to his own imaging information, including preoperative, intraoperative, or postoperative photographs, the question frequently arises as to how much of this information should be given voluntarily to the patient. Many patients are aware that some or all of these records exist and will request copies of them. Increasingly, patients are asking for their photographic file to be e-mailed to them. Often this contains intraoperative images of procedures and very explicit illustrations of open facial anatomy. Whether patients or their families can emotionally handle or should be exposed to such dramatic images of themselves is debatable. This situation creates an obvious ambiguity between what the patient is legally entitled to see and what the physician thinks is appropriate for patient viewing. Recognizable images of the patient and any use thereof are clearly within the release discretion of the patient. Unrecognizable images of intraoperative procedures, even if of the patient, are often thought to be within the province of the physician. The exact legal precedence on these issues remains to be established.

CONCLUSION

Facial injuries frequently result in medicolegal concerns due to the potential for resultant disfigurement and dysfunction. Most commonly, the treating physician becomes involved as a source of medical information to chronicle the history of care provided since the initial injury and the potential need for future reconstructive surgeries. In this role, the physician's involvement is as an ally of the patient in his effort to receive legal and financial recovery from the injuries.

More infrequently, the treating physician may become involved in an adversarial role in which his care is questioned or is believed to be a contributory factor in the less than desirable outcome. In the case of traumatic injuries, such physician involvement is usually rare. In any case, proper medical documentation, both written and photographic, is an invaluable asset.

With these potential roles in mind, the creation of written notes and dictated operative reports should be as thorough as possible, and they should never be altered subsequently. The objective medical facts should be recorded, and comments about the etiology of the facial injury should be confined to what can be substantiated. Digital facial photographs should be obtained before the initiation of any care, and, ideally, postoperative outcomes should be similarly documented.

THE ENGLISH LEGAL SYSTEM

Legal systems vary around the world. This part of the chapter is an overview of some medicolegal aspects of the legal system in England. Most doctors in England practice medicine in the state-run National Health Service (NHS). Some may also have a practice in the independent health care sector, and a small group work solely in the independent sector.

The circumstances in which a clinician may be brought before the courts in England are similar to those that pertain in the United States; that is, to give evidence at an inquest or in a civil or criminal action. In any of these situations, clinicians may be asked to give factual witness evidence or to give evidence and opinion as a medical expert witness. Whereas factual evidence is limited to the circumstances in which the injury came about, the nature and extent of the injury, and the observed course of recovery, expert evidence further gleans the opinion of the expert as to the likely mechanism or cause of the injury and the potential for partial or complete recovery in the future.

In a civil action for clinical negligence (medical malpractice), the clinician may be called on to give either factual evidence or expert evidence. Cases of alleged negligent treatment may be brought by patients against an NHS Trust in the public sector or against a clinician in the independent health care sector.

THE CLINICIAN'S ROLE IN THE LEGAL PROCESS

THE CRIMINAL CASE

A clinician who treats an individual who has suffered facial trauma may be asked to give factual or expert evidence in a criminal action if the trauma could have been the result of a criminal act. This usually follows an allegation of physical assault, although other common causes are road traffic accidents, attacks by animals, and, occasionally, accidents at work. The factual evidence required from the clinician will relate to the extent of injury at presentation, an opinion about the possible cause of the injury, and whether it is possible to use this "factual evidence" to determine that it was caused by

the alleged criminal act. In criminal law, the evidential standard is higher than in civil law, and the case must be proved beyond a reasonable doubt.

THE CIVIL CASE

To prove negligence in a civil action, the court has to be satisfied that there was a duty of care owed to the individual by the defendant, that the duty was breached, and that the breach caused loss or damage to the individual that was not so remote as to have been unforeseeable by the defendant. The evidential standard is lower than in a criminal case. The case has to be based on a balance of probabilities (i.e., that negligence is more likely to have occurred than not).

Allegations of negligence in a civil action may be made against one or more of the following:

- an employer, if the individual was injured at work (employer's liability)
- another individual, for example if the claimant was involved in a road traffic accident (Road Traffic Act) or an accident on another person's property (occupier's liability)
- the manufacturer of a defective product (manufacturer's liability)
- the owner of an animal that has caused injury (public liability)
- an NHS Trust (clinical negligence)
- a clinician treating patients in the independent health care sector (clinical negligence)

In relation to the first four of these categories, the clinician will be asked either to give factual evidence about the nature and extent of injury sustained or to give expert evidence about the probable mechanism or cause of the injury. Expert opinion on the extent to which the injury has affected the claimant, the potential for recovery, and the future effects on the individual's quality of life may also be needed by the court.

In relation to the last two categories, the clinician may be asked to give factual evidence concerning the medical treatment received by the claimant after an injury or during the course of an illness and the clinician's role in that treatment if he was personally involved. As an expert witness, the clinician may also be asked to give an opinion on the treatment in relation to the standard of care and whether it was appropriate in the particular circumstances. The factual witness cannot give expert opinion in an English legal case. A separate independent expert will be engaged for that purpose.

The most common allegations relating to clinical negligence are the following:

- There was inappropriate medical or surgical treatment (e.g., wrong or unnecessary surgery).
- There was a delay in diagnosis and treatment.
- There was incorrect interpretation of tests or results.
- There was an incorrect prescription or incorrect administration of medicines or other preparations.
- There was a lack of informed consent about the risks of treatment, and those risks ultimately materialized.
- The treatment was not performed to the standard expected from a reasonable body of practitioners working in the same field.

CONSIDERATIONS FOR THE TREATING CLINICIAN

Clinicians should consider the possibility of future litigation during every consultation with patients who have sustained facial injury. In the current atmosphere of an increasingly litigious society, clear and concise documentation of the nature and extent of injury is vital. The patient's version of the history of the injury is obviously important. Diagrams and photographs, where appropriate and where resources allow, are usually invaluable. They are particularly useful in criminal cases and in civil cases in which facial scarring could lead to a future allegation that the cosmetic outcome falls below the standard expected of a reasonably competent surgeon. Photographic evidence may also avoid a later dispute about the extent of the presenting injury.

ANATOMY OF THE LITIGATION PROCESS

The first indication of an impending claim is usually a letter detailing a complaint or requesting access to the patient's medical records. This may come from the patient or from his or her solicitor.

The Data Protection Act of 1998 governs the "obtaining, holding, use or disclosure of information." It makes provision for regulation of the processing of information[2] about individuals and recognizes the individual's right to be told what information is being processed about him and to have it disclosed. Under the Act, *data subjects* (in this case, patients) have the right to be told by any *data controller* (in this case, the doctor, the health authority, or the Trust) whenever personal data about them are being processed. The term *processed* is defined widely to cover every possible act relating to the data. The request for access must be made in writing, and the data controller must disclose the relevant information within 40 days after receiving the request. However, the data may be withheld in certain circumstances:

- if there has not been a reasonable interval since the individual last had access to his or her records
- if disclosure would be likely to cause serious harm to the physical or mental health or condition of the patient or any other individual[3]
- if disclosing the records would mean giving information about a third party

The NHS has a procedure operating within Trusts to deal with letters of complaint from patients before solicitors are involved.[4] The Department of Health places great emphasis on resolving complaints as quickly as possible.[5] This may be accomplished through a swift informal response from the clinician involved or through prompt action to open further investigations and seek conciliation. A properly handled complaints procedure can result in local resolution of many grievances and avoid expensive litigation.

It should be remembered that the complaints file is disclosable to the claimant (patient) or the claimant's solicitors in any subsequent litigation unless it can be argued that it was specifically created for the purposes of the litigation, in which case it attracts privilege from disclosure. However, it is rare that a complaints file is considered privileged in this way. Doctors need to think very carefully about their responses to complaints and should always have in mind that the patient is likely to see what they have written as well as any notes of conversations they may have had about the case.

If the claimant is not satisfied on completion of the internal complaints procedure, or if an internal investigation concludes that the standard of treatment was unacceptable, the claimant may instruct solicitors to pursue the complaint in a court of law.

If the patient does decide to proceed, a letter detailing the claim will be sent to the Trust's legal department or solicitors or to the individual doctor or his solicitors in the independent sector. The letter of claim is the first step in the legal process and is termed the *pre-action letter of claim*. There is a *pre-action protocol* that sets out the steps to be taken by both parties to attempt to resolve the dispute, if at all possible, before proceedings are issued in court. The aim is to encourage openness between the parties and to reduce delay, costs, and the need for litigation.

The letter of claim must set out the allegations and the alleged causal link with the injury and should also give an indication of the likely level of damages claimed. A *letter of response* must be provided within 3 months of receipt of the letter of claim. If there is no merit in the allegations, the claim may be denied, giving clear and detailed reasons, and the claimant may then decide to abandon any further legal proceedings.

If an agreement cannot be reached between the two parties, the claimant can issue a formal court document (a *claim form*) to begin legal proceedings. The claimant must submit particulars of the claim, detailing the specific allegations and the damage caused. If the clinician has been involved in the complaints procedure or during the pre-action protocol stage of proceedings, he will be asked to comment on the particulars of the claim. At this stage, a barrister (known legally as *counsel*) will become involved, and the clinician may be asked to attend a conference with counsel to examine the evidence obtained so far and to assess the probability of defending the claim successfully. Another clinician may be instructed to give an expert opinion at this stage.

ROLE OF THE FACTUAL WITNESS

In a civil action, the treating clinician may be approached by either the patient's solicitors or the solicitors for the defense to act as a factual witness. It is important to discover the exact nature of the proposed litigation immediately, because any potential for a clinical negligence claim will require early advice from solicitors acting for the NHS Trust or for a defense organization.

As a factual witness, the clinician is likely to be asked to give details of the extent of the initial injury or complaint. This will be in the form of a *witness statement*. The clinician should provide information only about facts that are within the scope of his knowledge, although such information may include a statement relating the patient's version of the cause of the injury. The witness statement should be clear and accurate; where there is no direct recollection of events, the clinician should state that the evidence is based on the contemporaneous recordings in the notes. He should refrain from giving an expert opinion. If for any reason the clinician refuses to give evidence, he may be subpoenaed. If he still refuses, he may be held in contempt of court, which can attract a fine or even a penal sentence.

If the allegations involve the quality of the treatment given to the patient, the factual witness is most likely to be approached by the hospital's solicitors or by those retained by a defense organization. There is a duty under the physician's contract with the NHS to assist with any such litigation. The evidence should be submitted as previously described (i.e., explaining only those facts within his knowledge or in the medical records). He may also comment on his usual clinical practice at the time, if this helps to clarify the evidence.

The process of giving evidence in England and Wales is different from that in the United States. The U.S. legal process frequently involves depositions, which often are given on video recordings, to answer questions from the lawyers acting for both parties. In England and Wales, the witness statement is written down in a specific format required by the court, and there are no questions from the opposing lawyers until the witness appears in court. The factual witness submits a written statement setting out the facts within his knowledge that are relevant to the allegations being made. He concludes by signing a *statement of truth,* which appears at the end, and he can be held in contempt of court if the statement is later proved to be false.

The witness statement is disclosed to the claimant's legal team and stands as the evidence of the factual witness at trial, although counsel for the defense may, with leave from the trial judge, raise some additional questions about it. The witness will be cross-examined by the opposing counsel, who may attempt to discredit the accuracy of the evidence submitted or to undermine the credibility of the witness. This can be prevented in part by good medical documentation and in some instances by photographic evidence. The trial judge may also question the witness, particularly for the purpose of clarifying any part of the evidence or understanding the medical terms.

The clinician as a factual witness should consider the questions carefully and give answers accordingly. Answers should be given only when the information is within the physician's personal knowledge, and the response should be unhurried. Answers are always addressed to the judge, and testimony should be slow and clear to give the judge time to take notes on the evidence.

ROLE OF THE EXPERT WITNESS

The expert witness has a duty directly to the court and not to those instructing him. He should be entirely independent, in accordance with Part 35 of the Civil Procedure Rules of 1998, which sets out the rules that apply to expert evidence.[2]

Wherever practical, the court will direct the use of a single joint expert witness who is instructed by both parties to the litigation. This is most appropriate when the expert is being asked to comment on the present condition of the claimant and the prognosis of the injury sustained. In a case of clinical negligence, the expert will also be asked to comment on any breach of duty and on causation. Although a single joint expert may still be appropriate in some cases, most defense solicitors will be concerned that the expert is being asked to arbitrate, which would be inappropriate. The legal test to be satisfied is whether a responsible body of doctors practicing in the same field would support the treatment given. It is not

difficult to imagine that one expert might be a proponent of the treatment in question and another might not. This obviously raises difficulties if a single expert is used to represent both sides, because it may be important for the judge to hear contrary views in order to decide whether the allegations of breach of duty and causation can be sustained. Therefore, the usual practice, subject to court approval, is to use separate experts to represent each side with regard to breach of duty and causation and to rely on joint experts only for condition and prognosis evidence.

Once expert evidence has been obtained, the next procedural step is for the solicitors acting for both parties to simultaneously exchange their reports. Both parties may submit written questions directly to the other party's expert within 28 days after this exchange for the purpose of clarifying the evidence contained therein. The expert witness receiving questions directly from the patient's solicitor may need to refer to his own solicitor for advice and clarification of the questions posed. For example, if a question relates to the factual evidence, it would be appropriate for the expert witness to decline to respond, on the basis that he was not present at the time of the alleged incident.

After the exchange of expert evidence and supplementary written questions, the court will direct the experts to meet in an attempt to narrow the areas in dispute and to reduce the time required for any subsequent trial. Even at this late stage, it may still be possible to resolve the matter altogether. A written statement must be produced after the meeting and should set out the areas of agreement and disagreement between the experts and the reasoning behind any remaining disagreements.

All of the statements and reports are signed and must contain a statement of truth. At trial, the expert's report should stand as his submission of evidence, although he may be taken through the report by counsel in order to summarize and clarify its contents for the benefit of the judge. As with the factual witness, experts should take time for careful consideration of the questions posed and should give unhurried answers based within the limits of their own knowledge. Answers are always directed to the judge and should be slow and clear to allow the judge time to record the evidence. Most courts of law have the facilities to record the evidence, but a transcript takes time to produce, and the Judge will make notes on key issues as the evidence is produced in court.

CONCLUSION

Many practicing clinicians have encountered a complaint from a patient, and some have become involved in the processes outlined here. Cases of facial trauma are most likely to involve allegations of criminal conduct or of clinical negligence related to the cosmetic result. As in the United States, excellent documentation and good communication with the patient and relatives will serve the treating clinician well in the avoidance of litigation. However, the increase in public expectations and a tendency to resort to litigation have resulted in a relentless rise in medical litigation.

Except for minor procedural differences in Scotland and Wales, the principles of law relating to clinical negligence are consistent throughout the United Kingdom, without the variations that occur among the states in America. For a claim to be successful, the patient must prove, on the balance of probabilities:

- that the doctor owed a duty of care
- that there was a breach of that duty of care
- that foreseeable harm followed as a result of that breach of duty of care

The standard of care is the standard of a responsible body of doctors practicing in the same field of medicine. However, it does not have to be the standard of the majority. This is known as the *Bolam test*.[6] Although this test was challenged in the case of *Bolitho v Hackney Health Authority*,[7] it remains essentially intact. Since *Bolitho*, a doctor needs to demonstrate not only that other doctors would have acted in a similar manner but that his course of action was reasonable in the circumstances (i.e., stands up to logical analysis). There is no equivalent of the locality rule in the United States.

With the further use of National Guidelines, audit, and clinical governance, the standard of treatment administered throughout the United Kingdom will inevitably become more regulated and as a consequence less varied, although there is always likely to be a range of techniques for different procedures. Whether this means that in the future the legal test will be held by the courts to have been satisfied by compliance with National Guidelines remains to be seen. At present, compliance is evidence of good practice, but noncompliance is not necessarily evidence of negligence.

REFERENCES

1. Data Protection Act, 1998. www.legislation.gov.uk/ukpga/1998/29/introduction
2. Civil Procedure Rules 1998, Part 35, Rule 35.3. www.justice.gov.uk/guidance/courts-and-tribunals/courts/procedure-rules
3. *Data Protection (Subject Access Modification) (Health) Order* (2000). www.ico.gov.uk
4. *The Hospital Complaints Procedure Act* (1985). www.legislation.gov.uk
5. http://www.doh.gov.uk. Accessed March 8, 2011.
6. *Bolam v Friern Hospital Management Committee,* 1 WLR 582 (1957).
7. *Bolitho v City and Hackney Area Health Authority,* AC 232 (1998).

CHAPTER 3

Immediate Care in the Emergency Room

David W. Macpherson, Roger M. Webb

Trauma is the leading cause of death from birth to age 44 years. It is third only to cancer and atherosclerosis in all age groups. It is a leading global public health problem, affecting 135 million people a year, and it is estimated that more than 5 million people died from trauma in the year 2004.[1] Of these, more than 1 million (20%) died from Road Traffic Accidents (RTAs) (Fig. 3-1). Other major causes of trauma are sports-related injuries, interpersonal violence, occupational injuries, and falls. In the United Kingdom, falls represent the biggest single group.

Worldwide, approximately 50 million people are severely or moderately disabled as a result of trauma and more than 180 million disability-adjusted life years are lost each year.[2] In the United Kingdom, across all age groups combined, trauma is a leading cause of death, and kills more than 16,000 people per year in England and Wales.[3] Trauma is one of the few disease categories in which mortality is increasing.

The burden of trauma constitutes 12% of the world's total disease load.[4] It is estimated that the global financial cost of trauma exceeds U.S.$500 billion annually. Apart from the emotional distress, a significant number of trauma victims are injured seriously enough that they are never able to work again. This converts them from productive, employed members of society, paying taxes and contributing to the state's finances, to net receivers of state aid, dependent on the welfare system for financial support, potentially for many years. This figure is further compounded when it is considered that trauma is largely a disease of younger people.

Since the full financial cost, as well as the physical and emotional suffering, major reviews of the field of trauma management have been carried out with the aim of improving the quality of service and reducing the mortality and morbidity. These reviews have focused both on improving the whole quality of care, from the time of trauma to eventual discharge, with full rehabilitation, and on prevention of the trauma in the first place.

The cost of trauma is escalating in all countries. In developed countries, the proportion of deaths from "preventable" trauma, such as RTAs, is declining but the proportion from other causes, such as falls and interpersonal violence, is increasing. The decrease in preventable deaths results from the twin approaches of prevention and better care. In these countries, society is moving forward from "managing illness" to "promoting wellness" and "preventing illness." This policy should eventually result in reduced health care costs. However,

both prevention and improved trauma management are very expensive to implement and may not be feasible in less developed countries. Consequently, more than 90% of RTA deaths worldwide now occur in the less developed countries.

Improved quality of care reduces both mortality and morbidity. A greater proportion of patients survive, and a greater proportion of survivors make a full recovery. This requires both national strategic planning and development of local provision of care. Experience from management of trauma on the battlefield is translated into more rapid evolution of improvements in civilian care as lessons continue to be learned from conflicts around the globe.

The earlier resuscitation can be initiated after injury and the quicker the victim can be transported to an appropriate care facility, the better. In war zones, this fact has led to immediate support by frontline medics and rapid helicopter evacuation, initially to a field hospital and then to a higher-level center.[5] In the civilian world, it has led to significant investment in prehospital care and in the emergency facilities that are provided at receiving hospitals.

The ideal hospital is a Level 1 Trauma Center where all medical specialties, with full back-up infrastructure, are on site 24 hours a day (Box 3-1). Because these facilities are extremely expensive to provide and maintain, it is more cost-effective to have centralized major trauma units. These need to be located in urban areas of high population, facilitating rapid access and high-quality care for the greatest number of people. Although this has been accomplished in the United States, trauma services in the United Kingdom are still largely designed around the district general hospital (DGH), which serves a population of 250,000 to 400,000. Although the services in these hospitals have been significantly improved, only one patient with major, life-threatening trauma (Injury Severity Score [ISS] >15) may be received in these hospitals on a weekly basis and additionally, the patient will still need to be transferred to a specialized unit if they have sustained cardiothoracic, neurosurgical, or burn injuries.

Work is now progressing to develop regional trauma systems in the United Kingdom. Major trauma cases would be taken directly to a Trauma Center, which would serve a population of 2 to 3 million. These units would expect to receive in excess of 400 major cases per year, leading to better outcomes.[6-9] Longer prehospital transfer times have been found to make little difference in mortality and morbidity if the destination is a fully staffed trauma center.[10] At present in

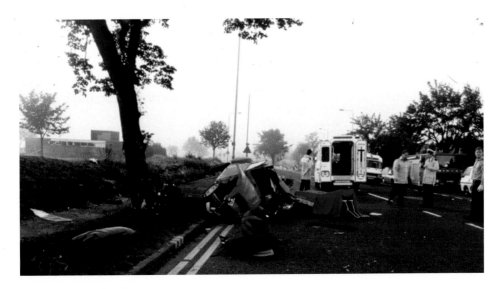

FIGURE 3-1   Road traffic accident scene. Emergency services are clearing up. The road will remain closed until the accident investigation team has assessed the scene fully.

BOX 3-1   **Aim of Trauma Care**

- Identification of major trauma patients at the scene of the incident
- Immediate intervention to allow safe transport
- Rapid transfer to appropriate trauma center for surgical management and critical care
- Coordinated specialist reconstruction
- Targeted comprehensive rehabilitation

the United Kingdom, the mortality rate for severely injured trauma patients who are alive on arrival at hospital is 40% greater than in the United States, where there is an established regional trauma system.[11]

The original paper showing that, in the absence of a trauma system, 30% of in-hospital trauma deaths are preventable was published more than 2 decades ago, in 1988.[12] However, the apparent downgrading of a local DGH Accident Center remains a politically very sensitive issue, and effective strategic communications will be required to help the local population understand the rationale behind reconfiguration of major trauma services.[13]

The whole ethos of patient care, from the arrival of the first emergency personnel at the scene through complete rehabilitation and discharge, must be to **"Do no further harm,"** and therefore appropriately trained personnel must provide the care (Fig. 3-2).

PREHOSPITAL CARE

The definition of an integrated trauma system incorporates prehospital care and the need to identify and deliver patients to a place of definitive care safely and quickly. It is essential that trauma services be thoroughly planned and funded to ensure provision of the most efficient and effective services to meet the predictable needs of the population within the capital budget available, because considerable numbers of

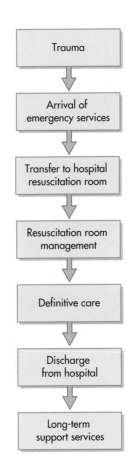

FIGURE 3-2   Seamless trauma care continuum.

trauma incidents occur at a significant distance from such facilities.

In the United Kingdom, this has resulted in significant investment in the ambulance services, upgrading their role essentially from first-aid hospital taxi services to first-line care providers. The vehicles themselves are outfitted with essential equipment necessary to provide immediate resuscitation. In addition, most regions have air ambulance facilities to expedite transfer of the victim from the scene of the accident to the hospital. The best environment for resuscitation is a safe, warm, dry, well-lit, fully staffed and equipped area with complete back-up resources—laboratory, imaging facilities, operating rooms, intensive care units, and so on—immediately available.

All emergency services personnel, including police and firefighters in addition to ambulance crews, are trained in basic life support techniques. The initial aim on arrival at the scene is to assess the situation in relation to the safety of both the victims and the service providers. Ambulance crews attending trauma scenes are now specifically trained paramedics; in addition to providing basic life support, they are able to assess the patient and carry out more advanced supportive techniques, concentrating on airway maintenance, respiratory support, immobilization of the patient, and control of external bleeding and shock during any delay that may occur in extricating and transporting the patient to the nearest appropriate facility.

Paramedic crews assess the victims and communicate with the planned receiving hospital, giving them advance warning of the number of patients, the severity of their injuries, and the estimated time of arrival. The crew also routinely carry digital cameras and take photographs at the scene to transport with the patient; these can help clarify the situation and assist in determining the "index of suspicion" of injuries incurred (Fig. 3-3).

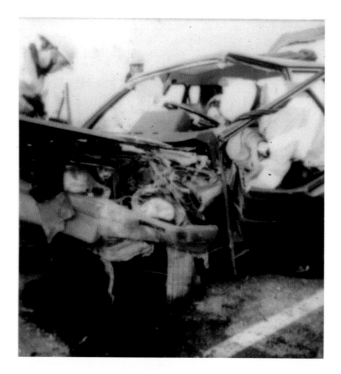

FIGURE 3-3 Typical Polaroid photograph brought in with the patient, taken by the paramedics at the scene. Although the image is out of focus, the severity of the accident can be pictured, enabling a more accurate assessment of "the index of suspicion" regarding the patient's injuries.

TRIAGE

Triage is the sorting of patients based on their need for treatment and the available resources to provide the treatment. This sorting may be carried out by the paramedic team at the accident scene, who decide what level of care is required and therefore to which hospital the patient needs to be transferred. Triage also may be done at the receiving hospital, if it is a small unit (e.g., a U.S. community hospital) with limited facilities and personnel. Triage in this situation may be based on which patients need immediate, life-saving intervention, which can wait, and which are, in fact, beyond saving.

There are two types of triage. *Multiple casualties* is the term used when the number of patients and the severity of their injuries do not exceed the ability of the facility to provide care. Patients with life-threatening problems and those who have sustained multiple-system injuries are treated first. *Mass casualties* is the term used to describe the situation in which the number of patients and the severity of their injuries exceed the capability of the facility and the staff. Those patients who have the greatest chance of survival with the least expenditure of time, supplies, equipment, and personnel are managed first.

PREPARATION AT THE RECEIVING HOSPITAL

Each hospital is capable of managing only a limited number of patients. If the number of trauma vicims exceeds the ability of the hospital to handle them, a *major incident* is called, and a pre-prepared and practiced action plan is implemented whereby neighboring hospitals are alerted and warned that they will also be receiving patients. Natural incidents such as floods, hurricanes, and tidal waves still account for most of the deaths worldwide, but manmade incidents resulting from technological or other human interactions are more common, especially in the urban setting. Terrorist actions in densely populated areas, such as in New York on 9/11/2001 and in London on 7/7/2005, test the best equipped and organized services.

However, under most circumstances, the receiving hospital should be capable of receiving the victims. The hospital must have a fully equipped and staffed *resuscitation room* with comprehensive back-up of all the necessary support teams, such as radiology, blood bank, and ICU.

A formally constituted *trauma team*, ideally comprising specialist anesthetic, surgical, and orthopedic components in addition to the emergency department staff, should be immediately available (Fig. 3-4), with the ability to summon extra specialist assistance (e.g., an obstetrician for a pregnant patient) if necessary. All members should have appropriate training, such as the Advanced Trauma Life Support (ATLS) course, which has become the gold standard and common language of trauma management.

The involvement of maxillofacial surgeons in trauma teams has significant benefits in terms of training and in the early identification and optimal management of craniofacial trauma. As a member of the trauma team, the maxillofacial surgeon must be skilled in trauma life support techniques and capable of dealing with both specialty-specific problems and other life-threatening conditions. In addition, expertise concerning midface injuries and any potential threat to eyesight from trauma and hemorrhage is invaluable.[14]

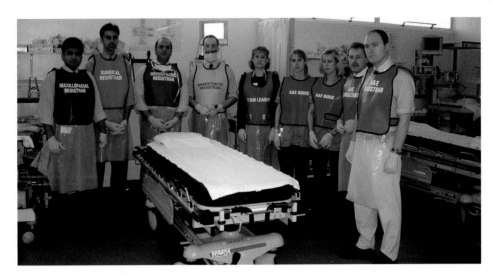

FIGURE 3-4   Full trauma team lined up in the resuscitation room before the arrival of the patient. The paramedical team telephones from the ambulance to enable the hospital team to be fully prepared for the victim's arrival. Medical and nursing staff work together as a team.

The team should assemble in the resuscitation room and put on protective clothing. The absolute minimum gear includes rubber latex gloves, plastic aprons, and eye protection, because all blood and body fluids should be considered to be infected with the human immunodeficiency virus (HIV) and hepatitis viruses. In addition, all members of the team should be immunized against tetanus and hepatitis B. Staff who undress the patients should initially wear more robust gloves, because trauma patients often have glass and other debris in their clothing, and ordinary surgical gloves do not provide enough protection.

The team leader should brief the team and assign specific duties, so that each member knows the task for which he or she is responsible (e.g., airway, circulation). To avoid chaos, no more than six people should be touching the patient at any one time. A final check of the equipment by the appropriate team members can then be made. Only minimal preparation of the resuscitation room should be necessary, because it should be kept fully stocked and ready for use at all times.

Once the patient arrives in the resuscitation room, a stop clock is started so that accurate times can be recorded. The patient should be transferred from the stretcher to the trolley in a coordinated fashion to avoid injury to the spinal column or exacerbation of preexisting injuries. The lines and leads should be checked so that they do not become tangled or disconnected.

INITIAL ASSESSMENT OF THE PATIENT

Deaths from trauma follow a trimodal distribution (Fig. 3-5). The first peak, constituting 40% to 50% of trauma deaths, occurs immediately or within minutes of the accident, at the scene. The causes are usually related to lacerations of the brain, brainstem, high spinal cord, heart, aorta, or other large blood vessels. Due to the severity of their injuries, very few of these patients survive. Only prevention—safer roads, speed restriction, air bags, and other measures—can significantly reduce this peak of trauma-related deaths, although the

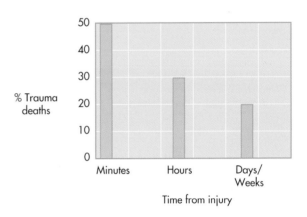

FIGURE 3-5   Trimodal death distribution. About 50% of victims die at the scene of the accident, and the remainder succumb soon after arrival in hospital (approximately 30%) or subsequently (approximately 20%).

speedy arrival of trained personnel who are able to begin immediate resuscitation may save some victims.

The second peak, representing approximately 30% of trauma-related deaths, consists of those patients who arrive alive in the hospital resuscitation room but succumb to their injuries over the next minutes or hours. This period is referred to as the *golden hour*. These patients die largely from hypoxia and hypovolemic shock as a result of severe chest injuries with hemothorax or cardiac tamponade, abdominal trauma with ruptured spleen or liver, or orthopedic injuries such as fractured pelvis or long bones associated with significant blood loss.

The third peak is made up of patients who succumb days or even weeks after the traumatic incident from causes such as multiple organ failure, sepsis, or respiratory distress (Box 3-2).

The immediate assessment and early management of the trauma patient is comprehensively covered by the ATLS course. ATLS focuses on the second peak, because

BOX 3-2 Causes of Trauma Death

- *Deaths at the scene*: brainstem injury, airway obstruction, heart or major vessel injury
- *Early deaths*: airway obstruction, uncontrolled blood loss, extradural or subdural hematoma
- *Late deaths*: multiple organ failure, respiratory distress, sepsis

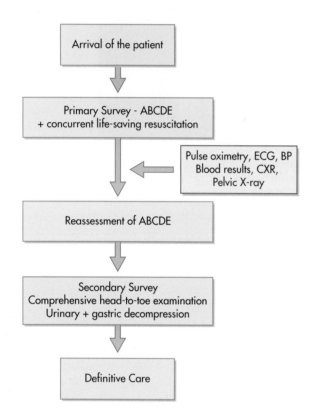

FIGURE 3-6 *Management of the trauma patient.*

appropriate and timely intervention in the resuscitation room will both save lives and minimize morbidity, thereby also reducing the third peak in the subsequent definitive care period lasting days or weeks.

PRIMARY SURVEY AND RESUSCITATION

The patient is transferred to the emergency (resuscitation) room where a rapid primary survey is carried out (Fig. 3-6). Care must follow the safest pathway, diagnosing and simultaneously treating life-threatening injuries in the order in which they would otherwise kill the patient. As each most pressing killer injury is treated, more resuscitation time is created to deal with the next most pressing problem.

Each patient should be assessed in the same way, and the appropriate tasks should be performed automatically and simultaneously by the team. To facilitate this, the primary survey of the patient follows a strict, sequential "ABCDE" protocol:

A: **Airway with Cervical Spine Control**
B: **Breathing and Ventilation**

C: **Circulation and Hemorrhage Control**
D: **Disability–(Neurological status**
E: **Exposure + environment – completely undress the patient, but prevent hypothermia**

To these, another point may be added:

F: **Frequent Reassessment must be made**

It is essential to ensure that prehospital personnel provide a comprehensive account of the accident scene. In addition to patient details, important information such as the time of the accident, weather conditions, ambient temperature, and other factors such as fires, explosions, hazardous chemicals, and injuries sustained by other victims must all be gathered. Photographs taken at the scene also provide vital information, giving clues to understanding the mechanism of injury and, from that, what injuries might be anticipated (index of suspicion).[15]

Maxillofacial injuries are addressed at this stage only if they have an impact on the airway, breathing, or circulation. Comprehensive assessment and definitive management of maxillofacial injuries occur later, away from the resuscitation room setting.

Priorities for care of the pediatric patient are the same as for adults, and priorities for care of the pregnant woman are similar to those for nonpregnant patients. Pregnancy should be identified early by palpation of the abdomen for a gravid uterus and by laboratory testing for human chorionic gonadotropin (HCG). Early fetal assessment is important for maternal and fetal survival.

Trauma is the fifth most common cause of death in the elderly. Comorbidities such as cardiac, respiratory, and metabolic diseases are more common, and, together with the aging process, they reduce the patient's functional reserve and ability to respond to injury. The chronic use of medications may also alter the usual physiological response to injury. The narrow therapeutic window frequently leads to overresuscitation or underresuscitation in the elderly, and early invasive monitoring is valuable.

A: AIRWAY AND CERVICAL SPINE CONTROL

There should be a high index of suspicion for cervical spine injury if the patient has maxillofacial injuries or multisystem trauma, if the level of consciousness is altered, or if there is a history of a high-speed impact. Approximately 15% of patients with supraclavicular injuries also have a cervical spine injury, and 5% of head-injured patients have some form of associated cervical, thoracic, lumbar, or sacral spinal injury. Although spinal injuries most commonly occur in the cervical region, other parts of the spine are affected in 45% of cases, and in 10% of cases, there is a second and completely separate spinal injury. Therefore, great care should be taken to prevent excessive movement of the cervical spine during assessment and management of a patient's airway (Fig. 3-7). Again, the overriding management principle should be, **"Do no further harm"** (Box 3-3).

An assessment must immediately be made as to whether the patient can maintain and protect his or her own airway. The team leader should talk to the patient while the neck is kept manually in a neutral position without longitudinal

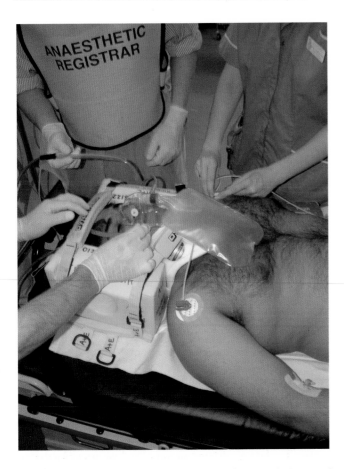

FIGURE 3-7 Cervical spine immobilization. A semirigid cervical collar with head blocks and tapes is being used. Supplementary oxygen is being supplied by a mask with reservoir bag.

BOX 3-3   Cervical Spine Assessment

Assume that the cervical spine may be injuried, particularly if any of the following is present:
- Blunt trauma above the clavicles
- Head injury (any patient with altered level of consciousness)
- Hypoxia, trauma, alcohol, drugs
- Maxillofacial trauma
- Multiple trauma (injury above and below the clavicles)
  Remember: SUSPECT, PROTECT, DETECT

"What happened?" If the patient gives an appropriate and coherent response, it suggests that the airway (A) is clear, that breathing and ventilation (B) are sufficiently effective to deliver enough oxygen into the circulation (C), which is functioning sufficiently to transport the oxygen to the brain (D), which in turn is functioning sufficiently to allow the patient to comprehend and respond. In addition, information about the patient, the medical history, and the details of the accident may be gathered. However, there is a significant caveat: Although the patient's ABCD factors may be functioning satisfactorily at the time of questioning, they may not be shortly, so that frequent re-examination is essential.

Basic Airway Maneuvers

Supplemental oxygen delivered through a well-fitted reservoir (rebreathing) mask, at a rate of 15 L/min to achieve maximum oxygenation of the tissues, should be given to every trauma patient.

If the patient fails to respond to questioning, formal airway assessment must be immediately instigated. As always, clinical assessment should follow the protocol, **"Look, Listen, and Feel."**

- **Look** to see if the patient is agitated or obtunded. Agitation suggests hypoxia, and obtundation suggests hypercarbia. Cyanosis indicates hypoxemia and can be seen in the lips and nailbeds. Look for the pattern of breathing and use of accessory muscles of ventilation.
- **Look** for facial burns; singed eyebrows, facial hair, or nasal vibrissae; and soot around the lips, in the mouth, or in the sputum (indicating burn injury, inhalational burns, and possibly impending airway obstruction).
- **Listen** for abnormal sounds. Noisy breathing is obstructed breathing. Snoring, gurgling, and crowing noises (stridor) may be associated with partial obstruction of the pharynx or larynx. Hoarseness implies functional laryngeal obstruction. The abusive or belligerent patient may be hypoxic and should not be presumed to be intoxicated.
- **Feel** for the location of the trachea and determine whether it is in the midline.
- The mouth should be opened and any foreign objects (e.g., fractured teeth, fillings, dentures) should be removed. The mouth is examined, and any fluid is sucked out. The nature and volume of the fluid (secretions, blood) and evidence of pooling in the oropharynx indicate loss of airway control by the patient.

In an unconscious patient who is lying supine on a gurney, the tongue may fall back and obstruct the airway; a simple chin lift or jaw thrust maneuver can be used to correct the tongue position and open the airway. Those patients with a gag reflex can maintain their own airway. The use of oropharyngeal (Guedel) airways in these patients can precipitate vomiting, neck movement, and a rise in intracranial pressure; therefore, a nasopharyngeal airway is preferred, provided there is no evidence to suggest a fracture of the base of the skull.

A **jaw thrust** is performed by grasping the angles of the mandible with one hand on each side and displacing the mandible forward. If the patient is breathing spontaneously, high-flow oxygen via the facemask and reservoir bag will provide good oxygenation and ventilation (Fig. 3-8). If the patient is not breathing, a facemask with a bag-valve device

compression or distraction. This can be achieved simply and quickly by placing one hand on either side of the patient's head and holding the head in a neutral position, taking care not to cover the ears. If the head is twisted to one side, it should be carefully straightened, ensuring that the neck is not extended or flexed in the process. In the motorcyclist, the neck should be supported from below while an assistant carefully expands the helmet laterally and removes it from above. Removal of the helmet using a cast cutter while stabilizing the head and neck minimizes cervical spine motion in a patient with a known cervical spine injury. The neck is then splinted with a rigid collar of appropriate size to grip the chin.

Much information can be gained very quickly by asking the patient a simple question such as "How are you?" or

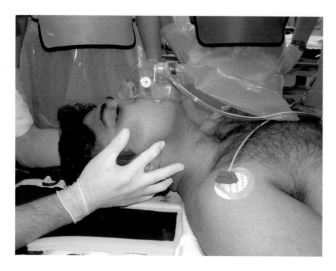

FIGURE 3-8 Jaw thrust is performed by one person who is also carrying out in-line immobilization.

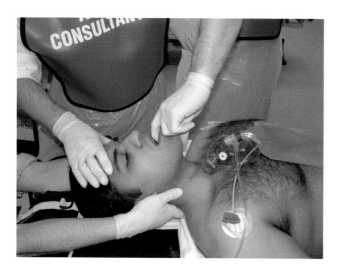

FIGURE 3-9 Chin lift is performed with an assistant who maintains in-line cervical spine immobilization.

(Ambu bag) connected to the oxygen supply and compressed by an assistant will work until formal management of the airway is achieved.

A **chin lift** should be performed without hyperextending the patient's neck. The mandible is gently lifted upward using the fingers of one hand placed under the chin. The thumb of the same hand lightly depresses the lower lip to open the mouth (Fig. 3-9).

The **oropharyngeal airway** must not be used in a conscious patient, because it may induce coughing, gagging, vomiting, and aspiration. During its insertion, care must be taken not to push the tongue backward and thereby block rather than clear the airway. The device is introduced upside-down so that its concavity is directed upward, until the soft palate is encountered. At that point, the device is rotated 180 degrees to direct the concavity caudad, and the airway is slipped into place over the tongue.

Alternatively, the oropharyngeal airway can be introduced directly by using a tongue spatula to depress the tongue, again ensuring that the tongue is not displaced backward as the tube is inserted. This method should be used in children to avoid knocking out loose primary teeth and, potentially, displacing them into the oropharynx.

If the patient vomits, the patient's head should not be moved to one side unless cervical spine injury has been excluded clinically and radiologically. If the patient is secured on a spinal board, the whole board can be turned. In the absence of a spinal board, the whole gurney should be tipped so that the head is down and the vomit sucked away with a rigid sucking device.

In a conscious patient, a well-lubricated **nasopharyngeal airway** is inserted in the nostril that appears to be unobstructed and passed gently into the posterior oropharynx. If obstruction is encountered during introduction of the airway, the procedure is stopped and then retried on the other side.

The **laryngeal mask airway** (LMA) has an established role in routine surgery to provide a protected airway and also in patients with difficult airways, particularly if orotracheal intubation has failed or bag-mask ventilation is not maintaining sufficient oxygenation. However, it is not a definitive airway because there is no cuffed tube in the trachea. Also, some training is required to use it, and it can be displaced relatively easily. If a patient presents with an LMA already in place, conversion to a definitive airway must be planned.

A **multilumen esophageal airway** is a form of LMA that has two tubes, enabling occlusion of the esophagus to reduce the risk of aspiration. However, it does not have a cuffed tube in the trachea and therefore does not constitute a definitive airway. The **laryngeal tube airway** also does not allow definitive airway protection; as with the LMA and the multilumen esophageal airway, plans must be made for it to be replaced by a definitive airway.

Maxillofacial Injuries

Up to 5% of patients presenting to the emergency department have facial injuries, and some may have airway compromise. Maxillofacial trauma demands aggressive airway management, and it may be appropriate for the maxillofacial surgeon to assist the anesthetist in assessing and securing the airway. The following problems may be encountered:

- A conscious patient will fight to maintain his own airway. If maxillofacial injuries are present, there is likely to be bleeding from those fractures, probably into the mouth or nose. ATLS principles advocate that the patient should be laid on his or her back with cervical spine control; this maneuver leads to pooling of blood in the nasopharynx and oropharynx, resulting in coughing or, in a more obtunded patient, airway obstruction.

It may be wise to leave such a patient sitting up, protecting the airway until a decision on airway management is made (Fig. 3-10). This decision must be made in the presence of a senior anesthetist and maxillofacial surgeon.[16] The only alternative is formal intubation by means of an orotracheal tube, which in the emergency setting requires general anesthesia, or a surgical cricothyroidotomy.

- The midface consists of a series of bony struts passing upward from the upper teeth to the base of skull (Fig. 3-11). These bone struts may fracture with severe impact,

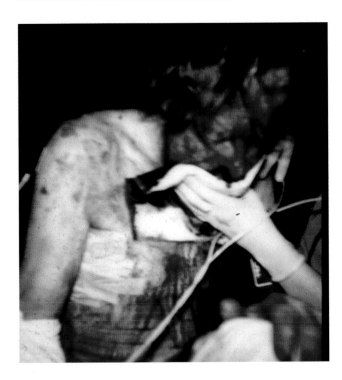

FIGURE 3-10 A photograph taken in the resuscitation room. The patient has had his lower face and anterior jaw shot away by a shotgun blast from above but is maintaining his own airway by sitting up with the head down and the tongue hanging loose.

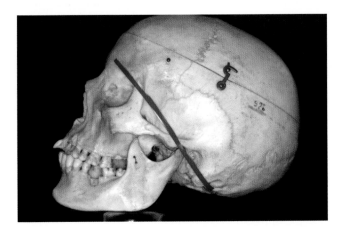

FIGURE 3-11 Skull showing the plane of the cranial base. With severe trauma to the midface, the facial bones shear off from the cranial base and are pushed down and backward.

and the middle third of the face can be sheared off the cranial base and forced downward and backward along the inclined plane formed by the frontal and sphenoid bones. It should be disimpacted by exerting upward and forward traction on the maxilla using the index and middle fingers of one hand, which are placed inside the mouth behind and above the soft palate, with the palm of the other hand braced against the forehead and applying countertraction.

- Voluntary tongue control is lost only when the patient's level of consciousness is depressed; it is only in such

circumstances that the tongue constitutes a threat to the airway. In these patients, a deep traction suture (0 black silk) may be inserted through the dorsum of the tongue and taped to the side of the face. Alternatively, the tongue may be pulled forward with the use of a towel clip. However, both of these techniques can cause additional bleeding, and insertion of an oropharyngeal airway or a definitive airway (if necessary) is preferable.

It is often said that in patients with bilateral symphyseal or parasymphyseal anterior mandibular fractures, the tongue may lose its anterior insertion and then, under the influence of the genial muscles, drop back in the supine patient, blocking the oropharynx. In fact, this is not the case if the patient is conscious, because the tongue is still firmly attached to the hyoid bone, which remains connected to the mandible by the posterior parts of the mylohyoid muscle. In addition, the intrinsic muscles of the tongue continue to exert control.

In elderly patients, it is not unusual to see bilateral fractures of the body of the edentulous mandible, each occurring near the posterior attachment of the mylohyoid diaphragm. Under these circumstances, extreme downward and backward angulation of the anterior part of the mandible may occur under the influence of the digastric and mylohyoid muscles and can compromise the airway. This so-called bucket-handle displacement should be reduced manually to unblock the airway.

- Teeth, dentures, vomitus, hematoma, or other foreign bodies may block the airway at any point from the oral cavity to the bronchi, with the right main bronchus being particularly susceptible. Early in the primary survey, the oral cavity should be cleared using a finger sweep followed by aspiration using a rigid sucker. If any teeth, crowns, or bits of denture are mssing, this fact should be recorded and the chest radiograph should be checked to be sure they have not been aspirated.
- Soft tissue swelling and edema resulting from trauma to the oral cavity may compromise the airway.

Rarely, maxillofacial trauma is associated with **injuries to the larynx** and trachea. Any neck swelling, dyspnea, voice alteration, or frothy hemorrhage should be noted, and the neck should be palpated for surgical emphysema, tenderness, and laryngeal or tracheal crepitus at the fracture site. Penetrating trauma to the neck may result in vascular injury with significant hemorrhage, which can cause displacement or obstruction of the airway. Endotracheal intubation should be attempted; if this is not possible, an urgent surgical airway may be necessary. Blunt or penetrating injury to the neck can cause disruption of the larynx or trachea, resulting in airway obstruction or severe bleeding into the tracheobronchial tree. A definitive airway is again urgently required.

Laryngeal fractures—indicated by hoarseness, subcutaneous emphysema, and palpable fracture—are rare but can manifest with acute airway obstruction. If the patient's airway is totally obstructed, an attempt at intubation is warranted. Flexible endoscopic intubation may be helpful, but only if it can be organized quickly. If intubation is unsuccessful, emergency tracheostomy is indicated, followed by operative repair. However, tracheostomy performed under these conditions can be difficult and time-consuming and may be associated with profuse bleeding. Under these circumstances, surgical cricothyroidotomy may be a life-saving option. If the injury is in the trachea below the potential tracheostomy site, the thoracic surgeons should be involved.

Advanced Airway Maneuvers: Definitive Airway

A *definitive airway* is defined as an inflated cuffed tube in the trachea. Definitive airways are of three types: the orotracheal tube, the nasotracheal tube, and the surgical airway (cricothyroidotomy or tracheostomy). A definitive airway should be considered if any of the following is present:

- Apnea
- Inability to maintain a patent airway by other means
- The need to protect the lower airway from blood or vomit
- Potential compromise of the airway (e.g., after burn injury, other inhalational injury, facial fractures, retropharyngeal hematoma, or sustained seizure activity)
- A closed-head injury requiring assisted ventilation (Glasgow Coma Scale [GCS] score of 8 or less)
- Inability to maintain adequate oxygenation by facemask oxygen supplementation

Patients who are without a gag reflex should be intubated with an appropriately sized endotracheal tube that has a low-pressure cuff, so that ventilation can be carried out safely. Attempts at ventilation with a bag and mask in these patients may lead to gastric distention with air and can precipitate vomiting. Orotracheal intubation with cervical in-line immobilization is recommended, rather than blind nasotracheal intubation, especially if a base-of-skull fracture is suspected. If this proves to be difficult, a surgical airway is then considered.

The most important determinant of whether to proceed with orotracheal or nasotracheal intubation is the experience of the doctor. Nasotracheal intubation should not be attempted in an apneic patient nor undertaken if a fracture of the base of the skull is suspected.

The route of choice for securing the airway depends on several factors. Between 5% and 10% of patients with blunt trauma of the head and neck have an associated fracture of the cervical spine. Laryngoscopy and orotracheal intubation are generally considered to be safe procedures and can be accomplished with minimal changes in the position of the neck when performed by a competent operator while an assistant immobilizes the patient's head. Visualization of the cords may require aids such as the gum elastic bougie. Another skilled assistant must provide pressure on the cricoid to protect the patient from aspiration of gastric contents. The stomach may already have been emptied by the passage of a nasogastric tube.

A fiberoptic intubating bronchoscope may facilitate difficult orotracheal or nasotracheal intubation if the patient's condition permits, but in the presence of distorted anatomy and hemorrhage, the procedure should be attempted only by an experienced anesthetist who is ready to abandon the procedure and proceed to establishment of a surgical airway if success is not achieved rapidly (Box 3-4).

Rapid-sequence induction with anesthetic agents, neuromuscular blocking drugs, and esophageal occlusion by cricoid pressure is best carried out by the anesthetist, who is

---

BOX 3-4	Airway: Patients at Risk

1. Altered level of consciousness
   - Hypoxia
   - Head injury
   - Hypoglycemia
   - Alcohol
   - Drugs
2. Maxillofacial injuries (patient in supine position)
   - Profuse bleeding
   - Displaced teeth, dentures, and so on
   - Facial fractures
3. Facial burns (inhalational injury): impending airway obstruction
4. Penetrating neck injury: potential compression of airway from closed hemorrhage
5. Direct laryngeal trauma

---

experienced in the use of these drugs. Before one embarks on intubation, the equipment must first be checked. Anesthetics with duplicate ampules should be ready in labeled syringes, and vasoactive drugs such as atropine should be at hand in case untoward bradycardia complicates extended laryngoscopy. A skilled assistant applies pressure to the cricoid while another assistant stabilizes the neck. Secure venous access and a pulse oximeter are essential.

Patients who have an intact gag reflex require induction of anesthesia and muscle paralysis for the airway to be secured by an oral or a nasotracheal tube. Preoxygenation is essential; while an assistant maintains pressure on the cricoid, neuromuscular blockade is produced with suxamethonium, and intubation proceeds with the onset of paralysis.

In deeply unconscious patients with a head injury, intubation should be preceded by the administration of a cerebral sedative and a muscle relaxant. This avoids dangerous increases in cerebral blood volume and intracranial pressure during laryngoscopy.

Orotracheal Intubation

In-line immobilization of the head must be maintained by an assistant to ensure that no extension of the cervical spine occurs. This is contrary to normal anesthetic practice in the non-trauma patient, where extension of the neck makes visualization of the vocal cords, and therefore intubation, easier.

The laryngoscope, held in the left hand, is inserted into the right side of the patient's mouth and over the back of the tongue, displacing it to the left. The back of the tongue is observed while the curved blade of the laryngoscope is advanced until the epiglottis comes into view. With care taken not to move the neck, the whole lower jaw is moved anteriorly as the tip of the blade is moved anterior to the epiglottis. Under direct vision, the anesthetist then advances the endotracheal tube through the vocal cords. If a gum elastic bougie is used, an endotracheal tube of the appropriate size is "railroaded" into the trachea. A size 8 tube is usually suitable for women and a size 9 tube for men. The cuff is then inflated, producing an airtight seal. Care must be taken to avoid trauma to the upper front teeth from the laryngoscope.

Proper placement of the tube is suggested but not confirmed by hearing equal breath sounds bilaterally on auscultation in both axillae and detecting no breath sounds in the epigastrium. An end-tidal carbon dioxide monitor will rapidly confirm the presence of the endotracheal tube in the airway. Pressure on the cricoid can only then be released and the tube secured with tapes. Proper positioning of the tube is best confirmed by a chest radiograph once the possibility of esophageal intubation has been excluded.

End-tidal carbon dioxide (CO_2) detectors are colorimetric devices that use a chemically treated indicator strip to reflect the CO_2 level. The indicator changes color from purple at low levels of CO_2 (e.g., atmospheric air) to yellow at higher levels. A tan color indicates levels of CO_2 that are generally lower than those found in the exhaled tracheal gases. Patients with gastric distention may have elevated CO_2 levels in their esophagus, which clear rapidly after several breaths, so care should be taken to avoid assessing the results until after at least six breaths. If the colorimetric device still shows an intermediate range, six additional breaths should be taken or given.

After intubation, the patient is appropriately ventilated. Although capnography and pulse oximetry may provide immediate noninvasive assessment of oxygenation and the adequacy of ventilation, arterial blood gas tension should be analyzed at the first opportunity.

Nasotracheal Intubation

Blind nasotracheal intubation requires spontaneous breathing and is therefore contraindicated in the apneic patient. The deeper the patient breathes, the easier it is to follow the air into the larynx. Facial fractures, frontal sinus fractures, base-of-skull fractures, and cribriform plate fractures are relative contraindications and are suggested clinically by the presence of nasal fractures, "panda eyes" (Fig. 3-12), Battle's sign (Fig. 3-13), and evidence of cerebrospinal fluid (CSF) leakage.

Endotracheal tubes can easily become displaced when patients are transported, so patients who arrive at the hospital with an endotracheal tube already in place must have the proper positioning of their tube confirmed.

Surgical Airway

Inability to intubate the trachea orally or nasally is a clear indication for creation of a surgical airway. If edema of the glottis, fracture of the larynx, or severe oropharyngeal hemorrhage obstructs the airway and an endotracheal tube cannot be placed through the cords, a surgical airway is performed. A surgical cricothyroidotomy is preferable to a tracheostomy for most patients. It is easier and requires less time to perform, and it is associated with less bleeding and fewer complications than an emergency tracheostomy.[17]

Needle Cricothyroidotomy Life-saving oxygenation can be provided through a large-bore (12- to 14-gauge) cannula (Venflon) that is connected to wall oxygen (at 15 L/min) and has a Y-connector or side hole in the tubing between the oxygen source and the cannula (Fig. 3-14).

Intermittent insufflation (1 second on and 4 seconds off) can be achieved by occluding and then uncovering the open end of the Y-connector or the side hole of the oxygen tubing. Although needle cricothyroidotomy can provide a life-saving supply of oxygen, there are associated problems:

- Although oxygenation may be adequate with this technique, ventilation is not, and there is a gradual rise in the

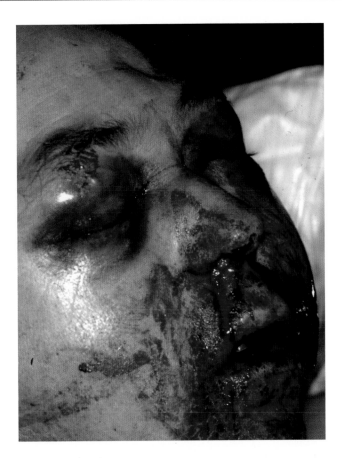

FIGURE 3-12 Severe facial trauma results in severe facial swelling, "football face," and bilateral "panda eyes" (or "raccoon eyes") associated with middle-third facial fractures.

P_{CO_2}. The patient can be ventilated by this technique for a maximum of 30 to 45 minutes. Jet insufflation must also be used with caution if obstruction by a foreign body in the glottic area is suspected. Although high pressure may expel the impacted material into the hypopharynx, from which it can be readily removed, significant barotrauma may occur, including pulmonary rupture with tension pneumothorax. Low flow rates (5-7 L/min) should be used if a persistent glottic obstruction is present. During the 4-second periods in which oxygen is not being delivered under pressure, some exhalation occurs. Because of the inadequate exhalation, carbon dioxide slowly accumulates. This limits the use of this technique, especially in head-injured patients.

- Patients in whom a surgical airway is required often have a head injury. A rise in P_{CO_2} must be avoided, because it will result in cerebral vasodilatation, a rise in cerebral blood flow, and possibly increased intracranial pressure.
- Needle cricothyroidotomy does not protect the airway. In cases of severe maxillofacial trauma with disruption of the normal anatomy and profuse bleeding, orotracheal intubation may fail, and a surgical airway may be necessary (Box 3-5).

Needle cricothyroidotomy should therefore be looked upon only as an immediate life-saving procedure. As soon as it has been completed and the P_{O_2} is improving,

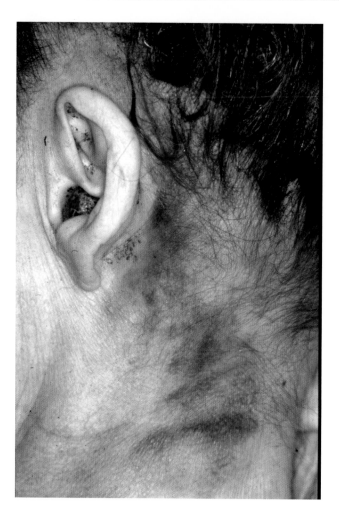

FIGURE 3-13 Battle's sign (bruising over the postauricular and mastoid area) usually indicates a base-of-skull fracture. It may take some hours before it becomes evident.

arrangements should commence to perform a surgical cricothyroidotomy to effect a definitive and secured airway. An experienced surgeon may elect to carry out a surgical cricothyroidotomy rather than first performing a needle cricothyroidotomy (Box 3-6).

Surgical Cricothyroidotomy Surgical cricothyroidotomy is performed by making a skin incision that extends through the cricothyroid membrane. Ideally, a tracheal dilator should be inserted to open up the incision, separating the thyroid and cricoid cartilages and enabling visualization of the trachea, suction with a Yankuer-type tube, and insertion of the tracheostomy tube under direct vision. A curved hemostat may be used if a tracheal dilator is not available. A small endotracheal tube or a tracheostomy tube (preferably 5-7 mm) should be inserted to avoid tearing the trachea or damaging the cricoid cartilage. Care must be taken, especially with children, to avoid damage to the cricoid cartilage, which is the only circumferential support to the upper trachea (Fig. 3-15; Boxes 3-7 and 3-8).

Percutaneous tracheostomy is not a technique designed for the emergency situation. The patient's neck must be extended to properly position the head to perform the

procedure safely. Percutaneous tracheostomy involves the use of a guidewire and multiple dilators (Seldinger technique), which is time-consuming and requires attention to detail; it is not advocated if a safer, more rapid technique is available.

Tracheostomy is rarely indicated as an emergency procedure. Severe distorting injury to the structures above or at the level of the larynx can render endotracheal intubation impossible, but in this setting cricothyroidotomy is preferred to emergency tracheostomy. Emergency tracheostomy is associated with high mortality and morbidity, often with profuse hemorrhage; cricothyroidotomy is quicker, easier, and safer to perform.[17-19]

Cervical Spine Control

Throughout the time that the airway is being secured, the patient must continue to have in-line immobilization of the cervical spine.

The patient may arrive with the cervical spine already immobilized on a long spine board with a semirigid cervical collar and head blocks. If not, definitive cervical spine control requires either in-line immobilization of the neck in the neutral position by having an assistant hold the head or the application of a semirigid cervical collar, sandbags placed on either side of the head, and tapes over the forehead and chin to immobilize the head and neck against the gurney. If these need to be removed temporarily, the head and neck should be immobilized by manual in-line immobilization. If the patient is restless and agitated, immobilizing the head and neck while allowing the rest of the body to move can damage the cervical spine; in such cases, just a semirigid collar is acceptable.

Stabilization must be maintained until cervical spine injury has been excluded. This may occur once the primary survey is completed and the patient is stabilized, but only if the patient is fully conscious, is not under the influence of alcohol or drugs, has no other "distracting" injuries that may prevent concentration on the neck, and is able to gently move the neck without any symptoms of pain or neurological abnormality. In the absence of any of these factors, the cervical spine may not be cleared until a magnetic resonance imaging (MRI) scan has been carried out and assessed by an expert. Plain cervical spine radiographs alone are not sufficient to exclude cervical spine injury.

B: BREATHING AND VENTILATION

Once the airway has been secured, breathing and ventilation must be assessed. Ventilation may be compromised not only by airway obstruction but also altered ventilatory mechanics or central nervous system depression. Therefore, if breathing is not improved by clearing of the airway, other factors must be considered:

- Direct trauma to the chest, especially with rib fractures, causes pain with breathing and leads to rapid, shallow breathing and hypoxemia. Elderly patients and those with preexisting pulmonary pathology are particularly vulnerable.
- Intracranial injury may cause abnormal patterns of breathing and compromise the adequacy of ventilation.
- Cervical spinal cord injury may result in diaphragmatic breathing and interfere with the ability to meet increased

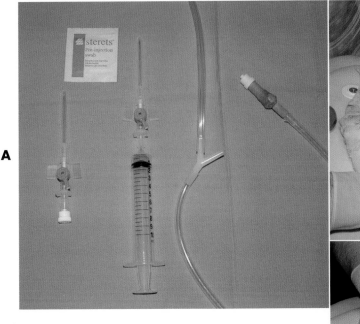
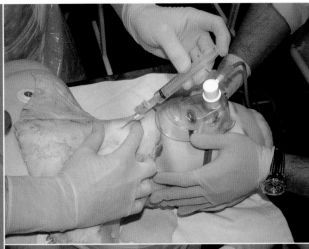
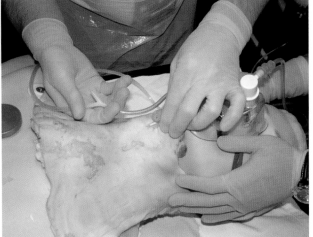

FIGURE 3-14 Technique of needle cricothyroidotomy. **A,** Assemble the required equipment: alcohol wipe, 12- to 14-gauge intravenous cannula with 10-mL syringe with 1 mL of air, and intravenous tubing with Luer lock connection to cannula and Y-connector. **B,** Insert cannula through the cricothyroid membrane, 45 degrees caudad; eject air from syringe and aspirate. Air indicates correct placement. **C,** Remove syringe and needle while fully inserting the cannula. Connect tubing to cannula. Connect the other end to the oxygen supply and run at 12 to 15 L/min, using intermittent insufflation (1 second of occlusion of the Y-connector and 4 seconds off).

BOX 3-5	Equipment for Needle Cricothyroidotomy

- Source of oxygen (up to 15 L/min)
- Connecting tube with either a Y-connector or a hole in the side
- 10-mL syringe
- 12- to 14-gauge Venflon + spare

BOX 3-6	Technique for Needle Cricothyroidotomy

1. Establish Universal Precautions against cross-infection.
2. Prepare skin quickly with antiseptic.
3. Attach syringe to Venflon with 1 mL of air in syringe.
4. Identify cricothyroid membrane.
5. Immobilize trachea with finger and thumb.
6. Insert Venflon in midline, through skin and membrane, at a 45-degree angle, aiming caudad, away from the larynx.
7. Eject air from syringe and aspirate through syringe; if air comes back, cannula must be in trachea.
8. Remove syringe and trocar.
9. Connect oxygen supply via tubing with Y-connector.
10. Jet insufflate: 1 second occluding the Y, followed by 4 seconds off.
11. Prepare for surgical cricothyroidotomy and call for an experienced surgeon to perform it, if possible.

oxygen demands. Complete cervical cord transection that spares the phrenic nerves (C3-4) results in abnormal breathing and paralysis of the intercostal muscles. Assisted ventilation may be required.

Thoracic injuries that are immediately life-threatening should be identified in the primary survey. They can be remembered by the mnemonic, ATOM FC:

A: Airway obstruction
T: Tension pneumothorax
O: Open pneumothorax

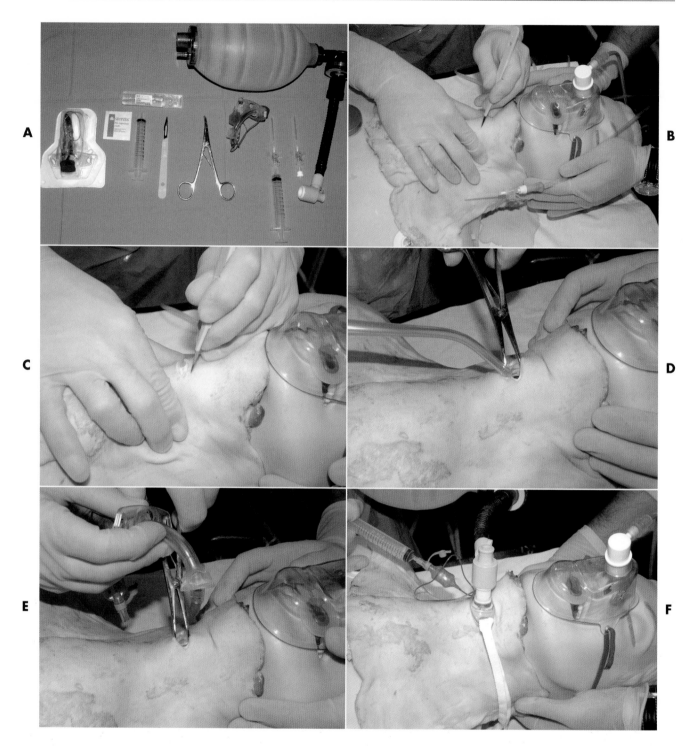

FIGURE 3-15 Technique of surgical cricothyroidotomy. **A,** Assemble the required equipment: local anesthetic with lido-caine (lignocaine) and epinephrine (adrenaline) for both anesthesia and vasoconstriction. **B,** Secure in-line immobilization of the patient's head by an assistant. Make a 3-cm horizontal incision through skin over cricothyroid membrane (having first removed the cannula if needle cricothyroidotomy was performed). **C,** Stab vertically down through membrane and make a 1-cm incision. **D,** Insert tracheal dilator horizontally and open it, separating the thyroid and cricoid cartilages. Suck out the trachea with a Yankeur-type sucker. **E,** Having checked that the cuff inflates, insert the tracheostomy tube into the trachea. **F,** Remove the introducer, inflate the cuff, and connect oxygen supply via Ambu bag. Reassess and monitor O_2 saturation and end-tidal CO_2; auscultate both sides of the chest for air entry.

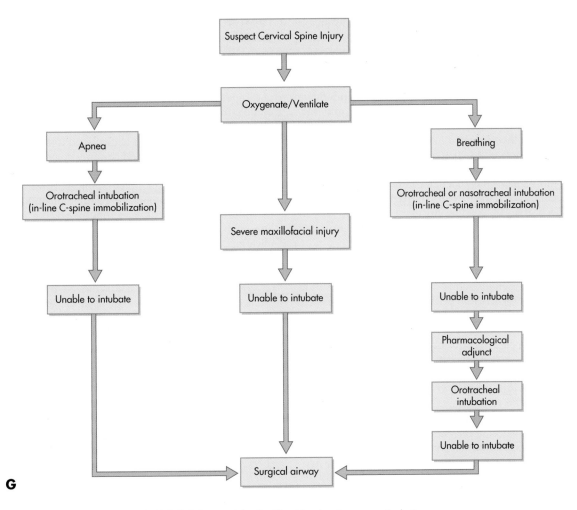

FIGURE 3-15, cont'd   **G,** Algorithm leading to surgical airway.

BOX 3-7	Equipment for Surgical Cricothyroidotomy

- Local anesthetic: lidocaine (lignocaine) + epinephrine (adrenaline)
- Scalpel
- Suction: rigid (Yankuer-type) tube
- Tracheal dilator
- Size 6 cuffed tracheostomy tube + spare
- 10-mL syringe
- 12- to 14-gauge Venflon + spare
- Ambu-type bag
- Oxygen supply
- Stethoscope

M: Massive hemothorax
F: Flail chest
C: Cardiac tamponade

Simple pneumothorax, hemothorax, fractured ribs, and pulmonary contusion may compromise ventilation to a lesser degree, are not immediately life-threatening, and are usually identified in the secondary survey.

Because ventilation requires adequate function of the lungs, chest wall, and diaphragm, each component must be examined and evaluated rapidly.

BOX 3-8	Technique for Surgical Cricothyroidotomy

1. Establish Universal Precautions.
2. Prepare skin with antiseptic.
3. Infiltrate local anesthetic and allow time for vasoconstrictor to work.
4. Check equipment (connections fit, cuff inflates).
5. Immobilize trachea between finger and thumb.
6. Remove jet-insufflation Venflon.
7. Make a 3-cm horizontal incision through skin so that skin edges part, using hole from Venflon to identify the level.
8. Stab vertically down with scalpel through cricothyroid membrane and incise a 1-cm cut.
9. Insert tracheal dilator and spread, separating thyroid and cricoid cartilages and creating an airway.
10. Insert suction to remove blood or other obstructions; view trachea (with or without application of oxygen), keeping tracheal dilator spread.
11. Insert tracheostomy tube; under direct vision, remove tracheal dilator, then remove introducer from tube.
12. Inflate cuff.
13. Connect oxygen supply via Ambu bag.
14. Auscultate chest.
15. Secure tracheostomy tube with tapes or stitches.
16. Monitor O_2 saturation and end-tidal CO_2.
17. If insertion fails, reinsert Venflon, reoxygenate, and reassess.

All of the patient's clothing must be removed to enable proper examination of the whole body.

Check that the trachea lies centrally in the suprasternal notch.

The respiratory rate, effort, and symmetry should be recorded, because these are sensitive indicators of underlying pulmonary contusion, hemothorax, pneumothorax, and fractured ribs. At the same time, both sides of the chest should be inspected and then palpated for bruising, abrasions, open wounds, and evidence of penetrating trauma. Cardiac tamponade is usually associated with a penetrating injury. Paradoxical breathing is seen with a flail chest only if the segment is large or central or if the patient's muscles become fatigued. After inspection and palpation, the chest should be auscultated and percussed to assess symmetry of ventilation and resonance.

Listening over the anterior chest detects air moving mainly in the large airways, and listening in the axillae gives an accurate assessment of pulmonary ventilation. This aids in the diagnosis of a tension pneumothorax or a massive hemothorax.

A tension pneumothorax should be relieved immediately by needle thoracocentesis and insertion of a chest drain. A pneumothorax or a hemothorax should be treated by the insertion of a chest drain with a gauge of 0.28 in the fifth intercostal space just anterior to the midaxillary line. This allows blood and air to be drained but should always be preceded by placement of intravenous lines.

During examination of the chest, a pulse oximeter should be used. This gives information regarding the patient's oxygen saturation and peripheral perfusion but does not assure adequate ventilation. Electrocardiographic (ECG) leads should also be attached.

Pulse Oximetry Monitoring

The pulse oximeter measures oxygen saturation and the pulse rate in the peripheral circulation. A microprocessor calculates the heart rate and also the percentage saturation of oxygen in each pulse of arterial blood that flows past a sensor. Two thin beams of light, one red and the other infrared, are transmitted from a light-emitting diode (LED) to a photodiode through blood and body tissue, which absorb a portion of this light. The photodiode measures that portion of the light that passes through the blood and body tissue. The relative amount of light absorbed by oxygenated hemoglobin differs from that absorbed by deoxygenated hemoglobin, and the microprocessor evaluates these differences in the arterial pulse and reports the values as a calculated oxyhemoglobin saturation value (% Sao_2).

The accuracy is unreliable when there is poor peripheral perfusion, whether from vasoconstriction, hypotension, a blood pressure cuff that is inflated above the sensor, hypothermia, or another cause of poor blood flow. Severe anemia and high levels of carboxyhemoglobin or methemoglobin may cause abnormalities, and circulating dye (methylene blue) may interfere with the measurement. Excessive patient movement, other electrical devices, or intense ambient light may also cause malfunction of the device; if the pulse oximeter has been attached to a finger, nail varnish will also affect accuracy.

Airway obstruction has already been discussed.

Tension Pneumothorax

Tension pneumothorax may develop when an air leak occurs from the lung or through the chest wall and acts as a one-way valve. With every breath, air is forced into the thoracic cavity, between the parietal and visceral pleurae, without any means of escape. The affected lung gradually collapses as the volume of the intrapleural space enlarges. The problem is exacerbated as ventilatory effort increases to overcome the increasing dyspnea. The mediastinum is displaced to the opposite side, decreasing venous return and compressing the opposite lung.

The most common cause is positive-pressure ventilation in a patient with a visceral pleural injury. However, a tension pneumothorax can complicate a simple pneumothorax after penetrating or blunt chest trauma in which a parenchymal lung injury has failed to seal, or it can even occur as a complication of insertion of a subclavian or internal jugular venous line. It is a clinical diagnosis, and treatment should not be delayed by waiting for radiological confirmation. A tension pneumothorax is characterized by chest pain, air hunger, respiratory distress, tachycardia, hypotension, tracheal deviation, unilateral absence of breath sounds, neck vein distention, and cyanosis as a late manifestation. It may be confused initially with cardiac tamponade, although a hyperresonant percussion note and absent breath sounds over the affected hemithorax distinguish a tension pneumothorax from cardiac tamponade.

Tension pneumothorax requires immediate decompression by insertion of a large-bore needle into the second intercostal space in the midclavicular line of the affected hemithorax. Definitive treatment requires the insertion of a chest drain into the fifth intercostal space (nipple level) just anterior to the midaxillary line (Box 3-9).

| BOX 3-9 | Needle Thoracocentesis |

1. Establish Universal Precautions.
2. Assess the patient's chest and respiratory status.
3. Administer high-flow oxygen and ventilate as necessary.
4. Identify the second intercostal space in the midclavicular line on the side of the tension pneumothorax. Find the angle of Louis and move out laterally.
5. Surgically prepare the chest.
6. Place the patient in an upright position if a cervical spine injury has been excluded.
7. Attach a 10-mL syringe, with 1 mL of air in it, to a large-bore (12- to 14-gauge) over-the-needle catheter.
8. Insert catheter into the skin and direct the needle just over the top of the rib into the intercostal space.
9. Puncture the parietal pleura.
10. Eject air from syringe into chest, ejecting plug of skin from catheter, and remove plunger from syringe.
11. Listen for a sudden escape of air when the needle enters the parietal pleura, indicating that the tension pneumothorax has been relieved.
12. Remove the needle. Leave the plastic catheter in place and secure it. Attach a three-way valve.
    Apply a small dressing over the insertion site.
13. Prepare for a chest drain insertion (see Box 3-10); it should be inserted at the nipple level anterior to the midaxillary line of the affected hemithorax.
14. Connect the chest drain to an underwater seal device, and remove the catheter used to relieve the tension pneumothorax initially.
15. Reassess breathing and respiration. Obtain a chest radiograph.

Open Pneumothorax

Large defects of the chest wall that remain open result in an open pneumothorax. Equilibration between intrathoracic pressure and atmospheric pressure is immediate. If the opening in the chest wall is approximately two-thirds the diameter of the trachea, air passes preferentially through the chest defect with each respiratory effort. Effective ventilation is thereby impaired, leading to hypoxia and hypercarbia.

Initial management is by prompt closure of the defect with a sterile occlusive dressing that is large enough to overlap the wound's edges and is taped securely on three sides to provide a flutter-type valve effect. A chest drain should be placed remote from the site of the open pneumothorax as soon as possible. Definitive surgical closure of the defect may be required later (Box 3-10).

Massive Hemothorax

Massive hemothorax results from a rapid accumulation of more than 1500 mL of blood in the chest cavity. It is most commonly caused by a penetrating wound that disrupts the systemic or hilar vessels, but it can also result from blunt trauma. The neck veins may be flat due to severe hypovolemia, but they may be distended if there is an associated tension pneumothorax or cardiac tamponade. Massive hemothorax is discovered when shock is associated with the absence of breath sounds or dullness to percussion on one side of the chest, or both.

It is initially managed by a simultaneous restoration of blood volume and decompression of the chest cavity. If 1500 mL is drained immediately, it is highly likely that the patient will require an early thoracotomy. Those patients who initially lose less than 1500 mL but continue to bleed may also require a thoracotomy. However, this decision is based not so much on the rate of blood loss (200 mL/hr for 2-4 hours) as on the patient's physiological status.

Penetrating anterior chest wounds medial to the nipple line and posterior chest wounds medial to the scapula should alert the examiner to the possible need for thoracotomy due to damage to the great vessels, hilar structures, and heart, with the associated potential for cardiac tamponade. Thoracotomy should be performed only by a surgeon who is qualified by training and experience.

Flail Chest

Flail chest occurs when a segment of the chest wall loses bony continuity with the rest of the thoracic cage; this is usually a result of trauma associated with multiple rib fractures with a number of ribs being fractured in two places. The presence of a flail chest segment results in severe disruption of the normal chest wall movement. Although chest wall instability leads to paradoxical movement with inspiration and expiration, this alone does not cause hypoxia. Serious hypoxia results from significant injury to the underlying lung parenchyma (pulmonary contusion). Associated pain with chest wall movement adds to the patient's hypoxia.

Flail chest may not be apparent initially because of splinting of the chest wall. The patient moves air poorly, and movement of the thorax is asymmetrical and uncoordinated. Palpation of abnormal respiratory motion and crepitus of rib or cartilage fractures aid the diagnosis. A chest radiograph shows multiple rib fractures, and arterial blood gas analysis shows respiratory failure with hypoxia.

Initial treatment includes provision of adequate ventilation, administration of humidified oxygen, and fluid resuscitation. In the absence of hypotension, fluid resuscitation should be carefully controlled to prevent overhydration. The definitive treatment is to re-expand the lung, ensure oxygenation as completely as possible, administer fluids judiciously, and provide analgesia with regional blocks to improve ventilation. Some patients can be managed without the use of a ventilator. However, prevention of hypoxia is important, and a short period of intubation and ventilation may be necessary.

Cardiac Tamponade

Cardiac tamponade results commonly from penetrating injuries, but blunt injury may also cause the pericardium to fill with blood from the heart, great vessels, or pericardial vessels. The human pericardial sac is an inelastic, fibrous structure, and only a relatively small amount of blood is required to restrict cardiac activity and interfere with cardiac filling. Removal of small amounts of blood, as little as 15 to 20 mL, by pericardiocentesis may result in immediate improvement.

The diagnosis can be difficult:

- The classic and diagnostic Beck's triad consists of venous pressure elevation causing distended neck veins, decline in arterial pressure, and muffled heart sounds. However, muffled heart sounds can be difficult to assess in a noisy resuscitation room; distended neck veins may be absent due to hypovolemia; and hypotension is most often caused by hypovolemia.
- Pulsus paradoxus (normal physiological decrease in systolic blood pressure during inspiration) greater than 10 mm Hg is another sign of cardiac tamponade, but this may also be absent in some patients and may be difficult to assess in the emergency setting.

BOX 3-10 | Chest Drain Insertion

1. Establish Universal Precautions.
2. Identify the insertion site; usually, it is at the nipple level (fifth intercostal space) anterior to the midaxillary line on the affected side. A second chest drain may be used for a hemothorax.
3. Prepare and drape the chest.
4. Administer local anesthetic with epinephrine (adrenaline) to the skin and rib periosteum.
5. Make a 3-cm transverse incision at the predetermined site, and bluntly dissect through the subcutaneous tissue just over the top of the rib.
6. Puncture the parietal pleura with the tip of a clamp and perform a finger sweep with a gloved finger through the incision, to avoid injury to other organs and to clear adhesions and clots.
7. Remove the trocar from the chest drain.
8. Clamp the proximal end of the chest drain tube and advance the tube into the pleural space to the desired length.
9. Look for "fogging" of the chest tube with expiration or listen for air movement.
10. Connect the end of the thoracostomy tube to an underwater seal.
11. Suture the tube in place.
12. Apply an occlusive dressing and tape the tube to the chest.
13. Reassess the chest. Obtain a chest radiograph.

- Tension pneumothorax on the left side may mimic cardiac tamponade.
- Kussmaul's sign (a rise in venous pressure with inspiration when breathing spontaneously) is a true abnormality associated with cardiac tamponade.
- Pulseless electrical activity (PEA) in the absence of hypovolemia and tension pneumothorax suggests cardiac tamponade.

A high index of suspicion regarding a patient who is unresponsive to resuscitation, most frequently in association with a penetrating injury to the chest, is all that is necessary to initiate pericardiocentesis by the subxiphoid method. If possible, an ultrasound examination of the pericardium (and the abdomen) should be urgently obtained to confirm the suspicion. The use of a plastic-sheathed needle or the Seldinger technique for insertion of a flexible catheter is ideal, but the urgent priority is to aspirate blood from the pericardial sac. ECG monitoring is mandatory and may identify traumatic (or preexisting) and needle-induced dysrhythmias. Because of the self-sealing qualities of the injured myocardium, aspiration of pericardial blood alone may relieve symptoms temporarily. However, all patients with positive pericardiocentesis resulting from trauma require open thoracotomy for inspection of the heart.

Pericardiocentesis may not be diagnostic or therapeutic because the blood in the pericardial sac may have clotted; open pericardiotomy can be life-saving but is indicated only if a qualified surgeon is available (Box 3-11).

Resuscitative Thoracotomy

Closed-heart massage for PEA or cardiac arrest is ineffective in the hypovolemic patient.

Patients with penetrating thoracic injuries who arrive pulseless but with myocardial electrical activity may be candidates for immediate resuscitative thoracotomy by a qualified surgeon. The patient must be intubated and ventilated, with appropriate fluid resuscitation running; access is then gained via a left anterior thoracotomy.

Resuscitative thoracotomy may enable:

- evacuation of pericardial blood causing tamponade.
- direct control of intrathoracic hemorrhage.
- open cardiac massage.
- cross-clamping of the descending aorta to slow blood loss below the diaphragm and increase perfusion to the brain and heart.

Despite the value of these maneuvers, open thoracotomy in the resuscitation room for patients with blunt trauma and cardiac arrest is rarely effective.

C: CIRCULATION AND HEMORRHAGE CONTROL

An adequate volume of blood in the circulation is essential to maintain cerebral perfusion and vital function of the heart, kidneys, lungs, and other organs. Acute blood loss resulting in hypovolemic shock is responsible for 30% to 40% of trauma deaths, up to half of which occur in the prehospital period.[20] Acute blood loss has been identified as one of the major causes of preventable deaths on arrival at hospital.[12] Early mortality in the resuscitation room is caused by continued

---

BOX 3-11   Pericardiocentesis

1. Establish Universal Precautions.
2. Monitor the patient's vital signs and ECG tracings before, during, and after the procedure.
3. Surgically prepare the xiphoid and subxiphoid area if time allows.
4. Administer local anesthetic if necessary.
5. Using a 16- to 18-gauge, 6-inch or longer over-the-needle catheter, attach a 20-mL empty syringe with a three-way stopcock.
6. Assess the patient for any mediastinal shift that may have caused the heart to shift significantly.
7. Puncture the skin 1 to 2 cm inferior and to the left of the xiphochondral junction, at a 45-degree angle to the skin.
8. Carefully advance the needle upward, aiming toward the tip of the left scapula.
9. If the needle is advanced too far, penetrating ventricular muscle, an injury pattern known as the current injury appears on the ECG monitor (i.e., extreme ST changes and widened or enlarged QRS complexes). This indicates that the needle should be withdrawn until the previous baseline ECG tracing appears. Premature ventricular contractions may also occur secondary to irritation of the ventricular myocardium.
10. After the needle enters the blood-filled pericardial space, withdraw as much nonclotted blood as possible.
11. During the aspiration, the epicardium approaches the inner pericardial surface, as does the needle tip. Subsequently, an ECG current injury pattern may reappear. Again, this indicates that the needle should be withdrawn slightly. If the pattern persists, withdraw the needle completely.
12. After aspiration, leave the catheter in place, remove the syringe and needle, and attach a three-way stopcock, leaving the stopcock closed. Secure the catheter in place.
13. If the cardiac tamponade symptoms persist, the stopcock may be opened and the pericardial sac reaspirated. The plastic pericardiocentesis catheter can be taped in place with a small dressing to allow for continued decompression en route to surgery.
14. Reassess.

Committee on Trauma, American College of Surgeons: *2008 Advanced Trauma Life Support manual*, Chicago, 2008, ACS, p 109.

---

hemorrhage, coagulopathy, and incomplete resuscitation; ATLS is directed toward this group of patients, among others.

Most injured patients who are in shock are suffering from hypovolemia, but there are also other forms of shock, such as cardiogenic, neurogenic, and septic shock. In addition, cardiac tamponade and tension pneumothorax reduce venous return to the heart and may produce shock. Neurogenic shock results from extensive injury to the central nervous system or spinal cord, which causes peripheral vasodilatation, and patients may present with shock from both hypovolemia and vasodilatation. Septic shock is unusual but must be considered in patients whose retrieval from the scene of trauma has been significantly delayed by many hours or days.

Pathophysiology of Shock

Shock is defined as "an abnormality of the circulatory system that results in inadequate organ perfusion and tissue oxygenation."[21] Left unchecked, it leads to the **"lethal triad" of metabolic acidosis, hypothermia, and coagulopathy**, resulting in end-organ dysfunction.[22] Metabolic acidosis is caused by inadequate tissue perfusion and oxygenation and the anaerobic glycolysis that results in lactic acid production. The acidosis leads to coagulation factor and platelet dysfunction, combined with coagulation factor consumption, resulting in a profound coagulopathy (Box 3-12).

Reperfusion Injury

Restoration of blood supply and oxygenation after a period of ischemia to the tissues may itself cause damage. The ischemic tissues produce an inflammatory response, and white cells arriving with the restoration of circulation release their own inflammatory factors, including interleukins and free radicals. In addition, the accumulation of white cells may block capillaries and lead to further ischemia. Reperfusion with oxygen may cause damage to cell proteins and cell membranes and may result in cell death.

Studies have demonstrated the following:

1. Coagulopathy of trauma is present at an early stage after trauma.[23]
2. Crystalloid transfusion may increase reperfusion injury and leukocyte adhesion.[24]
3. Increased transfusion is associated with increased risks.[25]
4. Massive transfusion is an independent risk factor for increased risk of death.[26]

Much research is being carried out in military and civilian areas on ways of reducing the number of deaths from hypovolemic shock in the prehospital setting. The aim of *damage control resuscitation* is to rapidly prevent further blood loss and urgently restore tissue perfusion.[27]

Control of hemorrhage—the most preventable cause of death on the battlefield—has significantly improved since the introduction of field-applied topical hemostatic agents such as Quikclot and HemCom Bandage and the improved use of prefashioned tourniquets. Other innovations, such as low-volume and hypertonic resuscitation, newer ratios of packed red cells to plasma in transfusions, availability of apheresis platelets, early resort to fresh whole blood, and possibly the use of human recombinant factor VIIa, are all being assessed for their benefits in military conflict zones.[28]

When in direct contact with an open wound, Quikclot adsorbs the water molecules from the blood. The larger platelet and clotting factor molecules remain in the wound in a highly concentrated form, promoting extremely rapid natural clotting. Hemcom Bandage is a positively charged polysaccharide (chitosan) that attracts negatively charged erythrocytes into the bandage, thereby forming a tight seal.

Damage Control Resuscitation

Research has led to a greater understanding of the physiology involved in the lethal triad and the need to treat early or even prophylactically, on expectation, patients who have severe injuries. Therefore, the principal aim of damage control resuscitation is to stop hemorrhage, minimize contamination, and restore near-normal physiology before embarking on definitive repair of injuries. The sooner this can be implemented and the quicker the patient can be transported to a center for definitive care, the better the outcome.

Hypothermia

Hypothermic patients with hemorrhagic shock do not respond normally to fluid resuscitation, and coagulopathy may develop. Aggressive measures should be taken to prevent the loss of body heat and to restore body temperature to normal. Hypothermia may be present when the patient arrives, or it may develop quickly in the emergency department in the uncovered patient or through rapid administration of room-temperature fluids and refrigerated blood.

The most efficient way to prevent hypothermia in any patient receiving large volumes of fluid is to heat crystalloids to 39° C before using them. The fluid may be stored in a warmer, or a microwave oven may be used. Blood products should not be warmed in a microwave oven, but they may be heated by passage through intravenous fluid warmers. In addition, the temperature of the resuscitation area should be increased to minimize the loss of body heat.

Coagulopathy

Together with metabolic acidosis and hypothermia, coagulopathy completes the lethal triad. Massive transfusion with resultant dilution of platelet and clotting factors and the adverse effect of hypothermia on platelet aggregation and the clotting cascade are the usual causes of coagulopathy in the injured patient.

Prothrombin time (PT), partial thromboplastin time (PTT), and platelet count are valuable baseline studies to obtain during the first hour, especially if the patient has a history of a coagulation disorder or takes medication that alters coagulation or if a reliable bleeding history cannot be obtained. Transfusion of platelets, cryoprecipitate, and fresh-frozen plasma should be guided by these coagulation parameters, including fibrinogen.

Patients who have a major closed-head injury are particularly prone to the development of coagulation abnormalities as a result of substances, especially tissue thromboplastin, that are released by damaged neural tissue. These patients should have their coagulation parameters closely monitored.

Hypotensive Resuscitation

When acute blood loss occurs, resulting in hypotension, baroreceptors in the carotid sinus release catecholamines which cause peripheral vasoconstriction, a narrowing of pulse pressure, increased myocardial contractility, and tachycardia. The tachycardia and increased myocardial contractility result in increased oxygen demand from the myocardium, and there is preferential perfusion to the vital organs (myocardium, cerebrum, and kidneys) at the expense of skin and peripheral tissues. Continuing uncontrolled hemorrhage results in shock (i.e., inadequate organ perfusion and oxygenation), anaerobic metabolism, and metabolic acidosis, resulting in further end-organ dysfunction.

Classic teaching in the management of hypovolemic shock requires aggressive fluid resuscitation to return the vital signs, particularly blood pressure, to normal pretrauma parameters. In some situations, however, this can be detrimental to the patient. Certainly in the prehospital setting, where immediate

BOX 3-12   Lethal Triad

- Metabolic acidosis
- Hypothermia
- Hypocoagulopathy

surgical intervention is not available, better results may be produced by *hypotensive resuscitation,* in which the aim is only to resuscitate to a level at which cerebral, myocardial, and renal perfusion is satisfactory.

A systolic blood pressure of 90 mm Hg should ensure adequate vital organ perfusion for the average adult but is not high enough to cause renewed bleeding from recently clotted vessels.[29] Children have a greater degree of hemodynamic compensation than adults. Elderly patients, who may have a higher pretrauma blood pressure, do not tolerate hypotension well, and a relatively higher blood pressure should be the target.

The ideal approach may be to manage airway and breathing immediately at the scene and then address circulation with hypotensive resuscitation until the patient reaches a hospital, where hemorrhage can be properly controlled and definitive treatment commenced. The concept of hypotensive resuscitation is appropriate for the prehospital setting or whenever definitive surgical intervention to stop continuing hemorrhage is delayed. If these concepts are to be formally implemented, it is essential that comprehensive training be provided to all parties involved in emergency medical care.

Recognition of Shock

Hypotension after injury must be considered to be hypovolemic shock until proved otherwise. Once airway and breathing have been stabilized, rapid evaluation of the patient's circulatory system is essential to identify the severity of the problem, prevent further blood loss, and resuscitate the patient.

There are several signs of shock:

- *Tachycardia:* Palpate a central pulse, either carotid or femoral. Check for rate, regularity, and quality. A slow, full, regular pulse indicates relative normovolemia, whereas a rapid, thready pulse (caused by catecholamine release) indicates hypovolemia. An irregular pulse may be a warning of impending cardiac dysfunction. Inability to palpate a central pulse mandates immediate resuscitation.
- *Skin color:* Cold, ashen-gray, diaphoretic (sweaty) skin indicates exsanguinated extremities and therefore likely hypovolemia.
- *Level of consciousness:* When circulating volume is reduced, cerebral perfusion may be impaired, resulting in hypoxia. This can cause confusion, aggression, drowsiness, or coma.
- *Respiratory rate:* Tachypnea indicates oxygen insufficiency and may be a result of hypovolemia.
- *Urine output:* In a catheterized patient, the urine output, in conjunction with the specific gravity, may give a good indication of circulating volume.

Because healthy elderly patients have a limited ability to increase their heart rate in response to blood loss, tachycardia, usually an early sign of volume depletion, may not reflect the true volume loss in these patients. Also, their blood pressure may have little correlation with cardiac output. Use of β-blockers and other drugs may further prevent tachycardia. Therefore, great care is required in assessing the "shock" state of the elderly.

Children, on the other hand, have enormous reserve of physiological function, and this may enable relatively normal physiological parameters despite significant blood loss.

However, when deterioration does occur, it can be precipitous. Well-trained athletes have similar compensatory mechanisms, are usually bradycardic at rest, and may not demonstrate the expected degree of tachycardia in the early stages of shock. Again, however, after compensatory mechanisms are no longer able to cope, precipitous deterioration can occur (Box 3-13).

Hemorrhage

Hemorrhage is an acute loss of circulating blood volume. The blood volume in a normal 70-kg adult is approximately 7% of the body weight (i.e., about 5 L). Classes of hemorrhage based on percentage of acute blood volume loss and the associated anticipated clinical signs have been described (Table 3-1). Volume replacement should be directed by the response to initial therapy rather than by relying solely on the initial classification. It is dangerous to wait until the trauma patient fits the precise physiological classification of shock before initiating aggressive volume restoration. Fluid resuscitation must be initiated when early signs and symptoms of blood loss are apparent, not when the blood pressure is falling or absent.

- *Class I hemorrhage*: up to 15% blood volume loss (up to 750 mL). This is the equivalent of donating 1 unit of blood. Minimal tachycardia may be seen. No measurable changes occur in blood pressure, pulse pressure, or respiratory rate. For healthy individuals, this amount does not require replacement; blood volume is restored within 24 hours.
- *Class II hemorrhage*: 15% to 30% blood volume loss. In a 70-kg man, this represents 750 to 1500 mL of blood. Clinical symptoms include tachycardia, tachypnea, and a decrease in pulse pressure, which makes the pulse less palpable. The latter sign is mainly related to a rise in the diastolic component due to increased circulating catecholamines, which cause constriction in the peripheral venous circulation. Despite the significant blood loss and cardiovascular changes, urine output is only mildly affected (i.e., it is usually 20 to 30 mL/h) in the adult. Some of these patients may eventually require a blood transfusion, but they may be stabilized initially with crystalloid solution.
- *Class III hemorrhage*: 30% to 40% blood volume loss. This is approximately 2000 mL in an adult and can be devastating. Patients present with the classic signs of inadequate perfusion, including marked tachycardia and tachypnea, changes in mental status, and a measurable fall in systolic pressure. This is the least amount of blood loss that consistently causes a drop in systolic blood pressure. Patients almost always require transfusion.
- *Class IV hemorrhage*: greater than 40% blood volume loss. This amount of blood loss is immediately life-threatening. Signs include marked tachycardia, a significant fall

BOX 3-13	Shock—Be Wary

- Athletes
- Children
- Elderly

TABLE 3-1	Classifications and Signs of Hypovolemic Shock*			
	Class I	Class II	Class III	Class IV
Blood loss				
Volume (mL)	750	800-1500	1500-2000	>2000
Percentage	<15	15-30	30-40	>40
Blood pressure				
Systolic	Unchanged	Normal	Reduced	Very low
Diastolic	Unchanged	Raised	Reduced	Unrecordable
Pulse (beats/min)	Slight tachycardia	100-120	120 (thready)	120 (very thready)
Capillary refill	Normal	Slow (0.2 s)	Slow (0.2 s)	Undetectable
Respiratory rate	Normal	Tachypnea	Tachypnea (0.20/min)	Tachypnea (0.20/min)
Urinary flow rate (mL/h)	>30	20-30	10-20	0-10
Extremities	Color normal	Pale	Pale	Pale, cold, clammy
Complexion	Normal	Pale	Pale	Ashen

*In an adult, assuming a 70-kg patient with normally 5 L of circulating volume.

in systolic blood pressure, and a narrow pulse pressure. Urine output is negligible, and mental status is markedly depressed. The skin is cold and pale. These patients require rapid transfusion and immediate surgical intervention. Loss of more than 50% of a patient's blood volume results in loss of consciousness, pulse, and blood pressure.

It is important to remember that, whereas loss of up to 30% of blood volume produces tachycardia and reduced pulse pressure, the blood pressure may remain within normal limits. There is a consistent fall in the systolic blood pressure only after more than 30% of the blood volume has been lost.

Initial Management of Hemorrhagic Shock

The twin goals in resuscitation of the shock patient are prevention of further blood loss and the earliest restoration of tissue perfusion (i.e., an adequate circulating volume).

The ability to reduce or prevent further blood loss depends on the circumstances. Local measures (described earlier) may be all that can be achieved in the prehospital setting, in conjunction with initiation of fluid replacement and rapid transport to an appropriate trauma care center. On arrival of the patient in the resuscitation room, airway and breathing must be addressed before circulation and hemorrhage control—or at the same time if a team is available.

External hemorrhage is identified and controlled by direct manual pressure on the wound. Tourniquets may be necessary in the prehospital setting but should be reassessed in the hospital, because they can lead to distal ischemia. Attempts should not be made to identify and clip vessels with hemostats in the resuscitation room, because this is time-consuming, is often unsuccessful, and may damage surrounding structures such as nerves.

Occult bleeding is more difficult to identify. However, there are a limited number of sites into which significant blood loss can occur. These are the thoracic and abdominal cavities, the pelvis, the retroperitoneal space, and

in association with closed fractures of the long bones. A fractured tibia or humerus can be associated with the loss of as much as 1.5 units (750 mL) of blood. Twice that amount (up to 1500 mL) is commonly associated with femoral fractures, and several liters of blood may accumulate in a retroperitoneal hematoma associated with a pelvic fracture. Life-threatening hemorrhage can occur in any one of these sites in association with a single penetrating injury and in a number of them at once in cases of high-velocity blunt trauma, such as RTAs or significant falls.

Two short, wide-bore (14- to 16-gauge) peripheral lines must be inserted, preferably in the antecubital fossae. The rate of flow is proportional to the fourth power of the radius of the cannula and is inversely related to its length (Poiseuille's law). If this is impossible, venous access should be gained by a venous cut-down, made 2 cm anterior and superior to the medial malleolus into the greater saphenous vein, or by insertion of a short, wide-bore central line into the femoral or subclavian vein by the Seldinger technique. If a subclavian approach is used and a chest drain is already in place, the central line must be inserted on the same side. In children younger than 6 years of age, the placement of an intraosseous needle should be performed before central line insertion. This technique may now also be used in adults, using a drill sytem (EZ-IO) that enables quick access and rapid fluid infusion; this system is now being used by the military[30] and increasingly in civilian practice.

Twenty milliliters of venous blood should be drawn off for group, type, or full crossmatch; full blood count; urea and electrolytes; blood sugar; a clotting screen; and a pregnancy test for women of child-bearing age. A sample of venous blood should be sent for toxicological analysis (alcohol and drugs). An arterial blood sample should also be taken for blood gas and pH analysis. The blood pressure and the rate, volume, and regularity of the pulse should be recorded. A blood pressure monitor and an ECG monitor should be attached to the patient.

Fluid Replacement

In a shocked, hypotensive patient, the aim of fluid resuscitation should be to restore critical organ perfusion until hemorrhage that is amenable to surgery is stemmed. In an adult trauma victim, 2 L of warmed isotonic crystalloid, preferably Ringer's lactate, should be given and the response assessed. In children, 20 mL/kg should be infused as the initial bolus.

There are three types of patient response:

- *Responder:* The vital signs return toward normality. These patients have probably lost less than 20% of their circulating volume and are probably not still actively bleeding.
- *Transient responder:* The vital signs initially improve but then deteriorate. These patients are still actively bleeding from either an open wound or, more likely, an occult site. They require transfusion with blood, identification of the source of continued bleeding, and probably surgery to halt it.
- *Nonresponders:* The vital signs do not improve. This implies that the blood loss is continuing at a rate at least equal to the rate of fluid replacement. The history, mechanism of injury, and physical findings will help identify the problem, and a central venous line should be inserted to exclude other potential causes such as neurogenic shock, tension pneumothorax, or cardiac tamponade. These patients need immediate blood transfusion and probably emergency surgery to identify and deal with the source of bleeding, which is usually within the thorax, abdomen, or pelvis.

Imaging may help to identify the source of occult bleeding, ideally with the patient remaining in the relative safety of the resuscitation room. Chest and pelvic radiographs may identify a hemothorax or a pelvic fracture. An ultrasound study (i.e., Focused Assessment with Sonography in Trauma [FAST]) may show free intraabdominal fluid and can also be used to check for cardiac tamponade in addition to visualizing the liver, spleen, and kidneys. Computed tomography (CT) may be necessary, but the patient must not be transferred from the resuscitation room until the primary survey is complete and the patient has been resuscitated and stabilized. If this is not possible, then surgery or even transfer to a more comprehensive trauma center may be necessary to enable stabilization before the patient is sufficiently well to undergo CT. Specific protocols for CT in severely injured trauma victims may help determine who needs a CT and when.[31]

Care must be taken to avoid overresuscitation, particularly in the presence of continuing hemorrhage. The aim must be only to restore critical organ perfusion until the hemorrhage can be controlled. Excess fluid may result in displacement of blood clots, counterintuitively leading to more bleeding; this compounds the problem and can lead to coagulopathy due to loss and dilution of clotting factors as well as being potentially harmful in patients who have traumatic brain injury or are at risk of developing respiratory distress syndrome. A critical balance is required to ensure adequate but not excess resuscitation, and this requires continuous reassessment, which is aided by the placement of a central line.

Crystalloid versus Colloid

ATLS teaches that if a patient needs colloid—that is, an agent that replaces intravascular loss and remains intravascular, thereby increasing circulating volume—blood should be given, because it is the only agent in general use that improves oxygen-carrying capacity.

Crystalloids such as Ringer's lactate are isotonic electrolyte solutions that pass freely between the intravascular and interstitial spaces; therefore, a three to four times greater volume is needed to produce a hemodynamic effect similar to that of colloids. Crystalloids also dilute clotting factors, and unless the patient is adequately warmed, they are more likely to cause hypothermia. Crystalloids are cheap and safe; however, in cases of severe uncontrolled hemorrhagic shock, damage control resuscitation must be considered.

Colloids are typically iso-oncotic and can be used to replace blood loss on a 1:1 volume basis; however, they do not directly improve the oxygen-carrying capacity. Polygelatins such as Hemaccel and Gelofusine are reasonably cheap, carry a relatively low anaphylactic risk, and have an intravascular half life of 6 to 8 hours. Care must be taken not to overload the patient with fluid if blood transfusion is necessary later. Hetastarch is more expensive; it has a longer half-life (about 12 hours) but still carries a relatively low anaphylactic risk.

However, in a systematic review comparing the mortality rates after fluid resuscitation with colloid or crystalloid solutions in critically ill patients, resuscitation with colloids was associated with an increased absolute risk of mortality. The authors stated that this finding "does not support the continued use of colloids for volume replacement in critically ill patients."[32]

Hypertonic Saline and Synthetic Fluids

A number of studies have suggested that early infusion of a limited volume (approximately 250 mL) of 7.5% hypertonic saline with 6% dextran 70 may be beneficial in patients with severe trauma and continuing hemorrhage, especially in the prehospital setting.[33] The hypertonic fluid osmotically draws fluid into the circulation, reducing viscosity; for this reason, it may also have a greater benefit than mannitol in reducing cerebral edema in head-injured patients.[34]

Because restoration of oxygenation to the tissues is essential to prevent metabolic acidosis and organ failure, new (fluorocarbon-based) synthetic fluids with oxygen-carrying capacity continue to be produced. Fluosol-DA20 was available in the United States in 1989 but had to be withdrawn due to limited success and side effects. More recently, trial results with Polyheme were not as promising as hoped. Given limited blood supplies, limited shelf life of blood, and the risks of cross-infection, a synthetic, sterile alternative would have a valuable role. Researchers are also looking at potential roles for stem cells, dendrimers, and placental umbilical cord blood.

Blood Replacement

Acute blood loss can be replaced either with fresh whole blood or by dividing the blood up into a number of separate components (e.g., packed red cells, platelets, fresh-frozen plasma), which allows greater use of a limited resource. Because of the significant cross-infection risks, transfusion of fresh whole blood is not used in a civilian setting nor as a primary treatment in the military. Initially, packed red blood cells may be given; if more than 4 units are required, fresh-frozen plasma, which contains clotting factors, must also be introduced to prevent development of a coagulopathy. Work has also been carried out on the use of recombinant factor VIIa, which initiates coagulation in conjunction with tissue factor; it has been used in isolated clinical settings with some benefit.[35]

In some circumstances, such as uncontaminated blood loss into the chest or abdominal cavity, it may be possible to retrieve the patient's own blood with a cell saver and auto-transfuse it back. The blood needs to be sterilely collected, anticoagulated, and retransfused.

Crossmatched, Type-Specific, and Type O Blood

Fully crossmatched blood is preferable, but crossmatching takes 1 hour in most blood banks. For patients who stabilize rapidly, crossmatched blood should be obtained and made available when indicated.

Type-specific blood can be provided by most blood banks within 10 minutes. This is compatible with ABO and Rhesus (Rh) blood types, but incompatibilities of other antibodies may exist. Type-specific blood is preferred for patients who are transient responders. If it is required, completion of the crossmatching should be performed by the blood bank.

If type-specific blood is unavailable, type O packed cells are indicated for patients with life-threatening hemorrhage. To avoid sensitization and future complications, Rh-negative cells are preferred for women of child-bearing age. For life-threatening blood loss, the use of unmatched, type-specific blood is preferred over type O blood. The exception is when multiple unidentified casualties are being treated simultaneously and the risk of inadvertent administration of the wrong unit of blood to a patient is great.

Maxillofacial Aspects

Despite the rich vascularity of the hard and soft tissues of the head and neck, life-threatening hemorrhage rarely originates in this region in isolation from sites in the thorax, abdomen, pelvis, or long bones. Bleeding from soft tissue lacerations can usually be controlled with direct pressure; for example, the facial artery can be compressed against the mandible and superficial temporal vessels against the skull vault. Extensive scalp lacerations, especially in patients at the extremes of age and in anticoagulated patients, are one exception. If unrecognized in an immobilized, supine patient, they can cause significant blood loss. Early application of full-thickness tension sutures to the scalp in the resuscitation room will control the majority of bleeding, but definitive exploration and closure with vacuum drains and pressure dressings will be required at a later stage to prevent hematoma formation (Fig. 3-16).

Bleeding from extensive midfacial fractures is problematic for two main reasons. The primary threat is to the airway, and this must be rapidly secured before any attempts are made at hemorrhage control, which will usually further occlude the mouth, nasal passages, and pharynx. In addition, bleeding from midface injuries is rarely from a single source; it is usually from a combination of lacerations to oronasal mucosa, bone edges, and the fragile pterygoid venous plexus behind the maxilla.

Because there is extensive collateral supply from the internal and external carotid systems, attempts to ligate single vessels are usually unsuccessful. The maxilla must be disimpacted and reduced against the skull base initially, using two

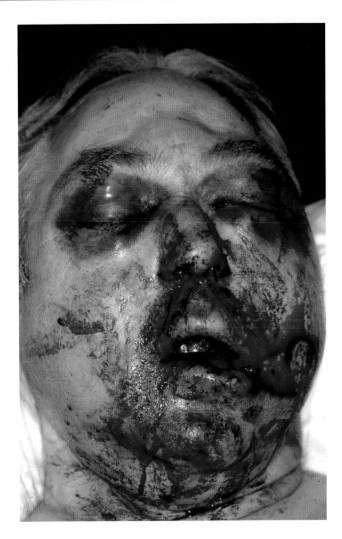

FIGURE 3-16 Severe maxillofacial trauma. In the resuscitation room, the patient has already developed a "football face" and "panda eyes." There is bilateral epistaxis with cerebrospinal fluid rhinorrhea.

mouth props placed between upper and lower molar teeth. The nasal cavities must then be packed bilaterally, using both posterior and anterior packing. Several custom-made, double-balloon devices are now available; after careful introduction into the nasal cavity, they are inflated to tamponade adjacent tissues. If these are unavailable, a 14-gauge Foley male urinary catheter can be introduced anteriorly into the nose and brought out into the oropharynx. The balloons are inflated with saline and pulled into the nasophaynx, where they impact, and the proximal ends are tied securely at the columella. Anterior packing can then be instituted with Merocel packs or ribbon gauze and bismuth subnitrate and iodoform paste (BIPP) against posterior support.

Whatever one places in the nasal cavitiy, great care must be exercised to prevent extention of mucosal lacerations or inadvertent entry into the cranial cavity via a base-of-skull fracture. All devices should be passed in a caudad direction, remembering the orientation of the plane of the nasal floor. Bleeding from mandibular fractures can be controlled with wire ligatures around adjacent teeth and compressive splint dressings.[36]

D: DISABILITY

A rapid evaluation is performed at the end of the primary survey, and this establishes the patient's level of consciousness.

The range of patient response can be remembered by a simple mnemonic, AVPU:

A: Alert
V: responds to Vocal stimuli
P: responds to Painful stimuli
U: Unresponsive to all stimuli

A more detailed neurological examination can be performed at this time. This includes recording a GCS score, pupillary size and reaction, lateralizing signs, and level of spinal cord injury (Table 3-2). The GCS is an objective, reproducible measure of brain injury severity based on the best reponses of eye opening, motor function, and voice to the examiner. It can be predictive of patient outcome, particularly with regard to best motor response. Should lateralizing neuropathy be present, the response of the better-scoring side should be recorded. If the GCS score is not determined in the primary survey, it should be performed in the secondary survey. It is generally accepted that a GCS score of 8 or less indicates coma or severe brain injury mandating elective intubation.

A decrease in level of consciousness may indicate decreased cerebral oxygenation or perfusion or both, or it may be caused by direct cerebral injury. An altered level of consciousness indicates an immediate need for reevaluation of the patient's oxygenation, ventilation, and perfusion. Alcohol and other drugs may also alter the patient's level of consciousness. However, if hypoxia and hypovolemia are excluded, changes in the level of consciousness should be considered to be of traumatic central nervous system origin until proved otherwise.

The lucid interval associated with acute extradural hematoma is an example in which the patient may talk yet subsequently die. Frequent reevaluation minimizes such problems by allowing early detection of changes. It may be necessary to return to the primary survey to confirm that the patient has a secure airway, adequate ventilation and oxygenation, and adequate cerebral perfusion. Early consultation with a neurosurgeon may be necessary to guide additional management efforts.

E: EXPOSURE AND ENVIRONMENTAL CONTROL

The patient should be completely undressed, usually by cutting off all garments with large, sharp scissors, to facilitate examination and assessment. Thorough examination must involve a formal, controlled logroll to assess the posterior surfaces of the head, neck, torso, and limbs. After the assessment is completed, it is important to cover the patient with warm blankets or an external warming device to prevent hypothermia in the emergency department. Intravenous fluids should be warmed before infusion, and a warm resuscitation room temperature should be maintained.

ADJUNCTS TO THE PRIMARY SURVEY AND RESUSCITATION

Regular assessment of pulse and respiratory rates; systolic, mean, and diastolic blood pressures; pulse oximetry; and core temperature are standard during the primary survey and are continued after the patient has left the resuscitation room. Trends are often more valuable than isolated readings. Pulse oximetry measures the percentage saturation of hemoglobin only; it can be affected by probe position and peripheral temperature. Partial pressures of oxygen and carbon dioxide to assess oxygenation and ventilation require arterial blood gas analysis. Capnography monitors the presence of carbon dioxide in exhaled gas and is vital for confirming initial and continuous correct endotracheal tube placement.

ECG monitoring of trauma patients is mandatory. If chest trauma is present, blunt cardiac injury may manifest in a variety of electrical rate, rhythm, and conduction abnormalities. These may include tachycardia in a normovolemic patient, atrial fibrillation, ventricular ectopic waveforms, and ischemic changes in the ST segment. PEA arrest may be the end point in cardiac tamponade, tension pneumothorax, or class IV hemorrhage. Myocardial hypoperfusion, hypoxia, and hypothermia may all produce both tachydysrhythmias and bradydysrhythmias and signs of aberrant conduction.

Placement of a urinary catheter and subsequent recording of urine output is a sensitive indicator of volume status and response to fluid resuscitation. The kidneys receive one fifth of the cardiac output, and urine output directly reflects renal perfusion. Transurethral bladder catheterization is potentially hazardous, and any patient with pelvic, abdominal, or lower limb injury should alert suspicion. Injury to the urethra

TABLE 3-2	Glasgow Coma Scale (GCS)*	
Assessment Area		**Score**
Eye Opening (E)		
Spontaneous		4
To speech		3
To pain		2
None		1
Best Motor Response (M)		
Obeys commands		6
Localizes pain		5
Normal flexion (withdrawal)		4
Abnormal flexion (decorticate)		3
Extension (decerebrate)		2
None (flaccid)		1
Verbal Response (V)		
Oriented		5
Confused conversation		4
Inappropriate words		3
Incomprehensible sounds		2
None		1

*GCS score = E + M + V. The best possible score is 15, and the worst possible score is 3.

should be presumed in the presence of any of the following signs after thorough pelvic, rectal, and genital examination:

- Blood at the urethral meatus
- Perineal ecchymosis
- Scrotal hematoma (Fig. 3-17)
- High-riding or impalpable prostate on per rectal (PR) examination
- Pelvic fracture

If urogenital injury is suspected, a retrograde urethrogram to assess urethral integrity should be performed together with formal urological review before catheterization.

Gastric stasis is inevitable after trauma, and gastric contents together with air potentially introduced by airway maneuvers are a cause of vomiting and aspiration. Orogastric and nasogastric tubes can decompress the stomach and reduce (but not completely prevent) this risk. Solid or semi-solid gastric contents will not be aspirated via standard wide-bore tubes. Introduction of tubes can also be hazardous, leading to mucosal trauma and perforation or actually causing

vomiting. Nasogastric passage should be avoided if there is a risk of anterior cranial fossa floor fracture; in such cases, the oral route is preferable. Once chest radiography has confirmed correct placement, the position of the tube must be secured and it must be attached to appropriate suction. Aspirated blood may indicate injury to the upper aerodigestive tract from the original trauma or from iatrogenic injury, or it may simply reflect swallowed blood from the nasopharynx.

Anteroposterior (AP) chest and pelvic radiographs can be performed in the resuscitation room and may aid the diagnosis of potentially life-threatening injuries, thus guiding resuscitation techniques. They should not delay resuscitation based on clinical information. A cervical spine series, once part of the standard primary survey radiographic triad, is now delayed until stabilization and secondary survey. Spinal trauma is presumed during the primary survey, and the patient remains in triple immobilization during this phase.

Contemporary use of fast spiral CT scanning to diagnose occult sources of abdominal, pelvic, and thoracic hemorrhage; spinal injury; and intracranial trauma is now routinely practiced. Its timing is critical, and the decision whether to move an unstable or potentially unstable patient to the CT scanner rather than directly to the operating room or to a distant center for definitive care is a key part of the ATLS doctrine. In an unstable, hypotensive patient, FAST ultrasound scanning in the resuscitation room to look for free fluid at common sites of intraabdominal collection and within the pericardial sac has its role but is dependent on the skill of the operator. Essential radiographic imaging using ionizing radiation should not be contraindicated in pregnancy.

During or on completion of the primary survey, it may be apparent that definitive treatment of the patient's injuries cannot be undertaken at the primary admitting facility. This is particularly relevant with regard to head, thoracic, or spinal trauma or significant burns. Early identification of the need to transfer, together with careful planning and communication with the receiving unit, are essential to minimize further injury. Once the decision is made, further nonessential investigations or interventions should not delay transfer.[37]

SECONDARY SURVEY

The secondary survey is a complete and comprehensive head-to-toe evaluation of the trauma patient that includes confirmation of the history and circumstances leading to the injury, a physical examination of the patient, and reassessment of all vital signs. It aims to identify and fully appreciate all other injuries that the polytraumatized patient may have suffered that might otherwise go unnoticed, particularly in the presence of a reduced GCS score. The secondary survey begins only after the primary survey has been completed, resuscitation is underway, and normalization of vital functions has been demonstrated.[4]

HISTORY

Many injuries and their prognosis can be predicted from a thorough history of premorbid events, the mechanism and energy involved in the injury itself, and its immediate sequelae. If the patient is moribund and has a reduced GCS

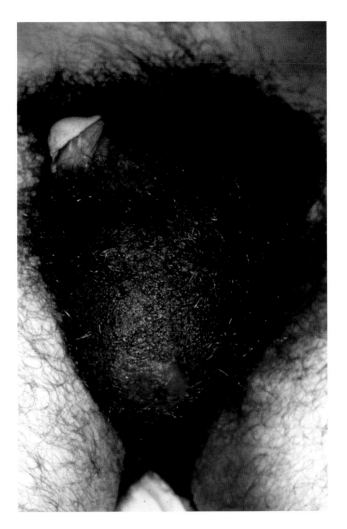

FIGURE 3-17 Scrotal hematoma may indicate urethral injury, and transurethral urinary catheterization is contraindicated until urethral trauma has been excluded. Suprapubic cathetherization should be performed instead.

score, this information must be obtained from prehospital personnel, family members, or witnesses at the scene.

The AMPLE history is a useful mnemonic:

A: Allergies
M: Medications currently used
P: Past illnesses and Pregnancy
L: Last meal
E: Events and Environment related to the injury

Blunt trauma results from RTAs, falls, sporting and occupation-related injuries. In relation to RTAs, important factors in the history include seat belt use, air-bag deployment, steering wheel deformation, direction of impact, damage to the vehicle in terms of major deformation or intrusion into the passenger compartment (Fig. 3-18), and ejection of the occupants from the vehicle.

Penetrating trauma includes injuries from firearms, stabbings, and impalement on objects. Its incidence is increasing. The type and extent of injury and its subsequent management depend on the region of the body injured, the organs in proximity to the path of the penetrating object, and the velocity of the missile. With firearm injuries, knowledge of the velocity, the caliber, the presumed path of the bullet, and the distance from the weapon to the wound provides important clues to the extent of the injury.

Burn injuries are especially significant and may occur in isolation or in concert with blunt or penetrating injury as the victim attempts to escape the burning source. Occult airway compromise and carbon monoxide poisoning often further complicate patient management. Burning agents (solvents, plastics, and other chemicals) may still be in contact with the patient in the resuscitation room and may be an active and continuous hazard to both the victim and the emergency department team. Other hazardous toxins, chemicals, and radiation may produce characteristic injury patterns and require immediate advice from a regional Poison Control Center.

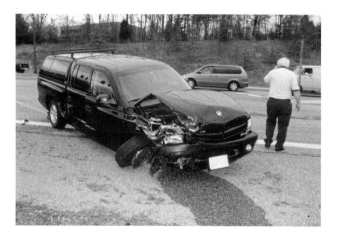

FIGURE 3-18 Modern automobiles have an engine-compartment crumple zone that absorbs the force of the impact. Intrusion into the passenger compartment indicates more severe trauma. *(From Chapleau W, Pons P:* Emergency medical technician, *St. Louis, 2007, Mosby.)*

Injury due to cold, particularly immersion in cold water, carries its own unique problems. Removal of wet clothing and active rewarming are essential.

PHYSICAL EXAMINATION

Scalp

Examine the entire scalp for lacerations, contusions, hematomas, and bone surface irregularities that may indicate underlying skull fracture. If spinal injury has not been excluded and the patient remains immobilized, the posterior scalp should be examined during logrolling.

Fractures may be seen in the base of lacerations, but wounds should not be probed blindly, because this may result in further damage to the underlying structures. Judicious exploration of small lacerations using local anesthetic and antiseptic skin preparation should be undertaken, if possible, to remove foreign bodies and cleanse the wound.

If the wound is uncomplicated, definitive primary closure can be achieved at this stage. More extensive injuries should be managed in the operating room as previously described. If an underlying skull fracture is found, the laceration should still be cleaned and closed, converting an open to a closed injury; then a CT scan of the head and a neurological reevaluation are performed as soon as possible.

Eyes

The examination of the eyes and visual pathways in a traumatized patient in the resuscitation room can be extremely challenging. Although pupillary response is routinely assessed at the Disability (D) stage of the primary survey, this assessment is largely directed to evaluation for brain shift and subsequent lateralizing signs. With other, more pressing A, B, and C problems taking priority, management of potentially vision-threatening eye injuries may be deferred or even overlooked. Patients who have a reduced level of consciousness may not be able to tell the examiner whether their vision has become impaired. If, as is often the case, an eye injury is associated with surrounding craniofacial injury, swelling of the periorbital soft tissues often develops rapidly, particularly if the patient is supine and is wearing a well-fitting hard collar that impedes venous return. Ocular assessment in the patient with a potentially reduced GCS score and other injuries must therefore focus on the rapid identification and treatment of vision-threatening injuries in concert with the overall management.

If the patient is conscious or relatives are present, a history of any preexisting eye problems can be obtained. Establishing whether the patient wears correcting lenses, has any history of glaucoma or ophthalmic surgery, or uses prescription eye drops is extremely useful. Again, details of the events and environment surrounding the injury may suggest blunt or penetrating trauma or exposure of the eyes to chemical or thermal burning agents. Inquiry should be made as to initial symptoms and whether these have changed, particularly with respect to visual acuity. Loss of sight after facial trauma may result from one or a combination of the following causes[14]:

1. Direct injury to the globe (blunt or penetrating injury)
2. Direct injury to the optic nerve (due to crush or transection via bony injury at the orbital apex)

3. Indirect injury to the optic nerve (from deceleration or shearing force)
4. Critical reduction in tissue perfusion, either generalized or local (systemic hypotension or orbital compartment syndrome)

Examination should proceed systematically, from without to within. The lids should be checked for ptosis, edema, laceration, burn, canalicular injury, and the integrity of the medial and lateral canthal ligament attachments. If the lids are grossly swollen, then an assistant is needed to part them, facilitating further examination. Visual acuity is tested by any means possible. The immobilized supine patient may be able to read a distance-modified, handheld Snellen chart or may simply be asked to read printed words. Failing this, record of the patient's ability to count fingers, see hand movement, or perceive light is made.

Globe position and external appearance are then noted. Subtle changes in globe position caused by orbital injury may be masked at this stage by soft tissue swelling. Posttraumatic proptosis is caused either by a reduction in orbital volume due to so-called blow-in fracture or by an increase in the volume of soft tissue behind the globe due to edema, air, blood, or anterior cranial fossa contents. Proptosis has been reported to be present in up to 3% of closed-head injuries.[38] Subsequent increases in retrobulbar pressure, termed *orbital compartment syndrome,* can result in rapid loss of vision due to ischemia of the optic nerve at the orbital apex.[39] Clinical signs include "A and 5 Ps":

- decreasing visual **A**cuity
- **P**ain
- ophthalmoplegia (**P**aralysis)
- tense **P**roptosis (the affected globe feels firmer compared with the normal side)
- development of a relative afferent **P**upillary defect
- swollen or **P**ale optic disc at fundoscopy

In a conscious patient in whom the first three of these signs can be assessed, the threat of increasing retrobulbar pressure is more readily identified. With agitated or unconscious patients who have a proptosed eye, one must rely on clinical acumen and a high degree of suspicion. CT of the orbits may help to identify pathology behind the globe and can be requested at the same time as a head scan.

In the presence of clinical signs and if vision is threatened, it may be necessary to decompress the orbit via a lateral canthotomy and cantholysis.[40] Medical management with the use of high-dose steroids (antiinflammatory), mannitol (an osmotic diuretic), and acetazolamide (carbonic anhydrase inhibitor reducing formation of vitreous) may buy time but can exacerbate hypotension and metabolic acidosis. Orbital compartment syndrome may manifest only after initial fluid resuscitation as the mean arterial pressure increases. Once again, the need for regular reassessment is critical.

The systematic ophthalmologic examination continues with assessment of shape, equality, and light reaction of the pupils. The cornea may appear opaque and may harbor foreign bodies. Abrasions are extremely painful and may be diagnosed with the use of fluoresceine drops and blue light. Successful examination of a painful eye when such an injury

is present may be made far more comfortable by the use of local anesthetic drops.

If the margins of a conjunctival hemorrhage are all readily seen, direct injury to the surface of the eye is suggested; a subconjunctival bleed that has no visible posterior limit indicates a fracture of one of the four orbital walls (Fig. 3-19). Examination of the anterior chamber for bleeding (hyphema) and depth anomalies, of the iris for tears, and of the lens for transparency and dislocation follows. Lastly, fundoscopy through a transparent vitreous assesses for hemorrhage, tears, or detachment of the retina. Blood in the posterior chamber may prevent this examination and demonstrate a black rather than a red reflex with the ophthalmoscope. An ophthalmology opinion must be sought in difficult cases.

Maxillofacial Structures

Most isolated maxillofacial injuries occur in conscious, hemodynamically stable patients who can protect their own airways. In the multiply injured patient whose maxillofacial injuries do not affect the primary survey, definitive management of these injuries can usually be deferred. However, it is vital for the secondary survey to identify the possibility of such injuries and prompt formal referral to the local or regional maxillofacial service for correct imaging, other adjunctive tests, and possible surgical intervention. Missed injuries can result in facial deformities and functional impairments that are generally much more difficult to manage late, leading to poor results and litigation. A description of the maxillofacial examination follows.

Examine the nose for deformity, pain, mobility, and difficulty in breathing, which suggest bony or cartilaginous fractures. A septal hematoma may cause nasal obstruction, which appears as swellings on both sides of the septum. If it is left untreated, there is a risk of cartilage necrosis and nasal collapse; therefore, the blood clot should be immediately

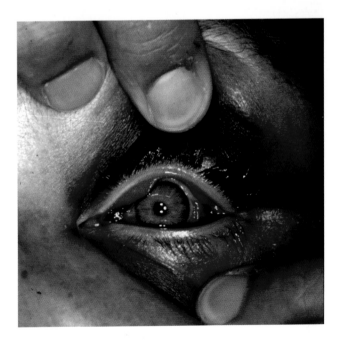

FIGURE 3-19 Subconjunctival hemorrhage may strongly suggest a fractured zygoma. If it is severe, the conjunctiva may herniate through the closed eyelids.

evacuated. Epistaxis and, in particular, CSF rhinorrhea may suggest an anterior cranial fossa fracture at the cranial base. If the patient is lying supine on a gurney, CSF may be trickling posteriorly into the nasopharynx rather than onto the face. Measure the intercanthal distance: If it is greater than 35 mm a nasoethmoid fracture should be suspected (Fig. 3-20).

Examine the ears for hemotympanum and CSF otorrhea. Bleeding from the external auditory canal soft tissue wall may be secondary to mandibular condylar fracture with or without glenoid fossa injury. Injuries to the pinna may involve both skin and cartilage and require accurate repair. It is important to recognize and drain subchondral hematomas to prevent the "cauliflower" deformity.

In the presence of any facial laceration or incised wound, knowledge of the surface anatomy of the facial nerve, parotid duct and capsule, and lacrimal apparatus is essential. Any laceration deep enough to involve the mimetic muscles in the territory of these structures should be assessed by a specialist and explored carefully with the use of local or general anesthesia, under good lighting, and with bipolar diathermy available. Facial nerve function must be assessed and documented before either form of anesthetic is administered.

Orbitozygomatic complex fractures may be difficult to formally assess at this stage because of soft tissue edema. Look for obvious asymmetry and facial flattening, and palpate for bony deformity if pain and edema allow. Periorbital emphysema may be seen after blowing of the nose when air escapes

via defects in the maxillary sinus walls into adjacent structures. The presence of subconjunctival blood is highly indicative of injury to the bony orbit. Document ophthalmoplegia and diplopia, which may be caused by soft tissue entrapment within a fracture or by bruising of the extraocular muscles only. Always consider the possibility of retrobulbar bleeding with the additional signs described previously. There may be numbness or altered sensation in the ophthalmic or maxillary divisions of the trigeminal nerve due to direct blunt trauma or fractures involving the roof and floor of the orbit, respectively. Mouth opening may be limited due to the entrapment of the coronoid process of the mandible and attached temporalis muscle beneath a medially displaced zygomatic arch fracture. Pure blowout fractures may have few signs, but in children their presence may be indicated by vagal symptoms of nausea, vomiting, and syncope on testing for ophthalmoplegia.

Lastly, examination of the mouth is performed. Any obvious bruising from bony injuries in the buccal vestibule (zygoma), the palate (maxilla), and the floor of the mouth (anterior mandible) is noted. Test for sensation in the mandibular division of the trigeminal nerve (mental and lingual nerves); abnormality may suggest mandibular fracture. Inspect intraorally for lacerations, bleeding, loose teeth, broken teeth and dentures, mobile bone segments, abnormal alignment of the jaw, step defects, and derangement of the occlusion. If possible, ask the patient to bite together on the back teeth and assess the range of mandibular movement. If recently missing teeth are not accounted for, a chest radiograph is mandatory.

Gripping the anterior maxillary teeth with one hand (with the thumb in front and the index finger on the palatal side) while applying the other hand across the forehead, followed by simple manipulation, will confirm whether the nose or cheekbones move, indicating a maxillary fracture at the Le Fort I, II, or III level. Any combination of Le Fort fractures can be present on one or both sides. Gagging of the occlusion often occurs, and gross displacement of the maxillary and mandibular midlines may be apparent. Percussion of the maxillary teeth may produce the "cracked cup" sound.

Imaging of the facial skeleton with plain radiographs or CT scanning is usually more helpful when the patient is conscious, sober, and compliant. Intraoral radiographs are useful if there are dental injuries. If the occlusion is deranged due to mandibular or mid third injury, impressions for study models to aid planning and the provision of arch bars are very useful.

Neck and Cervical Spine

Patients with maxillofacial or head trauma should be presumed to have an unstable cervical spine injury, and the neck should be immobilized until such an injury has been excluded. The absence of neurological deficit does not exclude injury to the cervical spine. Extreme care needs to be exercised when removing motorbike helmets; two operators are needed, one of whom ensures manual in-line cervical stabilization while the other removes the helmet.

Cervical spine tenderness, subcutaneous emphysema, and laryngeal fracture should be investigated. Suspicion of an injury to the upper cervical spine may be aroused by a retropharyngeal hematoma seen through the open mouth or by deviation of the trachea. The course of the carotid artery in

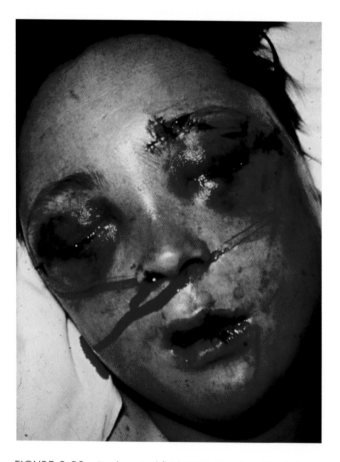

FIGURE 3-20   Cerebrospinal fluid (CSF) rhinorrhea. Blood clots at the sides, but the CSF in the middle does not clot. This produces the "rail-track" appearance.

the neck should be palpated for irregularity and auscultated for bruits, which may signify blunt injury. CT angiography or duplex ultrasound scanning may be required to exclude vascular occlusion or dissection. Vascular injury secondary to blunt trauma or traction injury from seat belts is rare and may initially be silent.

The majority of vascular trauma in the neck is associated with penetrating wounds and may involve injuries to nerves, trachea, pharynx, and thyroid gland. Wounds extending through the platysma should not be explored manually or probed in the emergency department by personnel not trained to deal with such injuries. A surgeon should evaluate these injuries either operatively or with specialized diagnostic procedures. Active arterial bleeding, expanding hematoma, arterial bruit, and airway compromise usually require surgical operative evaluation.

Cervical spine radiography is indicated in any trauma patient who describes neck pain, exhibits midline tenderness on palpation, or demonstrates any neurological signs referable to the cervical spine. Patients who demonstrate any reduction in GCS score or are intoxicated, have a distracting injury elsewhere, or are too young to describe their symptoms should also be imaged. Lateral and AP views showing all seven cervical vertebrae and the first thoracic vertebra (C1-C7/T1 junction), together with an open-mouth odontoid peg view are performed as part of the secondary survey. If these images are adequate, are of good quality, and are properly interpreted by an experienced doctor, unstable cervical spine injuries can be detected with a sensitivity of greater than 97%. Adequacy is frequently problematic, particularly at the C7/T1 junction, often becase of the patient's habitus. Traction on the shoulders or a swimmer's view may help to visualize this area.

Among patients in whom a fracture of the cervical spine is identified, approximately 10% have a second, noncontiguous fracture of the vertebral column. Increasingly, rapid spiral CT scanning of trauma patients, imaging the head, thorax, abdomen, and pelvis together with the whole spinal column, is replacing the traditional cervical spine series. It still may not exclude soft tissue injuries around the vertebrae or lesions within the cord itself, and MRI is routinely used.

It must be remembered that the purpose of the secondary survey is to identify and exclude all injuries, and in the case of spinal cord trauma, the potential consequences of missing an injury are huge. If there is any doubt surrounding the clearance of the spine, specialist orthopedic or neurosurgical opinion should be sought while the patient is kept immobilized.

Chest

The priority in the chest examination is to identify potentially life-threatening conditions. Pain, dyspnea, and hypoxia may suggest significant chest injury. Anterior and posterior inspection of the chest identifies open pneumothorax and large flail segments with their characteristic abnormality of chest wall movement. Contusions and hematomas suggest the possibility of occult pulmonary or cardiac injury. Distended neck veins may suggest cardiac tamponade or tension pneumothorax, although associated hypovolemia can minimize this finding. Palpation of the entire chest wall, including the clavicles, ribs, and sternum identifies bony deformity and localizes pain.

Reauscultation of the chest wall may pick up pathology not present at the time of the primary survey. Breath sounds are auscultated high on the anterior chest wall for pneumothorax and over the posterior bases for hemothorax. Muffled heart sounds and narrow pulse pressure may suggest cardiac tamponade. Decreased breath sounds, hyperresonance to percussion, and shock may be the only findings in tension pneumothorax.

The chest radiograph, which may have been done as part of the primary survey, confirms the presence of hemothorax or simple pneumothorax. Rib fractures may also be seen. A widened mediastinum or deviation of the gastric tube to the right may suggest an aortic rupture.

Abdomen

A specific diagnosis is not as important as recognizing that an injury exists and that surgical intervention may be necessary. Close observation and frequent reevaluation are important, preferably by the same observer. An intraabdominal bleed should be suspected if there are fractures of the ribs that overlie the liver and the spleen (i.e., ribs 5 through 11), if the patient is hemodynamically unstable, or if there are marks caused by seat belts or tires over the abdomen (Fig. 3-21). Fractures of the pelvis or the lower rib cage that cause guarding also may hinder accurate diagnostic examination of the abdomen.

Patients with unexplained hypotension, neurological injury, impaired sensorium secondary to consumption of alcohol or other drugs, or equivocal abdominal findings should be considered for diagnostic peritoneal lavage (DPL), FAST scan, or, if hemodynamically stable, abdominal CT. Ideally, DPL should be done by the surgeon who will be responsible for any subsequent laparotomy. There is no indication for DPL if laparotomy is already deemed necessary. Injury to the retroperitoneal organs (e.g., pancreas) may be difficult to identify even by CT.

Perineum, Rectum, and Vagina

Examine the perineum, rectum, and vagina for contusions, hematomas, lacerations, and urethral bleeding. A rectal examination should always be carried out before a urinary catheter is placed. Assess for the presence of blood within the rectum, a high-riding prostate, the presence of pelvic

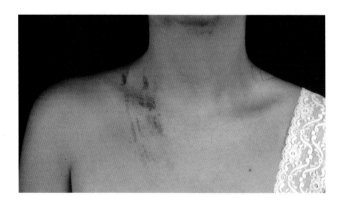

FIGURE 3-21 Bruising caused by a seat belt. Bruising over the shoulder may overlie a fractured clavicle and that over the abdomen may warn of intraabdominal trauma.

fractures, the integrity of the rectal wall, and the quality of the sphincter tone.

A vaginal examination is an essential part of the assessment in female patients. Look for the presence of blood in the vaginal vault and for vaginal lacerations. In addition, a pregnancy test should be performed on all women of childbearing age.

Musculoskeletal Assessment

Each limb must be inspected for bruising, wounds, and deformities. Vascular and neurological deficits are recorded by examination of the peripheral pulses and of motor and sensory impairments, respectively. These measurements, together with an assessment of the viability of the skin overlying fractures or dislocations, must be made before and after the deformity is reduced. The examiner must palpate all the bones in the limbs. Swabs should be taken for microbiological analysis from sites of open fractures. The wounds should then be covered with sterile dressings. Splinting of broken limbs is important because it reduces further damage to the soft tissues, pain, and, possibly, the production of fat emboli. A photograph or digital image taken before an open fracture is covered precludes the need for repeated inspection and reduces the risk of infection.

Pelvic fractures are suggested by:

- ecchymosis over the iliac wings, pubis, labia, or scrotum.
- pain on palpation of the pelvic ring in the alert patient.
- mobility of the pelvis in response to gentle anteroposterior. pressure in the unconscious patient. (This should be performed only once and preferably by the orthopedic surgeon taking responsibility for the injury.)

Significant limb injuries can exist without evident fractures on examination or on radiographs. In particular, ligament ruptures produce joint instability, and muscle-tendon injuries interfere with active motion of the affected structures. Impaired sensation or loss of voluntary muscle contraction strength may be caused by nerve injury or ischemia, including that due to compartment syndrome.

Spinal Cord Assessment

A detailed neurological examination, which includes testing for cranial nerves, sensation to fine touch and pinprick, proprioception, power, tone, coordination, and reflexes, is carried out at this stage to identify abnormalities in the peripheral nervous system. The patient should have a urinary catheter in place, because spinal injury may result in retention of urine. Immobilization of the patient with a long spinal board and a semirigid collar must be maintained until spinal injury is excluded. The common mistake of immobilizing the head and freeing the torso allows the cervical spine to flex with the body as a fulcrum. Any evidence of sensory or motor loss suggests major injury to the spinal column or peripheral nervous system and should never be disregarded, no matter how unimportant it may seem at the time.

The patient may complain of electrical shock–like pain radiating down the spine or into the limbs; this is caused by nerve root compression. In patients with partial cord lesions, some neurological function may be spared distal to the level of the injury (e.g., the sacral segments), and this may suggest a vascular lesion. The acute urinary retention seen in

paraplegic and tetraplegic patients may not be observed if there is sacral sparing. In patients with central cord syndromes, the zone of injury lies centrally and encroaches on the cervical segments of the long tracts, producing a flaccid weakness in the arms. Anterior contusions are associated with weakness and impaired pain and temperature sensation. Posterior injury results in loss of vibration sense and proprioception. In the Brown-Sequard syndrome, trauma is confined to one side of the cord, producing ipsilateral weakness and impaired contralateral pain and temperature sensation.

In the unconscious patient, there are no truly pathognomonic features of spinal cord injury, but important signs are flaccid paralysis, diaphragmatic breathing, priapism, and upward movement of the umbilicus on tensing of the abdomen. If the cord has been transected above the level of the sympathetic outflow, neurogenic shock results and hypotension without a corresponding tachycardia is observed.

Thoracic and lumbar spinal fractures and neurological injuries must be considered based on physical findings and mechanism of injury. If a spinal injury is suspected, the patient should be moved only by a well-coordinated logrolling technique. The back should be examined from the occiput to the heels. After palpation of the spinous processes and the paraspinal muscles, a rectal examination should be carried out to assess anal sphincter tone and the position of the prostate gland. The patient can then be logrolled back to the supine position.

Good-quality radiographs are essential for diagnosing spinal injuries. AP and lateral radiographs are the standard views of the thoracolumbar spine. Unlike a cervical hematoma, a paravertebral hematoma in this area is best seen in an AP view and may appear as mediastinal widening that may resemble aortic dissection. Subluxations, burst fractures, or potentially unstable injury affecting the posterior vertebral ligaments or bone may be seen on the lateral radiograph. Instability requires disruption of at least two of the three columns of the spine. The upper thoracic spine is usually difficult to assess; as with the neck, CT evaluation is now commonplace.

In some patients, decubitus ulcers develop quickly over the sacrum, heels, and other pressure areas after immobilization on a rigid spine board or in a cervical collar. Efforts to exclude the possibility of spinal injury and then remove these devices should be initiated as soon as practical. Removal can usually be achieved at the end of the secondary survey, when debris can also be removed from the back. If further radiographs have to be taken, the board provides a useful means of transfer to the radiology department. Patients should not be transferred to a tertiary center on a spinal board.

ADJUNCTS TO THE SECONDARY SURVEY

Pain control and alleviation of anxiety also form important parts of trauma care. Effective analgesia often warrants intravenous opioid therapy under close observation to prevent reduced levels of consciousness and respiratory depression. Regional anesthesia techniques such as femoral nerve blockade for femoral fracture are useful for patients awaiting access to the operating room, but the neurovascular status of the limb must be documented first. Pain persisting in a limb after what is considered a reasonable analgesic dose should always suggest compartment syndrome and need for urgent reassessment.

All adjuncts and further investigations of the secondary survey that require transportation of the patient to other areas of the hospital should be sanctioned only after the patient has been fully examined and deemed hemodynamically stable. It cannot be reiterated enough that ongoing monitoring and reassessment of trauma patients is critical, because a number of signs and symptoms related to injury may declare themselves only many hours or even days after the precipitating event.

RECORDS AND LEGAL CONSIDERATION

It is important to keep meticulous contemporaneous notes, including time notations. This is especially important in the trauma setting, because legal proceedings are frequently undertaken and multiple doctors can be caring for a patient over a short period of time. Photographs of injuries are ideal; alternatively, clear and accurate drawings, particularly in regard to facial injuries, must be made.

CONSENT FOR TREATMENT

In simple terms, consent is sought before treatment if possible. If this not possible, as in patients with life-threatening injuries or a reduced level of consciosness, treatment should be given first and formal consent obtained later.

FORENSIC EVIDENCE

Sometimes injury is thought to be a result of criminal activity. In such circumstances, it is important to preserve all of the evidence. Clothing and bullets should be saved for the police. In addition, laboratory determination of blood concentrations of alcohol and other drugs may be relevant.

CONCLUSION

Initial management of trauma patients requires a team approach in which each member is allocated a specific task, the overall aim being to identify and treat life-threatening conditions collectively. The ABC approach provides the doctor with one acceptable method for safe immediate management in which life-threatening injuries are identified and treated in the order in which they would otherwise kill the patient. Once the patient has been stabilized, a full assessment is carried out, during which an AMPLE history is taken and the patient is examined from top to toe, front to back, and side to side. Throughout this process, the emphasis is on continuous assessment and reevaluation, so that the response to any therapy can be monitored. If there is any deterioration, the primary survey is repeated.

REFERENCES

1. World Health Organization: *Disease and injury estimates for 2004*, Geneva, 2008, WHO.
2. Intercollegiate Group on Trauma Standards, Royal College of Surgeons of England: *Regional trauma systems: interim guidance for Commissioners*, London, 2009, RCS.
3. Office of National Statistics: *Mortality statistics for 2004, London*, London, 2006, Her Majesty's Stationery Office.
4. Committee on Trauma, American College of Surgeons: *2008 Advanced Trauma Life Support manual*, Chicago, 2008, ACS, p xviii.
5. Nessen SC, Lounsbury DE, Hetz SP: *War surgery in Afghanistan and Iraq: a series of cases, 2003-2007*, Washington, DC, 2008, Walter Reed Army Medical Center Borden Institute, 2008, pp 1-3.
6. Durham R, Pracht E, Orban B, et al: Evaluation of a mature trauma system. *Ann Surg* 243:775-785, 2006.
7. Nathens AB, Jurkovich GJ, Maier RV, et al: Relationship between trauma center volume and outcomes. *JAMA* 285:164-171, 2001.
8. London Severe Injuries Working Group: *Modernising major trauma services in London*, London, 2001, LSIWG.
9. Mackenzie EJ, Rivara FP, Jurkovich GJ, et al: A national evaluation of the effect of trauma-center care on mortality. *N Engl J Med* 354:366-378, 2006.
10. McGuffie AC, Graham CA, Beard D, et al: Scottish urban versus rural trauma outcome study. *J Trauma* 59:632-638, 2005.
11. UK Trauma Audit and Research Network: *TARN 2001-2004 dataset*, Chicago, 2004, American College of Surgeons, National Trauma Data Bank.
12. Anderson ID, Woodford M, de Dombal FT, et al: Retrospective study of 1000 deaths from injury in England and Wales. *BMJ (Clin Res Ed)* 296:305-308, 1988.
13. Office for Public Management: *Regional trauma networks: report to Department of Health*, London, 2010, OPM.
14. Perry M, Moutray T: Advanced Trauma Life Support (ATLS) and facial trauma: can one size fit all? part 4. *Int J Oral Maxillofac Surg* 37:505-514, 2008.
15. Scott SG, Belanger HG, Vanderploeg RD, et al: Mechanism-of-injury approach to evaluating patients with blast-related polytrauma. *J Am Osteopath Assoc* 1006:265-270, 2006.
16. Perry M, Morris C: Advanced Trauma Life Support (ATLS) and facial trauma: can one size fit all? part 2. *Int J Oral Maxillofac Surg* 37:309-320, 2008.
17. Wright MJ, Greenberg DE, Hunt JP, et al: Surgical cricothyroidotomy in trauma patients. *South Med J* 96:465-467, 2003.
18. Boyd AD, Conlan AA: Emergency cricothyroidotomy: is its use justified? *Surg Rounds* 12:19-23, 1979.
19. Kress TD, Balasubramaniam S: Cricothyroidotomy. *Ann Emerg Med* 11:197-201, 1982.
20. Wade CE, Kauvar DS, Lefering R: Impact of haemorrhage on trauma outcomes: an overview of epidemiology, clinical presentations and therapeutic considerations. *J Trauma* 60:s3-s11, 2006.
21. Committee on Trauma, American College of Surgeons: *2008 Advanced Trauma Life Support manual*, Chicago, 2008, ACS, p 56.
22. Keel M, Trentz O: Pathophysiology of polytrauma. *Injury* 36:691-709, 2005.
23. Schreiber MA, Perkins J, Kiraly L, et al: Early predictors of massive transfusion in combat casualties. *J Am Coll Surg* 205:541-545, 2007.
24. Cotton BA, Guy JS, Morris JA, et al: The cellular, metabolic and systemic consequences of aggressive fluid resuscitation strategies. *Shock* 26:115-121, 2006.
25. Rhee P, Wang D, Ruff P, et al: Human neutrophil activation and increased adhesion by various resuscitation fluids. *Crit Care Med* 28:74-78, 2000.
26. Como JJ, Dutton RP, Scalea TM, et al: Blood transfusion rates in the care of acute trauma. *Transfusion* 44:809-813, 2004.
27. Perry M, O'Hare J, Porter G: Advanced Trauma Life Support (ATLS) and facial trauma: can one size fit all? part 3. *Int J Oral Maxillofac Surg*, 37:405-414, 2008.
28. Nessen SC, Lounsbury DE, Hetz SP: *War surgery in Afghanistan and Iraq: a series of cases, 2003-2007*, Washington, DC, 2008, Walter Reed Army Medical Center Borden Institute, 2008, pp xix-xxi.
29. Dutton RP, Mackenzie CF, Scalea TM: Hypotensive resuscitation during active hemorrhage: impact on in-hospital mortality. *J Trauma* 52:1141-1146, 2002.
30. Cooper BR, Mahoney PF, Hodgetts TJ, et al: Intra-osseous access (EZ-IO(r)) for resuscitation: U.K. military combat experience. *J R Army Med Corps* 153:314-316, 2007.
31. Smith CM, Woolrich-Burt L, Wellings R, et al: Major trauma CT scanning: the experience of a regional trauma centre in the U.K. *Emerg Med J* 2010 Jun 1 [Epub ahead of print].
32. Schierhout G, Roberts I: Fluid resuscitation with colloid or crystalloid solutions in critically ill patients: a systematic review of randomised trials. *BMJ* 316:961-964, 1998.
33. Wade CE, Grady JJ, Kramer G: Efficacy of hypertonic saline dextran fluid resuscitation for patients with hypotension from penetrating trauma. *J Trauma* 54:s144-s148, 2003.
34. Battison C, Andrews PJD, Graham C, et al: Ramdomised controlled trial on the effect of a 20% mannitol solution and a 7.5% saline/6% dextran solution on increased intracranial pressure after brain injury. *Crit Care Med* 33:196-202, 2005.
35. Barletta JF, Ahrens CL, Tyburski JG, et al: A review of recombinant factor VII for refractory bleeding in non-hemophilic trauma patients. *J Trauma* 58:646-651, 2005.

36. Perry M, Dancey A, Mireskandari K, et al: Emergency care in facial trauma: a maxillofacial and ophthalmic perspective. *Injury* 36:875-896, 2005.

37. Price SJ, Suttner N, Aspoas AR: Have ATLS and national transfer guidelines improved the quality of resuscitation and transfer of head-injured patients? A prospective survey from a Regional Neurosurgical Unit. *Injury* 34:834-838, 2003.

38. Kulkarni AR, Aggarwal SP, Kulkarni RR, et al: Ocular manifestations of head injury: a clinical study. *Eye* 19:1257-1263, 2005.

39. Lindberg JV: Orbital compartment syndromes following trauma. *Adv Ophthal Plast Reconstr Surg* 6:51-62, 1987.

40. Vassallo S, Hartstein M, Howard D, et al: Traumatic retrobulbar haemorrhage: emergent decompression by lateral canthotomy and cantholysis. *J Emerg Med* 22:251-256, 2002.

CHAPTER 4

Management of Head Injury

John E. Crossman, Justin Nissen, Alistair Jenkins

Head injury is a major cause of preventable death and disability in the Western world among adults younger than 45 years of age[1] and carries a large cost in terms of manpower, resources and human suffering. The aims of those involved in the management of head injuries must be:

- to prevent or reduce the number of head injuries.
- to provide optimal care for those who suffer a head injury, and prevent secondary brain injury from further compounding primary brain injury.
- to produce an optimal environment in which rehabilitation from head injury can occur.

This chapter discusses the causes and mechanisms of head injury, the associated pathophysiology, the grading of the severity of injury, and the management of minor, moderate, and severe head injuries.

EPIDEMIOLOGY OF HEAD INJURY

About 200 of every 100,000 individuals in the Western world suffer a head injury each year. These range from a minor knock on the head without loss of consciousness or lasting neurological sequelae to a extremely severe head injury that leads directly to death. Collection of accurate data about the cause and seriousness of head injuries is difficult in the United Kingdom for several reasons[1]:

- Many head injuries are minor and are unreported to medical attendants.
- Many head injuries are part of a spectrum of serious injuries sustained during polytrauma and are classified as such.

A number of different classifications of head injury exist, and are not directly comparable, leading to difficulties with aggregation or comparison of data.

Most epidemiological studies have therefore had to rely on a classification based on eventual management of the patient, which within the United Kingdom is usually split into:

- seen in the emergency department but not admitted
- admitted for observation
- transferred to a regional neurosurgical unit
- operated on in a neurosurgical unit

Clearly, this categorization does not include those patients with very severe injuries who die before reaching the hospital nor those with apparently insignificant head injuries who do not seek medical attention. Additional confounding factors include differences in the management of head injuries among different neurosurgical units: Some units transfer most or all patients with serious head injuries, whereas others elect to manage at a distance those for whom neurosurgical intervention is not indicated.[2,3]

Most head injuries result from falls, vehicular accidents, pedestrian road accidents, or assaults. Cause of accident varies among different age groups. Young children and the elderly are most commonly injured by falls, whereas young men are more commonly victims of assault. Sports and other leisure activities are also an increasingly important cause of head injury.

Two peaks are observed in the incidence of death after head injury: in patients between 10 and 30 years of age and in those older than 70 years of age. Hospital admission rates follow a similar pattern. Men have a higher incidence of mortality and hospital admission after head injury than women do, and more patients with head injuries related to assault are admitted on weekends. Outcome following head injury has been demonstrated to be poorer in the elderly, deprived and in various racial/ethnic population groups.

Alcohol is undoubtedly an important factor in head injury in Western societies. In studies in which the influence of alcohol was assessed, high blood alcohol levels were associated with assault and road traffic accidents.

As a consequence of research on the causes of head injury, many Western countries have introduced legislation to enforce the wearing of seat belts and motorcycle crash helmets and to reduce vehicle speed limits, as well as controls on alcohol consumption by drivers. These preventive measures have contributed to a downward trend in the number of severe head injuries. However, in the developing world, an increasing number of head injuries are occurring as road traffic increases.

TABLE 4-1	Glasgow Coma Score: Motor Component

Action	Description	Score
Obeys command	Obeys spoken command	6
Localizes pain applied in area of sensation supplied by cranial nerves	Brings arm (or arms) up to stimulus	5
Withdrawal	Purposeful withdrawal from nailbed painful stimulus	4
Flexion	Flexion of the elbow on nailbed painful stimulus	3
Extension	Extension of the elbow on nailbed painful stimulus	2
None	No motor response to adequate painful stimulus	1

TABLE 4-2	Glasgow Coma Score: Verbal Component

Speech	Description	Score
Oriented	Knows place, time, location	5
Confused	Talks in sentences but does not know place, time, location	4
Words	Answers in words	3
Sounds	Utters incomprehensible sounds	2
None	No speech	1

TABLE 4-3	Glasgow Coma Score: Eye Component

Eye Opening	Stimulus	Score
Spontaneously	Eyes open normally	4
To speech	Eyes open only to speech	3
To pain	Eyes open only to pain	2
None	No eye opening	1

MEASUREMENT OF INJURY SEVERITY AND OUTCOME

GLASGOW COMA SCALE

The Glasgow Coma Scale (GCS) is the instrument most widely used to assess consciousness after a head injury.[4] Before its development, a series of loosely defined terms such as *obtunded, lethargy, stupor,* and *coma* were used to categorize the degree of unconsciousness.

A standardized method for scoring the level of consciousness, such as the GCS, is important in the management of head injuries for several reasons. A substantial number of head-injured patients present to hospitals that do not have resident neurosurgical support. A standardized scale of consciousness, together with image linking of the computed tomographic (CT) scan, allows a rapid evaluation of the severity of injury by the neurosurgeon and a swift decision as to whether transfer to the neurosurgical unit is required. The GCS also has been shown to have prognostic value regarding the eventual outcome of the injury.[5,6]

The development of the GCS permitted reliable and reproducible assessment with little interobserver variability across all classes of health care workers. The actual level of consciousness and the deterioration in that level are more clearly identifiable when regular GCS assessments are performed.

The GCS consists of three parts: a motor response, a verbal response, and an eye response. The motor component responses are given in Table 4-1. The motor response is scored as the best limb response. Failure of the patient to obey commands requires the observer to determine the patient's response to a painful stimulus—pressure on the supraorbital nerve or on the nailbed (see Table 4-1). Usually, the best response is elicited in the upper limbs. An asymmetrical response indicates a focal lesion of the central nervous system.

The verbal response is assessed as indicated in Table 4-2. Lack of a verbal response in an otherwise awake patient usually indicates damage to the speech center. The eye response (Table 4-3) assesses the integrity of the brain's arousal mechanisms. The eye response to pain should be elicited by limb stimulus, because reflex eye opening may occur with facial stimulation. Also vital are the pupillary response to light and pupillary size; these should be assessed along with the GCS score in head-injured patients.

The severity of a head injury is usually classified according to the best post-resuscitation GCS. A minor head injury has a GCS score of 15; a mild injury, 13 or 14; a moderate injury, between 9 and 12; and a severe head injury, between 3 and 8. Coma is defined as inability to obey commands, no intelligible speech, and no eye opening (M5 V2 E1). This classification is used to guide management and is prognostic of the eventual outcome.[7]

GLASGOW OUTCOME SCALE

To compare outcomes after a head injury and the beneficial effects (or otherwise) of interventions during the management of head injury, a standardized outcome measure must be used. The Glasgow Outcome Scale (GOS) was developed to measure global brain functioning rather than to specifically assess a particular mental or physical outcome.[8]

Improvement often occurs up to 6 months after head injury and may continue to occur for 1 to 2 years, so assessment of outcome should not be performed before 6 months after the injury.

The GOS assesses outcome based on the level of dependence or independence of the patient. There are five possible outcomes (Table 4-4).

Good recovery implies that the patient is able to resume his or her previous employment; neurological sequelae may exist, but the patient is able to maintain an independent existence. *Moderate disability* indicates that the patient is independent at home and can travel by public transport, but often there are significant persisting physical or mental neurological deficits. A patient with a *severe disability* is conscious but is dependent on the assistance of another person each day. *Persistent vegetative state* (PVS) allows normal respiration and sleep-wake states. A patient with PVS may occasionally follow

TABLE 4-4 Glasgow Outcome Scale

Category	Description	Score
Good outcome	Resumption of normal life despite minor neurological/psychological deficits	5
Moderate disability (disabled but independent)	Independent in daily life, but often significant disability remains (e.g., dysphasia, hemiparesis, cognitive dysfunction)	4
Severe disability (conscious but disabled)	Such patients are dependent on support for physical or mental activities	3
Persistent vegetative state	This is a difficult diagnosis; such patients often remain unresponsive after brain injury and may develop sleep-wake cycles	2
Death		1

a moving object or look toward a bright light or loud sound and also withdraws from a painful limb stimulus. The final category is *death*. The scale is often abbreviated by dividing outcomes into *favorable* (good recovery and moderate disability) and *unfavorable* (severe disability, PVS, and death).

As with the GCS, criticisms can be made that the GOS is too global an assessment; that a significant disability, either mental or physical, can exist despite an apparently favorable outcome; and that different levels of recovery are required to return to professional or managerial employment versus manual work, which may alter the outcome category.

PHYSIOLOGY OF HEAD INJURY

An understanding of the concepts of cerebral blood flow, cerebral perfusion pressure, and intracranial pressure is essential to comprehend the pathophysiology and management of head injury.

CEREBRAL BLOOD FLOW, INTRACRANIAL PRESSURE, AND CEREBRAL PERFUSION PRESSURE

The brain receives approximately one fifth of the total cardiac output—about 1 L/min at rest. This is equivalent to a mean *cerebral blood flow* (CBF) in gray matter of 49 mL per 100 g of brain per minute. The brain has little capacity to store either glucose or oxygen and is therefore dependent on continuous blood flow. Reduction in CBF to between 25 and 39 mL/100 g/min causes confusion and sometimes loss of consciousness. Reduction to 15 mL/100 g/min causes loss of measurable neuronal electrical activity, and flow of less than 8 mL/100 g/min causes neuronal death.[9,10]

Cerebral Blood Flow

The flow (Q) of a Newtonian fluid through a rigid vessel is described by Poiseuille's equation:

$$Q = \text{Pressure gradient} \times (\pi r^4 / 8\mu L)$$

where r is the radius, μ is the viscosity of the fluid, and L is the length of the pipe. Clearly in the physiological situation,

the pressure gradient and the blood vessel diameter have important effects on CBF. The pressure gradient is known as the *cerebral perfusion pressure* (CPP) and is usually calculated as follows:

$$CPP = \text{Mean arterial pressure} - ICP$$

Intracranial Pressure

The Monro-Kellie principle states that because the skull is a rigid structure and the skull contents of brain, cerebrospinal fluid (CSF), and blood are incompressible, an increase in any one or several of these, or development of a mass lesion such as a hematoma, will cause an increase in ICP.

Measurement of Intracranial Pressure

ICP can be measured by inserting a pressure transducer into the ventricular system, into the subarachnoid space, subdurally, or intraparenchymally. The "gold standard" measurement is that of ventricular pressure. The pressure is normally measured in centimeters of water relative to the foramen of Munro. Normal adult ICP ranges from 0 to 15 cm H_2O.

AUTOREGULATION

Autoregulation is defined as maintenance of a constant CBF over a range of CPPs. Constant CBF is maintained through variation in arterial diameter: The arterial diameter increases when the CPP falls and decreases when the CPP increases.

When the autoregulatory mechanism is exhausted or deficient, as may be the case after head injury, the CBF is dependent on the CPP and, consequently, on the blood pressure. Low blood pressure therefore decreases the CBF, and cerebral ischemia occurs as the CPP falls below 50 mm Hg. After brain injury, loss of autoregulation is usually patchy within the brain, and some areas retain normal autoregulation. Flow "steal" may then occur when blood vessels in normally functioning areas of brain dilate and therefore have a lower cerebrovascular resistance than the blood vessels in the abnormal area of brain.

BIOMECHANICS AND PATHOLOGY OF HEAD INJURY

Brain injury is usually classified as primary or secondary.[9,11] *Primary brain injury* is that which occurs at the time of the injury and is regarded as irreversible. *Secondary brain injury* occurs after the primary insult. It is the aim of head injury management to prevent or reduce damage occurring as a consequence of secondary brain injury. The mechanisms of secondary brain injury are:

- hematoma formation.
- brain swelling and cerebral herniation.
- cerebral infection.

A list of complications of head injury is given in Table 4-5.

PRIMARY BRAIN INJURY

The forces that cause primary brain injury can be categorized as inertial or contact, although there is overlap between the

TABLE 4-5	Complications of Head Injury	
Primary	Secondary	Extracranial
Scalp injury	Intracranial hematoma	Electrolyte disturbance
Skull fracture	Cerebral swelling	Chest or other sepsis
Perforating or penetrating wound	Cerebral herniation	Thromboembolism
Focal brain injury	Cerebral ischemia	Gastrointestinal bleeding
Diffuse brain injury	Infection (meningitis)	

groups. Most brain injury is a consequence of direct trauma to the skull, although facial injuries can also result in brain injury.

Inertial Brain Injury

Inertial forces are a consequence of differential acceleration within the brain and between the brain and the skull, usually resulting from a glancing blow to the head. Such a blow results in deformation of the brain substance and shear stresses throughout the brain, leading to axonal injury. Inertial injuries usually affect the whole of the brain and are termed *diffuse axonal injury*; they may also cause rupture of bridging veins and pial vessels with consequent hematoma formation. Because the center of the brain is most affected by the rotational forces, diffuse injury is most marked in the brainstem, corpus callosum, and other central brain areas.

Diffuse Axonal Injury

The shearing force causes stretching of the nerve fibers, and this results in axonal damage. In the early stages of injury, axonal injury is represented pathologically by axonal bulbs (retraction balls), which are seen particularly in the central structures such as the corpus callosum, the white matter on either side of the ventricle, and regions of the brainstem. Over time, atrophy and degeneration of the long white-matter tracts take place, and patchy formation of microglia occurs. Macroscopically in the early stages, small hemorrhagic lesions are seen in the sites of maximal stress. Rupture of the fornix may cause intraventricular hemorrhage. Later, brain matter atrophy with ventricular dilatation is the major finding.

The clinical consequence of this brain injury is a poor GCS from the outset, with lack of a lucid interval, low association with skull fractures, and, if the patient survives, often a high degree of residual brain dysfunction due to the widespread structural damage.

Contact Brain Injury

Contact injuries are usually caused by a direct blow to the skull; they result in skull fractures and contusions of the brain, both at the impact site and at a distance from the location of the injury. A blow to the skull results in inward movement of the skull at the point of impact; a fracture occurs if the degree of deformity exceeds the critical amount by which the skull is able to deform.

The morphology of the fracture depends on the size of the area of impact with the skull. A small contact area usually results in a relatively smaller, depressed fracture, whereas a larger contact area produces a greater dissipation of the force and usually results in a relatively larger, linear fracture.

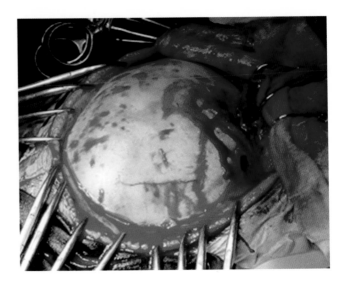

FIGURE 4-1 Intraoperative appearance of a linear skull fracture. This patient's computed tomography scan is illustrated in Figure 4-2, and the intraoperative appearance of the extradural hematoma is shown in Figure 4-4.

Cerebral Contusions

Cerebral contusions result from trauma to the brain that causes localized hemorrhagic swelling. Typically, cerebral contusions are found on the undersurface of the frontal lobes and temporal lobes and occur when these areas of the brain are damaged by the rough bone edges found in the region of the anterior and middle cranial fossae. The contusions may swell over several days, causing raised ICP, or bleeding into a contusion may result in the development of an intracranial hematoma.

Skull Fractures

A fracture is a discontinuity of the bones that form the skull surrounding the brain. A fracture usually occurs after a contact injury, when a large displacement of the bone at the point of impact has exceeded the limit of bone plasticity. Fractures may occur in the calvarial region and at the base of the skull.

A *stellate* skull fracture, one in which fracture lines radiate from the point of impact, occurs as a result of a blow that contacts only a small area of the skull surface, such as that from a hammer or missile. A *linear* fracture tends to occur after a blow during which the force is spread over a greater area of the skull surface. Stellate fractures occur only rarely in the skull base because of the protection afforded by the occipitocervical musculature, the pharynx, and the facial skeleton. Figure 4-1 demonstrates the intraoperative appearance of a linear skull fracture.

A skull fracture is *compound* if there is a potential conduit between the brain and the external environment through either a related scalp laceration or a paranasal sinus. This represents a route through which intracranial infection may occur, leading to abscess, empyema, or meningitis. A closed fracture has no such connection with the external environment.

A *depressed* skull fracture occurs when the fracture fragment lies deep to the surrounding bone, usually by a depth greater than the thickness of the surrounding bone. Depression of the fracture to this degree implies a dural laceration and, therefore, a potential route of infection. Depressed fractures may be closed or compound, and they may be linear or stellate.

Fractures may occur through the skull base, and potentially they can lead to disruption of the vessels and nerves that pass though the region of the fracture. CSF fistulae may occur with fractures through the frontal, sphenoidal, or ethmoidal sinuses or through the cribriform plate. CSF leakage through temporal bone fractures may manifest as rhinorrhea, if the fluid leaks into the nasopharynx through the middle ear and eustachian tube, or as otorrhea, if leakage occurs through a perforated eardrum into the external auditory canal.

Elevation of a depressed skull fracture does not appear to alter the incidence of posttraumatic epilepsy.

Penetrating and Perforating Brain Injury

Penetrating injury refers to those injuries caused by missiles or gunshot wounds, whereas *perforation* implies a puncture or stab wound by a knife or a nail. This type of injury results in a skull fracture with a tract hematoma. The severity of the injury depends on the area of brain damaged. The most common complications of perforating injury are infection (brain abscesses and meningitis) and hemorrhage. Vascular injury occurs in approximately one third of brain wounds and may lead to the formation of traumatic aneurysms.

SECONDARY BRAIN INJURY

Secondary brain injury is the most important cause of preventable morbidity and mortality.

Hematoma Formation

Hematoma formation or the formation of a lesion with mass effect (i.e., one that causes a rise in ICP) represents a neurosurgical emergency.

The type of hematoma that occurs after a head injury depends on the mechanism of the injury.

Extradural Hematoma

A focal injury associated with the formation of a skull fracture may result in the development of a hematoma in the extradural space. Typically, this occurs in the region of the temporal bone and results from damage to the middle meningeal artery, but extradural hematomas may also form in the frontal, parietal, or occipital regions or in the posterior fossa from lacerations to dural arteries or bleeding from the fracture itself. Because the source of the bleeding is usually arterial, these hematomas are usually under high pressure and cause mass effect. Typically, the size of the hematoma is limited by the dura, which is tightly bound to the skull at the cranial sutures. Figure 4-2 illustrates the CT appearance of an extradural hematoma.

Acute Subdural Hematoma

An acute subdural hematoma is usually the consequence of a widespread superficial cortical injury, with multiple resultant bleeding points. Occasionally, rupture of a cortical bridging vein between the brain and the cerebral venous sinus, as it passes through the potential subdural space between the dura and the arachnoid membranes, can result in a subdural

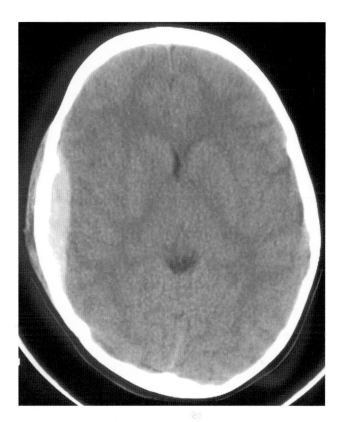

FIGURE 4-2 Computed tomography scan of an extradural hematoma. Notice the asymmetry of the lateral ventricles and the minor degree of midline shift, indicating that the hematoma has a mass effect.

hematoma. The bridging veins are most vulnerable when placed on stretch, as in young children and in those individuals with an atrophic brain (e.g., the elderly). Figure 4-3 illustrates the CT appearance of an acute subdural hematoma.

A rotational injury causing differential shearing between the skull and brain causes the veins to stretch beyond capacity and to rupture, with subsequent bleeding into the subdural space. Because the arachnoid and dura are tightly bound only at the cerebral sinuses, blood is able to track within the subdural space more extensively than with an extradural hematoma. Because these hematomas usually result from venous bleeding and because of the larger potential space into which they can spread, they are usually under low pressure and conform to the surface of the brain.

Chronic Subdural Hematoma

A chronic subdural hematoma also occurs in the space between the dura and the brain and is also found usually in the elderly. The origin of these hematomas is uncertain, but they probably arise as a result of minor, and often repeated, insignificant head injury. With time, the volume of the hematoma enlarges, either through repeated episodes of bleeding or because the high osmotic potential of the blood attracts water. Within the hematoma, the blood liquefies over a period of about 10 days, during which the hematoma consists of a mixture of fluid blood and organizing clot. This stage is often referred to as a *subacute subdural hematoma*. After about 3 weeks, the collection has usually liquefied. A fresh bleed can occur into a chronic subdural hematoma and may result in a

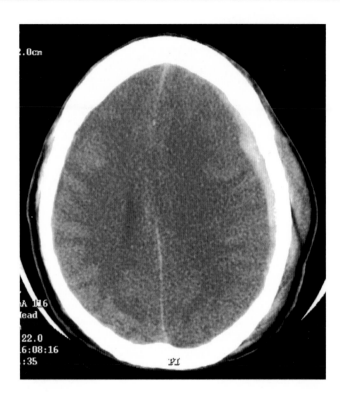

FIGURE 4-3 Computed tomography scan of an acute subdural hematoma.

rapid rise in the ICP with consequential neurological deterioration, which may prompt diagnosis of the previously unrecognized hematoma.

Often, a chronic subdural hematoma grows to a substantial size and results in a mass effect; this leads to compression of the ipsilateral cerebral hemisphere and a midline shift. However, there is relatively little neurological deficit, because the rise in ICP occurs over days rather than minutes to hours (as in an extradural or acute subdural hematoma), and this allows intracranial compensation to occur.

Intracerebral Hematoma

Intracerebral hematomas arise from two distinct mechanisms in relation to head injury. Deep-seated hematomas, usually within the basal ganglia, arise from rotational injury and are therefore indicative of diffuse axonal injury. They are often small and do not usually require surgical intervention. A hematoma may also occur in relation to a contusion, as discussed earlier. Such a hematoma may swell progressively over several days, develop a mass effect, and raise the ICP.

Burst Lobe

A burst lobe is distinct from an intracerebral hematoma in that the acute subdural collection occurs in continuity with the overlying contused brain. This injury occurs most frequently in the frontal and temporal lobes.

Intraventricular Hemorrhage

Intraventricular hemorrhage is a rare occurrence after head injury. The origin of the intraventricular blood is usually a tear in a central midline intraventricular structure such as

the fornix; this indicates that the brain has suffered a major rotational injury, and intraventricular blood is usually associated with severe diffuse axonal injury. Particularly if there is associated subarachnoid blood, it is important to consider whether the intraventricular bleed occurred as part of a primary event (e.g., rupture of a cerebral aneurysm), with the patient sustaining the head injury as a result of a collapse.

Traumatic Subarachnoid Hemorrhage

Traumatic subarachnoid hemorrhage results from injury to the cerebral vessels as they cross the subarachnoid space. Extensive subarachnoid hemorrhage can occur, with subsequent vasospasm. The distribution of the blood in traumatic subarachnoid hemorrhage is usually easily distinguishable from that observed in aneurysmal subarachnoid hemorrhage, but if uncertainty exists, cerebral angiography may be required to distinguish between the two causes.

Brain Swelling

Brain swelling may be caused by an increase in the brain water content, such as occurs in cerebral edema, or by increased blood due to cerebral hyperemia or development of an intracerebral mass lesion.

There are two main forms of cerebral edema. *Vasogenic* cerebral edema occurs when the blood-brain barrier has been disrupted and water, sodium, and protein molecules have been extravasated into the extracellular space. *Cytotoxic* cerebral edema occurs when the neurons lack energy to maintain the ionic gradient across the cell membrane; water passes into the cells, causing them to swell.

Cerebral hyperemia is more common in children than in adults. The causative mechanism is unknown, but the arterioles appear to dilate, and blood passes directly to the capillary bed.

As discussed earlier, brain swelling causes a rise in ICP, and in the absence of intact autoregulation, this leads to a reduction in the CBF.

Brain Herniation

The skull is divided into compartments by the infolding of the dura to form the cerebral falx and cerebral tentorium. Development of a mass lesion, such as an intracerebral or extradural hematoma, creates a pressure gradient across the different compartments. Brain herniation occurs in response to the pressure gradient.

Several different forms of herniation are described:

- *Subfalcine herniation* occurs when a unilateral supratentorial mass lesion causes brain to herniate under the falx. Compression of the anterior cerebral arteries is a possible consequence, but clinical symptoms and signs related to this are rare.
- *Lateral tentorial herniation* is also a consequence of a unilateral supratentorial mass lesion. The medial edge of the ipsilateral temporal lobe is forced medially and compresses the third cranial nerve. Clinically, this causes the pupil to dilate and become nonreactive to light. The brainstem can also become displaced and compressed, with deterioration in the level of consciousness and compression of the ipsilateral cerebral peduncle, causing contralateral hemiparesis.

- *Central tentorial herniation* occurs as a consequence of diffuse supratentorial swelling, when the contents of the supratentorial compartment are forced vertically through the tentorial hiatus. Pressure on the tectum causes loss of upgaze. Further downward movement of the brainstem leads to a deterioration in the level of consciousness, pupillary abnormalities, and eventually, as traction injury to the pituitary stalk occurs, diabetes insipidus.

A hematoma in the infratentorial compartment can cause herniation of the cerebellar tonsils through the foramen magnum and upward herniation of the cerebellum through the tentorial hiatus.

Cerebral Infection

Compound fractures represent a potential route of infection through which organisms may track and cause meningitis. Meningitis results in a purulent exudate that spreads throughout the subarachnoid space. Cerebritis and brain abscess formation may follow. The infection leads to vascular thrombosis, causing infarcts; occasionally, obstruction of CSF flow results in hydrocephalus.

Extracranial Complications

Many extracranial complications can occur, including hyponatremia, respiratory complications, and gastrointestinal hemorrhage. These compromise brain blood flow and oxygenation, to the detriment of the patient.

MANAGEMENT OF HEAD INJURIES

The overriding aim in the management of a head injury is to minimize the morbidity and mortality related to secondary brain injury. This requires rapid evaluation and triage of patients presenting with head injuries. Guidelines for the initial management of head injuries were first published in 1984.[12] The National Institute for Clinical Excellence (NICE) issued recommendations in 2003 and updated them in 2007.[13] The document outlines "best practice" for management of head injuries within the United Kingdom and sets timelines. The advice is outlined in the following sections, although the complete guidance should be consulted for recommended management.

Patients are usually transferred to the neurosurgical unit for specialized monitoring and observation or because an operation is indicated. Emphasis in the current NICE guidance is placed on detection of significant head injury by the early use of imaging and subsequent expedited management.

Other important evidence-based guidelines on the management of head injury include the following:

- *The Surgical Management of Traumatic Brain Injury*, published in 2006, discusses the role of surgery in the management of traumatic hematomas and skull fractures.[14]
- *Guidelines for Management of Severe Traumatic Brain Injury*, published by the Brain Trauma Foundation in 2007, covers intensive care management.[15]

NATIONAL INSTITUTE FOR CLINICAL EXCELLENCE GUIDELINES ON MANAGEMENT OF HEAD INJURIES

The guidance is comprehensive and covers the "triage, assessment, investigation and early management of head injury in infants, children and adults."[13] Best practice is described for patients with suspected clinically important brain or cervical spine injury. Indications and time scale for (1) CT scanning of the head and cervical spine, (2) admission and observation of head-injured patients, (3) transfer to a neurosurgical unit, and (4) patient discharge are presented.

INITIAL MANAGEMENT OF HEAD INJURIES

The initial management of any head injury is to ensure adequate resuscitation of the patient. Although most patients with minor head injuries do not require resuscitation, in a patient with a severe head injury it is vital to ensure that the airway is clear and that adequate respiration and circulation are established and maintained.

After resuscitation and stabilization of the patient, the history of the injury should be determined. In the case of a minor injury, this can be obtained from the patient; with a more severe injury, witness accounts should be sought. The most important information is the initial GCS, pupillary reaction and size, whether the patient's condition is improving or deteriorating, the blood pressure and pulse rate, and the presence of other associated injuries. Other factors include the period of unconsciousness, the period of posttraumatic amnesia, whether a seizure has occurred, and the presence or absence of a focal neurological deficit. The events surrounding the injury should also be determined, such as the degree of damage to the vehicle in a motor accident and the number of other victims and their injuries; this information can be used to gauge the seriousness of the accident.

The patient should then be examined. Obviously, the patient's level of consciousness will affect the examination performed, but in general, the following parameters should be assessed:

- level of consciousness (GCS score)
- presence or absence of lateralizing signs (e.g., pupillary abnormalities, hemiplegia/paresis, paraparesis)
- external evidence of head injury
- evidence suggesting a base-of-skull fracture (e.g., "raccoon eyes," subconjunctival hemorrhage, Battle's sign)
- presence of a CSF leak
- presence of spinal and other extracranial injuries

Investigation of the Head-Injured Patient

CT scanning is the investigation of choice for acute head injury, and the opportunity to scan for facial injuries at the same time should not be lost. Magnetic resonance imaging (MRI) is not advised because of the contraindications, potential delay in obtaining a scan, and difficulty observing the patient during scanning. Skull radiographs are no longer advised, because CT scanning should be available in all emergency departments and provides better information.

The CT scan provides information regarding (1) detection of life-threatening or potentially life-threatening primary or secondary brain injury and (2) the prognosis of the patient with a head injury.

The indications for immediate CT scanning in adults are given in Box 4-1.[13] These guidelines are modified in the elderly, in those patients with coagulopathy, and in those who have experienced a dangerous mechanism of injury. Corresponding advice for children is also given in the guidelines.[13]

Detection of Cervical Spine Injury

Patients with head injury may also have cervical spine injury. Failure to recognize a cervical spine injury can lead to catastrophic quadriparesis. NICE recommends that a potential cervical spine injury be considered along with management of the head injury. Although plain radiographs are the current investigation of choice for suspected cervical spine injury, CT of the cervical spine is often performed in patients who are already undergoing CT head scanning. In certain circumstances, MRI of the cervical spine is also performed.

Neurosurgical Referral and Management

If any patient has a raised ICP on radiological or clinical grounds or other significant surgical lesions, the local neurosurgical unit should be consulted. Other indications for neurosurgical advice on management include:

- presence of skull or base-of-skull fracture
- CSF leak
- persistently decreased GCS score or deterioration in GCS score
- seizure
- focal neurological deficit
- intracranial contusions or hemorrhage
- penetrating injury

However, the reader should refer to local guidelines for specific advice on management. Immediate neurosurgical management is usually limited to evacuation of mass lesions (e.g., extradural hematoma) and other treatment of raised ICP, including decompressive craniectomy and ICP monitoring.

Surgical Evacuation of Intracranial Hematomas

Mass lesions within the skull, such as intracranial hematomas, may cause a rise in the ICP and a consequent reduction in CPP. Locally raised pressure around the hematoma may also cause cerebral herniation. To minimize secondary brain damage, any hematoma with significant mass effect should be removed. Hematomas without significant mass effect may be treated conservatively with serial observation of the patient's condition. Invasive monitoring of the ICP may be required. Persistent elevation of the ICP or a decline in the level of consciousness indicates the need for a further CT brain scan to determine whether the hematoma has increased in size and requires operative removal. Exploratory bur holes are very seldom performed.

Extradural Hematoma

Extradural hematomas most commonly arise from tearing of a middle meningeal artery in the region of the squamous temporal bone. A craniotomy is performed over the site of the hematoma. The hematoma, which usually consists of a mixture of coagulated blood with some fresh blood, is aspirated and washed away, the bleeding vessel is found, and diathermy is performed. Hitch stitches are then placed around the edges of the dura, and the bone flap is replaced and fixed into position. If the ICP is markedly elevated, the bone may simply be placed back in the skull defect and allowed to ride, although this is rarely the case with an extradural hematoma. Figure 4-4 illustrates the operative appearance of an extradural hematoma.

BOX 4-1   **NICE Guidance for Immediate Scanning after Head Injury**

Criteria for immediate request for CT scan of head (adults):
- GCS <13 on initial assessment in the emergency department
- GCS <15 at 2 hours after injury on assessment in the emergency department
- Suspected open or depressed skull fracture
- Any sign of skull base fracture (e.g., hemotympanum, "panda eyes," CSF leakage from the ear or nose, Battle's sign)
- Posttraumatic seizure
- Focal neurological deficit
- More than one episode of vomiting
- Amnesia for events more than 30 minutes before the impact

  Also request immediate CT for adult patients who have experienced some loss of consciousness or amnesia since head injury and have any of the following:
- Age 65 years or older
- Coagulopathy (history of bleeding, clotting disorder, current treatment with warfarin)
- Dangerous mechanism of injury (pedestrian or cyclist struck by a motor vehicle, occupant ejected from a motor vehicle, fall from a height >1 m or five stairs)

From National Institute for Health and Clinical Excellence: *Head injury: triage, assessment, investigation and early management of head injury in infants, children and adults.* NICE Clinical Guideline 56. London, 2007, NICE.

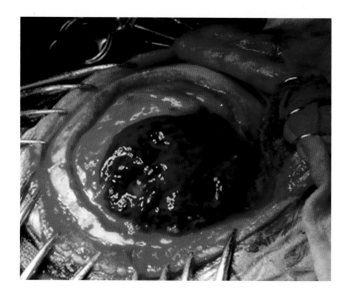

FIGURE 4-4 Intraoperative appearance of an extradural hematoma.

Acute Subdural Hematoma

Acute subdural hematomas are often larger than extradural hematomas and are frequently accompanied by extensive brain swelling. The hematoma lies between the dura and the cortical surface. Bleeding is usually the result of a widespread superficial cortical contusion with multiple bleeding points or, occasionally, a ruptured parafalcine or sylvian fissure cortical vein. A craniotomy is performed in the usual manner over the center of the clot. The dura is then opened, and the clot is washed away. Once hemostasis has been achieved, the bone is replaced as described previously, and the wound is closed in the usual manner.

Management of Skull Fractures

Most skull fractures do not require operative treatment. The indications for elevation of a depressed skull fracture are related to the presence of a dural tear and cosmesis. Fractures that are displaced beyond the inner table of the surrounding cortical bone indicate a dural tear; in the presence of a scalp wound, débridement and elevation of the fracture are required. Fractures outside the hair line are usually elevated for cosmesis.

Elevation of a Depressed Skull Fracture

In the case of a compound depressed skull fracture, the depressed fragments of bone are isolated from the skull and extracted from the fracture. The wound and bone fragments are cleaned, and the dural tear is repaired. The bone is then replaced if it is not too contaminated. The wound is closed, and the patient is given a course of intravenous antibiotics.

Treatment of Perforating or Penetrating Head Injury

Penetrating injury is usually a result of a gunshot wound. Several factors affect the degree of damage caused to the brain by a gunshot, the most important being the velocity of the projectile, because the kinetic energy is related to the square of the velocity. As the projectile passes through the brain, a pulsating cavity is created. This cavity often is many times larger than the projectile diameter and undergoes several cycles of dilatation and collapse. Shock waves created by the impact of the projectile against the skull also produce rapid and sudden compression and re-expansion of brain adjacent to the site of impact.

Penetrating and perforating injuries should be treated with prophylactic antibiotics. If the patient's condition warrants, a cerebral angiogram and wound débridement should be performed. Traumatic aneurysms are more likely to rupture than congenital aneurysms and should be managed operatively.

SUBSEQUENT MANAGEMENT OF MODERATE AND SEVERE HEAD INJURIES

Avoidance of secondary brain injury is of vital importance after the initial management of a head injury if the brain is to be given maximum potential for recovery and rehabilitation. Once control of the ICP has been obtained, the sedation is gradually reduced. The patient is extubated after his or her level of consciousness is good enough to maintain the airway and respiration. At this stage, the patient may still not be awake enough to obey commands or may have focal deficits (e.g., dysphasia) related to cerebral damage resulting from the trauma. Some patients require continued ventilation, either because of extracranial injuries (e.g., chest trauma, chest infection) or to control the ICP.

During this time, it is important to continue monitoring of the patient's blood pressure, oxygen saturation, ICP, and CPP to prevent secondary brain injury.

Control of Cerebral Perfusion Pressure and Intracranial Pressure

In order to minimize cerebral ischemia, an important cause of secondary brain injury, the brain must have an adequate blood flow. CBF is difficult to measure continuously on a routine basis, and in most centers the CPP is measured as a surrogate. CBF is related to CPP, as discussed earlier, although the autoregulation mechanism is often disrupted after brain injury.

That clinical outcome is related to ICP or CPP is debated. The ideal ICP and CPP after a head injury are unknown, but several studies have examined outcome in relation to CPP, and most authorities accept that an ICP of less than 20 to 25 mm Hg and a CPP greater than 70 mm Hg are required for optimal management.[16] Hyperventilation is rarely used in the management of head injury because it leads to vasoconstriction and a consequent reduction in the CPP.

Ischemic brain injury is found in about 90% of patients who die after head injury, and a single episode of hypotension is associated with an 85% increase in mortality. Experimental work in animals has suggested that higher perfusion pressures are beneficial in the presence of mass lesions, and reductions in perfusion pressure significantly increase the risk of brainstem ischemia.

Autoregulation maintains a constant blood flow to the brain over a wide range of CPPs and is therefore important in the prevention of cerebral ischemia. At CPPs of less than 50 mm Hg, cerebral arteriole vasodilatation is exhausted and the vessel collapses, with consequent cerebral ischemia. The upper limit of CPP autoregulation is 140 mm Hg. Above this level, the CPP increases with the CBF, causing damage to the blood-brain barrier and subsequent brain swelling. After head injury, the autoregulatory mechanism is often damaged, and experimental studies suggest that a perfusion pressure of between 60 and 70 mm Hg is required to achieve autoregulation.

The methods for managing persistently elevated ICP are:

- surgical evacuation of mass lesions
- head elevation
- control of $Paco_2$
- maintenance of a CPP greater than 70 mm Hg
- increased sedation and paralysis
- mannitol infusion or bolus
- ventricular drainage
- decompressive craniectomy

The initial measures are (1) to elevate the head to about 30 degrees with maintenance of the head in neutral position to increase venous return; (2) to maintain the CPP at a level greater than 70 mm Hg; and (3) to ensure that the $Paco_2$ is about 4 kPa. If these procedures are unsuccessful in lowering the ICP, further measures are instituted.

Failure to control the ICP is an indication for a repeat CT scan, because a traumatic hematoma may develop or enlarge with time; contusions or swelling also may worsen. If the ICP remains elevated, surgical decompression should be considered. In the absence of a mass lesion, the brain may be decompressed by a frontal or temporal lobectomy or a decompressive craniectomy.

Barbiturates

Barbiturates are rarely used for ICP control because of their deleterious effect on blood pressure and hence on CPP. Episodic rises in ICP may be caused by seizure activity; if present, this should be treated with an anticonvulsant drug.

Hyperventilation

Chronic hyperventilation in the management of ICP is no longer practiced, because it has a tendency to decrease the CPP. Conversely, Muizelaar et al. demonstrated that patients who are maintained in normocapnia, compared to those with hypocapnia, had a better outcome at 3 and 6 months although not at 1 year.[17] Usually, CBF is most severely decreased in the 24 hours immediately after a head injury, and hyperventilation during that time is most harmful.

Neuroprotective Agents

Trials involving steroids, free radical scavengers, and N-methyl-D-aspartic acid (NMDA) receptor antagonists have not shown any benefit in terms of patient outcome, although the search for neuroprotective agents continues.

MANAGEMENT OF EXTRACRANIAL COMPLICATIONS

Extracranial complications are common in head-injured patients, especially respiratory complications. If a patient remains intubated for longer than 10 days, a tracheostomy should be considered. Chest infection should be treated with antibiotics (guided by microbiological culture of sputum), suctioning as required, and physiotherapy. Nutritional support via nasogastric tube feeding should be commenced as soon as possible; this should be converted to a percutaneous gastrostomy if nutritional support is required for a longer period.

Hyponatremia may be caused by the syndrome of inappropriate secretion of antidiuretic hormone (SIADH) or by cerebral salt wasting. The best way to determine the cause is to measure the volume status. The dehydrated patient with hyponatremia due to cerebral salt wasting can be treated by sodium and volume replacement. Hyponatremia secondary to SIADH is normally responsive to fluid restriction. Hypernatremia is less common than hyponatremia and is usually a consequence of hypothalamic or pituitary injury causing diabetes insipidus. This is treated with desmopressin if required.

Deep vein thrombosis and pulmonary emboli occasionally occur and should be treated with anticoagulants. In the immobile patient, consideration should be given to heparin prophylaxis.

POSTTRAUMATIC SEIZURES

Posttraumatic seizures are a common accompaniment to head injury; they are of serious consequence to recovery, in that driving is disallowed and the side effects of anticonvulsant medication may delay cognitive recovery. Prevention of posttraumatic seizures and satisfactory management when they occur are essential for optimal management.[18]

Not all seizures occurring after a head injury are related to the head injury per se. Seizures can occur as a consequence of withdrawal from alcohol or illicit drugs, hypoxia, or therapeutic drugs.

CLASSIFICATION

Jennett defined early seizures as those occurring within 1 week of the injury and late seizures as those occurring thereafter.[19] Others have added an additional category of immediate seizures, although this adds little to prognosis and management.

Early Seizures

Early seizures occur in about 2% of unselected series of head injury. In pediatric series, the incidence approaches 7% to 9%. Risk factors for early seizures include skull fractures (especially depressed fractures), hematoma formation, contusions, a prolonged period of unconsciousness, focal signs, and young age.

One third of seizures occur within 1 hour, one third between 1 and 24 hours, and another third between 1 and 7 days after the injury. Seizures tend to occur later in adults than in children. Most early seizures are focal, and about 10% of adults and 20% of children younger than 5 years of age develop status epilepticus.

Late Seizures

Between 2% and 5% of patients suffer from late seizures after civilian head injury. The major risk factors are a penetrating missile wound, hematoma formation, depressed skull fracture, and early seizures. The risk of a late seizure is highest initially and decreases slowly with time, although seizures may occur even 10 to 15 years after a missile-related head injury. Most late seizures are either primary generalized seizures or secondary generalized seizures following focal onset.

MANAGEMENT OF POSTTRAUMATIC SEIZURES

Recurrent early seizures are typically managed with a loading dose of an anticonvulsant, usually valproate or phenytoin, followed by regular oral or intravenous doses. If status epilepticus occurs despite adequate anticonvulsant doses, serum electrolytes, glucose, calcium, and magnesium levels should be estimated and corrected. Further seizure activity requires intubation, sedation, and ventilation, usually with propofol in an intensive care unit, ideally with continuous electroencephalographic (EEG) monitoring. An ICP monitoring device may also be inserted, and the patient should undergo a CT brain scan to exclude the development of a treatable surgical cause. Continued epileptiform activity on EEG monitoring in a patient who is intubated, ventilated, and sedated requires specialist advice.

After control of early seizures has been obtained, anticonvulsant medication is usually continued for 6 weeks, after which the dose can be progressively decreased provided that no further seizures have occurred. Patients who suffer from two or more late seizures are usually started on long-term anticonvulsant medication. This may be continued for some years before gradual reduction and discontinuation of the anticonvulsant drug is considered.

PROPHYLAXIS

Despite several randomized, controlled trials of anticonvulsant drugs after head injury, no clear benefit or consensus opinion concerning their use as prophylaxis has emerged.

POSTCONCUSSION SYNDROME

The hallmarks of the postconcussion syndrome are a minor head injury, a normal neurological examination, and a variety of symptoms, usually out of proportion to the severity of the injury, most of which are difficult to substantiate.[20] The symptoms are variable but in the main consist of headache associated with dizziness and memory difficulties. A full list of symptoms is given in Box 4-2.

EPIDEMIOLOGY

Postconcussion syndrome occurs almost exclusively in patients who have had a minor head injury. Different studies have reported different incidences, possibly because the assessment was made at different times after occurrence of the injury. Rimel et al. monitored a group of patients for 3 months.[21] The inclusion criteria were hospital admission lasting less than 48 hours, mild head injury (i.e., GCS score between 13 and 15), and a period of unconsciousness lasting less than 20 minutes. They found that 79% of the patients complained of persistent headaches, and 59% complained of ongoing memory problems. Return to work was more likely in the professional, business, and managerial groups, and litigation was apparently not an important factor. Postconcussion syndrome is far less commonly observed in children than in adults.

PATHOPHYSIOLOGY

Elucidation of the pathophysiology of this disorder is difficult because of the vague nature of the symptoms and because the head injury is minor, so little formal neuropathological information is available. The syndrome is probably a consequence of microscopic structural changes, probably with related changes in neurotransmitter balance.

CLINICAL ASSESSMENT AND INVESTIGATION

A formal history, with full information about the accident and the patient's premorbid personality, is required. The symptom complex should be carefully delineated. Additional information may be provided by family members. A full neurological examination should be performed, and any abnormality that is apparent on clinical assessment should be confirmed with formal investigations.

Radiological imaging is important to exclude structural abnormality; it may reveal chronic subdural hematoma, atrophy (especially of the frontal lobes), or hydrocephalus. MRI may provide further evidence of subtle brain injury. An EEG should be performed in those patients whose symptoms could conceivably be caused by seizure activity.

Psychological assessment, using the Paced Auditory Serial Addition Task, has demonstrated an impairment in the rate of information processing, which improved with clinical improvement in the symptoms.[22] Other tests have demonstrated problems with memory recall.

MANAGEMENT

In most cases, reassurance that there are no abnormal findings on examination and investigation and education of the patient and the family about the syndrome help the symptoms to resolve, usually by 1 year after the injury. Symptomatic treatment of headache is indicated, as is treatment of proven seizures. If psychological testing demonstrates impaired processing, development of coping strategies is appropriate.

REFERENCES

1. Jennett B: Head injury. In Martyn C, Hughes RAC, editors: *Epidemiology of head injury*, London, 1998, BMJ Books.
2. Jennett B, MacMillan R: Epidemiology of head injury. *BMJ* 282:101-104, 1981.
3. Patel H, Bouamra O, Woodford M, et al: Trends in head injury outcome from 1989 to 2003 and the effect of neurosurgical care: an observational study. *Lancet* 366:1538-1544, 2005.
4. Jennett B, Teasdale G: Assessment of coma and impaired consciousness: a practical scale. *Lancet* 2:81-83, 1974.
5. Signorini DF, Andrews PJD, Jones PA, et al: Predicting survival using simple clinical variables: a case study in traumatic brain injury. *J Neurol Neurosurg Psychiatry* 66:20-25, 1999.
6. Mendelow AD, Teasdale G, Jennett B, et al: Risks of intracranial hematoma in head injured adults. *BMJ* 287:1173-1176, 1983.
7. Kelly DF, Nikas DL, Becker DP: Diagnosis and treatment of moderate and severe head injuries in adults. In Youmans JR, editor: *Neurological surgery*, Philadelphia, 1996, Saunders, pp 1618-1718.
8. Jennett B, Bond M: Assessment of outcome after severe brain damage: a practical scale. *Lancet* 1:480-484, 1973.
9. Liau LM, Bergsneider M, Becker DP: Pathology and pathophysiology of head injury. In Youmans JR, editor: *Neurological surgery*, Philadelphia, 1996, Saunders, pp 1549-1594.
10. Miller JD: Normal and increased intracranial pressure. In Miller JD, editor: *Northfield's surgery of the central nervous system*, Oxford, UK, 1987, Blackwell Science, pp 7-57.
11. Adams JH, Graham DI: Trauma. In Adams JH, Graham DI, editors: *An introduction to neuropathology*, Edinburgh, UK, 1994, Churchill Livingstone, pp 133-156.
12. Briggs M, Clarke P, Crockard A: Guidelines for the initial management after head injury in adults. *BMJ* 288:983-985, 1984.
13. National Institute for Health and Clinical Excellence: *Head injury: triage, assessment, investigation and early management of head injury in infants, children and adults.* NICE Clinical Guideline 56. London, 2007, NICE.

BOX 4-2   Symptoms after Minor Head Injury

- Headaches
- Dizziness
- Vertigo
- Tinnitus
- Visual blurring
- Reduced or absent taste and smell
- Irritability
- Anxiety
- Depression
- Fatigue
- Memory problems
- Impaired concentration
- Sensitivity to light and noise

14. Bullock MR, Chesnut R, Ghajar J, et al: Guidelines for the surgical management of traumatic brain injury. *Neurosurgery* 58(3 suppl):S25-S46, 2006.

15. Bullock MR, Povlishock JT: Guidelines for the management of severe traumatic brain injury. *J Neurotrauma* 24(suppl 1):S1-S106, 2007.

16. Reilly P: Management of intracranial pressure and cerebral perfusion pressure. In Reilly P, Bullock R, editors: *Head injury: pathophysiology and management*, London, 2005, Hodder Arnold, Chapter 16.

17. Muizelaar JP, Marmarou A, Ward JD: Adverse effects of prolonged hyperventilation in patients with severe head injury: a randomized clinical trial. *J Neurosurg* 75:731-739, 1991.

18. Temkin NR, Haglund MM, Winn HR: Post traumatic seizures. In Youmans JR, editor: *Neurological surgery*, Philadelphia, 1996, Saunders, pp 1834-1839.

19. Jennett WB: *Epilepsy after non missile head injuries*, London, 1975, Heinemann.

20. Miller JD, Ward BA, Alexander LF: Post traumatic syndrome. In Youmans JR, editor: *Neurological surgery*, Philadelphia, 1996, Saunders, pp 1825-1833.

21. Rimel RW, Giordani B, Barth JT, et al: Disability caused by minor head injury. *Neurosurgery* 9:221, 1981.

22. Gronwall DM: Paced auditory serial addition task: a measure of recovery from concussion. *Perceptual and Motor Skills* 44(2):367-373, 1977.

CHAPTER 5

Imaging

Mark S. Ballard, Ian Francis

In all cases of maxillofacial trauma, formal clinical appraisal, preferably by a specialist, should precede imaging. Some facial injuries require no imaging at all; others necessitate complex image investigation, so it is essential that the specialist's examination focus on the most appropriate imaging. Many factors are involved in the process, and success is heavily dependent on good teamwork among the surgeons, nursing staff, radiographers, and radiologists.

In deciding whether a patient requires imaging, it is important to remember that that there will be a radiation dose to the patient as well as a time and financial cost. Although the radiation dose from a simple orthopantomogram (OPG) is low, there are many glandular structures in the head with a high cell turnover. These have a higher susceptibility to radiation effect.[1] Patient presentation varies enormously, from an alert patient who has received a minor blow to a severely injured, comatose patient with polytrauma who may have extremity, abdominal, thoracic, spinal, and central nervous system injuries in addition to the facial fractures.

Acquiring images will inevitably introduce delay into a patient's treatment, and some may suffer as a result. It is essential to achieve balance between the need to identify all important lesions and the need to minimize radiation exposure and the time delay.

IMAGING MODALITIES AND TECHNIQUES

PLAIN RADIOGRAPHS

Plain radiographs provide the foundation of day-to-day imaging. They may on their own be sufficient to provide a radiological diagnosis, or they may need to be complemented by other modalities, such as computed tomography (CT). The general rule (anywhere in the body) is that fractures should be imaged in at least two planes, preferably at right angles to one another. However, although this is true in many circumstances in facial injury and is also true for locating foreign bodies, it is not a universal rule in the face.

Although a specialized skull radiographic unit is helpful, none of the plain film techniques (see "Radiography of Facial Injuries") requires it. Most can be quite adequately obtained with the use of an upright, bucky apparatus with an overhead gantry tube, provided the patient can sit up or stand.

For reasons of classification and convenience, the face is often divided into upper, middle, and lower thirds, and the middle third is further divided into central and lateral components. Suspected fractures of the upper third of the face require a Caldwell projection (Fig. 5-1) or, preferably, a modified Caldwell's view (Fig. 5-2) and a lateral projection. Middle-third injuries require occipitomental 10-degree (Figs 5-3 and 5-4) and 30-degree (Fig. 5-5) views, which can be supplemented by a lateral projection if the central middle third is involved (Fig. 5-6). Lower-third injuries require a posteroanterior (PA) mandible view and panoramic tomography (OPG) or, if the latter is not available, lateral oblique views of both sides (see "Radiography of Facial Injuries"). These views should be taken with the patient erect whenever possible, not only for comfort but to show fluid levels in the sinuses. Such plain film views may not be necessary if CT has been or needs to be done on an emergency basis or if there are adequate radiographs available from a primary referring hospital. Other projections (see "Radiography of Facial Injuries") are rarely needed.

COMPUTED TOMOGRAPHY

CT has almost entirely supplanted nonpanoramic tomography. It has the advantage of providing multiplanar thin-slice images of the facial skeleton, overcoming the problem of superimposition of structures that inevitably occurs on plain radiographs. The newest generation of multidetector CT scanners (MDCT) are able to acquire data very rapidly. Slice information obtained in one plane can be reconstructed to provide images in alternative planes, if such alternative image planes are not obtainable directly.

A small field of view should be used, and the scanning should be performed with a high-resolution bone algorithm. Soft tissue windows can then be obtained from this original dataset. Generally, a slice thickness of 2 to 4 mm is adequate in assessing facial trauma and has the advantage that the examination is faster than when thinner slices are acquired. However, if reformatting is needed, very thin slices are required: 1-mm axial slices should be obtained with subsequent coronal reformats. Sagittal reformats are not commonly required for facial imaging, and obtaining thinner axial slices, although technically possible, yields no significant improvement in resolution.

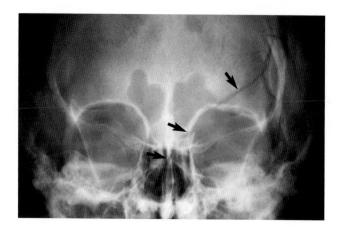

FIGURE 5-1   Caldwell's projection in a patient with a fracture of the frontal bone extending down to the superior orbital rim and crossing to the medial orbital wall in the region of the frontal sinus ostium to involve the upper nasal septum *(arrows)*.

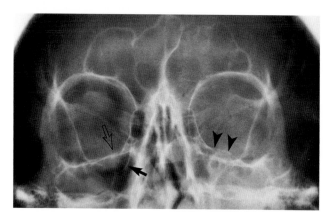

FIGURE 5-2   Modified Caldwell's projection illustrating a blowout fracture of the orbital floor. There is absence of the right orbital floor medial to the infraorbital groove and fissure *(open arrow)*. The corresponding segment of floor on the left is intact and normal in position *(arrowheads)*. There is a depressed fragment of bone on the right side *(closed arrow)* and mucosal thickening in the antrum on that side. The opacification in the left antrum is caused by coexisting and unrelated inflammatory disease. Notice also the air in the right upper orbit.

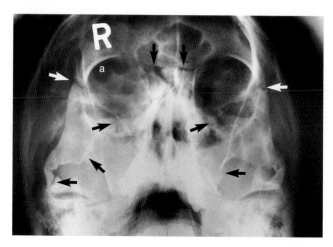

FIGURE 5-3   Fractures through the Le Fort II and III lines of weakness on an occipitomental 10-degree projection *(black arrows)*. There is slight separation of the frontozygomatic sutures *(white arrows)*. Step deformities are present at both inferior orbital margins. The pattern appears incomplete, because no fracture is evident in the left arch on this view. However, notice the decreased gap between the coronoid process tip and the buttress of the malar bone on the left side, compared to the right side. The ethmoidal air cells and the maxillary antra are opacified, with a fluid level in the left antrum. Air (a) is present in the right orbit.

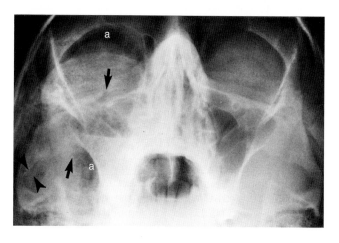

FIGURE 5-4   Fracture of the zygoma on an occipitomental 15-degree projection. Notice a fracture with a step deformity at the inferior orbital margin and at the medial part of the buttress *(arrows)*. There is a double shadow to the medial aspect of the arch *(arrowheads)*. Frontozygomatic suture separation is not evident. There is a fluid level in the right antrum. Air (a) is present in the orbit and lateral to the antral wall. The soft tissues of the cheek and lower lid are swollen.

In almost every case coming to CT scanning, axial-slice images are obtained (Figs. 5-7 through 5-9). The standard position for axial (transverse) slices is with the slice plane parallel to the anthropological baseline. This position is easy for the patient, and landmarks are easy to identify on the initial scanogram view. However, CT scanning protocols vary considerably with clinical circumstances. Coronal images are particularly helpful in orbital examination (Fig. 5-10) but are also useful in other situations. Coronal imaging has the benefit of visualizing the horizontal struts or plates of bone, which in standard axial slices lie parallel to the slice plane and therefore are poorly visualized. Such horizontal plates include the orbital roof, cribriform plate, orbital floor, and hard palate.

Direct coronal imaging is ideally performed in the true coronal plane, but two factors may require the gantry angle to be adjusted. First, many patients, particularly the elderly and those with a rigid spine, may not be able to extend their neck sufficiently. Indeed, in some patients, direct coronal scanning cannot be done at all (or, if the cervical spine is still under suspicion, should not be done). Second, dental amalgam and other fixed prosthodontic devices can produce serious streak-like artifacts that seriously diminish image quality.

Three-dimensional (3-D) datasets have become increasingly requested since the advent of navigational surgical techniques. These new approaches to surgery require CT information to accurately direct the navigational equipment.

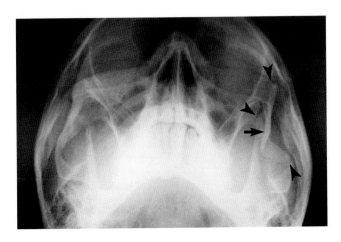

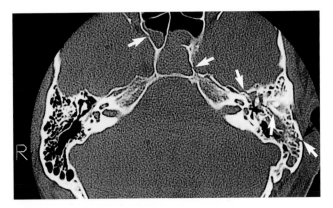

FIGURE 5-7 Axial computed tomogram of the skull base and petrous bones. There is longitudinal petrous fracture on the left side. This runs across the mastoid air cells and the middle ear cavity and anterior to the petrous apex, eventually crossing the walls of the sphenoid sinus (arrows). Notice the soft tissue shadow (blood and cerebrospinal fluid) in the mastoid air cells, the middle ear cavity, and the sphenoid sinus. Soft tissue swelling is present over the left mastoid. The normal right petrous bone structures help to demonstrate the asymmetry.

FIGURE 5-5 Occipitomental 30-degree projection showing a depressed left zygomatic arch fracture. Notice the rotated anterior arch fragment (arrow), the fracture in the posterior arch, and a fracture crossing the zygomatic buttress to reach the frontozygomatic suture (arrowheads).

When a CT is performed, the scanner ascribes a unit measurement to a 3-D pixel, called a *voxel,* that is representative of a portion of the area scanned. Many voxels make up an image (Fig. 5-11). The unit measurement ascribed is known as a *Hounsfield unit* and relates to the density of the tissue in that small area. The values of these measurements range from −1000 (fat) to more than +1000 (bone). If this range of values were translated directly into a gray scale, the human eye would not be able to differentiate all shades of gray from each other, and critical information would be lost. To allow complete assessment of the range of tissue densities, the viewing systems allow users to "window" the data. Based on a selection from the user, the computer sets a density middle value and a viewable range that the eye can appreciate. These settings allow certain tissues (e.g., bone, lung, brain) to be completely assessed according to the known density ranges they contain. It is critical to be aware of windowing and how to adjust the windows when assessing CT images so that image data are not missed (Fig. 5-12).

Conebeam Computed Tomography

Conebeam CT (CBCT) is a relatively new CT technique that uses a cone-shaped beam of radiation rather than the standard fan-shaped beam used in multislice scanners (on which most imaging is performed) (Fig. 5-13). These systems have been available since 2001 and allow for low-dose scanning of small areas of the body (Fig. 5-14). Current applications for this technology center on dentomaxillofacial imaging,[3] although its use is being explored in musculoskeletal imaging of the extremities. The technology is limited by poor soft tissue resolution in comparison to multislice CT scanners; however, fine discrimination of soft tissue detail is often of little relevance in the dentomaxillofacial and trauma settings, and technological improvements are paving the way for scanners with better tissue resolution.[4]

CBCT scanners are much smaller and less expensive than traditional multislice CT (MDCT) scanners (Fig. 5-15). Although their use is growing in the United States (where

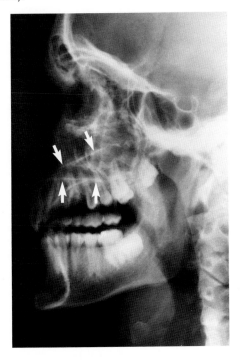

FIGURE 5-6 Lateral projection of the face in a patient with a unilateral Le Fort I–type fracture. The dentition on each side of the mandible superimpose, whereas the left upper dental arch is displaced upward and backward. The two halves of the split palate are widely separated and at an angle to one another (arrows).

Early published data from navigational surgery centers suggest these techniques confer improved functional and aesthetic results with reduced operating times.[2]

With the advent of digital image storage and Picture Archiving and Communication Systems (PACS), CT images are now routinely assessed on the computer rather than on the cut film of old. This has several advantages, because the software associated with the viewing computers allows for image manipulation (e.g., magnification) and direct calibrated measurement.

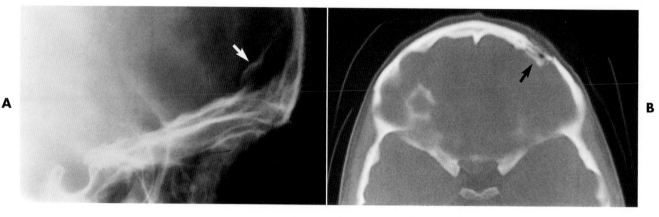

FIGURE 5-8 Depressed skull fracture. **A,** Part of a lateral skull projection showing a linear density caused by the depressed fragments *(arrow)*. **B,** Axial computed tomogram of the same patient showing depressed fragments *(arrow)*.

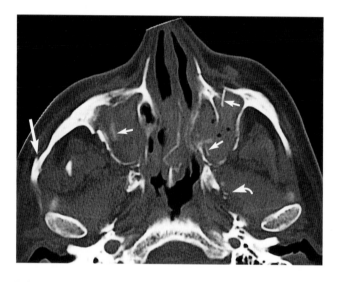

FIGURE 5-9 Axial computed tomogram of the face in a patient with Le Fort I and II level injuries and a right zygomatic fracture. There is extensive fracturing involving all of the walls of the maxillary antra with several bone fragments displaced into the antra *(small arrows)*. There is fracturing of the left nasal plate of the maxilla, fracturing and submucosal hemorrhage in the posterior nasal septum, and a fracture with lateral bowing of the right zygomatic arch *(large arrow)*. The maxillary antra are opaque from blood. There are fragments of bone avulsed from the left pterygoid plates *(curved arrow)*.

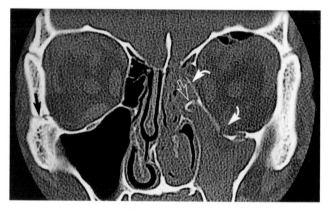

FIGURE 5-10 Coronal computed tomogram of the face in a patient with medial wall and orbital floor blowout fractures *(curved arrows)*. The left nasal cavity, ethmoidal air cells, and antrum are opaque from blood. There is air beneath the left orbital roof. The orbital floor fracture involves the inferior orbital canal. The major fragments of both fractures are hinged at the junction with the ethmomaxillary plate *(open arrow)*. The lucent line crossing the base of the frontal process of the right zygoma *(black arrow)* is the canal for the zygomaticotemporal nerve and is not a fracture.

there is much controversy regarding their predominantly office-based use), there has so far been little application in the United Kingdom. CBCT does, however, offer a viable alternative to MDCT, in which the dose is significantly higher and accessibility may be an issue.

When to Perform CT/CBCT Imaging of Facial Injuries

Although it may be convenient and sensible to expedite CT of the face in those patients who are undergoing a CT of the brain, most facially injured patients can be managed adequately without CT scanning. The decision to perform CT/CBCT imaging depends on both the initial radiographic evaluation and the clinical findings. If plain radiographs are negative, with no evidence of fracture, no fluid levels, no mucosal thickening of the sinuses, and no orbital or soft tissue emphysema and there is no evidence of penetrating injury, then the chance of finding a significant midface fracture on CT/CBCT imaging is negligible. However, *all* patients with upper-third fractures or suspected fractures should receive CT/CBCT evaluation. There is a very high incidence of intracranial damage in such patients, and there are important questions relating to the posterior wall of the frontal sinus, the nasofrontal duct, and the orbital roof, the answers to which affect the surgical approach and the long-term outlook. These questions are not reliably addressed by plain radiographs.

Many central middle-third fractures require CT/CBCT evaluation, although mild injury to the nasomaxillary complex (i.e., injury confined to the nasal bones and the nasal plates of the frontal process of the maxillae) does not, and the utility of CT/CBCT in Le Fort I level injury is highly debatable. Lateral middle-third injuries seldom require CT/CBCT imaging unless there is severe displacement or extension to the external angular process of the frontal bone or to the sphenoidal and temporal calvaria. There is no doubt that CT/CBCT shows displacement well, particularly displacement of the zygomatic arch; however, careful evaluation of unrotated PA, occipitomental 10-degree and occipitomental

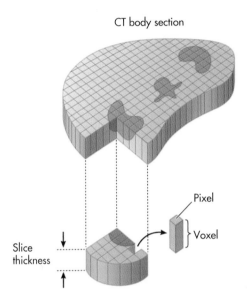

CT body section

Pixel

Voxel

Slice thickness

FIGURE 5-11 Voxel. The imaged slice of tissue is divided into volume elements called *voxels*. The x-ray attenuation in each voxel determines the shade of gray of the corresponding pixel in the final two-dimensional image. *(From Herring J:* Tachdjian's pediatric orthopaedics, *ed 4, St. Louis, 2007, Saunders.)*

30-degree radiographs is almost always sufficient for management, although the uncommon lateral bowing injury of the arch may be difficult to appreciate. Some orbital injuries require CT evaluation, but this decision should be guided clinically. Most patients with penetrating injury to the lids or conjunctiva should at least be considered for CT, because the risk of missing a foreign body in the orbit or anterior cranial fossa is significant. CT may also be needed later for evaluation of *some* patients with suspected blowout injury (see later discussion) and for evaluation of enophthalmos and other malpositions of the globe.

Evaluation of severe retrobulbar hemorrhage is a clinical emergency and one in which imaging has no role. Surgical orbital exploration should be carried out as soon as possible.

In the lower third of the face (the mandible and hyoid), CT/CBCT imaging is almost never needed, except in some cases of suspected condylar head fracture. Suspicion should arise only if a condylar fracture is not clinically or radiographically evident but there is otorrhagia or an apparent Battle's sign. CT/CBCT is then done primarily to exclude a petrous fracture. A significant number of patients with a condylar fracture have otorrhagia, and Battle's sign can be mimicked by seepage of blood back from the injury to the external auditory canal as a result of a condylar fracture.

MAGNETIC RESONANCE IMAGING

Magnetic resonance imaging (MRI) technology uses the manipulation of hydrogen atoms within the body to form images. Approximately two thirds of the total hydrogen atoms in the human body are located in water or fat molecules. MRI uses a strong electromagnetic field to line up the nuclei of these hydrogen atoms in a single plane. These atoms are then

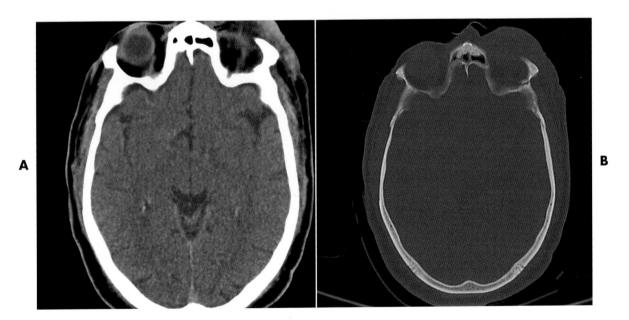

A   B

FIGURE 5-12 Windowing. **A,** An axial image through the head on a brain window allows assessment of the brain parenchyma, but bone detail is lost. **B,** An axial image in the same location on a bone window demonstrates a fracture through the left lateral orbital wall that would be easy to miss on the brain windows. This window allows assessment of bone, but the brain parenchymal detail is now lost.

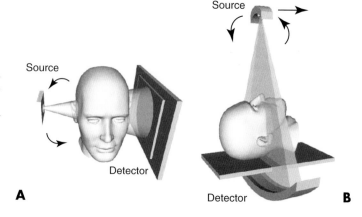

FIGURE 5-13 Conebeam computed tomography (CBCT) versus multidetector CT (MDCT). **A,** CBCT may be obtained with the patient either upright or supine and uses a cone-shaped x-ray beam. **B,** MDCT is obtained with the patient lying supine and uses a fan-shaped x-ray beam.

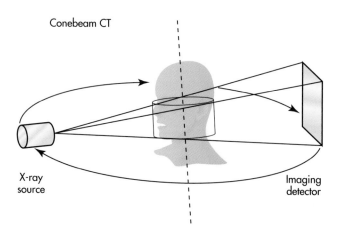

FIGURE 5-14 Conebeam computed tomography (CBCT) scan acquisition. CBCT imaging is accomplished by a rotating gantry to which an x-ray source and detector are attached. A divergent pyramid- or cone-shaped source of ionizing radiation is directed though the midsection of the area to be examined onto an x-ray detector on the opposite side. A rotation fulcrum is fixed within the center of the object of interest (e.g., facial skeleton) and the x-ray source and detector rotate around it. The entire field of view is encompassed during a single rotation, which is sufficient to acquire enough information to reconstruct the image.

knocked out of that plane by specific radiofrequency pulses. Once the radiofrequency energy is stopped, the hydrogen atoms return to the plane of the main magnetic field imposed by the electromagnet. This return to plane induces a radio signal that is measured by the MRI scanner and converted via a mathematical algorithm into a cross-sectional image. Although the image produced by an MRI scanner looks like an anatomical picture, it should not be considered as such and is more truly a representation of the strength of signal produced. Tissues with plentiful hydrogen atoms, such as cerebrospinal fluid (CSF) or fat, produce high (*bright*) signals, and those with little hydrogen, such as bone, produce low (*dark*) signal.

Because this technique does not depend on x-rays, it has an advantage over CT in that it minimizes exposure to radiation. However, because of the low number of hydrogen atoms in bone, the demonstration of fine bone detail in the face by MRI remains inferior to that of CT. Furthermore, ferromagnetic material in (or even outside) the patient, such as iron filings in the globe of the eye and some intracranial aneurysm clips, may move during MRI, with disastrous consequences. Such material can also produce spectacular artifacts, degrading the images. In addition, poor access and difficulty with some forms of monitoring equipment make MRI less attractive than CT in cases of acute maxillofacial injury.

However, MRI does have growing application in a number of specific areas. Most important is its ability to detect CSF fistulae and leaks (see later discussion) and its superior demonstration of posttraumatic meningoceles, encephaloceles, and, in children, leptomeningeal cysts (Fig. 5-16). It has increasing application in the orbit for injuries to the globe and optic nerve sheath complex, and it has a place in the evaluation of repair problems after blowout fractures. It can also be used to demonstrate acute soft tissue injury in the temporomandibular joint, although there is no conclusive evidence that such demonstration affects the early management and this examination is probably best reserved for those with persistent joint symptoms. MRI is also of assistance in estimating the vascularization of hydroxyapatite orbital implants after exenteration for trauma.

ULTRASONOGRAPHY

Ultrasonography has limited use in the assessment of bony trauma of the facial skeleton, although it has a well-defined role in the assessment of soft tissue injury and fluid collections. It is the modality of choice for assessment of the globe, particularly the posterior elements when anterior opacification (blood or cataract) prevents direct vision, and also for assessing intraocular foreign bodies. In patients with penetrating injuries, it can be used to detect nonmetallic foreign bodies in soft tissues with high accuracy.

OTHER MODALITIES

A number of other modalities, such as angiography (including therapeutic maneuvers), dacryocystography, sialography, and arthrography, very occasionally play a part in the management of maxillofacial injuries. Angiography may be required in the acute phase, and sialography has a place in the evaluation of suspected parotid duct transection. The

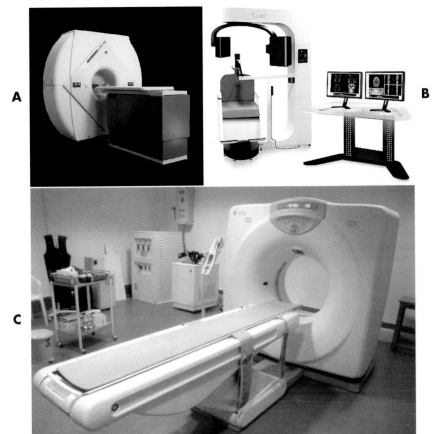

FIGURE 5-15 Comparison of conebeam computed tomography (CBCT) and multidetector computed tomography (MDCT) scanners. **A** and **B,** CBCT scanners have a small physical footprint; these are small enough for the office environment. **C,** A typical multislice CT scanner, which fills a whole room.

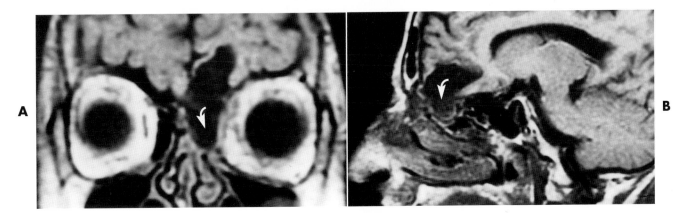

FIGURE 5-16 Magnetic resonance image of a patient with an encephalocele. Encephalomalacic brain tissue (darker than normal brain on image) originating from the rectus gyrus and part of the medial orbital gyrus has herniated through the left ethmoidal roof *(arrows)*. **A,** Coronal reconstruction. **B,** Parasagittal reconstruction. *(Courtesy of Dr. B.G. Conry, Kent and Sussex Hospitals, Tunbridge Wells.)*

others are usually reserved for assessing the delayed sequelae to trauma.

INITIAL ASSESSMENT

The imaging required for a given patient clearly depends on the pattern of injury and the affected anatomy. Less obvious, but equally important, is the physiological stability of the patient. Resuscitation of a patient on a CT gantry with limited monitoring equipment is suboptimal, and resuscitation in an MRI scanner is almost impossible.

THE STABLE PATIENT

There is almost always adequate time (hours, if not days) to take a measured view in assessing the facially injured patient. Most of these patients are stable, and, as Johnson has put it,

"Attempts at extensive plain radiographic evaluation under the direction of busy emergency room personnel often will not yield optimal results."[5]

In most cases, fractures are adequately demonstrated on a few plain films or with panoramic tomography or both; this is true of most isolated injuries to the zygoma and almost all mandibular injuries.

If any radiographic view is believed to be necessary for evaluation of midface injury in the early stages, a single occipitomental 10- or 15-degree view (see Figs. 5-3 and 5-4) is sufficient as a screening tool. This screening view is recommended if the clinical diagnosis is uncertain and there is no cervical injury. For suspected injuries to the mandible, a panoramic (OPG) view and a PA view of the mandible (Figs. 5-17 and 5-18) suffice in most cases, but again, as with the midface, specialist advice is preferable before imaging.

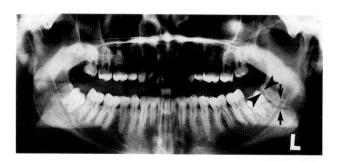

FIGURE 5-17   Fracture of the mandible on a panoramic tomogram. There is a lucent fracture line crossing the left angle of the mandible that involves the lamina dura of the third molar tooth. Slight separation of the fragments has caused apparent widening of the distal periodontal ligament (arrowheads). Notice that the fracture line appears to diverge into two limbs (arrows). These lines join together at both ends. The lower line is the fracture through the lingual cortex; it breaches the walls of the inferior dental canal, whereas the fracture through the buccal cortex (upper line) does not. The patient also sustained a fracture of the left zygoma: Notice the deformed arch on that side.

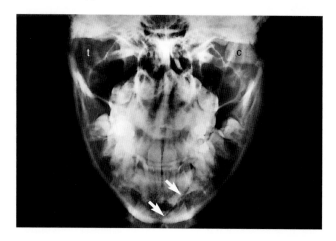

FIGURE 5-18   Posteroanterior projection of the mandible illustrating a left condylar neck fracture and a left parasymphysis fracture (arrows). The fracture at the condylar neck is not itself seen but is evident from the displaced and rotated condylar head (c). This is the classic condylar displacement. On this radiographic projection, the lucent triangle (t) bounded by the skull base, the zygomatic arch, and the posterolateral antral wall should always be closely inspected on both sides.

For certain injuries, imaging is not required at all or is needed only in very specific situations. For example, there is no evidence that patients with uncomplicated (isolated) nasal trauma benefit in any way from imaging. Patient management is determined purely on the basis of clinical examination and patient preference (i.e., a desire for improvement in function or appearance of the nose). The correlation between radiographic findings and external nasal deformity or need for surgical reduction is poor. Indeed, some 20% to 25% of patients who need some form of reduction of nasal fracture or dislocation have negative findings on radiology. Similarly, there is no place for a very urgent evaluation of most patients with diplopia and suspected blowout fractures with entrapment (see later discussion).

Patients with head injury who are fully oriented and have no history of loss of consciousness or amnesia need not be imaged, unless there are other clinical risk factors to indicate otherwise, because they are at negligible risk for clinically important brain injury.[6]

THE MULTIPLY INJURED PATIENT

The initial management of a multiply injured patient is usually performed according to the Advanced Trauma Life Support guidelines from the American College of Surgeons. Imaging should be performed as part of a secondary survey, after the patient is stabilized. Imaging should not be undertaken in patients who are inadequately ventilated or hemodynamically unstable, whatever their neurological status.

Injury to the cervical spine must be considered to be present in all patients who have depressed consciousness, are intoxicated, or have signs or symptoms related to the cervical spine. All such patients should have three-view radiographic assessment of the cervical spine. Unwise attempts to intubate or otherwise maneuver the patient can have catastrophic results.

Apart from such situations, no other imaging should take place until an adequate airway and ventilation have been established and the patient is hemodynamically stable.

SUSPECTED INTRACRANIAL INJURY

The primary study for investigation of suspected intracranial injury is a CT examination of the head. The skull radiographic series in the acute setting is now largely consigned to historical status, although there is still a role in the skeletal survey of children with suspected nonaccidental injury, for patients with penetrating injury to assist in deciding whether emergency angiography is required, in patients with calvarial fractures, and in the imaging of foreign bodies.

MRI of the head is of limited use in the acute trauma setting: The signal from acute blood spoils the image obtained from brain structures, the electromagnetic field of the scanner requires specialist life support equipment, and the imaging process takes significantly longer than a head CT.

Current clinical guidelines, from groups such as the National Institute of Clinical Excellence (NICE) in the United Kingdom, recommend early imaging rather than admission and observation for appropriate cases, with an aim to reduce the time to detection of life-threatening outcomes (Box 5-1).

BOX 5-1 | Criteria for Immediate Request for Computed Tomographic Scanning of the Head (Adults)

- Glasgow Coma Scale (GCS) score <13 on initial assessment in the emergency department
- GCS <15 at 2 hours after the injury on assessment in the emergency department
- Suspected open or depressed skull fracture
- Any sign of basal skull fracture (hemotympanum, "panda eyes," cerebrospinal fluid leakage from the ear or nose, Battle's sign)
- Posttraumatic seizure
- Focal neurological deficit
- More than one episode of vomiting
- Amnesia for events >30 minutes before impact
  In addition, in patients who have experienced some loss of consciousness or amnesia since the injury (adults):
- Age ≥65 years
- Coagulopathy (history of bleeding, clotting disorder, current treatment with warfarin)
- Dangerous mechanism of injury (pedestrian or cyclist struck by a motor vehicle, occupant ejected from a motor vehicle, fall from a height of >1 m or five stairs)

From National Institute of Clinical Excellence: *Head injury* (website): http://www.nice.org.uk/guidance/index.jsp?action=byID&o=11836. Accessed March 21, 2011.

BOX 5-2 | Criteria for Immediate Request for Computed Tomographic Scanning of the Head (Children)

- Loss of consciousness lasting >5 minutes (witnessed)
- Amnesia (antegrade or retrograde) lasting >5 minutes
- Abnormal drowsiness
- Three or more discrete episodes of vomiting
- Clinical suspicion of nonaccidental injury
- Posttraumatic seizure but no history of epilepsy
- Glasgow Coma Scale (GCS) score <14, or GCS (pediatric) score <15 for a baby <1 year old, on assessment in the emergency department
- Suspicion of open or depressed skull injury or tense fontanelle
- Any sign of basal skull fracture (hemotympanum, "panda eyes," cerebrospinal fluid leakage from the ear or nose, Battle's sign)
- Focal neurological deficit
- If <1 year of age, presence of bruise, swelling, or laceration >5 cm on the head
- Dangerous mechanism of injury (high-speed road traffic accident as pedestrian, cyclist, or vehicle occupant, fall from a height of >3 m, high-speed injury from a projectile or an object)

From National Institute of Clinical Excellence: *Head injury* (website): http://www.nice.org.uk/guidance/index.jsp?action=byID&o=11836. Accessed March 21, 2011.

There are significant differences between a head injury in a child and one in an adult. Although a large number of adults with intracranial hemorrhage have a fracture, most children do not. However, depressed fractures are more common in children (see Fig. 5-8). Such fractures are important but may be impossible to detect clinically. Heiskanen et al.[7] reported on 224 patients with depressed skull fractures and found that 7% eventually developed infection; the risk of this complication was greater if surgery was delayed beyond 24 hours from injury. Laceration of the scalp should also be taken seriously, because delayed recognition of a compound fracture can have profound consequences.

In children, the skull radiographic series is essentially limited to documentation of cases of suspected nonaccidental injury; however, in children younger than 6 months, CT of the head should be mandatory as part of the workup for nonaccidental injury, with either MRI or follow-up CT to further document the timing of the injury. CT is otherwise accepted as the first-line investigation to exclude brain injury, as in adults.[6] The indications for scanning the head of a child after trauma differ from the indications in an adult (Box 5-2), in part because of the different injury patterns but mainly because children present differently.

If time and the patient's condition permit, the brain CT scan examination can be usefully expanded to include other areas of interest. It is often appropriate to include the rest of the face, some of which will in any event be visible on the brain scan. Head-injured or multiply injured patients who require endotracheal intubation are difficult to assess clinically because the facial features are obscured and distorted by tubes and tapes and the response to painful stimuli is blunted or erased. Indeed, McAuley et al.[8] found that 16% of missed fractures involved the facial skeleton, and 21% of all missed injuries were accounted for by an impaired sensorium.

THE CERVICAL SPINE

The fact that a patient walks into the emergency department does not preclude serious cervical injury (Fig. 5-19). If there is any doubt, all patients, especially those who were involved in road traffic or other high-velocity accidents, should be given a collar until injury has been excluded. On the other hand, alert, cooperative, non-intoxicated patients who have a cervical spine injury *always* complain of pain or discomfort.

Routine cervical spine radiographs in all patients with isolated mandibular fractures is inappropriate, because the pick-up rate of cervical injury is likely to be negligible. Most patients with facial trauma have no cervical injury, and it is obviously preferable to be selective and not expose large numbers of patients to unnecessary irradiation. Velmahos et al. looked at this problem in relation to the blunt trauma victim who is alert and asymptomatic.[9] In a series of 549 alert, oriented, clinically non-intoxicated blunt trauma victims with no neck symptoms, no injury was missed when a careful three-step clinical examination was used. Therefore, in such patients, if there is no report of neck symptoms and no tenderness to palpation or on neck motion, the collar can be left off and no radiographic studies are necessary.

Conscious, alert patients with suspected neck injury and those with overt cord or root symptoms should have a three-view cervical plain film series, including a horizontal-beam (cross-table) lateral view of the cervical spine to the C7/T1 level, an AP view of the cervical spine, and an AP view of the odontoid peg taken as soon as possible, and this should be done with the cervical collar on.[10] Extreme caution should be used in maneuvering the patient. If other injuries have to take precedence, the patient must wear the collar until cervical injury can be ruled out. Because most injuries occur in the lower cervical spine, especially the C7/T1 level, the spine must be visualized down to these levels. If this fails, then CT or MRI must be performed. If the lateral cervical radiograph

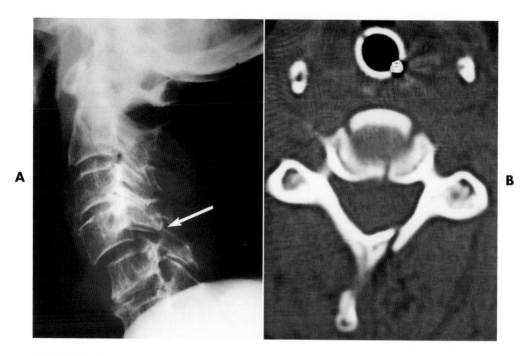

FIGURE 5-19 Injury to the cervical spine. **A,** Lateral cervical spine showing locked facets at C5-6 (arrow). **B,** Axial computed tomogram of the cervical spine showing a burst fracture of the vertebral body and fracture of the vertebral lamina.

does not demonstrate the C7/T1 junction adequately, further imaging is required. Historically, swimmer's views or oblique views were obtained, but these require manipulation and are ideally avoided in the trauma patient. Moreover, such images are difficult to interpret, so CT examination should be performed instead.

Additional (second) fractures occur in 5% of patients with spinal injury, and very subtle changes may be a sign of major injury. Missed cervical spine injury can occur in 15% to 30% of patients. Plain lateral views give a false-negative rate of 26% to 40%. For these reasons, the cervical spine radiographic series should be scrutinized for fractures. CT may not demonstrate fractures that are visible on x-ray examination,[11] so it is important to attempt radiography of the cervical spine before CT, whenever clinically feasible, to ensure complete radiological assessment.

If the patient is unconscious, sedated, or otherwise not alert, it is advisable to obtain images of the head and cervical spine at the same time with CT. CT images should be performed to the level of the T2 vertebral body unless the patient is intubated or unconscious, in which case the T4 level is preferred.[12] It is important to remember that a CT examination of the cervical spine does not clear it clinically, because ligamentous injury is not visible on CT[13,14] (see later discussion).

Although ligamentous injury can be identified on flexion/extension lateral views, this is a potentially hazardous procedure; it must be done under medical supervision and then only in alert, cooperative patients who have minimal spasm and no evidence of a potentially unstable fracture on plain radiographs or CT scans. Such views, if attempted at all, are best done under fluoroscopic control. MRI, however, can identify ligamentous and cord injury and should be considered in patients with focal neurological symptoms in cases

in which the cervical spine CT is normal, but there is ongoing clinical suspicion of injury. MRI in the acute phase should be mandatory in those patients who demonstrate abnormal neurology, but have no fracture seen on plain radiographs (to assess cord and soft tissue injury) and in patients who have ascending abnormal neurology (to exclude an epidural hematoma). It should also be performed after a set period of time if clinical evaluation of the patient remains impossible. MRI is also indicated if the neurological state is fluctuating or if the degree of neurological deficit appears out of proportion to the bony injury. In addition, it can assist in differentiating spinal cord edema (which has a greater capacity for neurological recovery) from cord hemorrhage, and it may be helpful in the later stages if there is further neurological deterioration.

It should be remembered that spinal cord injury can occur without a fracture in about 0.7% of cases. Spinal cord injury without radiographic abnormality (SCIWORA) was recognized in children by Pang and Wilberger in 1982.[15] They described trauma-related myelopathy with normal appearances on cervical spine radiographs, and this injury pattern also extends to the adult population.[16] Clinically, this explains why cervical spine radiographs and CT imaging cannot clear the spine. Ideally, all patients sustaining significant spinal injury should have MRI, but for practical purposes this is not possible. MRI should be performed with T1-weighted, T2-weighted, and fat-suppressed T2-weighted short tau inversion-recovery (STIR) images in the sagittal plane and T2-weighted images in the axial plane.

BLEEDING

In most hemodynamically unstable patients with facial trauma, the site of blood loss, whether overt or occult, is located outside the face. Nevertheless, bleeding related to the facial injury may rarely contribute to or constitute the sole cause of shock. Such bleeding may be presentational, or it may be delayed in onset, even occurring after fixation of facial fractures. It is most common after the more severe transfacial or panfacial fractures. It may originate from disruption of the anterior or posterior ethmoidal vessels or of the terminal branches of the maxillary artery. Nasal packing, clipping or ligation of obvious bleeding points, and arterial ligation may all be used. A few patients may need urgent temporary external reduction or fixation of their facial fractures. In a small group, bleeding is resistant to such treatments or recurs, and in these cases, arteriography and selective embolization should be considered.

More rarely, a mandibular fracture can cause a complete transection of the inferior alveolar artery. In this situation, if spasm and spontaneous arrest of bleeding do not occur, considerable hemorrhage may take place, requiring urgent temporary fixation with a bridle wire.

Angiography should be considered if there is penetrating injury to the neck. The face and neck have classically been divided into three zones: zone 1, from the sternal notch to the cricoid cartilage; zone 2, from the cricoid cartilage to the mandibular angle; and zone 3, from the mandibular angle to the skull base. In the case of penetrating trauma in zones 1 and 3, catheter angiography is widely accepted as the best measure of assessment of vascular injury.[17]

Zone 2 penetrating injuries were previously managed by routine surgical exploration in cases in which the penetration passed through platysma. However, the advent of CT angiography has allowed development of a different management approach; namely, CT angiography in the stable patient, with further management based on clinical status and imaging findings.[18,19] This approach has reduced the need for surgical intervention in such patients and virtually eliminated cases of negative neck exploration (which occurred in half of all trauma-related explorations in the past).[20]

VISUAL LOSS

Visual loss may result from a lesion anywhere along the path from the globe to the visual cortex. Loss that is instantaneous (i.e., from the moment of trauma) is usually considered irreversible and is not imaged. However, difficulty arises in patients who have been rendered unconscious for a period of time, because instantaneous loss cannot then be determined.

Causes arising within the globe, such as gross rupture and hemorrhage, are usually clinically obvious or can be investigated with ultrasound. CT done for other reasons, such as fracture assessment, may provide useful information: Rupture of the globe, lens dislocation, hemorrhage, and retinal detachment may be evident. Optic nerve damage at the canal level can occur, but assessment by imaging in this situation depends much on local practice, because surgery in these cases is controversial. Fractures at the canal are rare, but compression by bony fragments may be seen on CT images.

Visual loss may also occur as a result of lesions further forward in the extraocular intraorbital compartment. Bone fragments, foreign bodies, or a penetrating injury may involve the optic nerve and may be identified on CT. If there is a risk

of a foreign body, MRI should be avoided until radiography is performed to assess for the presence of metal.

Optic nerve avulsion or transection may be detectable on CT or MRI, but blindness will be permanent. Although acute optic nerve and optic nerve sheath hemorrhage can be identified on MRI, laser tomography with clinical examination is the current standard for assessing the optic nerve.[21]

Together with osseous compression of the optic nerve, these are the direct forms of traumatic optic neuropathy. Visual evoked potentials (VEP) using flashlight goggles provide valuable additional information about optic nerve injuries.

The indirect forms of visual loss are much more common and include contusion of the optic nerve leading to edema and compression of its vascular supply, hemorrhage into the optic nerve sheath, shearing of the nutrient vessels, and increase in intraorbital pressure. Nutrient vessel shearing is untreatable. Hemorrhage into the optic nerve sheath can be identified on CT or MRI but is rare: It is often accompanied by fundal appearances of central retinal vein occlusion and can be amenable to decompression. However, the most common treatable problem is increased intraorbital pressure resulting from bleeding or from the presence of air (see later discussion). Patients with trauma involving the optic nerve (i.e., traumatic optic neuropathy) can benefit from imaging, but in some circumstances it is useless and in others harmful. The danger is that imaging will delay urgent treatment. Careful patient selection is therefore essential.

RECOGNITION AND INTERPRETATION OF FACIAL INJURY

The skeletal anatomy of the face is the most complex in the body. The maximum amount of information will be gleaned from the radiographs and images if a few rules are followed and there is a methodical approach to searching the image for information: You see what you look for! A number of approaches to image assessment in the context of facial injury are suggested and described in this section, as are specific signs that should be sought.

Every film of the face should be examined, including any that may have been sent from a referring hospital or clinic. Radiographs made elsewhere should always be obtained; they may hold important information, even if badly done, and may obviate the need to obtain some or all of the radiographs one would normally acquire. Some patients habitually present to the emergency department: their previous radiographs should be reviewed. Every image should be checked for the date it was obtained, for the patient's name, and for orientation markers (left or right).

Since the advent of Picture Archiving and Communication Systems (PACS), images are stored as data on computer systems. These may be copied onto compact disks for transfer between medical institutions, and finding previous imaging is easier than with hard-copy film packets. The downside is that images that predate the introduction of PACS into a hospital are often not included on the digital archive, so hard copies still need to be obtained, often from off-site storage areas. Because of the adaptation of new technology, it is easy to miss potentially relevant historical images because they are not in the digital archive. Always bear in mind that there may be films you are not aware of unless you ask!

SEARCH PATTERNS AND REMINDERS

McGrigor and Campbell described a search pattern of four lines that the eye should follow when one is examining the frontal view of the face (occipitomental 10-degree projection).[22] These are known as Campbell's lines or sometimes as McGrigor's lines. A fifth line is known as Trapnell's line[23] (Fig. 5-20). Using these lines allows one to examine all those parts of the face where fractures and other signs are most likely to be found and reduces the chance of missing a fracture.

The first of these lines runs across the frontozygomatic sutures, the superior margins of the orbit, and the frontal sinuses. The second passes along the zygomatic arches, the zygomatic body, the inferior orbital margin, and the nasal bones. The third crosses the condyles, the coronoid processes, and the maxillary sinuses. The fourth crosses the mandibular ramus and the bite line (occlusal plane of the teeth), and the fifth runs along the inferior border of the mandible from angle to angle.

Dolan and Jacoby described three lines for evaluating occipitomental projections that can be used as an adjunct[24] (Fig. 5-21). These are known collectively as Dolan's lines:

- The *orbital line* extends along the inner margins of the lateral, inferior, and medial walls of the orbit, passing over the nasal arch to follow the same structures on the opposite side.
- The *zygomatic line* extends along the superior margin of the arch and body of the zygoma, passing along the lateral margin of the frontal process of the zygoma to the zygomaticofrontal suture.

- The *maxillary line* extends along the inferior margin of the zygomatic arch, the inferior margin of the body and buttress of the zygoma, and the lateral wall of the maxillary sinus.

The same authors described evaluation lines for the modified Caldwell's projection. The first of these extends along the outer margin of the orbital process of the frontal and zygomatic bones. The second is the innominate line or oblique orbital line. The third line extends along the inner margin of the orbit downward and breaks into two roughly parallel lines meeting at the inferior orbital foramen; the medial of these two lines is the posterior lacrimal crest, and the lateral is the lamina papyracea. The third line then continues along the orbital margin inferiorly, laterally, and superiorly (Fig. 5-22).

The "four S's" described by Delbalso et al. are a good reminder of what to look for on radiographs.[25] The four S's are Symmetry, Sharpness, Sinus, and Soft tissue.

Symmetry

With the exception of the frontal sinuses, the face is reasonably symmetrical in most people. Occasionally, a hypoplastic maxillary antrum or previous old trauma can cause confusion, but any asymmetry that is noticed should draw the examiner's attention to that area for further evaluation (see Figs. 5-2, 5-3, 5-4, and 5-7).

Sharpness

Sharpness refers to the accentuated sharpness brought about by fracture fragments' being rotated or displaced into tangency with the x-ray beam, which causes them to appear accentuated on the image (see Fig. 5-2). A number of radiographic signs have been described based on this principle, such as the bright sign, railroad track sign, and trapdoor sign,

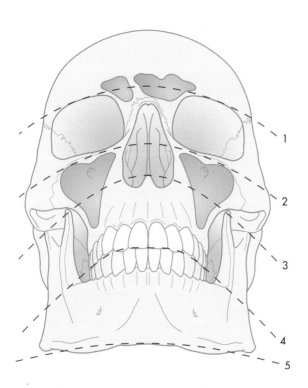

FIGURE 5-20 Campbell's and Trapnell's lines.

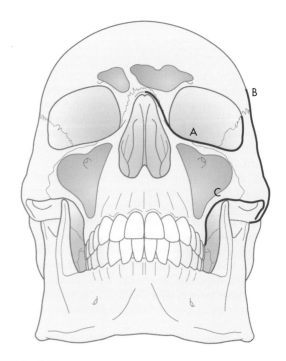

FIGURE 5-21 Dolan's lines for the occipitomental projection. **A,** Orbital line. **B,** Zygomatic line. **C,** Maxillary line.

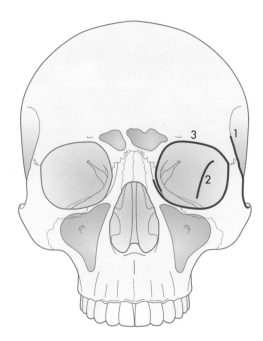

FIGURE 5-22 Dolan's lines for the modified Caldwell's projection.

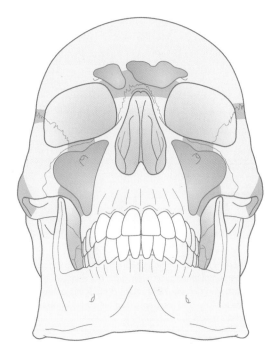

FIGURE 5-23 "Hot sites" for identifying fractures on the occipito-mental projection.

some of which are discussed later in this chapter. The converse of this principle is loss of normal sharp outline when a fragment is rotated out of tangency.

Sinus

Almost all of the midface fractures involve one or more of the paranasal sinuses (see Figs. 5-3 and 5-4). Valvassori and Hord used this fact to provide a classification scheme for midface injuries.[26] A number of abnormalities discussed in this section may be apparent in the sinuses.

Soft Tissues

Swelling, foreign bodies, and emphysema may all be apparent (see Fig. 5-4) and can help in the evaluation of the patient.

HOT SITES AND FRACTURE PATTERNS

Three fractures occurring along Le Fort's three great lines of weakness[27] have come to be known as the three great transfacial fractures: the Le Fort I, II, and III (although these are in reverse order to Le Fort's original assignation). These, together with the zygomatic fractures, orbital blowout fractures, and localized nasoethmoidal complex fractures, form the basis of most midface fracture classifications.

Two points should be emphasized. If these fracture lines or lines of weakness are mapped onto the image of an occipitomental 10-degree or modified Caldwell's projection in those areas where fractures are easily manifested to the observer (i.e., where bone is thick or is seen in tangent), then a pattern emerges, and certain sites (called *hot sites*) provide likely hunting grounds for recognizing injury. Second, these sites (Fig. 5-23) are not precise, because the lines of weakness vary slightly from individual to individual. Hence, they are indicated on the diagram as zones where fractures are most likely to be seen, and particular attention should be given to these areas. This approach speeds up and enhances the

discovery process. It does not, however, obviate the need for a complete study of the radiograph.

Allied to this notion is the idea of fracture patterns, which is inherent in the classifications of midface fractures. Use of these patterns allows the examiner, having identified a fracture, to direct attention to other likely sites. For example, having identified a fracture of an inferior orbital rim and knowing that this may not be localized but may be part of a tripod, Le Fort II, or nasomaxillary fracture (or some combination of these), the examiner can proceed to double-check the zygomatic arch, the frontozygomatic suture, the nasal arch, the lateral antral wall on the same side and the inferior orbital rim and lateral antral wall on the other side. Similarly, an arch fracture may be isolated, or it may be part of a tripod or Le Fort III fracture. A lateral antral wall fracture may be part of a tripod, Le Fort II, or Le Fort I fracture; it may be localized or dentoalveolar in origin; or it may be a combination of these.

That a fracture at a single site may occur as part of several different fracture types or patterns is important. Failure to appreciate this fact can lead to error (clinically as well as radiologically). For example, malar fractures are common, but not every inferior orbital rim fracture is a result of a malar injury. One of the most frequently misinterpreted fractures involving the inferior orbital rim is a fracture of the frontal process of the maxilla (Fig. 5-24).

One should not, however, be too rigid about such patterns or classifications, because hybrid and mixed forms, particularly in the Le Fort type of injuries, are more common than pure forms. Indeed, in severe, high-impact injuries, particularly of the panfacial type, the facial skeleton may split like an eggshell into dozens of fragments, making any attempt at ordered classification fruitless (Fig. 5-25). Concomitant injury patterns also occur, and identification of one should

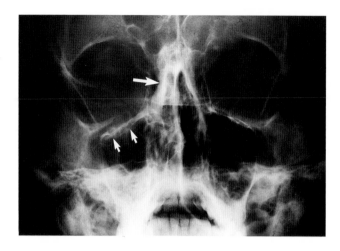

FIGURE 5-24   Fracture of the frontal process of the maxilla, as seen on an occipitomental projection with only 40 degrees of angulation. Notice the narrowing of the right nasal arch *(long arrow)*, compared with the opposite side, and the depressed medial portion of the inferior orbital rim *(short arrows)*.

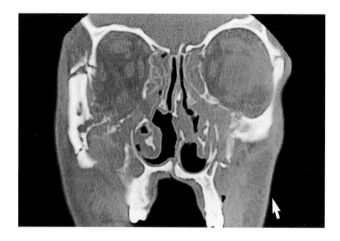

FIGURE 5-25   Coronal computed tomogram showing extensive fracturing at all the Le Fort levels with severe comminution and palatal splitting.

alert the examiner to check whether the other is present. Examples include the association of depressed zygomatic arch fracture with fracture of the coronoid process of the mandible; of Le Fort I and palatal fractures with mandibular injury; and of a parasymphysis fracture with a fracture of the opposite condylar neck or body.

THE CONCEPT OF COMPLETENESS AND INCOMPLETENESS

Not all fractures are apparent on clinical examination, and for a variety of reasons, not all will be discovered by either plain radiography (see Fig. 5-3) or CT scanning. What is important is whether the bone fragment is loose or displaced.

Some bone injury is only visible microscopically. Hairline fractures may become visible radiologically only after 7 to 10 days, when decalcification at the fracture edges occurs.

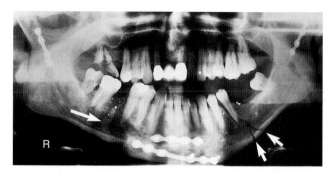

FIGURE 5-26   Bilateral mandibular body fractures. The fracture on the left shows true comminution *(short arrows)*, and there is widening of the periodontal membrane on the mesial aspect of the premolar. The fracture on the right is evident on this view only as an overlap sign of increased density *(long arrow)*. A fractured right upper molar is also present. There are plates for previous fractures in this patient, who had epilepsy.

Greenstick fracturing, in which there is a fracture through one side of the cortex with buckling on the other, and pure buckle fractures are common in children, particularly in the condylar neck. In these circumstances, only angular displacement may be seen, and the fragment is usually stable, albeit in an incorrect position.

In the skull vault, fractures commonly appear to give out, without ending at a bone edge. In addition, separation and movement may occur at sutures but be indiscernible radiologically. At certain suture sites, this can be a most difficult problem for the radiologist. The frontozygomatic suture is a case in point. It may be visible as a lucent line in some normal individuals, and in a few of them only on one side. The radiologist may therefore be unable to confirm a fracture or separation at that location, even though at surgery it is obviously loose and unstable.

DIRECT RADIOGRAPHIC SIGNS OF FRACTURE

All the signs of injury may be considered as being abnormal densities, either more lucent or more opaque than normal, or as being abnormalities of position, either incorrectly oriented or incorrectly located.

Separation Sign

The separation sign is sometimes called the cortical defect or crack (Figs. 5-26 and 5-27; see Figs. 5-1, 5-3, 5-5, 5-17, and 5-18). Fry et al.[28] pointed out that the radiographic appearance of fracture lines may vary in width, according to

- the amount of destruction
- the amount of displacement
- the angle of projection of the x-rays
- the stage of repair

Such a break in the continuity of bone allows x-rays to pass unimpeded and results in a lucent line on the image, but only if part of the fracture plane is oriented in tangent to the x-ray beam and there is sufficient depth (thickness) of bone. Many of the bones of the face are extremely thin plates. In the absence of other signs, the visibility of a fracture in such a

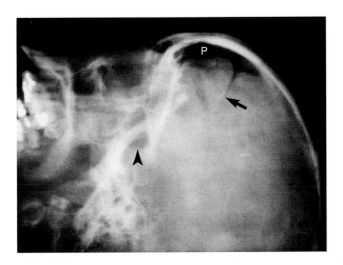

FIGURE 5-27 Horizontal-beam lateral skull radiograph (brow-up lateral skull). There is fracturing of the frontal calvaria (arrow), a pneumocephalus (p), and a fluid level in the sphenoid sinus (arrowhead). Notice also a fluid level in the maxillary antrum.

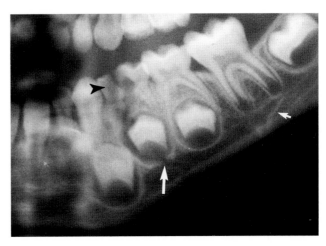

FIGURE 5-28 Fracture of the mandible, seen on part of a panoramic tomographic projection. There is a separation sign across the condensed bone of the lamina dura of a tooth bud (large arrow). A vertical fracture of the deciduous tooth above is present (arrowhead). The dense band distally (small arrow) is a pseudo-overlap sign caused by superimposition of the hyoid bone.

thin plate depends to a large degree on its orientation. Therefore, continuous fracture lines are rarely seen on radiographs of the midface. In a Le Fort I or II fracture, for example, the fracture line may be seen at the lateral antral wall on a frontal projection but not seen as it passes across the front and back walls of the antrum, where the bone is not only thin but oriented *en face* to the x-ray beam. When its plane of cleavage rotates or curls or suddenly alters direction, a fracture line may seem to disappear even though it continues farther in the bone in question. This accounts both for some fractures that appear to be incomplete and, to a lesser extent, for the pseudocomminution that is often seen in the mandible. In the latter situation, the fracture is visible as a lucent line on both the lingual and the buccal cortex (see Fig. 5-17); if these lines do not coincide geometrically, it can appear as if two fractures are present. Close examination usually reveals that the two lines approximate at a bone margin. Such changes in orientation also account for fractures in the frontal bone that appear to end at the orbital margin. These almost always continue into the orbital roof.

The margin of fracture lines should be inspected. In fresh fractures, the margins are well defined and sharp. Rounding off indicates either that it is not a fracture or that infection or nonunion is occurring. The width of a fracture line may increase slightly due to decalcification in the healing process, before ossification of the fracture callus. More extensive widening can be caused by displacement, intervening bone loss (e.g., ballistic injuries), or infection. However, this is a delayed feature and in any event takes at least 10 days to become apparent, because time is needed for removal of calcium salts.

If displacement is the cause, the width of a fracture provides additional information. Wide gaps indicate periosteal tearing and, in the calvaria, dural tearing. Cortical or condensed bone does not exist only at the perimeter of bone. The condensed bone of the mental foramen and the margins of the dental canal may demonstrate a separation sign. The lamina dura of tooth sockets and developing tooth buds should also be inspected for the presence of fracture lines. In

children, a fracture may be visible only as a lucency crossing the wall (lamina dura) of a developing tooth bud (Fig. 5-28).

A number of pitfalls exist for the unwary:

- Neurovascular channels produce lucent lines, as do sutures. Such channels and sutures can also cause confusion on CT scanning. Knowledge of anatomy is important here, but there are clues on the film: The margins of such anatomical lucent structures tend to be sclerotic (dense), unlike those of fresh fractures.
- A thin line of air between the tongue and palate (palatoglossal gap) can simulate a fracture on plain films, as can streaks of soft tissue emphysema. A clue to these and many other imitators is the bone margin: If the lucency goes beyond the bone margin, it is not a fracture of that particular bone and is therefore probably spurious. Some care is needed, however, because a lucent line projecting beyond a bone does not exclude a fracture, only a fracture of the bone in question. This problem occurs especially in the midface, where there is much superimposition of bone.
- An illusion of lucency may be identified where two different lightness gradients meet on an image due to the Mach effect. This often occurs at the overlap between soft tissue and bone and frequently leads to a false-positive diagnosis of fractures.

Sutural Diastasis

Separation of a fragment of bone from the rest of the facial skeleton may, in part or in whole, occur along a suture line. There are well-recognized sites in the face where such separation may be seen, such as the frontozygomatic suture (see Figs. 5-3 and 5-5), the frontonasal suture, the nasomaxillary suture, and, in young children, the internasal suture. Recognition of such suture separation is easy if the gap is well marked, but because such sutures in the normal patient may be seen as thin lucent lines, mild degrees of separation may be impossible to appreciate.

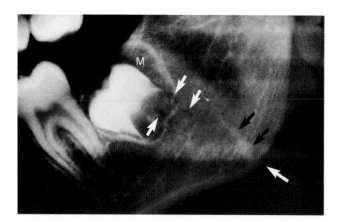

FIGURE 5-29 Left angular fracture of the mandible (part of a panoramic projection). The fracture is difficult to see, but several signs are present. There is widening of the periodontal ligament (M). Faint fracture lines cross the lamina dura and the region of the dental canal *(small white arrows)*. There is a linear density caused by overlap of fracture fragments *(black arrows)* and a tiny step deformity of the cortical margin *(large white arrow)*.

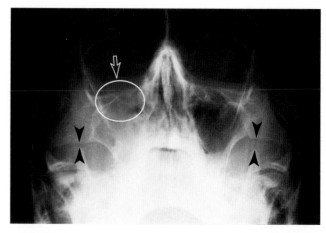

FIGURE 5-30 Abnormal linear density sign. An occipitomental 10-degree projection showing a subtle, minimally displaced malar fracture. The antrum is opaque, the soft tissues are slightly swollen *(open arrow)*, and there is a bright sign (abnormal linear density) projected over the inferior lateral antral wall *(circled)*. Notice also the reduced gap *(arrowheads)* between the tip of the coronoid process and the inferior margin of the buttress on the same side, which is caused by the displacement of the malar bone.

Overlap Sign

The overlap sign occurs when there is a displacement at the fracture site such that two fragments overlap, either wholly or in part. The thickness of bone is greater and shows as a band of increased opacity (Fig. 5-29; see Fig. 5-26). It may be the only sign of fracture. It is sometimes called the "double-density sign" or "cortical duplication," but these terms are misnomers, because, if the fracture plane is oblique and overriding is incomplete, the increase in thickness may be less than double. The margins of this band of increased opacity may be sharp or blurred, depending on the obliquity of the fracture line with respect to the x-ray beam. Care must be exercised with this sign, because normal structures such as the soft palate can produce a similar appearance. In addition, foreign bodies or displaced bone fragments from another site can project over the bone being examined.

Abnormal Linear Density

Abnormal linear density occurs when a fracture fragment is displaced or rotated (or both) so that it is seen "end on" in an abnormal position. This gives rise to a nonanatomical linear opacity. A common example occurs when a fragment of the antral wall rotates to produce a linear opacity projected over the antrum, the so-called bright sign (Fig. 5-30). Other examples include the trapdoor sign of an orbital floor fracture and the railroad or parallel line sign, which occurs when the lateral orbital wall is rotated to parallel the innominate (or oblique orbital) line. It is occasionally seen in high condylar neck fractures, when bone fragments may be seen projected over the sigmoid notch on panoramic, oblique, or lateral views. A further and important example is the increased density seen in the anterior fragment of a depressed zygomatic arch fracture on frontal projections (see Fig. 5-5). As with the overlap sign, foreign bodies (e.g., glass shards) may mimic this sign, as may normal antral septa and other superimposed anatomical structures.

Disappearing Fragment Sign

The absence of bone from an expected position is the opposite of the abnormal linear density (see Fig. 5-2). A bone structure that normally produces an image, such as the orbital floor or lateral antral wall, is displaced or rotated out of tangent to the beam, resulting in the appearance of a gap. The disappearing fragment sign is most commonly seen where there are thin bone plates. It too has its counterpart on CT images, and in CT there is a special example: the empty glenoid fossa, implying mandibular condylar neck fracture or dislocation.

Abnormal Angulation or Curvature

Abnormal angulation or curvature may be seen in children with greenstick or buckle fractures of the condylar neck, in the antral walls, and in the zygomatic arches (especially the outward bowing from frontal impact to the malar bone). It may be the only clue to injury, or it may be an obvious feature of an otherwise readily recognizable injury (Fig. 5-31).

Step Deformity

Step deformity is caused by displacement of bone in the plane at right angles to the x-ray beam, which gives rise to a sharp step in the contour of the outer margins of the bone cortex (see Figs. 5-4 and 5-29). It is seen notably in the mandible but can occur elsewhere in the face and is recognizable on CT and plain film images.

Displaced Bone

A large fragment or an entire osseous structure may change its location (see Figs. 5-6 and 5-18). Examples are depression of the orbital floor and margin in tripod injuries or of the midface with respect to the skull base and mandible in Le Fort fractures. This displacement may be the most immediate or obvious feature, but it is always seen in conjunction with other signs.

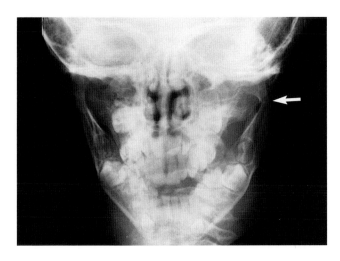

FIGURE 5-31 Greenstick injury. Note the angular deformity of the left condylar neck (arrow) on this PA projection of a child's mandible.

Widening of the Periodontal Ligament

Widening of the periodontal ligament is an important but often overlooked clue to fracture (see Figs. 5-17, 5-26, and 5-29). In any individual socket, the periodontal ligament has a uniform thickness all around the tooth, equivalent in thickness to that around adjacent teeth. The ligament may appear wider or thicker in some disease processes and in local injury, such as partial extrusion. However, in the absence of such extrusion, a periodontal ligament that appears wider on one side than the other (e.g., wider mesially than distally) should raise the possibility that a mandibular fracture passes into it.

INDIRECT RADIOGRAPHIC SIGNS OF FRACTURE

Soft Tissue Swelling

Soft tissue swelling is a common and fairly nonspecific sign (see Fig. 5-4) that is often present with no underlying fracture. Occasionally, if localized, it may direct the attention to a particular area of the face on the radiograph. For example, soft tissue swelling over one cheek directs attention to that side, and swelling over the nasal arch directs attention to the nasomaxillary structures. Swelling may also affect the airway, and this area should always be inspected on any lateral views and on CT images, bearing in mind that free blood may give a similar opacification.

Paranasal Sinus Opacification

Complete opacification, mucosal thickening (localized or general), and fluid levels in the sinuses may all be seen after trauma (see Figs. 5-3, 5-4, 5-27, and 5-30). These signs may be caused by preexisting disease (see Fig. 5-2) or just a severe nosebleed, but they should nevertheless be regarded with suspicion.

Recognition of a fluid level requires the x-ray beam to be horizontal (or nearly so—a tilt of up to about 10 degrees does not usually matter). A fluid level in the sphenoid sinus on a horizontal-beam lateral view of a severely injured patient should always be taken as indicating a fracture of the skull base (see Fig. 5-27), and further studies should be undertaken to prove or disprove the supposition.

Opacification of the frontal sinus can be problematic if there is much overlying soft tissue swelling; if the AP dimension of the frontal sinus is small, it can be impossible to determine from the PA films whether the sinus is fully aerated or full of blood or CSF unless a fluid level is seen. Opacification in the frontal or ethmoidal air cells may also be caused by herniation of brain tissue.

Air in the Soft Tissues

Soft tissue gas has several causes, including infection, penetrating injury, sinus fracture, and rupture of the trachea, larynx, or esophagus with dissection up to the face. Emphysema from facial fracture is fairly common, particularly if there has not been much delay between the time of the trauma and the acquisition of images. Abnormally located air is usefully divided into three groups: soft tissue, orbital, and intracranial. Very rarely, air may occur in the intravascular space (e.g., cavernous sinus) or in the spine (pneumorachis).

Soft Tissue Emphysema

Apart from superior dissection of air due to laryngeal, tracheal, or esophageal laceration, air in the soft tissue of the face is usually stated to be caused by communication via a fracture with a paranasal sinus (see Fig. 5-4). This can be misleading: Although uncommon, it is encountered from time to time in patients whose only injury is a fracture of the mandible, particularly a fracture around the angle. As with other signs, there are pitfalls. Air lateral to the maxillary antrum may be mimicked by lateral extensions of the sphenoid sinus and by pacchionian granulations in the skull vault. Rarely, air is localized and under tension within the soft tissues (i.e., soft tissue pneumatocele). Occasionally, air is seen in other sites, such as the temporomandibular joint. Soft tissue emphysema is always more extensive and widespread on CT images than one would expect from the plain radiographs.

Patients with facial fractures should be discouraged from nose blowing, sneezing, and so on, because increased air pressure can force large amounts of air into the soft tissues, increasing the risk of infection. This can also result in extension of emphysema down the neck, over the chest, and into the mediastinum. However, whenever air is seen in the soft tissues below the mandible (i.e., in the neck or lower), every effort should be made to exclude other causes, such as laryngeal, tracheal, or esophageal laceration.

Intraorbital Air

Intraorbital air, as seen on the plain film (see Figs. 5-2, 5-3, and 5-4), must be differentiated from the deep sulcus of the upper lid in an elderly or enophthalmic patient. Air is usually seen superiorly in the orbit but can occur anywhere, even within the globe. Large amounts can collect in the presental space and, on occasion, behind the globe. There are even a few reports of tension pneumo-orbitism presenting much like retrobulbar hemorrhage, with chemosis and threatened vision. Most cases of intraorbital air are said to be caused by medial orbital wall fractures, but air here can result from orbital floor injury. It can also occur as a delayed manifestation of an orbitoantral fistula, particularly in patients who have undergone repair of blowout floor fractures; these patients experience swelling and crepitus after nose blowing when they get colds.

Intracranial Air

Air may collect in any of the spaces where blood collects, namely in extradural (epidural), subdural, and subarachnoid (cortical, basal cistern, and intraventricular) spaces and in the brain substance (aerocele) (Figs. 5-32 and 5-33; see Fig. 5-27). Except in extradural sites, the presence of air implies tearing of the dura. Although pneumocephalus is only occasionally seen on plain films, and then usually in small amounts, it should nevertheless be looked for, particularly behind the frontal sinuses on the brow-up cross-table lateral projection obtained in the emergency department. The amount of air seen is highly variable, but even extremely small volumes (≤0.5 mL) can be recognized on CT, so it is not uncommonly encountered on CT images of patients with severe injury. Intracranial air may arise from the air cavities of the petrous bones but more commonly from breaches around the ethmoid roof, the sphenoid sinus, and, especially, the frontal sinus.

When very tiny amounts of air are seen immediately adjacent to bone, it may be impossible to determine whether it is extradural or subdural.

The rate of disappearance of intracranial air depends on the amount originally present and whether there is an ongoing leak. Small amounts disappear in a few days; large amounts may take a week or longer. If very large amounts are present, then the air may be under pressure, forming a tension pneumocephalus or aerocele. This is an emergency, because it acts much like a large intracranial blood collection. The appearance of pneumocephalus may be delayed—not just by a few days, but in some cases by years or decades after injury. This is often associated with unexpected CSF rhinorrhea, which may be profuse. Investigation of recurrent or delayed pneumocephalus is similar to that of recurrent or delayed CSF leak (see later discussion).

Changes to the Occlusal Plane

Changes in the occlusion are always best assessed clinically, but gross changes are visible radiologically (see Fig. 5-6) and

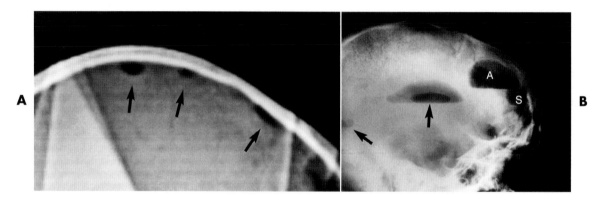

FIGURE 5-32   Examples of pneumocephalus. **A,** Computed tomogram (part of the lateral scanogram) in a patient with an orbitoethmoidal injury showing bubbles of subarachnoid air *(arrows)* beneath the calvaria. **B,** Lateral skull radiograph in a patient with delayed pneumocephalus after repair of fronto-ethmoidal injury. Notice the aerocele (A), air in the body and occipital horns of the lateral ventricles *(arrows)*, and air in the subdural space (S).

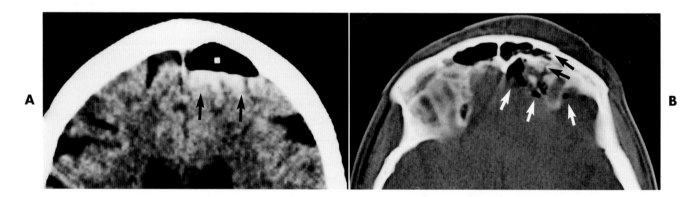

FIGURE 5-33   Examples of pneumocephalus. **A,** Axial computed tomogram (CT) obtained after orbitoethmoidal injury showing air in the subarachnoid space *(white cursor mark)* that is limited medially by the falx (unlike epidural air). The increase in density of the brain tissue immediately behind this air *(arrows)* is a beam-hardening artifact and should not be mistaken for brain contusion. **B,** Axial CT obtained after an injury to the frontal sinus. Notice the thickened soft tissues in front of the sinus, fracturing of anterior and posterior sinus walls *(black arrows)*, and small collections of intracranial air *(white arrows)* caused by dural tearing.

can aid the radiologist (who may have limited information on the request form). Premature occlusion on one side may suggest a unilateral Le Fort I or dentoalveolar injury. An open anterior bite may suggest one of the Le Fort or condylar neck fractures.

Dental Injury

Missing teeth and fractured teeth draw attention to areas of impact. Abnormal alignment of several adjacent teeth in the upper jaw may suggest the rotation of a dentoalveolar fragment.

COMPUTED TOMOGRAPHIC EVALUATION

CT imaging provides a series of slices through the facial skeleton. Assessment requires analysis of each image, with its soft tissue and bony abnormalities, together with an ability to stack up these images to provide a 3-D image in the mind. Gentry et al. developed the concept of a series of horizontal, coronal, and sagittal struts or buttresses.[29] These can be used to evaluate the CT images of patients with facial trauma (Box 5-3). Such an approach allows for a more thorough assessment of the CT images. With a few exceptions, these struts are best evaluated when the plane of the image slice is perpendicular to the strut plane.

Many of the specific changes described in relation to plain radiographs are also applicable to CT imaging (see Figs. 5-7, 5-9, 5-10, and 5-25). However, CT is very sensitive to soft tissue changes, which are often not readily visible on plain films. CT may demonstrate changes in the position of the globe, show the relationship of extraocular muscles to bone shards and blowout fractures, accurately locate foreign bodies, and demonstrate lens rupture or dislocation. CT can demonstrate hemorrhage at various intracranial sites, in the orbit, and in the globe (Fig. 5-34). It can identify fractures that would be difficult to see on plain radiographs, and it more accurately displays and localizes displaced bone fragments (Figs. 5-35 and 5-36; see Figs. 5-7, 5-9, 5-10). On the other hand, very thin walls located between structures of lower opacity may disappear on CT images because of partial voluming.

SPECIFIC PROBLEMS

DENTAL AND DENTOALVEOLAR INJURY

Dental injury may involve the relationship of the tooth to its socket, the substance of the tooth itself, or the surrounding bone. There is, of course, a lot of overlap—an injury to a tooth may result in changes in all three of these features, and in major trauma it frequently does.

The following are the purposes of radiography in the acute phase of dental injury:

- To assess the physiological development of the root apex. If the root formation is incomplete—that is, there is a wide open and funnel-shaped canal with a developmental sac still evident—the young tooth has marked healing potential. With advanced root development, the canal is narrow and there is a greater likelihood of vascular damage and pulp necrosis.

BOX 5-3 | Facial Struts

Horizontal Plane Struts
Superior
    Orbital roof
    Fovea ethmoidalis
    Cribriform plates

Middle
    Orbital floor
    Zygomatic arch

Inferior
    Hard palate
    Alveolar ridge

Sagittal Plane Struts
Midline
    Perpendicular plate of ethmoid
    Vomer
    Nasal septal cartilage

Parasagittal
    Medial orbital walls
    Medial walls of maxillary antra
    Pterygoid plates

Lateral
    Lateral orbital walls
    Lateral walls of maxillary antra

Coronal Plane Struts
Anterior
    Anterior wall of frontal sinus
    Anterior walls of maxillary antra
    Nasoethmoidal complex
    Frontozygomatic buttress
    Anterior maxillary alveolus

Posterior
    Posterior walls of maxillary antra
    Pterygoid plates

Adapted from Gentry LR, Manor WF, Turski PA, et al: High resolution computed tomographic analysis of facial struts in trauma. 1. Normal anatomy, *AJR Am J Roentgenol* 140:523-532, 1983.

- To assess the size of the pulp and its relationship to the fracture. However, one should be aware that a fracture here may appear to involve the pulp when it does not.
- To identify the presence of a root fracture.
- To identify the presence of foreign bodies such as tooth fragments in the soft tissues.
- To identify the presence of alveolar bone fracture.
- To assess any other abnormalities in the area and the condition of adjacent teeth.
- To obtain a baseline for prognosis.

FOREIGN BODIES AND MISSING TEETH

General

Every effort must be made to locate missing teeth (Figs. 5-37 and 5-38) and dentures, and all lacerations and penetrating

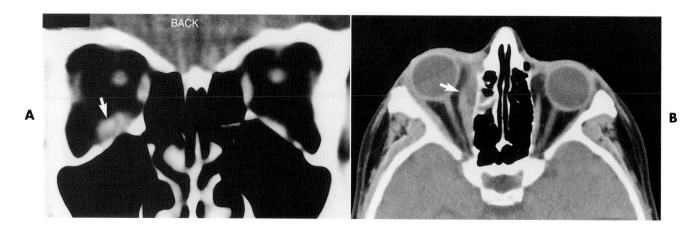

FIGURE 5-34 Orbital injuries. **A,** Coronal computed tomographic (CT) scan demonstrating hemorrhage in and around the right inferior rectus muscle sheath *(arrow)* caused by penetrating injury. A large wooden twig was removed but was not separately identifiable on the CT studies. **B,** Axial CT of the orbits. A posttraumatic, subperiosteal orbital hematoma is displacing the medial rectus muscle *(arrow)* and causing proptosis.

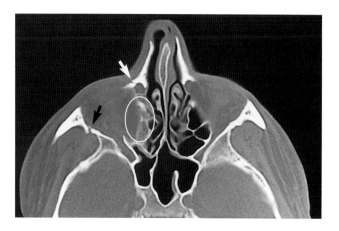

FIGURE 5-35 Axial computed tomogram in a patient with malar and maxillary trauma, part of a more extensive injury, showing a fracture of the lacrimal duct *(white arrow)* and sphenomalar suture diastasis *(black arrow)*. An inferomedial blowout fracture is also evident *(circle)*.

injuries must be suspected of harboring foreign bodies. In facial trauma, the most common foreign bodies are windshield glass and road grit. Teeth and foreign bodies may be ingested, inhaled, or implanted into soft tissues; foreign bodies may also impale the patient.

Foreign bodies may implant anywhere, even at a great distance from the mucosal or skin breach. A very high index of suspicion must be maintained with any laceration in or around the eye, including the lids, and particularly in children, who are often poor historians. Orbital roof penetration is a well-recognized injury and is all too often overlooked; the delayed results can be disastrous and can include CSF leak, orbital meningocele, meningitis, brain abscess, and death. CT should be considered in all suspicious cases, especially in children. Wooden objects are notorious for harboring organisms and producing abscesses, and they can be very difficult to detect (see Fig. 5-34A). If the history is appropriate and the

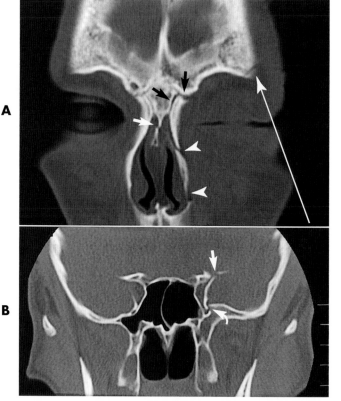

FIGURE 5-36 Coronal computed tomogram in a patient with a central, middle-third facial injury. **A,** Separation of the nasofrontal and nasomaxillary sutures *(black arrows)*. Fractures of the nasal septum *(short white arrow)*, the nasal plate of the frontal process of the maxilla *(arrowheads)*, and of the superior orbital rim *(long white arrow)*. **B,** A sphenoid fracture in the same patient involves the inferior part of the superior orbital fissure, the floor of the middle cranial fossa *(curved arrow)*, and the root of the anterior clinoid process *(straight arrow)*.

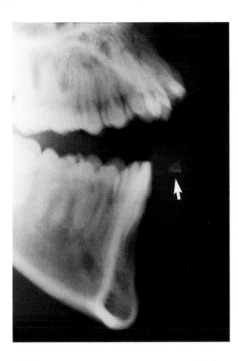

FIGURE 5-37   Missing dental fragment seen in the lower lip on a soft tissue lateral projection *(arrow)*.

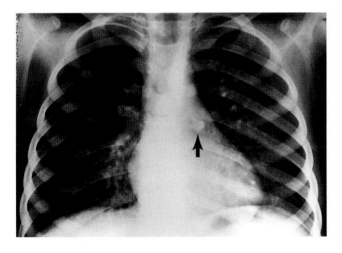

FIGURE 5-38   Inhaled tooth. This chest radiograph in a young child demonstrates a molar tooth *(arrow)* in the left main bronchus.

CT findings are negative, with no evidence of metallic foreign body, then MRI should be undertaken.

Avulsed teeth have been found implanted in the frontal sinus and as far away as the patient's forearm. The most common site for teeth or tooth fragments to become implanted is in the oral soft tissues—the gingiva, the floor of mouth, and the lips and tongue—but they may be propelled into the nasal cavity, palate, or maxillary sinus. If careful examination of routine plain radiographs of the face does not reveal their whereabouts and there are oral or lip lacerations, a soft tissue lateral radiograph should be obtained. If the tooth is still unlocated, a PA chest radiograph, and in some cases a CT chest scan, should be obtained (see Fig. 5-38). Inhaled teeth are distinctly uncommon, but the consequences can be grievous, with lung collapse, pneumonia, lung abscess, or

even death occurring. Delayed removal (beyond 24 hours) is associated with increased morbidity and hospital stay: imaging should be expeditious. Ingested teeth are rarely a problem once they have entered the esophagus; they are usually passed without problem. Large ingested foreign bodies and dentures may present a problem; if stuck in the esophagus, they may perforate into the mediastinum. Some foreign bodies and many dentures are not radiopaque, and a contrast swallow examination with fluoroscopy may be needed to confirm their presence and locate them. This should be done as soon as possible; otherwise, edema around the impacted foreign body can make removal difficult and increases the likelihood of esophageal perforation.

Long impaled foreign bodies in the esophagus should be left in place until CT and, if appropriate, angiography have demonstrated their exact anatomical relationships and any underlying vascular damage. Sharp, elongated, or pointed objects longer than 10 cm (6 cm in children) that are lodged in the stomach should be considered for removal, as should blunt round objects larger than 2.5 cm, because they may fail to pass the pylorus.

Orbital Foreign Bodies

Foreign bodies in the orbit may be isolated, or they may occur as part of more widespread facial injury. They can be intraocular or extraocular. Most extraocular intraorbital foreign bodies do not need removal except in special circumstances (e.g., organic material, impingement on the optic nerve). Projecting foreign bodies, whether intraocular or extraocular, require removal. Intraocular foreign bodies need removal because they can cause sympathetic ophthalmitis or premature cataract. Most intraocular foreign bodies that are clearly identifiable on ophthalmoscopy or slit-lamp examination do not require radiological imaging.

The purpose of imaging is twofold: to confirm that a foreign body is present and to demonstrate its approximate site. The methods used include plain radiography, special techniques (e.g., bone-free radiographs), ultrasonography, and CT. MRI should not be used in any patient who may have a metallic fragment in the orbit, because the magnetic field could displace the fragment and endanger sight; however, MRI has an important place in detecting wood fragments that have not been identified on CT. If the patient has undergone CT examination to assess facial or cranial fractures, that alone may provide all the information required, both to identify the presence of a foreign body in the orbit and to determine its exact location within the intraocular or extraocular compartment. CT is particularly useful when there are multiple foreign bodies, but it is less accurate than ultrasound in demonstrating intraocular damage.

If CT imaging is not otherwise being performed, the initial radiograph is a plain lateral view centered to the outer canthus, with the patient looking straight ahead. If no opaque foreign body is seen, then either no foreign body is present or it is a nonradiopaque foreign body requiring other imaging modalities to identify and locate it. If an opaque foreign body is seen, two views are taken: a PA projection with 35-degree elevation of the orbitomeatal line and a lateral view with a double exposure, one exposure in upward gaze and one in downward gaze. Those tiny fragments that lie in a very anterior position may be demonstrable on bone-free radiographs. This technique involves placement of a dental film in the inner canthus, with a central ray directed just behind the outer canthus to include as much of the globe (and lids) as possible.

Such simple views may provide all the information required. If further detail regarding the exact location of an intraocular foreign body is needed, then some special localizing technique is required. In these circumstances, the most appropriate imaging modality is ultrasonography. Extremely tiny (<0.3 mm) foreign bodies may not be visible with standard radiographic methods, and ultrasound is better, although CT is preferred for extraocular intraorbital foreign bodies.

Projectile extraocular metallic or glass foreign bodies located posterior to the equator are associated with a higher likelihood of ocular injury, but most do not need removal unless they are compromising the optic nerve (or unless it is done incidentally along with some other necessary surgical procedure). Anterior extraocular metallic or glass foreign bodies do not require imaging if they are clinically palpable, the history is reliable, and the eye examination is normal. CT should be considered if a ruptured globe is suspected, the foreign body is not palpable, there are significant ocular findings, the patient is a poor historian, or there is a possibility of multiple foreign bodies.

Organic matter such as wood or cotton incites an inflammatory reaction and can lead to a fungal cellulitis. In children especially, there may be no history of injury and little in the way of any physical evidence. The most common site is the superior orbit, and foreign body material in that site may lead to abnormal extraocular motility, proptosis, ptosis, acute cellulitis, and even osteomyelitis. Again especially in children, there is a risk that the injury may be orbitocranial, and this carries a high rate of mortality if unrecognized. Ultrasonography is helpful in assessing the globe but not elsewhere in the orbit. CT is probably the best modality. However, the appearance of organic matter on CT varies considerably: Wood may have densities ranging between −550 (pine) and +289 (ebony) Hounsfield units, with dry wood looking like air and green wood being isodense to orbital fat or even muscle.[30]

CT cannot be used to exclude organic material, because it correctly identifies the foreign body in only about half of all cases. CT does show well such secondary effects as abscess, osteomyelitis, periosteal thickening, optic nerve changes, and any fractures or intracranial damage. Success with MRI is also variable. Dry wood is hypointense to fat on T1 and T2 weighting, mimicking bone fragments and air. Green wood, which has a higher water content, is hypointense or isointense to fat on T1 and T2 weighting. The surroundings of the foreign body may enhance after contrast administration, and also some surrounding hyperintensity may be seen on T2 weighting. Plastic is seen variably on CT; like wood, it can be confused with air. It is more readily apparent on MRI, which demonstrates a signal void.[31]

MRI identification of the foreign body is somewhat better than what is possible with CT, but CT's added advantage in assessing bone and its ability to exclude metal (contraindicated with MRI) make it the first choice. The history and a high degree of suspicion are most important, and even if imaging is unhelpful, exploration may be necessary. Exploration without adequate imaging, however, courts disaster, because additional foreign body fragments and even an intracranial foreign body and intracranial damage may be missed.

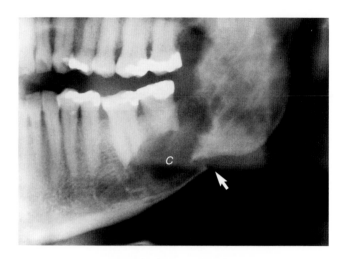

FIGURE 5-39 Pathological fracture. A fracture *(arrow)* occurred after surgery for a dentigerous cyst (c).

As mentioned earlier, a sensible approach would be to perform a CT scan and, if no foreign body is demonstrated, to proceed to MRI if clinical suspicion remains.

PATHOLOGICAL FRACTURES

A pathological fracture is one that occurs in bone that has been weakened by disease. The disease process may be local, widespread, or generalized. When such a process is present, fracture may result from less force than would normally be expected. Indeed, fracture often occurs with normal physiological loading (e.g., mastication) and sometimes spontaneously. Fracturing may occur during extirpation of teeth or during surgery for cysts (Fig. 5-39). The list of potential causes is as long as the list of diseases that weaken bone; it includes cysts, malignant tumors (primary or secondary), osteomyelitis, and osteoradionecrosis. Allied situations can also weaken bone (e.g., osseous implants). Developmental conditions such as ectopic teeth can also predispose to fracture. The patient may be aware of the traumatic incident, but occasionally a patient presents with no more than deranged occlusion. Clinically, there may be less—or no—crepitus on movement and less pain than expected.

Recognition that the fracture is pathological is usually easy, there being a cyst or destructive lesion involving the bone or a clinical history of irradiation with related bone changes adjacent to the fracture. Occasionally, the problem is not be so obvious, particularly if the disease is generalized (e.g., myeloma). In the face, the mandible is by far the most common bone to be involved. Because the site of fracture is determined by the disease, the pattern and location are often atypical: Fractures of the body and ramus are more common. Once a pathological fracture is recognized, further head and neck imaging is unlikely to be helpful, other than to stage malignancy and assess operability.

INJURY TO SECRETORY GLANDS AND THEIR DUCTS

Significant injury to the parotid gland is usually the result of penetrating injury and of itself does not usually require

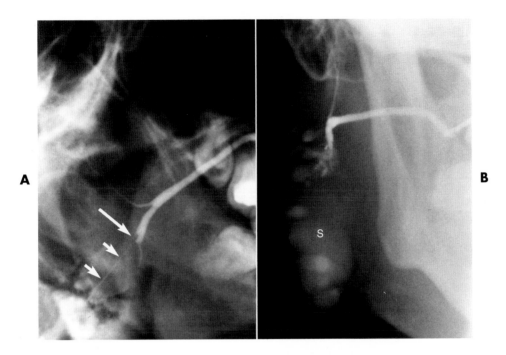

FIGURE 5-40   Parotid sialogram showing duct trauma. **A,** Lateral oblique projection. **B,** Posteroanterior projection. The patient fell through a plate glass door and developed swelling, having been sutured elsewhere. There is a laceration of a primary duct tributary *(long arrow)* with spurting of contrast medium *(short arrows)* into a large traumatic sialocele. Note the contrast puddling in the sialocele (s).

imaging. Stensen's duct and the major duct tributaries are most at risk. Sialography can be of some help in suspected cases by identifying and locating any disruption of the duct (Fig. 5-40). Injury to the other salivary ducts rarely requires imaging, except in late cases with stenosis.

Injury to the lacrimal drainage pathways is a fairly common sequela to severe fractures in the naso-orbitoethmoidal region. Injury may be direct, from laceration or penetration, or a result of shearing fractures in the bony canal. Imaging has a part to play in recognizing fractures of the bony canal and later in assessment of the lumen of the drainage apparatus. Fractures involving the bony canal are best identified on CT imaging with the use of bony windows (see Fig. 5-35). Fractures of the nasolacrimal fossa are usually avulsions of an intact fossa, comminution of the fossa itself being less frequent, although extensive comminution can occur in the surrounding bone. In contrast, most fractures involving the canal are comminuted, and especially so in the inferior canal. An important point to note on CT images of the nasolacrimal duct is that they are opaque in most normal people but can be aerated; no significance can be attached to this even if one side is aerated and the other opaque.

Dacryocystography is used to assess the lumen of the nasolacrimal canaliculi, sac, and duct; it involves introduction of contrast medium via the lower canaliculus, although the upper canaliculus (or, rarely, both canaliculi) may be used. Such dacryocystography is recorded by plain radiography or from fluoroscopy, but CT has been used by some workers. Unless repeated attacks of dacryocystitis have occurred, the majority of lesions will be found either at the bony ring or in the canal, rather than the sac, which usually escapes injury.

UPPER-THIRD FACIAL INJURIES

Upper-third injuries have more scope for disaster than anywhere else in the face. The upper third of the face comprises the frontal bone, which contains the frontal sinuses. These sinuses are undeveloped in early childhood and may remain so in a few adults. They are extremely variable, may show marked asymmetry, and may have extensions out to the external angular process and back along the orbital roof into the lesser wing of the sphenoid bone. These structures have an intimate relationship to the orbital contents and the brain. The lateral part of the frontal bone is exceptionally strong, but fracturing of the external angular process may occur, sometimes in association with a malar injury. Experiments with holographic interferometry show that supraorbital ridge loading causes stress in the form of surface perturbations in the orbital roof, some 5 to 8 mm in front of the optic foramen.[32] Blows to this part of the frontal bone are particularly associated with the onset of blindness (a fact noted by Hippocrates). Often, little is found on imaging, not even a local fracture, but isolated orbital roof fractures may be seen (Fig. 5-41), and in the very young these are more common than orbital floor fractures. Occasionally, ill-defined hemorrhage or a subperiosteal hematoma is identified close to the orbital apex.

Most orbital roof fractures extend to the orbital rim. The dura over the roof is thin and firmly attached, so dural tearing is common. However, because the frontal sinus may extend along the roof, not all roof fractures involve dura. When dura is torn, the usual problems arise: CSF may leak into the orbit, and large defects (greater than 1 to 1.5 cm) may allow dural herniation and pulsating exophthalmos. In addition,

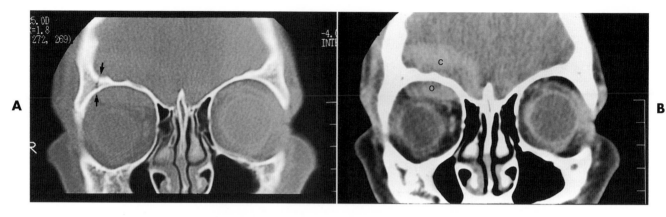

FIGURE 5-41 Coronal computed tomogram in a child with an isolated orbital roof fracture. Clinically, the patient was thought to have an orbital floor fracture because there was limitation of upward gaze with diplopia. **A,** Bone window setting shows an isolated fracture of the orbital roof *(arrows)*. **B,** Soft tissue window setting at the same level shows intracranial hemorrhage (c) and subperiosteal hemorrhage at the orbital roof (o). The orbital floor and the superior orbital rim are intact.

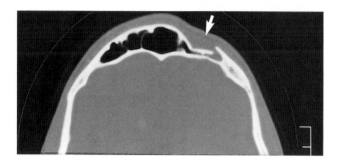

FIGURE 5-42 Frontal sinus injury seen on an axial computed tomographic scan. There is a depressed fracture of the anterior wall of the frontal sinus *(arrow).*

intraorbital hemorrhage or bone spicules may affect the action of extraocular muscles, including the levator apparatus.

Fractures of the frontal sinus may involve the anterior wall, the posterior wall, or the nasofrontal duct. Undisplaced fractures of the anterior wall require stabilization only if there are other adjacent fragments. Displaced fractures of the anterior wall are more common (Fig. 5-42) and require treatment, both for cosmetic reasons and because bone fragments or mucosal tears may block the nasofrontal duct and lead to mucocele or pyocele formation. Clear visualization of the nasofrontal duct is not always possible on imaging, but any injury in this area should be regarded as compromising frontal sinus drainage. Combined anterior and posterior wall fractures almost always involve the duct, unless the fracture is laterally placed. If the posterior wall is intact but the nasofrontal duct is involved or at risk, the sinus needs to be obliterated. It is essential to recognize and report the extent of pneumatization of the frontal sinus: If locules in the orbital roof or far laterally are not obliterated, mucocele and pyocele are likely to result (Fig. 5-43). Fractures of the posterior wall may involve the dura, leading to CSF leak. This is most likely if the fracture is displaced or comminuted. Undisplaced

fractures with no evidence of CSF leak may be treated as described previously, but otherwise the sinus needs to be cranialized. Good imaging and accurate assessment are essential.

Plain films (modified Caldwell's and lateral views), although useful for initial scout imaging, are notoriously unreliable and difficult to interpret. Some significant and severe injuries can be almost impossible to see. This is, in part, due to the curvature of the anterior and posterior walls of the frontal sinus: Only small portions of these walls are tangent to the x-ray beam. Additionally, apart from recognizing pneumocephalus, plain radiographs will not allow assessment of underlying soft tissues such as brain, meninges, and orbital contents. For this reason, CT is virtually mandatory.

DURAL TEARING AND CEREBROSPINAL FLUID LEAK

Severe blunt trauma or penetrating injury may breach the dura. CSF leak and pneumocephalus are the potential consequences, and they lead in turn to infection (e.g., meningitis) or, if brain tissue is involved, to abscess formation. Pneumocephalus has already been described, but the two conditions commonly coexist, although they may not be apparent at the same time. Fractures of the ethmoid and sphenoid sinuses with dural tearing and CSF leak commonly occur with Le Fort II, Le Fort III, and naso-orbitoethmoidal fractures, but the CSF leak in these cases is usually short-lived and ceases with fracture reduction and fixation. Leaks persists in only a few cases, and only those that persist for longer than 2 weeks, are recurrent or delayed, exhibit expanding pneumocephalus, or develop meningitis require detailed investigation. Recurrence can be delayed for decades.

The most common site of persistent CSF leaks is the frontal sinus. In patients with acute trauma to this sinus, CT is virtually mandatory, because plain films are notoriously unreliable in demonstrating fractures of the posterior table, let alone the commonly occurring coexistent intracranial damage. Wide fracture separation or displacement of fragments greater than

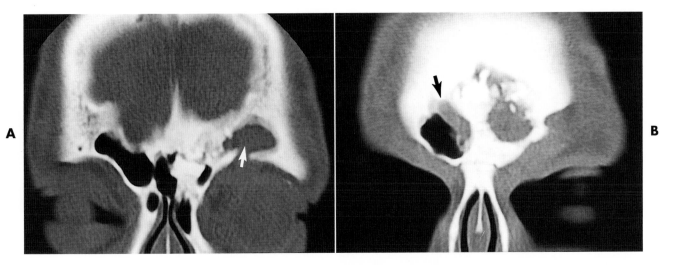

FIGURE 5-43 Coronal computed tomogram (CT) of a patient with a frontal sinus mucopyocele. There was a previous fracture with incomplete obliteration and bone chips. **A,** A far left loculus *(white arrow)* was left uncleared and unfilled, as was a right-sided loculus **(B)** which drained to the left *(black arrow)*. Eighteen months later, CT shows that these loculi have filled with pus, bone erosion is taking place, and the bone chips are being resorbed.

the thickness of the posterior table implies dural tearing; these signs should be sought on the CT images of patients with acute trauma. Rarely, CSF enters the orbit, forming a cyst, or, even more rarely, it leaks into the conjunctiva (orbitorrhea) and manifests similarly to epiphora.

Considerable ingenuity has been expended in developing tests to prove that leaking fluid is CSF and to locate the dural breach. Most of the location methods used in the past were superseded by the introduction of iodinated contrast media in the intrathecal space during CT (CT cisternography). This method is now rarely used because of the risks inherent in introducing such material into the CSF; moreover, as with almost all of the other methods, it is reliable only if the CSF is actively leaking at the time of the study. More recently, Lloyd et al.[33] showed that, with improvements in CT technology, high-definition CT is all that is required to demonstrate accurately the site of the leak (Fig. 5-44); this method does not depend on the presence of an active CSF leak at the time of the investigation. In their series, persistent bone defects were identified, and they were almost always accompanied by some soft tissue opacification in the adjacent sinus and, in about one quarter of the cases, by pneumocephalus.

However, the use of CT with or without intrathecal contrast media still exposes the patient to ionizing radiation. MRI avoids both radiation exposure and the injection of contrast medium. In 1994, el Gammal and Brooks,[34] as well as El Jamel et al.,[35] demonstrated that magnetic resonance cisternography provided an important alternative. CSF gives a high signal on T2-weighted images, providing its own contrast (Fig. 5-45). MRI can also display intracranial anatomy and trauma pathology in great detail, and images can readily be obtained in any plane.

The choice of modality remains controversial. Hegarty and Millar,[36] in 1997, looked at a control group having MRI for temporal lobe epilepsy and found that 42% fulfilled the criteria for diagnosis of CSF fistula! However, the year before their report, Stafford-Johnson et al.[37] published a study of 24

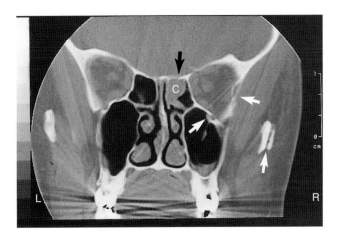

FIGURE 5-44 Coronal computed tomogram showing a cerebrospinal fluid leak into the sinuses (c). The floor of the anterior cranial fossa is fractured *(black arrow)*. Notice also the fractures of the orbital floor, lateral orbital wall, and malar arch *(white arrows)*. There is a fluid level in the antrum.

patients with CSF leaks and found the technique to be 100% reliable in identifying the site of leak (i.e., all were confirmed at surgery). High-resolution CT has a high incidence of false-positive findings, especially in the region of the cribriform plate. Both modalities may be helpful, but CT is likely to be used in most centers because it is faster and more widely available. Nevertheless, MRI should be considered if CT results are equivocal or unhelpful. Furthermore, MRI is the procedure of choice in evaluation of the rarer consequences of dural tearing, namely meningocele and encephalocele. These may present clinically with pulsating exophthalmos or hypoglobus (if through the orbital roof), as a soft tissue mass in the nasal cavity, or as soft tissue opacification of the frontal and ethmoid sinuses on plain radiographs.

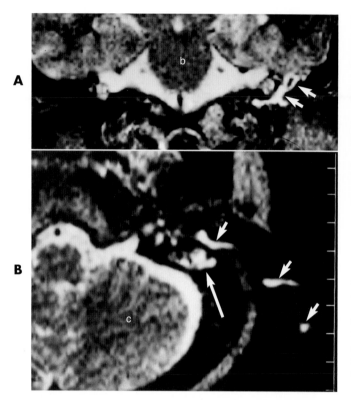

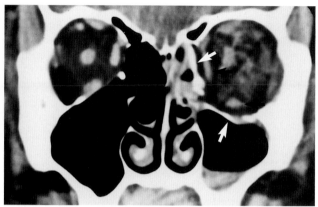

FIGURE 5-46 Coronal computed tomogram of the orbits in a patient who sustained blowout fractures and intraorbital hemorrhage (left/right orientation is reversed). Notice the fluid level in the maxillary antrum and opacification of the ethmoidal air cells on the affected side. There are medial wall, and orbital floor blowout fractures *(white arrows)*. There is a patchy increase in density within the orbital fat caused by widespread hemorrhage and edema. The inferior and medial rectus muscles are displaced downward *(black arrows)* on the affected side compared with the normal side, and there is apparent elongation of the cross-sectional image of the medial rectus. These changes are caused by septal tethering.

FIGURE 5-45 Magnetic resonance image showing a cerebrospinal fluid (CSF) leak. T2-weighted coronal **(A)** and axial **(B)** reconstructions. **A,** High-signal (white) CSF is seen leaking through a dural tear in the tegmen on the coronal study. The CSF fills the middle ear cavity *(white arrows)*, surrounding the ossicles *(black signal void)*. **B,** CSF is seen in the mastoid air cells *(long arrow)*, in the middle ear cavity *(large short arrow)*, and escaping through the tympanic membrane to pool in the scaphoid fossa of the pinna and drip off the helix margin *(small short arrows)*. (b = brain stem, c = cerebellum)

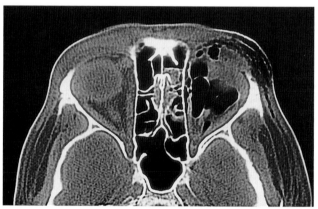

FIGURE 5-47 Axial computed tomogram in a patient with tension pneumo-orbitism. There is extensive air in the postseptal space as well as the preseptal space. *(Courtesy of P. Ayliffe, University College Hospital, London.)*

COMPARTMENT SYNDROMES

Acute Compartment Syndromes

The acute compartment syndromes comprise acute retrobulbar hemorrhage and tension pneumo-orbitism. Some degree of retrobulbar hemorrhage is common in orbital trauma and is recognizable on CT imaging as patchy areas of increased attenuation (Fig. 5-46). Most of these collections probably decompress, either because of the increased orbital capacity that occurs with coexistent blowout injury or through breaches into the sinuses. In other cases, hemorrhage is too small to be of significance to vision. Cadaver experiments in the young show that the orbital septum can withstand pressures between 70 and 100 mm Hg (rarely as high as 120 mm Hg) before rupture. In the elderly, the septum is weaker, and as little as 10 to 15 mm Hg of pressure may be enough to cause rupture.[38] Nose blowing can cause intranasal pressures as high as 114 mm Hg. If there is a wall defect in the orbit, air can be transmitted into the orbit at these high pressures, and with a valve mechanism, the air can remain trapped there. Similarly, bleeding into the orbit can produce high pressures. Retinal vessels and the optic nerve cannot withstand pressures of 65 to 70 mm Hg for long, and blindness may ensue. Higher pressures also cause central retinal artery occlusion, with irreversible damage.

The hemorrhage or air in such circumstances may be retrobulbar and within the fat or subperiosteal. Subperiosteal hemorrhage is more common in the young and is most often situated at the orbital roof. It is usually less of a problem, because the subperiosteal space is continuous with the preseptal space, and it becomes a problem only if the collection is very large or is directly compressing the optic nerve.

The cardinal clinical signs of acute retrobulbar hemorrhage causing a compartment syndrome are pain, progression of increasing proptosis, and decreasing visual acuity (leading to blindness). Signs indicating that active treatment is required are decreasing visual acuity and loss or impairment of the afferent pupillary reflex.

Tension pneumo-orbitism is exceedingly rare, but it manifests with clinical findings that are very similar to those of acute retrobulbar hemorrhage (Fig. 5-47). Preseptal air is never vision threatening. Air behind the globe is almost always innocuous and self-limited, with most of the intraorbital air resorbing within a few days to 1 week. However, there are enough cases in the literature to warrant a more cautious attitude.

Hunts et al.[39] suggested classifying orbital emphysema into four groups:

- Stage I: No proptosis/dystopia, no loss of vision, no increase in intraocular pressure, no central retinal artery occlusion
- Stage II: As in stage I, except proptosis/dystopia is present
- Stage III: Proptosis/dystopia is present, there is loss of vision, and there is a possible rise in intraocular pressure; no central retinal artery occlusion
- Stage IV: All of the above signs are positive, including central retinal artery occlusion

They suggested imaging as follows.

Stage I is common, and no special imaging is required; it is recognized radiologically. Stage II requires CT to rule out other intraorbital lesions. Stage III requires emergency CT, if available, to localize air and allow needle aspiration. Stage IV (suggested by no light perception) requires rapid orbital decompression, which should not be delayed by acquiring further images. However, the use of CT in stage III with loss of vision is debatable in this system.

The onset of blindness in acute compartment syndromes can be extremely rapid. Although these conditions are identifiable on CT, as a general rule no imaging should take place, because it merely prolongs the time to treatment and risks the blindness becoming permanent. Such cases require either immediate needle aspiration (if air is the cause) or a lateral cantholysis and canthotomy under local anesthesia in the emergency department. Only if these measures are unhelpful should CT be considered (to identify and locate the blood or air).

Chronic Compartment Syndromes

Chronic compartment syndromes occur very slowly, and manifestation may be delayed. They include hematocysts, posttraumatic cholesterol cysts, chronic abscess formation around foreign bodies, CSF cysts, meningoceles, encephaloceles, and posttraumatic frontal sinus mucoceles. Most are distinctly rare. They almost invariably cause dystopia—usually proptosis, sometimes hypoglobus, and occasionally other or mixed forms. They may also cause diplopia. When a chronic compartment syndrome is associated with a breach in the orbital roof, there may be a pulsating exophthalmos, which needs to be differentiated from the pulsating exophthalmos of a posttraumatic caroticocavernous fistula. CT is the usual method of investigation and is satisfactory; however, if it is not otherwise precluded, MRI is now the imaging modality of choice.

ENOPHTHALMOS

That posttraumatic enophthalmos (Fig. 5-48) is caused by orbital volume expansion has been repeatedly confirmed by CT imaging. Whitehouse et al.[40] attempted to predict the final degree of enophthalmos using CT to measure orbital

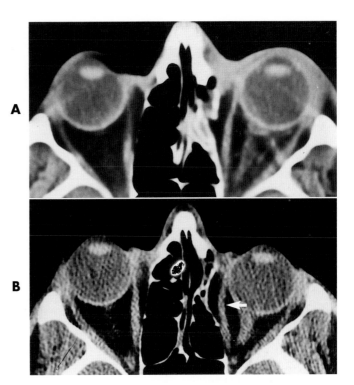

FIGURE 5-48 Orbital enlargement leading to enophthalmos. **A,** Axial computed tomogram (CT) with medial wall blowout fracture. Patchy hemorrhage in the orbital fat is not as obvious as on the coronal image. There is preseptal swelling and very slight proptosis. **B,** Axial CT obtained as part of a 3-D volumetric study 9 months after injury. Notice again the medial wall displacement. The edema and hemorrhage have resolved, and the patient has become slightly enophthalmic. The medial rectus muscle on the affected side appears slack (arrow) when compared with the opposite side.

volume. In 11 patients scanned more than 20 days after injury and 25 patients scanned within 20 days of injury, enophthalmos was less marked than would be predicted from orbital volume expansion when enophthalmus was measured within 20 days (due, no doubt, to hemorrhage and edema), but after 20 days, resolution of edema and hemorrhage permitted a good correlation between orbital volume expansion and the degree of enophthalmos, each 1 mL of increase in orbital volume corresponding to 0.8 mm enophthalmos. The authors suggested that orbital volume can be measured early by CT and that this will allow prediction of the expected final degree of enophthalmos, leading to appropriate early surgery.

In some patients, detailed imaging is not needed, other than that demanded to evaluate additional problems (e.g., diplopia) and to provide information about the integrity of the medial wall. However, many patients require volume-changing surgery. Detailed preoperative assessment of such cases is best provided by 3-D CT volumetric analysis, ideally with the use of a spiral (helical) technique. Volume changes can then be measured and their location identified, and models can be generated with the use of computerized milling, allowing more accurate placement and volume of implant material.

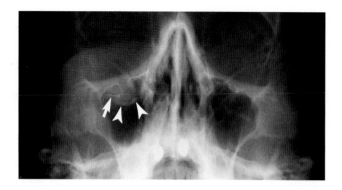

FIGURE 5-49 Blowout fracture of the right orbital floor seen on an occipitomental projection. Notice the soft tissue herniation *(arrowheads)* and displaced bone fragments *(arrow)*. Soft tissue swelling of the cheek is also present.

BLOWOUT AND BLOW-IN FRACTURES

Blowout Fractures

In patients with suspected blowout fractures (Fig. 5-49; see Figs. 5-2, 5-10, 5-46, and 5-48), three main questions have to be addressed by imaging:

1. Is a fracture present?
2. What is its effect?
3. If present, how extensive (how far posterior) is it?

Imaging in the initial stages has little part to play in the direct investigation of these disorders. In an article on the role of plain radiography in the management of suspected orbital blowout fractures, 100 consecutive patients were reviewed.[41] The plain films made no difference to patient management, the decision to operate being guided exclusively by clinical criteria. It was recommended that (1) patients in whom a competent clinician finds no direct evidence of an orbital fracture (orbital emphysema, enophthalmos, decreased infraorbital sensation, deformity, pseudoptosis, or certain types of eye movement disturbance) should not undergo plain radiography; (2) patients with minor degrees of these signs and symptoms should be given a follow-up clinical appointment, a request form and instructions to present for CT imaging after a given interval, or a delayed appointment for CT with the appointment being cancelled or the form torn up if the symptoms improve over a period to be determined by the clinician; and finally (3) patients who are found to have 3 mm or more of enophthalmos or diplopia (or both) strongly suggestive of orbital tissue entrapment or prolapse and those who have signs of a major or symptomatic fracture should be directly referred for CT. The authors made the point that all patients with diplopia should have formal orthoptic assessment.

In the adult, most small orbital floor blowout fractures are rather posteriorly situated, in the thinnest portion of the orbital floor, medial to the infraorbital groove and anterior to the inferior orbital fissure. An important aspect of imaging is the delineation of the posterior extent of the fracture. In one series, 95% of patients with diplopia persisting 6 months postoperatively had fractures extending more than 2 cm posterior to the orbital rim. The risk of such postoperative

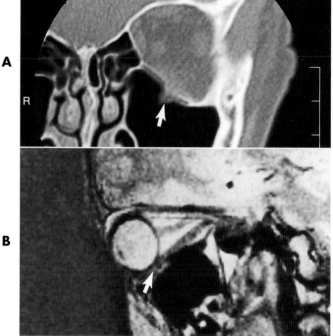

FIGURE 5-50 Tiny blowout fracture in a child. **A,** Coronal computed tomogram showing a tiny amount of soft tissue below the orbital floor *(arrow)*. No fracture can be reliably identified. **B,** Sagittal magnetic resonance image (STIR setting) showing high signal crossing the orbital floor *(arrow)*. At surgery, a minute (5-mm), undisplaced linear fracture was identified tethering the orbital septal apparatus.

diplopia was even greater in such cases than in patients with combined medial and floor injury.[42]

Large blowout (hammock-type) fractures, whether pure or impure (i.e., involving the orbital rim), are less likely to cause problems with orbital tissue tethering than the smaller ones (Fig. 5-50). In children and young adults, smaller fractures, particularly of the trapdoor type, are more common. Because of the greater elasticity of bone, they can be of greater clinical importance, despite being small, because incarceration and strangulation of even small amounts of prolapsed orbital tissue (not necessarily muscle) causes severe limitation in eye movement.

de Man et al.[43] recommended surgery as soon as possible in such cases. They described 15 patients younger than 15 years of age, almost all of whom had linear, closed trapdoor fractures, different from the open trapdoor or hammock-type fractures seen in older patients. These children had unequivocal forced duction tests, did not improve with conservative management, and required early surgery. Anderson and Poole,[44] in discussing two patients younger than 8 years old, emphasized the immature morphology of the antrum and orbit but pointed out that this did not prevent escape of orbital contents. Using logistic regression, Koltai et al.[45] demonstrated that the age at which the probability of lower orbital fracture exceeded that of orbital roof fracture was 7.1 years, noting that very young patients were more likely to have a roof fracture. In 1999, Cope et al.[46] reported on 45 patients and commented that such cases of floor fracture were especially rare before 8 years of age; children up to the age of 9 years were more likely to have small defects in the anterior orbital floor, which were of a linear trapdoor type, and more than half of these patients had persistent diplopia. From the age of 13 to 15 years, the fractures were more likely to be of an open-door type, and fewer than one third of the patients had persistent diplopia.

In 1998, Jordan et al.[47] pointed out that young patients may not exhibit all the usual signs. They described 20 patients who had no ecchymosis or edema but had marked motility restriction in up and down gaze. They termed this condition the *white-eyed* blowout fracture. In these patients, there was very minimal evidence of floor disruption on imaging, with CT showing a small crack in the floor or a small trapdoor defect with little bone displacement; some patients had a very small degree of tissue hematoma (teardrop sign). In this group, those having a 2- to 3-week wait for surgery had slower, and in some cases incomplete, resolution of gaze restriction. The authors, therefore, also recommended that surgery be done early, within 2 to 4 days after the injury.

Although plain films should not be requested to assess blowout fractures, it is reasonable to obtain plain radiographs in patients with clinically suspected orbital rim fractures, and this may reveal a blowout fracture (see Figs. 5-2 and 5-29). Although some authors claim a high degree of accuracy in diagnosing orbital floor blowout fractures with the use of plain radiography,[48] reports vary considerably. Furthermore, in most patients, diplopia resolves without intervention, not being caused by tethering. Selection for imaging, therefore, is based on clinical criteria and, in adults, on the evolution of signs and symptoms. In any event, few surgeons would be happy operating without the additional information available from CT.

Both CT and MRI may be used to address the questions posed at the beginning of this section. CT has the advantage of delineating the skeletal tissues more effectively than MRI, and in any event, it is frequently indicated for other concomitant facial injury outside the orbit. MRI, on the other hand, is more sensitive in assessing the soft tissue components, such as the orbital fat and its displacement; also, alternative imaging planes are easier to achieve with MRI.

CT imaging (Fig. 5-51; see Figs. 5-9, 5-46, and 5-50) is best done in the coronal position, because this displays the floor (where most injuries occur) better than the axial position, and it displays the medial wall as well as the axial position does. Coronal imaging can be done with the patient prone and the neck extended, supine with hyperflexion of the neck, supine with extension of the neck into the "hanging head" position, or by reconstruction from axial imaging. The first two methods are preferable because they place antral blood and fluid inferiorly, allowing more accurate assessment of soft tissue changes in the upper antrum.

All of the signs seen on plain radiographs may be evident on CT, and in addition, further important information is acquired regarding the position of the extraocular muscles relative to the fracture and the presence of hemorrhage and bone spicules. The coronal scans alone may provide adequate information, but direct sagittal images or sagittal reconstructions, in selected cases, may display the posterior extent of an orbital floor fracture and its relationship to the inferior rectus in a more readily appreciated way. On CT images, muscle can be difficult to see if there is much surrounding edema and

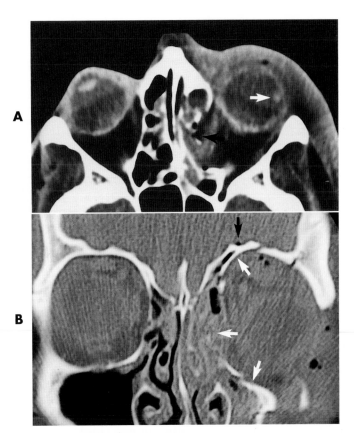

FIGURE 5-51   Orbital blowout fractures. **A,** Axial computed tomographic (CT) image showing preseptal soft tissue swelling with vitreal hemorrhage *(white arrow),* and a medial, orbital wall blowout fracture *(black arrow).* **B,** Coronal CT image of the same patient. There are further blowout fractures of the orbital roof and floor. Notice the opaque maxillary antrum and ethmoidal air cells and the air in the cranium *(black arrow),* orbit, and soft tissues. There are fractures of the medial orbital wall and the orbital floor with depression of these walls *(white arrows).* The base of the external angular process of the frontal bone and the roof of the orbit are fractured with cranial displacement of the medial segment of the roof. The orbital volume increase is obvious.

hemorrhage, but displacement can sometimes be inferred by the absence of a muscle from its usual position.

Blow-In Fractures

Blow-in fractures are common at the orbital roof. A high index of suspicion should be entertained, especially in children or in the presence of ptosis, which is evidence of restriction to the superior rectus muscle or hematoma confined to the upper lid. Bone fragments may involve not only the superior rectus and levator muscles but also the superior division of the oculomotor nerve. CSF may leak, and meningoceles and encephaloceles may cause proptosis (sometimes pulsating). Blow-in fractures also occur at the orbital floor due to buckling, again especially in children, and also at the medial wall in association with severe naso-orbitoethmoidal fractures (Fig. 5-52). If roof and floor blow-in fractures are suspected, coronal CT is the best projection; with medial wall fractures, axial or coronal CT is satisfactory.

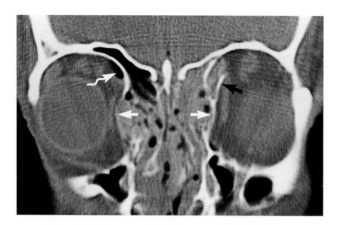

FIGURE 5-52 Blow-in fractures seen on a computed tomographic image of a patient who sustained a severe naso-orbitoethmoidal fracture. Both medial orbital walls have become displaced laterally, bulging into the orbital cavities *(white arrows)* as a result of the severe concertina effect of the primary injury. Notice the air in the right orbit *(curved arrow)*. There is a bone fragment in the left orbit which has displaced below the superior oblique muscle *(black arrow)*.

RADIOGRAPHY OF FACIAL INJURIES

DEFINITIONS

Orbitomeatal Baseline (Radiographic Baseline, Tragocanthal Line, Canthomeatal Line)

This line passes from the outer canthus of the eye to the middle of the external auditory meatus. The line projected forward passes through the nasion (which is helpful when the canthus reference point is uncertain). It is this line that is most often used in facial radiography.

Anthropological Baseline (Anatomical Baseline, Reid's Baseline, Line of Frankfurter)

This line passes from the infraorbital point to the superior border of the external auditory meatus. The orbitomeatal and anthropological baselines are approximately 10 to 12 degrees from each other.

Glabellomeatal Line

This line passes from the center of the external auditory meatus to the center of the glabella and makes an angle of about 15 degrees to the orbitomeatal line.

Sagittal Plane

A sagittal plane is any plane parallel to the median sagittal plane. The median sagittal plane is a vertical plane that divides the skull into left and right halves.

Coronal Plane

A coronal plane is any plane parallel to the meatal (or auricular) plane. The meatal plane is perpendicular to the anthropological baseline and passes through the external auditory meati.

Tube Angulation versus Orbitomeatal Line Elevation

Neck extension may be impossible because of concurrent spinal injury or preexisting disease (e.g., osteoarthrosis,

ankylosis) or because of a severe upper dorsal kyphosis or gibbus deformity. In such patients, the inability to elevate the orbitomeatal baseline can be compensated by an equivalent caudal tilt of the central ray. Severe degrees of tube tilt produce greater distortion, but this is usually acceptable.

Posteroanterior versus Anteroposterior

This terminology refers to the direction of the path taken by the x-ray beam. In the posteroanterior (PA) projection, the tube is posterior to the patient and the beam passes from back to front; in the anteroposterior (AP) projection, the reverse is true. In cases of facial trauma, frontal films should *always* be done in the PA projection, *never* the AP.

In the AP projection, on both Caldwell's or other occipitofrontal views, the lateral orbital margins can be superimposed over (and obscured by) the parietal and temporal bones, when these latter bones are seen in tangent. Similarly, on the AP Waters' and occipitomental group of views, including the occipitomental 30-degree view, both the lateral orbital margins and the zygomatic arches can be superimposed over the margins of the calvaria. Furthermore, there is a significantly higher radiation dose to the lens of the eye with AP than with PA projections. Finally, geometric sharpness is greatest in those anatomical parts closest to the film, which in a PA projection would be the face.

Imaging should always be delayed until the patient can cooperate with the radiographer to provide PA views.

PROJECTIONS FOR THE MIDDLE AND UPPER THIRDS OF THE FACE

The Occipitofrontal 15- to 20-Degree (Caldwell's) Projection

Caldwell's view is equivalent to an elevation of 15 to 20 degrees (standard, 17 degrees) in the orbitomeatal baseline, the glabellomeatal line used by Caldwell and the orbitomeatal line being about 8 degrees apart from one another. This view projects the petrous bones over the lower one quarter to one third of the orbit. It should be remembered that this view was designed for sinus imaging rather than trauma. For this reason, a modification is recommended: the occipitofrontal 25-degree projection or modified Caldwell's view.

The Occipitofrontal 25-Degree (Modified Caldwell's) Projection

With the orbitomeatal baseline horizontal (i.e., perpendicular to the film plane), the central ray is angled 25 degrees caudad, with a possible variation in some individuals of 26 or 27 degrees. The advantage of this view is that it provides good visualization of the orbital floor (projecting the petrous bones just below the orbit).

Waters' Projection

This projection was described by Waters and Waldron as a modification of the occipitofrontal positions and is designed to obtain a better view of the maxillary antra while retaining a view of the frontal and ethmoidal sinuses. The orbitomeatal baseline elevation (or tube depression) should be 37 degrees. This tilt will usually project the petrous bone over the inferior portion of the antra, obscuring it. Occasionally, the same problem occurs with the true occipitomental position

(45-degree elevation), and for this reason a modification is preferred: the occipitomental 10-degree projection.

The Occipitomental 10-Degree Projection

The orbitomeatal baseline is elevated 45 degrees, and the central ray is angled 10 degrees caudad and centered to the lower orbital margin. This projection provides a margin of safety, ensuring that the petrous bones are projected below the maxillary antra so that the whole of the lateral sinus wall is clear.

It is important in this and the occipitomental 30-degree projection to avoid any rotation of the patient from the sagittal plane.

The Occipitomental 30-Degree Projection

The orbitomeatal baseline is elevated 45 degrees, and the tube is angled 30 degrees caudad, centering to the lower orbital margins. This projection provides a superior view of the malar arches and the anterior aspect of the inferior orbital margins, allowing assessment of displacement of these structures. It is used in preference to the submentovertical projection for assessing the arches.

In the occipitomental 10- and 30-degree projections, it is very important not to allow any rotation of the patient from the sagittal plane. In some individuals, the arches can project very close to the image of the inner table of the lateral calvaria. If the latter is seen in tangent, slight rotation will superimpose one arch over the calvaria, diminishing the clarity with which the arch is seen.

The Occipitomental Projection View with Only 40 Degrees of Elevation of the Orbitomeatal Baseline

This is the best view to diagnose orbital blowout fracture on a plain film. Centering is to the inferior orbital margin. However, with CT scanning available, this projection should rarely be necessary.

The Lateral Projection

In the lateral projection, the median sagittal plane is parallel to the film plane and the central ray is perpendicular to the film plane. By convention, it is obtained as a left lateral view (i.e., the left side of the patient is closest to the film), but this is not essential in acute trauma work. Centering should be to the body of the zygoma, about 2.5 cm below the outer canthus of the eye.

The Lateral Soft Tissue Projection

This view provides useful information about foreign bodies, such as windshield glass. It also gives a good view of the nasal bones, the nasal plates of the frontal processes of the maxilla, and the nasal spine of the maxilla. However, it is not required for assessing isolated simple nasal trauma, which is better investigated clinically.

The Upper Occlusal Projection

An occlusal film is placed in the mouth as far back as possible. Positioning is more likely to be successful and gagging overcome if the equipment and patient position are set up beforehand, the patient is asked to swallow hard just before insertion of the film, and the film is placed gently, avoiding contact with the tongue and oral mucosa until the last moment. The central

ray is directed down 45 degrees to the film plane, centering to the anterior nasal spine. This view is occasionally useful to assess the palate, although palatal fractures are usually either clinically obvious or best demonstrated by CT scanning.

PROJECTIONS FOR THE LOWER THIRD OF THE FACE

Posteroanterior Projection of the Mandible

The PA mandible projection is standard and is performed as part of most mandibular trauma series, whether it be two views (PA mandible and OPG), three views (PA mandible and two lateral obliques) or five views (PA mandible, two rotated PA views, and two lateral obliques). For this projection, the patient faces the film cassette. The median sagittal plane and the orbitomeatal plane are perpendicular to the film plane. Centering is to the midpoint of the rami, with the central beam perpendicular to the cassette.

Lateral Oblique Group

The standard projection here is the 30-degree lateral oblique. For this, the patient's sagittal plane is parallel to the film plane, and the central ray is angled 30 degrees cranially, centered to the mandibular angle closest to the film. The head should be extended to throw the image of the mandible off the cervical spine. If more of the body of the mandible needs to be seen, the patient can be rotated so that the face is aimed toward the film cassette, to bring the body of the mandible parallel to the cassette. Some workers use a slightly higher angle, 35 to 40 degrees, for the central ray if the ramus is the main area of interest. An alternative to tube tilt is the use of an angle board.

Rotated Posteroanterior Mandible Projection

This projection is rarely used except when panoramic tomography is not available. The patient is turned from the PA position away from the parasymphyseal region of interest by 8 to 10 degrees, dropping the chin toward the cassette and centering 2.5 cm behind the opposite angle at the level of the midpoint of the rami, with the central beam perpendicular to the film plane.

Lower Occlusal Projection

An occlusal film is placed in the mouth, and a dental x-ray unit is used to expose the film from below the mandible. This projection is occasionally useful in the symphysis region, where both panoramic and PA mandible projections may be suboptimal.

Extraoral Submental Projection (Superoinferior Symphysis Projection)

This projection can be helpful in patients who will not be able to tolerate an occlusal film in the mouth. The film is placed underneath the chin and exposed from above with a dental x-ray unit.

Reverse Towne's Projection (Haas Position, Nuchofrontal Position)

This projection is a reverse of the half-axial or Towne's projection. The patient faces the cassette with both the median sagittal plane and the orbitomeatal line perpendicular to the film plane. The central ray is then directed at an angle of 30 degrees upward, centering to about 4 cm above the superior orbital margins. It is seldom that an injury is seen on this view that cannot be seen with careful inspection on the PA mandible view.

Frontal Open-Mouth Projection

The PA mandible projection taken with the mouth open undoubtedly gives a good view of the condyle. However, most patients with significant trauma have trismus and are reluctant to open the mouth far enough for this view to be useful. The central ray is angled up 12 degrees, centering to the nasion with the mouth open. Like the reverse Towne's view, and for the same reasons, this view should rarely be needed.

Panoramic Radiography

There are two forms of panoramic radiography: an intraoral and an extraoral technique. The intraoral technique, in which the tube and film are static, is seldom used for trauma and is not widely available. In the extraoral form, the tube and the film move relative to the patient to provide an image of a curved plane, usually the mandible (OPG). The extraoral panoramic systems thus provide a modified tomographic technique that takes into account the curvature of the mandible. The image layer is made to conform with the shape of the mandible, and objects outside the image layer are blurred.

Great care must be taken in positioning, because the image plane is thin, and even slight errors in positioning can result in parts of the mandible being outside the image plane and therefore blurred. This may, however, be unavoidable if there are grossly displaced fracture fragments.

Panoramic Zonography

Based on the well-established methods of panoramic radiography used for examination of the mandible, the panoramic principle has been extended to a variety of other image layer tracks to enable examination of the middle third of the face, the temporal bone, and the upper cervical spine and to provide additional imaging of the temporomandibular joints. A further advantage of this equipment is the ability to perform the examinations, including standard panoramic views of the mandible, on a supine patient.

ACKNOWLEDGMENTS

The authors would like to acknowledge the contribution of Dr. N. Bowley, DMRD, FRCR, who wrote the first edition of this chapter.

REFERENCES

1. International Commission on Radiological Protection (ICRP): Recommendation of the International Commission on Radiological Protection. Publication 103. *Ann ICRP* 37:1-332, 2007.
2. Mischkowski RA, Zinser MJ, Ritter L, et al: Intraoperative navigation in the maxillofacial area based on 3D imaging obtained by a cone-beam device. *Int J Oral Maxillofac Surg* 36:687-694, 2007.
3. Conebeam CT of the head and neck. Part 2. Clinical applications. *AJNR Am J Neuroradiol* 30:1285-1292, 2009.
4. Gupta R, Grasruck M, Suess C, et al: Ultra-high resolution flat-panel volume CT: fundamental principles, design architecture, and system characterization. *Eur Radiol* 16:1191-1205, 2006. Epub March 10, 2006.
5. Johnson DH: CT of maxillo-facial trauma. *Radiol Clin North Am* 22:131-144, 1984.
6. *Making best use of clinical radiology services (MBUR)*, ed 6, London, 2007, Royal College of Radiologists.
7. Heiskanen O, Marttila I, Valtonen S: Prognosis of depressed skull fracture. *Acta Chir Scand* 139:605-608, 1973.
8. McAuley CE, Sherman HF, Jones LM, et al: The "missed injury": a prospective evaluation of delayed diagnosis in blunt multisystem trauma. *J Trauma* 22:948, 1992.
9. Velmahos GC, Theodorou D, Tatevossian R, et al: Radiographic cervical spine evaluation in the alert asymptomatic blunt trauma victim: much ado about nothing? *J Trauma* 40:768-774, 1996.
10. Stiell IG, Wells GA, Vandemheen KL, et al: The Canadian C-spine rule for radiography in alert and stable trauma patients. *JAMA* 286:1841-1848, 2001.
11. Schenarts PJ, Diaz J, Kaiser C, et al: Prospective comparison of admission computed tomographic scan and plain films of the upper cervical spine in trauma patients with altered mental status. *J Trauma* 51:663-668, discussion 668-669, 2001.
12. Tins BJ, Cassar-Pullicino VN: Imaging of cervical spine injuries: review and outlook. *Clin Radiol* 59:865-880, 2004.
13. Schroder RJ, Vogl T, Hidajit N, et al: Comparison of the diagnostic value of CT and MRI in injuries of the cervical vertebrae. *Aktuelle Radiol* 5:197-202, 1995.
14. Holmes JF, Mirvis SE, Panacek EA, et al: Variability in computed tomography and magnetic resonance imaging in patients with cervical injuries. *J Trauma* 53:524-529, 2002.
15. Pang D, Wilberger JE: Spinal cord injury without radiographic abnormalities in children. *J Neurosurg* 57:114-129, 1982.
16. Hendey GW, Wolfson AB, Mower WR, et al: Spinal cord injury without radiographical abnormality: results of the National Emergency X-Radiography Utilization Study in blunt cervical trauma. *J Trauma* 53:1-4, 2002.
17. Rao PM, Ivatury RR, Sharma P, et al: Cervical vascular injuries: a trauma center experience. *Surgery* 114:527-531, 1993.
18. Woo K, Magner DP, Wilson MT, et al: CT angiography in penetrating neck trauma reduces the need for operative neck exploration. *Am Surg* 71:754-758, 2005.
19. Bell RB, Osborn T, Dierks EJ, et al: Management of penetrating neck injuries: a new paradigm for civilian trauma. *J Oral Maxillofac Surg* 65:691-705, 2007.
20. Múnera F, Soto JA, Palacia DM, et al: Penetrating neck injuries: helical CT angiography for initial evaluation. *Radiology* 224:366-372, 2002.
21. Dorey SE, Gillespie IH, Barton F, et al: Magnetic resonance image changes following optic nerve trauma from peribulbar anaesthetic. *Br J Ophthalmol* 82:584, 1998.
22. McGrigor DB, Campbell W: The radiology of war injuries. Part VI. Wounds of the face and jaw. *Br J Radiol* 23:685-696, 1950.
23. Trapnell DH: Diagnostic radiography. In Rowe NL, Williams JLI, editors: *Maxillofacial injuries*, Edinburgh, 1985, Churchill Livingstone.
24. Dolan KD, Jacoby CG: Facial fractures. *Semin Roentgenol* 13:37-51, 1978.
25. DelBalso AM, Hall RE, Margarone JE: Radiographic evaluation of maxillofacial trauma. In DelBalso AM, editor: *Maxillofacial imaging*, Philadelphia, 1990, Saunders.
26. Valvassori GE, Hord GE: Traumatic sinus disease. *Semin Roentgenol* 3:160-171, 1968.
27. Le Fort R: Étude experimentale sur les fractures de la machoire supérieure. *Rev Chir* 23:208-227, 360-379, 479-507, 1901.
28. Fry WK, Shepherd PR, McLeod AC, et al: *The dental treatment of maxillofacial injuries*, Oxford, 1942, Blackwell Scientific.
29. Gentry LR, Manor WF, Turski PA, et al: High resolution computed tomographic analysis of facial struts in trauma. 1. Normal anatomy. *Am J Roentgenol* 140:523-532, 1983.
30. Pyhtinen J, Ilkko E, Lähde S: Wooden foreign bodies in CT: case reports and experimental studies. *Acta Radiol* 36:148-151, 1995.
31. LoBue TD, Deutsch TA, Lobick J, et al: Detection and localization of nonmetallic intraocular foreign bodies by magnetic resonance imaging. *Arch Ophthalmol* 106:260-261, 1988.
32. Anderson RL, Panje WR, Gross CE: Optic nerve blindness following blunt forehead trauma. *Ophthalmology* 89:445-455, 1982.
33. Lloyd MNH, Kimber PM, Burrows EH: Post-traumatic cerebrospinal fluid rhinorrhoea: modern high-definition computed tomography is all that is required for the effective demonstration of the site of leakage. *Clin Radiol* 49:100-103, 1994.
34. el Gammal T, Brooks BS: MR cisternography: initial experience in 41 cases. *AJNR Am J Neuroradiol* 15:1647-1656, 1994.
35. El Jamel MS, Pidgeon CN, Toland J, et al: MRI cisternography and the localization of CSF fistulae. *Br J Neurosurg* 8:433-437, 1994.
36. Hegarty SE, Millar JS: MRI in the localization of CSF fistulae: is it of any value? *Clin Radiol* 52:768-770, 1997.
37. Stafford-Johnson DB, Brennan P, Toland J, et al: Magnetic resonance imaging in the evaluation of cerebrospinal fluid fistulae. *Clin Radiol* 51:837-841, 1996.
38. Muhammad JK, Simpson MT: Orbital emphysema and the medial orbital wall: a review of the literature with particular reference to that associated with indirect trauma and possible blindness. *J Craniomaxillofac Surg* 24:245-250, 1996.
39. Hunts JH, Patrinley JR, Holds JB, et al: Orbital emphysema: staging and acute management. *Ophthalmology* 101:960-966, 1994.

40. Whitehouse RW, Batterbury M, Jackson A, et al: Prediction of enophthalmos by computed tomography after "blow-out" orbital fracture. *Br J Ophthalmol* 78:618-620, 1994.

41. Bhattacharya J, Moseley IF, Fells P: The role of plain radiography in the management of suspected orbital blow-out fractures. *Br J Radiol* 70:29-33, 1997.

42. Biesman BS, Hornblass A, Lisman R, et al: Diplopia after surgical repair of orbital floor fractures. *Ophthal Plast Reconstr Surg* 12:9-16, 1996.

43. de Man K, Wijngaarde R, Hes T, et al: Influence of age on the management of blow-out fractures of the orbital floor. *Int J Oral Maxillofac Surg* 20:330-336, 1991.

44. Anderson PJ, Poole MD: Orbital floor fractures in young children. *J Craniomaxillofac Surg* 23:151-154, 1995.

45. Koltai PJ, Amjad I, Meyer D, et al: Orbital fractures in children. *Arch Otolaryngol Head Neck Surg* 121:1375-1379, 1995.

46. Cope MR, Moos KF, Speculand B: Does diplopia persist after blow-out fractures of the orbital floor in children? *Br J Oral Maxillofac Surg* 37:46-51, 1999.

47. Jordan DR, Allen LH, White J, et al: Intervention within days for some orbital floor fractures: the white-eyed blowout. *Ophthal Plast Reconstr Surg* 14:379-390, 1998.

48. Kim SH, Ahn KJ, Lea JM, et al: The usefulness of orbital lines in detecting blow-out fracture on plain radiography. *Br J Radiol* 73:1265-1269, 2000.

CHAPTER 6

Principles of Facial Soft Tissue Injury Repair

Barry L. Eppley

Injuries to the face commonly result in a significant psychological response that is unparalleled by the response to injury elsewhere on the body, especially if it is the result of interpersonal violence. The importance of facial appearance in modern society and its implication in vocational and social status makes changes to facial features, particularly by injury, an emotionally charged occurrence. Patients fear facial disfigurement and scars and risk loss of their self-esteem. Surgical repair of facial injuries is understandably associated with high expectations of a complete return to a normal facial appearance. Often the final result, fairly or unfairly, is judged to be a reflection of the surgeon's skill and ability.

In addition to the obvious skin and mucosal involvement, facial trauma frequently includes injury to the deeper hard and soft tissue structures. Understanding the mechanism of injury and the anatomy of the region is essential for satisfactory management.

WOUND ASSESSMENT

HISTORY AND EXAMINATION

Apart from general aspects of the history that are common to all patient contacts, a complete history of the incident leading to the injury should be taken, and if not available from the patient, the details should be obtained from anyone present at the time of the incident or those in immediate attendance after. Understanding the mechanism of injury will alert the surgeon to the possibility of associated injury or contamination (e.g., bacteria, viruses, foreign bodies) and sequelae that may not otherwise be apparent. For example, when dealing with a penetrating knife wound, it is necessary to know the type of weapon, the degree of force used, and the postures of the patient and the assailant when the injury was caused to assess the degree of tissue damage and possible contamination, the depth and direction of penetration, and the possibility of involvement of deeper structures. Similarly, when the injury results from a road traffic accident, the type of accident (e.g., motorcycle, car), the position of the patient in the accident (e.g., pedestrian, driver, passenger), and the circumstances and relative speeds of the vehicles involved alert the surgeon to the possibility of associated

injury underlying the presenting facial trauma or involving other systems.

The specialized nature of facial structures demand that particular attention be paid to injuries of different facial regions. Lacerations to the brow, eyelid, nose, lip, and ear require careful assessment and treatment to avoid deformity and potential interference with function. Lacerations to the lateral face, temple, and naso-orbital regions risk injury to branches of the facial nerve and to the parotid and lacrimal ducts. Injuries to the eyelid and orbit typically require ophthalmological evaluation to establish visual status and the presence or absence of corneal damage.

The tetanus immunization status of the patient is an essential part of the general medical history. Although facial wounds often appear to be clean, the patient is still at risk and requires tetanus prophylaxis. For clean minor wounds, no treatment is necessary if the immunization status is current. If more than 10 years has elapsed since the last booster injection, tetanus toxoid should be given. All patients with contaminated wounds should receive tetanus toxoid unless they have been immunized within the past 5 years.

BIOMECHANICS

An appreciation of the concept of relaxed skin tension lines (RSTLs) of the face is relevant to treatment and outcome. In a cadaver model exposed to blunt facial trauma, the induced soft tissue lacerations parallel the cleavage lines of the face (i.e., RSTLs) and were more severe on the forehead than on the zygoma or maxilla.[1] These injuries were inherent in the biomechanical and structural property of the dermis of the skin and independent of muscle or bony attachments. It has been postulated that the direction of skin lacerations in blunt trauma occurs as a protective mechanism to minimize injury to the underlying blood supply because the vessels and collagen bundles parallel the RSTLs (Fig. 6-1). The esthetic outcome of skin injuries is partially related to their relation to the RSTLs; scars have a better prognosis if they parallel the RSTLs or are in natural skin creases. With immediate repair and if the laceration is irregular but parallels the RSTLs, it can be excised and closed as a straight line. If it runs perpendicular or oblique to the RSTL, it should be closed as it manifests because the irregularities may offer better camouflage of the resultant scar.

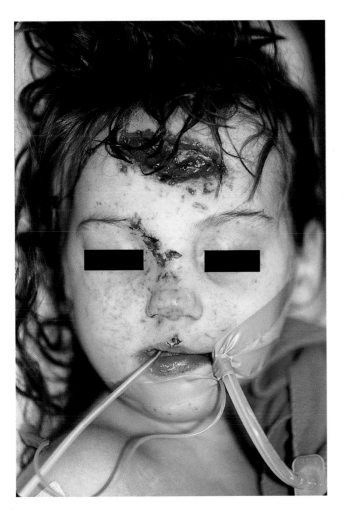

FIGURE 6-1 A 5-year-old girl's forehead impacted the windshield in a motor vehicle accident. The nose shows glass injuries, and the forehead skin separation parallels the relaxed skin tension lines.

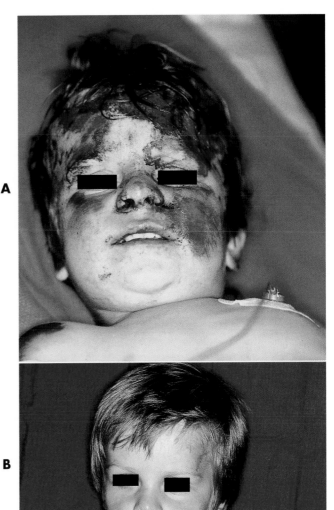

FIGURE 6-2 **A**, Four-year-old boy sustained multiple facial abrasions while falling from a moving car. **B**, With topical therapy, the superficial wounds healed completely and without scarring, as evident 3 months after the injury.

EXCLUDING FRACTURES DURING ASSESSMENT

Evaluation must exclude bone injuries. This failure can occur in busy trauma units when several specialists are involved in the patient's care and there is a desire to quickly treat the soft tissue injuries by a surgeon less familiar with hard tissue trauma.

CLASSIFICATION OF SOFT TISSUE INJURIES

Soft tissue trauma of the face may be classified according to the tissue insult (i.e., contusions, abrasions, lacerations, avulsions, and chemical or thermal burns) or the mechanism of injury (e.g., dog bite), which often involves a combination of the former elements.

Contusion

Blunt trauma to the face always results in some degree of swelling and bruising, depending on the area involved. Eyelids or lips, for example, develop a greater amount of swelling than forehead or cheek tissues. If subcutaneous vessels are ruptured, a hematoma may occur, which may or may not require primary or secondary management. Most facial contusions have no specific treatment, with the exception of ear or septal hematomas, which require immediate evacuation.

Many facial lacerations have contusions at their skin edges that require sharp débridement to minimize the long-term risks of adverse scarring, pigmented changes, and underlying soft tissue atrophy. Red dermal bleeding is the hallmark of viable skin, and these tissues usually should not be débrided.

Abrasion

Most abrasions that occur on the face are superficial and involve loss of the epithelium and exposed papillary dermis. These injuries will heal quite rapidly with topical agents (Fig. 6-2). Impact of the face against particulate surfaces (e.g., asphalt, gravel) or exposure to explosive charges (e.g., powder burns from gunshots) usually results in the implantation of foreign material. Frictional contact with otherwise benign

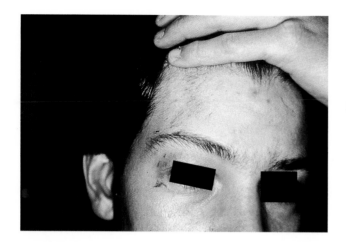

FIGURE 6-3 Traumatic tattooing that occurred from close-range discharge of a firearm and was not primarily treated.

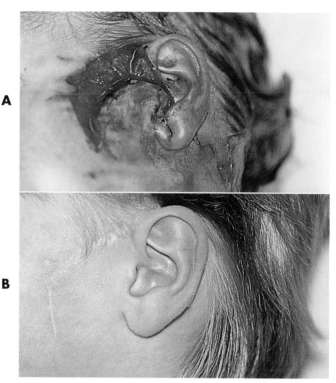

FIGURE 6-4 **A**, Laceration and preauricular skin avulsion from a dog bite in a 4-year-old boy. **B**, Scar revision cannot improve the resultant mature scar, which is shown 1 year after primary closure. Notice that the scar parallels the relaxed skin tension line and is quite narrow.

particulate matter results in dermal exposure and injury that may mimic a second- or third-degree burn, depending on the depth. If allowed to heal, the growth of new epithelium over the contamination results in the phenomenon known as *traumatic tattooing*, which leads to permanent discoloration (Fig. 6-3). Prevention requires meticulous débridement and occasionally may necessitate the use of a dermabrader. Petroleum-based liquids, such as grease and oil, can be removed with organic solvents such as acetone or ether. After adequate cleansing, the partially denuded dermis may be covered with antibiotic ointment alone or medicated nonadherent gauze dressing (e.g., Xeroform). Complete healing by re-epitheliazation occurs within 7 to 10 days, and erythema resolves within several months thereafter.

Lacerations

Facial lacerations occur as a variety of specific types, which affect the risks of scarring and eventual need for scar revision. Recognition of these forms permits modifications in the surgical repair techniques.

Sharp objects usually create wounds with clean, straight edges that are easy to repair and produce fine scars. Minimal or no débridement is necessary, and the apposition of tissues is done with a layered closure. Because sharp objects often penetrate deeper than initially perceived, careful exploration of the wound should be carried out in areas where vital structures lie underneath. Revision of linear scars often is not needed (Fig. 6-4) unless they violate the RSTL, in which case they may be improved by geometric rearrangement.

Stellate lacerations usually result from blunt injury, explosions, or crushing forces, which strike with enough force in a single area to "fracture" the surrounding tissue in noncleavage planes. Multiple flaps of skin are created, often with contused edges, around a more central area of tissue damage or loss (Fig. 6-5). The elastic recoil of the skin often gives the false perception of significant tissue loss. This type of laceration should be repaired as it is positioned, and only grossly nonviable tissue should be débrided. Despite the best initial repair, these lacerations often heal poorly, and many require secondary revision.

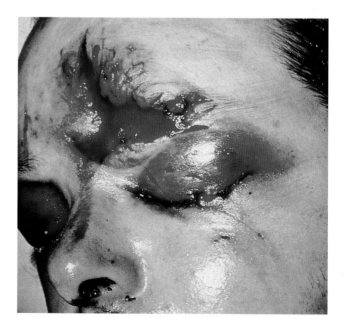

FIGURE 6-5 Direct impact of an unrestrained passenger's forehead on the dashboard in a motor vehicle accident. The significant blunt force has fractured the forehead and eyebrow tissues.

Tangential lacerations that undermine and lift up skin edges or lacerations that have a curvilinear or semicircular shape result in a trapdoor deformity. The laceration heals with a mound of tissue on its concave side due to contracture from unopposed fibrosis and from lymphatic and venous obstruction (Fig. 6-6). By creating a sharp, vertical edge on the flap side, undermining the undersurface of the side opposite to the flap, advancing it at the same level, and placing the initial suture support deep to the dermis between the flap and the surrounding tissue (see Fig. 6-6), the deformity may be averted or at least reduced.

Avulsions

Facial defects due to traumatic avulsion are relatively uncommon, occurring almost exclusively from gunshot or large, sharp-edged weapon injuries. For small defects, the surrounding tissue can be mobilized and the defect closed. The use of local random flaps or pedicle flaps should be discouraged during the initial repair, because the viability of surrounding tissues can be difficult to evaluate in the primary setting. For larger defects that are not amenable to primary closure, wet-to-dry dressings can be placed until the appropriate time for reconstruction. These dressings can be used for long periods as the zone of viability demarcates and granulation tissue develops. In more uncommon circumstances, the avulsion defect can initially be covered with a split-thickness skin graft. This allows the facial wound to heal before more complex methods of facial reconstruction with better esthetic outcome are carried out at a later time (e.g., tissue expansion, serial graft excision, local flaps) (Fig. 6-7).

Bites

Bite wounds, even on the well-vascularized face, have a significant risk of infection because of their high rate of contamination. They introduce highly infective bacterial flora, and the bite wound is often a combination of multiple types of damage, including penetrating, contusing, and avulsing injuries. Bites come from animals or humans, and each has its own distinctive bacterial content. Animal bites, particularly from dogs, are polymicrobial and include *Staphylococcus aureus*, β-hemolytic streptococci, and the anaerobes *Bacteroides* and *Fusobacterium*.[2] *Pasteurella multocida* also may be found, especially in cat bites. Human flora usually has a higher concentration of anaerobes such as *Bacteroides* and commonly contains *Staphylococcus* and α-hemolytic streptococci. Differences also exist in bite wound locations; human bites are far more prevalent on the lips, nose, and ear, whereas most animal bites are more random, involve more surface area, and are more avulsive due to the innate pull-back response of the victim.

For most wounds that are seen within 24 hours, primary treatment includes operative irrigation, limited débridement, and primary closure. With this approach, the infection risk is low, and the resultant scars are better[3] (Fig. 6-8). Only small puncture wounds are left to heal secondarily. For wounds that occurred more than 24 hours earlier or large avulsion

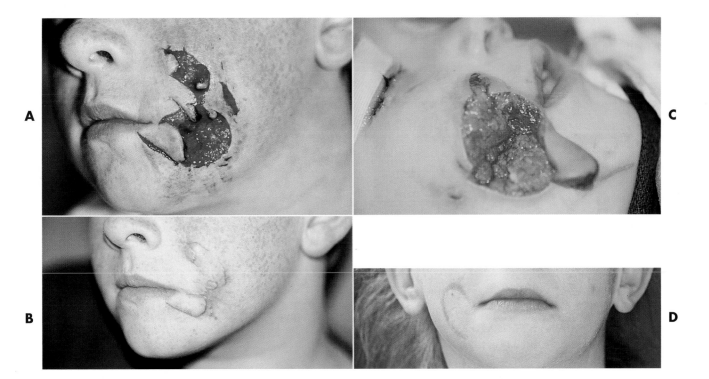

FIGURE 6-6 **A** and **B**, Semicircular-type lacerations frequently result in the classic trapdoor scar deformity. **C** and **D**, Several surgical maneuvers at the time of primary repair, such as deep suture support, same-level undermining on the side opposite the semicircular flap, and the creation of sharp vertical edges on the flap, may be helpful in its postoperative prevention. **A**, Dog bite in a 12-year-old boy. **B**, Repair with a trapdoor scar deformity 6 months postoperatively. **C**, Dog-bite flap avulsion in a 6-year-old girl. **D**, Repair without a trapdoor scar deformity 6 months postoperatively.

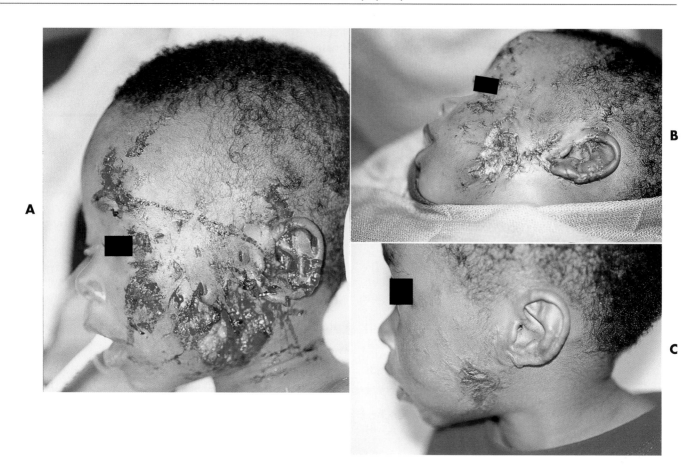

FIGURE 6-7   Facial lacerations and avulsion injury with pre-auricular tissue loss in a 4-year-old boy who was unrestrained in a motor vehicle accident. **A**, Immediately after injury. **B**, After closure of lacerations, the area of tissue loss is evident. The tissue was impossible to close primarily due to wound tension and would have resulted in significant distortion of the surrounding tissues. **C**, A split-thickness skin graft was placed for primary repair. Although it is hyperpigmented, it allowed time for the wound to heal and will be removed later by secondary tissue expansion.

injuries, closure is controversial. We prefer primary closure because the infection risk is higher and thereby hope to obtain more expeditious treatment and a better scar. Some surgeons prefer delaying closure of these wounds for up to 1 week, although whether this decreases the risk of infection is not clear. Adjunctive pharmacological treatment is essential, usually consisting of broad-spectrum (i.e., combined aerobe-anaerobic coverage) antibiotics (e.g., amoxicillin with clavulanic acid), tetanus immunization, and rabies prophylaxis as necessary.

DOCUMENTATION

Facial injuries should be documented because patients may benefit and cope better with the outcome if they are able to compare the outcome with the original injury and because the injury may at some point be the subject of a medicolegal action, and accurate recording, preferably with photographs, can facilitate the process.

Recording injuries on a handwritten facial cartoon is the most primitive method. One method of documenting facial information is the MCFONTZL classification system,[4] which represents a simplified method of recording blunt facial soft tissue injuries. The system divides the face into 12 esthetic

units (right and left in some cases) using the mnemonic MCFONTZL: *maxilla, chin, forehead, orbit, nose, temple, zygoma, lips.* The soft tissue laceration is recorded using an ASTERISK notation scheme: area (MCFONTZL esthetic unit designation), side, thickness (depth of penetration), extension (branching), relaxed skin tension conformation (directionality), index laceration (laceration with the maximal continuous skin interruption), soft tissue defect (presence or absence), and coding (current procedural terminology). The information is recorded along the rays of the asterisk symbol in a clockwise direction. However, conventional color slides or prints document the injuries in such a graphic and detailed manner that they should be the method of choice when possible. Digital photography may gradually replace conventional light photography, although it may be more prone to exploitation.

SOFT TISSUE HANDLING

OPERATIVE SETTING

The patient with facial lacerations should always be treated promptly—in an ideal world, as soon as an assessment has

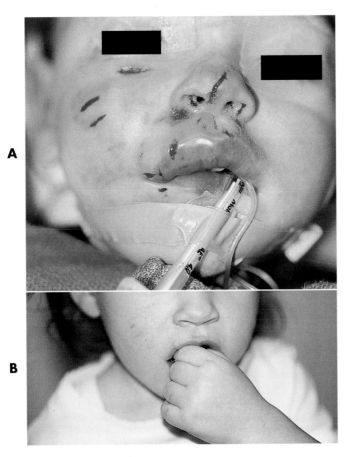

FIGURE 6-8 Almost all dog-bite injuries to the face can be primarily repaired without a significant risk of postoperative infection. **A**, Multiple small lacerations and puncture wounds from a dog bite in a 2-year-old girl. **B**, Uncomplicated wound healing at 6 months postoperatively.

been made to eliminate other injuries. Most facial injuries requiring soft tissue repair are not extensive and may be treated in an outpatient setting under local anesthesia. Although this usually is the quickest way, it has some disadvantages. The local anesthetic solution distorts the tissues, and infiltration may be painful. There is a risk that incomplete anesthesia is achieved, which may prevent careful cleaning and suturing. More extensive injuries or complex repairs involving the eyelids, nose, lips, or ears should be managed in the operating room under local anesthesia with sedation or general anesthesia. If the procedure is expected to take longer than an hour, complex facial structures are involved, or there is any question of involvement of deeper structures, the procedure should be carried out in the operating room.

Children more frequently require management in the operating room because of their greater anxiety and the level of their cooperation and understanding is more limited. If the repair is expected to take more than 15 minutes and is more than a simple laceration, it should be carried out in the operating room.[5]

ANESTHESIA

Administration of local anesthesia for the repair of facial wounds serves three purposes: to anesthetize the wound during an awake procedure, to provide postoperative analgesia at the repair site, and to facilitate hemostasis, irrespective of the surgical setting. Several technical points should be considered:

1. The local infiltration agent should be injected through the existing wound edges, where there may already be reduced sensation resulting from the injury.
2. The volume of the syringe should be matched to the needle size. It is least painful to use a 30-gauge needle with a 1- or 3-mL syringe. The small needle combined with the low pressure of infiltration from the low-volume reservoir provides the most comfort (Fig. 6-9A). Although a larger

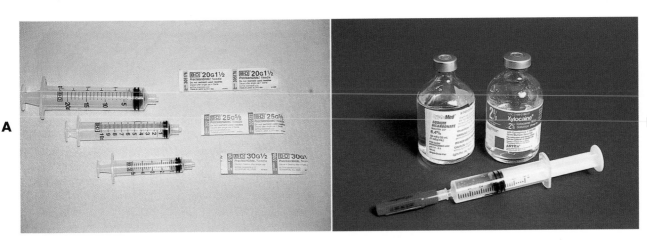

FIGURE 6-9 **A**, To lessen injection pain in the face in the awake patient, the smallest needle (30 gauge) in a small syringe (1 or 3 mL) is the most effective. It creates a small puncture wound and causes little pain by fluid pressure and tissue distention. Large syringes require larger needles and are best used for the administration of regional blocks. **B**, Using bicarbonate to buffer a local anesthetic that contains epinephrine neutralizes the acidic pH and contributes to less injection pain.

25-gauge needle with a 10-mL syringe is appropriate for intraoral and facial blocks (because of the need for longer needle length), it causes more discomfort during direct local infiltration.

3. Buffering of the pH of the local anesthetic reduces discomfort during infiltration.[3] Because all local anesthetics containing epinephrine are acidic (pH < 4), they cause a burning sensation on contact with the subcutaneous tissues. For large-volume infiltrations, adding a small amount of bicarbonate eliminates this source of immediate tissue pain (see Fig. 6-9B).[6]

4. The use of regional nerve blocks can be invaluable when there is extensive injury. They expedite the onset and distribution of the anesthetic, and they lessen the total volume of solution required. The supraorbital, infraorbital, and mental nerves are the ones most commonly blocked.

5. Consideration should be given to the use of long-acting local anesthetics for postoperative pain relief. The infiltration of bupivacaine (Marcaine) in and around the wound site gives up to 24 hours of pain relief, which is particularly useful in children.

A full understanding of the pharmacology and pharmacokinetics of the drugs used is essential. The safe limits of local anesthetic volumes include 7 mg/kg for lidocaine with epinephrine, 4 mg/kg for lidocaine without epinephrine, and 1 mg/kg for bupivacaine.

Several topical anesthetics can provide skin anesthesia in cream formulations.[7] The two best known are EMLA (eutectic mixture of two local anesthetics, 2.5% prilocaine and 2.5% lidocaine) and TAC (mixture of 0.5% tetracaine, epinephrine at a concentration of 1 : 2000, and 11.8% cocaine). Both preparations need to be applied to the skin a significant length of time before injection or manipulation to achieve dermal penetrations of 3 to 4 mm (Fig. 6-10). They should not be applied to open wounds or around mucous membranes or the eyes. Although both achieve some degree of skin anesthesia and are often promulgated for use in small lacerations in children, they have some practical limitations that severely limit their use in facial wound repair. The time lapse before onset of

anesthesia, difficulty in keeping the topical creams confined to the desired area, and lack of anesthesia of the deeper tissues often make their use less than practical.

WOUND PREPARATION AND DÉBRIDEMENT

Fortunately, most facial wounds are seen early, usually within hours after their occurrence, but even after 24 hours, the wounds usually can be closed after thorough irrigation and débridement.

Initial cleansing of the wound should be carried out using a gentle soap (e.g., Ivory soap) or a dilute Betadine (5% ophthalmic) solution. Use of either agent causes little or no cellular damage to open wounds but reduces bacterial counts. Most other cutaneous preparatory agents, including alcohol, hydrogen peroxide, benzalkonium chloride, and hexachlorophene, are quite toxic to cells. A general rule is never to use any solution that is not well tolerated by the conjunctival lining of the eye.

Hair usually does not need to be removed, and its presence can be a guide to good anatomical reconstruction. Eyebrow and eyelash hair should never be removed because regrowth cannot be ensured. Scalp and associated hair removal should be limited to facilitate tissue repositioning only. Facial hair (e.g., beard, moustache, goatee) can freely be removed because it impedes good skin repair and always regrows. The wounds should be meticulously examined for the presence of foreign bodies, especially if the history of the injury suggests that foreign bodies may be present. The facial wounds of road traffic accident victims commonly contain embedded glass. In many instances, the glass is better identified by listening for the "chink" of a metallic instrument against the glass than trying to visualize it. In wounds that are contaminated with dirt and other debris, pressure irrigation with an 18-gauge needle and 20-mL syringe generates sufficient pressure to dislodge implanted particles and reduce the bacterial count. Because there is no convincing evidence that antibiotic irrigations in the facial region are advantageous and that there is a risk of toxicity to the cornea, saline irrigation should be sufficient in most cases.

An abrasion may contain particulate material that can cause a traumatic tattoo if not removed. Light scrubbing of the wounds can be carried out using a surgical scrub brush or a toothbrush. However, a dermabrader with a very fine diamond wheel is usually much more effective because some removal of the papillary dermis is necessary to remove or expose many of the embedded particles (Fig. 6-11).[8] Particles not removed with the dermabrader can be systematically removed with a No. 11 blade. It is important not to dermabrade too deeply into the reticular dermis or expose the underlying fat, because this likely will result in hypertrophic scarring. It is better to perform a secondary laser or dermabrasion procedure than manage hypertrophic scarring. A light dermabrasion heals within 5 to 7 days, particularly in men because of the epithelial contributions from the beard skin.

Excision of the wound edges usually is not advised unless the tissues are obviously crushed and nonviable. Because the blood flow to the facial skin is extensive and receives contributions from the dermis and underlying perforators, it is often remarkable how little soft tissue attachment may be needed for survival (Fig. 6-12). It is always easier to remove

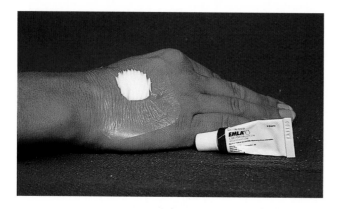

FIGURE 6-10 Topical anesthetics, such as a eutectic mixture of local anesthetics (EMLA), are commonly used to prevent pain from the insertion of venous catheters. Their effectiveness and practicality in the closure of facial lacerations are questionable.

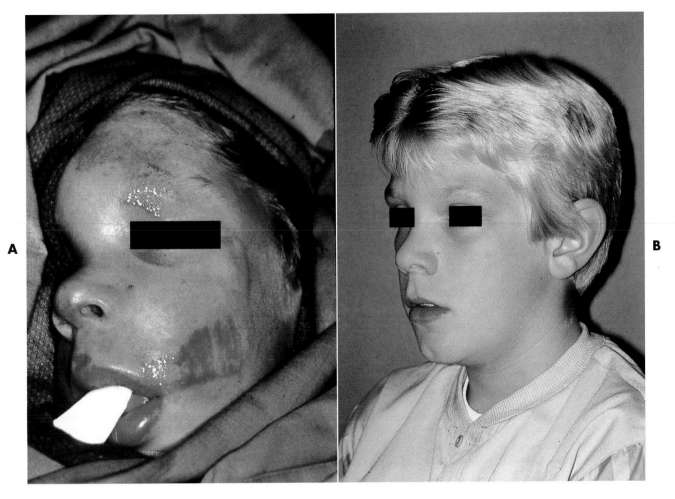

FIGURE 6-11 Dermabrasion into the papillary dermis is a reliable method for removing impregnated material and preventing traumatic tattooing. **A,** Dermabrasion removal of asphalt debris. **B,** Scarless healing at 9 months after surgery.

excess scar and tissue secondarily than it is to recruit replacement tissue.

WOUND CLOSURE TECHNIQUES

The face is unique among all other tissues in the body. It merits an approach different from many aspects of traditional wound care.

Tissue Handling Principles

Several guidelines for tissue handling should be followed:

1. Reduce operative tissue damage. The tissues should be handled gently with fine instruments, and if necessary, loupes should be used.
2. Minimize sharp débridement. Most facial wounds require minimal excision, but when needed, it should be carried out with the scalpel held at right angles to the skin surface. In hair-bearing areas, the incision should parallel the hair follicles to reduce the possibility of damage.
3. Repair wounds as they are positioned. The classic instruction is to close wounds along tension lines and the natural folds (i.e., RSTLs) of the facial skin. In reality, facial wounds tend to be random, and adherence to this concept is frequently impractical. Important facial landmarks should be aligned and the wounds repaired as they are found. Allow for natural healing and wound maturation to make the first attempt at optimizing scars.
4. Close in layers. Good dermal support is one of the primary keys to flat, narrow scars. When skin sutures are removed early to prevent track marks, a lack of dermal support may allow scars to widen, particularly if they cross the RSTLs. If necessary, the surgeon should undermine the wound margins to create a deeper layer for suturing and eversion of the wound edges. Tension across the wound should be reduced to a minimum.
5. Use fine sutures and remove early. With good dermal support and the rapid epithelialization of facial tissues, the sutures should be removed 5 to 7 days after insertion. Alternate sutures may be removed after 3 days.

Instrumentation

The finest and most precise instruments should be used. A large number of instruments is unnecessary (Fig. 6-13).

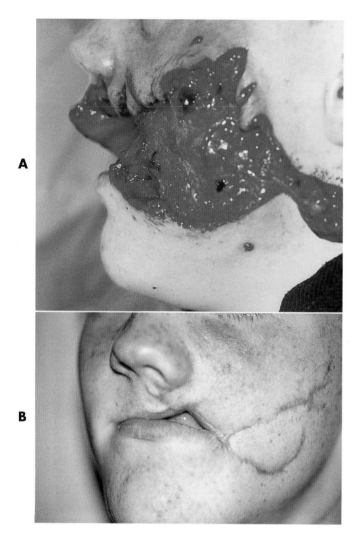

FIGURE 6-12 Gunshot wound to the face with lateral facial flap avulsion. **A**, The lateral facial skin flap is hanging on by a small skin pedicle. **B**, Complete survival of the hanging skin flap followed primary repair.

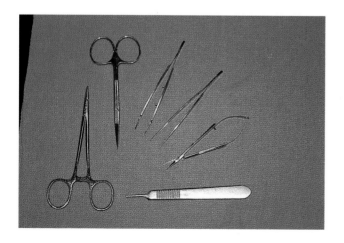

FIGURE 6-13 Instrument set for facial soft tissue repair.

Suture Types

There are two fundamental suture types: absorbable and permanent.[9] Although used by surgeons of all specialties, their composition and technical details are frequently not known or are misunderstood.

Absorbable Sutures

Sutures that are absorbed include gut (plain or chromic), Dexon, Vicryl, Maxon, and PDS. A plain gut suture is composed of twisted collagenous strands of sheep or beef intestinal wall. Because of its animal origins, it is being with drawn from use in Europe. This suture is rapidly absorbed by phagocytosis, maintaining strength for up to 10 days with complete absorption within 70 days. When heat treated, a fast-absorbing gut suture is created with accelerated tensile strength loss and absorption. Wound support is provided for only 5 to 7 days, and it is used primarily for epidermal suturing. When gut is coated with a chromium salt solution, chromic gut suture is created, which is more resistant to body enzymes, resulting in slower absorption and maintenance of strength for up to 14 days. It also has better tensile strength and knotting capability. A mild chromic gut suture is made that is absorbed between 3 and 5 days. The other absorbable sutures are synthetically derived and have much longer retention.

Dexon is a braided suture composed of a glycolic acid polymer, which breaks down by hydrolysis and maintains strength for up to 30 days. Vicryl (polyglactin 910) is a polymer but incorporates lactide and calcium stearate (lubricant) with the glycolic acids. Because of the lactide, which is hydrophobic, hydrolysis is slowed, and complete absorption takes up to 70 days to occur. Significant strength is maintained at 21 days after placement. Maxon is also of glycolic acid composition but has the addition of trimethylene carbonate in a monofilament form; the tensile strength is prolonged, and complete absorption can take up to 180 days. PDS is a synthetic monofilament made from the polyester derivative polydioxanone. It glides easily through tissue, has significant memory, takes about 180 days to absorb, and has extended wound strength for up to 6 weeks. These features account for its frequent use as an absorbable subcuticular suture. Monocryl (poliglecaprone 25) is a monofilament suture that is used for subcuticular closure and that maintains its strength for several weeks, with complete absorption occurring by 120 days.

Practically, the types of absorbable sutures used in the face are limited to the gut and Vicryl or Dexon sutures. Closure of the skin when suture removal is not desired, as can be the case in young children, should be performed with 5-0 or 6-0 plain gut. Any of the other absorbable sutures cause too much inflammation and take too long to dissolve. Plain or fast-absorbing gut sutures are suitable for closure of the mucous membranes of the eye, nose, and mouth.

Dermal closure should be carried with 5-0 gut or 5-0 Dexon and Vicryl. Although some postoperative suture extrusion occurs with the longer-lasting absorbables, it is not as significant as in other areas of the body, probably because the smaller-sized sutures are used in the facial region. Deeper structure apposition, including fascia and muscle, can be performed using the larger 3-0 and 4-0 longer-absorbing sutures, and closure benefits from their increased strength retention.

Nonabsorbable Sutures

Monofilaments have replaced the traditional braided silk suture materials. They offer smooth tissue passage, minimal tissue reactivity, and easy handling by virtue of their elasticity. These features make them well suited for retention and skin closure. Nylon, derived from the synthesis of polyamide polymers, and polypropylene (Prolene), a linear hydrocarbon polymer, are commonly used in the facial region. They are extremely inert and can hold tensile strength for years. The flexibility of the polypropylene is superior to nylon and accounts for its popularity in the pullout subcuticular technique of skin closure.

Either of these sutures, ranging in sizes from 5-0 to 7-0, can be used for facial skin closure, depending on the specific site. In the scalp, the blue coloring of Prolene makes it easier to remove.

Suturing Techniques

Although all techniques, including simple, continuous, subcuticular, horizontal, and vertical mattress methods (Fig. 6-14), occasionally are used, the simple and continuous techniques are most often used. The vascularity of the wound edges, already compromised as a result of the injury, should not be further jeopardized by the suturing technique. The simple interrupted or the continuous non-interlocking suture techniques provide the least strangulation of tissue (Fig. 6-15). There is no real advantage to a running interlocking suture, but if used, the suture loops should not be too tight (Fig. 6-16). Occasionally, an interrupted vertical mattress suture may be of value to evert the skin edges, but good dermal support usually makes the use of this suture technique unnecessary.

For the skin, 6-0 or 7-0 sutures should be used. Sutures should be placed close enough to the wound margin (1 to 2 mm) to optimally relieve wound tension. The suture should be tied with an allowance for postoperative edema and without blanching of the wound margins. Suture track marks usually result from the suture being tied too tightly, causing tissue necrosis, or delayed removal, resulting in epithelialization of the suture track.

On the scalp, a larger suture, usually 3-0 or 4-0, is used, and the sutures are placed farther from the wound margins. Because of the structure and vascularity of the scalp, the tissues can tolerate a tighter closure if required for hemostasis. Dermal sutures should not be used because they may injure hair follicles. Deep support comes from closure of the galea. Metallic staples can be used and are probably the least compromising approach to vascularity, because they do not completely encircle the apposed tissues. Their use, however, typically is retained for rapid closure and ease of removal in the hair-bearing scalp, where track marks are less relevant. The importance of layered closure in facial wounds cannot be overemphasized.

Skin Adhesives

The use of glue for epidermal repair has great appeal. Previous attempts at developing a skin adhesive have been fraught with handling problems and cytotoxicity, but a cyanoacrylate derivative, octyl-2-cyanoacrylate (Dermabond, Ethicon, Somerville, NJ), has had significant success without the previous problems (Fig. 6-17). The adhesive is quite durable but

Interrupted sutures

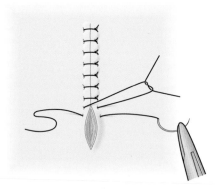

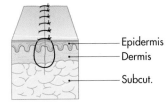

Epidermis
Dermis
Subcut.

Continuous sutures

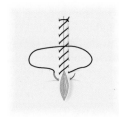

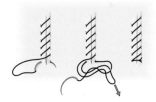

Intracuticular sutures

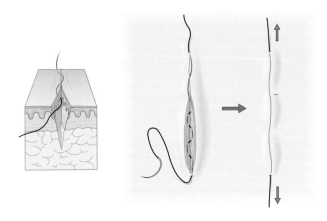

FIGURE 6-14 Commonly used facial suturing techniques.

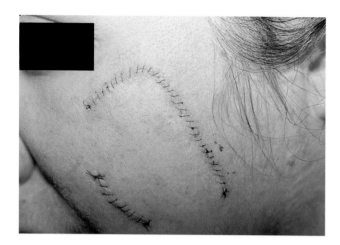

FIGURE 6-15 Running, non-interlocking, 6-0 nylon skin suture repair.

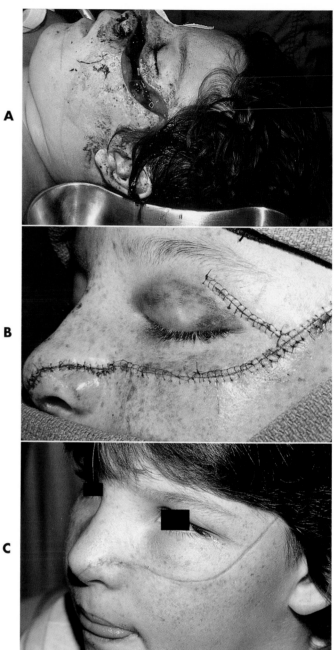

FIGURE 6-16 Knife laceration of the face. **A**, Preoperative status. **B**, Multilayer wound repair of skin with running, interlocking, 6-0 nylon. **C**, One year postoperatively.

flexes with the skin. Multiple studies have demonstrated its equivalency to 5-0 and 6-0 skin sutures in facial surgery.[10,11] It is still important to provide dermal suture support (Fig. 6-18), and care must be taken to seal the epithelium without allowing the liquid to flow between the wound margins, where it will harden and block epithelial and dermal healing. It is particularly useful after suture removal instead of taping because it secures the wound edges better and does so in a near-invisible fashion.

POSTOPERATIVE CARE

Dressings other than a line of an ointment to prevent drying of the tissues are usually not required. Some surgeons use antibiotic creams, but the use of chloramphenicol (Chloromycetin) has a possible risk of producing aplastic anemia and is best avoided, although it is still used widely. Extensive taping obscures the wound margins and does not allow the wound exudate to be cleaned from the edges. Crusting is removed with dilute hydrogen peroxide, and antibiotic ointment is reapplied two or three times per day. Face and hair washing can be performed within 48 hours, because it has been shown that wetting of sutures with soap and water, particularly on the face, does not increase the incidence of wound infection. Keeping the suture line clean and soft without crusting makes it easier to remove the sutures.

There is good evidence that more rapid healing can be achieved by applying negative-pressure dressing over the wound. This removes inflammatory exudates and speeds healing. It has little place in routine closure, but in difficult areas with abrasions or tissue loss, it may have a place.

Facial sutures are usually removed 5 to 7 days after placement, whereas those in the scalp are removed 2 to 3 weeks later. Removal of sutures, although rarely discussed, can be uncomfortable and cause anxiety for the patient. Fine instruments, a delicate touch, and several simple maneuvers can make the experience more tolerable for the patient (Fig. 6-19).

After suture removal, the wound can be supported using Steri-Strips (brown paper strips) or cyanoacrylate adhesive. Postoperative care should include clear (ideally, written) instructions about the natural history of wound healing and maturation. The patients need to know about healing time; for example, wound maturation may take up to 18 months in young patients. They must be aware that scar revision can be considered only after maturation has taken place.

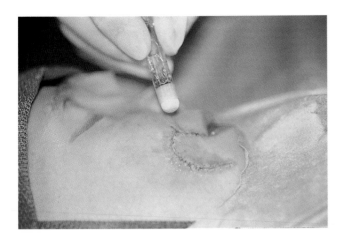

FIGURE 6-17 Cyanoacrylate adhesive (Dermabond) for skin closure comes in a bullet-shaped ampule dispenser.

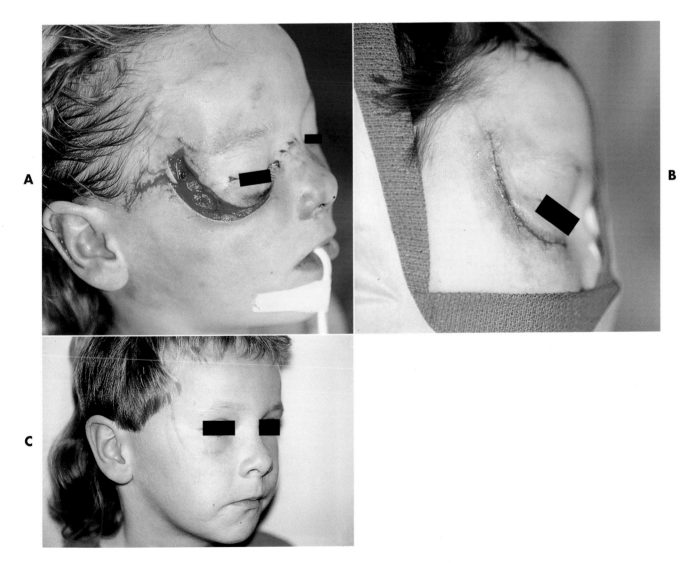

FIGURE 6-18 Closure of a dog-bite facial wound with topical skin adhesive. **A**, Preoperative status. **B**, Skin closure with good dermal support. **C**, One year postoperatively.

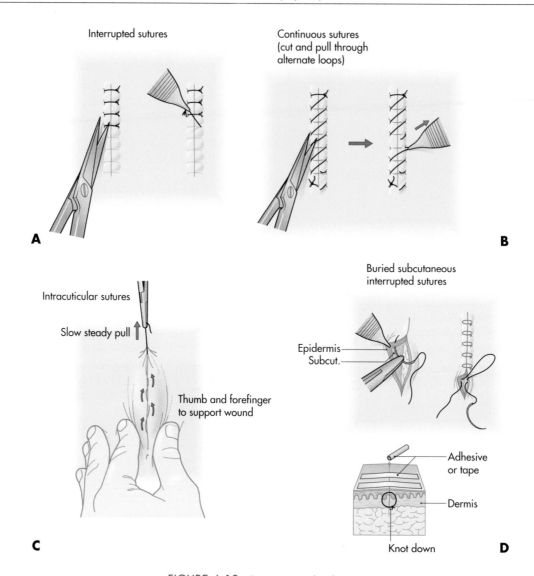

FIGURE 6-19   Suture removal techniques.

ACKNOWLEDGMENT

We would like to acknowledge Dr. Bhuller for his previous contributions to this chapter.

REFERENCES

1. Lee RH, Gamble WB, Robertson B, Manson P: Patterns of facial lacerations from blunt trauma. *Plast Reconstr Surg* 99:1544-1554, 1997.
2. Wolff KD: Management of animal bites to the face. Experience in 94 cases. *J Oral Maxillofac Surg* 56:838-843, 1998.
3. Donkor P: A study of primary closure of human bite injuries to the face. *J Oral Maxillofac Surg* 55:479-481, 1997.
4. Lee RH, Gamble WB, Robertson B, Manson P: The MCFONTZL classification system for soft tissue injuries to the face. *Plast Reconstr Surg* 103:1150-1157, 1999.
5. Kolta PJ: Management of facial trauma in children. *Pediatr Clin North Am* 43:1253-1275, 1996.
6. Eppley BL, Sadove AM: Reduction in injection pain by buffering of local anesthetic solutions. *J Oral Maxillofac Surg* 47:762-763, 1989.
7. Hirko MK, Lin PH, Greisler HP, Chu CC: Biologic properties of suture materials. In Chu C, von Fraunhofer J, Greisler H, editors: *Wound closure biomaterials and devices*, New York, 1996, CRC Press, pp 237-288.
8. Cronin ED: A new technique of dermabrasion for traumatic tattoos. *Ann Plast Surg* 36:401-402, 1996.
9. Ratner D: Basic suture materials and suturing techniques. *Semin Dermatol* 13:20-26, 1994.
10. Spotnitz WD: The role of sutures and fibrin sealants in wound healing. *Surg Clin North Am* 77:651-659, 1997.
11. Toriumi DM, O'Grady K, Desai D, Bagal A: Use of octyl-2-cyanoacrylate for skin closure in facial plastic surgery. *Plast Reconstr Surg* 102:2209-2215, 1998.

CHAPTER 7

Principles of Reduction of Fractures and Methods of Fixation

Malcolm Cameron, Peter Ward Booth

The maxillofacial region is in many ways anatomically unique. In the past, failure to appreciate its differences from the rest of the bony skeleton led to poor outcomes and unnecessary morbidity, particularly in the management of trauma. Although maxillofacial surgeons have used experience and research from general orthopedics to great effect, the mindless transfer of orthopedic techniques and principles is sometimes unhelpful. It must be recognized that surgeons are vulnerable to the market forces created by the manufacturers of fixation devices, although the same companies have, of course, introduced highly effective innovations. Proper evaluation of fixation techniques takes many years, so it is a long time before the shortcomings of some devices become apparent. Surgeons must not be seduced by the latest innovations but should always critically assess new devices and ideas and scrutinize relevant supporting publications. A thorough audit of outcomes by surgeons free from commercial pressures should allow well-informed decisions about new techniques.

Two innovations from general orthopedics—osteogenic distraction and bioresorbable fixation devices—have much to offer the maxillofacial traumatologist, and they are strongly promoted by the supply industry. They may not, however, be the ultimate answer to our surgical requirements in the way that the sales teams would have us believe. Although innovation is the precursor of progress, many new techniques, instruments, and materials do not stand the test of time.

The stigma of unreduced, unstable facial fractures can be severe. Minor cosmetic changes after facial injuries are common, and in modern societies, good results are often not enough: Perfection is demanded. For the surgeon, a less than perfect outcome is always unsatisfactory. Poor cosmetic and functional outcomes have several causes:

- Incorrect choice of surgical access. Because all skin incisions have the potential to form bad scars, hidden or mucosal incisions should be used wherever possible (Figs. 7-1 through 7-4).
- Inability to operate early. Normal skin draping is prevented if early healing has begun.
- Poor timing of surgery. For example, excessive swelling makes the precise placement of incisions difficult (Fig. 7-5).
- Poor reduction of bone fractures. Closed reduction always has the risk of poor reduction.

- Poor understanding of the fracture sites. Lack of knowledge, usually because of inadequate clinical and radiological examinations, can lead to poor reduction and stabilization.

Posttraumatic functional problems may be more significant than any esthetic considerations, and these patients often feel markedly disabled. Typical functional problems include the following:

- Excessive scar tissue after poor primary care; inadequate wound cleaning and suturing
- Disabling visual problems, such as loss of vision or diplopia, with or without enophthalmos
- Loss of masticatory efficiency from iatrogenic malocclusion
- Impairment of speech and swallowing (rare)
- Persistent epiphora after ectropion
- Troublesome anosmia after midface fractures (rare)
- Motor or sensory neurological damage, which is common early after trauma and can persist, producing significant problems

Inadequate reduction and stabilization are the most common causes of esthetic and functional problems, even in less severe cases. These problems may also be associated with pain or chronic infection, although less often than in general orthopedic practice. Inadequate reduction and stabilization may not be as rare as we would like, but only careful follow-up and evaluation can establish the incidence.

Poor outcomes may result from patients' not seeking treatment (Fig. 7-6). In less severe cases, it is sometimes difficult to determine what constitutes a perfect result. The aim of reduction and stabilization is to return the patient to the pre-injury status. The morbidity of the surgery must not exceed that of the traumatic injury itself (e.g., inappropriate and overzealous open reduction of an uncomplicated, minimally displaced orbital rim fracture). It is important to remember that bone is a living structure that will remodel, especially in young patients.

More difficult decisions have to be made in third world countries, where resources and manpower are limited. Is it reasonable to undertake a 1-hour open reduction of a fractured malar or to accept the less than perfect reduction achieved by a closed lift procedure? Similarly in the

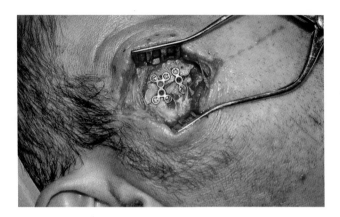

FIGURE 7-1   Use of an existing laceration is desirable, especially in this position which is difficult to access by other routes.

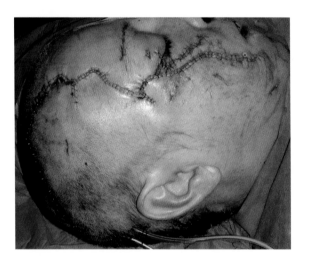

FIGURE 7-2   This laceration gave excellent access, and a good scar resulted from careful closure. (Copyright Media Studio, Cambridge University Hospitals NHS Foundation Trust.)

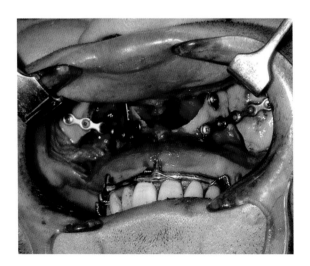

FIGURE 7-3   This intraoral incision provided excellent access to the extensive midfacial injuries, but further incisions were necessary to repair the periorbital fractures.

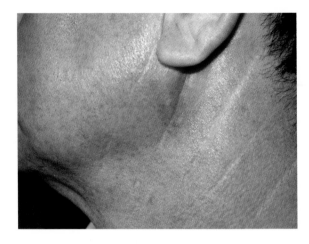

FIGURE 7-4   This retromandibular scar has healed well after open reduction and internal fixation of a condylar fracture. It demonstrates the appropriate use of a skin crease incision.

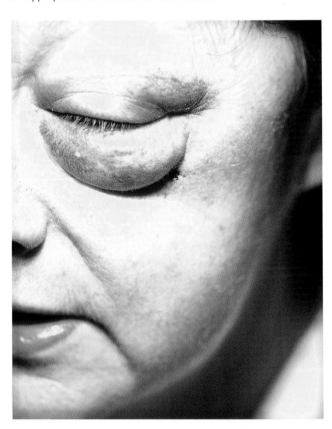

FIGURE 7-5   Excessive swelling will make it difficult to get a good result with any periorbital scar, and delay may be the best course.

industrialized world, should surgeons spend a long time reducing a nasal fracture in a pugilist who will probably reappear with a fractured nose again in 3 months? The senior physician must make these decisions on an individual basis, with full consultation with the patient and or family. It is, however, important to have targets of excellence, which may be modified in light of an individual patient's circumstances.

Suboptimal outcomes that are unrelated to socioeconomic factors (e.g., failing to present for care after a fracture) are not

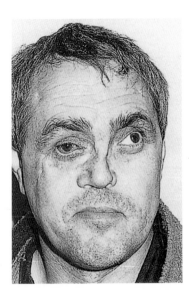

FIGURE 7-6   This patient, who had multiple assaults, rarely attended appointments for treatment. Failure to treat facial trauma can result in functional and cosmetic disaster.

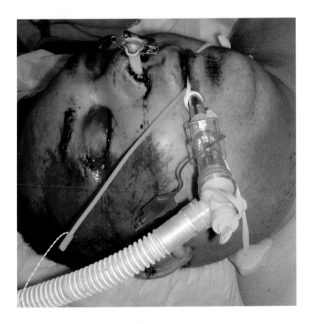

FIGURE 7-7   In addition to his facial injuries, this patient suffered intracranial trauma, which necessarily delayed treatment. In the end, his injuries were managed nonoperatively. *(Copyright Media Studio, Cambridge University Hospitals NHS Foundation Trust.)*

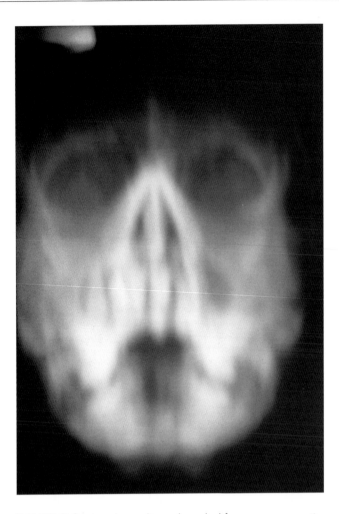

FIGURE 7-8   A useless radiograph resulted from an uncooperative patient who moved during imaging.

uncommon, but only by careful follow-up and evaluation can the outcome be fully established.[1] Poor outcomes may occur for a variety of other reasons, which may be beyond the control of the maxillofacial surgeon:

- Coexisting medical problems, particularly head injuries (Fig. 7-7), may delay definitive surgery, making it difficult to achieve good reduction. Secondary correction of initial problems is rarely as good as primary surgery.
- Inadequate preoperative investigations, particularly if there is lack of appropriate imaging, may fail to reveal the true extent of the bony injuries. It is acceptable to delay surgery until adequate plain radiographs and scans are available (Figs 7-8 and 7-9).
- Inadequate surgical planning, notably failing to plan the surgical access or the need for bone for grafting, affects results. Adequate patient consent requires that these important eventualities be considered and discussed before any procedure is initiated.
- Very severe fractures, particularly grossly comminuted fractures, can be extremely difficult to reduce and stabilize. These technical difficulties can be overcome only by experienced surgeons with a special interest in facial trauma.
- Some surgeons (often from anatomically related specialties) with limited experience in facial trauma may not fully appreciate the structure and function of the oral and maxillofacial region and may therefore attain less than ideal results.
- Patients who are from poor socioeconomic backgrounds or who abuse alcohol or drugs may refuse or fail to present for treatment. These patients then may require secondary procedures.

We believe that if there is a logical approach to reduction and fixation many of these poor outcomes can be minimized.

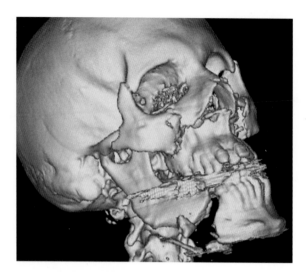

FIGURE 7-9 A three-dimensional computed tomogram provides good information about the number and pattern of facial fractures, but it must be interpreted in light of the clinical findings, and its shortfalls must be appreciated. In this case, the artifact caused by amalgam dental restorations obscure the mandibular ramus. *(Copyright Media Studio, Cambridge University Hospitals NHS Foundation Trust.)*

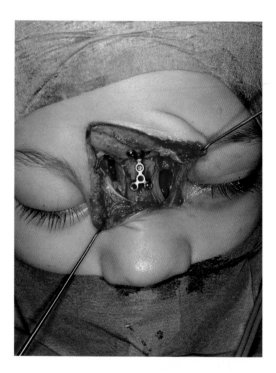

FIGURE 7-10 A small laceration allowed excellent access to place a plate and provide a stable reduction, far superior to that possible with nasal packs and plaster of Paris splints. *(Copyright Media Studio, Cambridge University Hospitals NHS Foundation Trust.)*

PRINCIPLES OF REDUCTION

OPEN OR CLOSED?

Terminology in this field can be confusing. The terms *closed* and *open* treatment are preferred to *conservative* and *operative*. *Open* refers to deliberate surgical intervention to open and directly explore the fracture site, normally by means of a surgical incision or a laceration. Fractures involving the teeth-bearing areas are biologically open, although this does not normally afford surgical access. Some surgeons refer to intermaxillary wiring as conservative treatment, but others refer to a soft diet alone as conservative management. The use of intermaxillary fixation (IMF) (also called mandibular maxillary fixation [MMF]) has well-documented morbidity and mortality rates that do not fit with the concept of conservative management.

The term *open* refers to exposure, reduction, and fixation of the fracture under direct vision. *Closed* refers to no direct visualization of the fracture site; that is, blind fixation, which usually is achieved indirectly or by relying on nonsurgical stabilization, like IMF (MMF).

The vague term *conservative* may mean no treatment of any kind, no surgical treatment, or, for some surgeons, the use of IMF. It is better to use more specific terms such as *wait and watch*, *nonsurgical*, or, preferably, *closed* treatment.

Not all displaced fractures need reduction. However, only severe medical problems obviating general anesthesia should prevent open reduction if it is otherwise indicated. Many fractures can be treated by open reduction with the use of sedation and local anesthesia. Open reduction involves exposure of the fracture through the skin or mucosa (surgical exposure is discussed later). Once opened, the fracture can be reduced and directly fixed through the incision (Fig. 7-10). Closed reduction is blind reduction and relies on

the fragments' locking together. This is more likely to be successful if the periosteum is largely intact. Examples of closed reduction include fixation of the teeth in occlusion (i.e., IMF), elevation of a fractured zygoma, and use of an arch bar to stabilize dentoalveolar fractures. In these circumstances, reduction usually occurs without direct visualization of the fragments in their final position.

In maxillofacial surgery, the most common method of closed treatment is IMF, which relies on the correct positioning of the teeth to control the reduction. For mandibular fractures, open reduction with internal fixation (ORIF) has traditionally been performed with the use of temporary intraoperative IMF to secure the occlusion before plate placement. Although the IMF is released at the end of the operation, it may be reapplied if necessary. This belt-and-braces approach may be questioned for several reasons.[2] First, operating time is reduced if IMF is not used. Second, although this is a more certain reduction for the surgeon,[3] is it more comfortable for the patient? Moreover, there is ample evidence of short- and long-term risk to the patient when IMF is used. Evidence indicates it may damage the periodontium and reduce airflow, and weight loss and long-term temporomandibular joint (TMJ) function may be adversely affected.[4]

Fifty years ago, facial fractures were typically managed by closed methods. Open reduction was reserved for cutaneous compound fractures or certain unstable mandibular fractures. This evolution toward open reduction has improved the precision of the reduction, because the fragments can be carefully examined and manipulated. What led to this change in philosophy?

In the pre-antibiotic era and before modern aseptic techniques, surgeons were extremely cautious about open reduction. Experience, particularly from general orthopedic practice, suggested that open reduction almost invariably led to local infection, severe osteomyelitis, and even death of the patient. Caution about open reduction and internal fixation (ORIF) was fueled by the lack of suitable implant material with which to stabilize the fracture. This problem continued beyond the introduction of modern sterile techniques and antibiotics. Although more suitable implants became available, the biomechanics of the systems often lacked a scientific basis. Bad experiences created a climate of antipathy toward routine open reduction.

Historically, the avoidance of ORIF was based on sound surgical principles that were difficult to achieve for a variety of reasons. In modern surgery, with excellent plating and fixation systems and with safe, largely infection-free surgical procedures, these principles are relatively easy to achieve:

- Open reduction should be used only if the procedure itself does not have a significant or unacceptable morbidity.
- Open reduction should be followed by direct fixation of the fracture to ensure that the full benefits of the procedure are gained.

CLOSED REDUCTION

Disadvantages of Closed Reduction

Closed reduction can be problematic. With this method, the position of the teeth, palpation, and postoperative radiographs are used as guides to the accuracy of reduction. The most common problem with closed reduction is poor fracture alignment. In many cases, closed reduction relies on correct positioning of the teeth, on the assumption that this produces correct orientation of the bony fragments. Although the occlusion must be correctly restored, the teeth have only a limited effect on the final position of the bones. This influence significantly diminishes as fractures extend away from the dental arches, such as in the zygomatic complex, which is not related to the teeth. Even in mandibular fractures, muscle tone and activity may displace bone fragments despite firm location of the teeth.

This problem becomes compounded in cases of preexisting malocclusion, which is a common predisposition to mandibular fractures. In cases of a depleted dentition or injury to the teeth themselves, reduction of the occlusion becomes a less reliable method of reducing the bony fractures. Errors of reduction are tolerated much less in facial fractures than in other orthopedic procedures. Inadequate reduction, even in the presence of a normal occlusion, may be associated with poor esthetics and functional problems. Facial fractures are most common in the young, and it is unacceptable to leave these patients with long-standing facial deformity or dysfunction.

Closed reduction for maxillary and mandibular fractures demands IMF. This is a technically simple procedure that may not require general anesthesia, although it has several disadvantages Patients dislike IMF, and it can be dangerous by obstructing the airway.

Closed reduction relying on the dentition has little value in the treatment of upper facial injuries and none in isolated zygoma, orbital, or nasal fractures. Closed reduction of upper facial fractures relies on palpation to ensure reduction and on periosteal attachment to provide stability, neither of which can be guaranteed preoperatively or intraoperatively. In the past, external fixation, typically pin fixation, was performed, with antral or nasal packs used in an attempt to provide stability. However, the nature of these gauze packs ensured only limited stability, and even if the surgeon was optimistic, the experience of having these packs removed usually failed to persuade the patient of their value.

External pin fixation, which is still used in general orthopedics and in treatment of facial continuity defects, can provide stability. The 3 to 6 weeks of fixation pins often leaves ugly scars, and it is difficult for patients to work or lead normal lives during this period.

Advantages of Closed Reduction

Perhaps the greatest advantage of closed reduction has been demonstrated in war zones, in the treatment of maxillary and mandibular fractures. In the United Kingdom, particularly during World War II, this technique was important. Custom-made cast silver splints were constructed and sectioned at the fracture site. IMF was applied slowly through the splints, and a slow reduction and then fixation of the fractures was achieved. This procedure was predominantly carried out away from the front line, often without the need for anesthesia. Closed reduction also worked well in patients with missile injuries, stabilizing continuity defects. With the available technology and limited facilities at that time, it proved to be an adequate method.

In many third world countries, with limitations imposed by too many patients, too few maxillofacial surgeons, and inadequate resources, these basic techniques still have a place. Cast silver splints have been replaced by simple arch bars, which are much easier and cheaper to manufacture. However, in some developing countries, local manufacturers can economically produce plating systems for internal fixation, although not necessarily out of exotic materials. The costs of the plating system should not prevent their use. There are significant hidden costs for closed reductions with IMF, including the costs of extra patient supervision, which often involves intensive care; increased morbidity (e.g., poor ventilation, persistent trismus); and delayed return to work.

Closed treatment may be an acceptable compromise, such as for a patient with medical problems that preclude general anesthesia or sedation. IMF may be used to treat simple, minimally displaced fractures very effectively. However, conditions that preclude general anesthesia (e.g., uncontrolled epilepsy, chronic respiratory disease) may also contraindicate IMF. Patients dislike having their teeth wired together and may not comply with prolonged treatment. Alternatively, open reduction is possible under local anesthesia with supplementary awake sedation.

The choice between open and closed reduction may be clear in some cases, but there are many instances in which both are equally acceptable. With good outcomes from surgery and anesthesia, open reduction offers the chance of better reduction and direct osteosynthesis. This means a safer postoperative recovery, earlier return to normal function, and prompt discharge to home in most cases.

The debate over open versus closed treatment of facial fractures is no more sharply focused than in condylar fractures. Those in favor of closed reduction point to the good results obtained with IMF conducted over 2 weeks and supplemented by physiotherapy using a controlled protocol and a highly compliant group of patients. For example, in a large series, Marker et al.[5] obtained excellent results with a closed treatment regimen in patients with a full range of severity of injury and condylar neck sites. Union always occurs, and surgical complications are rare. Those in favor of open reduction think that modern techniques and surgical experience enable safe reduction, quicker discharge from the hospital, and quicker return to work. They emphasize that closed reduction is frequently associated with poor long-term function. Problems include reduced mouth opening, malocclusions, and deviation on opening. TMJ pain and clicking are also cited as problems, but they are unreliable indicators of outcome because they are such common symptoms. At a symposium in 1999,[6] many controversies and disagreements were highlighted, but certain areas of agreement were reached (Fig. 7-11). Terminology applied to condylar neck and condyle trauma can add to the confusion, and the following guidelines may be more appropriate:

- It is best to refer to closed or open treatment rather than using the term *conservative*, which has different meanings for different surgeons. The use of IMF should also be qualified as *rigid (fixed) IMF* or *training elastics*, which allow guided opening of the jaws.
- The terms *displaced* and *dislocated* (from the fossa) are best used to describe the position of the condylar head. These terms are less confusing than descriptors such as *subluxated*.
- Description of the level of the fracture can be limited to intracapsular, high, or low condylar neck. Fractures may extend to more than one site.

More prospective studies are needed to evaluate the best methods of treatment. Although areas of controversy still exist, there are areas of general agreement:

- Closed treatment is not always associated with good results, whereas open reduction in experienced hands has a low morbidity rate and more predictably good outcomes.
- Closed treatment seems to be an effective method of treating any type of condylar fractures in children.
- Currently, pure intracapsular fractures are treated by closed methods. Research suggests that open treatment may be indicated, but further work is needed.
- Immobilization for 6 to 8 weeks by rigid IMF is not ideal for closed treatment. The use of *function*-guided elastics as a method of closed treatment has a more therapeutic role. In some studies enrolling cooperative patients, closed treatment has been as effective as open procedures for a wide range of fracture types and severity.
- Clinical and radiological evaluations may not define those who will get a poor result from closed treatment (except in cases of no or minimal displacement). This reflects the range of pericapsular and intracapsular soft tissue damage.

Increasing numbers of reports show that open reduction can produce excellent outcomes with low morbidity.[6a] There is inadequate evidence to identify which surgical approach or type of fixator is the best. However, it does seem that single microplate fixation is inadequate and is associated with plate fracture.

There is little doubt that the innovation of open reduction and miniplate fixation has improved outcomes, patient safety, and comfort. The focus on innovation in fixation devices has largely replaced the debate about open versus closed treatment. The open approach has become the gold standard, but innovation never ceases, and minimally invasive approaches are challenging the simple open approach. Minimally invasive approaches include totally endoscopic procedures and endoscopically assisted procedures. Whereas a totally endoscopic approach potentially offers a great advantage, an endoscopically assisted approach may muddy the waters because it still requires a surgical incision, albeit a less extensive opening. Advocates point to the inevitable progress toward a much less invasive procedure with less morbidity. However, advocates must show good outcomes and reasonable operating times in the hands of most trauma surgeons.

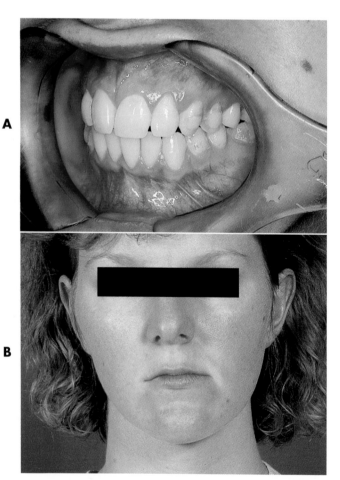

FIGURE 7-11 Two teenagers who had similar displaced fractures of the condylar neck. **A,** Perfectly symmetrical opening and a normal occlusion. **B,** Mandibular asymmetry and deviations on opening. Both patients were treated with a closed approach without intermaxillary fixation. These two cases reflect the confusion in the literature.

TIMING OF REDUCTION

The best time to reduce fractures is not clearly defined in the literature. For open injuries, it is assumed that the longer the delay, the more the wound becomes contaminated and the greater the risk of poor outcome due to infection. This seems logical, but the time frame over which this principle applies is unclear. There is an obvious difference between 5 hours and 5 days, but is there a significant difference between, for instance, 2 hours and 24 hours after fracture? Few studies have been able to quantify these variations, although some[7] have failed to show any difference in complications between fractures treated at less than 24 hours and those treated more than 24 hours after injury.

More worrying are the assumptions based on the orthopedic literature that reduction, if applied too inflexibly to maxillofacial injuries without due thought for function and form, results in unsatisfactory conclusions. The rich blood supply and rapid mucosal healing make comparison of outcomes between long bone and mandible fractures unrealistic.

In the case of a long delay (about 14 days), there is little doubt that initial healing is well established, and this makes mobilization and reduction difficult. Soft tissues become adherent to the displaced bones, making reduction even harder to achieve. This is particularly important in the canthal region of the eye. After displacement is established, the canthal ligament is unlikely ever to settle into its correct position.

Delays inevitably occur, and life-threatening conditions must take precedence. For patients with associated head injuries, fears about extensive maxillofacial reconstruction may lead to a delay in definitive surgery. Some maxillofacial surgery units have shown that early intervention is possible without any significant morbidity. For this to be possible, anesthetists and neurosurgeons must work closely together.

In summary, there is strong evidence that an open approach to fixation leads to better, more accurate reductions of fractures. This approach allows for adequate fixation, leading to early mobilization and return to normal function. The greater use of surgical incisions can be mitigated by a wise choice of mucosal and skin incision sites, which may be further mitigated by greater use of minimally invasive procedures in the future.

FIXATION

As new ideas and philosophies develop, the controversies move on to new areas. In the past, heated discussions raged over which type of IMF gave the best results. After osteosynthesis became the gold standard, the site and size of the implants became the subject of debate. It has become accepted by the mainstream that "small is good" in maxillofacial surgery. The use of biological, semirigid miniplate or microplate fixation leads to excellent outcomes in terms of good bone healing and reduced surgical morbidity. The use of orthopedic, heavy compression plates has no role in routine facial trauma management. Miniplates and microplates are used, with an emphasis on careful placement of the plates to maximize their biomechanical potential. Heavy-reconstruction, noncompression plates have only a temporary role in cases of mandibular continuity defects or gross fragmentation of the mandible, because they will eventually fracture.

Whereas the previous debate was about how best to achieve fixation, the current controversy concerns resorbable plates made of various materials versus non-resorbable plates (discussed later). Although the benefits of resorbable materials are being debated, most of the true controversy about fixation devices is historical.

After good exposure of the fracture is obtained, stabilization is best achieved by the smallest appropriate fixation device. The fixation or osteosynthesis device is a plate, and the plates used for most facial fractures are miniplates or microplates. Miniplates have various dimensions, but the term is used to distinguish them from the heavy plates that are used to provide compression osteosynthesis, which requires bicortical screws that prevent the correct biomechanical placement of the plate, along the line of tension. In modern maxillofacial surgery, these heavy plates are used only in rare cases. Osteosynthesis with plates having two screws, usually on either side of the fracture, can provide three-dimensional stability of the fracture, unlike wire osteosynthesis, which provides no more than monoplane traction, with no useful two- or three-dimensional stability except in a few sites (e.g., a frontozygomatic suture fracture). The smallest suitable device is used to minimize periosteal stripping around the fracture, which is helpful for fast healing, and the smaller devices are less likely to be felt by the patient.

There is a certain latitude in the size of the device used. For example, a grossly comminuted fracture may require a heavy (but noncompression) plate that is long enough to span the comminution. Bicortical or monocortical screws can retain these plates. A mandibular fracture in a young adult or a child may require only a microplate. In certain sites, such as the parasymphyseal area and particularly the mandible, the muscular vectors demand more than one plate to provide stability.

The materials used for the plates have been a source of debate. Currently, titanium alloys are most widely used. The decision to remove plates after their function has ceased (e.g., after 3 months) is still controversial. The Strasbourg Osteosynthesis Research Group (SORG) has produced guidelines that advocate removal of nonfunctional devices after healing is complete. However, removal is undertaken only if the perceived risk is insignificant compared with the risk of retention of the plate. For example, if there is chronic infection around a plate, the risk of morbidity for removal of the plate is less than that of leaving a focus of chronic infection. In contrast, in an adult, the complications of raising a coronal flap to remove a titanium plate on the zygomatic arch that is not palpable and is not infected, are greater than those of leaving it in situ. For most patients, removal of asymptomatic plates requires general anesthesia, which to many represents an unnecessary risk of morbidity compared with leaving the plate. For most surgeons in the United Kingdom and the United States, elective plate removal is not routinely undertaken. In Germany, however, demand from patients to remove nonfunctional devices pushes the equation toward elective plate removal.

How Rigid Should Rigid Fixation be?

Stabilization and its effect on bone healing have been controversial, and dogmatic views have been expressed. It is reassuring to know that a similar debate rages in orthopedics with equal vigor. The debate is relatively new, because it is only recently that biomechanical products have become available to stabilize fractures and anesthesia and reliable infection control have allowed these procedures to be carried out with low morbidity rates. Until the 19th century, only crude external devices, if any, were applied to stabilize fractures and achieve some kind of union. Limited function was considered successful treatment. In the 20th century, a few isolated reports of stabilization of facial fractures began to appear. Fixation mostly relied on use of the dentition with crude forms of IMF, and this technique persisted, with few exceptions, until the 1950s.

In orthopedics in the 19th century, it was recognized that any attempt to open a fracture was accompanied by a significant rise in mortality. Death mainly resulted from the use of nonsterile instruments and a lack of aseptic technique. After the fundamentals of sterility were applied and safe anesthesia became possible, the desire to develop improved methods of fixation increased. Centuries of caution meant for many that the idea of open reduction and placement of foreign bodies (plates) was unacceptable. This was the general view despite early reports of internal plate fixation as early as 1886. It was left to enthusiastic individuals to develop the modern concept of osteosynthesis. Roberts and Battersby[8] in the United Kingdom and Speissl[9] in Basel, Switzerland, made significant contributions. General acceptance of open osteosynthesis did not appear in the maxillofacial literature until the organized research of the Arbeitsgemeinschaft für Osteosynthesefragen (Association for Osteosynthesis [AO]) group in the 1950s. Even then, the work was accepted only in the German-speaking countries. The first osteosynthesis courses in maxillofacial surgery conducted in English occurred in the 1970s.

Although many surgeons continued to avoid open approaches, they became frustrated by the shortcomings of poorly reduced and unstable fractures. The debate about poor results frequently was blurred by confusion between poor *reduction* and poor *stabilization*. Even the best fixation device is of little value if reduction is inadequate. On the other hand, an anatomically reduced fracture will become displaced if it is inadequately stabilized. This is particularly important in the maxillofacial region, where a well-healed but displaced fracture may carry significant morbidity (e.g., malocclusion, diplopia, "flat face"). Such outcomes are clearly unacceptable. Maxillofacial surgery has significantly benefited from the research carried out in orthopedics, but the transfer of orthopedic concepts and techniques to the maxillofacial region still has problems.

Anatomical peculiarities of the facial skeleton can make the application of some orthopedic concepts and techniques very difficult. The excellent blood supply to the bones, overlying skin, and mucosa provides favorable conditions for healing and enables the placement of plates with low morbidity rates. This is at variance with general orthopedic procedures, where blood supply may be poor, especially in the distal extremities in elderly patients. Degloving injuries of the fractured mandible often heal uneventfully, a situation rarely seen in the lower limbs after a comparable soft tissue insult. Many parts of the facial skeleton are paper-thin, and this precludes rigid fixation, but the mechanical loads (e.g., displacing forces created by the muscles of mastication) do not compare with those in the limbs.

In maxillofacial surgery, the use of rigid fixation has several goals:

- To maintain reduction
- To restore early function at the fracture site, surrounding muscles, and joints, which in the case of the jaws means restoration of normal mastication, deglutition, and speech
- To minimize healing time
- To prevent infection by allowing movement at unstable fracture sites

What is the effect of no fixation? There are many examples of untreated fractures found in specimen jars in medical museums, but they are rarely seen in modern practice. Animal studies have yielded much more information. The work of the AO group provided much of the earlier data. These studies traced the progress of untreated radius fractures in dogs to a displaced fibrous union. Although it is reasonable to question the relationship between young animals and human patients, particularly elderly osteoporotic patients with mandibular fracture, animal models do provide some useful data.

From this animal work, a better understanding of fracture healing was developed. The AO group divided the bone-healing process into direct and indirect types. *Direct healing* was seen to occur, for example, after a 1-mm hole was cut into bone. Because there was complete stability, there was immediate growth of bone into the hematoma, which was then replaced and remodeled into trabecular bone. No intermediate cartilage formation occurred, nor was there proliferative callus formation.

Indirect healing classically occurred across a mobile long bone fracture, following a quite different process. Initial hematoma formation preceded ingrowth of fibrous tissue and blood vessels. This tissue underwent remodeling accompanied by proliferative osteoid growth at the periosteum (i.e., callus formation) (Fig. 7-12). Callus provided early stability for osteoid formation across the fracture. Once union was achieved, remodeling of the callus and the osteoid produced trabecular bone. However, in both humans and animals, if mobility was excessive, there was proliferative but incomplete formation of callus. The resulting callus was unable to stabilize the fracture; it failed to bridge the fracture site. At best, malunion was the final result, but other complications frequently intervened, including osteomyelitis. Indirect healing therefore became associated with the traditional problems of fracture management:

- Infection
- Malunion
- Nonunion
- Excess callus formation
- Prolonged hospitalization
- Prolonged immobilization
- Prolonged antibiotic regimens
- Joint dysfunction
- Secondary surgery to encourage union or eliminate infection
- Opening of a second donor site for bone grafting

Researchers and clinicians contrasted these problems with those of animal models of direct healing, in which perfect reduction led to production of osteoid and trabecular bone without callus formation and, ultimately, to early healing and restoration of normal function. With hindsight, it is easy to see that such comparisons involved unlike starting points:

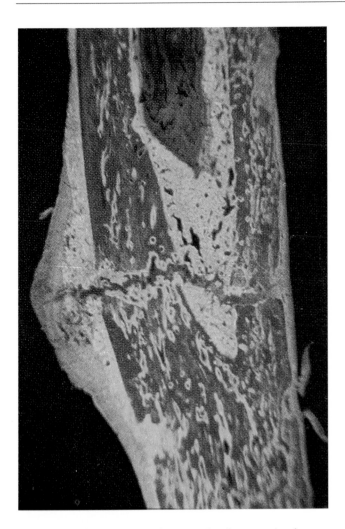

FIGURE 7-12 Normal development of callus around a fracture. Although excessive callus formation occurs with excessive motion, it is not necessarily a sign of abnormal healing. In the past, futile attempts to prevent any callus formation produced increasingly rigid fixation systems. Champy's work with miniplates demonstrated that complete rigidity is actually a disadvantage.

They did not recognize that there are many degrees of rigidity between fixation achieved with adequate stability and that achieved with inadequate stability. Although the argument at first may appear to be one between direct and indirect healing, it is actually a question of stability during the healing period. Indirect healing does not necessarily lead to instability and failure; the problems listed earlier are the result of *inadequate stability*.

Thirty years ago, research workers decided that direct healing had to be the goal, and this led to the artificial situation of absolute stability. The engineers set about providing methods of fixation that would produce sufficient stability for direct healing to take place. Even the early enthusiasts recognized that in a biological system in which bone itself has some flexibility, absolute rigidity is not possible. To highlight the inadequate stability of some systems, such as wire ligatures used alone, the AO workers referred to the need for absolute stability; they thought that only this method would achieve direct healing. However, such thinking was muddled, because the achievement of stability in a mandible required

compression plates (by their rules), and for these plates to work, bicortical screws were needed. Use of bicortical screws in a dentate patient required the plate to be moved to the lower border of the mandible, which is biomechanically the wrong site.

The philosophies of dynamic compression osteosynthesis had an enormous impact on orthopedic trauma services as the concept became established practice in most trauma units. This was not the case in maxillofacial surgery, however. Although several large maxillofacial units in the German-speaking countries wholeheartedly accepted this philosophy, the technique did not become widely accepted around the world for several reasons:

- Even the strongest advocates of the system did not apply heavy compression plates to all facial fractures. Only mandibular fractures were treated in this way.
- The complex curvature of the mandible creates difficulties for a system designed to provide straight-line compression.
- The presence of teeth and the inferior alveolar nerve forces placement of the compression plates in zones that are already exposed to compression by muscle activity and not in tension.
- Too much compression (especially in comminuted fractures), inadequate compression at the upper border, and straightening of the natural curvature of the mandible may produce malocclusions.
- The precision of reduction in maxillofacial surgery is far in excess of anything demanded in orthopedic surgery.
- Skin incisions are required in most cases (intraoral incisions do not allow enough access), resulting in scarring and a small risk of damage to the mandibular branch of the facial nerve. IMF may be unpleasant, but it is only temporary, with no risk of scarring or permanent nerve damage. These aspects, however, are not discussed in the Association for Osteosynthesis/Association for the Study of Internal Fixation (AO/ASIF) manual.
- Dynamic compression plating (DCP) is an unforgiving and difficult technique. Although it can be applied, the benefits of this technique usually can be achieved by a simpler procedure with less morbidity.
- Some feared (without scientific proof) that the plates were so rigid that stress shielding would diminish healing strength.
- Contact with these long, wide plates reduced the periosteal blood supply, which can be important in the elderly atrophic mandible with an already impaired blood supply.
- A second, often extraoral operation is required to remove these thick bulky plates.

Overall, there was a significant complication rate with use of the AO system for mandibular fractures—as high as 13% in one series.[10] Despite many modifications, the use of heavy compression systems has failed to become universally acceptable, although it has provided valuable research data. Its current influence lies in the limited use of lag screws, which are particularly useful in condylar neck fractures, as popularized by Ecklet[11] et al. Even for maxillofacial units in which the AO system was accepted, there has been a move away from compression to monocortical, noncompression miniplates.

Miniplates

Miniplates found almost universal acceptance because they provided a well-engineered system that achieved stable bone union without the technical difficulties of other systems and with lower morbidity rates.

In maxillofacial surgery, two separate events were responsible for the cessation of dynamic compression. First, Michelet et al.[14] and then Lodde et al.[12] developed an osteosynthesis system using smaller plates, which were inserted along the lines of tension. Lodde was working with Maxine Champy, who was aware of the need to publish and disseminate this information. Dieter Pape,[13] who was schooled in the use of traditional heavy compression plates, provided thorough evaluation of the new systems and championed the concept in Germany. Because of his background, this gave the system much credibility, and successful audits of long-term results were published.[1] Second, studies of semirigid or biological fixation in animal models showed that micromovement produced earlier healing, as measured by strength at the fracture site.

Noncompression and the use of smaller plates (i.e., miniplates) now comprise the standard method of internal fixation in many maxillofacial trauma units. This approach has effectively demonstrated that indirect healing, if combined with adequate fixation leading to good stability, can produce excellent bone healing comparable to that produced by systems aiming to generate direct healing. Because miniplates are placed transorally using monocortical screws, they are associated with much less morbidity than was seen with the compression systems.

The work of Michelet et al.[14] was essentially intuitive, but it was developed by Lodde and Champy,[12] who undertook animal studies and made measurements in human volunteers that supported the concept. This work was initially confined to the mandible.

The principle that forms the basis of the miniplate technique is to identify the line of tension within the mandible at the site of the fracture and apply the plate without compression across the fracture along this line. In a way analogous to suspension bridges, huge loads can be controlled by relatively small structures through reliance on the tensile strength of the materials. Miniplates can control relatively large loads. More importantly, because compression is unnecessary, the plate can be anchored to the bone using only monocortical screws. As a result, the plate can be placed where it is biomechanically desirable, rather than only where there is room to place a bicortical screw. Monocortical screws can be safely placed in the outer cortex over dental roots and the inferior alveolar nerve as long as care is taken in drilling.

Champy's studies examined the loads at different parts of the mandible, particularly the forces in play anteriorly. They are complicated in part by the curve of the bone and in part by the attachment of the muscles, with each pulling in a different direction. These displacing forces need to be controlled for a small plating system to work. Posterior to the canine, the mylohyoid muscle pulls medially, whereas anterior to the canine, the genial and digastric muscles tend to pull posteroinferiorly, resulting in additional rotational forces. In this region, a single miniplate can provide inadequate fixation, but two plates are necessary to prevent displacement.

For comminuted or sagittal fractures, miniplating must be modified. In both circumstances, although the plate may be correctly placed along the lines of tension, the fragments slip past each other, and tension is not generated because the fractures do not have solid contact in the area of compression. The plate then functions as the only means of fixation in all directions. The plates are not designed to take these kinds of loads. Such scenarios can occur if there is a sagittal split of the mandible or if there is gross comminution, particularly at the lower border. In the former example, a position or lag screw placed at the lower border can control the rotatory element and generate the appropriate forces. In comminuted fractures, careful repositioning and fixation of all of the fragments are needed, although smaller fragments may become devitalized.

The simplicity of miniplate application has reduced the risks of malocclusion compared with the very rigid and unforgiving heavy compression plates. Champy and Pape[13] evaluated hundreds of cases and demonstrated an exceptionally low complication rate. The technique is carried out entirely by the transoral route, with no need for skin incisions or trocar punctures. The plates are small and can be left in situ if desired. Light elastics can be used to fine-tune the occlusion if necessary. The technique, although originally not recommended by Champy, has been extended to the treatment of all fractures of the facial skeleton. With better understanding of the biomechanics, smaller plates are now recommended for the upper face and cranium.

As is often the case, full scientific explanation follows clinical success, and to some extent this is true of the small plate systems. Although Lodde and Champy[12] undertook biomechanical studies that were later complemented by the assessments of Champy and Pape, further studies added to understanding of these systems. Kroon et al.[15] demonstrated that at a certain angle, there are circumstances in which tension and compression are reversed. Bos et al.,[6] using finite element analysis, accurately documented the forces and directions within the functioning mandible. However, the forces generated in a noninjured jaw are significantly different from the smaller loads generated in the fractured mandible. Mathematical models have not confirmed Kroon's work[15] but have suggested greater torsional movements in body fractures.

Extensive evaluations of miniplates have confirmed their effectiveness. Miniplate fixation using Champy's principles has been compared with transosseous wiring. Miniplates are associated with fewer complications, especially when Champy's principles are adhered to.

Despite the trend in the orthopedic literature toward biological or semirigid fixation, it must not be forgotten that *excessive* movements are associated with excessive callus formation, less strength, and delayed union. Excellent, predictable results are obtained with the use of miniplates.

The literature suggests that an optimal number of micromovements at the fracture site are ideal for healing; 10,000 cycles per day produces nonunion, but 10 cycles per day produces good union. However, the optimal number of cycles is unclear even in animal models, and translation into use for humans with fractures is extremely difficult. Carter et al.[16] reviewed the mechanobiology of bony healing. Huge variations in the site and nature of the fractures and in variables such as age, nutrition, muscle bulk, and hormonal status may significantly affect the healing process. The precise degree of stability still eludes researchers, but the miniplating concept, which is associated with minimal morbidity, has sound biological principles to account for its effectiveness. Semirigidity imparts some advantages to the bone-healing process, including some degree of fracture mobility.

This approach has been the source of much controversy, although the need for reduction is not in doubt. The controversy concerns the balance between maintaining perfect reduction during the healing process and inadequate reduction, which may lead to nonunion (including fibrous union) or malunion. Perfect reduction may be biologically impossible in microscopic terms, except during the first few days of the reduction. Even then, the price of a perfect reduction may be the need for very heavy, rigid, and large implant devices that can have adverse effects:

- Rigidity causes stress shielding at the fracture site and on the adjacent normal bone. Without the normal stresses and strains of function, bone becomes osteoporotic.
- The heavy devices deprive the periosteum of its blood supply.
- Even if the reduction is initially perfect, the pressure between the bone ends and around the implant-retaining screws quickly leads to bone resorption, and the stability and reduction are lost.
- Perfect reduction initially obtained with the use of heavy implants is technically difficult and eventually leads to a poor reduction. A large skin incision usually is required.

Much of the controversy has been the result of the greater choice offered by ORIF and the plethora of fixation devices. Closed techniques offered only limited opportunities to perfectly reduce and stabilize a fracture. In the pre-antibiotic era and before better access surgery was available, closed reduction was effective at least for obtaining union of bone ends. As safe open techniques became available, the emphasis was on avoiding the problems of closed treatment, particularly malunion and nonunion. Early in the ORIF era, the approach was to produce perfect reduction maintained by heavy compression plates. In the maxillofacial region, this technique was associated with a high morbidity rate. The surgical access (usually an extraoral approach) produced scarring and nerve damage; fixation devices produced poor reduction, nerve damage, and infections and required multiple operations.

Subsequent development of osteogenic distraction and a better understanding of the role of callus formation have enhanced the move toward biological reduction and stability. Achieving these goals means creating an environment that maximizes healing without allowing malunion, nonunion, or fibrous union to occur. This is in marked contrast to the earlier pronouncements of study groups such as the AO, who proposed heavy, rigid fixation and compression reduction. Although its work was innovative, this is not a principle normally used in current maxillofacial surgery.

Some European centers continue to advocate the use of the AO system for mandibular fractures, pointing out that thoroughly experienced operators have a low complication rate in a compliant population. However, even in these groups, the overall complication rate is 7% using the AO system.[9] Extensive studies by Pape,[13] involving thousands of patients, proved the effectiveness of miniplate fixation. In a later prospective study, Ellis et al.[17] demonstrated higher complication rates for heavy plate fixation and the disadvantage of two miniplates

in mandibular angle fractures. These studies ended the debate about routine osteosynthesis for facial fractures, showing that there is little place for heavy orthopedic plates.[1,9,17,18]

Intermaxillary Fixation

Virtually all maxillofacial units in the developed world favor plate fixation. However, most facial fractures worldwide do not occur in industrialized societies. It is from emerging nations, which see the greatest volume and range of facial injuries, that many of the future developments will come. However, many of these countries do not have the resources to pay for expensive plating systems. They are therefore obliged to use more traditional methods of fixation, particularly IMF. In developed countries, it was recognized a decade ago that use of miniplates was actually cheaper than IMF when the hidden costs of care were considered.[16]

IMF was first reported in the 17th century, and it is most commonly used for fractures of the mandible. Its principle is simple. The teeth arise from the bone fragments to which they are firmly attached. By securing them in occlusion with the upper, intact arch, the fracture is stabilized and reduced to the correct position. However, IMF cannot be applied to all fractures:

- Fractured jaws are often associated with preexisting malocclusions, which may be difficult to define accurately.
- There may be an inadequate number of teeth to provide stability.
- Although the teeth may appear to be in the correct position, muscle attachments may still displace the bony fragments.
- This approach is unsuitable for fractures that do not involve teeth-bearing structures, such as malar and naso-ethmoidal fractures.
- In combined lower and upper face fractures, neither jaw is capable of stabilizing or accurately reducing the fractures.
- IMF is not without risk, especially in the early postoperative period, when the patient may vomit and intraoral swelling may not be detected. Patients who have undergone general anesthesia frequently must spend the first postoperative night in an intensive care unit. In the United Kingdom, this costs about £1000 per night and offsets any savings realized by not using expensive plating systems.
- Patients may lose weight, and those with respiratory disorders such as asthma have had respiratory function deterioration.
- Patients dislike it.

The disadvantages of osteosynthesis are of a technical nature, and to abandon it in favor of a less satisfactory method because of technical errors is not in the best interest of the patients. The fundamental problem of IMF is the unpleasant nature of the procedure and its poor results, especially in treating midface trauma. Many believe that it is inappropriate even for simple fractures.

Other Methods of Fixation

Before plating, extraoral pin fixation was an important method of fixation. It was used in two main ways. In fractures of the midface, it can be used to indirectly secure upper and lower arch bars to another fixed point, usually the cranium.

Alternatively, it can be used as a direct fixator across a fracture, commonly the mandible or malar. However, patients dislike the bulky apparatus, and they must exercise care not to injure themselves with it. Even modern miniature devices are very intrusive. Placement normally involves skin punctures, which can leave unsightly scars. The external fixator has had a new lease on life as a means of callus distraction, and although it is a very successful technique, the cutaneous scarring and awkwardness of the fixator remain important problems.

As a means of securing the dental arches to a fixed point, external fixators have been quite successful. Fixation involves the use of a halo frame around the skull. The halo frame, which was initially developed for traction of unstable cervical injuries, is mechanically very stable. However, the system of rods and joints that link the halo to the jaws is less rigid. Previously, cast silver cap splints were used to secure the apparatus to the dental arches. The main advantage of this system is that it can provide anterior traction to a fractured maxilla. It also acts as a guide in establishing the correct vertical height in patients with multiple facial fractures, particularly those with bilateral condylar neck fractures. The cranial attachment may be modified to attach posteriorly if a craniotomy is necessary. Levant developed a very compact, efficient modification by creating a bar attached to two supraorbital pins.

Fixators placed across fractures, usually in the mandible, have several attractions. They can be quickly applied, and there is minimal exposure and stripping of the periosteum around the fracture. The degree of rigidity can be modified during healing (dynamization), thereby reducing the potential effects of stress shielding. The position of the fixators can also be adjusted if postoperative radiology shows inadequate reduction. These fixators can be used to provide callus distraction in appropriate cases.

The main role of this type of treatment is to provide rapid stabilization in the multiply injured patient or for use where there are limited facilities before transfer to a definitive care center. In areas where gunshot wounds are common, this method provides good fixation until the contaminated wounds have healed. The external fixator is particularly useful in maintaining space and orientation in continuity defects.

The obvious problems around the face are the unacceptable inconvenience of these devices in the short term and cosmetic defects in the long term. Pin sites frequently become infected and leave unsightly scars. After 6 to 8 weeks, the pins in the bone loosen. To obtain effective stability, two pins are required on each side of the fracture.

Locking screws attached to small plates are becoming popular, but this system constitutes an "internal" external fixator, because contact between the bone and the plate is not important. It is hoped this can make the fixation easier to use and equally rigid. These plates are larger and much more expensive than others. Although well-designed studies have shown that the system works,[19] a randomized study comparing this system with existing systems is not available. Caution must be exercised to ensure that the innovation is treating the existing problems and not just a manufacturer's marketing gimmick. These plates are bulkier than a miniplate and must be removed more often, but they have a place in the treatment of difficult fractures with comminution, because these fractures can behave like a continuity defect.

OUTCOMES

Outcome assessment of reduction and fixation is not perfect because it concentrates on measurable benefits. Studies have documented complications of various surgical access approaches, and outcomes of miniplate osteosynthesis have been reported.[11,17] Most of these studies evaluated the mandible, because it is easier to measure occlusion than, for instance, cosmetic outcomes after zygoma fractures. These studies also looked at complications such as plate infection, screw loosening, and wound infection. Many animal studies[12] have investigated the biomechanics of miniplate fixation, reaction of the tissues to the devices, and material toxicity. Little evidence exists concerning the quality of open versus closed reduction, and randomized studies of osteosynthesis are rare.

SPECIAL CONSIDERATIONS

Fractures in children and fractures of the severely atrophic mandible or the condylar neck do not behave in the same way as more typical fractures, and a different approach is needed.

CHILDREN

Rapid healing and rapid remodeling mark childhood facial fractures. In many ways, these fractures are easy to treat and have minimal complications. These factors are a function of growth and excellent blood supply. In most fractures, reduction and fixation is not necessary. However, there is a risk of ankylosis in intracapsular mandibular joint fractures, and early mobilization is desirable. If fixation is required, microplating systems are usully adequate. The problem of plate removal is heightened in this patient group because of the fear of impairing further growth.

Another conundrum is determining when a child is not a child. The simple determinant is cessation of growth, but we know from orthognathic surgery that this period can extend into the late teens. A more clinically relevant definition is provided by dental maturity: After children are beyond mixed dentition, they can be treated as adults in most trauma cases. The exception is trauma of the condyles or the nose, because continued growth may affect outcomes. In the former case, remodeling and continued growth may allow a closed approach in a 16 year old but may be a contraindication to surgery for fear of damaging normal development.

Severely Atrophic Edentulous Mandibular Fractures

Treatment of the severely atrophic edentulous mandible often has a poor outcome, especially in those patients in whom the radiographic height of the mandible is 10 mm or less (Fig. 7-13). The bone is characterized by a poor blood supply and slow reparative efforts. Older patients may be in poor general health, which sometimes precludes prolonged general anesthesia. Patients are commonly female with osteoporotic bones, making screw fixation difficult and unreliable. The thin, atrophic mandible has very little separation between compressive and tension zones, and this often demands greater strength in the osteosynthesis, which has to control

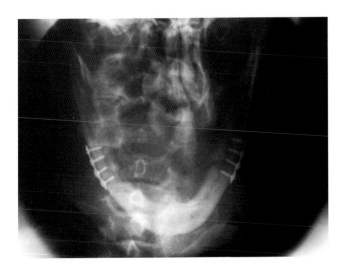

FIGURE 7-13 This typical severely atrophic mandible was successfully treated with small plate fixation and good patient compliance. (*Copyright Media Studio, Cambridge University Hospitals NHS Foundation Trust.*)

both. Interfragmentary contact is poor, brittle, and unstable. The poor blood supply within the central cancellous bone places greater demands on an intact periosteal blood supply, making use of heavy large plates less desirable. Therefore, it is not surprising that these fractures are some of the most demanding to treat.

Management of the edentulous mandible is discussed in detail in Chapter 15. Despite the absence of well-designed studies reporting treatment outcomes, the literature appears to suggest that equally good results can be obtained by very different methods. Two retrospective studies[20,21] showed that most problems arise in patients with mandibles less than 10 mm high at the fracture site. These cases are rare, with both studies reporting about 15 patients in 10 years. Both articles drew attention to anecdotal reports of poor results from traditional methods, particularly the use of Gunning splints. It appears from these studies that equally good results were achieved by heavy rigid fixation and by minimal stabilization. In the latter approach, fresh rib bone grafts were used to provide stabilization and bone morphogenic protein to hasten healing. This finding warrants further investigation.

Less Severely Atrophic Edentulous Jaws

The not severely atrophic edentulous jaw (fracture height >10 mm) is of special interest because traditional methods of fixation are severely compromised by the lack of teeth. Gunning splints are useful. This approach consists of the use of modified dentures secured to the upper and lower jaws to provide IMF and stabilization. Splints are wired to the jaws, passing in the maxilla through the alveolus and passing in the mandible around the lower border. In the maxilla, the wires frequently cut through the atrophic, edentulous alveolus and are therefore modified by wires passed higher up the facial skeleton—through the piriform rim or around the zygomatic arch, or both. In midface fractures, the wire tends to pull posteriorly. This is highly undesirable if the fracture has been displaced posteriorly. In the mandible, the solid bone makes the fixation much more rigid. Problems also arise with oblique

fractures, because it may be difficult to have a good distribution of the wires around the jaws.

This system is inherently unstable because the wires stretch and then become loose. The use of screws to locate the Gunning splints has helped somewhat, especially in the lower jaw. The use of open reduction with appropriately sized plates has greatly improved the management of these fractures.

CONDYLAR NECK FRACTURES

Controversy abounds in this area of traumatology. Is it better to treat with a closed approach, relying on the activity of the musculature and dental occlusion to allow return to normal function, or should ORIF be applied? The closed approach has been shown in some studies to have poor outcomes, but others showed good results.[10] ORIF ensures that the correct posterior facial height is restored, but it has complications[15] related to the surgical access, requires a long operative time, and in some cases, produces avascular necrosis of the condylar head. There appears to be a trend toward surgical therapy, especially when the condylar head is displaced from the fossa.[2]

The controversy will remain until there is clear evidence for and against these two methods, but agreement does exist in some areas:

- In children, conservative, nonoperative approaches are the norm.
- For condylar neck fractures occurring in combination with displaced midface fractures, there is a need to establish the posterior vertical height of the face. Because at least one of the condylar necks must be intact, open surgery is needed if there is a bilateral fracture.
- If IMF is used, it should allow opening of the jaws, and guiding elastics should be used.
- Opening of intracapsular fractures carries a high risk of leading to avascular necrosis of the condylar head.
- Low subcondylar neck fractures are least likely to need open reduction.
- Grossly displaced neck fractures are most likely to need open reduction.

Classification of Condylar Fractures

There are many classification systems for condylar fractures, but a simple one seems to provide good comparisons with outcomes:

- Intracapsular condylar fractures
- Extracapsular condylar fractures
  - Neck
  - Low
- Isolated condylar fractures and those associated with other mandibular fractures
- Adult or child

Open Treatment

Although open treatment allows direct visualization of the fracture, improved reduction, and better fixation,[22] these factors must be balanced against the potential risks to the facial nerve and maxillary artery. Even through an optimally placed access incision, the approach to the condyle is often difficult and leaves a facial scar. Several cosmetically acceptable approaches have been suggested, such as the widely used retromandibular approach.[23]

ORIF ideally leads to an improved outcome in terms of function, preservation of posterior facial height, and reduced risk of malocclusion. However, the surgeon also must consider the risks of postoperative infection, fixation device failure or fracture, and avascular necrosis of the condylar head.

An advantage of closed treatment of condylar head fractures is that it is simple, and in some surgeons' hands, it is very effective.[5] However, if the outcome is suboptimal, the patient may be left with a poor occlusion or an anterior open bite if a bilateral condylar injury has been sustained. Deviation on mouth opening is another unwanted consequence of inadequately treated condylar fractures.[25] The data are inadequate to help decide protocol, and clinical decisions must be made on an individual basis.

REMOVAL OF FIXATION DEVICES

Plates are foreign bodies, and they should ideally be removed after they have assisted fracture healing. Most plates are made of titanium, which is considered to be inert but is bioactive,[26,27] especially where the plates contact bone or screws.

Plate removal is commonly undertaken in orthopedic practices and in many maxillofacial units in mainland Europe. However, in the United Kingdom and the United States, plates are not routinely removed. Removal is undertaken in the event of symptoms, which occur in 5% to 20% of cases. Fewer plates need removal in the midface and in patients having elective orthognathic surgery.[7] Removal often requires the added risks of another general anesthesia or further surgery, which usually are considered too great to justify routine removal.

Debate has become more vigorous with the introduction of new materials. Titanium, for example, is thought to be more biocompatible than many traditional materials, such as Vitallium and stainless steel, which corrode. However, no plate is completely bioinert, and studies of patients with dental or other implants have demonstrated titanium in the lymphatic system.[24]

There has been a move toward development of biodegradable materials. These materials do not have the range of properties to substitute for all desirable characteristics of the metallic plating systems. Further understanding about how these materials are actively degraded is required. The process seems to involve active phagocytosis or enzymatic degradation, or both. Neither process is truly inert. This is a rapidly developing field,[19] and although some animal studies suggest that complete degradation occurs, great caution is needed. The degree of degradation also depends on how carefully the local tissues are examined for degradation products; for example, with electron microscopy (EM) or simple light microscopy. EM studies suggest that these products remain, but the relevance of these fragments is not understood. However, as with the successful litigation regarding certain types of breast implants despite scientific evidence, EM deposits from resorbable plates may some day be implicated in a variety of apparently unrelated conditions.

Ideal Properties of Biodegradable Materials

Resorbable or biodegradable plates and screws must exhibit several features before they become an accepted alternative to the various metal miniplates and screws currently available. They must be nontoxic, but this cannot be measured only in terms of local tissue reaction. They must be nonallergenic and, in the long term, noncarcinogenic and nonteratogenic. Data on the latter two features are not available for humans. Equally important, the degradation products must also be nontoxic.

Surgeons can most closely scrutinize the physical properties of these materials. Good strength and ease of handling are of paramount importance.[28] These devices must provide adequate stability, enabling some movement but permitting reliable bone healing. They should have limited memory to allow correct adaptation and bending. The plates and screws should degrade completely within an acceptable time scale. One advantage of biodegradable materials over their metal counterparts is their noninterference with imaging.

Several biodegradable materials have been assessed in trials[28]:

- Polylactic acid (PLA)—four types depending on the L and D configurations (e.g., poly-L-lactide [PLLA], poly-D-lactide [PDLA])
- Polyglycolic acid (PGA)
- Polydioxanone (PDS)
- Copolymers of PLA and PGA and self-reinforcing polymers of PLLA and poly-DL-lactide (PDLLA)

Pure PGA and PLLA cause adverse reactions, and they are no longer used. There is much interest in the self-reinforcing copolymers of PLLA and PDLLA. These plates can be sterilized by γ-radiation, which improves the resorption characteristics, enabling them to resorb faster. This has the benefit of avoiding the ethylene oxide remnants found on metallic fixation devices. These devices can easily be manipulated into the desired shape, typically using hot water baths at 70° C. They do not require a second operation for removal.

CONCLUSIONS

Through research and experience, maxillofacial surgeons have advanced the management of facial fractures during the past 2 decades. It is important that the specialty keep abreast of developments in the management of fractures from other disciplines, but we also should remain critical and ensure that we accurately appraise new techniques and materials.

It is essential that management continue to be based on the sound principles of care used throughout surgery. Accurate diagnosis by a careful history, thorough examination, and carefully chosen special tests should lead to evidence-based treatment plans. The treatment plan should take account of the patient's general medical condition and type of injury. It is reasonable to delay treatment until all of the required information is available, especially adequate imaging studies.

In our litigious society, experienced surgeons should discuss the treatment options with the patient so that informed consent can be obtained. Equally, experienced surgeons should perform or direct any operation so that the benefit of the experience is appreciated by the patient or passed on to a trainee. The only way to ensure good outcomes is to audit our activity carefully.

Open reduction is associated with low morbidity rates in terms of cosmesis and risk of infection, and it should be considered the technique of choice for facial fractures unless there is an overriding reason for using the closed method. Internal fixation with miniplates has become the gold standard, although this standard may change over the next few years as the use of biodegradable plates becomes more common.

Problem areas of facial fracture management include childhood bony injuries and edentulous lower jaws. The threshold for ORIF is higher in children than in adults, because immature facial bones have a greater capacity to heal without intervention and because the use of plating systems, although they may initially assist healing, can impair later growth. Treatment of edentulous jaws has been improved by the use of miniplates, but the severely atrophic mandible requires extra care in management.

The management of condylar fractures is likely to remain controversial for some time; the fact that these injuries are treated in so many different ways is testament to this. Prospective research is required to establish the optimal choices for condylar fractures in any given circumstance.

REFERENCES

1. Sneddon KJ: Audit of 40 consecutive subconjunctival approaches to the orbital floor. Personal Communication 2003.
2. Fordyce AM, Lalani Z, Songra AK, et al: Intermaxillary fixation is not usually necessary to reduce mandibular fractures. *Br J Oral Maxillofac Surg* 37:52-57, 1999.
3. Avery C, Johnson P: Surgical glove perforation and maxillofacial trauma: to plate or wire? *Br J Oral Maxillofac Surg* 30:31-35, 1992.
4. Hayter JP, Cawood JI: The functional case for miniplates in maxillofacial surgery. *Int J Oral Maxillofac Surg* 22:91-96, 1993.
5. Marker P, Nielsen A, Bastian HL: Fractures of the mandibular condyle. Part 2: Results of treatment of 348 patients. *Br J Oral Maxillofac Surg* 38:422-426, 2000.
6. Bos RR, Ward Booth RP, de Bont LG: Mandibular condyle fractures: a consensus. *Br J Oral Maxillofac Surg* 37:87-89, 1999.
6a. Schneider M, Erasmus F, Gerlach KL, et al: Open reduction and internal fixation versus closed treatment and mandibulomaxillary fixation of fractures of the mandibular condylar process: a randomized, prospective, multicenter study with special evaluation of fracture level. *J Oral Maxillofac Surg* Dec;66(12):2537-2544, 2008.
7. Brown JC, Trotter M, Cliffe J, et al: The fate of miniplates in facial trauma and orthognathic surgery. *Br J Oral Maxillofac Surg* 27:306-315, 1989.
8. Battersby TG: The plating of mandibular fractures. *Br J Surg* 1:79, 1974.
9. In Spiessl B., Rahn B; *Internal Fixation of the Mandible*, Springer-Verlag, 1989.
10. Zachariades N, Papademetriou I: Complications of treatment of mandibular fractures with compression plates. *Oral Surg Oral Med Oral Pathol Oral Radiol Endod* 79:150-153, 1995.
11. Eckelt U, Hlawitschka M. Clinical and radiological evaluation following surgical treatment of condylar neck fractures with lag screws. *J Craniomaxillofac Surg* 27(4):235-242, 1999.
12. Lodde JP, Champy M: Justification biomecanique d'un nouveau materiel d'osteosynthese en chirurgie faciale. *Ann Chir Plast* 21:115-121, 1976.
13. Pape HD: Microplate osteosynthesis: 5 Years of clinical use of a new technique. *Int J Oral Maxillofac Surg* 26:65, 1997.
14. Michelet FX, Deymes J, Dessus B: Osteosynthesis with miniature screwed plates in maxillofacial surgery. *J Maxillofac Surg* 1:79-84, 1973.
15. Kroon FH, Mathisson M, Cordey JR, Rahn BA: The use of miniplates in mandibular fractures. An in vitro study. *J Craniomaxillofac Surg* 19:199-204, 1991.
16. Carter DR, Blenman PR, Beaupre GS: Correlations between mechanical stress history and tissue differentiation in initial fracture healing. *J Orthop Res* 6:736-748, 1988.
17 Ellis E 3rd: Treatment methods for fractures of the mandibular angle. *Int J Oral Maxillofac Surg* 28:243-252, 1999.
18. Brown JS, Grew N, Taylor C, Millar BG: Intermaxillary fixation compared to miniplate osteosynthesis in the management of the fractured mandible: an audit. *Br J Oral Maxillofac Surg* 29:308-311, 1991.
19. Ellis E, Graham J: Use of a 2.0 mm locking plate/screw system for mandibular fracture surgery. *J Oral Maxillofac Surg* 60:642-645, 2002.
20. Newman L: The role of autologous primary rib grafts in the treatment of fractures of the atrophic mandible. *Br J Oral Maxillofac Surg* 33:386-387, 1995.
21. Luhr HG, Reidick T, Merten HA: Results of treatment of fractures of the atrophic mandible by compression plating: evaluation of 84 cases. *J Oral Maxillofac Surg* 54:250-254, 1996.
22. Rasse M: Recent developments in therapy of condylar fractures of the mandible. *Mund Kiefer Gesichtschir* 4:69-87, 2000.
23. Cheynet F, Aldegheri A, Chossegros C, et al: The retromandibular approach in fractures of the mandibular condyle. *Rev Stomatol Chir Maxillofac (Paris)* 98:288-294, 1997.
24. Kim YK, Yeo HH, Lim SC: Tissue response to titanium plates: a transmitted electron microscopic study. *J Oral Maxillofac Surg* 55:322-326, 1997.
25. Brandt MT, Haug RH: Open versus closed reduction of adult mandibular condyle fractures: a review of the literature regarding the evolution of current thoughts on management. *J Oral Maxillofac Surg* 61:1324-1332, 2003.
26. Undt KG, Rasse M: Surgical reduction and fixation of intracapsular condylar fractures: a follow up study. *Int J Oral Maxillofac Surg* 27: 191-194, 1998.
27. Mosbah MR, Oloyede D, Koppel DA, et al: Miniplate removal in trauma and orthognathic surgery—a retrospective study. *Int J Oral Maxillofac Surg* 32: 148-151, 2003.
28. Laughlin RM, Block MS, Wilk R, et al: Resorbable plates for the fixation of mandibular fractures: a prospective study. *J Oral Maxillofac Surg* 65:89-96, 2007.

CHAPTER 8

Alloplastic Biomaterials for Facial Reconstruction

Barry L. Eppley

The use of implantable biomaterials and devices plays a critical role in reconstruction of most traumatic facial injuries, particularly those of the underlying bony skeleton. Significant advances in materials science and engineering during the latter half of the 20th century have made the internal use of alloplastic implants an integral part of many primary and secondary facial procedures. Their use can also be traced to the simultaneous development of broad-spectrum antibiotics, an improved understanding of the healing of bone and soft tissues, and the remarkable tolerance of well-vascularized facial tissues to alloplastic materials.

Alloplastic implants are made from a wide array of biomaterials and have diverse physical structures and properties, principally dictated by their role, broadly those used for short term use to aid healing, or long term deformity. The facial surgeon may have difficulty interpreting the merits of the particular biomaterial and its appropriateness for the specific facial site. In the future, novel biomaterials will be fabricated, and pharmacological technology (e.g., antibiotics, growth factors) will be merged with existing biomaterials to produce new types of surgical implants. Selection of a synthetic implant should be based on knowledge of its chemical composition, its physical structure, and the proposed site of tissue implantation. Surgeons must also look critically at manufacturer's claims, recognizing that the implant will be in place for many years.

ALLOPLASTIC MATERIALS, BIOCOMPATIBILITY, AND WOUND HEALING

Alloplastic materials can be described by the term *synthetic*, indicating that they are manufactured from nonorganic sources. They should not be confused with allografts, heterografts, or xenogeneic materials, which are derived from organic sources and represent a completely different type of surgical implant that carries different risks from those of alloplastic materials (e.g., immunological rejection, transmission of viral diseases). Alloplastic implants provide an array of reconstructive materials that offer solutions to many facial needs, and their use often simplifies the operative procedure in terms of time and complexity of technique.

For an alloplastic material to be clinically successful, it must be biocompatible, entailing an acceptable interaction between the host and the implanted material. The level of material biocompatibility is influenced by several major factors, including the host reaction to the physical characteristics of the implant material, the tissue site of implantation, and the surgical technique of placement.[1] The difficulty in developing consistent and long-term biomaterial success after implantation underscores the complex interactions between an implant and the body and explains why so few safe and effective biomaterials exist despite the tremendous advances that have been made in biomaterial development and engineering during the past 50 years.

The end-stage healing response to most biomaterials is the formation of an enveloping fibroconnective tissue scar or fibrous encapsulation. This reaction is initiated with the surgical implantation procedure, which generates an acute inflammatory response due to the induced tissue damage; this is followed by a cascade of events, including chronic inflammation, granulation tissue development, foreign body reaction, and ultimately an enveloping fibrosis. The fibrous capsule represents the body's reparative response, which is to separate the body from the foreign material, and is essentially a biologic barrier between self and nonself. Almost all biomaterials implanted in the face develop a surrounding fibrous scar, with the one exception of metallic plates used for bone fixation, which can develop bone attachment directly to the implant.

PRINCIPLES OF FACIAL ALLOPLASTIC MATERIAL SELECTION AND SURGICAL PLACEMENT

Although the composition of implanted alloplastic material has an impact on biocompatibility, the anatomic location of placement and the surgical technique used to place the implant have an equal or greater effect on long-term clinical success. Ensuring that the biomaterial is appropriately matched to the tissue plane within which it will be implanted is ultimately the responsibility of the surgeon.

When the tissue quality of the recipient site is initially assessed, emphasis is placed on vascularity and adequacy of soft tissue coverage. Decreased vascularity due to scar or prior operations or irradiation compromises the establishment of a normal fibrovascular tissue encapsulation and significantly limits a proper inflammatory response if the surface of the biomaterial becomes inoculated or infected secondarily. Soft tissue coverage over an implant should be as thick as possible, because the thinner the overlying tissue coverage, the greater the likelihood over time that implant exposure or extrusion may occur. Alloplastic implants that are more deeply placed (e.g., subperiosteal, submuscular plane) rarely develop exposure. Implants placed immediately under the skin or with thin overlying subcutaneous fat eventually may develop thinning of the skin, particularly if the material lacks sufficient flexibility or if it is placed in an area of significant tissue mobility. In either case, the overlying dermis of the skin thins due to pressure of the underlying avascular implant. Placement of an implant into or through a tissue plane of existing or recent contamination significantly increases the risk of subsequent infection. Because most alloplastic implants never establish an intramaterial vascular supply and have an affinity for bacterial adhesion, alloplastic tolerance is very low for wounds that are contaminated or are in contact with facial sinuses. Fortunately, implant placement in the face is fairly forgiving.

The size of the implant should be considered in relation to that of the tissue pocket or wound cavity. An implant that places the surrounding soft tissue under tension is more likely to extrude or become exposed, particularly if there are other adverse tissue or implant characteristics. In certain clinical situations, the overlying soft tissue can safely stretch and expand to accommodate large biomaterial placements. However, this is most safely done when the implant has a thick overlying soft tissue layer or is placed in the submuscular plane.

Implant mobility should be minimized by fixation to the most stable adjacent structure whenever practical or be placed in a well-contained, healthy tissue pocket. This ensures the desired postoperative implant position and prevents migration or exposure of the implant to other, less desirable tissue planes.

Patients undergoing alloplastic facial implantation should receive an intravenous antibiotic infusion during placement, followed by an oral course postoperatively. Other than coverage for *Staphylococcus* or *Streptococcus*, depending on the path of insertion (e.g., intraoral, transcutaneous, transconjunctival), no specific antibiotic or duration of administration has been shown to have a superior clinical advantage. The rationale for antibiotic coverage is to prevent or eliminate any bacterial inoculation that may have occurred on the implant surface. No large clinical trials have been conducted to confirm that this is true, but it appears to have no compelling disadvantage. Additional antibiotic coverage for certain types of facial implants is often sought by washing or soaking of the implant before intraoperative insertion. The value of this technique is best determined by the hydrophilicity or wetting ability of the implant material. Increased hydrophilic capacity of a biomaterial allows more antibiotic solution to be drawn into the implant. Whether this antibiotic impregnation lowers the postoperative infection rate is unknown, but this intraoperative technique is widely used, particularly for nonmetal implants. With less hydrophilic or overtly hydrophobic biomaterials, antibiotic soaking only mechanically removes any bacteria or contamination that has inadvertently become attached to the implant surface during the placement process, and it is likely to be no more effective than washing with any nonantibiotic solution.

Intraoperative handling of the implant is associated with the risk of postoperative infection. Extensive handling or exposure of the implant before insertion should be avoided.

The implant should not be removed from its sterile packaging until the pocket or recipient site has been fully dissected and irrigated. Once removed from its sterile package or container, the implant should be handled by instruments and have minimal contact with the contaminated gloved hand. Ideally, new gloves should be used if the implant is to be manually handled. Implant contact with the surrounding skin or oral cavity should be minimized to prevent a final source of bacterial transmission onto the implant surface. Whether these intraoperative techniques decrease the risk of postoperative infection is difficult to prove, but they are reasonable and prudent precautions to decrease potential postoperative complications.

ALLOPLASTIC IMPLANT TYPES

Although many types of implants have been used over the past 25 years, only some classifications of biomaterials have a significant clinical history of successful use for soft or hard tissue replacement and repair. Several biomaterials are commercially available for surgical implantation: dimethylsiloxane, polytetrafluoroethylene, polyethylene, polyester, polyamide, and acrylic polymers; titanium and gold metals; calcium phosphate–based biomaterials; and cyanoacrylate adhesives.

SILICONE

The use of dimethylsiloxane (silicone) is widespread throughout many areas of medicine and surgery and is associated with a remarkable paucity of significant adverse tissue reactivity. It is used in the face primarily as onlay implants for reconstruction of zygomatic, maxillary, nasal, and mandibular contours (Fig. 8-1).

Silicone is a polymer created from interlinking of silicon and oxygen (positions 14 and 8, respectively, on the periodic table of chemical elements) with methyl side groups; it is the only noncarbon chain polymer used in medical implantation devices. The backbone of this polymer has alternating monomers of dimethylsiloxane, $SiO(CH_3)_2$, and is extremely resistant to degradation in the body due to the very strong and stable silicon-oxygen bonds. When the monomers of dimethylsiloxane are linked together, polydimethylsiloxane is formed, and the amount of crosslinking between different strands of polydimethylsiloxane results in various physical forms. Minimal crosslinking produces a gel, which was commonly used in the past as the filler material for breast implants. When combined with silica particles and other chemical reagents, a silicone gel can be converted (i.e., vulcanized) into a solid rubber. The varying elasticity of silicone rubber gives it great clinical versatility for use as various facial implants. The excellent biocompatibility of silicone materials in the body may have some relation to its proximity to carbon (position number 6) on the periodic table of chemical elements.[2]

Implants composed of solid silicone represent one of the earliest alloplastic materials used with extensive applications for facial skeletal augmentation procedures.[3] Although the material was initially developed for use in the chin, an extensive array of implants have become available for every conceivable facial site, including the parasymphysis; inferior

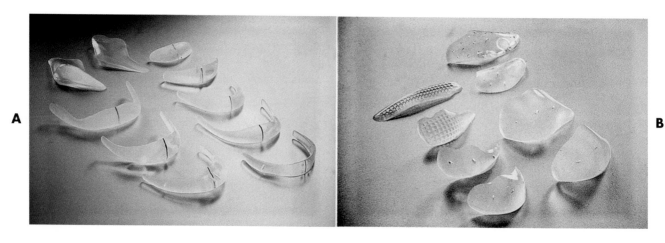

FIGURE 8-1   Silicone (Silastic) implants are available for a wide variety of onlay facial contouring procedures. **A**, Mandibular chin implants. **B**, Midfacial malar implants.

border and mandibular ramus (angle); paranasal, infraorbital, maxillary, and malar sites; orbital floor and globe; nasal dorsum and columella; and ear (see Fig. 8-1). Solid silicone offers several advantages: it is easy to sterilize by steam autoclaving or irradiation without degradation of the implant; it is easily modified intraoperatively by scalpel or scissors; it retains its flexibility through a wide temperature range; it can be stabilized by suture or screw fixation through the implant; and it is economical.

Solid silicone has a high degree of chemical inertness, is hydrophobic, and is extremely resistant to degradation. No significant clinical toxicity or allergic reactions appear to exist. Tissue ingrowth or attachment to the implant does not occur, and it acts as a relatively inert filler with a predictable surrounding fibrous encapsulation that may change very little or not at all over a long period of implantation. When the implant is exposed to mechanical loading, fragmentation of the material and a synovitis may occur because of its poor mechanical properties. Therefore, it should not be used in the temporomandibular joint as an arthroplastic or interface material.

POLYTETRAFLUOROETHYLENE

The perfluorocarbons represent a very biocompatible group of carbon-based biomaterials that are used in almost every specialty of surgery and in dentistry. They have an ethylene (carbon) backbone to which is attached four fluorine molecules, producing polytetrafluoroethylene (PTFE).

The bonding of highly reactive fluorine to carbon creates an extremely stable biomaterial that is not biodegradable in the body due to the lack of any known human enzyme that can disrupt the fluorine-carbon bonds.[2,3] In addition to its chemical stability, its surface is very nonadherent, with significant antifrictional properties. Because of the lack of crosslinking in its molecular structure, it is very flexible and has a low tensile strength.

PTFE was originally introduced in facial surgery in the 1980s as a skeletal augmentation material known as Proplast; it was combined with graphite (Proplast I), alumina (Proplast II), or hydroxyapatite (Proplast-HA) as preformed or block facial implants. It is no longer available in the United States.

It was withdrawn after a misconceived approach of using it in the temporomandibular joint as a meniscal replacement or as part of a glenoid fossa or condylar joint prosthesis, where it was exposed to mechanical loads resulting in delamination, material fragmentation, particulation, and subsequent foreign body reactions.

However, PTFE has been reborn as a subcutaneous augmentation material (SAM) (W.L. Gore and Associates, Flagstaff, Ariz). Based on the manufacturer's extensive experience with other surgical implants composed of PTFE (e.g., vascular prostheses, soft tissue patches, sutures), a variety of blocks, preformed implants, strips, and strands are available for facial augmentation from subperiosteal to subdermal placement (Fig. 8-2). The material is composed of fine, expanded PTFE fibrils that are oriented and held together by solid pieces of the same material. The fibrillar composition results in noninterconnected surface openings with pore sizes of 10 to 30 μm. This allows for some soft tissue ingrowth, less fibrous encapsulation, and little tendency for migration. The material is easily shaped with scalpel and scissors, may be resterilized (stable at temperatures up to 325° F) if not used, threads easily through subcutaneous tissue and into tissue pockets, and can be anchored to adjacent tissues by sutures or screws.

With its long history of use as a vascular prosthesis since 1975 and in other abdominal and thoracic surgery applications, its clinical safety is well established, and extensive histologic evaluations of its tissue response have been done. It has been approved as an implant material for facial applications since 1994 and has been widely employed for subdermal implantation in the lip, nasolabial folds, glabella, nasal dorsum, and other subcutaneous facial defects; as slings for ptotic tissues of the eyelid and face; and for bony augmentation of the midface, malar, and mandibular areas.[4,5] In block form, its compressive deformability by handling has been improved by the addition of reinforcement layers. Its ease of removal in subcutaneous sites due to the lack of significant ingrowth offers an advantage in the event of infection or if additional augmentation or modification of the material is required secondarily. In areas of thin skin with little subcutaneous substance (e.g., nasal dorsum), PTFE, like all other inorganic materials, should be used cautiously because of the higher potential for complications.[6]

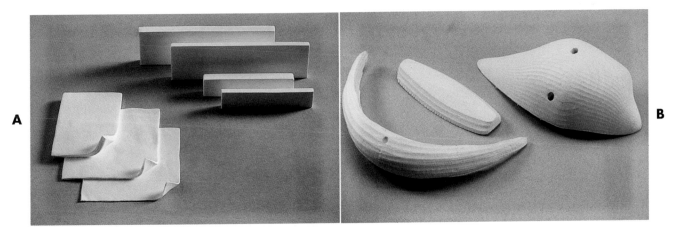

FIGURE 8-2   Gore-Tex subcutaneous augmentation material (SAM) implants are available as strands and cords for subdermal implantation and as blocks (**A**) and preformed implants (**B**) for subperiosteal onlay implantation.

POLYETHYLENE

Polyethylene has a simple carbon chain structure and is differentiated from PTFE by lack of fluorination of the ethylene monomer. It is available commercially in three major grades: low-density, high-density, and ultrahigh-molecular-weight polyethylene. Ultrahigh-molecular-weight polyethylene is used for load-bearing orthopedic implant fabrications due to its superior mechanical properties and low propensity for creep. High-density polyethylene (HDPE) is used in facial surgery because of its higher tensile strength compared with low-density grades. Like PTFE, it is non-resorbable and highly biocompatible, with no tendency for chronic inflammatory reactions. HDPE and PTFE are chemically similar, but HDPE has a much firmer consistency that resists material compression but permits a degree of flexibility. In addition, it has an intramaterial porosity with a pore size between 125 and 250 μm, which permits extensive fibrovascular ingrowth throughout the implant. Limited bone ingrowth may occur in some clinical circumstances, but the material should not be considered osteoconductive.

Although it can be produced in a variety of physical forms, it initially experienced significant use as a mesh for abdominal and chest wall reconstruction (Marlex) and is still favored by some surgeons because of its superior tensile strength. HDPE has been used successfully as a facial augmentation material, and a variety of preformed facial, ear, orbital, and cranial implants are available[7,8] (Medpor, Porex Medical, Fairburn, Ga) (Fig. 8-3). Fibrous ingrowth into HDPE has several important clinical manifestations: eventual stabilization of the implant to the recipient site, greater difficulty with secondary removal, and minimal settling of the implant (i.e., underlying bone resorption) in areas of overlying soft tissue tension (e.g., chin). HDPE can be shaped intraoperatively with some difficulty compared with other softer biomaterials; it can be loaded with antibiotics by syringe vacuum impregnation (which displaces the air within the material; the material itself is hydrophobic); and it accepts drilling and fixation techniques without fracture of the implant. Care should be taken when placing the material immediately underneath a thin soft tissue cover because it can be exposed by trauma or lead to infection.

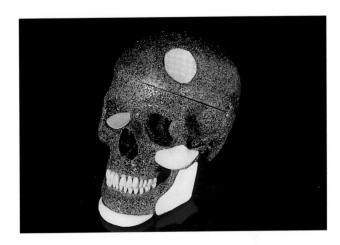

FIGURE 8-3   Polyethylene craniofacial implants demonstrate the porous surface of the material and a variety of onlay facial applications.

POLYESTERS

The polyester compounds are one of the most widely used families of biomaterials in surgery. They comprise a diverse group of surgical devices that have a wide range of shapes (e.g., suture, mesh, vascular conduits, plates, screws) and sites of tissue implantation, with physical properties that extend from resorbable to permanent implants. They are composed of large, linear, aromatic (permanent) or aliphatic (resorbable) thermoplastic polymers created by the establishment of ester linkages between the carbon bonds.

Polyethylene Terephthalate

Besides suture materials, the most widely recognized surgical implants of the polyethylene terephthalate (PET) group are the synthetic meshes such as Dacron (DuPont Chemical, Philadelphia, PA) and Mersilene (Ethicon, Somerville, NJ). This material has a long history of use as knitted and woven prostheses for arterial vessel replacement. Like Marlex, PET mesh is used for abdominal and chest wall replacement. The knitted multifilament mesh material is essentially nonreactive, becomes encased in an interwoven fibrous tissue matrix, and should be non-resorbable. It has found limited applications in facial surgery but has some proponents as an onlay facial and nasal augmentation material. It is primarily used in genioplasty procedures, for which it is rolled onto itself, sutured, shaped, and inserted as an onlay to the symphyseal region.[9] Because of the fibrous ingrowth and its soft flexible nature, fixation to the implantation site without palpable edges is usually ensured. Secondary removal can be difficult, however, and it is often necessary to remove a cuff of surrounding tissue. For this reason, use of PET mesh in areas of thin overlying skin (e.g., nose) should be avoided.

A special use of PET mesh in the past was its application as a craniofacial reconstructive material, which was reinforced with polyurethane (Xomed, Jacksonville, FL). Available in a mandibular reconstructive tray or as a sheet for cranial coverage, it provided a porous material for bone graft containment or defect coverage. Because of the development of metallic mesh and other, more stable metal reconstructive systems, Dacron-polyurethane implants are rarely used now.

Resorbable Polymers

The aliphatic polyesters are the most widely used class of resorbable polymers in surgery, and the poly(α-hydroxy) acids (PHAs), consisting of six-membered lactone rings known as *lactide* and *glycolide*, comprise most resorbable implantable devices commercially sold. Through ring opening polymerization of lactide and glycolide, the homopolymers polylactic acid (PLA) and polyglycolic acid (PGA) are created. With more than 20 years of human use, these resorbable polymers have a very safe history, accounting for the wide array of surgical devices available.

The clinical applications for these polymers extend from tissue repair and regeneration to drug delivery in a wide range of medical and dental specialties, but they initially achieved awareness in surgery as braided, resorbable suture material. The introduction of Dexon suture (pure PGA, Davis & Geck, Wayne, NJ) in 1971 was followed by the development of suture material from a copolymer of PGA and PLA (Vicryl [90% PGA, 10% PLA], Ethicon, Somerville, NJ). Improvements in handling properties were obtained by the development of smooth, resorbable, monofilament sutures composed of new PHAs, including Maxon (polyglyconate, a glycolide and trimethylene carbonate copolymer, Davis & Geck) and Monocryl (polyglecaprone 25, a glycolide and ϵ-caprolactone copolymer, Ethicon).

From the standpoint of a nonsuture implant, the most common application of copolymers in facial surgery is as bone fixation devices. Plates and screws composed of 82% PLA and 18% PGA (LactoSorb, Walter Lorenz Surgical, Jacksonville, FL) became available for craniomaxillofacial applications in 1996. This copolymer combination combines the more hydrophilic and rapidly resorbing PGA with the more hydrophobic and very slowly resorbing PLA to produce workable fixation devices that maintain strength long enough for craniofacial bone healing (6-8 weeks) while ensuring eventual complete resorption (approximately 1 year, depending on polymer mass and site of implantation) without inflammatory reactions.

As with suture material, resorption of these devices is a two-phase process, beginning with a physicochemical process of absorption of water (hydrolysis), which separates the ester linkages, followed by a metabolic cellular response through fibrovascular ingrowth that permits macrophages to clear the monomeric debris.[10] Molecular weight reduction by hydrolysis usually precedes strength loss, which precedes mass loss. A resorbable implant loses its mechanical strength long before the polymer material is resorbed. The use of essentially amorphous polymeric materials (i.e., those with little or no crystallinity and low molecular weight) appears to be the primary reason why previous negative experiences in orthopedic and maxillofacial surgery (inflammation and lack of device resorption) have not occurred with these contemporary resorbable implants. Some so-called amorphous materials may form crystals during the resorption process. Because the process is a foreign body reaction, patients should be warned that redness and sterile abscess formation may occur.

Implants were initially used in immature bone in pediatric craniofacial surgery, and their use has been successfully extended to midfacial fracture sites[11,12] (Fig. 8-4). Further work is needed to determine their potential effectiveness in more load-bearing applications for the mandible. Given the large number of resorbable implants (e.g., suture anchors, bone pins, meniscal staples, bone plates, bone screws) in use in orthopedic surgery and the diverse number of new poly(α)-esters and manufacturing methods available, novel polymeric varieties of resorbable implants for craniomaxillofacial surgery from various manufacturers are likely in the immediate future.

POLYAMIDE

Polyamides are organopolymer derivatives of nylon that are chemically related to the polyester family of materials. They are best known clinically as a mesh material (Supramid, S. Jackson. Alexandria, VA).[3] They are very hydroscopic, are structurally unstable in vivo, and undergo hydrolytic degradation. Histologically, the material is degraded with a mild foreign body reaction. They were once used for nasal contouring and augmentation genioplasty, but clinical experience demonstrated that fibrosis and resorption of the material occurred over time. Although still used by some surgeons for orbital floor reconstruction, this material is now largely of historical interest.

ACRYLIC

Acrylic biomaterials are derived from polymerized esters of acrylic or methylacrylic acids. With a long history of use in orthopedic surgery as a bone cement for joint prostheses, polymethylmethacrylate resin (PMMA) is fabricated intraoperatively (cold curing) by mixing a liquid monomer with a powdered polymer. An exothermic reaction results (temperatures can be as high as 80° C) as the two polymers cure over 8 to 10 minutes, creating a rigid, almost translucent plastic. Although the monomer is extremely allergenic and cytotoxic, the mixing and initial polymerization process occurs outside the body, and very little free monomer comes into contact with tissue. Once formed, PMMA is impervious, nonbiodegradable, and tolerated in the body by the development of a relatively avascular fibrous capsule. It has a long history of use in orthopedic surgery as a bone cement for fixation of joint replacements, but it has achieved its greatest use in plastic surgery for cranioplasty procedures in filling full-thickness

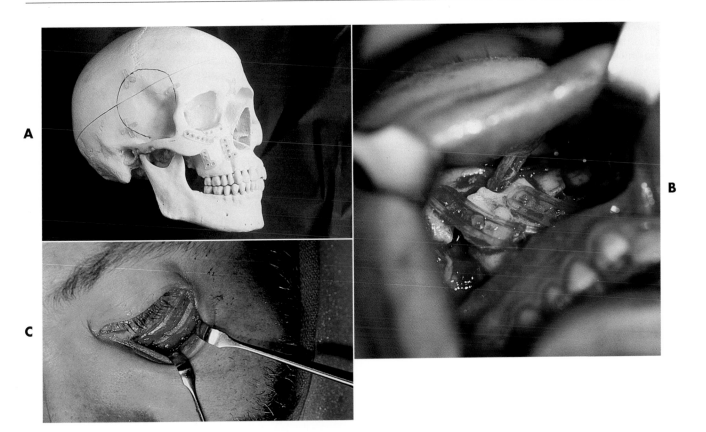

FIGURE 8-4 **A**, Resorbable polymer (LactoSorb) craniomaxillofacial bone plate and screw fixation devices are used in the fixation of facial fractures. **B**, Zygomatic fracture fixation with cranial bone grafts across the face of the maxilla. **C**, Infraorbital rim fracture fixation.

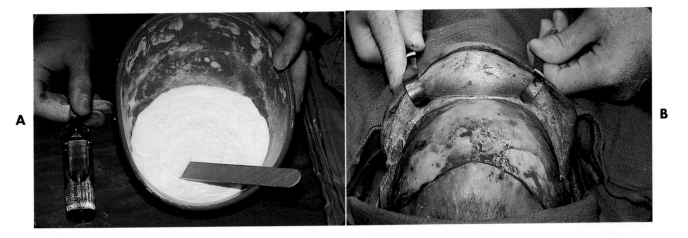

FIGURE 8-5 Liquid monomer and powdered polymethylmethacrylate resin (PMMA) polymer are mixed and cured intraoperatively for a frontal cranioplasty. **A**, Liquid and powder components. **B**, Cured in situ for frontal cranioplasty.

cranial defects or in secondary forehead contouring[13] (Fig. 8-5).

PMMA is a powdered mixture of methylmethacrylate polymer and methylmethacrylate-styrene copolymer and a benzyl peroxide monomer; it essentially is identical to the acrylic materials used in dentistry (Cranioplastic, Codman and Shurleff, Randolph, MA). This mixture offers numerous advantages for these procedures, including a very low cost,

intraoperative fabrication, and adaptation (contourable with a handpiece and bur after curing). It can be loaded with antibiotics by mixing antibiotic powder in the acrylic resin, is very durable, and can be heated or autoclaved without change in its physical form. Although PMMA is rigid, the adjunctive use of metal mesh reinforcement decreases the risk of fracture on impact and more closely approximates the strength of cranial bone. Because of antibiotic impregnation and its documented postoperative release, PMMA beads have been used in the treatment of infected craniofacial fractures and reconstructions.

PMMA has several unique disadvantages. It has a profound and offensive odor when mixed, which has caused allergic reactions to its fumes among operative room personnel; female support staff who are pregnant or are trying to become pregnant should be asked to leave the operating room. The high cure temperatures require cool irrigation after placement until the material sets to prevent thermal damage to adjacent tissues. It has a very high bacterial adhesion property, which makes it poorly tolerated in the body once infected or in proximity to the oral cavity, air-filled sinuses, or tissues with recent infection.[14] Thinning of the overlying skin, implant exposure, and infection can occur with long-term implantation in pediatric cranioplasties.

A distinct variation of PMMA with some different physical properties is a hard tissue replacement (HTR). It is a composite of PMMA and polyhydroxyethylmethacrylate (pHEMA) and has significant strength, interconnected porosity, marked hydrophilicity, and a calcium hydroxide coating that imparts a negative surface charge. Although it has a long clinical history of use in dentistry and jaw implantation as a granular bone replacement material, it is also available as a preformed (heat-cured) craniofacial implant (HTR-PMI, Walter Lorenz Surgical, Jacksonville, FL) that is custom manufactured to the patient's defect from a computed tomography (CT) study. It is useful as a replacement for large, full-thickness defects involving the cranial, frontal, and orbital regions, where sufficient autologous material may not be available or there is significant morbidity due to the size of the donor defect (Fig. 8-6). This typically occurs when craniotomy bone flaps are lost due to postoperative infection or when significant cranial bone is lost due to trauma. Unlike traditional PMMA, the interconnected porosity of the material allows extensive fibrovascular ingrowth throughout the implant and may allow for some limited bony ingrowth at the implant-tissue interface.[15] The custom design of the implant enables a reconstructive procedure that produces an optimal

cranial contour in a short operative period. Precise interlocking of the implant to the defect allows for good stabilization, or the material may be drilled and fixation hardware applied. Cost of this reconstructive approach is significantly higher than with pure PMMA due to the CT scan and preoperative implant fabrication time.

METALS

Metals have been used in facial surgery for the past 30 years for skull reconstruction, for repair and reconstruction of craniofacial and upper extremity skeletal injuries, and as an adjunct to oral and craniofacial prosthetic rehabilitation. The biocompatibility of metal implants is primarily determined by their surface properties and corrosion (i.e., electrochemical conversion of a metal to its base compounds) resistance. After implantation, an oxide layer quickly forms on the metal's surface that determines its resistance to corrosion and the amount of leaching of metals or oxides into the adjacent tissues.[16] The combination of corrosion and metal ion release may cause pain and localized tissue reactions around the implant, necessitating its removal. Migration of metal ions to distant tissue and organ sites has been reported, but their long-term implications are unknown.

Stainless steel, Vitallium, and titanium have been used successfully for implantation in humans. Stainless steel implants (i.e., alloy of iron, nickel, and molybdenum, with a surface layer of chromium oxide), however, have a higher corrosion potential, have a greater amount of metal ion release, and are more likely to require secondary removal. The nickel content also contributes to an increased incidence of allergic reactions. As a result, the use of stainless steel for craniofacial implants has dramatically decreased. Vitallium was introduced in the 1930s to help overcome the corrosion problem with stainless steel. It is a cobalt-chromium alloy that has strength comparable to that of stainless steel, and its development as a bone-plating system in the 1980s helped revolutionize facial skeletal surgery.[17] Although it also forms a chromium oxide surface layer, it is much more highly resistant to corrosion than stainless steel due to the higher concentration of chromium in the alloy. Because of concerns about radiographic imaging and artifact scatter, Vitallium has lost favor for most craniofacial indications. It has been replaced by titanium, for which these issues are not a concern.

Unlike other metals manufactured for medical devices, titanium is a pure material (element 22 on the periodic table), and there have been no reports of titanium allergy, toxicity, or tumorigenesis. It is most commonly manufactured and available clinically as pure titanium or as an alloy with small amounts of other metals (e.g., Ti-6A-4V: 6% aluminum and 4% vanadium), which improve the strength of the material considerably. Titanium forms a titanium oxide surface layer that is very adherent and highly resistant to corrosion, and even if the oxide layer is damaged, it reforms in milliseconds. This superior corrosion resistance makes titanium highly biocompatible. The low density of the metal allows it to have minimal x-ray attenuation, and it does not produce artifact on CT or magnetic resonance images. These properties, combined with its strength, make titanium the best metal available for the requirements of craniomaxillofacial bone stabilization[18] (Fig. 8-7).

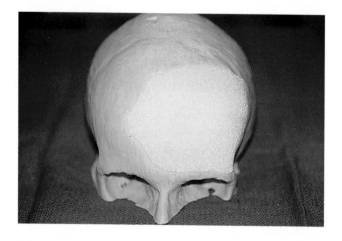

FIGURE 8-6 Computer-generated cranial implant is composed of sintered hard tissue replacement (HTR) granules, creating an anatomic prosthesis with interconnected porosity for reconstruction of a large frontal-orbital defect.

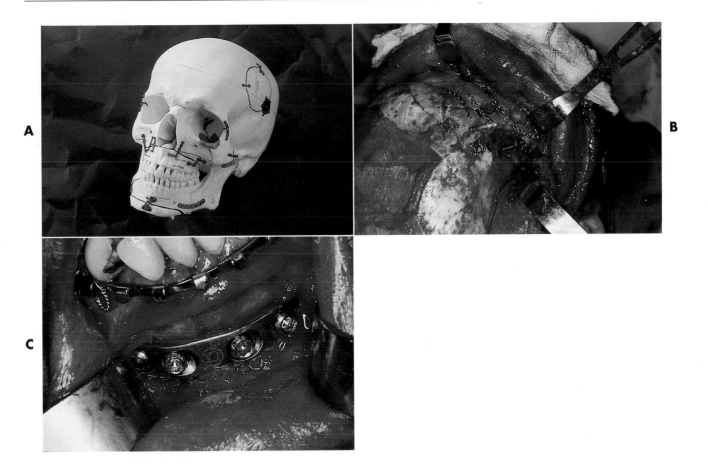

FIGURE 8-7 **A**, Titanium plates and screws are the standard method of metal fixation of all facial fractures. **B**, Complex fronto-orbital zygomatic fracture fixation. **C**, Mandibular symphyseal fracture fixation.

Titanium has a unique role in *osseo-integration*, which is defined as direct contact between metal and bone, without a fibrous interface, at the light microscopic level. This healing response provides the needed stability for long-term retention of bone-anchored dental prostheses. Although the biocompatibility of titanium for this purpose is important, other parameters contribute, including surgical technique (e.g., keeping the thermal insult to the bone during drilling to less than 44° C), osseous quality of the implant bed, implant design, and exposure to the amount and duration of postoperative loading conditions.[19] The scientific principle of osseo-integration of titanium implants has revolutionized prosthetic reconstruction of the edentulous mandible and maxilla, as well as single tooth replacement. Its success in the demanding intraoral environment has led to numerous craniofacial applications for extraoral retention of facial prostheses and hearing aids, which have a reasonable retention rate even in irradiated bone (Fig. 8-8).

The newest application of titanium is in the form of bone-anchored suturing devices. Used as a titanium anchor screw or a self-deploying barbed anchor, the devices are designed to be implanted into bone onto which resorbable or permanent sutures are placed. The suture anchor is composed of a titanium body with internal wire arcs (which spring apart after anchor insertion) composed of a titanium-nickel alloy (Nitinol). This provides a secure method for attaching soft tissue to a bone site. Although used mainly in orthopedic surgery, their continued refinement and miniaturization have led to certain facial surgery applications, such as orbital canthal repositioning and facial soft tissue reattachment and suspensions.[20]

Although gold was used for one of the first surgical implants, it is commonly used today only in dentistry. Unlike other pure metals, gold is a noble element (number 79 on the periodic table) that does not develop a layer of oxide on its surface after implantation. As a result, it is exceptionally well tolerated in the body but typically is not used as a conventional metal implant due to its lack of strength (i.e., softness) and expense. It has one surgical use as an upper eyelid implant for the treatment of acquired ptosis in facial nerve palsies.[21] It is produced from 99.99% pure gold and is available in different spherically shaped sizes, with weights between 0.6 and 1.6 g (MedDev, Palo Alto, CA). The gold weights are placed in a subcutaneous plane above the tarsus and have a low rate of postoperative exposure or extrusion (Fig. 8-9).

CALCIUM PHOSPHATE

Implants composed of calcium phosphate have been commercially available for almost 20 years as bone replacement or augmentation materials. Unlike most other alloplasts that are inert, these materials are bioactive (i.e., capable of

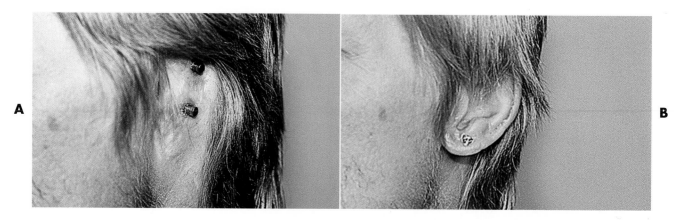

FIGURE 8-8   Titanium endosseous implants placed into the mastoid for retention of an ear prosthesis after traumatic ear loss. **A**, Preoperative ear loss. **B**, Postoperative prosthetic ear in place.

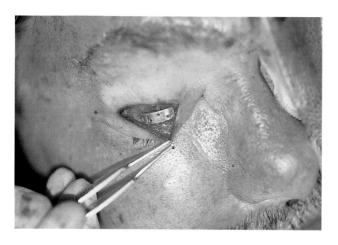

FIGURE 8-9   A gold weight is inserted into the upper eyelid for treatment of lagophthalmos in a patient with traumatic facial nerve palsy.

osteoconduction) and have the potential for tissue ingrowth and integration into the recipient site after placement. As a result, they are very well tolerated, with essentially no inflammatory response, minimal fibrous encapsulation, and no negative effects on local bone mineralization. Calcium phosphate materials are not osteo-inductive by themselves, but they do provide a physical substrate onto which new bone from adjacent surfaces may be deposited and potentially guided into areas occupied by the material.

Most calcium phosphate materials are manufactured as hydroxyapatite, $Ca_{10}(PO_4)_6(OH)_2$, which is the principal inorganic component of bone, accounting for up to 70% of the calcified skeleton. It can be manufactured as ceramic or nonceramic apatites and can be formed into a wide variety of physical configurations.

Ceramic hydroxyapatite is made from crystals that are sintered at high temperatures into a hard, non-resorbable solid. Appearing initially as dense granules or blocks, they became available in the early 1980s and were used in maxillofacial reconstruction, particularly alveolar ridge augmentation. The dense form of the granules was prone to migration before significant fibro-osseous ingrowth, and the dense blocks were difficult to shape and prone to extrusion. Dense hydroxyapatite was replaced by a different physical structure. Porous forms of hydroxyapatite are based on the structure of marine corals (i.e., calcium carbonate skeletons) and have an interconnecting porosity of a size (50-200 μm) that permits fibrovascular and osseous ingrowth and the potential for cell-mediated resorption and osseous replacement. Of the available porous hydroxyapatite forms, the granules have achieved the greatest use as an augmentation material for the craniofacial skeleton[22] (Fig. 8-10). The block forms have been primarily used as an interpositional graft material in facial skeletal osteotomies, are shaped and contoured with some difficulty due to potential fracturing, and should not be used in load-bearing facial areas. After tissue ingrowth is complete, almost one half of the block implant remains as residual hydroxyapatite that does appear to resorb, albeit very slowly at approximately 1% per year. Although very biocompatible and well tolerated after placement, preformed hydroxyapatite has been of less value than initially perceived due to continued handling and recipient site containment issues, an inability to tolerate any significant load bearing, and incomplete or no bony replacement.

Nonceramic (i.e., not sintered to make a stable physical structure) forms of hydroxyapatite are available as powder and liquid mixtures that are mixed intraoperatively, filled or contoured into the bony defect, and subsequently converted in vivo by direct crystallization without heat formation to pure hydroxyapatite.[23] Multiple varieties of these mixtures form a dense cement that sets in 5 to 30 minutes, depending on the types of calcium phosphate powders and liquid solvents used. After intraoperative setting, the material converts to hydroxyapatite within hours to days. Due to its limited shear resistance, its use is restricted to non–stress-bearing craniofacial regions as an onlay contouring material[24] (Fig. 8-11). Experimental animal work indicates that initial fibrovascular ingrowth is followed by slow material resorption without change in shape and by bone replacement. In humans, however, significant bony ingrowth and replacement has yet to be confirmed. Whether this biologic behavior changes with a longer period of implantation (e.g., 5-10 years) is unknown because of its short clinical history. The lack of shape changes postoperatively makes it ideal as an onlay reconstructive material.

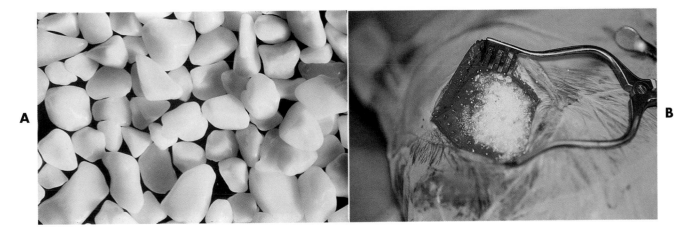

FIGURE 8-10 **A**, Porous hydroxyapatite granules are used to fill in a small outer table defect in the frontal calvarium. Granules, 103. **B**, Granules are used to cover a small partial-thickness cranial defect that is held in place by a resorbable mesh cover to prevent migration.

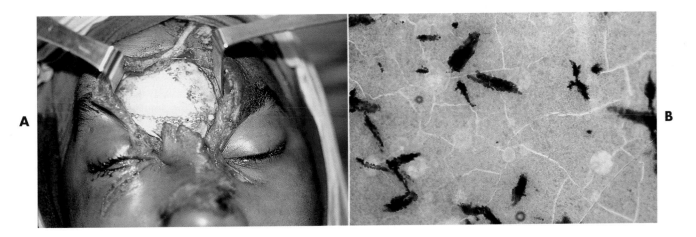

FIGURE 8-11 **A**, Hydroxyapatite liquid and powder composite is used to reconstruct a traumatic impaction of the frontal bone after surrounding bone stabilization. **B**, Histologic assessment demonstrates the nonporous nature of the set material, which is undecalcified *(Goldner's stain, original magnification ×10)*.

CALCIUM CARBONATE

Calcium carbonate is a cranioplasty material (bone cement). It is a porous and adhesive mixture that is composed of naturally occurring fatty acids and calcium carbonate. (Kryptonite, Danbury, CT). The synthesis of the material requires mixing of three components: two castor oil–derived fatty acids (prepolymer and polyol) and a calcium carbonate powder. When mixed together, two reactions occur. The release of calcium dioxide occurs from the interaction of the fatty acids, which creates the material's porosity and expands the volume of the final filler. The mixing and setting-up phase goes through three distinct phases, from very liquid to a firm solid. The second liquid phase, which lasts 4 to 8 minutes after mixing, makes it possible for the material to be injected through small-bore tubes or needles. Once polymerized, this bone cement becomes a predominantly closed pore (cell) scaffold that provides bonelike rigidity and strength. Laboratory and animal studies have shown that osteoclasts are able to penetrate this closed pore structure over time and create an interconnected network.

CYANOACRYLATE

The use of tissue adhesives in surgery has been studied for almost 3 decades for diverse applications, including tissue adhesion and wound closure, vascular embolization, hemostasis, closure of cerebrospinal fluid leaks, and skin grafting. Historically, the autologous and homologous fibrin tissue adhesives have achieved the most use for these applications due to their safety and reliability. First described in 1949, synthetic cyanoacrylate derivatives, despite tremendous success for nonmedical uses, have not been as successful for surgical purposes because of their handling problems and associated cytotoxicity. Adverse tissue reactions result from the byproducts of cyanoacrylate polymer degradation: cyanoacetate and formaldehyde. Degradation is affected by the length of the alkyl (R) group of the cyanoacrylate derivative.

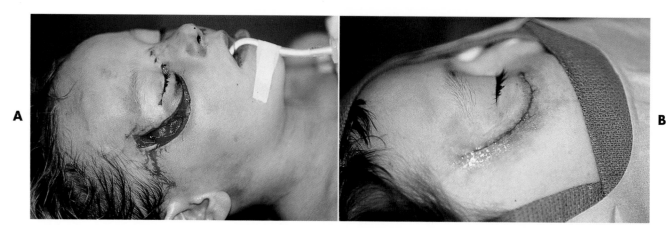

FIGURE 8-12   Dermabond skin adhesive is used on a large facial laceration caused by glass from a motor vehicle accident. **A**, Open laceration. **B**, Epidermis closed with adhesive after placement of dermal sutures.

Shorter chain derivatives such as methylcyanoacrylates and ethylcyanoacrylates degrade quickly but have more tissue toxicity than longer-chain derivatives such as butyl-2-cyanoacrylate (Histoacryl, TriHawk International, Montreal, Canada). Histoacryl has sufficient strength and reliability for skin closure and is approved for use in Europe and Canada but not in the United States.

Another cyanoacrylate derivative, octyl-2-cyanoacrylate (Dermabond, Ethicon, Somerville, NJ), has been approved for skin closure in the United States. It has an 8-carbon alkyl constituent off the carboxyl group that slows degradation and byproduct release into the surrounding tissues. Plasticizers have been added that make the adhesive bond stronger (three times stronger than butyl-2-cyanoacrylate) and more durable but allow flexion with the skin. Multiple studies have demonstrated its equivalence to 5-0 and 6-0 skin sutures in esthetic facial surgery and repair of traumatic facial wounds[25] (Fig. 8-12). However, dermal suture support is still needed (in wounds that traverse the full thickness of the dermis), and the superficial skin must be held together as the adhesive is applied to prevent deposition of the cyanoacrylate polymer into the wound, potentially delaying or preventing healing. The cost of a single ampule of the material (enough to cover 15-20 cm of wound closure) is roughly twice that of conventional nylon suture for the same-sized wound.

MANAGEMENT OF ALLOPLASTIC INFECTION

Several complications (e.g., migration, extrusion, palpability) can occur with any implant-related procedure,[1] but one factor that is shared by all biomaterials is the risk of infection. Adhesion of bacteria to an implanted biomaterial surface is an essential step in the pathogenesis of infection and has been described as a two-phase process. There is an initial reversible physical phase (i.e., physicochemical interaction between bacteria and material surface) and an irreversible cellular phase (i.e., cellular interactions between bacteria and material surface). The initial attachment of bacteria to the material surface is the beginning of adhesion, and it occurs through the contact between the two initiated by a variety of physical forces and may be reversed by mechanical washing or

irrigation. In the second phase, a firmer adhesion of the bacteria to the surface occurs through a variety of bacterial surface polymeric structures, including capsules, pili, or slime. After it becomes strongly adherent, this biofilm results in colonization, protection against phagocytosis, interference with the cellular immune response, and reduction of antimicrobial agent effectiveness. It is likely that the reversible phase occurs intraoperatively during implantation and that the second phase occurs in the early postoperative period, which coincides with the timing of a large number of implant infections, typically appearing within weeks to months after the initial surgery.[26] Alloplast infections that occur years after implantation are initiated by hematogenous spread or by direct violation of the surrounding capsule (e.g., needle injection, secondary surgery).

When a purulent infection occurs, antibiotics and drainage alone usually do not provide a permanent solution. The established bacterial biofilm is essentially impenetrable by antibiotics. At this point, drainage and removal of the material is advised. Reimplantation should not be done for at least 3 to 6 months to allow complete resolution of infection and inflammation in the adjacent tissues. Salvage of the alloplastic implant can be considered by its removal, extensive irrigation of the anatomic site, mechanical scrubbing or sterilizing the implant to remove the biofilm, reinsertion, and a prolonged postoperative antibiotic course, providing the patient understands the inherent risk of recurrent infection with this approach.

Numerous biomaterial characteristics influence bacterial adhesion, including chemical composition of the material (e.g., *Staphylococcus epidermidis* often causes polymer implant infection; *Staphylococcus aureus* is usually found in metal implant infections), surface roughness (e.g., irregular surfaces typically promote bacterial adhesion), surface configuration (e.g., bacteria colonize porous material surfaces preferentially), and surface hydrophobicity (e.g., hydrophilic materials are more resistant to bacterial adhesion than hydrophobic materials).[27] This suggests that smooth, nonporous, nonresorbable biomaterials have lower rates of infection. However, alloplastic implant infections are multifactorial, and the host-material interactions are far more complex than explained by these factors. It remains unclear whether any infectious risk differences exist among the different alloplastic materials available and the various clinical problems that they are designed to treat.

REFERENCES

1. Rubin JP, Yaremchuk MJ: Complications and toxicities of implantable biomaterials used in facial reconstructive and aesthetic surgery: a comprehensive review of the literature. *Plast Reconstr Surg* 100:1336, 1997.
2. Constantino PD: Synthetic biomaterials for soft-tissue augmentation and replacement in the head and neck. *Otolaryngol Clin North Am* 27:223, 1994.
3. Eppley BL: Alloplastic implantation. *Plast Reconstr Surg* 104:1761, 1999.
4. Lassus C: Expanded PTFE in the treatment of facial wrinkles. *Aesthetic Plast Surg* 15:167, 1991.
5. Maas CS, Gnepp DR, Bumpous J: Expanded polytetrafluoroethylene (Gore-Tex soft tissue patch) in facial augmentation. *Arch Otolaryngol Head Neck Surg* 119:1008, 1993.
6. Daniel RK: The use of Gore-Tex for nasal augmentation: a retrospective analysis of 106 patients. *Plast Reconstr Surg* 94:228, 1994.
7. Bikhazi HB, van Antwerp R: The use of Medpor in cosmetic and reconstructive surgery: experimental and clinical evidence. In Stucker F, editor: *Plastic and reconstructive surgery of the head and neck*, St Louis, 1990, Mosby, pp 271.
8. Wellisz T: Clinical experience with the Medpor porous polyethylene implant. *Aesthetic Plast Surg* 17:339, 1993.
9. McCullough EG, Hom DH, Weigel MT, Anderson JR: Augmentation mentoplasty using Mersilene mesh. *Otolaryngol Head Neck Surg* 116:1154, 1990.
10. Pietrzak WS, Sarver DS, Verstynen ML: Bioabsorbable polymer science for the practicing surgeon. *J Craniofac Surg* 8:87, 1997.
11. Eppley BL, Prevel CD, Sadove AM, Sarver D: Resorbable bone fixation: its potential role in cranio-maxillofacial trauma. *J Craniomaxillofac Trauma* 2:56, 1996.
12. Eppley BL: Zygomaticomaxillary fracture repair with resorbable plates and screws. *J Craniofac Surg* 11:377, 2000.
13. Prolo D: Cranial defects and cranioplasty. In Wilkins RH, Rengachary SS, editors: *Neurosurgery*, vol. 2, New York, 1985, McGraw-Hill, pp 1647.
14. Manson PN, Crawley WA, Hoopes JE: Frontal cranioplasty: risk factors and choice of cranial vault reconstructive material. *Plast Reconstr Surg* 77:888, 1986.
15. Eppley BL, Sadove AM, German RB: Evaluation of HTR polymer as a craniomaxillofacial graft material. *Plast Reconstr Surg* 86:1085, 1990.
16. Altobelli DE: Implant materials in rigid fixation: physical, mechanical, corrosion, and biocompatibility considerations. In Yaremchuk AJ, Gruss JS, Manson PN, editors: *Rigid fixation of the craniomaxillofacial skeleton*, Boston, 1992, Butterworth-Heinemann.
17. Munro IR: The Luhr fixation system for the craniofacial skeleton. *Clin Plast Surg* 16:41, 1989.
18. Mercuri MR: Titanium implants in maxillofacial reconstruction. *Otolaryngol Clin North Am* 28:351, 1995.
19. Holt GR: Osseointegrated implants in oro-dental and facial prosthetic rehabilitation. *Otolaryngol Clin North Am* 27:1001, 1994.
20. Antonyshon OM, Weinberg MJ, Dagum AB: Use of a new anchoring device for tendon reinsertion in medial canthopexy. *Plast Reconstr Surg* 98:520, 1996.
21. Kelly SA, Sharpe DT: Gold eyelid weights in patients with facial palsy: a review. *Plast Reconstr Surg* 89:436, 1992.
22. Byrd HS, Hobar PC, Shewmake K: Augmentation of the craniofacial skeleton with porous hydroxyapatite granules. *Plast Reconstr Surg* 91:15, 1993.
23. Costantino PD, Friedman CD, Jones K: Hydroxyapatite cement. I. Basic chemistry and histologic properties. *Arch Otolaryngol Head Neck Surg* 117:379, 1991.
24. Costantino PD, Friedman CD, Chow LC, Sisson GA: Experimental hydroxyapatite cement cranioplasty. *Plast Reconstr Surg* 90:174, 1992.
25. Toriumi DM, O'Grady K, Desai D, Bagal A: Use of octyl-2-cyanoacrylate for skin closure in facial plastic surgery. *Plast Reconstructr Surg* 102:2209, 1998.
26. An YH, Friedman RJ: Concise review of mechanisms of bacterial adhesion to biomaterial surfaces. *J Biomed Mater Res* 43:338, 1998.

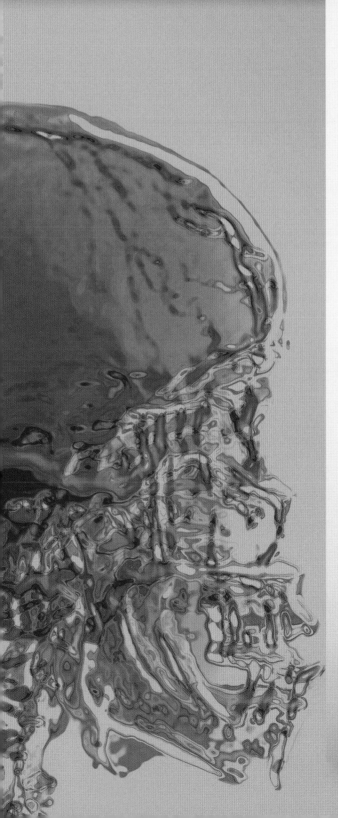

Definitive Management

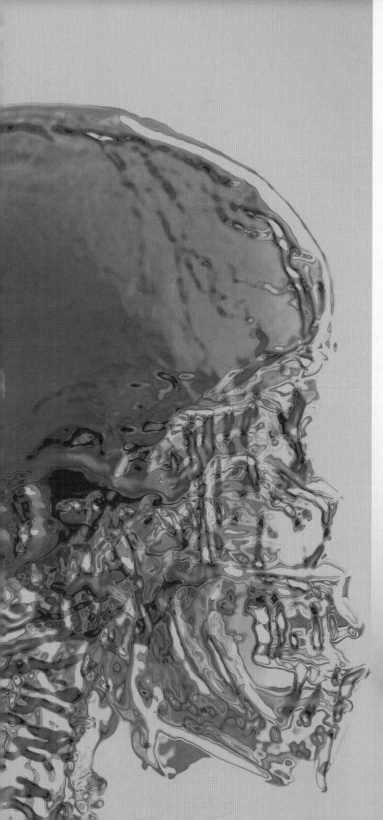

Soft Tissues

CHAPTER 9

Surgical Access

Barry L. Eppley

A long with understanding the technical details of a specific facial surgical procedure, proper access through the skin or mucosa must be obtained. Access provides critical exposure of the injury site. Proper exposure is needed to accomplish the contemporary techniques of rigid fixation, placement of bone grafts or biomaterials, and alteration of regional bony or soft tissue anatomy. It can be argued that a thorough understanding of the various methods of contemporary surgical access has permitted many of these advances in facial reconstructive surgery to be realized.

In traumatic injuries, a laceration often provides the access to complete the necessary repair of underlying facial structures. More commonly, however, additional facial or intraoral incisions are needed. In secondary reconstructions, the use of old lacerations or new incisions is required. Either approach adds scar burden and potential associated morbidity, which in the facial area may be as potentially deforming or visually noticeable as the original injury. It is therefore important that the surgical approach and its anatomical and technical aspects be understood and well executed. In facial reconstruction, getting there often is far more difficult than executing the procedure once there.

Many areas of the facial skeleton can be accessed by an intraoral approach, and it should be the first choice. Areas not accessed through the mouth can usually be reached by means of a coronal incision that is made within the hair. Both approaches minimize the risk of visible scars. Isolated periorbital fractures can be accessed by a transconjunctival approach, and virtually all common zygomatic fracture sites can be visualized with a lateral canthopexy.

PRINCIPLES

The face is composed of many intricate, delicate, and vital structures from the scalp to the neck. Rearranging and repairing many of these facial components is often not difficult, but exposing and finding them without producing additional morbidity can be. Unlike most surgical disciplines in which a direct cut-down to the defect site is usually done, facial surgery often requires remote incisions with great emphasis on their healed esthetic result. The appearance of the incisional scar or revised laceration can add or detract from the facial result as much as the original traumatic problem.

Three factors distinguish facial access from that in the remainder of the body. First, the prominent location and social importance of the face mandates that incisions be placed in locations that are as inconspicuous as possible. Second, the presence of peripheral nerves makes the location of the incisions and the dissection around them critically important. Loss of sensory input and, more importantly, weakness or loss of facial movement can be devastating for many patients and difficult to correct secondarily. Third, the compact nature of facial structures exposes structures in the path of dissection to injury, especially as the incision is located more remotely from the defect site. Complete knowledge of facial muscles, nerves, tendons, bones, and dental anatomy is important to avoid injuries. The intraoral approach should be used whenever possible to avoid skin incisions.

INCISION PLACEMENT

RELAXED SKIN TENSION LINES

The concept of relaxed skin tension lines (RSTLs) is obvious in the older face, and these lines of minimal tension are good choices for incision placement because they heal with less chance of scar hypertrophy and may be less noticeable due to decreased skin shadowing. In the younger face and in most cases of surgical access, this concept has less utility than is often perceived. RSTLs are of most value in scar revision and reconstruction of local defects due to resection of skin cancer. In most cases of facial access, no surgeon would think of using any conspicuous skin area for incision placement. The first principle is to use a remote incision that lies in the nearest hidden skin crease. This creates a list of 14 basic facial incisions, including 1 coronal, 4 periorbital (upper eyelid crease, supraorbital, lower eyelid subciliary, lower eyelid transconjunctival), 5 cervicofacial (high cervical, submental, retromandibular, rhytidectomy, preauricular), 2 transoral (maxillary and mandibular vestibular), and 2 nasal (endonasal, external open) incisions.

SHORT VERSUS LONG INCISIONS

In theory, a shorter incision results in less scar burden. Many surgeons therefore limit the incisional length, often at the expense of adequate exposure. Because the skin can stretch and slide over the surface of deeper structures, a short incision may be capable of moving a considerable distance, permitting the necessary manipulation of the underlying structures. In a limited number of facial procedures (e.g., repair of zygomatic arch fractures, endoscopic brow lift, subcondylar mandibular fracture repair), the short incision can serve as a remote portal for insertion of an endoscope or other instrument.

On a practical basis, the use of remote skin creases permits their full length to be used without excessive scar formation because the crease is already hidden. A longer incision is permitted because there is no disadvantage to using the full crease as long as the surgeon does not extend the incision beyond the anatomical boundary of the skin crease. For example, the full length of the preauricular incision can be used from the temporal hairline to the bottom of the earlobe, or a subciliary incision can be used from the medial punctum to the lateral canthal crease, as long as it does not extend beyond the lateral orbital rim.

COLD VERSUS HOT CUTTING

The use of "cold steel" (scalpel) causes the least skin injury, with only sharp cutting of the epidermal and dermal surfaces. Bleeding of the dermal edges may prompt cauterization of some of the edges, increasing the potential for scar formation. This temptation can be avoided by the use of preincisional infiltration with a local anesthetic containing epinephrine. High concentrations work best, and 1:100,000 epinephrine solutions work very well, provided that the surgeon waits the obligatory 7 to 10 minutes for maximal vasoconstrictive effect. Not all skin edges need to be immediately cauterized, because most bleeding stops with some pressure and time.

Despite these basic steps, it remains appealing to use a thermal instrument to cut the skin and for subcutaneous cutting because of the immediate hemostatic effect. Traditionally, the use of cautery was associated with significant burning of skin edges because of the width of the blade and the energies used. Contemporary fine-tip needle cautery (e.g., Colorado needle, Colorado Biomedical, Evergreen, CO) uses better metals and low energies and makes it possible to significantly reduce the zone of the thermal injury on the skin edges. It is particularly useful for periorbital and preauricular incisions without any increase in adverse scarring. It should not be used in hair-bearing areas due to follicular injury and

hair loss immediately adjacent to the incision. Hot cutting should never be used in the scalp, because it inevitably results in a wider, more noticeable scar due to traumatic alopecia along the incision line.

CORONAL ACCESS

An incision in the hairline between the temporal regions provides unparalleled exposure of the upper craniofacial skeleton and much of the orbitozygomatic region. In trauma cases, it is mainly used for fractures of the frontal bone and sinus or the naso-orbital ethmoid region and for Le Fort II and III patterns. In exceptional cases, complex fractures of the zygomatic arch may justify the use of coronal access. Its major advantages include the relative simplicity of execution, the negligible rate of complications, and the hidden location of the scar within the hairline.

TECHNICAL POINTS

- The location of the incision in female and non-alopecic male patients is 3 to 4 cm behind the frontal and temporal hairline. In balding men, more of a W-shaped pattern is chosen across the frontal component in anticipation of further recession. In the completely bald patient, the incision is made as if there were hair. It is remarkable how well bald scalp skin heals with minimal scarring (Fig. 9-1).
- The ability to turn the scalp flap and attain the desired skeletal exposure depends on the inferior extent of the incisions in the temporal and auricular areas. The inferior extent of the incision can run in the preauricular or postauricular areas without compromising anterior exposure. When placing the incision in the preauricular area, retrotragal positioning is used to further hide the scar (see Fig. 9-1).
- Shaving of the incision site is optional. Shaving the hair offers no significant improvement on postoperative wound infections. It does help speed closure and is more comfortable for the patient during suture removal; ideally, it should be a narrow-strip shave.
- A large, running W-plasty or zigzag pattern hides the scar better by intermingling the hair pattern around the scar (Figs. 9-2 and 9-3).

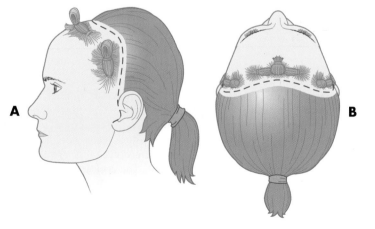

FIGURE 9-1   Location of a coronal incision 3 to 4 cm behind the frontal hairline.   **A**   **B**

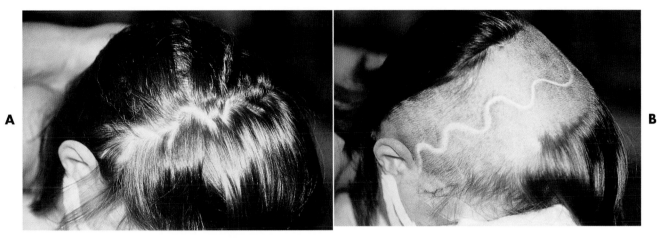

FIGURE 9-2 Wavy coronal incision used in pediatric cranial vault surgery. **A,** Preoperative view of secondary surgery shows intermingling of the hair and hiding of the scar. **B,** The scalp is shaved, showing the width and pattern of the scar that is fairly well hidden despite being wider than desired.

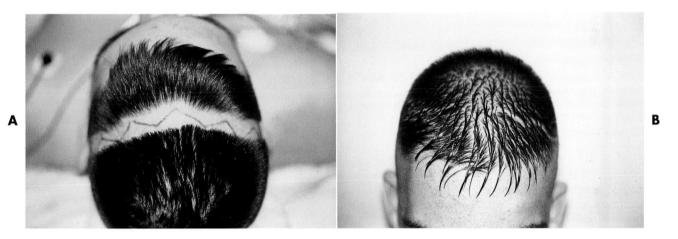

FIGURE 9-3 A broken-line, irregular coronal incision makes the hair intermingle, producing improved camouflage of the scar. **A,** Preoperative incision marking for frontal access. **B,** Six-month postoperative view through short hair.

- The incision is cut with a scalpel down to the galea below the hair follicles. A thermal cautery may be used thereafter without increasing postoperative alopecia around the scar. Injectable vasoconstriction, clamps, or running sutures are hemostatic measures that are preferable to electrocautery for the skin edges.
- The scalp flap is raised forward in the subgaleal level. The periosteum is incised only directly above the bone area to be treated. This limits the amount of bleeding bone surface (Fig. 9-4).
- To avoid injury to the frontal branch of the facial nerve, the surgeon stays at the deep temporal fascial level. The nerve lies lateral to the superficial layer of the temporalis fascia (Fig. 9-5). The periosteum is incised on the superior surface of the zygoma and zygomatic arch, which then reflects the superficial fascia outward, protecting the nerve (Fig. 9-6; see Fig. 9-5).
- Across the supraorbital rim, the neurovascular bundle is dissected from the notch. When it is a foramen, an

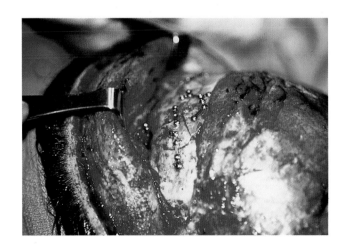

FIGURE 9-4 Frontal sinus fracture repair. The periosteum is incised and raised only directly above the operative site; this limits bone bleeding in the repair site.

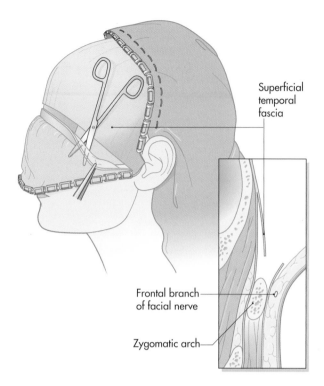

Superficial
temporal
fascia

Frontal branch
of facial nerve

Zygomatic arch

FIGURE 9-5   Location of the frontal branch of the facial nerve in the temporal area. Incision of the deep temporal fascia 1 to 2 cm above the zygomatic arch with dissection directly onto the arch protects the nerve branch superiorly.

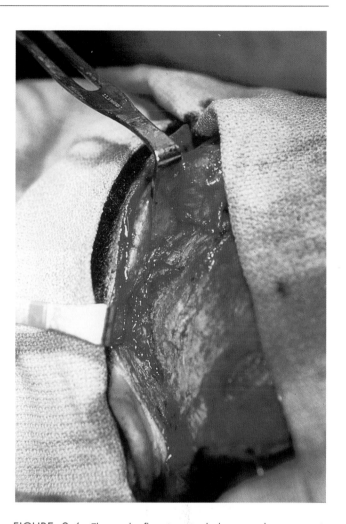

FIGURE 9-6   The scalp flap is raised down to the zygomatic arch. The frontal branch of the facial nerve is protected by incising the deep temporal fascia above the arch and then continuing toward the bone.

ostectomy is done to release the bundle. Dissection can be carried onto the nasal bones and medial orbits easily. The lacrimal sac and medial canthal tendons provide landmarks (Fig. 9-7).
- Before closure, all soft tissues are resuspended if necessary, including the lateral canthal tendon and the temporalis muscle.
- The scalp skin closure should be done in two layers with nonstrangulating (noninterlocking) sutures or staples.

Endoscopic scalp access is of limited value in facial trauma and is used almost exclusively in endoscopic brow lifting, but this approach may achieve wider application in the future as endoscopic techniques and instrumentation improve. At least two incisions are required; the endoscope (nondominant hand) is placed through one and instruments (dominant hand) through the second incision. These incisions are small (1-2 cm long) and are placed immediately behind and perpendicular to the frontal or temporal hairline (Fig. 9-8). Two or four incisions may be used, depending on the extent of dissection needed across the supraorbital and frontal areas.

TEMPORAL ACCESS

The smallest incision used for facial fracture repair is the transtemporal or classic Gilles approach. Its use is limited strictly to repair of zygomatic fractures, most commonly the zygomatic arch. Traditionally, its very small size was used for blind manual instrumentation of the arch or zygomatic body.

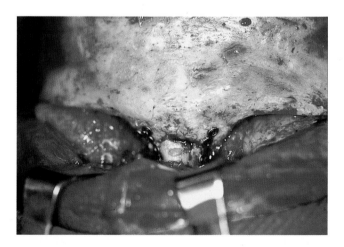

FIGURE 9-7   The scalp flap can be elevated easily and safely over the bony nose and medial orbits for access, as in this Le Fort III fracture repair.

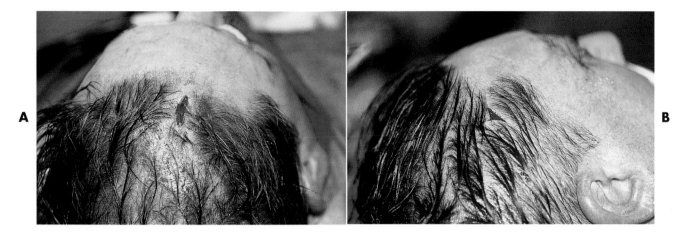

FIGURE 9-8 Frontal and temporal incisions for endoscopic brow lifting. **A,** Parasagittal frontal incisions. **B,** Temporal incision for lateral brow access.

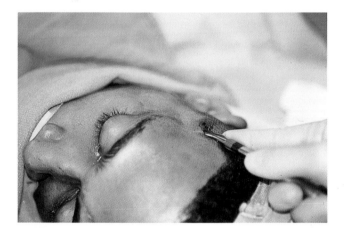

FIGURE 9-9 Small temporal incision for instrument manipulation of the zygomatic arch.

With the advent of endoscopic techniques, it can also serve as a portal for instrument or endoscope insertion.

TECHNICAL POINTS

- The incision is placed several centimeters behind the frontotemporal hairline.
- Dissection proceeds directly down to and through the deep temporal fascia. This permits instruments to be directed along the temporal bone inferiorly (Fig. 9-9). The superior branches of the facial nerve are vulnerable in this approach. The incision should be high and posterior to allow the nerves to be lifted out of the surgical field by remaining deep to the deep temporal fascia.

PERIORBITAL ACCESS

Surgical access to the entire orbit is not possible through any single incision. A series of standard incisions (two upper and two lower) must be used, and even these do not always provide complete access to medial orbital structures. Because of the thin and delicate structures of the eye and its relative intolerance to poor surgical technique, these incisions must be well placed, and superb attention to small detail is necessary to avoid postoperative scar problems. Intraoperative globe protection is important, and corneal protectors and an ophthalmic lubricating ointment should always be used.

UPPER EYELID

The upper eyelid usually offers a well-defined supratarsal crease that permits access to the superolateral orbital bone, lacrimal gland, and lateral canthal tendon. This is a natural location for an incision, and it heals inconspicuously, as is demonstrated in the commonly performed blepharoplasty procedure. In addition to skin and the orbicularis muscle that overlies the tarsus and conjunctiva, the upper eyelid contains the levator superioris aponeurosis, which must not be cut or postoperative ptosis will develop.

Technical Points

- The incision should be made either in the well-defined supratarsal crease or at least 10 mm above the upper lid margin. An extension can be carried out laterally in a skin crease, but it should not extend beyond the lateral orbital rim.
- A skin-muscle (orbicularis) flap is raised superiorly and laterally without violation of the underlying levator aponeurosis or orbital septum (Fig. 9-10).
- Use of the full length of the supratarsal crease incision extends exposure from the medial supraorbital rim to the lateral canthus (Fig. 9-11).

SUPRAORBITAL EYEBROW

The very limited supraorbital eyebrow incision offers simplicity by direct access to the supraorbital rim, portions of the frontal sinus, and the frontozygomatic region. When it is made laterally, there is no potential involvement of branches of the supraorbital nerve. When it is made more centrally, the branches of the supraorbital nerve are often in the way, limiting access. Care should be taken to dissect and preserve these nerves whenever possible.

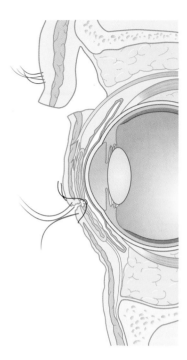

FIGURE 9-10   Sagittal section through the orbit with the plane of dissection between the orbicularis muscle and the levator in the upper eyelid incision.

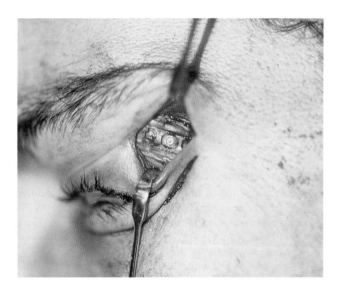

FIGURE 9-11   Lateral portion of the upper eyelid crease incision used for access to frontozygomatic fixation.

Technical Points

- The incision can be made at the junction of the eyebrow and skin or within the eyebrow itself. When it is made in the brow itself, hair loss is common. An incision in this area should not extend beyond the medial or lateral tail of the brow unless the patient is made aware that a postoperative scar is likely (Fig. 9-12).
- When undermined above or below the periosteum, the skin can slide along the brow, improving the amount of access.

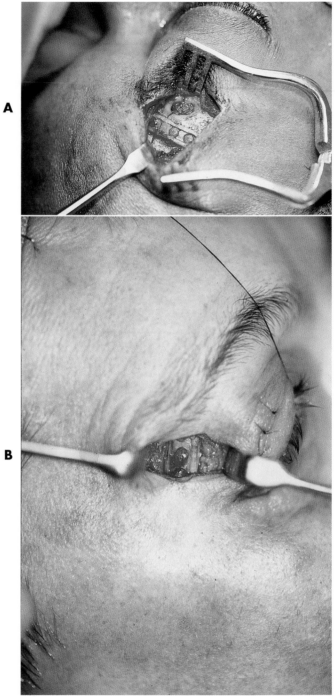

FIGURE 9-12   Supraorbital rim incisions produce more noticeable scars but provide direct access to the supraorbital portions of the lateral orbital rim. **A,** Medial supraorbital rim incision for frontal sinus fracture repair. **B,** Lateral supraorbital rim incision for frontozygomatic fixation.

EXTERNAL LOWER EYELID

The lower eyelid offers numerous incisional opportunities for exposure to the lower orbit extending from the medial orbital rim and wall, orbital floor, and lateral orbit. All of these incisions are based on skin creases in the lower eyelid, some of which are most obvious in older patients. From superior to

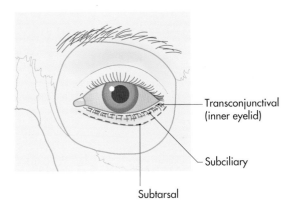

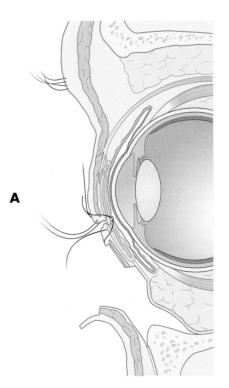

FIGURE 9-13   Location of lower eyelid skin incisional approaches.

inferior, they include the subciliary, lower lid or subtarsal, and infraorbital incisions. Except for the infraorbital incision, which lies at the orbital-cheek groove and always leaves a conspicuous scar, advocates exist for the remaining two. Because of the very thin skin of the eyelids and the usual presence of some skin laxity, healing is superb, with almost no chance of hypertrophic scar formation with any of these choices. Because the lower eyelid is essentially a static structure and is suspended by the medial and lateral canthal tendons, a preoperative appreciation of lower lid laxity is essential. Understanding of lid tightening and canthal manipulation procedures is necessary to postoperatively treat or, more importantly, to intraoperatively prevent ectropion.

Technical Points

- The external skin incision may be placed at two levels: subciliary or lower blepharoplasty (subtarsal) (Fig. 9-13). For incision selection, the surgeon considers the presence of a prominent skin crease to guide incision placement, the risk of postoperative ectropion (with increased risk factors, the incision should be placed farther from the lashline), and the age of the patient. Extended access can be gained by lengthening the incision beyond the lid margin in a skin crease, which is almost always done.
- Regardless of the incision used, a skin-muscle flap should be raised. This is technically easier to perform and maintains good blood supply to the skin. Some limited subcutaneous dissection can be done inferiorly (3-5 mm), and the muscle can then be transected if desired (i.e., stepped incision). Whether this lessens the risk of ectropion is controversial.
- If possible, the surgeon should stay in the preseptal plane down to the rim, which avoids the nuisance of orbital fat herniation into the wound (Fig. 9-14A).
- At the infraorbital rim level, the surgeon makes the periosteal incision on its anterior surface. This allows the periosteum to be raised without directly cutting through the orbital septum.
- Wide subperiosteal undermining throughout the orbit can then be done. In this process, the inferior oblique muscle, which is the only orbital muscle that does not originate from the apex, is stripped from its anterior attachment. If this muscle is not seen, it means that the periosteal incision was adequately anteriorly placed (see Fig. 9-14B).

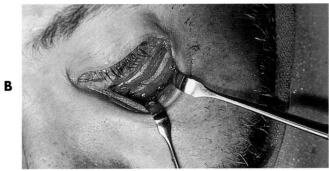

FIGURE 9-14   Subciliary and subtarsal incisional approaches. **A,** Sagittal plane through orbit demonstrates a lower eyelid skin-muscle flap raised anterior to the orbital septum. **B,** A subciliary incision with lateral canthal extension is used for infraorbital rim and floor access in zygomatic-orbital fracture repair.

- With extended periosteal elevation on the lateral orbital wall, the lateral canthus may be inadvertently or intentionally stripped for exposure. It must be reattached before closure.
- Closure consists of closing the dermis and skin. Suturing of the periosteum, muscle, or septum is likely to encourage ectropion. Suture suspension to the forehead is helpful for several days after surgery to prevent vertical lid shortening. A suture is placed below the lower eyelashes and taped to the forehead.

TRANSCONJUNCTIVAL APPROACH

The transconjunctival approach to the inferior orbit is performed through the inner lower eyelid at the inferior fornix level. It has become popular because of the lack of any external skin scar and the belief that ectropion risk is significantly reduced with its use. The technique is fairly rapid to perform and does not involve any skin or muscle dissection. Its main disadvantage is that exposure to the medial orbit is limited due to the presence of the lacrimal drainage system. If extended by a lateral canthotomy, it provides access to all the fracture sites in zygomatic complex injuries.

Technical Points

- The incision is made midway between the lower margin of the tarsal plate and the inferior conjunctival fornix.
- Two paths of dissection down to the orbit exist: the preseptal and the retroseptal. The retroseptal approach is more direct and easier to perform, but orbital fat will be encountered (Fig. 9-15A).
- A lateral canthotomy is frequently needed with a lateral canthal skin incision for maximal exposure (see Fig. 9-15B and C).
- Periosteal incision and elevation is done and is aided by a traction suture through the cut end of the conjunctiva.
- Closure consists of a lateral canthopexy suture and dermal and skin closure of the lateral canthal skin incision. Reattachment of the lateral portion of the tarsal plate to the superior portion of the lateral canthal tendon is a critical element in the closure of this approach. It is not necessary to close the conjunctiva, and the cornea may be abraded if any sutures are placed.

TRANSORAL APPROACHES

Intraoral incisions through the mucosa provide excellent exposure to the midface and mandibular structures. These approaches are easy to perform and have minimal morbidity, other than some risk of trigeminal nerve damage and postoperative loss of sensation of facial skin, mucosa, and the anterior dentition. These are essentially scarless approaches for wide degloving of the lower two thirds of the facial skeleton.

MAXILLARY VESTIBULAR APPROACH

The maxillary vestibular approach is probably the simplest of all facial approaches to perform and has the least morbidity. This intraoral approach allows complete exposure from the anterior zygomatic arches, infraorbital rim, and piriform aperture down to the alveolus. The only nerve structure exposed is the infraorbital nerve, which is easy to find, is always in the same location below the infraorbital rim, and has quick sensory recovery. As long as dissection is in the subperiosteal plane, it can proceed safely and rapidly.

The other potential problem with midfacial degloving is the detachment and superolateral retraction of the nasolabial musculature. Some patients have adverse facial effects, including widening of the alar bases, rolling inward of the upper lip, and slight loss of tip projection. Proper closure technique can avoid these problems in patients at risk.

Technical Points

- The incision is made at least 5 to 6 mm above the mucogingival junction. It is important to leave an inferior cuff of mucosa and muscle to facilitate closure. The incision does not need to extend posterior to the maxillary first

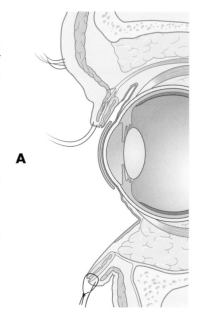

A

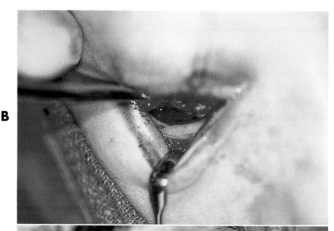

B

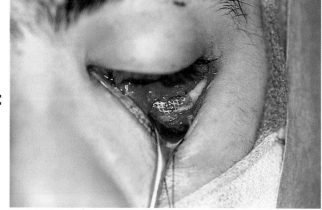

C

FIGURE 9-15 Transconjunctival incisional approach. **A,** Sagittal plane through orbit demonstrates the transconjunctival approach. **B,** The transconjunctival approach is used for orbital floor repair. **C,** The transconjunctival approach with lateral canthal extension is used for wider access to the orbital floor.

molar. The stretch of the mucosa allows adequate exposure without risk of injury to the parotid duct from long, posterior incisional extensions.

- Wide subperiosteal dissection can be done to provide extensive midfacial exposure (Fig. 9-16).
- Closure should incorporate a muscle layer with medial advancement of the superior tissues and a V-Y mucosal

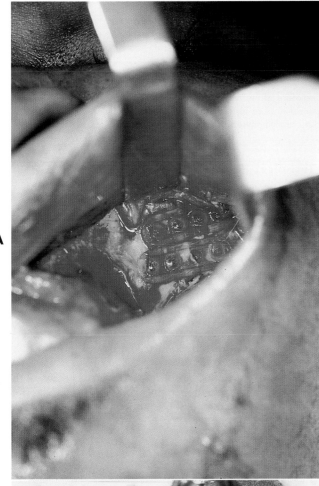

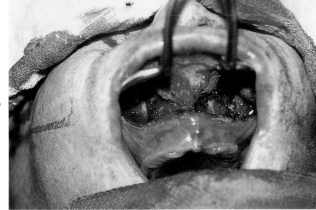

FIGURE 9-16   Maxillary vestibular incision and wide degloving of the midface. **A,** Unilateral maxillary vestibular incision provides access for zygomatic fracture repair. **B,** Complete maxillary vestibular incision is used for extensive intraoral exposure in a Le Fort I fracture repair.

closure. In some patients (with normal to wide preoperative alar base width), an alar cinch suture technique can be used.

MANDIBULAR VESTIBULAR APPROACH

The mandibular vestibular approach, like the maxillary vestibular approach, is relatively easy to perform and produces little morbidity. It differs in the amount of exposure of the anterior surfaces of the bone. Because of the mental nerve and the curvilinear structure of the mandible, access is more limited to the anterior body and the lower border of the ramus of the mandible. The issue of muscle detachment and retraction also influences this approach at the anterior mandible, where detachment of the mentalis, without proper reattachment, may result in postoperative ptosis of the chin tissues.

Technical Points

- The incision anteriorly runs between the canines and is placed slightly up on the lip side of the vestibule to leave an ample cuff of mucosa and muscle for closure.
- Wide subperiosteal dissection is done with attention to the exit of the mental nerve from its foramen, which is situated between the first and second premolars. The mental nerve and its branches can be dissected for greater exposure without significantly increasing the risk of permanent nerve injury (Fig. 9-17).
- The incision can be extended posteriorly, or a separate incision can be made along the ascending ramus of the mandible, where the entire lateral body and ramus can be widely dissected in the subperiosteal plane (Fig. 9-18).
- Anterior closure requires good mentalis muscle reapproximation to prevent postoperative chin ptosis. Posteriorly, a single-layer closure over the body and ramus is adequate.

TRANSFACIAL APPROACHES

Seven basic transfacial incisions can be used: Five access the mandible, and two access the nose. Incisional access to the mandible and soft tissues of the lateral face and upper neck is complicated primarily by the presence of branches of the facial nerve. Aside from the importance of the esthetics of the visible scar, access and closure would be almost as easy as in the intraoral vestibular approaches if it were not for these structures. Because of cross-innervation of the buccal branches of the facial nerve and their increased size, the real risks are to the marginal mandibular and frontal branches, which are small and have little chance of recovery if significantly stretched or cut.

PREAURICULAR APPROACH

The preauricular incision is primarily used for access to the temporomandibular joint (TMJ). Its limited length and exposure mean that it is less useful for the more anterior structures. In the pathway to the joint are the parotid gland, superficial temporal vessels, the auriculotemporal nerve, and branches of the facial nerve. Although it would be ideal to save all of these structures during the dissection, it is most important to preserve the frontal or temporal branch of the

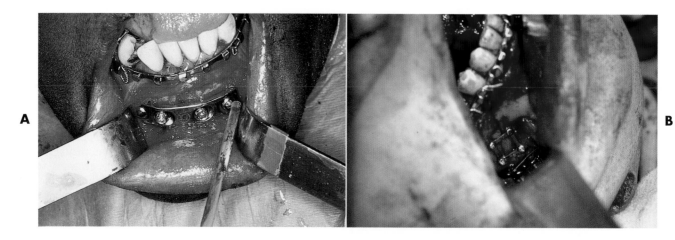

FIGURE 9-17 Mandibular vestibular incision for exposure of the mandible. **A,** Anterior vestibular incision between the mental nerves is used for symphyseal fracture repair. **B,** Anterolateral vestibular incision with the mental nerve dissected out is used in a parasymphyseal fracture repair.

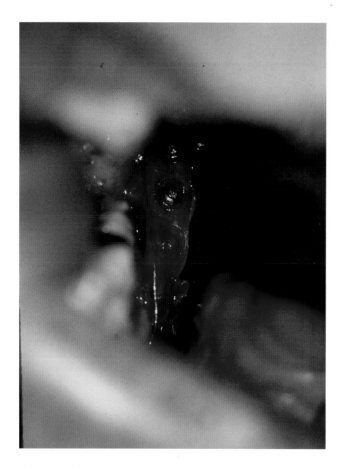

FIGURE 9-18 Posterior mucosal incision along the ascending ramus for access to superior border plate fixation.

facial nerve. One or two temporal branches cross the lateral surface of the zygomatic arch at the level of the superficial temporal fascia. The crossing point is highly variable and can be anywhere from 10 to 30 mm in front of the external auditory canal. A safe plane of dissection to the TMJ is to stay on the cartilaginous anterior surface of the canal and retract all soft tissue forward; this also protects the temporal vessels and the auriculotemporal nerve.

Technical Points

- The incision follows the junction of the skin and ear from the temporal area down to the earlobe, with the exception of the tragus. Extending the incision retrotragally hides the scar better and carries no risk of tragal deformity because this is not a skin excisional procedure (Fig. 9-19).
- Dissection above the zygomatic arch continues down to the superficial temporal fascia. Below the arch, the dissection proceeds along the external auditory canal.
- The joint is entered by incising the temporal fascia and developing a subperiosteal plane down into the superior joint space with retraction of the tissues in front of the canal (Fig. 9-20).
- Closure of the joint capsule is controversial because it may contribute to postoperative formation of adhesions. Closure of the temporal fascia should be done before skin closure.

RHYTIDECTOMY

The facelift approach is an extension of the preauricular approach and inferiorly incorporates the retromandibular approach. Calling it a facelift denotes only the location of the skin incision and has nothing to do with dissection or manipulation of the superficial facial fascial planes. It primarily places the great auricular nerve, which is the most commonly injured structure in a facelift, and the marginal mandibular branch of the facial nerve at risk. Elevation of the skin flap may injure the greater auricular nerve inferiorly as it emerges from the deep fascia at the middle of the posterior border of the neck to cross over the sternocleidomastoid muscle at a 45-degree angle toward the posterior border of the mandible. The deeper dissection to approach the mandible places the facial nerve branch at risk.

Technical Points

- The incision is identical to the preauricular incision with a retrotragal extension until it reaches the earlobe. At that point, the posterior extension can take one of two routes. A traditional rhytidectomy incision is carried onto the

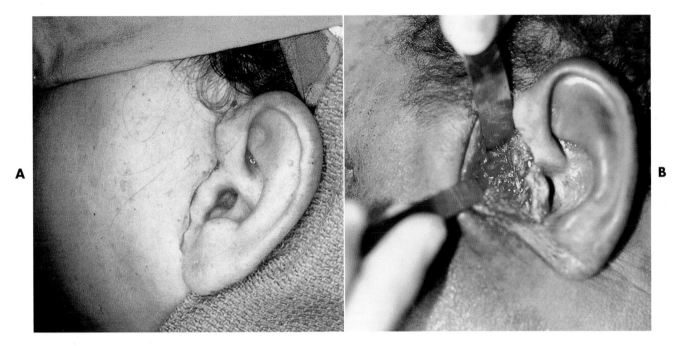

FIGURE 9-19   Preauricular incisional approach. **A,** The preauricular incision should go retrotragal and not pretragal, as in this patient. **B,** The retrotragal preauricular incision hides the scar better, with no increased morbidity.

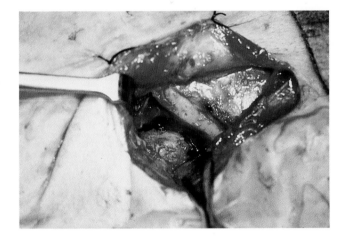

FIGURE 9-20   Preauricular approach with exposure into the superior joint space of the temporomandibular joint.

back of the ear and cut into the hairline at the level of the tragus (Fig. 9-21A). An alternative and preferable approach is to curve the incision back and downward from the earlobe into a high cervical crease (see Fig. 9-21B). Although this makes a slightly more visible scar, the anterior exposure obtained by the neck extension is greatly improved.
- The skin flap is quickly raised and is best done with blunt scissors pointed upward with a spreading and pushing maneuver.
- Access to the mandible is done as for the retromandibular approach.
- Skin closure should be performed over a drain that exits posteriorly.

RETROMANDIBULAR APPROACH

The retromandibular approach is commonly used for exposure of the posterior ramus of the mandible and for low subcondylar and condylar neck fractures. It is the shortest distance from the skin to that area but requires identification of the marginal mandibular branch of the facial nerve. The path of dissection to the posterior mandible lies between the superior and inferior divisions of the facial nerve. Short of the angular region, access to the superior and anterior ramus is somewhat limited by the mass of the overlying parotid gland and soft tissue. Blunt dissection is recommended after the skin incision has been made.

Technical Points
- The incision is placed in a vertical orientation directly beneath the earlobe, paralleling the posterior border of the ramus. The incision may be placed more posteriorly in a skin crease, but access then becomes farther away.
- Dissection cuts through the parotid gland with exposure of the facial nerve. A more posterior incision avoids the inferior branch of the facial nerve and the parotid gland, but exposure is more limited.
- Division of the pterygomasseteric sling is necessary to approach the bone.
- Once the subperiosteal plane of the mandible is reached, retractors placed in the sigmoid notch or the anterior ramus, or both, aid greatly in exposure.
- Closure of the pterygomasseteric sling, parotid capsule, and platysma layer should be done before skin closure.

SUBMANDIBULAR APPROACH

Approach from a high cervical incision, historically referred to as a Risdon incision, is a standard method for procedures

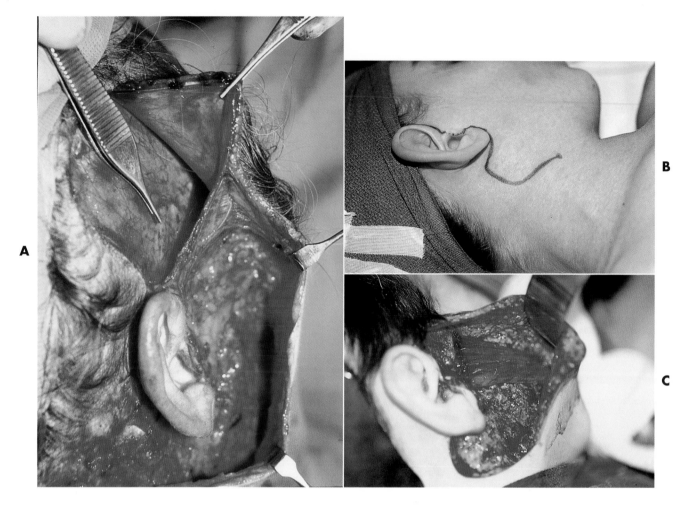

FIGURE 9-21 Facelift-type approaches. **A,** Traditional full facelift with the temporal fascial plane *(forceps)* separated from the submusculoaponeurotic plane inferiorly. **B** and **C,** The traditional superior facelift approach combined with an anterior neck incision for improved access to facial vessels is necessary in this free gracilis facial reanimation procedure.

involving the posterior body and ramus of the mandible. The exact location of the incision varies, but all descriptions place it below the inferior border of the mandible. The single greatest obstacle in the dissection is the marginal mandibular branch of the facial nerve. Although its course varies somewhat, this branch is below the inferior border of the mandible in many cases when it is posterior to the crossing of the facial artery. Anterior to the facial artery, it is almost always above the inferior border. It is rarely lower than 1 to 1.5 cm below the inferior border, and for this reason, the incision is often placed two fingerbreadths or 2 cm below the inferior border.

Technical Points

- A skin crease that is 1.5 to 2.0 cm below the inferior border is chosen for the incision. It may be horizontally more posterior or anterior, depending on what part of the mandible is to be treated. Turning the head away from the side to be treated helps move the nerve more superiorly.
- Below the platysma, the underlying cervical fascia, the facial artery and vein, and the marginal mandibular nerve are found. The facial vessels often need to be ligated in more anterior approaches (Fig. 9-22). The nerve should be

stimulated to confirm its location, and it should lie superiorly.

- Division of the pterygomasseteric sling, subperiosteal dissection, and exposure of the mandible are then performed (Fig. 9-23). Closure proceeds as in the retromandibular approach.

SUBMENTAL APPROACH

The most anterior-inferior border approach to the mandible and midline neck structures is an extension of the submandibular approach. It is used for access to the anterior mandible for symphyseal manipulation. It differs from all other cervicofacial approaches by having no significant anatomic structures between the skin and the bone. Sharp dissection may be performed with impunity.

Technical Points

- The submental skin crease is chosen for the incision. In young patients, a skin crease may not be present, and the incision should be placed behind the inferior border, because the neck will be at some degree of extension.

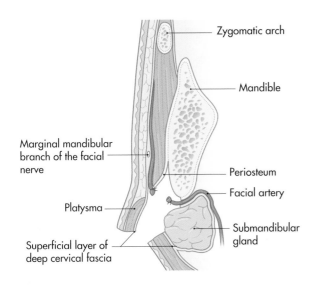

Zygomatic arch

Mandible

Marginal mandibular branch of the facial nerve

Periosteum

Facial artery

Platysma

Submandibular gland

Superficial layer of deep cervical fascia

FIGURE 9-22 Coronal illustration of the path of dissection in the submandibular approach. The initial dissection goes through the platysma muscle to the superficial layer of the deep cervical fascia. It then moves above the submandibular gland to the periosteum of the mandible.

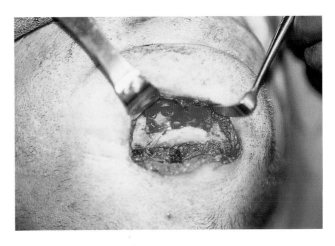

FIGURE 9-24 Submental approach for a symphyseal fracture repair.

- Direct access is provided to the bone, where good exposure can be achieved for fracture repair or implant placement (Fig. 9-24).

NASAL APPROACHES

The nasal bones and cartilages are addressed through two basic approaches: an endonasal approach, in which all the incisions are within the nasal cavity, and an external open method, which incorporates a columellar skin incision. Either approach can be effective in experienced hands. They differ primarily by the amount of exposure and visualization of the nasal structures. These unique facial incisions provide access to a structure composed of bone and cartilage.

ENDONASAL APPROACH

A variety of mucosal incisions exist for intranasal access for treatment of dorsal, tip, and septal deformities. They include the marginal, intercartilaginous, and transfixion incisions (Fig. 9-25), which represent standard closed approaches to nasal surgery. An intercartilaginous incision permits approach to the nasal dorsum. A unilateral transfixion incision alone (i.e., hemitransfixion) allows access to the septum. The combination of the marginal, intercartilaginous, and transfixion incisions allows complete delivery of the lower lateral cartilages. There is little use for the isolated marginal incision, except in secondary cases for graft placement for the treatment of alar retraction.

Technical Points

- A marginal incision follows the caudal margin of the lower lateral cartilage rather than the margin of the nostril. It is important to appreciate the relationship of these two structures; the caudal cartilaginous margin and the rim are closer together medially than laterally (see Fig. 9-25). The incision diverges from the rim as it goes laterally. It is important to avoid traversing the soft triangle, a medial alar rim zone formed by two juxtaposed layers of skin unsupported by cartilage, to avoid postoperative alar rim notching.

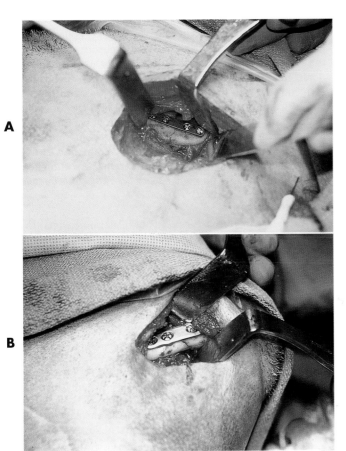

A

B

FIGURE 9-23 Surgical procedures with a submandibular approach. **A,** More posterior approach for access to an angle fracture. **B,** More anterior approach for access to a body fracture.

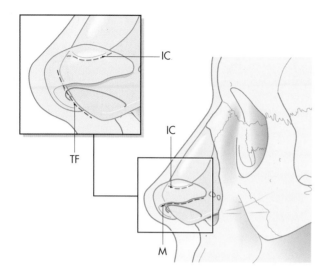

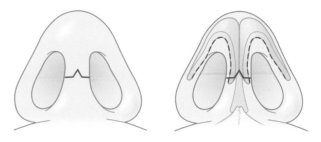

FIGURE 9-27   Transcolumellar incisional designs.

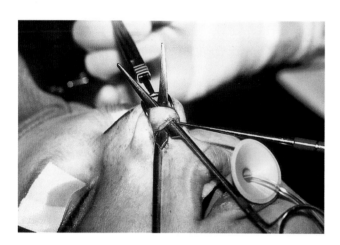

FIGURE 9-25   Sagittal view of intranasal incisions. IC, intercartilaginous incision; M, marginal incision; TF, transfixion incision that follows the caudal border of the septum (inset).

FIGURE 9-26   Technique of lower lateral cartilage delivery through intranasal incisions.

with vestibular skin based medially and laterally for its vascularity.

- Isolated septal exposure is done through a transfixion incision. For septal manipulation, the incision is placed at the caudal end of the septum. For cartilage graft harvest, the incision may be placed more posteriorly, directly over the septum. In either case, wide subperichondrial dissection is done.
- Closure of the septum and intranasal incisions is done with small resorbable sutures and with external taping or splints, or both. Quilting resorbable sutures are used through the septum to close dead space. No intranasal packing is used.

EXTERNAL (OPEN) APPROACHES

The popularity of the external rhinoplasty approach has resulted primarily from the amount of exposure obtained and the resultant increased ease and reliability of nasal tip and dorsal manipulation. It caused considerable debate during its early introduction and quickly became the most controversial 6 mm of skin incision in the entire face. However, its ability to guide surgeons in rhinoplasty and to improve the postoperative results, particularly in the tip and dome area, have rightly confirmed its place as a recognized method of nasal access. With some experience and careful dissection technique, the resultant columellar scar is of little consequence.

Technical Points

- The external approach consists of bilateral marginal incisions connected by a midcolumellar incision. The marginal incision follows the caudal margin of the lower lateral cartilage rather than the margin of the nostril. The columellar incision is made at the narrowest portion of the columella between the columella-lobule junction and the flare of the feet of the medial crura. Many types of skin incisions are used, most commonly an inverted V and stairstep pattern (Fig. 9-27).
- The two incisions are connected, with care taken not to transect the medial crura, which are quite superficial, particularly in the transition from the columella to the dome.
- The skin is dissected off the dome and lower lateral cartilages and up onto the upper lateral cartilages to the dorsum, providing wide exposure of the lower two thirds of the nasal framework (Fig. 9-28).
- Closure is done with small permanent sutures on the columellar skin (no dermal suturing) and small resorbable sutures for the nasal mucosa. External taping or splinting is done to adapt the skin to the underlying skeleton.

- The intercartilaginous incision is placed at the junction of the upper and lower lateral cartilages. With the lower lateral cartilage everted, the inferior edge of the upper lateral cartilage can be seen protruding into the vestibule. The incision is made parallel to the cephalic margin of the lower lateral cartilage, avoiding the nasal valve area (see Fig. 9-25).
- A transfixion incision is made at the caudal end of the septum. A hemitransfixion incision is made only through one nostril, leaving the membranous septum intact on the opposite side. A full transfixion incision traverses both sides, extends inferiorly to sever the columella and lip from the septal cartilage and anterior nasal spine, and connects superiorly to the intercartilaginous incision for complete separation of the soft tissues overlying the dorsum and columella from the septum. This allows complete exposure of the septum and delivery of the lower lateral cartilages (Fig. 9-26). These incisions and dissection create a bipedicled flap of lower lateral cartilages lined

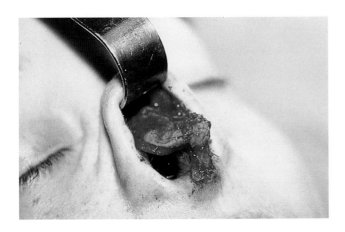

FIGURE 9-28 Complete exposure of the lower two thirds of the nose through the open approach.

ENDOSCOPIC ACCESS

A new and alternative approach for the treatment of maxillofacial trauma can be offered by endoscopic techniques. Potentially, this approach can minimize the incisions and scars, decrease the risk of a sensory or motor nerve injury, and help the surgeon to better visualize the reduction of the fractures. There is still no general agreement among surgeons regarding the practicality of these procedures. The results and the efficiency of these techniques depend on the experience and training of the surgeon, the nature of the procedure, and the instrumentation that is used. The literature contains descriptions of endoscopic or minimally invasive techniques that can assist in the exposure of fractures of the zygomatic arch, the orbital floor, or the frontal sinus and the subcondylar fracture of the mandible.

Endoscope-assisted zygomatic arch repair represents an advance in midfacial trauma management and has the potential to avoid the use of coronal incision. It has been proposed for the repair of Le Fort III, complex zygoma, and isolated arch fractures. Early use of preauricular incisions for placement of the endoscope to follow the arch has been associated with possible damage to the frontal branch of the facial nerve. Most accepted techniques combine the Keen or Gilles approach with intraoperative radiographic techniques (i.e., mini-C arm, special three-dimensional C-arm, or intraoperative computed tomographic imaging). Disadvantages are the

steep learning curve, the loss of tactile perception, and the need for expensive special surgical instruments and devices.

The main approach used in the various endoscopic techniques for treatment of orbital trauma is a Caldwell-Luc approach to the anterior maxillary sinus. The maxillary sinus represents a real cavity that can be used to enhance visualization of the fracture defect. This approach can facilitate the repair of certain orbital floor fractures with release of periorbital tissue trapped in a hinged or small blowout defect. It can also determine the need to repair the floor after reduction of displaced orbitozygomatic fractures. Placement of an orbital floor implant with this approach has been described. It can be pushed into the orbit to span the orbital defect or anchored within the maxillary sinus and secured in place with screws.

Endoscopic techniques have been used in the management of selected frontal sinus fractures (e.g., anterior wall frontal sinus fractures) that involve several large segments without extensive comminution. Reduction of these fractures can be facilitated with the use of an endoscope, similar to an endoscopic forehead lifting technique. Forehead soft tissues are elevated subperiosteally, and the fractures are visualized by means of a 30-degree endoscope with an external sheath for soft tissue retraction. After the fracture site is visualized, small external incisions are made directly over the fractures to allow the surgeon to apply anterior force for anatomical reduction of the fracture segments. The fractures are elevated with the use of percutaneous nerve hooks or by drilling into the fragments and grabbing them with threaded Steinmann pins. With gentle retraction, the fragments often elevate into a reduced position and are frequently stable without the need for rigid fixation. It is common to have residual surface irregularities, which can be camouflaged with patches of overlying synthetic materials.

One of the most controversial applications of endoscopic techniques in the management of facial fractures is the use of the endoscope in the management of subcondylar fractures. This technique uses an intraoral approach to create a wide exposure of the posterior portion of the subcondylar region and ramus. A 30-degree endoscope and a 4-mm endoscopic brow lift sheath that maintains the optical cavity are inserted through the incision. After fracture reduction, fixation is accomplished with the use of transcutaneous trocars for drilling the holes and placing the screws, or right-angled drills and screwdrivers that can be inserted through the intraoral incision are used. This is a technically difficult procedure, and there is a risk of injury to the vein or the facial nerve branch that runs immediately behind the condyle.

CHAPTER 10

A Logical Approach to Orbital Trauma

Leo F.A. Stassen, Nils-Claudius Gellrich

The management of orbital injuries is one of the most interesting and difficult areas in facial trauma. The consequences of an orbital injury are dramatic. They vary from a loss of vision to diplopia, loss of an eye, epiphora, a disturbing loss of facial sensation, and an unsightly and unacceptable appearance of the eye and the hard and soft tissues around it (Fig. 10-1). These injuries demand a careful attention to detail, but the difficulties are often underestimated and therefore undertreated.

When we look at each other, all areas of the face are important, but there is no doubt that the eyes and how they appear play a very important part in how we initially perceive each other. The eyes are the outward expression of our minds (Fig. 10-2).

Persistent enophthalmos (sunken eye), hypoglobus or hyperglobus (dropped or raised level of the globe, respectively), strabismus (squint), diplopia (double vision), deteriorated visual acuity or blindness, a false eye, ectropion (eyelid turned out), entropion (eyelid turned in), scarring, fat atrophy, zygomatic malalignment, and canthal dystopia are all significant and debilitating problems (Fig. 10-3). They are common complications of orbital and zygomatic surgery. All lead to distress and to a loss of function (vision) or esthetics or both. Psychological support and counseling may be required.[1]

It is essential to take both the soft and hard tissues into consideration. If either is ignored, patient care will be compromised. Treatment must avoid exacerbation of the problem by the poor positioning of facial access incisions (Figs. 10-4 through 10-6).[2,3] It is possible to expose most of the face and orbit with esthetic incisions: coronal, transconjunctival (sometimes with lateral extension), transcaruncular, lower lid, and intraoral.[2-5] Endoscopic assessment of injuries and orbital fracture repair is becoming more common.[6-8]

How do we ensure that we get the best results for our patients? The controversies surrounding orbital injuries include the following:

- The type, detail, and extent of preoperative clinical examination and investigations that are required
- The timing of primary surgery (early or late)
- Incisions for fracture exposure
- The type of fixation at primary and secondary surgery (i.e., none, multiple, resorbable plates, or non-resorbable plates)
- Role of intraoperative guidance (navigation systems)
- Bone grafting versus alloplastic materials

- The management and prevention of diplopia
- The prevention of enophthalmos
- The management of infraorbital nerve numbness or dysesthesia
- The management of decreasing visual acuity or an acutely blind eye
- The management of ocular injuries
- Length of follow-up and use of postoperative imaging (computed tomographic [CT] scans)

Assessment, preoperative investigations, collaboration with others, timing of surgery, and methods of treatment, follow-up, and secondary management all demand consideration.

Orbital injuries can occur alone, but most often they are associated with other injuries, such as zygomatic (malar), frontal sinus, naso-orbitoethmoidal, or Le Fort II/III fractures and skull fractures. They are a mixture of low-force injuries (zygomatic fracture, orbital floor, naso-orbitoethmoidal) and high-force injuries (supraorbital rim, orbital roof, frontal sinus) (Fig. 10-7). Orbital injuries are complicated by their proximity to the brain, eye, nasolacrimal apparatus, facial nerve, and sinuses.

The etiology of orbital injuries varies by geographic location. In the United Kingdom, orbital injuries are most often caused by assaults, usually in association with alcohol, but they also occur as a result of road traffic accidents, horse riding accidents, falls, sports, and industrial accidents. Gunshot injuries are rare but are becoming more common. The greater the force, the more comminuted and displaced the fracture and the greater the association with other serious injuries. High-force injuries (e.g., orbital roof, supraorbital rim) have a mortality rate of 12% from associated injuries of the head, neck, and chest. Zygomatic and orbital injuries involving the floor and medial wall are low-impact (low-force) injuries. Injuries involving the medial canthal area (naso-orbitoethmoidal) are associated with intermediate force.

The principles of acute trauma life support for maxillofacial surgery must not be forgotten and are similar to those for any injury (Fig. 10-8):

Airway
Breathing
Circulation, **c**ervical spine

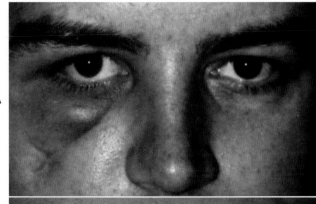

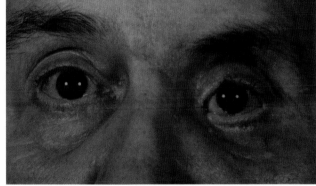

FIGURE 10-1 Long-term consequences of an orbital injury. **A,** Severe right orbital injury to the soft and hard tissues. **B,** Severe left orbital injury: soft and hard tissues, diplopia, loss of vision, enophthalmos, hypoglobus, canthal dystopia.

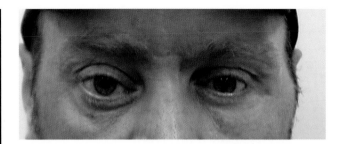

FIGURE 10-3 Canthal dystopia.

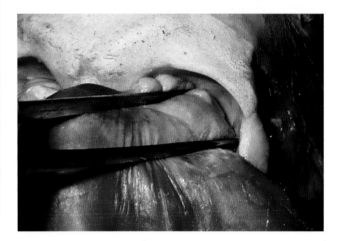

FIGURE 10-4 Coronal exposure.

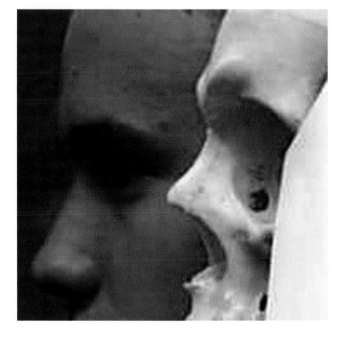

FIGURE 10-2 Soft and hard tissue relationship.

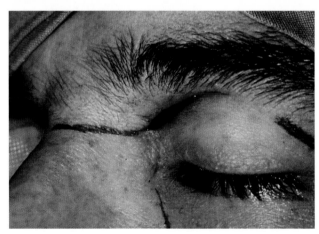

FIGURE 10-5 Orbital access incisions: medial blepharoplasty to explore medial wall.

Go over it all again
Help

Disability, **d**rainage (intracranial hematoma, retrobulbar hemorrhage), **d**rugs (for cerebrospinal leak, fractures)
Expose and **e**xamine **e**yes, **e**ars, and the back of the head
Facial nerve

Facial injuries are sometimes considered to be less important than other injuries in the severely injured patient. After any life-threatening injuries have been dealt with, facial injuries should be treated in conjunction with any other procedures (e.g., orthopedic, surgical) rather than left unattended. If a CT scan is requested to rule out an intracranial injury, it is sensible to use that opportunity to assess the orbit and the

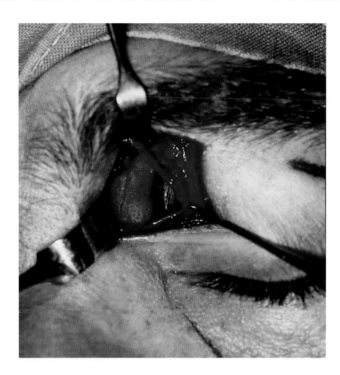

FIGURE 10-6   Medial wall exposure via upper blepharoplasty with extensive subperiosteal dissection and preservation of nerves and vessels.

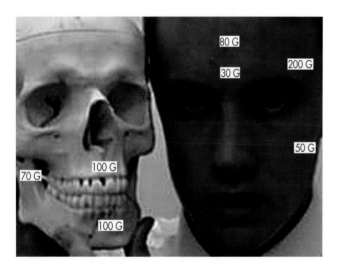

FIGURE 10-7   Forces required to fracture facial bones.

naso-orbital area, if injury is suspected. Facial lacerations demand attention to detail, and a maxillofacial surgeon should be part of the acute trauma team. Once the patient is stable, lacerations should be explored and sutured within the first few hours.

Blindness is a serious complication of orbital injury. In a prospective study undertaken by al-Qurainy et al., the incidence of severe ocular injury in 438 zygomatic fractures was 12%, with 2.5% of the patients having a significant traumatic optic neuropathy.[9] The incidence of diplopia was 20%, and even with early surgery, long-term diplopia occurred in 1% of the patients.[10] These prospective studies led to the development of a scoring system for eye injuries and highlighted the

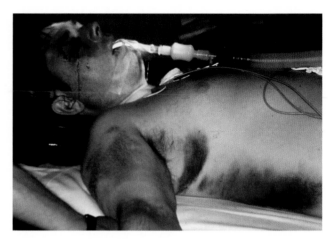

FIGURE 10-8   Acute trauma life support.

acronym "BAD ACT": **b**lowout fracture, **a**cuity, **d**iplopia, **a**mnesia, and **c**omminuted **t**rauma (Appendix 1). If a serious eye injury is suspected or identified, urgent collaboration with an ophthalmologist is required, and consideration of urgent exploration is essential.[11]

Visual acuity must be assessed and recorded. If the patient is conscious but has swelling around the eyes, the assessment can be made easier by explaining to the patient that you need to examine his eyes and that you will be helping him to open his eyes and then asking him to open his eyes while you gently elevate the upper lid and depress the lower lid. If an attempt is made to pry open the eyes, the orbicularis oculi will spontaneously contract and resist the attempt.

Edema of the retina (Berlin's edema) is the most common cause of decreased visual acuity, but an intraocular injury, retrobulbar hemorrhage, and optic nerve lesion must be ruled out. Among patients with head and neck trauma, optic nerve injury is the third most common major cranial nerve injury after olfactory and facial nerve injuries. If severe facial injuries are present, these potentially serious problems must be identified during the secondary survey. Traumatic optic nerve lesions (TONL) often occur acutely and are missed or ignored because of other, potentially more serious injuries. Approximately 2% (0.7%-5.0%) of all closed-head injuries and 20% of all frontobasal injuries show some kind of visual pathway damage. In these injuries, it is usually the intracanalicular part of the optic nerve that is affected (Figs. 10-9 and 10-10); and TONLs most commonly are found with frontal (72%) or frontotemporal (12%) injuries.

The first orbital surgery should give the best outcome, and it needs to be thorough. The main aim of orbital surgery is restoration of the anatomy to its normal and esthetic form with preservation of vision, movement, globe position, esthetics, and lacrimation. It is essential to address the whole problem. It is wise to remember the morbidity of surgery, as well as its advantages, but also to consider the problems of neglected treatment. A patient who survives is likely to do better from all aspects if he or she is not left with severe deformities. If there are significant soft tissue injuries, it often is not possible to return the face to its pre-injury state.

Assessment and investigations should be thorough, including access to plain radiography, CT, magnetic resonance imaging (MRI), ultrasonography, and spiral three-dimensional

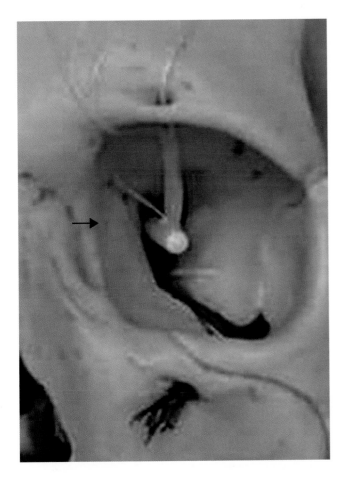

FIGURE 10-9 Orbital apex: optic nerve (arrow).

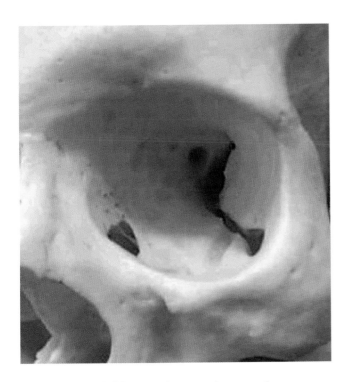

FIGURE 10-10 Orbital apex to show optic foramen.

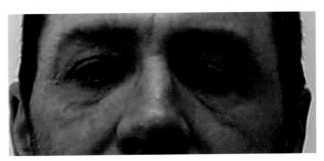

FIGURE 10-11 Inadequate fixation leading to flat left zygoma with lateral canthal drift.

(3-D) reconstruction.[12-18] Usually, more than one type of investigation is required to get a clear picture. A provisional surgical plan is made, but the final assessment can be made only after open surgical exposure and exploration of the injuries.[19]

Orbital surgery requires a multidisciplinary team including a maxillofacial surgeon, a surgeon with facial plastic surgical experience, an ophthalmic surgeon with access to orthoptists, a neurosurgeon, and a radiologist. Intraoperative fluoroscopy, cameras, and CT screening are becoming more common and are likely to influence the direction of future treatment in this area.[20-22] Radiological screening helps assess the position of the zygoma and its arch, the correction of enophthalmos, orbital wall and optic canal exploration, and extensive orbital reconstruction. The zygomatic arch, infraorbital rim, and buttress positions are of paramount importance in supporting the zygoma and ensuring optimal orbital reconstruction.[19,23,24] Endoscopic assessment of the arch, rim, and orbital floor at the time of surgery is relatively straightforward and is likely to influence future treatment.[6,7,8,17]

Secondary problems are usually related to one or more of the following:

- The complexity of the initial soft and hard tissue injury
- Delayed treatment
- Excessive scarring, including within the orbital fat
- Failure of adequate support of soft tissues
- Fat atrophy
- Inadequate exposure, reduction or fixation of orbital/ zygomatic fractures[23-29]
- Comminuted zygomatic fractures (Fig. 10-11), missed medial and floor injuries
- Bone loss

CLINICAL ASSESSMENT OF ORBITAL INJURY

A thorough history and clinical examination are undertaken (Appendix 2) to determine the possibility of a penetrating, chemical, or blunt injury to the eye or soft tissues. Evidence of a head injury (amnesia), a neck injury (10% of cases), loss of smell (anosmia), deterioration or loss of vision, development of double vision (diplopia—vertical, horizontal, or rotatory), eye movements (painful or not), and eye position in all three planes (proptosis or enophthalmos, hypoglobus or hyperglobus, or an orbital dystopia) should be recorded.

Orbital trauma can result in displacement of the globe in any direction. Proptosis occurs in the acute phase due to hematoma or swelling of orbital tissues, or both. As the swelling subsides, proptosis resolves and may become enophthalmos. Persistent proptosis may be caused by subperiosteal hematoma or intraorbital bone fragments. Enophthalmos is a common late sequela and may result from a combination of expansion of the orbit, prolapse of soft tissue through a blowout fracture, necrosis of soft tissue (rare), and intraorbital fibrosis. There is often an associated impairment of ocular motility. Vertical displacement of the globe is common. Upward displacement may result from hematoma or edema in the acute phase or from orbital floor impaction causing a reduction in orbital volume. Downward displacement (hypoglobus) is far more common, particularly in patients with comminuted orbital floor or lateral wall fractures or roof fractures. Horizontal lateral displacement of the globe can result particularly from naso-orbitoethmoidal fractures and from severing of the medial canthal ligament. Traumatic herniation of the globe into the maxillary sinus can occur. Good recovery of visual function and esthetics is achievable after effective repair.

Eye position can be measured with the use of an exophthalmometer but is best assessed from CT or MRI scans. The exophthalmometer is of little benefit for patients with lateral orbital disruption, the most common orbital injury. Surgeons have developed exophthalmometers based on the ear canals and supraorbital positions, but these are less accurate than CT scan assessment, which also allows an assessment of orbital fat volume and helps determine the need for surgery.[12,13,16,22,30-32]

Facial sensation is tested. Altered facial sensation around the orbit may be the only initial clinical sign of a blowout fracture. The alar of the nose should be gently touched, and the patient should be asked if she can feel one side and then the other and whether they feel the same. Swelling can give a false impression of true nerve damage.

Facial nerve injury compounds any orbital injury and should be actively sought. If the nerve is severed through a laceration, the laceration should be explored and the nerve primarily repaired with the aid of a microscope, unless it is a peripheral injury.

Intercanthal (medial and lateral) and interpupillary measurements are taken (see Appendix 2). The use of a local anesthetic to enable a full clinical assessment for medial canthal disruption is advised.

Mouth opening should be assessed, because any displacement of the zygomatic complex can impinge on the temporalis muscle or coronoid process and interfere with jaw movement. Trismus is not an uncommon complication of a zygoma or orbital fracture.

It is an advantage to have a diagram or photograph in the notes to demonstrate grazes, bruises, and the presence of periorbital or lid lacerations and to record any loss of soft or hard tissue.

Forced duction tests under local anesthesia can be helpful but are not necessary in the conscious patient (Figs. 10-12 through 10-14). The clinical sign of pain on looking up or laterally with diplopia is evidence of entrapment. The pain is thought to be caused by disturbance of the periosteum by the entrapped tissue. A Hess test helps display any restriction, but it is important to look for the clinical sign of

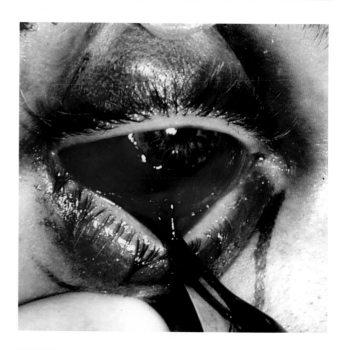

FIGURE 10-12 Forced duction test, picking up adventitial tissue around the inferior rectus muscle.

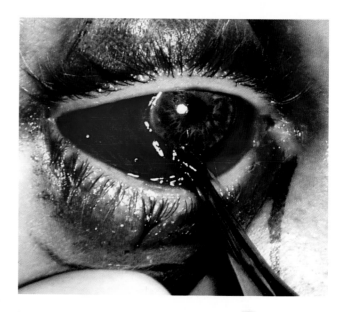

FIGURE 10-13 Forced duction test, picking up attached conjunctiva at the margin of the cornea.

pain (i.e., slight grimace) and retraction of the globe on eye movement.

APPLIED SURGICAL ANATOMY

The orbit (Figs. 10-15 through 10-17) has several important anatomical features. Knowledge and appreciation of the anatomy enables one to understand the injuries and to postulate how to reconstruct them. The orbital skeleton should be returned to its norm with enough strength to resist

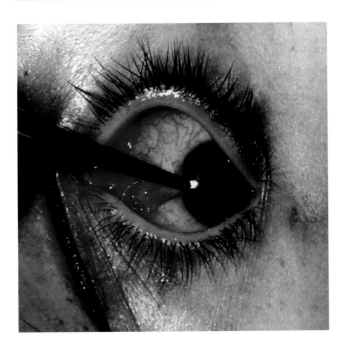

FIGURE 10-14 Medial forced duction test, preoperatively.

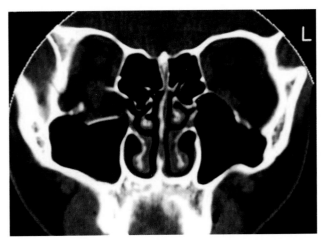

FIGURE 10-16 Computed tomographic scan showing orbital floor fracture.

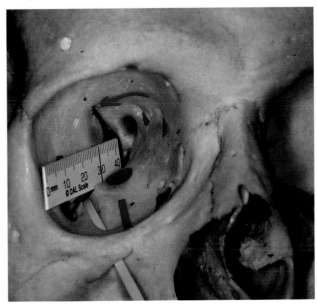

FIGURE 10-17 Measurements to aid orbital dissection. *Orange arrow,* superior fissure. *Red arrow,* inferior fissure. *Green ring,* posterior floor, retrobulbar bulge. *Red line,* anterior floor (concave). *Yellow line,* infraorbital nerve in groove and exiting from canal through infraorbital foramen. *Red triangles,* anterior and posterior ethmoidal arteries.

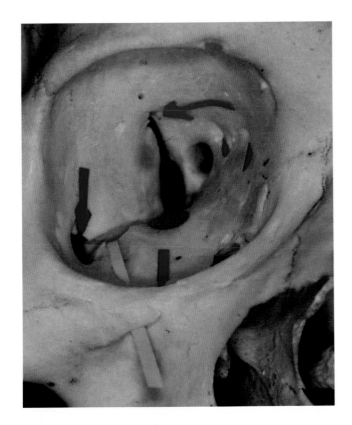

FIGURE 10-15 Orbit anatomy. *Orange arrow,* superior fissure. *Red arrow,* inferior fissure. *Green ring,* posterior floor, retrobulbar bulge. *Red line,* anterior floor (concave). *Yellow line,* infraorbital nerve in groove and exiting from canal through infraorbital foramen. *Red triangles,* anterior and posterior ethmoidal arteries.

disrupting forces. There is argument about simple elevation and single, two-point, and three-point fixation approaches.[23,24] It is recognized that even with frontozygomatic and infraorbital rim fixation, posterolateral orbital rim rotation can be missed. It is advisable with unstable zygoma fractures to view the frontozygomatic fracture and either the buttress (intraoral) or the zygoma/sphenoidal fracture line to prevent the development of enophthalmos.[33]

The orbit can be anatomically classified in many ways. It has been described in relation to its bony components; it is made up of seven bones. It has been divided into anterior, middle, and posterior thirds to help differentiate the sites related to hypoglobus (anterior orbital floor), enophthalmos (middle), and visual or neurological problems (posterior) (see Fig. 10-9). Correction of hypoglobus requires lifting of the globe and repair (with or without bone grafting) of the anterior half of the orbit. Prevention or correction of enophthalmos requires the globe to be pushed forward with repair of the lateral and medial walls and reconstruction of the retrobulbar bulge.[34]

The orbit has also been described according to its anatomical walls: it has a floor, a medial wall, a roof, a lateral wall, an apex, and an orbital rim. This method is the easiest to comprehend, and combined with the other classifications, it allows for a logical anatomical assessment and a logical treatment of orbital injuries.

The orbit is a quadrangular pyramid with its base on the facial surface. Its apex is the optic foramen and the medial end of the superior orbital fissure.

The orbital rim is composed of cortical bone. Its strength arises from its circumorbital continuity. If the rim is broken, the strength—particularly of the inferior, medial, and lateral walls of the orbit—is significantly decreased. Dissipation of the impact required to fracture the rim often transmits the forces to the floor and medial wall, leading to concomitant damage to the floor and wall, while leaving the rim intact.[35] A patient with an isolated orbital rim fracture may initially have few symptoms, exhibiting only infraorbital anesthesia, but may present later with enophthalmos or dysesthesia, epiphora (secondary to nasolacrimal obstruction), or dacryocystorhinitis. These patients should be monitored for at least 6 weeks before discharge (see Fig. 10-16). Symptomatic infraorbital nerve problems warrant treatment.[36,37]

The floor of the orbit is very thin and S-shaped. It is concave anteriorly and convex posteriorly (see Figs. 10-15 and 10-17). It is traversed anteriorly by the infraorbital groove and canal (lateral to medial). The infraorbital canal is suspended from the floor. This groove and canal carry the infraorbital nerve from the pterygopalatine fissure below the inferior orbital fissure to the infraorbital foramen and further weaken the floor. This anatomical relationship accounts for the clinical sign of facial numbness, paresthesia, or dysesthesia affecting the alar of the nose, cheek, upper lip, and anterior teeth after an orbital floor or zygomatic fracture. The floor is fractured either by buckling (dissipation of orbital rim forces) or by rapid expansion of the orbital contents, which leads to a fracture of the floor or the medial orbital wall.[35] Floor fractures are usually medial to the nerve. If a fracture involves the whole floor, the infraorbital nerve supports the floor like a piece of string, camouflaging the initial clinical signs of hypoglobus and enophthalmos.

The anatomy of the postbulbar bulge (maxillary sinus expansion posterior to the globe) is important in maintaining the eye's anterior-posterior position (assuming that the soft tissue support is damaged) and must be reconstructed to prevent enophthalmos. Volume changes on CT examination illustrate clearly the importance of this area in the development of enophthalmos. This area is often not explored because of a reluctance to dissect far enough into the orbit. It is essential to dissect the inferior fissure free from the orbital contents, at least to behind the infraorbital nerve (see Fig. 10-16). The inferior orbital fissure is traversed by only minor vessels, lymphatic channels, and fibrofatty tissue. The infraorbital nerve passes below the fissure to enter the infraorbital groove. These tissues are carefully dissected under magnification by a combination of bipolar diathermy and knife dissection. The floor must be fully explored, and in the adult this usually requires a dissection along the floor and lateral wall for at least 35 mm (see Fig. 10-17).

Most failed explorations are caused by a reluctance to adequately free up this area and get completely around any floor fracture or defect (navigation systems may be helpful). The difficult areas are (1) the junction of the infraorbital groove and the inferior fissure and (2) identification of the posterior aspect of the retrobulbar bulge as it passes posteriorly and medially to the inferior fissure. The periosteum needs to be incised on either side of the fissure and elevated gently. Care must be taken at the junction of the infraorbital groove and fissure to dissect the infraorbital nerve free from the orbital tissues. This subperiosteal dissection, using careful eye retraction, magnification, and a light source (head light), enables a full exploration of the orbital floor and its lateral and medial walls. The transconjunctival or lower eyelid skin incision does not need to be extended if the orbital periosteum is well mobilized. The inferior rectus and inferior oblique muscles are protected by remaining in a subperiosteal plane. The anatomy of the nasolacrimal sac and canal should be kept in mind.

It has been suggested that an inferior orbitotomy may help in exploring large blowout fractures. In our experience, an inferior orbitotomy is used occasionally in secondary procedures but usually is not necessary in the acute situation. An inferior orbitotomy may be useful to decompress the infraorbital nerve in patients with infraorbital nerve dysesthesia or persistent numbness (Figs. 10-18 through 10-22). Resolution and protection of cheek and lip sensation is best achieved, even with minimal infraorbital rim disruption, by reduction and fixation of the fractured bone at the frontozygomatic or infraorbital rim or both.[36,37]

The anterior floor supporting the globe is reconstructed (usually with bone grafting) to prevent hypoglobus. It is our preference to use autogenous bone from the cranium, mandible, or opposite lateral maxillary sinus wall, although nasal septum, ear cartilage, and fascia lata have also been used with success.[38,39] Alloplastic material (Silastic) has a tendency to

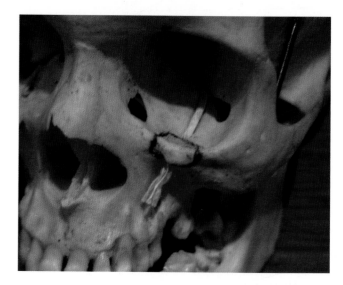

FIGURE 10-18   Inferior orbitotomy to explore the orbital floor or decompress the infraorbital nerve.

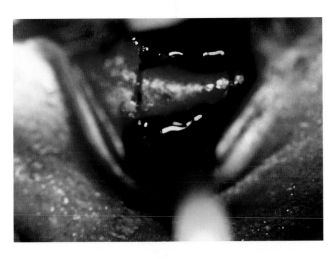

FIGURE 10-19   Clinical picture of inferior orbitotomy.

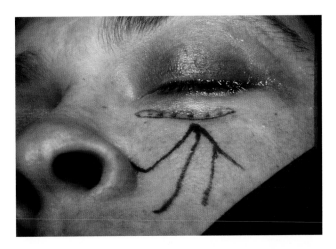

FIGURE 10-21   Position of plate for inferior orbitotomy.

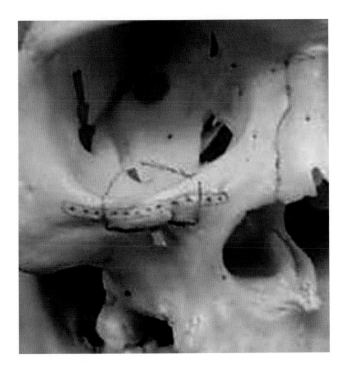

FIGURE 10-20   Plate on inferior orbitotomy for reconstruction of orbital rim.

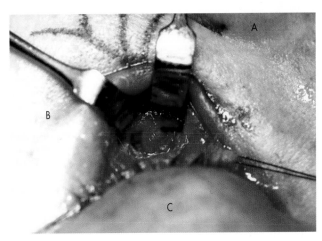

FIGURE 10-22   Infraorbital nerve exposed. A, nose; B, cheek; C, eyelid.

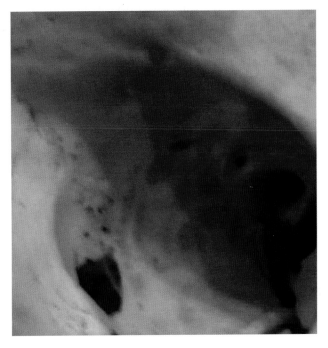

FIGURE 10-23   Thinness of medial wall.

extrude, but Silastic remains the most frequently used material in the United Kingdom.[40,41] Resorbable material, although useful in small defects, potentially leaves the patient with late enophthalmos after resorption. Very large defects are well restored with a combination of metal (titanium or Vitallium) and autogenous bone. The posterior floor (bulbar bulge) is reconstructed with layers of bone to correct and prevent enophthalmos. There is still a reluctance to undertake bone grafting in the acute management of these injuries. Primary bone grafting in facial injuries has been shown to give good long-term results.[27,38,39,41,42]

The medial wall is paper thin (Fig. 10-23). It obtains its strength from the continuity of the ethmoidal air cells and

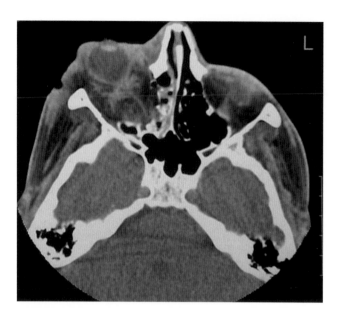

FIGURE 10-24   Computed tomogram showing retrobulbar hemorrhage in the right eye.

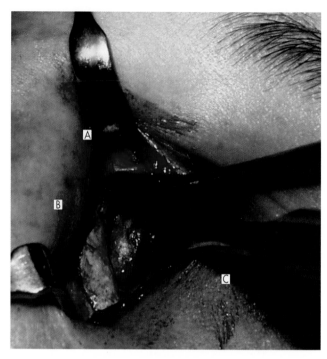

FIGURE 10-25   Dissection of lacrimal fossa. A, medial canthus; B, fossa; C, nasolacrimal sac retracted.

from their multiple septa. When it is fractured, the forces of injury are rapidly dissipated, thus protecting the brain and eye. Nasal fractures frequently involve the medial wall and the inferior orbital rim.

Although nasal radiographs are not usually taken, there should be a high index of suspicion of medial wall injuries in cases of anterior collapsed nasal fracture. If there is any clinical indication of nasal or cheek numbness, radiographs should be taken. Medial wall defects tend to be small and minimally displaced, and they are easily missed. There is a high incidence (30%-50%) of medial wall fractures associated with floor fractures.[13,28] Medial wall injuries contribute to enophthalmos and can cause horizontal diplopia. The medial wall is traversed by the anterior and posterior ethmoidal arteries at about 24 and 34 mm, respectively, from the anterior lacrimal crest (orbital rim). If the medial wall is being explored, these arteries should be identified and coagulated. Bleeding can easily be arrested by bipolar diathermy. Although these are relatively low-pressure vessels, they do contribute to the problems of visual impairment, ophthalmoplegia, and proptosis after retrobulbar hemorrhage (Fig. 10-24).

The nasolacrimal sac is sited anteriorly between the orbital rim and the posterior lacrimal crest. It is protected by the anterior and posterior bands of the medial canthal ligament (Figs. 10-25 and 10-26) and drains through the nasolacrimal duct to the inferior meatus of the nose. In the treatment of orbital injuries, it is important to protect the canaliculi, the sac, and the duct when placing incisions and for osteosynthesis. Obstruction in the duct or damage to the sac can cause epiphora and recurrent dacryocystorhinitis.

Telecanthus, medial canthal dystopia, nasal deformity, epiphora, and dacryocystitis are also complications of medial orbital wall and nasal injuries; they can be addressed only by considering them in the acute phase and reconstructing the areas anatomically.

The lateral orbital wall is fairly strong. It is supported by the temporalis muscle but weakened inferiorly by the inferior

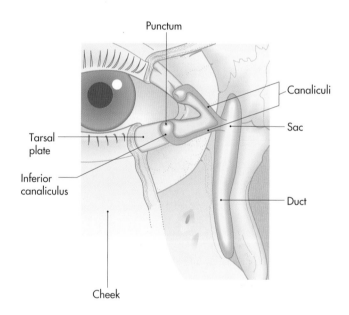

FIGURE 10-26   Nasolacrimal anatomy.

orbital fissure and posterosuperiorly by the superior orbital fissure. It is sensible to understand the relationship between these two fissures (see Figs. 10-9 and 10-15). Fractures in the lateral wall and displacement are usually associated with zygomatic fractures. Inferior displacement of the zygoma leads to displacement of the lateral canthus and to a unilateral mongoloid slant to the palpebral fissure (see Fig. 10-11). Undercorrected or overcorrected lateral displacement (lateral wall) is the most common cause of enophthalmos and hypoglobus. If zygomatic fixation at the frontozygomatic suture is

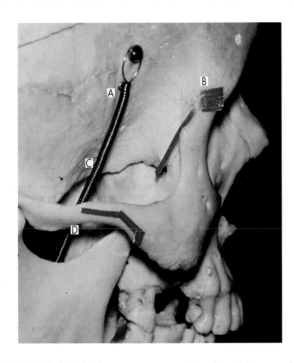

FIGURE 10-27 Malar osteotomy cuts. A, calvarial bone graft to augment the floor, retrobulbar area, and any bone defects; B, resection (5 mm); C, osteotomy into inferior fissure; D, arch osteotomy.

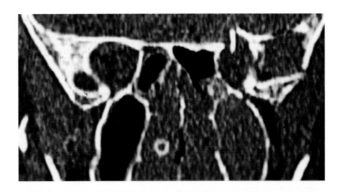

FIGURE 10-28 Orbital blow-in fracture.

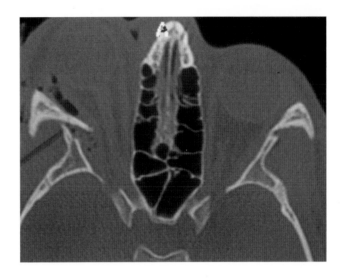

FIGURE 10-29 Lateral blow-in fracture leading to proptosis with impingement on the lateral rectus and, indirectly, on the optic nerve.

not secure, the masseteric and temporalis muscles can pull the zygoma inferiorly, leading to an osteodistraction force at the frontozygomatic suture with elongation of the lateral wall. This is a very important concept in secondary reconstruction and explains the need to resect a measured piece (usually 5 mm) of the lateral orbital rim in a malar (zygomatic) osteotomy (Fig. 10-27).

Adequate reduction of the zygoma is difficult to determine on the table, in particular the final volume of the orbit. As a result supplementary methods like that of ultrasonography, fluoroscopy, CT navigation, or endoscopy have become more popular.[6,7,8,20,21] CT navigation is currently the "gold standard" to ensure a perfect reduction and correction of the orbital volume. Postoperative radiographs or some accurate analysis are an integral part of assessment of the postoperative positions of the zygoma and orbit. Reoperation should be undertaken earlier rather than later to avoid the long-term sequelae. In some countries (United States, Australia), postoperative spiral CT scans are taken for moderate to complex orbital reconstructions to assess orbital volume, zygoma and bone graft position, and orbital wall reconstruction. This is the gold standard and enables clinicians to improve future treatment for these patients, but of course there are concerns about the radiation given to this sensitive area, without any clear evidence of an audited benefit.

The orbital roof is protected by the very strong supraorbital rim, but fractures of the roof are commonly seen in association with frontal sinus and naso-orbitoethmoidal fractures (Figs. 10-28 and 10-29). These can be blowout fractures but more commonly are blow-in fractures, leading to hypoglobus and proptosis.[32] This injury is also associated with diplopia due to displacement of the trochlea, which transmits the tendon of the superior oblique muscle of the eye.[43] Consideration of the orbital roof is essential in any craniofacial injury. The orbit's relationship with the frontal sinus is a natural defense mechanism against injury to the brain or eye, because the forces are dissipated through fracturing of the walls of the air-filled sinus. If injured, this area warrants reconstruction, because damage to the frontonasal duct can lead to mucoceles, sinusitis, and possible meningitis. An isolated blow-in fracture with proptosis is relatively easily treated. This is best done in collaboration with a neurosurgeon and by means of a subcranial or transcranial approach.

The orbital apex is not well understood (see Figs. 10-9, 10-10, 10-15, and 10-17). It transmits the optic nerve with its retinal artery, which is an end artery. Injury or constriction of this vessel may lead to acute or insidious blindness after an orbital injury (i.e., TONL) and development of traumatic optic atrophy (Fig. 10-30). There is an increasing tendency, although unproven need, to explore this area to decompress the optic nerve (see later discussion of ocular injuries).

Other important anatomical factors in the apical area include the posterior aspects of the inferior and superior orbital fissures, the tendinous ring origin of the ocular muscles, and the oculomotor, trochlear, abducens, and ophthalmic nerve branches. Injury to this area leads to a number of well-recognized syndromes. The orbital apex syndrome is blindness (optic nerve injury). The clinical signs of superior orbital fissure syndrome are:

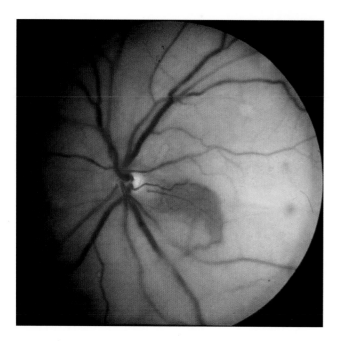

FIGURE 10-30   Traumatic optic atrophy with preservation of a small retinal artery (normal color in that area).

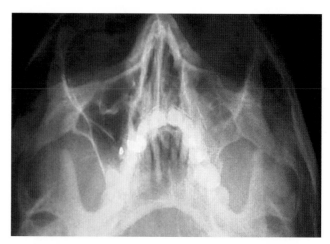

FIGURE 10-31   Occipitomental view of a fractured left zygoma, not suitable for simple elevation. Notice the radiopacity and decreased size of the triangle (maxillary sinus), the decreased distance between the coronoid tip and zygoma body on the left compared with the right side, the left zygomatic arch (two fractures with distal disruption), and multiple fractures along the infraorbital rim with naso-orbital disruption.

- gross and persistent periorbital edema.
- proptosis (due to loss of tone of muscles of the eye).
- ophthalmoplegia and ptosis (third, fourth, and sixth cranial nerves).
- subconjunctival hemorrhage.
- pupil dilatation.
- an absent direct light reflex but a persistent indirect light reflex (i.e., second nerve is normal).
- loss of accommodation, corneal reflex, and sensation to the forehead (frontal nerve).

Treatment for these symptoms has been conservative in the past. It is now advisable to consider orbital apex exploration if the patient has an acute visual loss with no intraocular cause, in an effort to save vision.

It is necessary when operating to understand the dimensions of the orbit and how far it is safe to dissect down any individual wall.[34,44] For this reason, the availability of a dried or plastic skull in the operating room is advocated to facilitate understanding of orbital dissection. It is possible through orbital incisions to mobilize the orbital contents so that they are free except for the superior fissure, the tendinous muscle origin and optic nerve, and the nasolacrimal and medial canthal area.[2,3] This allows for a thorough exploration of all the orbital walls, floor, and roof. It is also a good use of a navigation system to ensure precise access to the damaged area.

In the case of avulsive orbital defects, the remaining orbit should be reconstructed. The bony defect should be reconstructed with primary autogenous bone grafting, supported with rigid fixation (low-profile plates), and covered with soft tissue through local rotation flaps or free vascular tissue, rather than waiting for the scarring process to proceed. Scarring will further compromise the orbital outcome.

ASSESSMENT

Orbital injuries require a thorough investigation that includes an ophthalmic assessment,[9-11] an orthoptic assessment, photographs (pre-injury, before repair, and postoperative), plain radiographs, CT assessment with or without MRI, occasionally 3-D reconstruction, and possibly stereolithic models. Ultrasonography has been shown to be useful in the emergency department and in the operating room for assessment of zygomatic and orbital fractures, particularly medial and floor blowout fractures.

Radiology is covered in Chapter 5. Briefly, plain radiographs are very useful and, if carefully assessed, can yield good information. Comparison in a noninjured patient between the left and right zygoma, orbit, and maxillary sinus usually reveals symmetry. Comparison in an injured patient can provide an accurate assessment of the displacement, accepting that there may have been a previous injury.

Occipitomental views at 10 and 30 degrees, a submento-vertex projection (if there is no neck injury), and a lateral face view give the most information. It is advisable to look at the zygomatic arch (particularly posteriorly), the orbital rim (for buckling and separate fragments), the frontozygomatic junction (frontozygomatic distraction and diathesis), the lateral maxillary buttress (displacement), the body of the zygoma (comminution), and the distance between the coronoid tip and the buttress to assess the amount of displacement (Figs. 10-31 and 10-32). A comparison and estimation of the size and shape of the quadrangular orbit and the maxillary sinus (black triangle) can help in both the acute and the secondary assessment. The lateral face radiograph is examined mainly in terms of the nasal projection, the frontal sinus, and height changes in those patients with associated maxillary fractures.

Tomography is rarely used but can be helpful to identify the position of metallic foreign bodies. This assessment should be done with some external metallic marker.

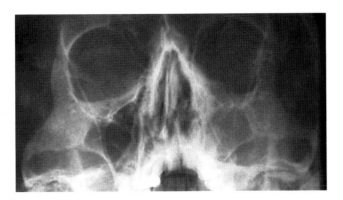

FIGURE 10-32 Occipitomental view of a fractured left zygoma, not suitable for simple elevation. Notice the altered axis (horizontal to vertical) of the orbital quadrangle, the radiopacity and decreased size of the triangle (maxillary sinus), the left zygomatic arch (two fractures with distal disruption), loss of the gentle curve of the lateral maxillary sinus wall on the left, and the decreased distance between the coronoid tip and zygoma body on the left (overlap) compared with the right side.

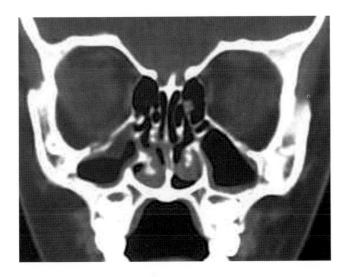

FIGURE 10-33 Computed tomogram showing right orbital floor crack fracture in a child.

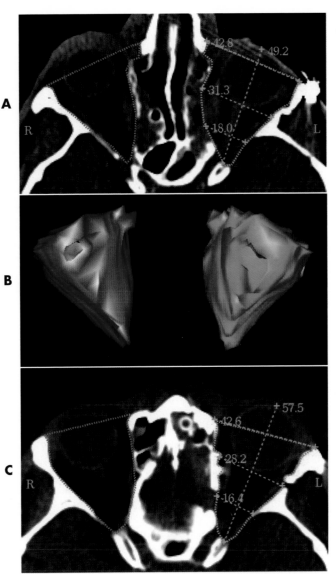

FIGURE 10-34 Computed tomogram of left orbital injury. **A,** Computer measurements. **B,** Computer-generated volume 3-D assessments. **C,** Postoperative measurements.

CT assessment is the investigation of choice for any patient with a blowout fracture, diplopia, or a comminuted orbital fracture and before secondary reconstruction (Figs. 10-33 and 10-34; see Figs. 10-16, 10-24, 10-28, 10-29). To see the floor and the medial wall, coronal and transverse images (1-2 mm) are required. CT allows the clinician to look at the bony orbit, the air sinuses around the orbit (frontal, ethmoidal, and maxillary), the soft tissues for evidence of edema and hematoma, and the muscles for edema and fibrosis. Conventional 3-D CT scans can be misleading (Fig. 10-35). Spiral 3-D CT scans are much more accurate but still lack definition because of the very thin bones that make up the orbit. Stereolithic models have been used and are helpful, but they are expensive and have not been accurate enough to allow for planning of plate positioning and bending.[18]

CT is very useful for orbital volume assessment in orbital blowout fractures in the acute situation and after the swelling

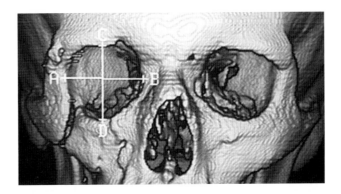

FIGURE 10-35 Three-dimensional computed tomographic scan showing difficulty in interpretation because of thinness and computer reconstruction of the floor and medial wall; it does, however, show displacement of the body of the right zygoma.

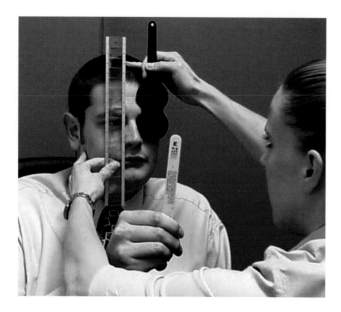

FIGURE 10-36   Cover test and assessment of hypoglobus.

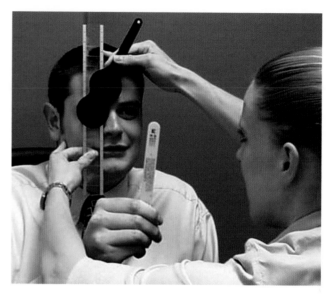

FIGURE 10-37   Cover test and assessment of hypoglobus.

has settled; it gives an idea of the amount of augmentation required and whether surgery is indicated (see Fig. 10-34). It is advisable in all cases of enophthalmos to determine the presence of any bony defects, the lateral displacement, and the amount of bone required to restore the orbit to normal. CT navigation devices are very useful in helping reconstruct orbital fractures and determining the position and amount of bone grafting required.[15,20,29,45] Orbital bone grafting should be combined with some assessment of intraocular pressure.[39]

MRI scans can be very helpful, particularly for looking at soft tissues, and they have been shown to be just as accurate as CT scans in identifying blowout fractures of the medial wall.[13,14,34] The combination of MRI and CT scanning can improve the information gained, particularly for assessment before secondary correction.[30,31] Spiral CT scanning remains the gold standard. Ultrasonography is particularly useful in the acute situation in the emergency department or with a severely injured patient in the intensive care unit to assess for an orbital injury.[17] It is particularly good at picking up buttress wall, medial wall, and zygomatic arch fractures. Fluoroscopy can be used to assess the bony positions and the vascular supply.[21] Soft tissue scarring of the orbital septa may be a cause of poor motility, independent of the bony injuries. This seems very important in children.

Orthoptic tests (Figs. 10-36 through 10-41) include the cover test, diplopia test, Hess test, binocular fixation tests, and field tests. Ocular pressure is also assessed.

The Hess test is very useful for assessment and review of patients with diplopia. It allows clinicians to distinguish between edema, entrapment, neurological impairments, and a previous strabismus. It is important to recognize that, if entrapment is present, the noninjured eye will overreact, because of the muscle straining in both eyes, in an attempt to get the injured eye to move (see Fig. 10-38); this makes the discrepancy in eye movements appear greater than it really is.

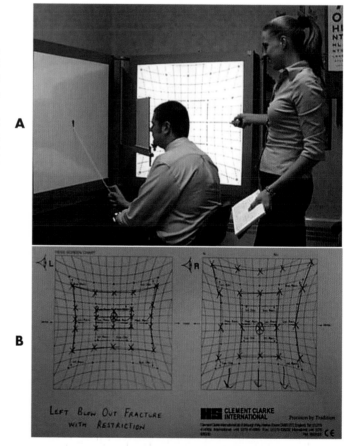

FIGURE 10-38   Hess test. **A,** Test in progress. **B,** Printout showing decreased movement of the left eye and overaction of the right.

The diplopia test should be increased from the 9 cardinal positions to 25, to allow the testing of central gaze, peripheral gaze (<25 degrees) and extreme peripheral gaze (>25 degrees). The type of separation (vertical or horizontal) should be indicated on the form (see Fig. 10-41).

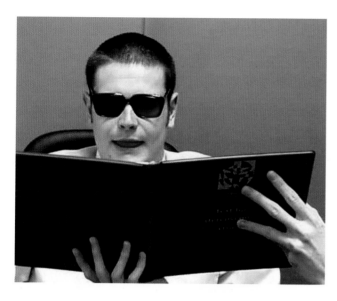

FIGURE 10-39   Test for stereotactic vision.

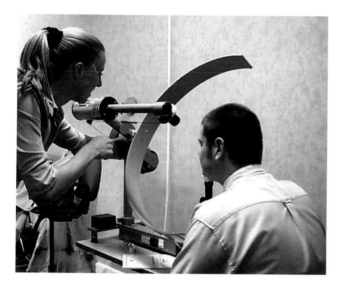

FIGURE 10-40   Visual field testing.

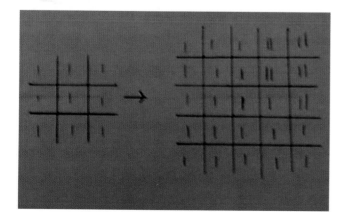

FIGURE 10-41   Diplopia test showing double vision on looking up and to the left at extreme vision.

It is essential to work closely with an ophthalmology department to enable assessment of these patients for ocular injury and to have access to orthoptists and to an ophthalmologist with a particular interest in managing diplopia.[9,10,11,29,46,47]

THE TIMING OF SURGERY

The timing of surgery is controversial for a number of reasons. Are the facilities available for accurate assessment, stabilization, intensive care, and treatment? Is the surgical team available (surgeons, anesthetists, nurses)? Will the patient survive the severity of the head injury or other injuries? Are CT and neurosurgical support available for an accurate assessment? Many of these problems have been resolved with the universal availability of CT and the development of telemedicine, which enable neurosurgical, ophthalmological, and other consultations to proceed. If the patient has a Glasgow Coma Scale score greater than 6, no evidence of an intracranial hemorrhage or midline shift, and intracranial pressure lower than 15 mm Hg lying down, facial surgery can proceed early and at the same time as other surgical procedures (e.g., orthopedic fixation).[48-50]

It is probably best for the definitive surgery to proceed as soon as investigations are complete and the team can be brought together, ideally before the swelling becomes too severe. This should be done early or within 5 to 14 days at the latest. Soft tissue results appear to be better with early surgery.[26] The results for severe orbital and craniofacial fracture reconstruction have also been shown to be better from an esthetic and functional point of view if the surgery (i.e., full reconstruction) can be undertaken early. If there is a considerable threat to life from chest injury, abdominal bleeding, or severe head injury, facial surgery should be delayed for a few days. It is inappropriate to keep patients waiting 2 to 3 weeks before providing definitive treatment, because the surgery becomes more difficult and the eventual outcome is worse. An advantage of early surgery appears to be the ability to limit the amount of fibrosis by limiting ingrowth of fibroblasts and avoiding the need for two insults (i.e., the injury and the delayed repair). Surgery is usually performed under steroid and antibiotic cover.[51]

Swelling of the soft tissues can make assessment more difficult, but the development of CT scanning and the acceptance of the need to explore these injuries more thoroughly through coronal, facial, and oral incisions have led to a better understanding of the extent of facial injuries. Surgical correction has been further improved by the acceptance of primary bone grafting with rigid low-profile fixation for bony defects, orbital wall fractures, and naso-orbital injuries. It is important to control any mobilized facial soft tissue by reattaching the periosteum supporting the facial soft tissue envelope to the facial bones. This prevents the unsightly facial soft tissue ptosis that is often associated with panfacial fractures.[26] The periosteum is supported with non-resorbable monofilament sutures to the orbital rim and temporalis muscle fascia. Careful attention to a layered closure of any soft tissue lacerations or incisions and to facial suturing is essential.[25] All facial sutures should be removed by 5 days at the latest.

There is a view that more simple orbital injuries (blowout fractures) should be allowed to settle before surgery

(<10 days) to enable ophthalmological, orthoptic, and radiographic investigations to be completed. Waiting a few days allows for the diplopia occurring secondary to edema or hematoma to settle. Early surgery (<10 days) has been shown to give better results than delayed surgery (>3 months), particularly in children.[10,46,52-54] Orbital (lower lid) incisions are easier if there is less swelling and enable the identification of a crease line. The latter problem can be avoided by the use of a transconjunctival or transcaruncular incision with adequate subperiosteal dissection to enable satisfactory access.

PREVENTION AND MANAGEMENT OF ENOPHTHALMOS

Prevention of enophthalmos is much easier than cure. The cause of enophthalmos is an increased orbital volume postoperatively; the soft tissue support is damaged, including the periorbita and suspension ligaments.[30,31] Enophthalmos may also occur if the orbital content is decreased by loss of orbital contents (fat) through the floor or the medial wall (or both) or by loss of the globe or its rupture. Fat atrophy was considered to be a major cause of enophthalmos and was previously thought to result from a vascular insult due to the trauma or the surgery. This is no longer considered to be a significant cause, although cicatricial enophthalmos is well described.

It is not uncommon for an orbital blowout fracture to be missed. The signs may be subtle because of orbital swelling; in some cases, the only sign is some numbness of the cheek and nose. Radiographs are difficult for those who are not maxillofacial surgeons to interpret, but the late signs are very obvious: enophthalmos, hypoglobus, supratarsal hollowing, supratarsal hooding, diplopia, numbness of the cheek, and an altered palpebral fissure (see Fig. 10-1). The palpebral aperture (opening and width) should be measured. The altered palpebral fissure manifests as an asymmetry and is classically described as being almond shaped, but it can have different shapes (e.g., rounded, widened, narrowed).

An accurate assessment of the extent of the orbital injury with plain radiographs and CT scanning, adequate exposure, anatomical reconstruction, and primary bone grafting should prevent the development of enophthalmos (see Chapter 12). The extent of surgery and the exposure required are proportional to the severity of the injury. The common problems relate to comminution of the zygomatic arch or infraorbital rim, failure to augment the orbital floor posteriorly or to explore the medial wall, and inadequate stabilization.[23,24] It is advisable to monitor patients for at least 6 months after an orbital injury to rule out the possibility of late enophthalmos and for at least 12 months to assess the outcome of infraorbital nerve anesthesia.[36,37]

DISORDERS OF OCULAR MOTILITY

Acute disturbance in eye movement after trauma (Fig. 10-42) may be caused by orbital edema; hematoma; direct orbital injury with associated extraocular muscle injury; periorbital fat entrapment; injuries to the third, fourth, and sixth cranial nerves; or disorders of the central control of eye movement.[10,11,16,28,29,43,46,47,52,54,55] Persistent diplopia is usually caused

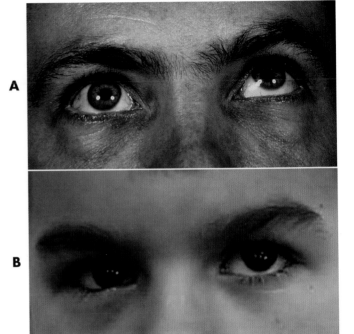

A

B

FIGURE 10-42   Limitation of movement of the right eye. **A,** Movement. **B,** Hypoglobus. Both patients complained of pain on looking up. The difference in level of light reflex allows for a clinical measurement and an assessment in time.

by entrapment of the periorbital fat or fibrosis around the extraocular muscles.

DIPLOPIA

Double vision (diplopia) is a common and debilitating sequela to orbital injury. Diplopia is usually associated with a blowout fracture of the floor or medial wall but can occur after roof or lateral wall injuries.[10] Hematoma, edema of extraocular muscles or their surrounding fascia, and entrapment of the orbital fat septa are the principal causes (Fig. 10-43; see Fig. 10-33). Entrapment of extraocular muscles is no longer considered to be the cause of diplopia in the acute phase, but ischemic injury leading to fibrosis is considered important in secondary surgery. This ischemia may be a consequence of the initial trauma or surgery. Cranial nerve palsies must be distinguished from these causes, and this is relatively easily done with the advantage of orthoptic tests (Fig. 10-44). After trauma, a previous latent squint can break down and become manifest; this is easily detected by orthoptic testing.

It is necessary to test visual acuity in each eye before testing for diplopia. Double vision usually does not occur in patients with poor vision in one eye or in those who have received successful patching for amblyopia in the past and effectively use only one eye at a time. Testing for diplopia should be done with the patient's reading glasses in place. If visual acuity is so bad that diplopia is not a problem, surgical repair may not be required unless the limited eye movement is esthetically unacceptable. Although monocular diplopia can occur, it is rare and warrants ophthalmological

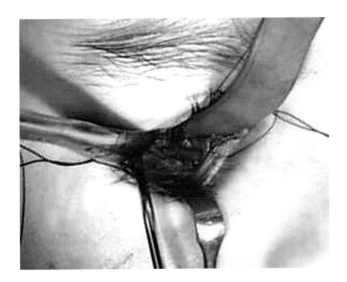

FIGURE 10-43   Orbital floor crack fracture with fascial entrapment (computed tomogram of the same patient as in Fig. 10-33).

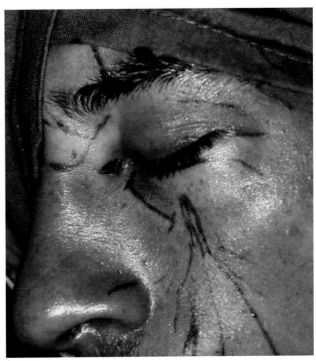

FIGURE 10-45   Multiple access incisions: medial blepharoplasty (dissecting supraorbital nerve), lateral blepharoplasty, medial canthal, lower blepharoplasty, lower lid, and lateral orbital.

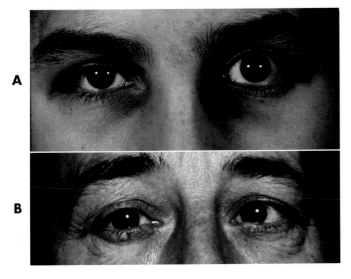

A

B

FIGURE 10-44   Cranial nerve palsy. **A,** Right oculomotor (third) nerve palsy. **B,** Left abducens palsy secondary to caroticocavernous sinus fistula.

assessment. Corneal scarring, lens dislocation, cataract formation, or retinal detachment usually causes it.

ORBITAL FLOOR BLOWOUT FRACTURE

Diplopia may be vertical, horizontal, or both. There may be restriction of upward and downward gaze with a sudden onset of pain engendered by eye movement. The clinician should look for a slight retraction of the globe on attempts at upward gaze. A positive forced duction test may be elicited. Orbital emphysema may be present for 24 hours after injury. Enophthalmos may occur but is often camouflaged for 24 to 48 hours. It is associated with an asymmetrical palpebral fissure, compared with the normal eye. Ptosis of the upper eyelid due to enophthalmos may occur. When the patient

attempts to lift that eyelid, the other lid is also elevated (i.e., there is pseudoretraction of the lid on the contralateral side). Fast up-and-down eye movements (saccades) help to differentiate between muscle bruising and entrapment. In muscle bruising, a slower eye movement occurs; with entrapment, a rapid movement occurs but is of incomplete amplitude. Increased intraocular pressure occurs on attempts at upward gaze due to tethering of the globe. Infraorbital nerve anesthesia may occur and may be accompanied by persistent pain and dysesthesia. Patients with an orbital injury and altered infraorbital sensation should be presumed to have a blowout fracture until proven otherwise by review a few days later.

In the literature, there is an apparent difference in the way these patients are treated depending on whether they are seen by an ophthalmology service or in an oral and maxillofacial surgery unit.[10,54,55] Cooperative practice in a joint clinic has helped resolve some of the gray areas.[10,46] All patients have a thorough maxillofacial and ophthalmic assessment. Surgery depends on the severity of the problem. If the injury is severe, there is little controversy. If there is clinical entrapment (diplopia), enophthalmos, hypoglobus, or infraorbital nerve anesthesia, both specialties, after investigations, advise surgery. If there is entrapment but no enophthalmos, no hypoglobus, and no infraorbital anesthesia, ophthalmologists prefer to wait and, if diplopia persists, to correct it with muscle surgery.[55] We have found that the best results for persistent diplopia (>3 days with orthoptic evidence of entrapment) are achieved with early surgery.[10,46,54]

There are many surgical approaches to the orbital floor, each with advantages and disadvantages (Fig. 10-45). These are the infraorbital, lower lid, blepharoplasty, transconjunctival, medial canthal, transcaruncular, transmaxillary sinus, and coronal approaches. All approaches have their place.[34] It is important to be comfortable with all of these incisions so as to give the patient the best available treatment.

Correction of enophthalmos alone is a decision that the team makes with patient involvement. Enophthalmos of greater than 2 mm is noticeable, and greater than 4 mm is clinically obvious. Patients must be aware of the risks of surgery: the incidence of blindness is 3/1000 in the acute repair and 1/1800 after delayed corrective surgery.[42]

There is an indication for immediate infraorbital nerve decompression in cases of acute or persistent dysesthesia. This is achieved more easily through a lower eyelid or transconjunctival incision with an inferior orbital rim orbitotomy, rather than using an intraoral incision and attempting to decompress the nerve with a bur from below (see Figs. 10-18 through 10-22). Access is better, and it is easier to free the whole nerve. Transconjunctival incisions and those in eyelid skin heal very well and are imperceptible at 1 month.

MEDIAL WALL BLOWOUT FRACTURE

Medial wall blowout fractures accompany orbital floor blowout fractures in about 50% of cases. Entrapment of the orbital fat septa medially results in horizontal diplopia and restriction of abduction with retraction of the globe. Early surgical repair is indicated in these cases. These are usually small defects and are easily repaired with a thin piece of bone (maxillary sinus) or some alloplastic material. Access to the medial wall is through the transcaruncular, medial canthotomy (see Fig. 10-25), medial upper blepharoplasty, or coronal approach.

BLOW-IN FRACTURE

Fractures of the orbital roof may be undisplaced, or the bone may blow in or blow out.[32] Symptoms after blow-in fractures of the orbital roof, floor, and medial wall vary. These injuries can interfere with eye position, motility, and optic nerve function. If symptoms persist, treatment is by open reduction and fixation. Perforating injuries of the orbital roof can lead to displacement of bone fragments into brain tissue. Injuries to the levator palpebrae superioris and to the superior rectus muscle lead to ptosis and impaired upward gaze, respectively. Fracture at the posterior aspect of the orbital roof, where it is weakest, and in the region of the optic canal and superior orbital fissure can result in profound damage to the optic and oculomotor nerves. Prolapse of orbital tissue into the frontal sinus has been described.

TRAUMA TO THE TROCHLEA

The superior oblique muscle passes through the trochlea, which is close to the medial superior orbital margin. Injury in this area can lead to entrapment of the superior oblique tendon, which causes restriction of elevation of the eye in adduction.[43] Simple stripping of the periosteum and repair of the bony skeleton in the area seem to resolve the problem. Detachment of the trochlea at the time of coronal dissection does not carry any long-term problems.[3]

CRANIAL NERVE INJURY

In severe head injury, damage to the third, fourth, and sixth cranial nerves is commonly seen. Postmortem studies have shown that the nerves may even be avulsed from the brainstem.

Oculomotor (third cranial) nerve injury results in ptosis, dilatation of the pupil, and abduction with slight depression of the globe due to the unopposed actions of the remaining lateral rectus and superior oblique muscles (see Fig. 10-44). There may be no recovery, normal recovery, or recovery with aberrant regeneration. This injury leads to paradoxical eye movement. Eyelid elevation occurs on adduction or looking down. Spontaneous recovery may take 4 to 6 months.

Trochlear (fourth cranial) nerve palsy may result from a contrecoup injury against the tentorium cerebelli. The superior oblique muscle causes depression of the globe in adduction, resulting in vertical double vision. There may be a torsional element in which the two images appear to be rotated with respect to each other. Torsional diplopia usually occurs after bilateral fourth nerve injuries. Spontaneous recovery may take 4 to 6 months. Surgical repair of the squint is deferred to allow spontaneous recovery to take place.

Abducens (sixth cranial) nerve injury causes loss of abduction. The sixth cranial nerve passes very close to the lateral orbital wall and the lateral rectus muscle. It is prone to injury after zygomatic or orbital fractures or orbital reconstruction. It usually recovers spontaneously. The sixth cranial nerve passes through the cavernous sinus and therefore may also be injured after the development of a traumatic caroticocavernous sinus fistula (see Fig. 10-44). Surgery is deferred to allow spontaneous recovery to take place after treatment of the fistula.

Surgery for persistent diplopia after entrapment or nerve injury depends on what is possible. Surgery may be undertaken on the healthy eye to weaken a muscle pull and is best performed with the use of an adjustable suture technique. The major surgery is done with the patient under general anesthesia, and the final adjustment (tightening or relaxation) is completed with the patient sitting up and awake with the use of a local anesthetic and a little sedation to enable fine adjustments to be made.

DISORDERS OF CENTRAL CONTROL OF EYE MOVEMENTS

IMPAIRMENT OF CONVERGENCE

Impaired convergence may result from a closed-head injury. The presumed cause is an upper midbrain injury. Treatment is with prisms on glasses.

LOSS OF FUSION

Fusion of the images provided by the two eyes is required for single vision. Patients who have undergone orthoptic treatment for squint during childhood may have a reduced fusional capacity, and a head injury can result in double vision if fusion is lost. Spontaneous recovery may occur. The subjective nature of double vision due to fusion loss can make it difficult to analyze objectively when compensation is involved. Treatment is with prisms on glasses.

SKEW DEVIATION

Skew deviation is characterized by vertical deviation of the eyes on lateral gaze. This can result from closed-head injury and produces double vision on lateral gaze. Spontaneous recovery usually occurs.

PARINAUD'S SYNDROME

Injury to the region of the superior tectal plate can lead to Parinaud's syndrome: dilated pupils, impairment of accommodation and convergence, and impaired upward gaze.

POSTTRAUMATIC NYSTAGMUS

Posttraumatic nystagmus may result from damage to the labyrinthine system or from brainstem trauma. This can be very difficult to treat and is outside the scope of this chapter.

EYE INJURIES

Decreasing visual acuity or blindness demands urgent assessment. The differential diagnosis includes TONL, retrobulbar hemorrhage, and vitreal hemorrhage.

RETROBULBAR HEMORRHAGE

Retrobulbar hemorrhage is an eye-saving diagnosis, but it is underdiagnosed in serious orbital injuries.[56] The patient presents with an orbital injury, proptosis, pain, developing ophthalmoplegia, decreasing visual acuity, and dilating pupil; on ophthalmoscopy, pallor (arterial compression) or venous dilatation (venous compression) of the disc is seen. If time allows, with the support of medical treatment, an ultrasound study or preferably a CT scan should be obtained to determine the site of the hemorrhage and to facilitate urgent decompression (see Fig. 10-24). Medical treatment involves the use of:

- mannitol 20%, 2 g/kg IV over 5 minutes.
- dexamethasone, 8 mg IV.
- acetazolamide, 500 mg IV and then 1000 mg orally over 24 hours.
- surgical decompression, which remains the most certain option.

If visual acuity is deteriorating rapidly, a four-wall decompression under local anesthesia is required to prevent a permanent loss of vision. It is probably easier in the non-operated patient to decompress initially through a medial blepharoplasty rather than the usually recommended lateral canthotomy (see Fig. 10-5).

TRAUMATIC OPTIC NERVE LESIONS

The optic nerve may be damaged at the junction of the eye, within the orbit, or within the optic canal. This is a common long-term cause of decreased visual acuity after an orbital injury.[57] A significant percentage (2%) of patients with an orbital injury have an ocular injury severe enough to render them blind in that eye.[9,11] The incidence of blindness in those patients with more severe orbital fractures (fronto-orbital) is significantly higher.

Partial tearing of the optic nerve from the eye leads to tearing of nerve fiber bundles with a corresponding visual field defect. Hemorrhage at the optic nerve head is seen initially and evolves into optic nerve pallor (see Fig. 10-30). As the pigment epithelium of the retina heals, a crescent of pigmented change may be seen in the late stages. The distribution of the nerve fiber loss dictates whether central vision is lost. The mechanism of damage is probably torsion of the globe with respect to the optic nerve.

TONLs typically occur acutely. About 2% (0.7%-5.0%) of all closed-head injuries and 20% of all frontobasal injuries show some kind of visual pathway damage in which the intracanalicular part of the optic nerve is affected (see Figs. 10-28 and 10-29).

As stated earlier, TONLs most commonly are secondary to frontal or frontotemporal injuries (72% and 12%, respectively). These patients often have associated complex general injuries. In about 60% of patients with severe midface or skull base fractures, a routine neuro-ophthalmological investigation with evaluation of optic nerve function is not possible because of swelling or the patient's level of consciousness. Some means of testing is required to distinguish permanent from temporary TONLs. Electrophysiological testing of the visual pathways with a flash electroretinogram (ERG) and visual evoked potentials (VEPs) is a known method in the nonacute situation but is not frequently used in acute care to assess TONLs. This testing allows diagnostic assessment of vision and facilitates the decision on whether to operate (decompress) (Fig. 10-46). Total avulsion of the optic nerve is very rare but occurs with severe orbital injuries and results in immediate blindness (Fig. 10-47). Decompressive surgery is not indicated in avulsion injuries.

The first clinical step is the assessment of vision, followed by gross visual field testing and, if necessary, the swinging flashlight test. If the patient is unconscious and a decision on visual pathway function or a diagnosis of visual pathway damage cannot be made, electrophysiological testing with flash ERG/VEP is undertaken. Visual pathway function is classified as *normal*, *pathological*, or *absent*, and treatment decisions are made on that basis. The checkerboard VEP investigation is superior for the detection of TONL but is not applicable in the unconscious or uncooperative patient.

If decreased visual acuity is detected, an axial spiral CT scan of the midface and the frontal skull base with reconstructed coronal planes is performed. This enables visualization of the orbit, optic canal, optic chiasma, and displaced bones and identification of the origin of the TONL. This helps in the decision whether to treat surgically. A compressive TONL does not necessarily require a displaced fracture in the optic canal. A whiplash-type injury with no displacement, an occult fracture, or simply edema can result in compression and may require decompression (Fig. 10-48). Most patients with a confirmed posttraumatic afferent disorder of the visual pathway (i.e., TONL) have a fracture in the bony optic canal or the posterior third of the orbit or a space-occupying intraorbital lesion (retrobulbar hemorrhage).

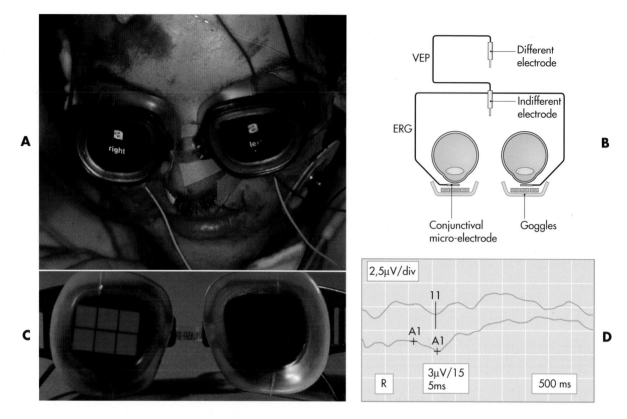

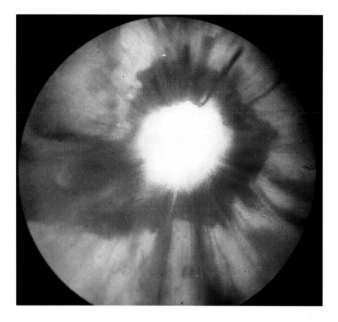

FIGURE 10-46   Electrophysiological testing. **A,** Patient with goggles. **B,** Electrical setup. **C.** Goggles. **D,** Printout, ERG, electroretinogram; VEP, visual evoked potential.

FIGURE 10-47   Traumatic optic avulsion with immediate loss of vision and decreased intraocular pressure.

In these cases, 3-D CT reconstructions are of no additional diagnostic value and might be misleading because of the window threshold normally used and the thinness of the bony structures in the area. MRI is better than CT at showing optic nerve edema or hematoma, but CT is still preferred to assess for bony injuries. High-resolution axial spiral CT with coronal reconstruction is the gold standard to detect midface and skull base fractures. Plain radiographs are usually of little value in detecting the bony lesions responsible for visual pathway damage. Ultrasonography is a valid method, especially for detection of retrobulbar hematoma, but is of limited value for optic nerve injuries.

Therapy for TONL

In the treatment of TONLs, there are basically four options with research support:

- wait and see
- conservative treatment
- surgical treatment
- combined conservative and surgical treatment

The diagnosis of TONL is important. Orbital injuries associated with severe midface or skull base fractures should be investigated on a routine basis. If there is no evidence of a TONL in an unconscious patient, a wait-and-see policy is acceptable. It is the delay to onset of treatment that limits the prognosis for a successful visual pathway treatment.

Glucocorticoids dominate the conservative treatment. Their therapeutic effect is related to their antiedematous, antiinflammatory, and antioxidative effects. They prevent vasospasm, which in turn helps prevent neuronal death. They inhibit gliofibrillary scarring of the traumatized optic nerve.

There has been one study advocating the use of high-dose steroids; it was undertaken in the United States in 1994. Treatment with methylprednisolone must be started not later

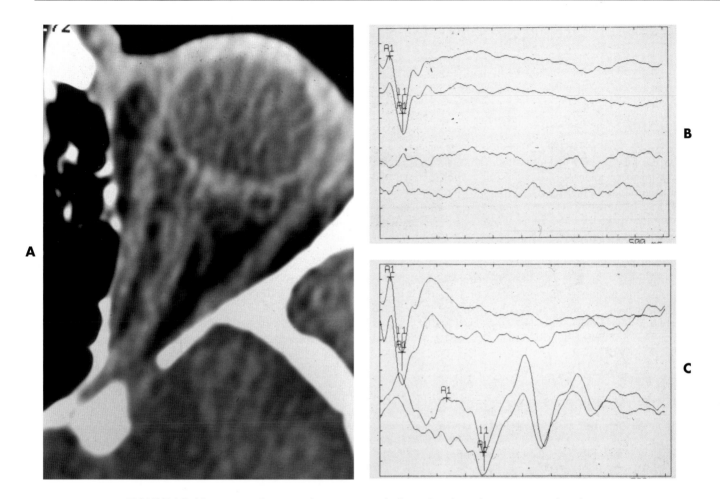

FIGURE 10-48   Computed tomographic scan (**A**) with electrophysiological printouts (**B** and **C**) displaying neurotmetic injury to the optic nerve.

than 8 hours after the trauma, with an initial IV bolus of 30 mg/kg bodyweight, followed by 5.4 mg/kg bodyweight over the next 48 hours. This protocol originated from the National Acute Spinal Cord Injury Study (NASCIS). The rationale for the methylprednisolone megadose is the reduction it produces in free radicals, the decrease in secondary posttraumatic lesions due to impaired lipid peroxidation, and the improved perfusion of the central nervous system. With this dose of steroid, blood glucose levels need to be monitored and antacid therapy commenced prophylactically. Treatment with acetazolamide and mannitol infusion has been described, although there is still no evidence for the value of this therapy.

Joseph's team correlated the severity of the external trauma, the location and extent of the fracture, and TONL with the amount of brain contusion, swelling, hematoma, and intracranial bleeding.[58] In combination with neuro-ophthalmologic findings, they undertook a prospective study, but despite early promise, they were unable to define the need for early optic nerve decompression. They concluded that optic nerve decompression must be a case-oriented decision, based on the clinical and CT findings.

Clinical findings have been correlated with individual fractures and show that the prognosis for the afferent disorder of the visual pathway depends on whether the optic canal is involved.

A retrobulbar hematoma needs to be differentiated from a bone-related TONL. If posttraumatic globe protrusion is present together with an ipsilateral afferent disorder of the visual pathway, the intraorbital pressure within the orbital compartment has to be released by opening the orbital septum. This should be done in conjunction with medical treatment and an urgent CT scan. If there is any delay in obtaining a CT, treatment should be started. Decompression depends on the site of the bleed. In our experience, this is usually medial, and a medial blepharoplasty approach is preferred. This is easily performed with local anesthesia and sedation in the emergency department. The only contraindication for this emergency operation is a pulsating exophthalmos, which may be caused by a caroticocavernous sinus fistula. In this rare case, pretherapeutic imaging is performed, including angiographic investigations.

The controversy with regard to surgical treatment of TONL relates to the extent of surgery, the surgical approach, and its timing. The aim of surgical therapy is to mechanically release the nerve along the optic tract but especially in the optic canal area, where bone fragments might impinge on the nerve or where relative narrowing of the canal (from hematoma or edema) might be present. If there is evidence of TONL, an urgent decompression procedure is considered to relieve the optic nerve in its canal. The dura over the optic nerve or chiasma is not incised.

Surgical approaches vary, and all have some advantages. Besides the transethmoidal approach, transcranial, sublabial, transsphenoidal, and endonasal microsurgical approaches are now possible to reach the area of interest. The method chosen depends on previous surgical experience.

TONL in Craniofacial Reconstruction

There is a danger of visual loss with any orbital procedure, in both primary and secondary orbital reconstruction, and patients should be warned about it. The risk can be reduced by the use of computer-assisted surgery (Fig. 10-49). Modern navigation systems allow for precise preoperative planning and intraoperative control of any contour changes; all changes close to the optic canal can be directly controlled. This is important in defining the most posterior position of bone transplants or alloplastic grafts to augment the orbit.[20,22,39,59] During the operation, three infrared cameras are used to detect the position of preset markers by means of integrated light-emitting diodes (LEDs), and changes in the patient's position are monitored with LEDs attached to a Mayfield clamp.

Changes in pupillary diameter or shape are not uncommon during complex orbital reconstructions. Obviously, optic nerve injury needs to be ruled out. Because the patient is under general anesthesia, the function of the visual pathway cannot be judged clinically. Flash ERG and VEP can be used intraoperatively to assess vision and to confirm lack of compression of the optic nerve by the grafting procedure.

EYELID INJURY

The most common eyelid injury is a bruise. The pattern of bruising depends on whether the leakage of blood is superficial or deep. Superficial bruising extends down onto the face.

Deep bruising gives rise to a demarcation line resembling the eye of a panda, with blood constrained behind the septum, and this type of bruising usually follows an orbital fracture. A subconjunctival hemorrhage with a posterior limit is usually caused by direct ocular injury, whereas a subconjunctival hemorrhage with no posterior limit is a common sequela to an orbital fracture (Fig. 10-50). Swelling of the eyelids is very common and is exacerbated if a patient with an orbital fracture blows her nose, leading to the clinical sign of crepitus. Massive swelling can be a sign of a retrobulbar hemorrhage or orbital vein obstruction.

Lacerations need special care, particularly those affecting the medial eyelids that have the potential for injury to the nasolacrimal apparatus and canthal area (Fig. 10-51). These lacerations should be examined under magnification and with good lighting. The canthal area should be assessed. Lid margins must be accurately realigned. The layers of the eyelid should be identified and repaired with 5-0 or 6-0 resorbable sutures in the deep layers, ensuring proper apposition of the orbicularis oculi, and fine monofilament sutures in the skin of the eyelid. Tears of the medial canthus should be identified and primarily repaired with non-resorbable sutures. The nasolacrimal apparatus, if injured, should be repaired over appropriate stents.

CORNEAL ABRASION

Corneal injury causes severe pain, blurring of vision, photophobia, and lacrimation. Damage to the corneal epithelium may be caused by direct injury or may result from inadequate eyelid closure due to facial palsy or loss of eyelid tissue. Alcohol-based skin preparations must never be used on the eyelids before surgery, because they can cause corneal epithelial loss. Incomplete eyelid closure during surgery is another hazard to be avoided. Fluorescein staining of the cornea identifies the pathology (green). Antibiotic ointment is instilled as prophylaxis against secondary infection.

CORNEAL FOREIGN BODY

Superficial corneal foreign bodies can be lifted off with the pointed end of a hypodermic needle, preferably under

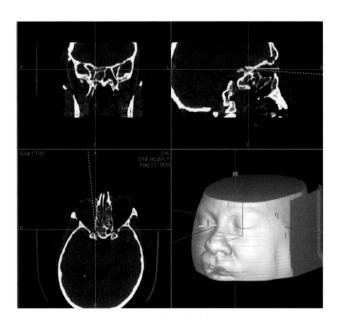

FIGURE 10-49   Three-dimensional spiral computed tomographic preoperative reconstruction with probe identifying the surgical area under investigation (compare Fig. 10-34).

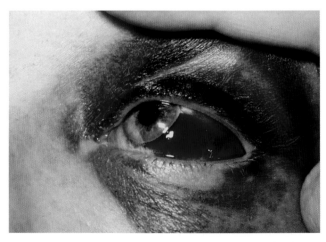

FIGURE 10-50   Bruising and subconjunctival hemorrhage.

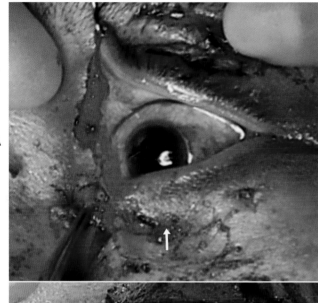

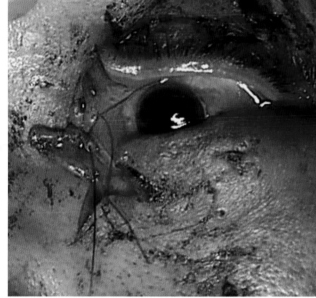

FIGURE 10-51 Nasolacrimal laceration. **A,** Laceration with probable nasolacrimal injury (*arrow* indicates the punctum). **B,** Exploration of canalicular system with fine nylon sutures.

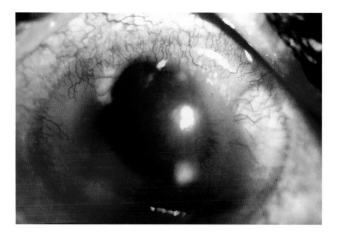

FIGURE 10-52 Anterior chamber hemorrhage with hyphema.

sclera has been described. Distortional injury can also cause tearing of the choroid, which is associated with subretinal hemorrhage, and in very severe cases, avulsion of the optic nerve.

The concussional component of the injury can damage the cornea, lens, retina, choroid, and optic nerve, all of which are susceptible to transient or permanent damage. These injuries are best assessed by an ophthalmologist.

Conjunctiva

Swelling of the conjunctiva is commonly associated with subconjunctival hemorrhage and resolves spontaneously.

Cornea

The cornea is made up of five layers: the epithelium and its basement membrane, the stroma, and the endothelium with its basement membrane. Damage to the epithelium results in an erosion, which requires the topical application of a long-acting anesthetic and a topical antibiotic.

Stromal and endothelial damage causes corneal edema. This occurs because the pumping action of the endothelium, which retains the cornea's transparency, ceases to function after the injury. In most cases, corneal edema clears spontaneously.

Anterior Chamber, Iris, and Anterior Chamber Angle

Ripping of the iris from its root is a common sequela to blunt injury. Tearing of fine vessels in the iridocorneal angle results in bleeding in the anterior chamber and hyphema (Fig. 10-52). The hyphema is managed conservatively in most cases. Spontaneous rebleeding into the eye is rare but is more likely to occur in those patients who are given aspirin, which is contraindicated in ocular hemorrhage. Severe hemorrhage can impair the drainage of aqueous humor, which leads to a raised intraocular pressure. A hemorrhage in the anterior chamber may be complicated by blood staining of the cornea.

Traumatic iritis is common. An injury to the iris causes the release of protein and inflammatory cells into the anterior chamber. These are seen on slit-lamp microscopy. Treatment is with topical steroids to diminish the inflammation and with pupil dilatation (cyclopentolate), to decrease the probability

binocular magnification, using one drop of topical local anesthetic. A short-acting cycloplegic agent such as cyclopentolate 1% (which diminishes pain from ciliary spasm) and a topical antibiotic are instilled. Topical diclofenac has been shown to afford good pain relief.

BLUNT EYE INJURIES

Closed injury causes damage from both distortion and concussion of the globe (during the brief duration of the injury). Both types of injury can be seen. A high-speed blow to the eye causes marked globe distortion. The eye is compressed, resulting in anteroposterior shortening and coronal distention. Because the cornea and sclera are unable to distend, the iris, ciliary body, zonule of the lens, and peripheral retina may be torn from their insertions. In severe cases, rupture of the of the iris' sticking to the lens (posterior synechiae). Deepening of the anterior chamber suggests that the lens may have been subluxated or may even have become dislocated.

Iridodialysis (tear in the iris) results when the iris is ripped from its root (Fig. 10-53). Traumatic mydriasis is common. The dilated pupil does not react directly or consensually. In severe cases, pupil sphincter ruptures can be seen on the slit lamp, and this results in permanent wide dilatation of the pupil. More commonly, the result is a moderately dilated pupil, and spontaneous recovery can take place.

Angle recession occurs when the iris is partially stripped from its root without being torn completely. Rarely, severe injuries can lead to 360-degree recession. The iridocorneal angle contains Schlemm's canal. The healing response can give rise to fibrosis and scarring in this area, diminishing the outflow of aqueous humor, and can cause raised intraocular pressure, either acutely or many years later. Angle recession takes place at the time of injury and can be visualized by gonioscopy (slit-lamp examination using a mirror or prism system to see into the angle). This pathology can easily be missed if detailed slit-lamp eye examination is not carried out and can lead to glaucoma in the long term.

Lens

The lens can be damaged in several ways. Subluxation of the lens is a common sequela to a severe blunt injury. Macroscopically, the principal clinical sign is wobbling of the iris, or iridodonesis. Dislocation of the lens into the vitreous is less common. Occasionally, the lens is dislocated into the anterior chamber. This is an acute ophthalmic emergency and is more common in people with underlying spontaneous lens subluxation, such as those with Marfan syndrome. Such lens injuries cause changes in refraction, both because the lens is moved and because it does not accommodate for near vision so well. Traumatic cataract can be the result of severe concussional injury. In cases of severe injury, the pupil margin impacts the anterior surface of the lens, leaving a permanent pigmented ring.

Rarely, rupture of the lens capsule can take place. Aqueous fluid then enters the lens and causes opacification or cataract formation, for which the only effective treatment is cataract surgery after the acute effects of the injury (e.g., traumatic iritis) have resolved.

Ciliary Body

The ciliary body performs two principal functions: production of aqueous humor and accommodation of the lens. Damage to the ciliary body can lead to reduction in aqueous humor formation and a reduced intraocular pressure.

Impaired accommodation is common after blunt eye injury. Patients complain of blurring of vision and eye strain, particularly when reading. Reading matter held in front of the affected eye cannot be seen in focus as close as by the unaffected eye, and in some cases, reading glasses that give balance to the focusing system are required.

Tearing of the ciliary body from its root is rare and is called *traumatic cyclodialysis*. A persistent, very low intraocular pressure results and may necessitate surgical repair of the injury.

Retina

The distortional effects of blunt injury can lead to tearing of the peripheral retina (known as *retinal dialysis*) or peripheral retinal hole formation. The vitreous gel adheres firmly to the peripheral retina. The acute coronal distention of the injury distorts the vitreous, which can pull and tear the peripheral retina. Most cases of retinal dialysis occur secondary to trauma. Water from within the vitreous can pass through the tear and lift off the retina, resulting in progressive retinal detachment (Fig. 10-54). Patients who are short-sighted or who have conditions predisposing to retinal detachment (e.g., myopia, Stickler's syndrome, Marfan syndrome) are at a significant risk. Approximately 10% of traumatic retinal detachments occur at the time of the injury, 70% within 2 years, and 20% more than 2 years after injury. If the tear passes through a retinal vessel, bleeding into the vitreous can take place. This gives rise to the sensation of seeing "floaters" in the visual field. Blunt injury to the globe can also cause damage to the vitreous humor, which can collapse; this leads to the formation of strands in the vitreous, which can also give rise to floaters.

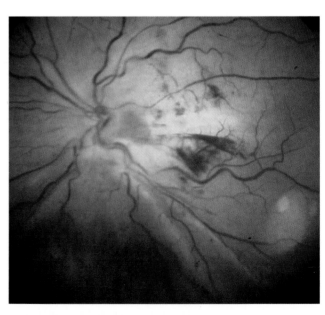

FIGURE 10-54   Retinal detachment.

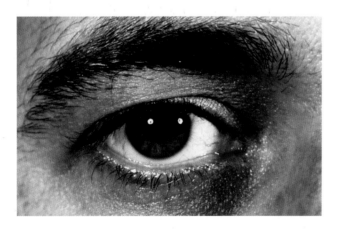

FIGURE 10-53   Iridodialysis.

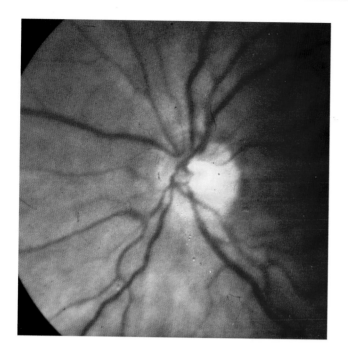

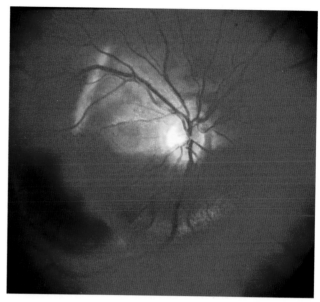

FIGURE 10-56 Choroidal tear with choroidal effusion.

FIGURE 10-55 Traumatic retinal edema or commotio retinae (Berlin's edema).

Treatment of retinal detachment is complex and not always successful. Therefore, it is important to prevent retinal detachment by identifying and treating dialysis and retinal holes with photocoagulation or cryotherapy or both. Exudative retinal detachment can occur as a rare sequela to blunt eye trauma. In such cases, spontaneous flattening of the retina takes place, but the prognosis for recovery of vision is poor.

Traumatic retinal edema is also known as *commotio retinae* or Berlin's edema (Fig. 10-55). Whitening of the retina is seen. If the edema takes place at the posterior pole, blurring of vision occurs. Peripheral edema, which causes peripheral visual field impairment, may not be symptomatic and may be missed. Most patients report rapid improvement in vision during the first 40 minutes after injury. In some cases of severe injury, improvement does not take place, and fluorescein angiography reveals breakdown in function of the pigment epithelium in the retina. Permanent visual impairment can ensue, and such pathology may be accompanied by the development of a traumatic retinal hole or pigmentary changes in the retina, known as *traumatic pigmentary retinopathy*. This clinical pattern is very similar to that of retinitis pigmentosa.

Choroidal Tears

Choroidal tears due to blunt injury characteristically occur circumferential to the optic disc (Fig. 10-56). Initially, extensive subretinal hemorrhage is seen, but as the hemorrhage resolves, the tear becomes apparent. If the tear passes through the fovea, central vision is lost; the prognosis is much better for tears that do not affect the fovea. Occasionally, the healing response can include the development of new blood vessels, which can grow under the macula and cause secondary visual loss.

Choroidal effusion looks very similar to retinal detachment. However, there are no holes in the retina, and the appearance is more ballooned in nature. Severe hypotonia (which may be caused by cyclodialysis) is the principal underlying cause.

Injury to the Sclera

Injury to the sclera is most common in the superonasal quadrant and is present in 18% of scleral tears associated with an orbital fracture. If an eye has a very low intraocular pressure, rupture of the sclera posteriorly may be present, and imaging studies are required to diagnose this injury.

If a scleral rupture is not repaired, persistent hypotonia or ingrowth of fibrous tissue can develop. Surgical exploration is indicated in most cases of persistent hypotonia for which there is no clear explanation. Repair of the scleral rupture is usually accompanied by restoration of intraocular pressure and prevents the complication of fibrous ingrowth. In addition, sympathetic ophthalmia, in which inflammation of the other eye occurs, can rarely complicate scleral rupture.

PERFORATING EYE INJURIES

Orbital and facial fractures may rarely be accompanied by perforating eye injury, particularly after road traffic accidents. The presence of multiple facial lacerations increases the index of suspicion of an underlying perforating eye injury.

Visual function is determined, if possible. The eyes are examined by gentle retraction of the eyelids without direct pressure on the bottom of the eye. There may be an obvious perforation or some irregularity of the pupil, opacification of the anterior chamber due to intraocular hemorrhage, or a shallow anterior chamber. Prolapse of the iris, ciliary body, or vitreous may be observed. Loss of vision secondary to a

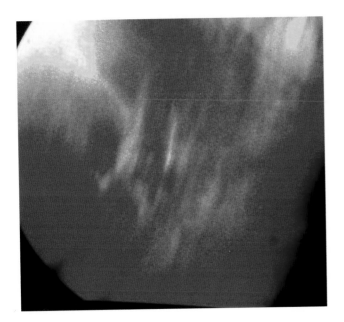

FIGURE 10-57   Vitreal hemorrhage secondary to a perforating eye injury.

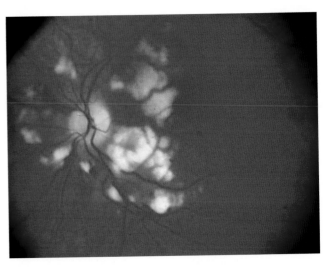

FIGURE 10-58   Traumatic retinal angiopathy.

vitreal hemorrhage may be the only clinical sign of the injury (Fig. 10-57).

Perforation of the globe by a small, fast, flying missile necessitates appropriate radiological examination. Immediate transfer to the care of an ophthalmologist is indicated. A pad is applied to the eye, and pressure to the globe is avoided. Primary surgical repair is carried out within 24 hours. If surgical treatment is delayed, prophylactic intravenous broad-spectrum antibiotic treatment is indicated.

INDIRECT OPHTHALMIC SEQUELAE TO INJURY

Traumatic Retinal Angiopathy (Purtscher's Retinopathy)

In traumatic retinal angiopathy, multiple cotton-wool spots are observed at the posterior pole of the eye (Fig. 10-58). A sudden increase in intravenous pressure due to severe head or chest injury is thought to give rise to a reactive precapillary arteriolar spasm in the retina, which causes multiple small retinal infarcts. A similar appearance is observed in patients who sustain long bone fractures with secondary fat emboli. Impairment or loss of central vision ensues in one or both eyes. There is no specific treatment, but spontaneous resolution with return of normal visual function takes place in most cases.[59]

Caroticocavernous Sinus Fistula and Arteriovenous Anastomosis

The formation of a fistula between the arterial and venous systems may occur a few days after a severe skull injury (see Fig. 10-44). The ophthalmic features include pulsating exophthalmos, ophthalmoplegia, chemosis, and markedly dilated blood vessels on the conjunctivae and eyelids. The intraocular

pressure is raised. Loss of vision may ensue without treatment.

Papilledema

Swelling of the optic nerve head due to raised intracranial pressure may be observed. In the acute phase, swelling does not take place, but the absence of spontaneous venous pulsation and failure of the retinal veins to collapse when pressure is applied the upper eyelid during ophthalmoscopy is a useful clinical sign.

Facial Palsy

Incomplete eyelid closure as a sequela to traumatic facial palsy can give rise to corneal ulceration and infection. Patients who do not manifest Bell's phenomenon (in which the eye rolls up when the eyelids are closed) are particularly at risk. Eye ointment is required to prevent drying of the cornea. Tarsorrhaphy or injection of the levator palpebrae superioris with botulinum toxin to produce eyelid closure may be required if ulceration has developed.

CONCLUSION

The management of orbital injuries is a challenging area. It requires an ability to collaborate with others and to understand the surgical anatomy, pathophysiology, and potential complications. A thorough assessment (Fig. 10-59), full investigations, satisfactory exposure, anatomical reconstruction with appropriate material, and audit of results will improve the lot of these patients.

ACKNOWLEDGMENT

The authors wish to acknowledge Dr. Gordon Dutton for his previous contribution to this chapter.

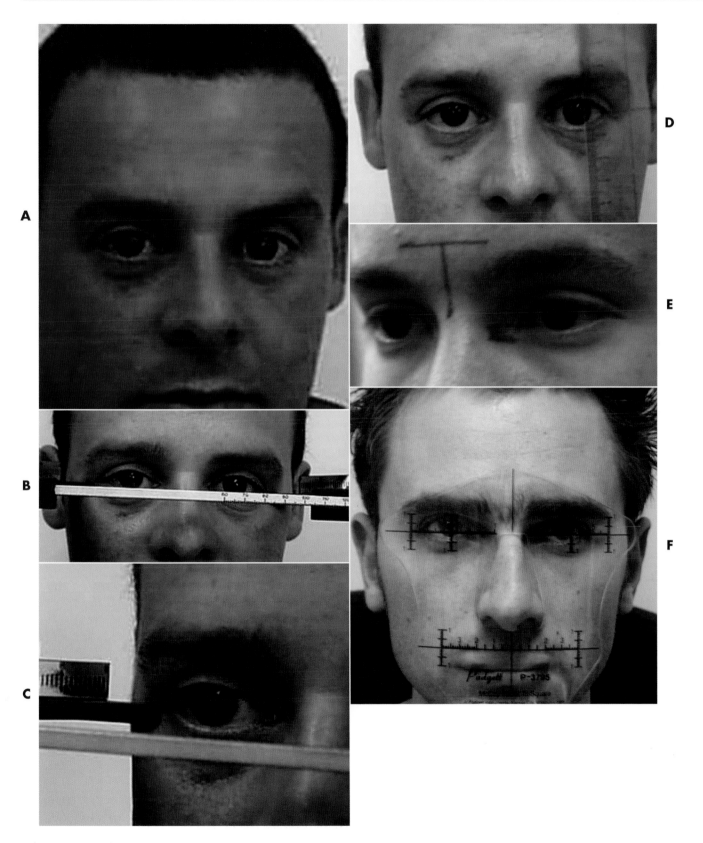

FIGURE 10-59 Measurements. **A,** Left orbital injury, enophthalmos, hypoglobus. **B,** Hertel exophthalmometer, unsuitable to use because of lateral wall dystopia. **C,** Assessing enophthalmos. **D,** Pseudocorrection of orbital dystopia by rotating head allows measurement of the hypoglobus (see Figs. 10-36 and 10-37). **E.** Measurement of canthal area. **F,** Facial measurements using the McCoy facial square.

Continued

Name: DOB: Age: Sex: M/F

Injury: Date: Time: Location:

Drugs: alcohol / other

How: assault / road traffic accident / fall / sport / industrial / firearm / other

Others involved:

Amnesia Retrograde / Antegrade / Both

Visual acuity:	Right eye 6/6, 6/12, 6/36, NPL	Left eye 6/6, 6/12, 6/36, NPL
Pupil size:	Symmetrical /asymmetrical, Size: Reaction to light:	right pinpoint, 3mm, 5mm, >8mm left pinpoint, 3mm, 5mm, >8mm right direct / indirect left direct / indirect
Eye movements:	Right eye: normal / limited / globe retraction Left eye: normal / limited / globe retraction Diplopia yes / no Specify:	
Right eye:	Normal	proptosis / enophthalmos hypoglobus / hyperglobus lateral dystopia / medial dystopia
Left eye:	Normal	proptosis / enophthalmos hypoglobus / hyperglobus lateral dystopia/medial dystopia
Canthal area:	Intercanthal distance: Intercanthal level: Intercanthal distance: Intercanthal level:	medial____mm Right____Left____ medial Right 5 Left asymmetric____mm lateral____mm Right____Left____ lateral Right 5 Left asymmetric____mm level / mongoloid / anti-mongoloid
Palpebral fissure:	Width:	Right:____ Height: Right:____ Left:____ Left: ____
Facial nerve function:	Right Left	normal weak Specify____ normal weak Specify____
Eye closure:	Right Left	complete, incomplete, Bell's phenomenon Y / N complete, incomplete, Bell's phenomenon Y / N
Jaw movement:	Mouth opening mm R (lateral) L (lateral)	____ ____ ____

G

FIGURE 10-59, cont'd   **G,** Orbitofacial evaluation form.

REFERENCES

1. Errington J: Facing the future. *Br J Oral Maxillofac Surg* 37:161-163, 1999 (editorial).
2. Ellis E III, Zide MF: *Surgical approaches to the facial skeleton*, Baltimore, 1995, Williams & Wilkins, pp 7-65.
3. Kerawala CJ, Grime RJ, Stassen LFA, et al: The bicoronal flap (craniofacial access): an audit of morbidity and a proposed surgical modification in male pattern baldness. *Br J Oral Maxillofac Surg* 38:441-444, 2000.
4. Baumann A, Ewers R: Transcaruncular approach for reconstruction of medial orbital wall fracture. *Int J Oral Maxillofac Surg* 29:264-267, 2000.
5. Ilankovan V: Transconjunctival approach to the orbital region: a cadaveric and clinical study. *Br J Oral Maxillofac Surg* 129:169-172, 1991.
6. Jin HR, Shin SO, Choo MJ, et al: Endonasal endoscopic reduction of blowout fractures of the medial orbital wall. *J Oral Maxillofac Surg* 58:847-851, 2000.
7. Chen CT, Lai JP, Chen YR, et al: Application of endoscope in zygomatic fracture repair. *Br J Plast Surg* 53:100-105, 2000.
8. Lee CH, Lee C, Trabulsy PP, et al: A cadaveric and clinical evaluation of endoscopically assisted zygomatic fracture repair. *Plast Reconstr Surg* 101:333-345; discussion 346-347, 1998.
9. al-Qurainy IA, Stassen LF, Dutton GN, et al: The characteristics of midfacial fractures and the association with ocular injury: a prospective study. *Br J Oral Maxillofac Surg* 29:291-301, 1991.
10. al-Qurainy IA, Stassen LF, Dutton GN, et al: Diplopia following midfacial fractures. *Br J Oral Maxillofac Surg* 29:302-307, 1991.
11. al-Qurainy IA, Titterington DM, Dutton GN, et al: Midfacial fractures and the eye: the development of a system for detecting patients at risk of eye injury. *Br J Oral Maxillofac Surg* 29:363-367, 1991.
12. Fox LA, Vannier MW, West OC, et al: Diagnostic performance of CT, MPR and 3DCT imaging in maxillofacial trauma. *Comput Med Imag Graphics* 19:385-395, 1995.
13. Ilankovan V, Hadley D, Moos K, et al: A comparison of imaging techniques with surgical experience in orbital injuries: a prospective study. *J Craniomaxillofac Surg* 19:348-352, 1991.
14. Maya MM, Heier LA: Orbital CT: current use in the MR era. *Neuroimag Clin North Am* 8:651-683, 1998.
15. Mauriello JA Jr, Lee HJ, Nguyen L: CT of soft tissue injury and orbital fractures. *Radiol Clin North Am* 37:241-252, xii, 1999.
16. Cahan MA, Fischer B, Iliff NT, et al: Less common orbital fracture patterns: the role of computed tomography in the management of depression of the inferior oblique origin and lateral rectus involvement in blow-in fractures. *J Craniofac Surg* 7:449-459, 1996.
17. McCann PJ, Brocklebank LM, Ayoub AF: Assessment of zygomaticoorbital complex fractures using ultrasonography. *Br J Oral Maxillofac Surg* 38:525-529, 2000.
18. Holck DE, Boyd EM Jr, Ng J, et al: Benefits of stereolithography in orbital reconstruction. *Ophthalmology* 106:1214-1218, 1999.
19. Gruss JS, Van Wyck L, Phillips JH, et al: The importance of the zygomatic arch in complex midfacial fracture repair and correction of posttraumatic orbitozygomatic deformities. *Plast Reconstr Surg* 85:878-890, 1990.
20. Stanley RB Jr: Use of intraoperative computed tomography during repair of orbitozygomatic fractures. *Arch Facial Plast Surg* 1:19-24, 1999.
21. Kobienia BJ, Sultz JR, Migliori MR, et al: Portable fluoroscopy in the management of zygomatic arch fractures. *Ann Plast Surg* 40:260-264, 1998.
22. Watzinger F, Wanschitz F, Wagner A, et al: Computer-aided navigation in secondary reconstruction of post-traumatic deformities of the zygoma. *J Craniomaxillofac Surg* 25:198-202, 1997.
23. Kasrai L, Hearn T, Gur E, et al: A biomechanical analysis of the orbital zygomatic complex in human cadavers: examination of load sharing and failure patterns after fixation with titanium and bioresorbable systems. *J Craniomaxillofac Surg* 10:400-403, 1999.
24. Kasrai L, Hearn T, Gur E, et al: A biomechanical analysis of the orbitozygomatic complex in human cadavers: examination of load sharing and failure patterns following fixation with titanium and bioresorbable plating systems. *J Craniomaxillofac Surg* 10:237-243, 1999.
25. Key SJ, Thomas DW, Shepherd JP: The management of soft tissue facial wounds. *Br J Oral Maxillofac Surg* 33:76-85, 1995.
26. Phillips JH, Gruss JS, Wells MD, et al: Periosteal suspension of the lower eyelid and cheek following subciliary exposure of facial fractures. *Plast Reconstr Surg* 88:145-148, 1991.
27. Dufresne CR: The use of immediate grafting in facial fracture management: indications and clinical considerations. *Clin Plast Surg* 19:207-217, 1992.
28. Burm JS, Chung CH, Oh SJ: Pure orbital blowout fracture: new concepts and importance of medial orbital blowout fracture. *Plast Reconstr Surg* 103:1839-1849, 1999.
29. Harris GJ, Garcia GH, Logani SC, et al: Orbital blowout fractures: correlation of preoperative computed tomography and postoperative ocular motility. *Trans Am Ophthalmol Soc* 96:329-347, discussion 347-353, 1998.
30. Ramieri G, Spada MC, Bianchi SD, et al: Dimensions and volumes of the orbit and orbital fat in posttraumatic enophthalmos. *Dentomaxillofac Radiol* 29:302-311, 2000.
31. Raskin EM, Millman AL, Lubkin V, et al: Prediction of late enophthalmos by volumetric analysis of orbital fractures. *Ophthal Plast Reconstr Surg* 14:19-26, 1998.
32. Penfold CN, Lang D, Evans BT: The management of orbital roof fractures. *Br J Maxillofac Surg* 30:97-103, 1992.
33. Burns JA, Park SS: The zygomatic-sphenoid fracture line in malar reduction: a cadaver study. *Arch Otolaryngol Head Neck Surg* 123:1308-1311, 1997.
34. Stassen LFA, Kerawala C: Peri- and intraorbital trauma and orbital reconstruction. In Ward-Booth P, Schendel SA, Hausamen J, editors: *Maxillofacial surgery*, vol 1, Edinburgh, 1999, Churchill Livingstone.
35. Bullock JD, Warwar RE, Ballal DR, et al: Mechanisms of orbital floor fractures: a clinical, experimental, and theoretical study. *Trans Am Ophthalmol Soc* 97:87-110; discussion 110-113, 1999.
36. Vriens JP, Van Der Glas HW, Moos KF, et al: Infraorbital nerve function following treatment of orbitozygomatic complex fractures: a multitest approach. *Int J Oral Maxillofac Surg* 27:27-32, 1998.
37. Tengtrisorn S, McNab AA, Elder JE: Persistent infra-orbital nerve hyperaesthesia after blunt orbital trauma. *Austr N Z J Ophthalmol* 26:259-260, 1998.
38. Lee HH, Alcaraz N, Reino A, et al: Reconstruction of orbital floor fractures with maxillary bone. *Arch Otolaryngol Head Neck Surg* 124:56-59, 1998.
39. Forrest CR, Khairallah E, Kuzon WM: Intraocular and intraorbital compartment pressure changes following orbital bone grafting: a clinical and laboratory study. *J Plast Reconstr Surg* 104:48-54, 1999.
40. Morrison AD, Sanderson RC, Moos KF: The use of Silastic as an orbital implant for reconstruction of orbital wall defects: review of 311 cases treated over 20 years. *J Oral Maxillofac Surg* 53:412-417, 1995.
41. Courtney DJ, Thomas S, Whitfield PH: Isolated orbital blowout fractures: survey and review. *Br J Oral Maxillofac Surg* 38:496-503, 2000.
42. McGurk M: Blow-out fractures of the orbit and enophthalmos. In Langdon JD, Patel MF, editors: *Operative maxillofacial surgery*, part 7, London, 1998, Chapman & Hall Medical.
43. Haug RH: Management of the trochlea of the superior oblique muscle in the repair of orbital roof trauma. *J Oral Maxillofac Surg* 58:602-606, 2000.
44. Karampatakis V, Natsis K, Gigis P, et al: Orbital depth measurements of human skulls in relation to retrobulbar anesthesia. *Eur J Ophthalmol* 8:118-120, 1998.
45. Gellrich N-C, Schramm A, Hammer B, et al: Computer-assisted reconstruction of unilateral posttraumatic orbital deformities. *Plast Reconstr Surg* 110:1417-1429, 2002.
46. Cope MR, Moos KF, Speculand B: Does diplopia persist after blowout fractures of the orbital floor in children? *Br J Oral Maxillofac Surg* 37:46-51, 1999.
47. Iliff N, Manson PN, Katz J, et al: Mechanisms of extraocular muscle injury in orbital fractures. *Plast Reconstr Surg* 103:787-799, 1999.
48. Derdyn C, Persing JA, Broaddus WC, et al: Craniofacial trauma: an assessment of risk related to timing of surgery. *Plast Reconstr Surg* 86:238-245, 1990.
49. Jordan DR, Allen LH, White J, et al: Intervention within days for some orbital floor fractures: the white-eyed blowout. *Ophthalmol Plast Reconstr Surg* 14:379-390, 1998.
50. Verhoeff K, Grootendorst RJ, Wijngaarde R, et al: Surgical repair of orbital fractures: how soon after trauma? *Strabismus* 6:77-80, 1998.
51. Flood TR, McManners J, el-Attar A, et al: Randomised prospective study of the influence of steroids on postoperative eye-opening after exploration of the orbital floor. *Br J Oral Maxillofac Surg* 37:312-315, 1999.
52. Egbert JE, May K, Kersten RC, et al: Pediatric orbital floor fracture, direct extraocular muscle involvement. *Ophthalmology* 107:1875-1879, 2000.
53. Bansagi ZC, Meyer DR: Internal orbital fractures in the paediatric age group: characterisation and management. *Ophthalmology* 107:829-836, 2000.
54. Manson PN, Iliff N: Management of blowout fractures of the orbital floor. II. Early repair of selected injuries. *Surv Ophthalmol* 35:280-292, 1991.
55. Putterman AM: Management of blowout fractures of the orbital floor. III. The conservative approach. *Surv Ophthalmol* 35:292-298, 1991.
56. Steinsapir KD, Goldberg RA: Traumatic optic neuropathy. *Surv Ophthalmol* 38:487-518, 1994.
57. Girotto JA, Gamble WB, Robertson B, et al: Blindness after reduction of facial fractures. *Plast Reconstr Surg* 102:1821-1834, 1998.
58. Levin LA, Beck RW, Joseph MP, et al: The treatment of traumatic optic neuropathy: the International Optic Nerve Trauma Study. *Ophthalmology* 106:1268-1277, 1999.
59. Stassen LFA, Goel R, Moos KF: Purtscher's retinopathy: an unusual association with a complicated malar fracture. *Br J Oral Maxillofac Surg* 27:296-300, 1989.

APPENDIX 1:   EYE SCORING SYSTEM (BAD ACT) AND REFERRAL TO OPHTHALMOLOGIST

Total Score			Amnesia		
0	4	Do not refer	Yes	5	(retrograde or antegrade)
5	11	Routine referral	No	0	
11	14	URGENT referral			
Visual Acuity			Female		
6/12	4		Yes	1	
6/24	8		No	0	
6/36	12				
NPL	16				
Fracture Type			Age		
Comminuted	3		>35	1	
Blowout	3				
Other	0				
Diplopia			RTA		
Yes	3		Yes	1	
No	0		No	0	
			Total	_____	

BAD ACT: Blowout, Acuity, Diplopia, Amnesia, Comminuted Trauma.

APPENDIX 2: CLINICAL HISTORY AND EXAMINATION

Name:	DOB:	Age:	Sex: M/F
Injury:	Date:	Time:	Location:

Drugs: alcohol / other

How: assault / road traffic accident / fall / sport / industrial / firearm / other

Others involved:

Amnesia: retrograde / antegrade / both

Visual acuity:	Right eye	Left eye		
	6/6, 6/12, 6/36, NPL	6/6, 6/12, 6/36, NPL		
Pupil size:	Symmetrical / asymmetrical			
	Size:	right pinpoint, 3 mm, 5 mm, 8 mm		
		left pinpoint, 3 mm, 5 mm, 8 mm		
	Reaction to light:	right direct / indirect		
		left direct / indirect		
Eye movements:	Right eye: normal / limited / globe retraction			
	Left eye: normal / limited / globe retraction			
	Diplopia: yes / no			
	Specify:			
Right eye:	Normal	proptosis / enophthalmos		
		hypoglobus / hyperglobus		
		lateral dystopia / medial dystopia		
Left eye:	Normal	proptosis / enophthalmos		
		hypoglobus / hyperglobus		
		lateral dystopia/medial dystopia		
Canthal area:	Intercanthal distance:	medial_____mm	Right_____Left_____	
	Intercanthal level:	medial Right Left	asymmetric_____mm	
	Intercanthal distance:	lateral_____mm	Right_____Left_____	
	Intercanthal level:	lateral Right Left	asymmetric_____mm	
		level / mongoloid / anti-mongoloid		
Palpebral fissure:	Width:	Right:_____	Left:_____	
	Height:	Right:_____	Left:_____	
Facial nerve function:	Right	normal / weak	Specify_____	
	Left	normal / weak	Specify_____	
Eye closure:	Right	complete, incomplete, Bell's phenomenon Y / N		
	Left	complete, incomplete, Bell's phenomenon Y / N		
Jaw movement:	Mouth opening mm	_____		
	R (lateral)	_____		
	L (lateral)	_____		

CHAPTER 11

Craniofacial and Frontal Sinus Fractures

Nicholas J. Baker, Barrie T. Evans, Dorothy A. Lang

The treatment of fractures of the frontal sinus has become less contentious as the contemporary principles of modern maxillofacial trauma management have become more widely adopted. The key rationale to treat fractures of the frontal sinus has always been to produce a "safe" sinus and reduce the long-term risks of complications. Early treatment was based on experience from the management of infective frontal sinus disease extrapolated to equate with the frontal sinus involved in trauma. The difficulty has been in predicting exactly which patients are at risk for these complications. Progress has been hampered by studies of small numbers of patients in retrospective reviews. Complications may develop many years after the initial trauma, with patients often presenting to teams not involved in the initial management. We will suggest that management of dural tears is the key to a "safe" sinus and has been under emphasized in the past.

The aim of this chapter is to provide an overview of currently accepted principles of management of frontal sinus fractures based on the experience of others and our own experience of more than 163 consecutive cases of craniofacial trauma managed between 1988 and 2008.

HISTORICAL PERSPECTIVES

Traditionally, in view of the perceived risk of infection and neurological deterioration, craniofacial injuries have been managed in at least two separate stages. These injuries were treated as separate entities by neurosurgeons and maxillofacial surgeons often working in isolation. Understanding of the aims of other specialties was limited, and the overall management of these injuries suffered as a result of the fragmented nature of the treatment.

Initial treatment usually consisted of urgent craniotomy for the evacuation of intracranial clots, elevation of depressed bone fragments, and repair of the dura over the convexity of the brain. Wounds were débrided, and loose bone fragments were discarded. Facial fracture repair was carried out 7 to 14 days or longer after the initial neurosurgical management. Formal exploration and reconstruction of the anterior cranial fossa (ACF) was seldom done, basal repair being limited to cases of persistent cerebrospinal fluid (CSF) rhinorrhea. Fixation of facial fractures was usually achieved with closed techniques by means of bone pins, halo frames, and internal suspension wires, which were usually attached to the teeth with the patient placed into intermaxillary fixation. Direct visualization of fracture sites by elevation of the periosteum was kept to a minimum for fear of devitalizing bone fragments. Primary bone grafting was rarely, if ever, performed. Contour defects of the forehead were treated secondarily, often with the use of alloplastic material such as methyl methacrylate.

The limitations of traditional frontobasal repair, combined with the lack of coordinated treatment, resulted in inadequate functional and cosmetic results, particularly in the critical frontal nasoethmoidal and orbital regions. Late secondary correction of these posttraumatic sequelae was difficult and often produced unsatisfactory results.

Management of the frontal sinus was based on historical experience in the treatment of acute and chronic frontal sinusitis. Initial techniques were based on the Reidel procedure of sinus ablation with excision of the bony walls. This approach resulted in severe frontal deformity and was later replaced by several modifications intended to exenterate the sinus mucosa while preserving the bony anatomy of the sinus. All of these techniques carried a significant failure rate. They were subsequently replaced by techniques to obliterate the sinus by excising the sinus mucosa, plugging the frontonasal ducts (FNDs), and obliterating the sinus with autogenous or alloplastic materials.

Fractures of the frontal sinus form an integral part of craniofacial fracture management and cannot be considered in isolation. This chapter examines the contemporary principles of craniofacial fracture management with particular reference to management of the frontal sinus.

CLASSIFICATION OF CRANIOFACIAL FRACTURES

Fractures of the naso-fronto-orbital region account for approximately 5% of facial fractures.[1] Fractures involving the anterior or posterior wall of the frontal sinus occur in 2% to 12% of cranial fractures.[2] Combined frontobasilar and facial injuries may be isolated to the cranio-orbital area, or they may be part of more extensive injuries involving the upper, middle, and lower facial regions. Craniofacial fractures may be divided into central and lateral groups.

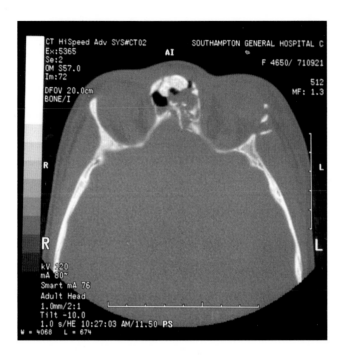

FIGURE 11-1 Axial computed tomogram shows a type I central craniofacial injury with disruption at the level of the cribriform plate.

CENTRAL INJURIES

Central injuries are those that involve the skull base adjacent to the paranasal sinuses: the frontal, ethmoid, and sphenoid sinuses. Central injuries are subdivided into two types depending on the location of the fracture.

Type I Cribriform Fracture

A type I cribriform fracture is a linear fracture that extends through the cribriform plate without involvement of the ethmoid or frontal sinuses. These fractures may result from relatively low-energy injuries that would not cause fractures in stronger areas of the anterior skull base. The dura covers this area with the arachnoid layer, and together they form tubular sheaths around the branches of the olfactory nerves, with the dura being continued into the periosteum of the nose and the arachnoid into the neurolemma of the nerve. The cribriform plate is thin, is easily fractured, and may be difficult to repair, resulting in a high propensity for the development of CSF fistulae (Fig. 11-1).

Type II Frontoethmoidal Fracture

Type II frontoethmoidal fractures involve the medial portion of the ACF and directly involve the frontal or the ethmoid sinuses or both. As with type I fractures, CSF pools toward the midline, and this may prevent brain herniation and seal by brain or adjacent tissues[3] (Fig. 11-2).

LATERAL INJURIES

Lateral injuries involve the frontal bone and the orbital roof. These fractures may lie lateral to the frontal sinus, or they may involve the superior or inferior walls of the lateral frontal sinus. In this area, the brain is completely invested in dura, and the brain lies superior to the fracture site, in contrast

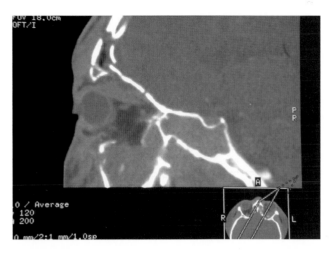

FIGURE 11-2 Sagittal computed tomogram shows a type II central craniofacial injury with fractures involving the anterior and posterior walls of the frontal sinus.

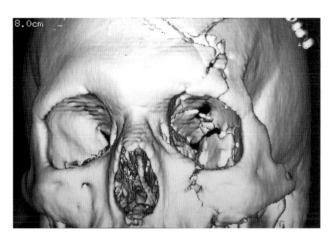

FIGURE 11-3 Three-dimensional computed tomographic reconstruction shows a lateral craniofacial injury with fractures of the frontal bone, orbital roof, and zygomatic complex.

to the situation with central injuries. CSF fistulae are therefore more likely to subside spontaneously as a result of gravity and brain herniation through the dural laceration (Fig. 11-3).

Complex injuries can occur in which a combination of central and lateral fracture patterns occurs (Fig. 11-4).

CLINICAL FEATURES

Up to one third of patients with a head injury and a Glasgow Coma Scale (GCS) score of 8 or less can be expected to have a major injury elsewhere in the body.[4] All life-threatening conditions must be treated and stabilized before a full assessment of other injuries is undertaken. In addition, patients who are unconscious, particularly if they have sustained facial injuries, are unable to protect their own airway and should be intubated. The nature and severity of the craniofacial injuries are assessed once the patient has been stabilized after emergency treatment.

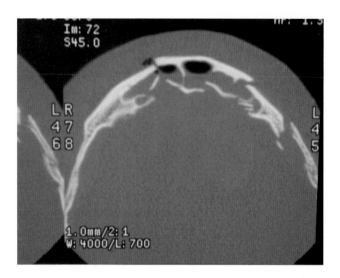

FIGURE 11-4   Axial computed tomogram shows a combination of central and lateral craniofacial fractures.

The risk of cervical spine injury in the unconscious patient with craniofacial injuries must be assumed until the spine can be "cleared" radiologically. The cervical spine should be stabilized with a hard cervical collar as part of the management of the airway, and the collar must be left in position until the cervical spine has been imaged. Radiographs should be taken to visualize the cervical spine from a lateral and an anteroposterior direction and a further film to visualize the odontoid peg. All seven cervical vertebrae must be visualized, including the cervicothoracic junction. If there is any doubt based on the plain radiographs, or if a soft tissue injury is suspected, computed tomography (CT) or magnetic resonance imaging (MRI) of the cervical spine (or both) must be obtained in the unconscious patient.

CLINICAL EXAMINATION

An initial assessment of the level of consciousness can be made using the acronym AVPU: **a**wake, responds to **v**ocal commands, responds to **p**ain, or **u**nresponsive. This provides a baseline against which more detailed assessment of the level of consciousness may subsequently be made.[5]

Once the patient has been stabilized, a more detailed assessment of the level of consciousness is made and a thorough examination of the head and neck is performed. A full neurological assessment looking for focal or general neurological signs should also be included. The assessment of the level of consciousness should be repeated and recorded at regular intervals to detect any deterioration in the patient's condition. The GCS provides a means of rapid and repeated assessment of the level of consciousness by individual or multiple clinicians and direct comparison of clinical findings. Any deterioration in the level of consciousness as evidenced by the GCS is an indication for an urgent CT scan. The GCS has three components: eye opening, best verbal response, and best motor response. The score in each group is totaled to give a final score of between 3 and 15. A score of 8 or less indicates that the patient is unconscious.[6]

After assessment of the level of consciousness, examination of the head and neck should be undertaken, including the cervical spine if the patient is conscious. This should be performed in a systematic manner, starting with inspection of the scalp and working downward, noting any physical signs and palpating all bony margins. The eyes should be examined and the visual acuity, pupillary responses, range of eye movement, and presence of diplopia or restricted eye movements recorded. Visual fields should be tested to confrontation. The intercanthal distance should be recorded, particularly if nasoethmoidal injury is suspected. Sensation to light touch and pinprick should be tested in all three divisions of the trigeminal nerve. Facial nerve function should be assessed, particularly if a base-of-skull fracture is suspected or in the presence of facial lacerations that may involve the peripheral branches of the nerve. If the patient is conscious, it is important to inquire about loss of smell or hearing; if necessary, these should be formally tested. Initial assessment may be difficult in the acute situation because of the presence of blood in the nasal airway or external meatus.

The external auditory meatus should be inspected for the presence of hemotympanum, lacerations, damage to the tympanic membrane, and the presence of otorrhea.

Anterior rhinoscopy should be undertaken to examine for the presence of CSF rhinorrhea and nasal septal hematoma. This area may be difficult to visualize in the presence of blood. Clear secretions from the nose can be tested for glucose by the glucose oxidase test. This should be used only to confirm that the secretion is *not* CSF, because both nasal and lacrimal secretions may contain glucose.[7] This test is unreliable and has been replaced by immunoelectrophoresis of the secretions for β_2 transferrin, which identifies CSF and does not produce false-positive results in the presence of nasal or lacrimal secretions or blood.[8] β_2 transferrin is present in CSF but absent in tears, saliva, nasal secretions, and serum except perhaps in neonates and individuals with deranged liver function.

Intraoral examination should be performed to examine for bruising, swelling, and mobility of the tooth-bearing segments. The patient's occlusion should be checked for evidence of derangement.

CLINICAL FINDINGS

Skull vault fractures may manifest with localized scalp swelling and bruising with varying levels of consciousness. A range of neurological signs may also be present. The presence of an underlying intracranial hemorrhage correlates with the presence of a skull fracture and with the patient's level of consciousness.[9]

Fractures involving the ACF may show bilateral circumorbital ecchymoses, nasal epistaxis, and CSF rhinorrhea. A variety of eye signs may be demonstrated, including visual loss, and the patient may complain of loss of smell. Middle fossa fractures may demonstrate Battle's sign (bruising around the mastoid process), blood in the external auditory meatus, and CSF otorrhea. There may be evidence of hearing loss or facial nerve weakness.

In craniofacial fractures, bruising around the eyes is common, and there may be evidence of subconjunctival hemorrhage. Subconjunctival hemorrhage as a physical sign merely demonstrates that bleeding has occurred deep to the orbital periosteum. Visual loss may occur as a result of the intracerebral insult or from direct trauma to the optic nerve itself, usually within the optic canal. Fractures extending into the orbital apex are rare because this area is the strongest part of the orbital skeleton. Fractures of the optic canal may occur, particularly with severe, high-energy injuries.[10] Orbital fractures involving the superior orbital fissure may also occur and give rise to a range of physical signs depending on the individual nerves involved (*superior orbital fissure syndrome*).[11] The oculomotor, trochlear, and ophthalmic divisions of the trigeminal and abducens nerves all pass through the superior orbital fissure and may produce limitation of eye movement, pupillary dilatation (mydriasis), and sensory disturbances in the frontal region (the supraorbital and supratrochlear branches of the ophthalmic division of the trigeminal nerve). The superior orbital fissure syndrome secondary to trauma is also a rare occurrence.

Pupillary mydriasis may be an indication of rising intracranial pressure as a result of its effect on the oculomotor nerve as it passes forward from the posterior aspect of the brainstem on its intracranial course. This occurs as a result of transtentorial herniation and is always secondary to a fall in the GCS.[12] The oculomotor nerve contains parasympathetic fibers to the iris of the eye and is responsible for pupillary constriction (miosis). Direct damage to the oculomotor nerve may occur either intracranially or extracranially to produce an isolated third nerve palsy. The eye takes an abducted and depressed position with an associated mydriasis and upper eyelid ptosis. The direct pupillary reflex is absent, but is the consensual pupillary reflex are present if the ipsilateral optic nerve and the contralateral oculomotor nerve are both functioning normally. This is in contrast to an isolated optic nerve lesion, in which the ipsilateral direct and contralateral consensual pupillary reflexes are both absent.

Damage to the abducens and trochlear cranial nerves occurs less frequently. An isolated abducens nerve palsy produces an inability to abduct the eye, and an isolated trochlear nerve palsy produces an inability to abduct the eye in downward gaze. In all cases of damage to the third, fourth, and sixth cranial nerves, diplopia is present when the range of eye movements is assessed. With any suspected orbital or globe injury, an ophthalmic opinion must be sought. If eye signs are present, particularly restricted eye movements or diplopia, an orthoptic assessment should be performed, including a Hess chart.

The eyes should be assessed for the presence of enophthalmos. Assessment of enophthalmos in the acute situation may be difficult if its presence is masked by swelling of the periorbital tissues. Enophthalmos may occur with either orbital floor or medial wall blowout fractures if there is also rupture of the periorbita. Disruption of the medial orbital walls is invariably present in severe nasoethmoidal injuries and is therefore often present in craniofacial injuries.

Disruption of the attachments of the medial canthal tendons may also occur with nasoethmoidal injuries. The medial canthal tendon has an anterior limb that attaches to the anterior lacrimal crest and a posterior limb that lies posterior to the lacrimal sac. Disruption of the anterior limb of the tendon alone does not produce telecanthus (increase in the intercanthal distance). Telecanthus is a sign of disruption of both anterior and posterior limbs of the tendon and necessitates reattachment of the anterior limb to prevent

persistence of the deformity postoperatively. The intercanthal distance should be checked in patients with suspected nasoethmoidal and craniofacial injuries. The normal intercanthal distance is 25.5 to 37.5 mm in women and 26.5 to 38.7 mm in men. Injuries to the medial canthal tendon may also occur with lacerations to the area in the absence of underlying fracture.

A fracture involving the frontal sinus may be suggested by the presence of a laceration in the region of the supraorbital ridge, glabella, or lower forehead.[13]

Traumatic hypertelorism (increased inter-pupillary distance) may also occur in severe fronto-orbito-nasoethmoidal injuries with a true increase in the interorbital distance. Failure to appreciate the distinction between traumatic telecanthus and hypertelorism leads to inadequate treatment with a poor functional and cosmetic result.

RADIOLOGICAL ASSESSMENT

CT scanning has revolutionized the management of craniofacial trauma by allowing precise delineation of injuries and exact preoperative planning before intervention. Assessment of both skeletal and soft tissue elements is possible with the use of appropriate bone and soft tissue windows. Scanning is performed in both the axial and coronal planes to allow visualization of all anatomical structures. The coronal views are essential for assessment of the orbital and frontal sinus roof and floor and for detailed assessment of the cribriform plate, the roofs of the ethmoid sinuses, the jugum sphenoidale, and the optic canals (Fig. 11-5). All other fractures are usually demonstrated on the axial views. One-millimeter slices are required to allow adequate evaluation of the skull base and orbits. Three-dimensional (3-D) CT reconstruction often adds little in the way of practical information in the assessment of patients with craniofacial trauma but may be of benefit in selected complex cases[14] (Fig. 11-6).

INDICATIONS FOR COMPUTED TOMOGRAPHY

CT scanning should be performed in all patients with suspected craniofacial injuries. In addition, a CT scan must also be obtained under any of the following circumstances:

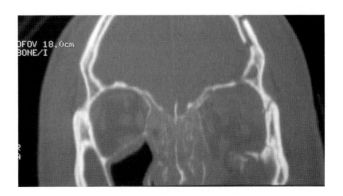

FIGURE 11-5 Coronal computed tomogram demonstrates an increase in left orbital volume secondary to disruption of the orbital roof and floor and the zygomatic complex.

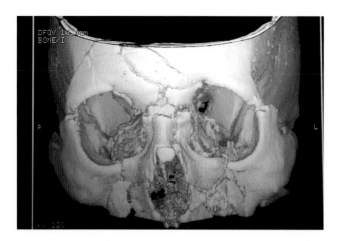

FIGURE 11-6 Three-dimensional computed tomographic reconstruction demonstrates complex frontal, nasoethmoidal, orbital floor, and midface injuries.

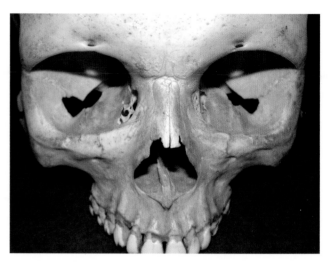

FIGURE 11-7 Precise appreciation of premorbid anatomy is essential in craniofacial trauma management to allow accurate reconstruction and prevention of posttraumatic deformity.

- Basal skull fracture
- GCS <8
- Confusion persisting after resuscitation
- Deteriorating level of consciousness or progressive focal neurological deficit
- Seizure
- Neurological symptoms or signs including headache or vomiting
- CSF rhinorrhea or otorrhea

CT scanning is essential to precisely delineate the site and extent of injury associated with the frontal sinus. CT scanning may be used to assess injury to the ostia or ducts of the sinus. Fine-cut axial views will demonstrate disruption of the anterior and posterior walls of the sinus. Coronal views are necessary for adequate examination of the horizontal aspect of the frontal sinuses, the cribriform plates, the roofs of the ethmoid sinuses, and the orbits. It has been suggested that the level of fracture and degree of disruption of the base of the sinus predict the probability of ductal obstruction.[13] We would question this. Our view is that it is not possible to predict with any degree of accuracy whether a sinus will continue to function after injury, based on imaging appearance alone.

Plain skull radiographs do not add to the information gained from CT scanning and are unnecessary in patients who are already undergoing CT.

Plain radiographs of the midface may give an extra overall dimension to information gained from the CT scan. It can be difficult to obtain satisfactory views in the unconscious patient, but plain films are of particular benefit in assessing facial symmetry after internal fixation of fractures.

If mandibular injury is suspected, the mandible may be imaged on plain films or as part of the overall CT scan.

RATIONALE FOR THE TREATMENT OF CRANIOFACIAL FRACTURES

Current management of craniofacial trauma is based on the principles of pediatric craniofacial surgery pioneered by Paul

Tessier in 1967 and adopted to apply to craniofacial trauma by Merville in 1978.[15] This was the first approach that addressed combined injuries in a definitive, single-stage repair. A frontal bone flap is raised to allow inspection of the dura, both convexity and basal, and its repair. The frontal sinus is cranialized, and the fronto-orbital and facial injuries are treated during the same anesthesia.[15]

The aims of treatment for craniofacial injuries are twofold: (1) the restoration of satisfactory form and function and (2) the prevention of early and late complications, and in particular, infective sequelae.

RESTORATION OF SATISFACTORY FORM AND FUNCTION

The key to achieving accurate 3-D reconstruction in combined skull base and facial injuries is complete simultaneous exposure of the cranial vault, skull base, and facial fractures.

Accurate 3-D reconstruction of the frontal bandeau and orbital roofs is a prerequisite to satisfactory orbitofacial reconstruction. This may be achieved by reproducing the precise premorbid projection and convex curvature of the supraorbital rims. Laterally, the temporal buttresses of the frontal bone determine the projection and width of the upper midface. The position of the glabella in the midline determines the projection of the nasoethmoidal complex and may necessitate primary bone grafting in comminuted injuries or when bone is lost (Fig. 11-7).

The convexity of the orbital roof in the anteroposterior and lateral planes must be reproduced to prevent globe displacement and disturbed ocular motility. Inaccurate reconstruction of the superior orbital rim and orbital roof resulting in inferior globe displacement is one of the most difficult posttraumatic deformities to correct satisfactorily. The premorbid ocular position can be reestablished by wide exposure and accurate reduction of the zygomatic arch and lateral orbital rim. The inner orbital skeleton can be reconstructed secondarily to the lateral position.[16,17]

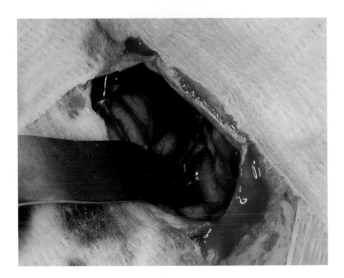

FIGURE 11-8 Intradural exploration reveals brain plugging a dural tear. Although there is no cerebrospinal leak, failure to repair this type of injury places the patient at a lifelong risk of infection.

PREVENTION OF EARLY AND LATE INFECTIVE SEQUELAE

Dural tears that communicate with the nasal cavity and paranasal sinuses are common in craniofacial fractures; if untreated, they may leave the patient at significant risk for either meningitis or a cerebral abscess. Importantly, the absence of an overt CSF leak does not indicate the absence of a dural tear. In the presence of a dural tear, the brain may act to plug the hole in the dura and prevent the CSF leak (Fig. 11-8).

In 1954, Lewin showed the risk of meningitis to be at least 25% in patients with CSF rhinorrhea and cranial base fractures communicating with the paranasal sinuses in the absence of dural repair.[18] In 1990, Eljamel and Foy reported on a series of patients with acute traumatic CSF fistulae. They found an overall incidence of meningitis of 30.6% before dural repair with a 10-year cumulative risk in excess of 80.5%.[19] Surgical repair of the dura reduced the overall risk of meningitis from 30.6% before surgery to 4% after surgery; the cumulative risk at 10 years was reduced from 80.5% before dural repair to 7% after dural repair.[20]

In 1989, Poole and Briggs published their approach to the management of craniofacial trauma based on their experience of 48 patients over a 7-year period.[21] Their indications for combined craniofacial repair were:

- radiological evidence of displaced fractures involving the posterior wall of the frontal sinus, the cribriform plates, or the orbital roofs with or without the presence of CSF rhinorrhea.
- displaced fractures of the frontal bone or upper orbital skeleton.
- extensive bone loss as a result of the injury or the initial débridement procedure.

Sakas et al. outlined the need for surgical intervention in patients with or without CSF rhinorrhea based on the results of detailed neuroimaging.[3] They identified certain factors that

were linked to a high long-term risk of developing posttraumatic meningitis:

- Proximity to the midline, particularly central type I cribriform fractures
- Large fracture displacement (≥1 cm)
- Prolonged rhinorrhea (≥8 days)

The effects were shown to be cumulative, and fracture patterns exhibiting a combination of these features carried particular risk.[3]

Our group has refined Sakas' criteria to determine the indications for combined craniofacial repair.[16] A combination of clinical and CT criteria are employed as follows:

1. Central injuries that show clinical or radiological evidence of displaced fractures of the posterior wall of the frontal sinus, the cribriform plate, or the roof of the ethmoid sinus (or some combination of these) with or without a CSF leak. The fractures are considered to be *displaced* if the degree of disruption is equal to or greater than the width of the lamella of bone forming the posterior wall of the frontal sinus, cribriform plate, and roof of the ethmoid sinus. These fractures are considered to be *internally compound* fractures because the intracranial contents are in contact with the nasal cavity or the paranasal sinuses or both.
2. Lateral injuries with displaced fractures producing contour deformity, globe displacement, or ocular motility disturbance.
3. Extensive bone loss in the supraorbital rim or orbital roof resulting from the injury or the débridement procedure.
4. Growing skull fractures in association with the orbital roof or frontal sinuses. This is a rare complication that occurs in 0.6% of linear skull fractures in pediatric patients. The fracture is associated with a dural laceration with arachnoid herniating into the dural tear, which prevents primary dural healing and results in progressive enlargement and eversion of the fracture line. Ninety percent of these fractures occur in children younger than 3 years of age. These fractures may result in significant functional and cosmetic disturbances.

We have reviewed 163 consecutive cases of craniofacial trauma managed jointly in the Maxillofacial Unit, Southampton University NHS Trust, Southampton, UK, over the 20-year period from 1988 to 2008. The cases were selected for treatment based on the previously mentioned criteria. An additional 18 cases of penetrating injuries were not included in this series.

Considering the predictive value of the CT criteria alone, our results demonstrated a dural tear in direct communication with the nasal cavity or paranasal sinuses, irrespective of the presence of a CSF leak, in 89% of the 163 patients.[22] The sensitivity of pure CT criteria in this series is increased to 93% if the degree of fracture displacement is greater than the width (thickness) of the lamella of bone forming the posterior wall of the frontal sinus, roof of the ethmoid sinus, or cribriform plate. Only about 30% of the patients had a CSF leak, confirming that CSF leakage is a very poor indicator of a basal dural tear.

Further refining of the CT criteria for case selection is being considered to bring their sensitivity as a predictor of a dural tear as close to 100% as possible. Nevertheless, we believe that these CT criteria represent a very significant improvement over CSF leakage as a predictor of dural disruption, although the latter remains the gold standard for exploration and repair in many centers.

The key to reducing, and potentially eliminating, the risk of intracranial infection after treatment of fractures of the skull base is to effectively isolate the intracranial contents from the frontal, ethmoid, and sphenoid sinuses. This is achieved by watertight dural repair, appropriate management of the frontal sinus, and vascularized soft tissue flaps (pericranial/galeal frontalis) inserted between the dural repair and the underlying nasal cavity and paranasal sinuses. Very infrequently, the degree of disruption of the forehead skin precludes the use of vascularized (pedicled) soft tissue flaps. Nonvascularized autologous soft tissue such as fascia lata or temporalis fascia may be employed under these circumstances.

TIMING OF SURGERY

Early combined repair of craniofacial injuries has been demonstrated to be effective in improving functional and cosmetic results with acceptable morbidity and mortality and no adverse effect on neurosurgical outcome in selected patients.[23] The advocates of early intervention cite a better outcome in terms of functional and cosmetic results. This must be balanced against unacceptable morbidity from the surgical procedure itself. Benzil et al. looked at a series of patients with craniofacial trauma who underwent a single-stage combined surgical repair within 24 hours after injury and demonstrated a 15% rate of postoperative CSF fistula and an 8% rate of meningitis.[24]

Other series have reported a mortality rate as high as 11.8% in patients undergoing early surgical intervention, but this was apparently balanced by a good neurosurgical, functional, and cosmetic outcome in 79.2% of patients.[25] When early intervention is excluded based on certain clinical criteria—elevated intracranial pressure, severe associated injury or medical condition, or poor prognosis for survival due to cerebral injury—there is no significant difference in survival between patients who undergo early versus middle or late surgical repair.[23]

Our criteria for case selection for early surgery are based on:

- GCS >13 after resuscitation.
- A stable intracranial pressure ≤15 mm Hg in a cardiovascularly stable patient.
- No CT evidence of midline shift or effacement of the basal cisterns or third ventricle.

PRINCIPLES OF SURGICAL MANAGEMENT OF CRANIOFACIAL FRACTURES[16,17]

ORDER OF TREATMENT

Usually, reduction and fixation of fractures of the cranial vault and ACF should precede the treatment of the facial fractures; that is, the treatment proceeds from above downward. With severe comminution or bone loss in the frontobasal region,

the reconstruction may have to commence with the facial fractures. The full extent of any bone loss in the cranial vault and anterior skull base may then be determined and any missing bone replaced with primary autogenous bone grafts.

ADEQUATE EXPOSURE

Management of craniofacial fractures requires complete subperiosteal exposure of all fracture sites and complete exposure of the basal dura in relation to the fractures. Although endoscopic frontal sinus surgery is well established, there is only a limited role for endoscopic surgery in the management of frontal sinus trauma. There are few reports in the literature describing the use of this technique, and most are anecdotal. Access to the frontal sinus via the endoscope requires a significant amount of experience with endonasal surgery and is technically difficult. Access to the frontal sinus via the transcranial route, via a standard coronal flap or a limited eyebrow incision, is straightforward and allows repair of the dura and management of the frontal sinus in an effective manner while minimizing the risk of missing dural tears.

The standard approach is to combine a coronal flap with a low bifrontal craniotomy (Fig. 11-9). Raveh et al. reported on a series of 395 patients and advocated an extracranial-subcranial approach to repair craniofacial fractures and associated dural tears.[26] This is achieved by incisions confined to the hair borders of the eyebrows with no nasal extension. Dural repair is performed microsurgically along the ethmoid, sellar, and temporal planes via an extracranial approach. The naso-fronto-orbital injuries, including the injuries to the frontal sinus, are also treated by this approach. In Raveh's series, the surgery was performed within 48 hours after the injury and with the aim of avoiding frontal lobe retraction and anosmia. Despite a low incidence of postoperative CSF fistula and no cases of meningitis, there were five postoperative deaths in this series.

Endoscopic repair of CSF fistulae has been reported with the aim of reducing the morbidity of standard approaches.[27] Given the nature of dural tears and their unpredictable

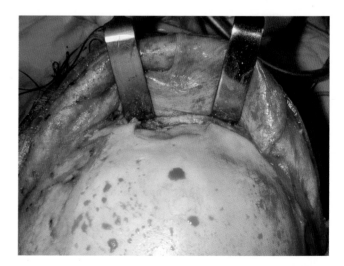

FIGURE 11-9 A coronal flap allows wide access to a fracture involving the anterior wall of the frontal sinus.

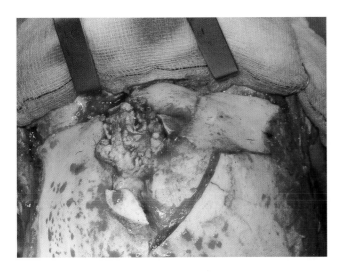

FIGURE 11-10   A comminuted fracture of the frontal bone is widely exposed to assess the fracture pattern before craniotomy.

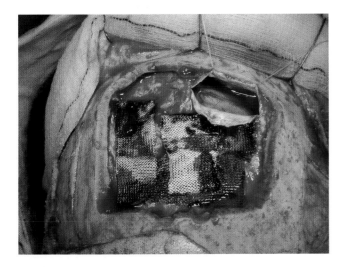

FIGURE 11-11   Intradural dural exploration allows direct inspection of the basal dura and detection of dural tears that may otherwise be missed.

pattern, the risk of missing tears by this approach must place the patient at long-term risk of infective sequelae.

The standard approach combining a coronal incision with a low bifrontal craniotomy allows wide access to the entire craniofacial skeleton. Fracture patterns may be directly assessed and repaired (Fig. 11-10). Convexity and basal dural repair can be performed under direct vision with easy access. Dural tears that are not easily appreciable can be addressed via intradural exploration and repair (Fig. 11-11). This was our approach for all of the 163 patients in our current series.

Access to the entire craniofacial skeleton can be achieved with a combination of esthetically acceptable incisions. A coronal incision extended into the preauricular or postauricular region on each side to the level of the tragus allows access to the frontal and temporal bones and upper facial skeleton, particularly the zygoma, lateral orbit, orbital roof, and nasoethmoidal regions. The supraorbital neurovascular

bundles should be identified and freed from their bony canals in the supraorbital rim, because they provide sensation to the skin of the forehead up to the vertex and can provide the vascular pedicle for any subsequent pericranial or galeal frontalis flap used for ACF repair. The temporalis fascia should be split above the root of the zygomatic process of the temporal bone. In splitting the fascia, an incision oriented superiorly at 45 degrees to the base of the zygomatic arch is necessary to preserve the frontal branch of the facial nerve, which runs in the plane between the two layers of the temporalis fascia. Dissection may then continue deep to the nerve.[28] The coronal flap may be combined with lower eyelid incisions (transconjunctival with or without lateral extension, subtarsal, or subciliary) to gain access to the inferior orbital rim and floor and the medial and lateral orbital walls. Ideally, the eyelid incisions should be made before the coronal flap is raised; if this is left until later in the procedure, the lower eyelid may become edematous. An alternative to a lower eyelid incision is performance of a lateral orbitotomy via the coronal flap, which gives excellent access to the orbital floor and medial wall by retracting the globe laterally.

The projection and width of the upper midface are determined by accurate restoration of the position of the body of the zygoma in three dimensions in relation to the cranial base. The key to this task is accurate restoration of the length of the zygomatic arches. The accurate positioning of the body of the zygoma in three dimensions is also a critical factor in restoring the correct orbital volume and, hence, the correct position of the ocular globe. If there is disruption to the medial canthus but there is still attachment to bone, this can be reduced and plated back into position. If there is no bony attachment, the ligament can be picked up with a permanent suture. This can be passed transnasally and fixed to the contralateral posterior lacrimal crest. After extensive lateral orbital subperiosteal dissection, the lateral canthus should be reattached to a fixed reference point just below the frontozygomatic suture.

An intraoral vestibular incision allows access to the lower midface. All of these incisions may be linked subperiosteally, and no attempt should be made to retain the periosteal attachment of small pieces of bone fragments. Occasionally, large facial lacerations may be used to gain access to fracture sites, but often the access is inadequate without unacceptable extension of the laceration.

A low bifrontal craniotomy allows access to the ACF and basal dura as far posteriorly as the lesser wing of the sphenoid and jugum sphenoidale. Exposure of the basal dura does not necessitate sectioning of intact olfactory nerve filaments. Intradural exploration allows identification and preservation of the olfactory tracts.

Definitive reduction and fixation of fractures should be undertaken only after the entire fracture pattern has been assessed by direct inspection. This is of particular importance when one is attempting to mobilize fractures of the orbital roof, because mobilization can be potentially dangerous if the optic canal is involved.

MINIMAL BRAIN RETRACTION

A low subfrontal exposure minimizes frontal lobe retraction. It may be reduced further by removal of the supraorbital fracture fragments or by performance of an osteotomy of the superior orbital margin, so that any additional retraction is at the expense of the orbital contents rather than the frontal lobe. Spinal drainage may be used in selected cases to further reduce frontal lobe retraction.

STABLE FIXATION OF FRACTURES

Current fixation systems have been specifically designed to allow accurate and stable 3-D reconstruction of the craniofacial skeleton (Fig. 11-12). Stable reconstruction of hard tissues

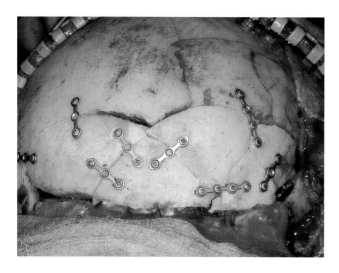

FIGURE 11-12 Accurate reduction of a comminuted frontal bone fracture and internal fixation with multiple monocortical plates and screws.

after fracture resists later distortion due to muscle pull and scar contracture.

The number of plates and screws used should be kept to a minimum, and they should be placed at sites where they may easily be removed, if necessary, without significant morbidity. Plates should be placed on the convexity of the outer table of the skull, if possible, avoiding intracranial plates.[29]

PRIMARY BONE GRAFTING

Primary autogenous bone grafting may be necessary to replace severely comminuted or missing bone segments. It has been suggested that bone gaps greater than 5 mm should be replaced with bone grafts.[29] The need for a bone graft depends on the site of the defect and the extent to which it is subject to the forces of muscle pull and soft tissue contracture. Bone grafting is most commonly required for fractures involving the orbital roofs, the frontal bandeau, the anterior wall of the frontal sinus, the orbital floor, the medial and lateral orbital walls, the nasal skeleton, and the anterior aspect of the maxilla (Fig. 11-13).

In the management of craniofacial fractures, the usual donor sites for bone graft harvest are the calvaria, iliac crest, and ribs. Calvarial bone is a particularly attractive option for craniofacial fractures because there is no additional donor wound, and if the inner table is harvested, there is no visible donor site defect. Limited full-thickness calvarial grafts may be harvested from children younger than 1 year of age without the need to reconstruct the donor site, because bone regeneration can be expected to occur. Inner table calvarial bone may be used to provide a satisfactory volume of bone to reconstruct craniofacial fractures in most patients. The outer table is split from the inner table of the calvaria to provide the graft material, and the outer table can then be

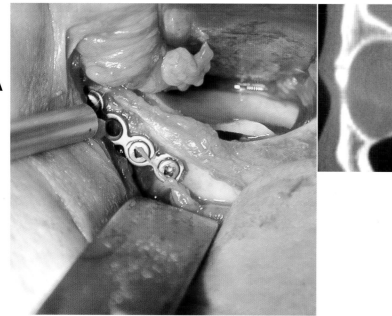
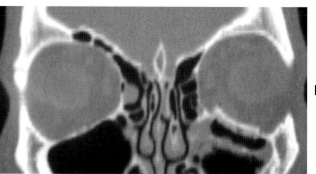

FIGURE 11-13 **A,** Split inner table calvarial bone graft has been harvested for reconstruction of a large orbital floor defect. **B,** Postoperative coronal computed tomogram shows satisfactory graft position; the graft lies passively across the orbital floor defect.

repositioned to avoid a defect at the site of the craniotomy (Fig. 11-14). Calvarial bone can be difficult to contour satisfactorily; in complex defects such as the orbital floor and walls, iliac crest may be the graft material of choice.

Rigid fixation of primary autogenous bone grafts reduces subsequent resorption and volume depletion (Fig. 11-15). The combination of bone grafting and rigid fixation allows complete and stable reconstruction of the craniofacial skeleton after trauma.

Titanium mesh and other alloplastic materials are now commonly used in orbital reconstruction and provide excellent results. The material used depends on the preference of the individual surgeon, but in our unit, autologous bone remains the reconstructive material of choice.

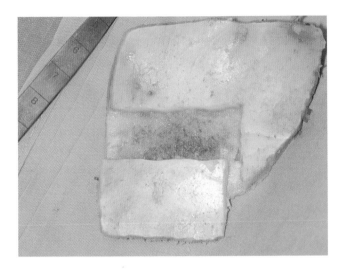

FIGURE 11-14   Split calvarial inner table taken from the craniotomy bone flap can yield a large volume of autologous bone for primary grafting. The bone flap can be repositioned without contour deformity.

STUDY OF PATIENTS TREATED AT SOUTHAMPTON, 1988-2008

A total of 163 consecutive patients were treated. Emergency neurosurgical procedures within the first 24 hours were required in 15% of these patients, and 27% required preliminary procedures for orthopedic and abdominal injuries.

The mean time from injury to combined craniofacial repair was 10 days in the group of patients who fit our criteria (discussed earlier) and 20 days in those patients who failed to meet the criteria for early surgical repair. There was no detriment to neurological, functional, or cosmetic outcome in the former group, and there appeared to be no significant disadvantage in delaying surgery for up to 3 weeks in the latter.[30]

The rate for revisional facial surgery in our series was 14% with 87% showing a good recovery according to the Glasgow Outcome Score (GOS).

There were two cases of postoperative meningitis in this series, both occurring within 3 months after the initial procedure. In one of these cases, a synthetic dural substitute was used for basal dural repair, going against our policy of using only autologous soft tissue. This was the only patient in our series who was not treated by the skull base surgical team. The second patient who developed meningitis had very extensive bilateral dural disruption that required further intervention to achieve an adequate basal dural seal. Both patients recovered well with no neurological deterioration and no further infective sequelae after repeat repair, and neither case of infection was related to concerns with the frontal sinuses.

There have been no cases of cerebral abscess.

A single case of postoperative CSF leakage from the convexity of the dura required reoperation for closure. Considering the findings of Eljamel and Foy mentioned earlier,[19] if cases had been selected based purely on the presence of a persistent CSF leak regardless of the degree of

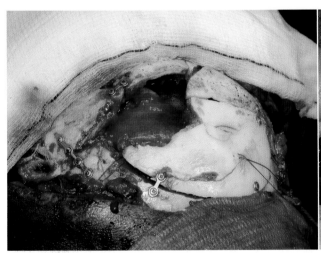
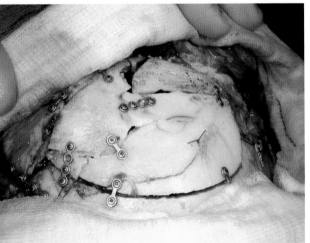

FIGURE 11-15   **A,** Large residual defect in the frontal region after removal of multiple comminuted bone fragments and replacement of the craniotomy bone flap. **B,** Reconstruction of the defect with split inner table calvarial bone taken from the craniotomy bone flap.

fracture displacement in central injuries, the predicted rate of meningitis would have been significantly higher over the 20-year period. The mortality rate for this series of patients was 0%.[22]

In our view, these results confirm the validity of our original CT and clinical criteria for combined craniofacial repair, accepting that further refinement of the CT case selection criteria is necessary to increase their sensitivity as a predictor of dural disruption in the region of the base of the skull. The approach adopted for timing of surgery in patients with significant head injuries combined with other injuries also appears to be sound, considering both the outcome in terms GOS and the 0% mortality rate. Finally, the rate of revisional surgery compared favorably with that in published series.

MANAGEMENT OF FRONTAL SINUS INJURIES

SURGICAL ANATOMY

The frontal sinuses are derived from the frontal recess portion of the middle meatus or occasionally from an air cell of the ethmoid infundibulum. The sinuses are radiologically evident at 5 to 6 years of age and reach adult size by 10 to 12 years of age.[13]

The common description of the frontal sinus as a pyramidal, air-filled cavity that lies within the lamina of the frontal bone and creates an anterior and posterior wall for the sinus considers only that portion of the frontal sinus that is related to the skull vault. It fails to take into account the considerable element of the frontal sinus that is situated in the skull base—the horizontal aspect of the frontal sinus. As with the vertical component, this aspect varies considerably in size, is unique to the individual, and may extend as far posteriorly as the sphenoid wing and laterally to incorporate the entire orbital roof. It may also be intimately associated with the anterior ethmoid air cells.[31,32] The size and shape of the sinus varies among individuals and on right and left sides in the same individual.

The anterior wall of the sinus is stronger than the posterior wall, but it also has low resistance to either low-energy or high-energy impact. The brows and buttress of the supraorbital rims demarcate the lower anterior border of the frontal sinus and offer some protection to the anterior wall of the sinus. The posterior wall of the sinus is thinner and weaker and separates the sinus from the dural covering of the brain in the ACF. The sinus floor consists of membranous bone and is the thinnest of the sinus boundaries. A thin septum usually arises from the midline of the sinus floor and partially or completely separates the two sides of the sinus. The horizontal aspect of the sinus is intimately related to the orbits, cribriform plates, ethmoid sinuses, and nasal cavity (Fig. 11-16).

Drainage of the frontal sinus is variable. A true FND exists in only 15% of the population, varying from a few millimeters to 1 cm in length.[31] In the remaining 85%, the frontal sinus drains directly into the anterosuperior portion of the middle meatus via an ostium without a true duct or occasionally by a communication through the ethmoids via the ethmoidal infundibulum.[13] The proximal opening is a more constant feature; it lies in the posteromedial aspect of the frontal sinus floor.[33]

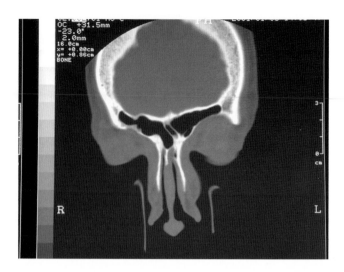

FIGURE 11-16 Coronal computed tomogram shows the position of the frontal sinus and its immediate relationships. Notice the septum dividing the sinus in the midline.

Importantly, the floor of the frontal sinus is on average 3.1 mm below the nasion (i.e., the frontonasal suture).[31,32] As a result, it is reasonable to assume that in severely displaced nasoethmoidal fractures, disruption of the drainage of the frontal sinus is a distinct possibility.

RATIONALE FOR MANAGEMENT OF FRONTAL SINUS INJURIES

Injury to the frontal sinus is an integral part of most central craniofacial injuries and some lateral craniofacial injuries. The principles involved in the management of the frontal sinus are essentially no different from those used in the overall management of the craniofacial fracture: to avoid infective sequelae and to restore satisfactory restoration of form and function. However, its unique anatomical position and physiological function mean that the frontal sinus is usually assessed and managed as a separate entity within the overall fracture pattern. Adverse outcomes such as acute and chronic sinusitis, mucocele, mucopyocele, osteomyelitis, meningitis, and cerebral abscess have all been reported after treated and untreated frontal sinus fractures.[2]

With the exception of displaced fractures of the anterior wall, which are purely a cosmetic problem, injuries to the frontal sinus are treated with the explicit aim of reducing or eliminating the risks of infection and mucocele development.

Historically, the risk of infection after damage to the frontal sinus was believed to be caused principally by disruption of the drainage of the sinus, leading to retained secretions that become infected or to the formation of a mucocele, or both. A mucocele is a collection of mucus within the sinus that gradually enlarges and destroys the bony walls; it is an expansile lesion, not simply a sinus filled with mucus. A minority of frontal sinus mucoceles are the result of trauma.[34] Infection in a mucocele results in a mucopyocele.

Localized osteomyelitis and intracranial complications such as meningitis and epidural or subdural abscesses have also been attributed to injury to the frontal sinus. Because these complications can occur many years after the initial injury, the actual risk of complications after apparent disturbance of frontal sinus drainage is unclear.

In our view, the more likely cause of intracranial infection after trauma to the anterior skull base is untreated dural tears that are in communication with the nasal cavity and the frontal and ethmoid sinuses, rather than infection purely related to the frontal sinus. In the treatment of nasoethmoidal injuries, it is not usual practice to address drainage of the frontal sinus despite the high risk of disruption of the drainage in these injuries. Considering the relative lack of frontal sinus morbidity after treatment of nasoethmoidal fractures in which the frontal sinus is not addressed, the role of disrupted frontal sinus drainage in any subsequent infective sequelae can be questioned.

Historically, management of frontal sinus injury was extrapolated from experience gained in treating acute and chronic frontal sinusitis. This led to confusion and controversy regarding the management of frontal sinus injuries that still exists today.

Our experience and that of other contemporary units treating large numbers of craniofacial injuries suggest that the frontal sinus can be managed reliably and effectively with minimal long-term risk of morbidity. This is based on clinical and radiological evaluation of each case combined with planned surgical intervention based on the findings.

CLASSIFICATION OF FRONTAL SINUS FRACTURES

There are multiple classifications of frontal sinus fractures in the literature. Luce divided frontal sinus fractures into anterior fractures, anterobasilar fractures, and frontal skull fractures with extension into the sinus. The fractures were further classified as closed or open, depending on the presence of an overlying laceration and whether there was an associated CSF leak.[13] Gonty et al. classified frontal sinus fractures into four groups based on the fracture pattern[2] (Box 11-1). Each of these systems has its merits, particularly in descriptive terms, but they are not particularly helpful in terms of management.

We believe that frontal sinus fractures can be categorized into one of four groups related to management:

1. Fracture of the anterior wall
2. Fracture of the sinus with disruption of the posterior wall
3. Fracture involving the floor of the frontal sinus
4. Through-and-through injuries

SURGICAL MANAGEMENT OF FRONTAL SINUS INJURIES

Safe surgical management of the frontal sinus is based on thorough clinical and radiological evaluation of the nature of the injury, which allows precise preoperative surgical planning. Patients are fully assessed in terms of the risks of developing late complications, and this in turn determines management of the frontal sinus injuries.

FRACTURES OF THE ANTERIOR WALL OF THE FRONTAL SINUS

Cosmesis is the only consideration in fractures of the anterior wall of the frontal sinus. Treatment is indicated only for those patients with displaced fractures resulting in cosmetic deformity that is of concern to the patient.

In a series of 72 frontal sinus fractures, isolated fractures of the anterior wall of the frontal sinus occurred in 18% of patients.[35] These fractures may occur with relatively minimal trauma and few clinical signs. Bruising and tenderness over the region of the sinus and the presence of a laceration may all be indicative of an underlying fracture. Fine-cut axial CT imaging demonstrates the degree of displacement.

Undisplaced fractures of the anterior wall require no surgical intervention. Minimally displaced fractures with no evidence of clinical deformity after any edema has subsided may also be managed conservatively. Displaced fractures requiring treatment should be explored via a coronal incision. An overlying laceration is not ideal for surgical exploration and is best avoided. The anterior wall should be reduced and fixed in the anatomical position to restore normal forehead contour (Fig. 11-17). Occasionally in severely comminuted fractures, primary bone grafting is required. If a concomitant craniotomy has been performed, a split inner table calvarial bone graft is ideal. Otherwise, outer table calvarial or iliac crest bone may be harvested. Titanium mesh may be used to advantage in selected cases to avoid the need for harvesting an autologous bone graft.

FRACTURES OF THE FRONTAL SINUS WITH DISRUPTION OF THE POSTERIOR WALL

When there is a fracture involving the frontal sinus, involvement of the posterior wall is relatively common. In a series of 72 fractures of the frontal sinus, the posterior wall was involved in almost 80% of cases.[35] If the frontal sinus is large, it may absorb much of the force, leaving the posterior wall intact even if there is gross comminution of the anterior wall. If the sinus is small, there is a greater likelihood of posterior wall involvement.[36] Occasionally, a high-energy injury to the nasoethmoidal area produces relatively minimal primary deformity at the site of impact; the energy is transmitted to the weaker posterior wall of the frontal sinus, and disruption occurs at that site (Fig. 11-18). This "burst" phenomenon may also occur with skull fractures. The etiology is analogous to that of orbital floor fractures: the energy of

---

BOX 11-1 | **Gonty's Classification of Frontal Sinus Fractures**

Type I—Anterior Table Fractures
  1. Isolated to anterior table
  2. Accompanied by supraorbital rim fractures
  3. Accompanied by nasoethmoidal complex fractures
Type II—Anterior and Posterior Table Fractures
  1. Linear fractures
    A. Transverse
    B. Vertical
  2. Comminuted fractures
    A. Involving both tables
    B. Accompanied by nasoethmoidal complex fractures
Type III—Posterior Table Fractures
Type IV—Through-and-Through Frontal Sinus Fracture

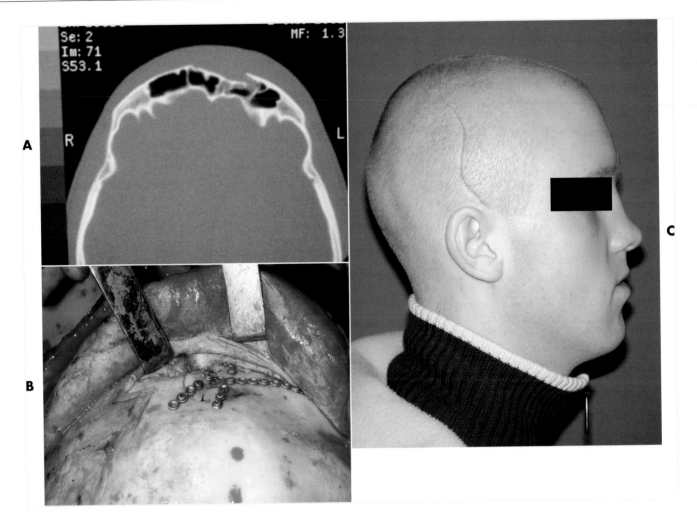

FIGURE 11-17 **A,** Axial computed tomogram shows a displaced fracture involving the anterior wall of the frontal sinus. **B,** Reduction and fixation of the anterior wall of the frontal sinus fracture shown in Figure 11-8. **C,** Early postoperative view shows satisfactory restoration of forehead contour.

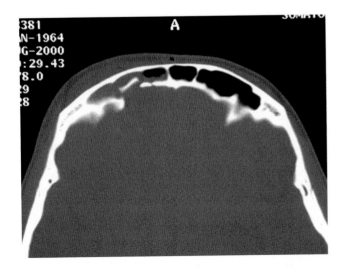

FIGURE 11-18 Axial computed tomogram shows isolated displaced fracture involving the posterior wall of the frontal sinus with no disruption of the anterior wall.

the force is transmitted through the infraorbital margin to the relatively weaker area of the orbital floor, producing a fracture remote from the point of impact. These injuries can easily be missed without appropriate imaging, thereby placing the patient at lifelong risk of developing infective complications.

Significant complications of intracranial sepsis have been demonstrated in cases in which posterior sinus wall fractures were treated conservatively.[37] This is not surprising in light of the incidence of dural tears associated with disruption of the posterior wall of the frontal sinus and the implicit long-term risk associated with leaving a dural tear in communication with the nasal cavity via the frontal sinus.

Our approach to displaced fractures of the posterior wall of the frontal sinus has always been as part of the management of the ACF in trauma rather than as treatment of the frontal sinus per se. The CT and clinical criteria for combined ACF exploration and repair are listed earlier. The CT criteria (i.e., displaced fractures of the posterior wall of the frontal sinus, cribriform plate, and roof of the ethmoid sinuses with or without a CSF leak) are associated with a high (89%)

likelihood of dural tears in communication with the nasal cavity and paranasal sinuses, including the frontal sinus.

Undisplaced fractures are managed expectantly (i.e., not treated).

When there are displaced fractures of the posterior wall of the frontal sinus (as defined in the criteria), the frontal sinus is cranialized as part of the ACF exploration, dural repair, and isolation of the contents of the ACF from the underlying nasal cavity and sinuses.

A craniotomy is mandatory, because adequate dural exploration and ACF exploration and repair cannot be reliably performed through the sinus itself. A low bifrontal craniotomy is performed and provides access to the entire ACF back to the sphenoid wing and the jugum sphenoidale if necessary, with minimal brain retraction. The convexity and basal dura are explored; intradural exploration is ideal for the latter because it permits preservation of olfaction.

Importantly, dural tears are not necessarily confined to the dura immediately behind the fracture. Moreover, in our experience, the size of the fracture on CT is a poor indicator of the extent of dural disruption; the dural tears are usually larger than the fracture. Direct dural repair using purely the sinus for access without a formal craniotomy is both technically difficult and potentially hazardous if the repair is performed inadequately.

A further advantage of a formal craniotomy is that it permits complete removal of both the posterior wall of the vertical component of the sinus and the "roof" of the horizontal portion of the sinus (i.e., that portion of the sinus that is in contact with the basal dura) without difficulty. Complete removal of the sinus lining is also greatly facilitated regardless of the size of the sinus (Fig. 11-19).

Dural tears can be closed primarily or, if they are complex, a pericranial patch can be sutured across the defect and sealed with fibrin glue. In our experience, the remnants of the FND in severe injuries are frequently not identifiable. If still present, they can be plugged with antibiotic-impregnated sponge. Sealing of the remnants of the FNDs is not a critical element in the ACF repair. The nasal cavity and adjacent sinuses are

then separated from the cranial cavity and intracranial contents with a vascularized pericranial or galeal/frontalis flap raised with the coronal flap (Fig. 11-20). The flap is inlaid over the sinus floor via the inferior aspect of the craniotomy. Care should be taken when repositioning the bone flap at the end of the procedure not to damage or inhibit the vascularity of the flap (Fig. 11-21).

It is our firm opinion that there is no place for nonautologous materials (e.g., synthetic dural substitutes) in the repair of the basal dura. In our series, the only instance in which a synthetic dural substitute was employed resulted in the patient's developing meningitis, necessitating further surgery. We have not found the need to reconstruct the central skull base (i.e., the region of the cribriform plate and the roofs of

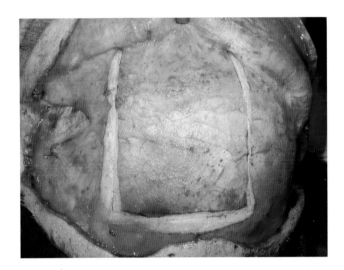

FIGURE 11-20 A pericranial flap has been raised with the coronal flap for later use after cranialization of the frontal sinus. Notice the split in the temporalis fascia that was made to preserve the frontal branch of the facial nerve.

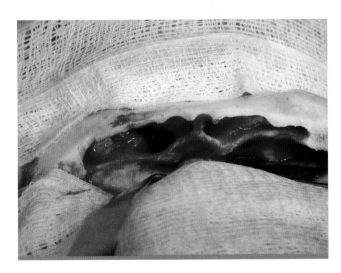

FIGURE 11-19 The posterior wall of the frontal sinus has been removed to the level of the floor of the anterior cranial fossa, and all mucosa has been removed.

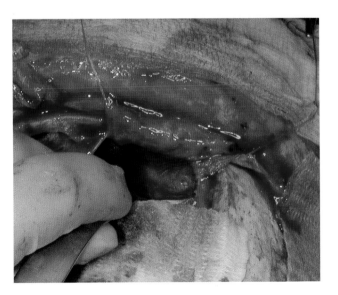

FIGURE 11-21 A pericranial flap is being inlaid to separate the repaired dura from the cranialized frontal sinus.

the ethmoid sinuses) with autologous bone grafts. The soft tissue flaps described earlier are adequate in this region.

Cranialization of the frontal sinus effectively eliminates this structure as an entity. This procedure is, however, only part of the treatment of the ACF, the most important elements being identification and repair of dural tears and isolation of the contents of the ACF from the underlying nasal cavity and sinuses.

FRACTURE INVOLVING THE FLOOR OF THE FRONTAL SINUS

Isolated frontal sinus fractures without concomitant involvement of the anterior or posterior walls of the sinus are uncommon. In a series of 72 fractures of the frontal sinus, only two patients (1.44%) had isolated fractures involving the floor of the frontal sinus.[35]

The most common source of isolated fractures of the floor of the frontal sinus are displaced fractures of the nasoethmoidal complex. This is not an expected finding, because the floor of the frontal sinus is situated below the nasion.[32]

The rationale for treating injuries to the floor of the frontal sinus has been to prevent the later development of a frontal sinus mucocele or infection in any retained secretions in the sinus as a result of presumed disruption to the frontal sinus drainage.

Patency of the FND has been considered to be important in preventing infection of the frontal sinus and the development of a mucocele. This is certainly the case when one considers acute and chronic frontal sinusitis. However, the role of the FND in trauma appears to have been overstated, based, as it has been, on previous experience with inflammatory sinus disease.

Mucocele is a rare complication of trauma to the frontal sinus.[38] In like measure, infection of the frontal sinus after treatment of isolated displaced nasoethmoidal fractures appears to be a rare finding based on the absence of significant numbers of case reports in the literature.

Despite suggestions that the CT appearance of the FND[13] or its appearance at operation (with or without the use of methylene blue dye) can be used to assess whether the duct will function adequately, the reality is that there is no reliable method of assessing whether the sinus will resume normal drainage after disruption by trauma.

Active treatments undertaken to address presumed disruption of the drainage of the frontal sinus have taken three forms:

• Stenting of the FND for varying periods in an attempt to reestablish sinus drainage
• Obliteration of the sinus with a variety of materials after removal of the sinus mucosa, the aim being to eliminate any residual sinus activity
• Stripping of the sinus lining with the hope of new bone formation, so-called osteoneogenesis

Each of these methods is considered in turn.

Stenting of the Frontonasal Duct

There is no reliable evidence for the use of stenting in reestablishing adequate sinus drainage. Evidence for its efficacy is at best anecdotal. Attempts to surgically reestablish the function of an incompetent FND have a failure rate of almost 30% due to subsequent scar formation and stenosis.[39] It is our view, therefore, that there is no place for attempts to reestablish drainage of the sinus.

Obliteration of the Sinus

Obliteration of the frontal sinus with autologous materials such as fat, muscle, or bone or with synthetic materials such as hydroxyapatite or lyophilized cartilage has been described. The list of materials used is very extensive. Fat appears to be the most popular choice for attempts to obliterate the frontal sinus, but failure rates of up to 25% have been reported.[40] In a series of 46 fractures of the frontal sinus treated by obliteration with fat, only 28% of patients developed no postoperative complications. Two patients in this series developed meningitis, and one patient developed a cerebral abscess after treatment.[39] Other series have demonstrated variable rates of complication and success with sinus obliteration. Free fat grafts can be expected to undergo a significant rate of necrosis when used to obliterate the frontal sinus, because any nonvascularized graft is dependent on the vascularity of the recipient site to survive.

Obliteration is an absolute term, and it is clear complete obliteration cannot possibly be achieved with substances such as fat or temporalis fascia. The lesson to be learned from the various techniques is perhaps not the supposed therapeutic effect of the obliteration procedure or the choice of material used, but rather the forgiveness of the frontal sinus to insult. Resort to the "unobliteration" procedure advocated in cases of failure of frontal sinus obliteration supports this suggestion.[41]

Osteoneogenesis

Osteoneogenesis is a fascinating concept, but it has no basis in fact. It arose as a method of treating chronic sinus infection. It is, in effect, an attempt to obliterate the frontal sinus by stripping it of its mucosa, plugging the FND and "allowing" the sinus to fill with new bone. The sinus is expected to obliterate itself; hence, the term *osteoneogenesis*.[13] Although no such obliteration of the maxillary sinus by new bone formation would be expected if a similar procedure were carried out there, nonetheless this is advocated for the frontal sinus. Enthusiasm for obliteration of the frontal sinus with bone grafts, whatever the source, appears to be inversely related to the size of the sinus, with the simpler procedure of "osteoneogenesis" being adopted in patients with large frontal sinuses.[42]

Our approach to injuries to the floor of the frontal sinus is to do nothing. This is in keeping with the current method of treatment of nasoethmoidal fractures.

This aspect of the management of frontal sinus fractures is perhaps the most contentious, with strong advocates for every approach. To date, however, there have been no controlled studies comparing operative intervention versus observation alone. The literature suggests that the complication rate of operative intervention is on the order of 9%, with a range of 0% to 50%, whereas that of observation alone is approximately 3%, with a range of 0% to 12%.[43] This is reasonable grounds for a conservative approach to these injuries if management is to be evidence based.

BOX 11-2   Southampton Protocol for the Treatment of Fractures of the Frontal Sinus

Anterior Wall Fractures
- Undisplaced: no treatment
- Displaced with cosmetic deformity of concern to the patient: open reduction and internal fixation via coronal flap; autologous bone graft or titanium mesh, or both, in selected cases

Posterior Wall Fractures
- Undisplaced: no treatment
- Displaced: craniotomy, cranialization of the sinus, and dural repair with isolation of the anterior cranial fossa with pedicled flaps (pericranial or galeal frontalis)

Floor Fractures
- No treatment

Through-and-through Fractures
- As for fractures of the posterior wall

SOUTHAMPTON PROTOCOL

The Southampton protocol for the treatment of fractures of the frontal sinus is presented in Box 11-2.

USE OF PROPHYLACTIC ANTIBIOTICS

The question of prophylactic antibiotics remains. Retrospective analyses of the use of antibiotics in patients with traumatic CSF leaks have given conflicting results in attempting to demonstrate a benefit. There is no strong evidence for prophylactic antibiotic therapy in these patients.[44,45]

Patients who have suffered one episode of meningitis are liable to experience further instances of infection. This group may benefit from the provision of prophylactic antibiotics.

OUTCOMES

The rationale for the treatment of craniofacial fractures is the prevention of late infective complications and of late cranio-orbital deformity. At Southampton, we have followed the criteria described earlier for more than 20 years and treated more than 163 patients. Of these, 87% have made a good recovery according to their GOS, and the revisional facial surgery rate is 14%.

We have had two cases of postoperative meningitis (including one in which our policy of using only autologous materials for basal dural repair was violated), a single case of loss of frontal bone flap, no cases of postoperative late intracranial abscess, and one case of postprocedure repair because of convexity dura CSF leakage. There have been no cases of mucocele to date, and the postoperative mortality rate for the series is 0%. These results compare very favorably with all published series to date. Our approach using a dedicated skull base and craniofacial trauma team with defined criteria for case selection, rigorous follow-up, and auditing of results would appear to be justified. Of course, there is always potential for improvement. Teamwork is essential in the management of these challenging patients.

KEY POINTS

- Craniofacial fractures are classified as central, lateral, or complex injuries depending on the site of the fracture.
- Preoperative computed tomographic imaging in axial and coronal planes allows precise delineation of fractures and accurate planning for management.
- The rationale for the management of craniofacial injuries is to prevent late infective sequelae and cranio-orbital deformity.
- Untreated dural tears have an unacceptably high risk for the long-term development of meningitis.
- Early combined repair of craniofacial injuries is effective in improving functional and cosmetic results with acceptable morbidity and mortality and no adverse effect on neurosurgical outcome in selected patients.
- The principles of the surgical management of craniofacial fractures are based on adequate exposure, minimal brain retraction, rigid fixation of fractures, and primary bone grafting where necessary.
- Fractures involving the anterior wall of the frontal sinus are treated on the basis of cosmesis.
- Displaced fractures of the posterior wall of the frontal sinus have a high risk of dural tear and are treated by cranialization of the sinus and isolation of the sinus contents from the nasal cavity with a vascularized pericranial flap.
- The risk of mucocele development is minimal in adequately treated fractures of the frontal sinus.
- There is no place for obliteration of the frontal sinus or attempts to reestablish drainage of the frontonasal duct in contemporary management of frontal sinus fractures.

REFERENCES

1. Ionnides CH, Freihofer HP, Friens J: Fractures of the frontal sinus: a rationale of treatment. *Br J Plast Surg* 46:208-214, 1993.
2. Gonty AA, Marciani RD, Adornato DC: Management of frontal sinus fractures: a review of 33 cases. *J Oral Maxillofac Surg* 57:372-379, 1999.
3. Sakas DE, Beale DJ, Ameen AA et al: Compound anterior cranial base fractures: classification using computerized tomography scanning as a basis for selection of patients for dural repair. *J Neurosurg* 88:471-477, 1998.
4. Jones N: *Craniofacial trauma*, New York, 1997, Oxford University Press.
5. American College of Surgeons: *Advanced trauma life support course manual*, Chicago, 1993, ACS.
6. Teasdale G, Jennet B: Assessment of coma and impaired consciousness: a practical scale. *Lancet* 2:81-84, 1974.
7. Kirsch AP: Diagnosis of cerebrospinal fluid rhinorrhoea: lack of specificity of the glucose-oxidase test tape. *J Pediatr* 71:718-719, 1967.
8. Meurman OH, Irjala K, Suonpaa J et al: A new method for the identification of cerebrospinal fluid leakage. *Acta Otolaryngol* 87:366-369, 1979.
9. Teasdale GM, Murray G, Anderson E et al: Risks of acute traumatic intracranial haematoma in children and adults: implications for managing head injuries. *BMJ* 300:363-367, 1990.
10. Zacharides N, Vairaktaris E, Papavassiliou D et al: Orbital apex syndrome. *Int J Oral Maxillofac Surg* 16:352-354, 1987.
11. Bowerman JE: The superior orbital fissure syndrome complicating fractures of the facial skeleton. *Br J Oral Surg* 7:1-6, 1969.
12. Palmer JD: *Neurosurgery*. New York, 1996, Churchill Livingstone.
13. Luce EA: Frontal sinus fractures: guidelines to management. *Plast Reconstr Surg* 80:500-508, 1987.
14. Broumand SR, Labs JD, Novelline RA et al: The role of three dimensional computed tomography in the evaluation of acute craniofacial trauma. *Ann Plast Surg* 31:488-494, 1993.
15. Merville LC, Derome P: Concomittant dislocations of the face and skull. *J Maxillofac Surg* 6:2-14, 1978.
16. Evans BT, Lang D, Neil-Dwyer G: Current management of craniofacial trauma. In Palmer JD, editor: *Neurosurgery*, Edinburgh, 1996, Churchill Livingstone.
17. Baker NJ, Evans BT, Neil-Dwyer G et al: The surgical management of craniofacial trauma. In Ward-Booth P, Schendel SA, Hausamen J, editors: *Maxillofacial surgery*, London, 1999, Harcourt Brace.
18. Lewin W: Cerebrospinal fluid rhinorrhoea in closed head injuries. *Br J Surg* 42:1-18, 1954.

19. Eljamel MS, Foy PM: Acute traumatic CSF fistulae: the risk of intracranial infection. *Br J Neurosurg* 4:381-385, 1990.

20. Eljamel MSM, Foy PM: Post-traumatic CSF fistulae: the case for surgical repair. *Br J Neurosurg* 4:479-483, 1990.

21. Poole MD, Briggs M: Cranio-orbital trauma: a team approach to management. *Ann R Coll Surg* 71:187-194, 1989.

22. Webb AAC, Evans BT, Baker NJ et al: Craniofacial injuries: indications for combined repair. *J Craniomaxillofac Surg* 28:106-109, 2000.

23. Derdyn C, Persing JA, Broaddus WC et al: Craniofacial trauma: an assessment of risk related to timing of surgery. *Plast Reconstr Surg* 86:238-245, 1990.

24. Benzil DL, Robotti E, Dagi TF et al: Early single-stage repair of complex craniofacial trauma. *Neurosurgery* 30:166-171, 1992.

25. Piotowski WP, Beck-Mannagetta J: Surgical techniques in orbital roof fractures: early treatment and results. *J Craniomaxillofac Surg* 23:6-11, 1995.

26. Raveh J, Vuillemin T, Sutter F: Subcranial management of 395 combined frontobasal-midface fractures. *Arch Otolaryngol Head Neck Surg* 114:1114-1122, 1988.

27. Jones NS, Becker DG: Advances in the management of CSF leaks. *BMJ* 322:122-123, 2001.

28. Al-Kayat A, Bramley P: A modified pre-auricular approach to the temporomandibular joint and malar arch. *Br J Oral Surg* 17:91-103, 1978.

29. Yaremchuk MJ, Gruss JS, Manson PN: *Rigid fixation of the craniomaxillofacial skeleton*, Boston, 1992, Butterworth-Heinemann.

30. Webb AAC, Evans BT, Baker NJ et al: Case selection and timing of surgery in craniofacial trauma. *Br J Oral Maxillofac Surg* 38:386, 2000.

31. Gross CL: Pathophysiology and evaluation of frontoethmoid fractures. In Mathog RH, editor: *Maxillofacial trauma*, Baltimore, 1984, Williams & Wilkins.

32. Lang J: *Clinical anatomy of the nose, nasal cavity and paranasal sinuses*, Stuttgart, 1989, George Thieme Verlag, pp 62-84.

33. Heller EM, Jacobs JB, Holliday RA: Evaluation of the frontonasal duct in frontal sinus fractures. *Head Neck* 11:46-50, 1989.

34. Schenk NL, Rauchbach E, Ogura J: Frontal sinus disease. II. Development of the frontal sinus model: occlusion of the nasofrontal duct. *Laryngoscope* 84:1233-1247, 1974.

35. Wallis A, Donald PJ: Frontal sinus fractures: a review of 72 cases. *Laryngoscope* 98:593-598, 1988.

36. Gruss JS, Pollock RA, Phillips JH et al: Combined injuries of the cranium and face. *Br J Plast Surg* 42:385-398, 1989.

37. Newman MH, Travis LW: Frontal sinus fractures. *Laryngoscope* 83:1281-1292, 1973.

38. Koudstaal MJ, van der Wal KG, Bijvoet HW et al: Post-trauma mucocele formation in the frontal sinus: a rationale of follow-up. *Int J Oral Maxillofac Surg* 33:751-754, 2004.

39. Wilson BC, Davidson B, Corey JP et al: Comparison of complications following frontal sinus fractures managed with exploration with or without obliteration over 10 years. *Laryngoscope* 98:516-520, 1988.

40. Sailer HF, Grätz KW, Kalavrezos ND: Frontal sinus fractures: principles of treatment and long term results after sinus obliteration with the use of lyophilized cartilage. *J Craniomaxillofac Surg* 26:235-242, 1998.

41. Javer AR, Sillers MJ, Kuhn FA: The frontal sinus unobliteration procedure. *Otolaryngol Clin North Am* 34:193-210, 2001.

42. Leipziger LS, Glasberg SB: Acute management of frontal sinus fractures. *Tech Plast Reconst Surg* 5:257-265, 1998.

43. Chuang SK, Dodson TB: Evaluation and management of frontal sinus injuries. In Fonseca RJ, Walker RV, Betts N et al, editors: *Oral and maxillofacial trauma*, vol. 2, ed 3, Philadelphia, 2005, Saunders, pp 721-735.

44. Klastersky J, Sadeghi M, Brihaye N: Antimicrobial prophylaxis in patients with rhinorrhea or otorrhea: a double-blind study. *Surg Neurol* 6:111-1145, 1976.

45. MacGee EE, Cauthen JC, Bracken CE: Meningitis following acute traumatic cerebrospinal fistula. *J Neurosurg* 33:312-316, 1970.

CHAPTER 12

Nasoethmoid Fractures

Peter Ayliffe, Peter Ward Booth

The nasoethmoid region is an important area of the face for cosmesis and determining facial projection and width. The region relies for form and strength on a complex interrelationship between uniquely specialized soft tissues and bones formed into buttresses and thin plates.

Nasoethmoid fractures represent a spectrum of injury from simple nasal fractures with minimal ethmoidal involvement to grossly comminuted fractures with displacement. The complex anatomy and direction of the force, together with the degree of development of the paranasal sinuses and related structures, often mean that the fracture patterns extend posteriorly into the orbit, the skull base, and the frontal sinus. Fractures of the frontonasal duct as it traverses the anterior part of the labyrinth of the ethmoid should be considered in all nasoethmoid fractures. In more than 50% of individuals, the frontonasal duct is continuous with the anterior ethmoidal sinus through the infundibulum, which means that all nasoethmoid fractures should be considered to be compound fractures. Nasoethmoid injuries should also be considered as fractures of the orbit, with all their associated problems.

STATE OF THE ART

Management of these injuries requires a thorough understanding of the anatomy. Because standard textbooks do not emphasize certain important aspects of surgical anatomy, it is a controversial area. The surgical anatomy is extensively reviewed later in this chapter (see "Controversies").

The gold standard of care of patients with nasoethmoid injuries begins with a careful clinical evaluation, which includes a detailed radiologic examination and careful ophthalmic examination. Rarely, secondary examinations are done, particularly to verify the function of the lacrimal apparatus. This protocol should establish a precise diagnosis. With this information, typically using an open approach, precise reduction and stabilization should be possible, leading to a good outcome.

CLINICAL EXAMINATION

The clinical findings are related to the time of examination of the patient after injury. Soft tissue injuries usually can be

readily evaluated by clinical examination, but gross edema or emphysema initially may mask the full extent of the injuries. If the patient is examined soon after the injury, gross swelling may mask canthal detachment (Fig. 12-1).

Nasoethmoid fractures may manifest with traumatic telecanthus and impaction of the bridge of the nose, producing the characteristic appearance (Fig. 12-2). Telescoping of the nasal dorsum into the ethmoidal region (Fig. 12-3) and the lack of distal support lead to nasal tip elevation. Depression of the nasal bridge with lack of normal form in the frontonasal angle projects the nostrils almost horizontally, producing a pig snout appearance when the swelling has subsided (Fig. 12-4).

Some workers[1] have attempted to classify these bony fractures. The classifications are infrequently used because they have not proved useful in clinical practice and do not correlate well with outcome. It is, however, important to determine the severity of the fracture. Greater problems occur with compound, comminuted fractures with gross displacement than with simple fractures.[2] In nasoethmoid trauma, comminution and detachment from bone of the canthus represent important, poor prognostic criteria for a satisfactory outcome. Even later classifications do not consider damage to the lacrimal apparatus.[3]

In trauma to this region, the bones most commonly fracture in such a way as to leave a fragment with the medial canthal ligament attached. However, the oblique slope of the nasal bones and their concavoconvexity from above down and their concavity anteroposteriorly mean that anterior forces can cause overriding of bony fragments. The fragments can be pushed posteriorly and disrupt the lacrimal sac (Fig. 12-5) or guillotine the canthal ligament. This can be seen on computed tomography (CT) (Fig. 12-6) and clinically, and careful exploration of lacerations in this area can reveal the extent of the damage to the canthal attachment (Fig. 12-7) or lacrimal system, or both.

The eyelids should be held and distracted laterally. This maneuver is particularly directed at pulling the canthus to ensure it is still attached to stable bone. If the canthus is detached or the canthal-bearing bone fragment is small, the canthal apex will move laterally, and the canthal angle will be blunted (Fig. 12-8). When the nasoethmoid fragments are severely impacted, the canthal-bearing fragment can become wedged in an incorrect position, and the distraction test result will be falsely negative.

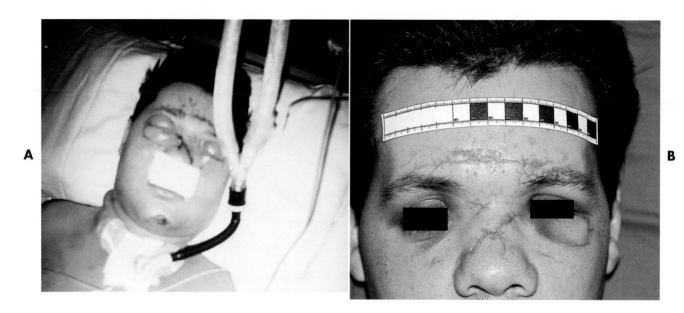

FIGURE 12-1 **A,** Severe injuries and the problems of immediate care may allow a traumatic telecanthus from a nasoethmoid fracture to be overlooked. **B,** After the swelling has decreased, the fracture
and displacement of the canthi are obvious. A delay in diagnosis can by prevented by a careful initial
examination. This patient first was seen in a nonspecialist environment.

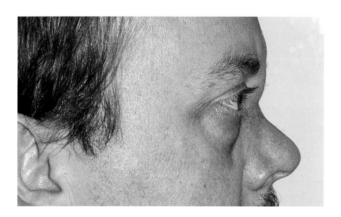

FIGURE 12-2 Displacement of the nasal bridge into the ethmoids
causes this characteristic pig snout appearance, which is caused by
relative upturning of the nasal tip.

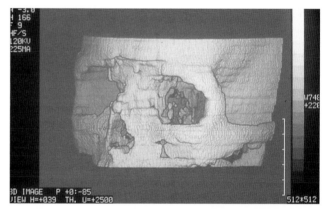

FIGURE 12-4 Computed tomography of the patient described in
Figure 12-2 demonstrates displacement of the nasal bridge, causing
the soft tissue appearance.

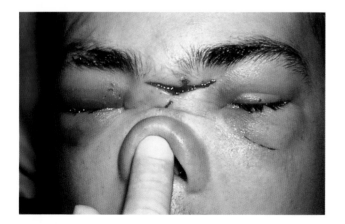

FIGURE 12-3 Comminution of nasal bones adds to the problem of
no support, and the soft tissue is easily depressed.

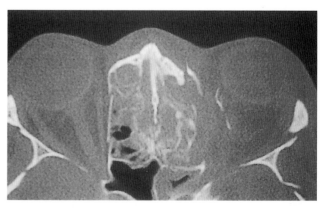

FIGURE 12-5 Overriding of the bony fragments can cause sectioning of the canthal ligament.

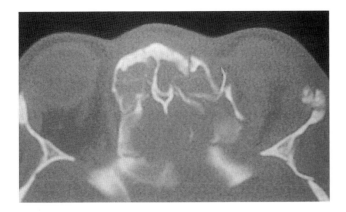

FIGURE 12-6 Computed tomography demonstrates bony fragments.

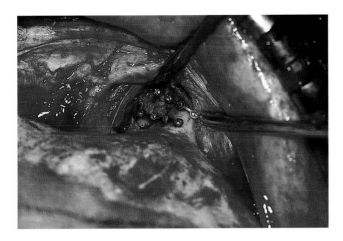

FIGURE 12-7 In this case, the ligament is still attached to a piece of bone that has been plated.

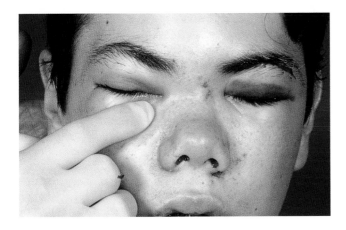

FIGURE 12-8 Applied lateral tension demonstrates the lateral movement caused by damage to the medical canthal attachment.

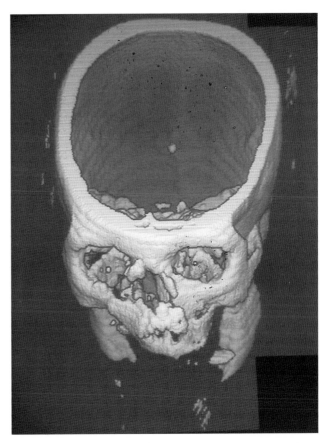

FIGURE 12-9 Three-dimensional computed tomography shows severe impaction and comminution involving the cribriform plate.

More severe forces may extend the fractures into the base of skull (Fig. 12-9) through the cribriform plate of the ethmoid; this frequently is associated with a cerebrospinal fluid leak. Tears in the dura may occur if a fragment of misplaced bone punctures the membrane. Shearing forces may tear the dura, particularly if the crista galli is fractured, as often occurs with severely displaced nasoethmoid fractures. The energy of impact may also be dissipated through the frontal sinus, and fractures of the posterior wall of the frontal sinus are commonly associated with high-energy trauma, causing severely displaced nasoethmoid fractures that extend into the skull base and anterior cranial fossa.

The midline of the patient's face and asymmetry of the canthi are important indicators. The intercanthal and interpupillary distances should be measured. Although a gross increase in the intercanthal distance (range in whites, 24-39 mm) is diagnostic, borderline cases can be difficult. A better guide in clinical practice is to relate the intercanthal distance to the interpupillary distance, provided there is no globe displacement due to gross orbital disruption. The intercanthal distance typically is twice the interpupillary distance. If the bone attachment has been fractured and displaced laterally with the canthus, the situation needs to be explored more formally at the time of surgery in order to fix the medial canthus and prevent late complications of canthal drift.

A full ophthalmic examination is essential, but it may be compromised by the neurological status of the patient. The function of the optic nerve and the ocular reflexes must be examined. In a posteriorly impacted nasoethmoid fracture, the optic nerve can be compressed by collapse of the bony complex into the sphenoid sinus and direct compression of the nerve in the canal. In the unconscious patient, the swinging flashlight test is particularly important, and the fundus should be examined thoroughly for signs of optic nerve compression. Among patients who have sustained sufficient trauma to cause compression of the optic nerve, there is a high incidence of globe injuries.

The lacrimal apparatus is damaged infrequently, usually as a result of direct penetrating trauma or overriding fragments of sharp bone. Lacerations in this area must be carefully explored. Dye can be introduced into either of the lacrimal puncta, and backflow usually demonstrates the leak. If doubt remains, radiological confirmation may be needed.

Bony injuries are frequently difficult to examine well enough to give a precise diagnosis. Even in the most swollen patients, however, it is usually possible to gauge the extent of the fractures by careful clinical examination. This information is important for obtaining well-targeted radiographic examinations.

RADIOLOGICAL EXAMINATION

Good-quality radiographs are normally required, but in patients with marked swelling, the fine bones of the nasoethmoid region may be effaced by soft tissue shadows. Careful examination of the orbital and other facial bones is required. Occipitomental views (10- and 45-degree projections) are most helpful as an initial screening examination. Lateral face or skull radiographs are usually disappointing for evaluation of nasoethmoid trauma; occasionally, an occlusal film shows disruption of the ethmoid.

Good-quality CT scans are extremely valuable and can be essential, particularly for assessing high-energy trauma cases in which the frontal sinus and base of skull may be disrupted (Fig. 12-10). Because reconstructed and three-dimensional images contain artifacts, it is helpful if the patient is fit enough to allow axial and coronal views to be made. These images must be used to exclude related fractures or injuries, particularly orbital wall fractures. Special radiological methods, such as a dacryocystogram, are not commonly used for primary surgery, because direct examination usually is possible during the operation.

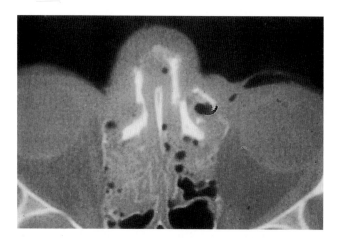

FIGURE 12-10   Good-quality computed tomography provides unrivaled detail, which is essential for nasoethmoid fractures, in this case even showing damage to the lacrimal sac.

TIMING OF TREATMENT

The timing of facial surgery is a difficult problem, especially in cases of nasoethmoid trauma. Delays in treatment can lead to difficulty in repositioning the soft tissues, particularly the canthal ligaments, and in identifying damage to the lacrimal duct system. However, early treatment may be impossible because of other injuries, commonly head injuries. Edema poses significant problems for operating in this region, and delay can allow it to resolve. Many patients with these injuries can be treated at 7 to 10 days, but the earlier surgery can be undertaken, allowing for other injuries and swelling, the more satisfactory.

ANATOMY

A thorough understanding of normal anatomy is essential to achieve a satisfactory treatment result. Certain anatomical structures are disproportionately important.

BONY ANATOMY

The nose is the most conspicuous feature of the bony skeleton in the nasoethmoid region. The two nasal bones and the vertical midline bony septum form its major structural components. The nasal bones superiorly articulate through a serrated joint with the nasal part of the frontal bone. Laterally, they articulate with the frontal process of the maxilla. Superiorly, the bones are thick; they gradually thin to the notched inferior borders that are continuous with the lateral nasal cartilages. The medial borders are thicker above than below, and the two nasal bones articulate with each other around the midline of the nose. The paired nasal bones have a vertical crest on their posterior surface that forms part of the midline septum of the nose. They articulate with the nasal spine of the frontal bone, the perpendicular plate of the ethmoid bone, and the cartilage of the nasal septum from above downward.

The nasal skeleton is a pyramidal form and the frontal process of each maxilla form the major buttresses of the anterior midface. They provide strength and protect the relatively thin sheets of the lacrimal bone, the cribriform, and perpendicular and orbital plates of the ethmoid bone more posteriorly. The frontonasal buttresses provide considerable strength to resist the energy transmitted from a direct anterior blow, but there is relatively little strength to resist a lateral blow. After the thick nasal bridge collapses, the forces are dissipated into the air cells. Although this mechanically protects the base of the skull as a natural "crumple zone," relatively small forces in patients with large pneumatized air cells can collapse the whole complex.

The bones of this region provide the area of insertion to the part of the medial canthal ligament that attaches anterior to the lacrimal sac. The medial canthal ligament provides the primary functional support of the eyelids medially by connecting the orbicularis muscle to the medial orbit, lateral nose, and lacrimal diaphragm.

EYELIDS

The skin of the eyelids, at less than 1 mm thick, is the thinnest in the body[3,4] and almost transparent. The skin over the medial canthal ligament is smooth and shiny, unlike the skin of the temporal eyelids. It is firmly attached to the underlying structures in this region and has very few hairs. The few that are present are fine and have only rudimentary sebaceous glands. In the medial part of the lower lid, bundles of muscle fibers fan out from the underlying preseptal muscle and insert directly into the skin, and they are responsible for the vertical wrinkles seen in this area (muscles of Merkel).[5] There are no such muscle fibers in the upper lid.

The axis of the palpebral fissure is not horizontal; the lateral angle is about 2 mm above and behind the medial angle. An increase in the obliquity of the palpebral fissure is characteristic of Mongolian racial groups, as is a fold of skin passing from the medial end of the upper lid to the lower and obscuring the caruncle, a feature known as *epicanthus*. Epicanthus occurs in the human fetus but disappears with nasal development in whites. It persists in some cases of congenital ptosis.

The palpebral fissure at the lateral canthus is more acute than the medial counterpart, is 3.0 to 4.08 mm long, and is positioned directly against the globe. At the medial canthus, the fissure is more rounded; the lower margin is horizontal, and the upper passes downward and medially (Fig. 12-11). It is separated from the globe by a little recess, the lacus lacrimalis. Within this is a yellowish elevation, the lacrimal caruncle, an area of skin containing modified sweat and sebaceous glands. Lateral to the caruncle is the plica semilunaris, a reddish, narrow, crescentic fold of conjunctiva lying vertically with its concavity facing laterally. It lies partly under cover of the caruncle, and its lower horn reaches to the middle of the lower fornix; the upper horn does not extend quite so far. This fold represents the third eyelid, or membrana nictitans, of lower animals. The connective tissue stroma of the plica contains numerous vessels, a lobule of fat, and some muscle. Similar structures are found within the caruncle and arise from the medial capsulopalpebral muscle of Hesser, whereas some arise from the medial rectus.[1]

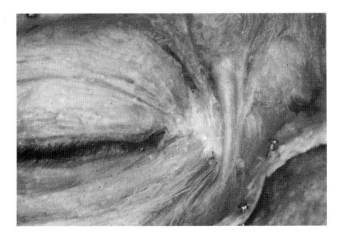

FIGURE 12-11 Superficial dissection of the ligament. The angular artery and fat have been removed to reveal the muscles and the extent of attachment of the ligament over the frontonasal buttress.

LACRIMAL DRAINAGE SYSTEM

The lacrimal papillae are elevations at the medial end of the lid margins just lateral to the plica semilunaris. They are pierced by the small, round or transversely oval apertures of the lacrimal puncta. The puncta are situated in line with the openings of the tarsal gland ducts and lie about 1 mm medial to the nearest opening, dividing the lids into ciliary and lacrimal parts. The superior punctum is slightly nearer to the nasal side (6 mm from the medial canthus), and the lower punctum is 6.5 mm from the canthus. Each punctum is surrounded by dense fibrous tissue continuous with the tarsus. This tissue keeps the punctum patent and is surrounded by fibers of the orbicularis, which pass onto and attach to the medial canthal ligament.

Each lacrimal canaliculus is lined by stratified squamous epithelium on an extensive corium of elastic tissue. Macroscopically, they consist of a vertical and a horizontal part; the vertical components are about 2 mm long and then bend medially almost at right angles to become the horizontal portions. At the junction of the two is a dilatation, or ampulla. Both horizontal components of the canaliculi slope toward the common medial canthal ligament within the substance of the pretarsal components of the upper and lower eyelids. They take a convergent course, with the lower in a slight upward inclination for 8 mm and the lower in a downward inclination for 7.5 mm within the lid margins. They have pretarsal fibers of the orbicularis in superficial and deep relationships over the medial third of their course. The tarsal glands lie below the canaliculi, and the ciliary glands of Moll and the ciliary glands of Zeiss lie superficially. The canaliculi pierce the lacrimal fascia separately or in common. They enter the lacrimal sac through the fossa of Rosemüller at a small diverticulum, the sinus of Maier. This lies behind the middle of the lateral surface of the lacrimal sac about 2.5 mm from its apex.

The membranous lacrimal sac lies in the lacrimal fossa formed by the frontal process of the maxilla and lacrimal bone. The sac is open and continuous below with the nasolacrimal duct; a constriction marks the junction between the two. The sac is enclosed by a splitting of the orbital fascia, called the *lacrimal fascia* or *lacrimal diaphragm*; the action of the attached muscles is in part responsible for the normal aspiration of tear fluid.[6] The lacrimal fascia adheres to the sac around the fundus, but it is otherwise separated by a thin layer of areolar tissue. The medial canthal ligament is attached to the lacrimal fascia in front and behind the sac. The lacrimal sac extends for 3 to 5 mm above the horizontal component of the ligament. A thin layer of orbicularis covers the sac below the medial canthal ligament, and it is therefore in this region that herniations, abscesses, and fistulae tend to come to the surface.

MEDIAL CANTHAL LIGAMENT

The medial canthal ligament, when viewed from the anterior aspect, is a diamond-shaped fibrous band that is longer in its horizontal dimension. It has a superficial anterior limb with an average length of 11.7 mm and an average width of 4.9 mm.[7,8] It is attached to the frontal process of the maxilla just lateral to its suture, with the nasal bone behind the angular vein and the angular artery positioned more medially. This anterior attachment extends laterally to the anterior lacrimal crest (Figs. 12-12 and 12-13). The area of this insertion averages 25.3 mm². This forms an extensive attachment to the frontonasal buttress. The angular vein lies 8 mm from the medial canthal apex. The extent of medial aspect of the ligament beyond the anterior lacrimal crest is demonstrated by the fact that the crest is only 2 to 3 mm from the medial commissure of the eyelids and lies just lateral to the canthal apex.

The medial canthal ligament may require reconstruction or replacement after nasoethmoid trauma, resection for neoplastic disease, congenital deformity, or detachment during craniofacial surgery. The anatomical arrangement of the individual components is important to the functional role of the ligament and the cosmetic appearance of the face. An understanding of the three-dimensional arrangement is essential for satisfactory management of this region.

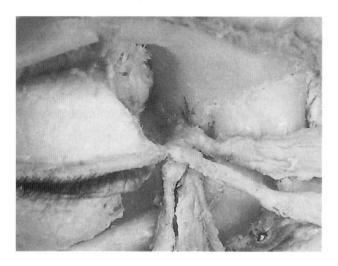

FIGURE 12-12   The major muscle components of the ligament are displayed. Riolan's muscle and the strong attachment to the posterior lacrimal crest and medial orbital periosteum can be seen.

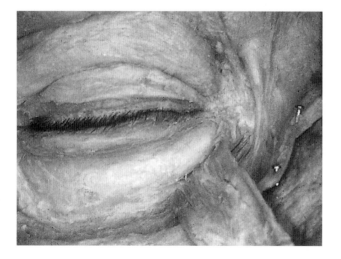

FIGURE 12-13   The vertical component of the ligament can be seen lateral to the angular vein. The inferior orbicularis muscle has been retracted medially to show the orbital septum. The orbital fat can be seen bulging forward from below.

Historically, the eponym *Horner's muscle* was applied to the muscularis orbicularis oculi pars lacrimalis or tensor tarsi, as described by William Edmonds Horner (1793-1853) in 1822.[9,10] Reiffler[11] showed that the muscle was first discovered by Jacques Francois-Marie Duvernay approximately a century earlier. The first published description appeared in 1730 in a manuscript by Johann Caspar Schobinger, one of Duvernay's pupils,[11] who credited Duvernay with the discovery. The first published illustration of the muscularis orbicularis oculi pars lacrimalis was in the second plate of the first atlas published by Duvernay in collaboration with the engraver Jacques-Fabian Gautier d'Agoty in 1745,[12] in which Duvernay described the structure as "le petit muscle des paupières."

Reconstruction of the medial canthal ligament remains a challenging clinical problem and is associated with a significant failure rate.[13] Debate continues about the best surgical method and techniques for its reconstruction.[7,14-25] Much of this is probably related historically to a poor understanding of the anatomy and physiological function of this area, as demonstrated by the confusion about the nomenclature that was employed in the past. The structure has been referred to in the published literature by many names, including the medial canthal tendon, medial canthal ligament, tensor tarsi, medial palpebral tendon, and medial palpebral ligament. In their experimental work, Dagum et al.[25] showed that the structure behaves biomechanically as a ligament and demonstrated the extensibility and strain behavior that is typical of a ligament rather than of a tendon. Histologically, the structure is composed of fibrous tissue that is more characteristic of a ligament than a tendon, and it seems more appropriate to call the structure the *medial canthal ligament.*

Several modern contributions have been made to our understanding of the medial canthal ligament, many of them based on anatomical studies. Duke Elder published comprehensive descriptions of the anatomy and histology of the orbital region in 1931 and 1961.[26,27] For many years, these remained the standard authoritative texts, and much of his work remains relevant today. Wolfe's 1954 textbook[6] contributed to our three-dimensional understanding of the ligament, but the meticulous dissections and precise descriptions of the anatomy by Jones remain outstanding references.[28-32] In 1961, he published a paper that included photographs of his dissections, displaying the muscular origins of the medial canthal ligament.[33] He described a deep head of the preseptal orbicularis muscle,[33] which was subsequently referred to as *Jones' muscle* by Edelstein[24] and others.

Edelstein postulated that the deep attachments of the orbicularis muscle provide the major positional support for the eyelid medially and activate the lacrimal pump by generating negative pressure in the lacrimal sac during blinking. Edelstein said, "The primary functional support for the medial eyelid is from the deep attachments of the orbicularis muscle to the posterior lacrimal crest and lacrimal diaphragm." This contradicts many earlier observations that the posterior component of the ligament was thin and insignificant.

Robinson et al.[8] dissected the medial canthal ligament in six cadavers and found it to be a band of fibrous tissue, which acts as an insertion for the orbicularis oculi muscle to the medial orbit, into the lacrimal bone and the frontal process of the maxilla. The most lateral parts of the medial canthal ligament act through the upper and lower palpebral extensions, and they attach to the margins of the tarsal plates lateral to the caruncle. Medial to the caruncle, the ligament bifurcates into superficial anterior and deep posterior limbs. The investigators found the posterior limb difficult to define and suggested it consisted of lacrimal fascia, Horner's muscle, and areolar tissue. They concluded that the posterior limb lacked strength because of its weak fibers and that the underlying bone was thin and incapable of providing solid anchorage.

In 1976, Warwick[4] provided one of the most comprehensive descriptions of the medial canthal region. He used many of Wolff's dissections and histological preparations, and he detailed the relationship of the ligament with the lacrimal system.

In a cadaveric study in 1977, Anderson[34] demonstrated a superior branch of the medial canthal ligament that attaches to the periosteum of the frontal bone. He postulated that by attaching to the frontal bone, it gave additional support to the ligament when the anterior limb was accidentally or surgically detached (e.g., dacryocystorhinostomy). This vertical component had been demonstrated before and labeled as the corrugator superciliaris muscle,[35] and it can be seen in the anatomical preparations by Jones,[7] in which it is labeled as the superficial and deep origins of the upper part of the orbital muscle. It is clear that it attaches to the anterior aspect of the ligament and lacrimal fascia just posterior to the angular vein and lateral to the procerus muscle. These illustrations show that the muscle would lose its attachment to the medial canthal ligament when the anterior portion is resected and is therefore unlikely to be the sole reason for stability of the canthal ligament after disruption of the anterior limb.

In 1983, Zide et al.[21] dissected 12 medial canthi in fresh human cadavers under magnification. They found that the medial canthus attached to the medial bony orbit in a tripartite manner. The vertical and horizontal components comprise two parts, and the deep heads of the pretarsal and preseptal muscles arise from the posterior lacrimal crest as described by previous investigators.[5,23,34] However, they emphasize that the medial canthal ligament attaches far beyond the anterior lacrimal crest as depicted in most anatomical texts. This gives support to the empirical observation by Converse et al.,[16,18] made before this tripartite arrangement was widely known, that the optimal position for surgical replacement of the medial canthal ligament was posterior and superior to the insertion.

Manson et al.[36] published an anatomical study of the region in 1986. They substantiated the gross anatomical findings of the anterior limb described by previous investigators. They further described the association of the posterior ligamentous attachments to the medial check ligament, the medial horn of the levator aponeurosis as described by Koorneef[37,38] and to Lockwood's ligament[39,40] as they insert with the orbital septum into the lacrimal bone.

Ayliffe[9] discussed the importance of the three-dimensional arrangement of the muscles that attach to the medial canthal ligament. He demonstrated the relative complexity of the posterior components of the structure, particularly the posterior insertion of the superior orbital part of the orbicularis oculi, a previously undescribed arrangement. He demonstrated the thickening of the periosteum of the medial orbital wall, which reinforces the triangular nature of the ligament in the third dimension. By broadening the base of the triangle in the

horizontal plane, it makes the posterior attachment of the ligament strong and strengthens the whole structure. This observation emphasizes the importance of reconstructing the posterior attachment. Our current understanding of the anatomy and relationships of the medial canthal ligament is one of a complex, three-dimensional association between highly specialized structures.

Laterally, the ligament is attached to the tarsus through a small strip or bands of fibrous tissue. The pretarsal orbicularis runs superficial and deep to the canaliculi at the lid margin and is referred to as *Riolan's muscle*.[35] The superficial fibers form the anterior crus of the medial canthal ligament and insert into the frontal process of the maxilla and anterior lacrimal crest. The posterior crus or deeper limb of the pretarsal orbicularis arises from the posterior lacrimal crest and lacrimal bone behind the lacrimal sac.

The preseptal muscle forms the horizontal raphe. It decussates to insert into the anterior and posterior limbs of the medial canthal ligament, sometimes referred to as Jones' muscle and Horner's muscle, respectively. The inferior part of the orbital orbicularis attaches medially to the lower border of the medial canthal ligament, the nasal part of the frontal bone, and the medial orbital margin inferiorly.[35] The superior orbital orbicularis attaches to the medial canthal ligament, into the posterior lacrimal fascia,[8] and into the upper half of the posterior lacrimal crest.[7] A discrete vertical muscular component is inserted into the cephalic aspect of the medial canthal ligament and anterior aspect of the lacrimal fascia; it attaches superiorly to the frontal bone.[20,34] This vertical stabilizing muscular element is 1 to 2 mm thick and 5 to 7 mm long, and it lies just lateral to the angular vein. It is separated from the orbital part of the orbicularis by adipose tissue.

In the past, the deeper reflected part of the ligament was described as a thin fascial expansion,[7,41] but it is now known to be a more substantial part of the ligament,[8,23,33] having a thickness of 1 to 3.3 mm.[7] It extends more posteriorly over the medial orbital wall as a thickening of the orbital periosteum.[8] It is important for maintaining the medial aspect of the palpebral fissure close to the globe, and its position is significant for lacrimal drainage.[23] The deep crus is a strong component of the ligament and the reason why a posterosuperior position has been advocated when reattaching or reconstructing the ligament.[16,18] Behind the sac, the ligament attaches to the lacrimal fascia and the posterior lacrimal crest. The superior orbicularis muscle makes part of its insertion into the ligament and the posterior lacrimal fascia at this point. It runs posterosuperiorly behind the sac and behind the posterior aspect of the medial third of the superior canaliculus.

Behind the orbicularis lie the orbital septum and the check ligament of the medial rectus. The inferior oblique arises from the floor of the orbit just lateral to the lacrimal fossa. A few fibers take origin from the lacrimal fascia and the posterior lacrimal crest. Lockwood's ligament is a fascial sling and an important component of the global support mechanism; it extends from the zygomatic bone in around the lateral canthus and the lateral check ligament. It inserts into the inferior border of the medial canthal ligament with the medial check ligament[36] and inserts into the lacrimal bone at the posterior lacrimal crest.

The medial canthal ligament is a strong, interlocking, three-dimensional arrangement of many individual components and structures. The skin over the lateral nose and eyelids is unique to this site in its structure and its relationship with the underlying structures. The lacrimal drainage apparatus is intimately related to the ligament. The insertions of the many individual muscular components into the frontal process of the maxilla, those into the lacrimal bone, and their attachments and relationship with the ligament are complex. Lockwood's suspensory ligament and the orbital and capsulopalpebral fascia are important structures for support of the globe, and they are intimately related to the medial canthal ligament. All of the individual structures affect the overall integrity of the ligament. The complex, three-dimensional, interlocking, triangular arrangement of the muscular and ligamentous components described by Ayliffe[9] gives the structure its strength. It is therefore not appropriate to dismiss any individual component as unimportant. Each component should be considered when dealing with the pathology and reconstruction of this region.

TREATMENT

Treatment should begin only when the surgeon has a clear understanding of the injuries and has a precise plan and objective based on findings from the clinical and radiological examinations. The plan must integrate surgery for the nasoethmoid fracture with treatment of any other facial injuries. Because these fractures are often part of panfacial fractures, the more peripheral facial injuries are treated first.

Classification of nasoethmoid injuries can be helpful in executing a coherent plan. A useful practical classification was published by Ayliffe.

- Type I: en bloc, minimally displaced fracture of the entire nasoethmoid complex (Fig. 12-14)
- Type II: en bloc, displaced fracture, usually associated with a large pneumatized sinus and minimal fragmentation (Fig. 12-15)

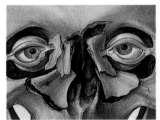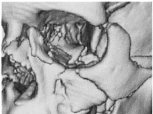

FIGURE 12-14   Bone plating for a type I fracture.

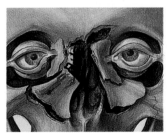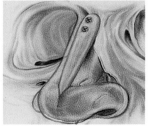

FIGURE 12-15   Bone grafting for a type II fracture.

- Type III: comminuted fracture but canthal ligaments firmly attached with bone fragments that are big enough to plate (Fig. 12-16)
- Type IV: comminuted fracture with free canthal ligaments not large enough to capture by bone plating (Fig. 12-17)
- Type V: gross comminution needing bone grafting (Fig. 12-18)

The introduction of miniplates and microplates revolutionized the treatment of these injuries. The principal benefit is the ability of the bone plate to provide three-dimensional stability to the fractures and maintain the projection of the nose.

The aims of treatment should be to restore normal anatomy and physiological function, particularly with respect to a patent functioning lacrimal system, and to prevent complications due to involvement of the frontal sinus and nasolacrimal duct. Symmetrical fixation of the bones, restoration of orbital

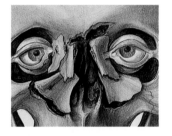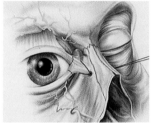

FIGURE 12-16   Canthopexy for a type III fracture.

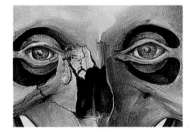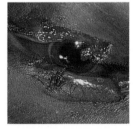

FIGURE 12-17   Lacrimal repair for a type IV fracture.

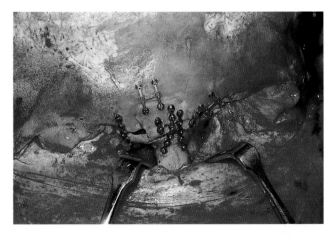

FIGURE 12-18   Microplates placed through a coronal incision provide good reduction and stability.

volume, globe position, frontonasal angle, and nasal projection are essential for a satisfactory cosmetic outcome. Stable, symmetrical fixation of the canthus in three dimensions with good apposition of the eyelids against the ocular globe and a pleasant cosmetic curve to the medial canthal angle are essential for a satisfactory esthetic and functional result.

SURGICAL SEQUENCING

1. Determine access, and complete exposure
2. Reconstruct the cranial base, frontal bandeau, and outer orbital frame; manage the frontal sinus; and decompress the optic canal, if necessary
3. Address the frontonasal buttress and orbital rim. These fragments usually are easy to locate and reduce.
4. Reconstruct the nasal dorsum and restore the nasal projection, ideally by plating the bone fragments or using grafts that can be cantilevered from the glabella with miniplates. It is important to contour the frontonasal angle.
5. Reconstruct the medial orbits. When the nasoethmoid complex is disrupted in a patient with panfacial trauma, the projection of the face will be restored if surgical treatment is sequenced correctly. After reconstruction of the mandible, zygomas, frontonasal buttress, and maxilla and location of the correct occlusion, the outer orbital frame will be correct, and it is only at this stage that the true nature and size of the medial orbital defect can be accurately assessed and reconstructed.
6. Assess and correct medial canthal ligament defects.
7. Assess and correct lacrimal system defects.
8. Close, and place a drain.
9. Consider secondary external support of the medial canthal ligament.
10. Apply nasal plaster.
11. Apply dressings and antibiotic eye drops.

HARD TISSUES

The principle is simple: Reduce and stabilize the fractured fragments to stable, normal bone.[42] In practice, there is a significant difference between achieving this in a noncomminuted, minimally displaced fracture or a grossly compound, comminuted "bag of bones" fracture. However, the best results are achieved for any fracture using the following principles:

1. Prompt treatment aids good reduction and reduces complications.
2. Good surgical exposure should be achieved through existing lacerations or a coronal flap, or both.
3. Bone fragments are reduced and stabilized with the use of small, low-profile osteosynthesis plates.
4. Immediate bone grafting may be indicated if there is gross comminution of key bone buttresses or the orbital walls.

Surgical Exposure and Access

The aims of surgical exposure are to explore the injuries to diagnose the nature of the injuries, expose all fracture sites, preserve all bone fragments, give access to reconstruct the area, and preserve function or esthetics. Excessive subperiosteal dissection, especially in children, may lead to subperiosteal new bone formation in the postoperative period. In the canthal area, this can cause blunting of the canthal angle and the appearance of pseudotelecanthus. No individual approach fulfills all of these criteria. An existing laceration may be used, but this approach can cause contamination. In these circumstances, surgery should be carried out as soon as the patient is fit for anesthesia.

Few skin incisions around the nose and forehead are satisfactory. This is in marked contrast to the excellent cosmetic results and wide access produced by a coronal flap.[42] The coronal approach has the advantage of providing access to harvest outer calvarial bone for primary reconstruction of bony deformities. Even with this flap, care must be taken to place it well into the hairline or as posteriorly as possible in male patients to avoid exposure of the scar if recession of the hairline occurs; incisions at the hairline leave unsatisfactory scars, particularly as the hair thins. A simple strip shave or no shave is required to make this incision. A full-head shave is not indicated or justified.

Reduction and Stabilization

Microplates can stabilize very small fragments and provide three-dimensional stability. Care must be taken to identify and stabilize bone fragments that have the canthi attached without stripping the medial canthal ligament from them. In cases of gross comminution or in patients who have a midline split of the nose, it may be helpful to place a plate over the bridge of the nose horizontally to pull the fragments into a sharp, narrow arch (Fig. 12-19).

Bone Grafting

Bone grafting is infrequently required, but in cases of gross comminution, particularly of structurally important bones, an immediate bone graft is indicated. It is critically important that both onlay grafts and any plates used to correct comminution of the nasal dorsum be contoured to reconstruct the frontonasal angle (Figs. 12-20 and 12-21).

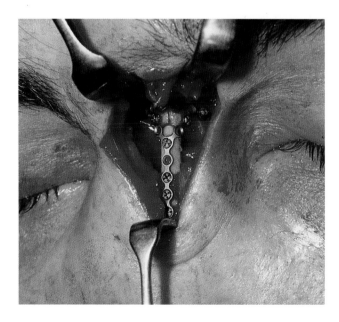

FIGURE 12-19 Bone grafting and microplate stabilization of a bone graft were needed because there was gross comminution. Access was gained through an existing laceration.

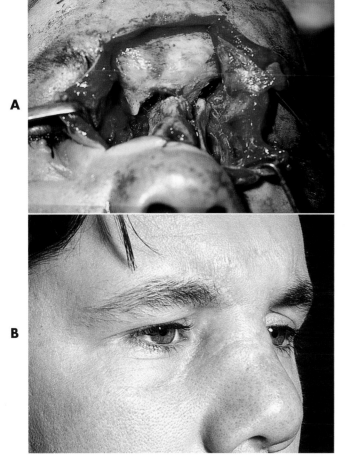

FIGURE 12-20 **A,** Late treatment was undertaken with a bone graft. **B,** The final result is poor, and scarring can be seen on the dorsum of the nose, which was caused by some skin breakdown over the bone graft. This case illustrates the problems of late secondary treatment.

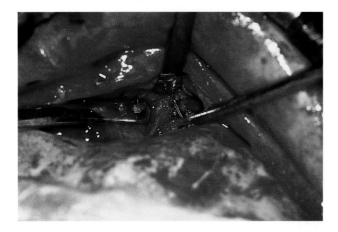

FIGURE 12-21 The canthal ligament is attached to a small fragment of bone. Modern microplates allow even these small fragments to be reduced and stabilized, avoiding much less successful treatments such as wire canthopexy.

If bone grafting is to be delayed, the soft tissues may contract, making later secondary grafting difficult and possibly leading to erosion through the tight skin. Unfortunately, these grossly comminuted fractures are often compound, making a less than ideal environment for immediate grafting.

SOFT TISSUES

Treatment of soft tissue injuries consists of several phases:

- Examination
- Débridement
- Management of specialized structures
- Closure, drainage, and dressings
- Postoperative care

Lacrimal Drainage System

Pure soft tissue damage to the lids may result in lacrimal system damage, particularly shearing injuries to the eyelids medial to the lacrimal puncta that may transect the canaliculi. Lacrimal damage is underdiagnosed in nasoethmoid trauma, with 3% to 18% of patients subsequently requiring dacryocystorhinostomies. Careful exploration and suturing are required at the time of initial repair.

The vulnerable parts in lid lacerations are the canaliculi, particularly the short medial segment lying between the medial canthi before it enters the sac, because the lid margin is particularly vulnerable in this site. Careful approximation of the severed ends of the canaliculi should be performed, and the duct should be cannulated with fine-bore polyethylene or silicone tubes through the puncta along the length of the canaliculus into the lacrimal sac to prevent stenosis. Careful identification of both ends of the canaliculus is essential. The use of pigtail probes should be avoided in unicanalicular injuries because this can damage the normal canaliculus. Repair of the canaliculus may be carried out secondarily with a dacryocystorhinostomy if necessary, but scar tissue and technical difficulties make this a difficult endeavor. The evidence suggests that primary repair leads to better results.

The whole lacrimal system, including the intrabony lacrimal sac and duct, are at risk in displaced nasoethmoid fractures. In patients with bicanalicular lesions and gross disruption of the region, intubation of both puncta can be carried out, and the soft silicone tubes should be left in situ for at least 6 months.

Detached Medial Canthus

In cases of trauma to the nasoethmoid area, care must be taken to diagnose any damage to the canthi and lacrimal system. The nature of the reconstructive problem depends on the type of lesion. If the canthus is attached to a small fragment of bone, it should be identified. With modern microplates, it is possible to fix the bone fragment in its normal anatomical position, and this usually gives excellent and stable results, provided the fixation is solid enough.

The ligament is usually attached to a fragment of bone (see Fig. 12-21). The canthi rarely can be detached or avulsed from the bone, and this presents a difficult problem. Complete detachment is unusual in the absence of damage to the underlying bone or in the absence of penetrating injuries. One cause of complete detachment is careless surgical exploration,

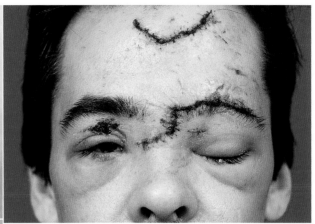

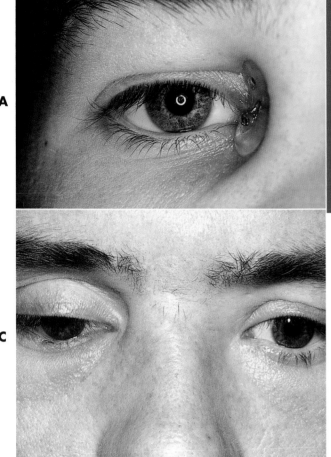

FIGURE 12-22 **A,** The clear acrylic button supports the wire canthopexy but is not a substitute for wiring if there is no bone to plate. Without these buttons, the wires frequently cut through the canthus. **B,** Preoperative appearance of a late presentation. **C,** A satisfactory postoperative appearance is possible even for late presentations. The enophthalmus is caused by a prosthetic globe.

which should be guarded against because subsequent identification and reattachment may be difficult and lead to disappointing results.

When the ligament is detached from the bone, it can be located lateral to the lacrimal sac by passing a needle through the canthal angle and identifying the needle on the deep surface posterior to the lacrimal sac. A fine wire suture then is passed through the surface of the canthal ligament deep to the lacrimal canaliculi and sac. This wire is passed transnasally[14] to the opposing canthus if it is attached or passed through a bony point on the other side of the nose. The wire is directed to pull the ligament medially and posteriorly. The use of tendon anchor screws can be considered, provided there is a large enough fragment of bone of sufficient strength in the appropriate position to fix the screw. In our experience, this leads to a sharp medial canthal angle, but this technique does have the advantage of making a posterior attachment easy to attain, and good positioning of the lid margin against the globe of the eye can be achieved. It also has the advantage of minimal subperiosteal dissection. The technique of transnasal canthopexy is easily described, but those experienced in the procedure recognize its shortcomings.

After capture of the canthus, it may be possible to reduce and fix it directly to plates placed on the anterior and posterior lacrimal crests. Direct canthopexy does give stable results, but it is important to position the attachment posteriorly enough to maintain the medial eyelid in close approximation to the globe and to restore a normal lacus. Failure to do this may lead to problems with lacrimal drainage and recurrent inflammation. Direct canthopexy may involve extensive subperiosteal stripping to attach the canthopexy plates.

In a case of true detachment, it is difficult to maintain the canthus. The fine wire very easily cuts through the delicate ligament, especially if edema puts any significant pressure on the repair or the treatment is delayed and undue strain is applied when tightening the wire. It may be helpful to support the canthal reattachment from the cutaneous surface. This can be carried out using a preformed, clear acrylic button (Fig. 12-22). The risk of this procedure is skin necrosis, but with clear acrylic, the status of the skin can be monitored.

PEDIATRIC CONSIDERATIONS

In children, the paranasal air sinuses may not be fully developed, and direct blows to the nasoethmoid region tend to concentrate the energy in the area of the primary force. This tends to cause gross comminution and collapse of the nasoethmoid region.

Before the frontal sinus has developed, dissemination of energy through the cranial base is different in children, and the fracture pattern consequently does not follow that of adults. The nasoethmoid fragment often is disrupted in continuity with the frontal bone in its entirety (Fig. 12-23) or

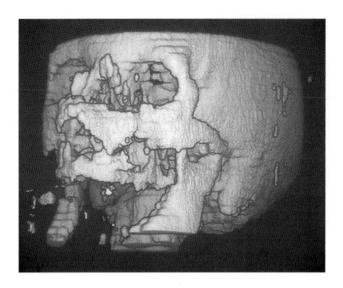

FIGURE 12-23 Computed tomography shows extensive involvement of the frontal sinus.

extends superiorly. In these cases, the nasoethmoid component is rotated in the direction of the frontal bone. The whole complex needs to be fully exposed through a coronal approach, allowing the nature of the distortion to be accurately diagnosed. It is often not possible to relocate the fragment in its correct anatomical position because a small discrepancy in the frontal bone is magnified in the nasoethmoid region and distal nose. There is a risk of leaving the nasoethmoid fragment angled incorrectly. A better approach in these cases may be to formally osteotomize the nasoethmoid bone fragment from the frontal bone at the frontonasal suture and relocate and fix it formally after relocation of the frontal bandeau, taking care to maintain the frontonasal angle, nasal projection, and symmetry.

During direct canthopexy, extensive subperiosteal stripping, particularly in children, may cause the deposition of subperiosteal new bone, leading to blunting of the canthal angle. In children, it is useful to provide secondary external support to the reconstruction to prevent canthal drift, and the acrylic buttons approximate the soft tissues and help to prevent subperiosteal new bone deposition.

OUTCOMES

There are few reviews comparing different methods of repair. Anosmia is a severely debilitating sequela of nasoethmoid trauma, and it can result from fractures in which there is gross comminution of the cranial base or severe posterior displacement of the nasoethmoid complex, causing shearing of the olfactory system. Inappropriate removal of bone fragments or aggressive dissection to repair dural tears at the time of reconstruction can cause postoperative anosmia.

Late drift of the canthus can occur if the canthal-bearing bone fragment is not fixed properly or if the ligament is not captured or attached to the bone adequately in cases of complete detachment. Subperiosteal new bone formation is a problem when it is necessary to strip the periosteum widely

to fix the bony fragments; it is a particular problem in younger patients.

Lacerations resulting from the initial trauma will cause scarring. Sometimes, these lacerations can be used to give access to the fractures, but they rarely provide access to the whole complex and rarely allow for the complete management of the injury. The use of lacerations in isolation usually leads to compromises in the surgical treatment of nasoethmoid fractures and to disappointing results. Few surgical incisions in the local area can give direct access to the more common nasoethmoid fractures, and they usually lead to conspicuous scars. Delayed surgery allows scarring to develop, impeding reduction of the fractures.

CONTROVERSIES

Two main areas of controversy are timing and reduction.

TIMING

Surgery on an established, partly healed fracture rarely produces a good result. The main problem is difficulty in mobilizing the soft tissue and identifying soft tissue structures such as the canthal ligament and lacrimal drainage system. However, delay does allow the swelling to resolve. This is an entirely valid argument, because open reduction or placement of incisions is less satisfactory in the presence of gross edema. Nerves may not be seen, and incisions on the skin may turn out to be poorly placed after the swelling resolves.

Other systemic factors, particularly head injuries, may preclude early surgery. A frontal injury is much more likely to be associated with a head injury than a mandibular injury. Unfortunately, there is no uniform international approach by neurosurgeons to early intervention for nonhead injuries. In some units, early intervention has been successfully undertaken, but in most cases, neurosurgeons think early intervention for non–life-threatening conditions poses a greater risk than benefit for the patient. Each case is addressed on its merits. In any event, resolution of edema and systemic stability often follow the same time frame.

Timing of surgery is largely driven by events and is not negotiable. However, this does not justify the long delays that can occur, often because of poor communication between surgical teams. Long delays generate poor outcomes. In most cases, delays of up to 10 days do not significantly damage the final result.

REDUCTION

Arguments can be made for and against open reduction. Closed reduction is superficially attractive because it is quick and avoids skin incisions. The argument against closed reduction, which applies to the whole facial skeleton, is inadequate reduction and fixation, producing poor functional and esthetic outcomes.

These arguments are especially valid for surgery in the nasoethmoid and orbital regions. They are complex, three-dimensional structures made of fine bones. In the nasoethmoid region, closed reduction means the use of large lead plates placed over the complex to squeeze the bones into the correct shape. The position can sometimes be improved by running wires through the lead plates to pull the complex forward to an external fixator, such as a halo. In the rare case of an intact nasoethmoid complex that has been displaced en bloc, results may be satisfactory, but in most cases, this approach produces poor esthetic and functional outcomes.

Incisions in the face are needed for proper open reduction, but if well-placed coronal incisions are used, most nasoethmoid incisions can be easily reduced and fixed with no other incisions. This means that raising this flap must be executed with care and forethought. It must be placed high, especially in male patients, and with minimal damage to hair follicles. Most importantly, sensory and motor nerves must be seen, isolated, and protected from damage.

In summary, surgical delays of more than 10 days should be avoided, and the well-established open reduction and fixation approach should be adopted.

REFERENCES

1. Markowitz BL, Manson PN, Sargent L CA et al: Management of the medial canthal tendon in nasoethmoid-orbital fractures: the importance of the central fragment in classification and treatment. *Plast Reconstr Surg* 87:843-853, 1991.
2. Sheperd DE, Ward Booth P, Moos KF: The morbidity of bicoronal flaps in maxillofacial surgery. *Br J Oral Maxillofac Surg* 23:1-8, 1985.
3. Sargent LA: Nasoethmoid orbital fractures: diagnosis and treatment. *Plast Reconstr Surg* 120(suppl 2):716s-730s, 2007.
4. Warwick R, editor: *Eugene Wolff's anatomy of the eye and orbit*, ed 7, Philadelphia, 1976, WB Saunders, pp 182-237.
5. Jakobiec FA: *Ocular anatomy and teratology*, Philadelphia, 1982, Harper & Row, pp 677-731.
6. Wolff E: *The anatomy of the eye and orbit*, ed 4, Philadelphia, 1954, Blakiston.
7. Jones LT: An anatomical approach to problems of the eyelids and lacrimal apparatus. *Arch Ophthalmol* 66:111-124, 1961.
8. Robinson MD, Stranc MF: The anatomy of the medial canthal ligament. *Br J Plast Surg* 23:1-7, 1970.
9. Ayliffe PR: The anatomy of the medial canthal ligament, personal communication, 2002.
10. Horner WE: A description of a muscle connected with the eye lately discovered by W.E. Horner, M.D., one of the Professors of Anatomy in Philadelphia. *Lond Med Rep Rev* 18:32-33, 1822.
11. Reifler DM: Early descriptions of Horner's muscle and the lacrimal pump. *Surv Ophthalmol* 41:127-134, 1996.
12. Schobinger JC: Sur la fistule lacrymale [abridged translation by Macquart HJ]. In Haller A, editor: *Collection de theses medico-chirurgicales, sur les points les plus importans de la chirurgie theorique et pratique*, vol 4, Paris, 1757, Vincent, pp 240-262.
13. Duvernay JFM, Gautier d'Agoty JF: *Essai d'anatomie, en tableaux imprimes, qui representent au naturel tous les muscles de la face, de col, de la tete, de la langue, it du larinx*, Paris, 1745, Chez Gautier.
14. Freihofer HPM: Experience with transnasal canthopexy. *J Maxillofac Surg* 8:119-124, 1980.
15. Callahan A: Secondary reattachment of the medial canthal ligament. In Scheie HG, editor: *Surgical techniques*, Philadelphia, 1962, University of Pennsylvania Hospital, pp 240-241.
16. Converse JM, Smith B: Naso-orbital fractures and traumatic deformities of the medial canthal region. *Plast Reconstr Surg* 38:147-162, 1966.
17. Bostwick J, Jurkiewicz MJ: Functional anatomy of the eyelids as related to reconstruction. *Am Surgeon* 42:696-700, 1976.
18. Converse JM, Smith B, Wood-Smith D: Malunited fractures of the orbit. In Converse JM, editor: *Reconstructive plastic surgery*, Philadelphia, 1977, WB Saunders, p 1016.
19. Munro IR, Das JK: Improving results in orbital hypertelorism correction. *Ann Plast Surg* 2:499-507, 1979.
20. Bass CB: Medial canthal ligament reconstruction. *Ann Plast Surg* 3:182-185, 1979.
21. Zide BM, McCarthy JG: The medial canthus revisited—an anatomical basis for canthopexy. *Ann Plast Surg* 11:1-9, 1983.
22. Callahan A, Callahan MA: Fixation of the medial canthal structures: evolution of the best method. *Ann Plast Surg* 11:242-245, 1983.
23. Rodriguez RL, Zide BM: Reconstruction of the medial canthus. *Clin Plast Surg* 15:255-262, 1988.
24. Edelstein JP, Dryden RM: Medial palpebral tendon repair for medial ectropion of the lower eyelid. *Ophthal Plast Reconstr Surg* 6:28-37, 1990.
25. Dagum BD, Antonyshyn O, Hearn T: Medial canthopexy: an experimental and biomechanical study. *Ann Plast Surg* 35:262-265, 1995.
26. Duke-Elder WS: *Textbook of ophthalmology*, vol 1, St Louis, 1938, Mosby.
27. Duke-Elder WS, Wybar KC: The anatomy of the visual system. In Duke-Elder WS, editor: *System of ophthalmology*, vol 2, Mosby, St Louis, 1961, Mosby.
28. Jones LT: Epiphora: its relation to the anatomic structures and surgery of the medial canthal region. *Trans Pac Coast Ophthalmol Soc* 37:31, 1956.
29. Jones LT: The anatomy and physiology of the ocular appendages. In Reeh MJ, editor: *Treatment of lid and epibulbar tumors*, Springfield, 1963, Charles C Thomas, pp 16-21.
30. Jones LT: The anatomy of the upper eyelid and its relation to ptosis surgery. *Am J Ophthalmol* 57:943-959, 1964.
31. Jones LT: New anatomical concepts of the ocular adnexa. In Mustardé JC, Jones LT, Callahan A, editors: *Ophthalmic plastic surgery up-to-date*, Birmingham, Ala, 1970, Aesculapius Publishing, pp 3-6.
32. Jones LT, Reeh MJ, Wirttschafter JD: *Ophthalmic anatomy*, 1970, Rochester, NY, American Academy of Ophthalmology and Otolaryngology, pp 39-48.
33. Jones LT: New concepts of orbital anatomy. In Tessier P, Callahan A, Mustardé JC et al, editors: *Symposium on plastic surgery in the orbital region*, St Louis, 1976, Mosby, p 11.
34. Anderson RL: Medial canthal tendon branches out. *Arch Ophthalmol* 95:2051-2052, 1977.
35. Bergin DJ: Anatomy of the eyelids, lacrimal system and orbit. In McCord C, Tanenbaum M, editors: *Oculoplastic surgery*, ed 2, New York, 1987, Raven Press, pp 41-71.
36. Manson PN, Clifford CM, Su CT et al: Mechanisms of global support and posttraumatic enophthalmos. I. The anatomy of the ligament sling and its relation to intramuscular cone orbital fat. *Plast Reconstr Surg* 77:193-202, 1986.
37. Koorneef L: *Sectional anatomy of the orbit*, Amsterdam, 1981, Aeolus Press, pp 1-29.
38. Koorneef L: *Spatial aspects of the orbital musculo-fibrous tissue in man*, Amsterdam, 1987, Swets & Zeitlinger.
39. Lockwood CB: The anatomy of the muscles, ligaments, and fascia of the orbit, including an account of the capsule of Tenon, the check ligaments of the recti, and of the suspensory ligament of the eye. *J Anat Physiol* 20:1, 1886.
40. Whitnall SE: *Anatomy of the human orbit and accessory organs of vision*, ed 2, London, 1932, Oxford University Press, p 152.
41. Leipziger LS, Manson PN: Nasoethmoid orbital fractures. *Clin Plast Surg* 19:167-193, 1992.
42. Champy M, Lodde AW, Wilk A, Grasset D: Plate osteosynthesis in midface fractures and osteotomies. *Dtsch Z Mund Kiefer Gesichtschir* 8:26-36, 1978.

CHAPTER 13

Nasal Fractures

Barry L. Eppley

The nose is the most prominent feature of the face and has little protection from trauma. It is the most easily fractured of the facial bones[1] and, not surprisingly, the most commonly fractured.[2] Fractures occur twice as often in men as in women and are often the result of automotive accidents, interpersonal violence, or sporting injuries. One report indicates that more than one third of nasal fractures are associated with alcohol use.[2]

Despite a relatively low incidence of facial fractures in children, an estimated 25% of nasal fractures occur in patients younger than 12 years of age.[3] Fractures can occur in newborns due to malposition in utero and during birth, in infants and toddlers as a result of bumps and falls as they begin to crawl or walk, and in children and teenagers as they participate in competitive sports. Because the child's nose is more cartilaginous than bony, fractures can be difficult to diagnose, and they frequently remain undiagnosed until a deformity develops with growth.

Repair of nasal fractures is a simple procedure,[4] but it is associated with relatively high revision rates.[5,6] Results of inappropriate treatment include cosmetic external deformity and internal nasal airway obstruction, with resultant snoring and sinusitis. Delayed or abnormal growth of the nose and midface and disturbance of the dentition can occur in children.

CLASSIFICATION

The type of nasal injury sustained depends on the age of the patient and the direction and intensity of the forces applied. Most nasal fractures in adults result from a lateral blunt force. Typically, the nasal bone and the frontal process of the maxilla are involved unilaterally (Fig. 13-1A). With greater force, bilateral displacement of the nasal bones is seen. Because the nasal bones increase in thickness from their inferior aspect upward toward the junction with the frontal process, most nasal fractures occur in the midsection below the thicker portion, with the base of the nasal pyramid remaining in situ. Frontal rather than lateral blows result in posterior displacement or impaction of the nasal bones. The fracture line is located along the midsection (see Fig. 13-1B). More severe force disrupts the frontonasal suture, and as the impact force increases, nasal, orbital, and ethmoidal fractures occur in combination. In children, the relatively large amount of cartilage and open suture lines predisposes to an open book–type fracture, which results in a flattened appearance of the nose (see Fig. 13-1C). The bony component of these fractures is classified as type I (simple unilateral), type II (simple bilateral), and type III (comminuted unilateral, bilateral, or frontal).[5]

The septal component, the most important but often undiagnosed feature, requires accurate reduction and alignment if secondary deformities are to be avoided.[7] The septum tends to follow the displacement of the nasal bone fractures, and the nasal bones tend to unite in the direction of the deviated septum. The extent of the septal injury determines the appropriate technique for septal correction.[5] Lateral force results in displacement or a low fracture of the septal cartilage from the maxillary crest, producing a partial or complete obstruction on one side of the nasal cavity. The fracture dislocation usually occurs along the vomerine groove (Fig. 13-2A). Greater force, particularly when associated with frontal impact, may extensively fracture the septum in a more vertical direction through the thin central region of the quadrangular cartilage, which extends between the perpendicular plate of the ethmoid above and the upper edge of the vomer below[5] (see Fig. 13-2B). Most septal fractures result in some telescoping of the cartilages, loss of vertical central support, and widening of the base of the septum. The septal component of these fractures is classified as type IV (nasal bone and septal dislocation), which is subdivided into type IVa (associated with a septal hematoma) and type IVb (associated with an open nasal laceration).[5]

ASSESSMENT

Understanding the mechanism and direction of the forces involved should provide an accurate three-dimensional mental image of the disrupted nasal anatomy. Examination includes a visual assessment of the nasal deviation, location of any lacerations, and assessment of the degree of swelling and bruising. Palpation may reveal specific areas of tenderness, crepitus, or a bony step. Simple nasal fractures should be differentiated from more complex facial fractures. Complex nasal fractures predominantly involve extension of the fracture into the nasoethmoidal complex. These fractures may be associated with much more serious complications, are more difficult to treat, and often are accompanied by other injuries,

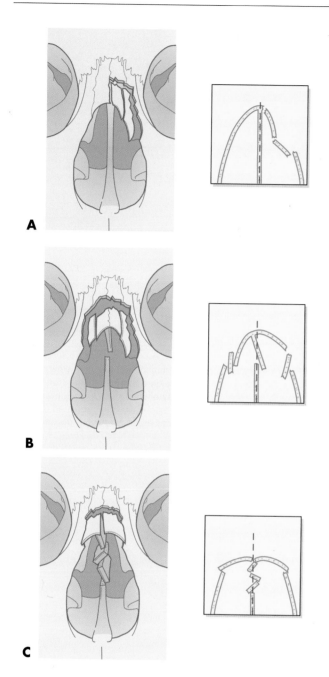

FIGURE 13-1 Nasal bone fracture patterns. **A,** Simple, unilateral fracture (type I). **B,** Comminuted, bilateral fracture (type III). **C,** Open book–type fracture (children).

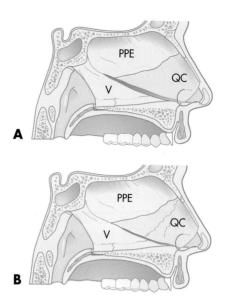

FIGURE 13-2 Sagittal views of nasal septal fracture patterns. **A,** Fracture and dislocation of the septum from the maxillary crest typically are caused by low-impact forces. **B,** Vertical fractures through the quadrangular plate typically are caused by higher-impact, particularly frontal, forces. V, vomer; PPE, perpendicular plate of the ethmoid; QC, quadrangular cartilage.

such as head injuries. For example, after the nasoethmoidal complex is fractured, there may be detachment of the medial canthal ligament or fractures extending into the frontal sinus or cribriform plate. These fractures require assessment with computed tomography (CT) and treatment by open reduction. The intercanthal distance may be increased in severe injuries, indicating a more complex nasoethmoidal injury.

An intranasal examination to determine the status of the septum should be carried out under adequate lighting and using a nasal speculum. A septal hematoma requires immediate evacuation. Decongesting the nose with a topical decongestant can be beneficial to the examination. A full endoscopic examination is advised for a complete assessment of the septum (particularly at the posteroinferior junction with the perpendicular plate of the ethmoid), turbinates, and inferior meati. This examination may have to be delayed until the operating room. Airway patency is in part determined by the patient's own assessment of his or her breathing before and after injury.

Radiographic examination, although routinely performed, is often of questionable value.[8] Plain films are of little benefit other than for medicolegal reasons, because they are rarely helpful in determining the need for surgery or the type of surgical intervention required (Fig. 13-3A). A CT scan provides better information, particularly of the position of the septum and patency of the airway, but it is costly and does not replace a thorough history and physical examination, particularly if an endoscopic assessment is performed (see Fig. 13-3C).

MANAGEMENT

Not all nasal fractures require surgical manipulation. The main criteria for surgery are the obvious presence of or risk of later, cosmetic deformity and a functional (breathing) impairment that is not primarily caused by intranasal swelling (mucosal edema or bruising) or retained blood. If either exists, surgery is justified, and it should be carried out as soon as the precise deformity is evident. The extent of the bony or cartilaginous deformity determines the appropriate treatment. Murray et al.[9] have described poor outcomes for the treatment of simple nasal fractures (albeit with a small number of patients returning for review), and they suggested that more aggressive treatment is indicated. In many cases with significant deviation of the septum (i.e., more than one half of the nostril width), small fractures occur in the septum

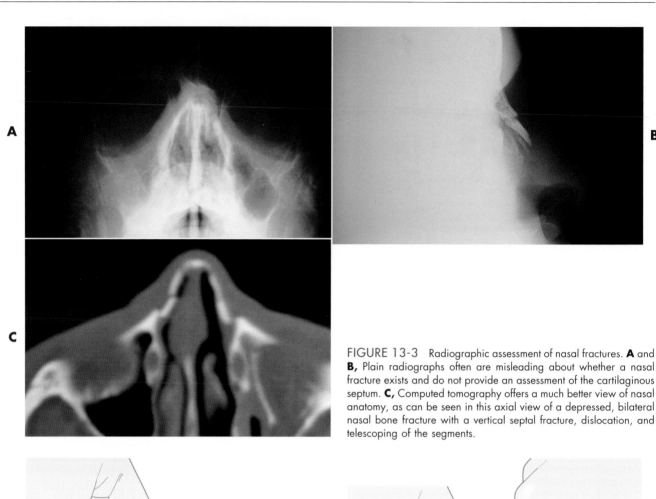

FIGURE 13-3   Radiographic assessment of nasal fractures. **A** and **B,** Plain radiographs often are misleading about whether a nasal fracture exists and do not provide an assessment of the cartilaginous septum. **C,** Computed tomography offers a much better view of nasal anatomy, as can be seen in this axial view of a depressed, bilateral nasal bone fracture with a vertical septal fracture, dislocation, and telescoping of the segments.

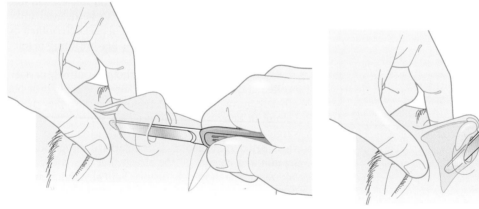

FIGURE 13-4   Technique of bimanual closed reduction of nasal fractures. **A,** The straight elevator is used internally to push out or over the displaced nasal bone while the external fingers mold it into the proper position. **B,** Septal relocation is done by pushing the septum over and then immediately evaluating with a speculum.

close to the rigid support of the palatal groove. The investigators suggested a miniseptoplasty be carried out acutely to prevent late deformation of the septum at the fracture site. This study, like many posttraumatic reviews, had a low follow-up rate.

CLOSED REDUCTION

General anesthesia greatly facilitates a successful closed reduction. Although local anesthesia alone is often used, this

practice seems unduly punitive to the patient, and it probably limits the thoroughness of the technique.[10] I prefer to carry out the reduction under general anesthesia supplemented by a 4% solution of topical cocaine and an injectable solution of 2% Xylocaine with 1:50,000 epinephrine.

The nasal bones usually can be manually manipulated back into a midline position. If required, depressed nasal fragments can be elevated using the Boies (straight) elevator internally and digital manipulation externally (Fig. 13-4). Minor dislocations of the septum along the vomerine groove

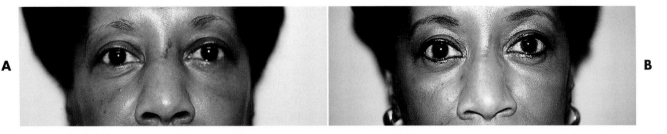

FIGURE 13-5   A 52-year-old woman sustained a type II nasal fracture caused by high frontal impact. **A,** One week after injury. **B,** One month after closed reduction.

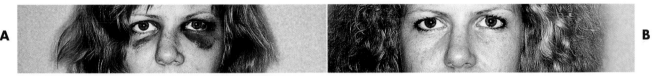

FIGURE 13-6   A 30-year-old woman had a type III nasal fracture caused by domestic violence. **A,** One week after injury. **B,** Three months after closed reduction.

can be reduced with the same instrument. Walsham forceps may be required for severe impactions as a method of grasping the septum and lifting. When using Walsham forceps to reposition the nasal bones, compression or crushing of the skin should be avoided. Support for the nasal bones and septum is usually provided by gel foam packing, which also aids hemostasis.

After reduction, the nose is taped and splinted for 1 week. A small piece of Telfa is placed in the nasal vestibule overnight to absorb any drainage. Because of the well-documented reports of recurrent deviation after closed reduction, patients are followed closely for 1 year (Figs. 13-5 and 13-6).

OPEN REDUCTION

Open reduction is reserved for patients who have an unstable intraoperative result after closed reduction, have failed previous attempts at closed reduction, or have presented more than 4 weeks from the time of injury. The key to successful open reduction is management of the septum.[7] Persistent deviation of the septum is the most common cause of misalignment of the nasal bones.

The septum is approached through a hemitransfixion incision. A mucoperichondrial flap is usually elevated on one side of the septum only, but both sides can be raised if necessary. The cartilage segments are repositioned, with resection done only if it aids the repositioning of the remaining fragments. When the quadrangular cartilage is dislocated from the maxillary crest, removal of an inferior strip of cartilage may be necessary to permit reduction (Fig. 13-7A). In common with the traditional septoplasty, at least 1 cm of cartilage must be preserved along the caudal border and dorsum for adequate support (see Fig. 13-7B). Bent cartilage may be crosshatched on the concave side to aid straightening. Caudal septal dislocations are fixed to the anterior nasal spine with a permanent figure-of-eight suture. When the septum is fractured and unstable, an internal straight splint composed of resorbable polymers may be placed submucosally on one side of the septum and the overlying mucosa repositioned and adapted by sewing through it.[11] More commonly, the cartilage is

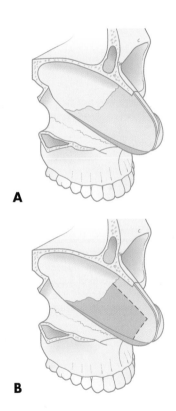

FIGURE 13-7   Management of the septum in open reduction. **A,** Resection of the inferior end of the cartilaginous septum permits repositioning in the midline. **B,** More extensive cartilage resection can be done if necessary (although not preferred), but 1 cm of dorsal and caudal support must be maintained.

secured into position, and the mucosal flaps are adapted with through-and-through sutures of 4-0 plain gut on a straight needle. If the mucosa is significantly torn, Silastic splints are placed on each side and sewn into place for support (Fig. 13-8).

Open reduction of the nasal bones is usually carried out after the septal support is reestablished through an

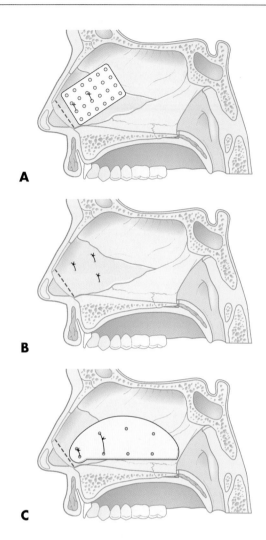

FIGURE 13-8 Septal support techniques in open reductions. **A,** An internal rigid splint composed of resorbable polymers can be placed directly against the cartilage and secured into position with external transmucosal sutures. **B,** Through-and-through sutures coapt the mucosa to the septum and provide structural support. **C,** When the external mucosa is severely torn, extramucosal internal Silastic splints can be bilaterally placed and sutured into position.

intercartilaginous incision. Lateral and, if necessary, medial osteotomies are performed to facilitate the reduction of the fracture. Appropriate reduction of the bones usually corrects any deformities of the tip or supratip cartilages. Dressings are applied and follow-up is carried out as for closed reductions (Fig. 13-9).

The treatment of nasal fractures in children is different from that in adults. Because unrecognized injuries can result in nasal and midface deformities later in life, accurate diagnosis and treatment remain important. Care must be taken to avoid damage to the growth centers. Because these injuries are often greenstick fractures, the use of closed reduction techniques is effective in most cases (Fig. 13-10). When

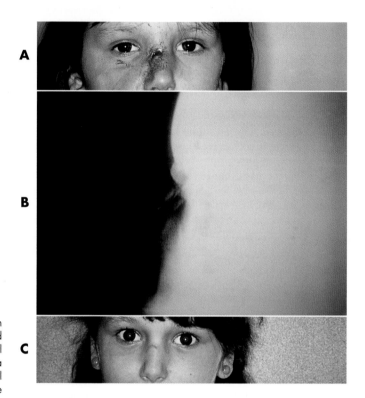

FIGURE 13-10 A 5-year-old girl had a nasal fracture caused by a bicycle accident. **A,** Preoperative status. **B,** Preoperative plain radiograph. **C,** Result 3 months postoperatively.

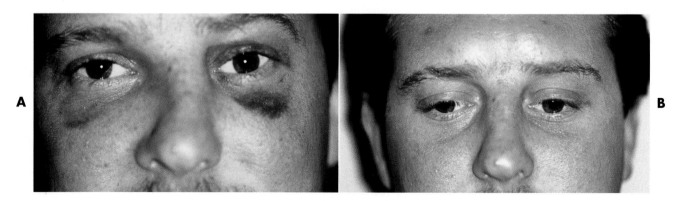

FIGURE 13-9 A 30-year-old man had a nasal fracture that was treated with open reduction. **A,** Preoperative status. **B,** Result 6 months postoperatively.

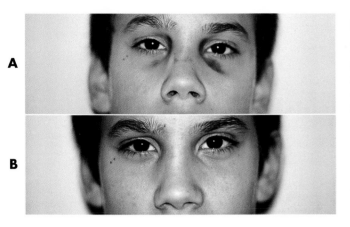

A

B

FIGURE 13-11   A 10-year-old boy had a nasal fracture caused by a sporting accident. **A,** Preoperative status. **B,** Result 6 weeks postoperatively after open reduction with no cartilage resection.

required, open reduction is performed but without removal of bone or cartilage (Fig. 13-11).

OUTCOMES

Treatment of the relatively simple nasal fracture is perceived to be highly successful, but postoperative results often are disappointing. The need for revision is historically high, ranging from 10% to 50% in reported series. Using the approaches previously described, the need for revision in the more severe type III fractures should not exceed 10% to 20%. Results obtained for treatment of type I and II fractures should include no more than a 10% revision rate.[2,5]

COMPLICATIONS

Closed and open reductions of nasal fractures are associated with few complications.

EPISTAXIS

Epistaxis can occur but is usually controlled with conservative measures, including upright positioning, mild sedation, and topical vasoconstrictive agents. Packing can dislocate the reduction and should be used only as a last resort.

SEPTAL HEMATOMA

Septal hematomas can occur at the time of injury or after reduction. Unrecognized septal hematomas can lead to necrosis of the cartilage and occasionally to saddling of the middle third of the nose in severe cases. Immediate evacuation is always indicated.

INFECTION

Infection is uncommon. Prophylactic antibiotics are routinely given, although their benefit is often debated. A septal abscess requires drainage and additional antibiotics. Osteitis of the nasal bones, which is rare, requires bony débridement and intravenous antibiotics.

SYNECHIAE

Synechiae can result from lacerations of the nasal mucosa. This problem can most often be treated under local anesthesia by incising the scar band and placing packing between the septum and the lateral nasal wall.

REVISION SURGERY

Posttraumatic rhinoplasty can have a poor outcome. Careful patient selection is needed to ensure growth has ceased and lifestyle changes have occurred so that further trauma will not take place. This is topic discussed in more detail in Chapter 26 of this text.

> **KEY POINTS**
> Nasal fractures are the most common facial bone injury. Despite perceptions that they are relatively easy to treat, revision frequently is needed because of secondary deformity. These poor outcomes can be improved by careful assessment of the injury, an understanding of the underlying bony or cartilaginous deformity (including the important role of the septum), and proactive, and in appropriate cases more aggressive open, treatment to produce the best cosmetic and functional outcomes.

REFERENCES

1. Swearington JJ: *Tolerance of human face to crash impact*, Oklahoma City, OK, 1965 Federal Aviation Agency.
2. Wang TD, Facer GW, Kern EB: Nasal fractures. In Gates GA, editor: *Current therapy in otolaryngology: head and neck surgery*, vol 4, Philadelphia, 1990, BC Decker, pp 105-109.
3. Goode RL, Spooner TR: Management of nasal fractures in children. *Clin Pediatr* 11:526, 1972.
4. Verwoerd CDA: Present day treatment of nasal fractures: closed versus open reduction. *Facial Plast Surg* 8:220, 1992.
5. Rohrich RJ, Adams Jr WP: Nasal fracture management: minimizing secondary nasal deformities. *Plast Reconstr Surg* 106:266, 2000.
6. Murray JAM, Maran AGD: The treatment of nasal injuries by manipulation. *J Laryngol Otol* 94:1405, 1980.
7. Gunter JP, Rohrich RJ: Management of the deviated nose: the importance of septal reconstruction. *Clin Plast Surg* 15:43, 1988.
8. Logan M, O'Driscoll K, Masterson J: The utility of nasal bone radiographs in nasal trauma. *Clin Radiol* 49:192, 1994.
9. Murray JA, Maran AG, Busuttil A, Vaughan G: A pathological classification of nasal fractures. *Injury* 17:338, 1986.
10. Cook JA, McRae DR, Irving RM, Dowie LN: A randomized comparison of manipulation of the fractured nose under local anesthesia and general anesthesia. *Clin Otolaryngol* 15:343, 1990.
11. Eppley BL: The use of resorbable spacers for nasal spreader grafts [discussion]. *Plast Reconstr Surg* 106:922, 2000.

Ian S. Holland, Jeremy D. McMahon, David A. Koppel, Mark F. Devlin, Khursheed F. Moos

In 1968, Rowe and Killey,[1] in the second edition of their text on facial fractures, distilled the experience of half a century in the management of facial trauma. The lessons came primarily from an unforgiving teacher—the theater of war. What evolved from this experience was a management protocol that was safe and provided resource-efficient treatment. The largely closed treatment techniques allowed a return to satisfactory function for most patients. Persistent deformity in many was accepted.

The last 4 decades of relative peace and prosperity for much of the developed world have seen major developments in the field of facial trauma, with advances in resuscitation techniques, imaging, other diagnostic tools, anesthesia, and instrumentation. Concomitantly, there has occurred an increase in the available resources to manage the trauma that occurs in peacetime. Innovative surgeons have exploited these changes in an attempt to achieve much improved results in facial form and function after trauma. A paradigm shift has occurred, with the emphasis now placed on adequate exposure with precise, usually "open", reduction and fixation of fractured segments. The direct antecedent of this change was the experience gained in the management of craniofacial deformity through wide exposure and osteotomy with direct osteosynthesis of mobilized fragments.[2] At the same time and in part as a result of these advances, patient expectations have also steadily risen.

We believe there has been a steady improvement in outcome; however, validation of this belief with objective data has not always been achieved. What has emerged is a treatment protocol that aims to deliver excellent results but is resource expensive. However, the techniques learned in the preceding era must not be lost, because it is evident from the experience of current conflicts that those techniques will still be required in some form by today's and tomorrow's surgeons.

This chapter presents a management protocol that is applicable to civilian peacetime practice, where considerable resources are available and can be brought to bear on the management of relatively small numbers of individuals at any one time.

CLASSIFICATION OF MIDFACE FRACTURES AND OUTCOMES

Le Fort's 1901 classic treatise describing experimentally induced midfacial fracture patterns has remained in use for more than a century and continues to have utility (Fig. 14-1). However, a satisfactory classification schema should accurately describe the major clinical features present and allow the stratification of patients presenting according to severity, for the purposes of measuring outcome. Le Fort's simple classification has important deficiencies in both respects. It fails to adequately account for fractures at multiple levels—including asymmetrical fracture patterns, separation of major fragments, comminution of vulnerable areas, concurrent anterior cranial fossa (ACF) and mandibular fractures.[3] All of these features have a bearing on management protocols and outcome and are seen in many cases of panfacial trauma (see Fig. 14-1C).

A number of workers have made useful contributions in an attempt to provide more comprehensive classification systems for the mid and upper face. Developments in the 1980s incorporated and recognized the significance of sagittal palatal fractures,[4] naso-orbitoethmoid comminution,[5] and involvement of the ACF.[6] In addition, varying degrees of zygomatic complex involvement have been classified, as have frontal injuries. These descriptions have the virtue of being clinically significant, with classification of fractures of each of the major midfacial subunits facilitating communication among clinicians and planning of surgical intervention. However, if several subunits are involved, it is descriptively cumbersome. For example, a patient with a frontal sinus fracture, a naso-orbitoethmoidal fracture with traumatic telecanthus, pyramidal maxillary fracture, and displaced zygomatic complex would have a number of different classification labels applied.

Guerrissi devised a maxillofacial trauma scoring system that aims to identify patients with potentially life-threatening maxillofacial injuries, allowing appropriate triage as well as quantifying the severity of facial injuries for the purpose of

A 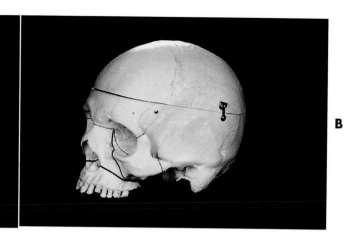 **B**

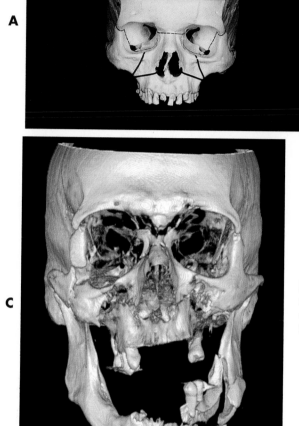 **C**

FIGURE 14-1 **A** and **B,** Le Fort's 1901 description of experimentally induced midfacial fractures: Le Fort I *(black line),* Le Fort II *(red line),* and Le Fort III *(green dashes).* **C,** Compliacted fracture patterns that are often seen in panfacial trauma.

stratification according to functional and esthetic impact.[7] This scoring system has the disadvantage of being descriptive of both bony injuries and soft tissue injuries, which can lead to potential difficulties with interpretation. Furthermore, it has not, to our knowledge, been validated in a prospective study.

More recently, comprehensive scoring systems[8] applicable to facial trauma have been described, some with validation of the proposed system[9] for reproducibility and correlation with complexity of injury. As might be expected, the more severe the scores, the worse the degree of injury; none of these scoring systems can accurately predict outcome from a functional or esthetic point of view.

An alphanumeric scoring system has been devised by Cooter and David, and a prospective evaluation of this method has been reported.[3] This instrument expresses the degree of facial disruption as a percentage. The authors claim that it offers a detailed analysis of fracture pattern and accurately represents the severity of bony injuries. That contention is supported by the published data. In 100 patients studied prospectively, both the maxillary fracture score and the total

facial fracture score demonstrated a strong correlation with complications or adverse sequelae.

Although it is hardly surprising that greater degrees of facial disruption are associated with less favorable outcomes, the strong correlation coefficient suggests that Cooter and David's method provides a useful objective stratification instrument. Accurate stratification of the severity of injury allows comparison of outcomes among centers even if variations exist in treatment methodology. Moreover, the pattern of adverse results observed in this study is revealing. Most of the posttreatment problems were seen in the orbital region (20% of patients) and principally comprised enophthalmos, orbital dystopia, and canthal deformities. Eight percent of the patients had occlusal abnormalities after treatment, 8% had nasal problems, and wound and implant-related problems occurred in 9%. The overall adverse sequelae rate was 36% in this group of patients who, for the most part, had sustained high-energy injuries. These data, from a major craniofacial surgical center, emphasize that residual deformity after treatment of midfacial trauma of more than moderate severity is commonplace.

A publication from two major North American centers also found worse outcomes with respect to physical problems and psychosocial well-being in patients with severe midface injuries. Patients with severe midface disruption were compared to patients with less severe facial disruption and with a second control group of patients who had sustained injuries other than to the facial region.[10] Specifically excluded from all three groups were individuals with severe brain injury, spinal cord injury, major burns, or an extremity requiring amputation. Only 55% of those subjects with more severe Le Fort–type fractures returned to work, compared with 70% of those with less severe midface fractures and those in the age- and sex-matched group with general injuries.

There was a 23% incidence of persistent diplopia (minimum follow-up, 18 months) after Le Fort–type fractures, similar to the 20% incidence of diplopia reported after midface fracture in a sample of 363 patients from the West of Scotland.[11] In the American study, 35% of patients reported epiphora, and the prevalence of this problem increased with severity of facial injury. Difficulty with mastication was reported in 31% (trismus, malocclusion, pain, residual nerve injury). Subjectively reported altered smell and taste occurred in 35%, and one third of patients reported persistent areas of facial numbness. This work emphasizes that the functional and psychosocial costs of midfacial injuries are high. Minimizing long-term disability requires early intervention of the highest standard and follow-up care that seeks to rectify remediable problems, together with appropriate referrals to other health care professionals when necessary.

Haug et al.[12] also reported that more superior levels of midfacial fracture resulted in a higher incidence of adverse sequelae. Their study sought, retrospectively, to compare largely closed management of maxillary fractures with open reduction and internal fixation, using the rate of complications and of adverse sequelae as the outcome measure. No difference was observed between the groups, and the authors concluded that, "given the advantage of airway protection, enhanced nutrition, and a more rapid return to pretraumatic functioning, open reduction with rigid internal fixation may be the preferred modality of treatment."[12]

The lack of a demonstrable benefit from techniques that employ wide exposure and direct fixation in Haug's study is disappointing and surprising. It is clear that less invasive management strategies leave substantial fragments malpositioned (Fig. 14-2), and it has been assumed that more precise reduction and fixation would lead to improved outcomes. There are two possible explanations. Either the method of outcome measurement was insufficiently sensitive to detect a difference, or the extended exposure required to effect precise reduction and fixation of all fragments was associated with adverse effects, nullifying a potential benefit. These explanations are not mutually exclusive, but it is our belief that the former is the more significant factor.

What is currently lacking are objective methods by which to assess both functional and esthetic outcomes. Measurement of complication rates and the requirement for revisional surgery provides only limited information. Adverse outcomes vary from the trivial and transitory to the functionally and esthetically disabling, and thresholds for revision procedures vary widely among patients and among surgeons.

The diverse functions performed by the facial region (e.g., special senses, mastication, verbal and nonverbal

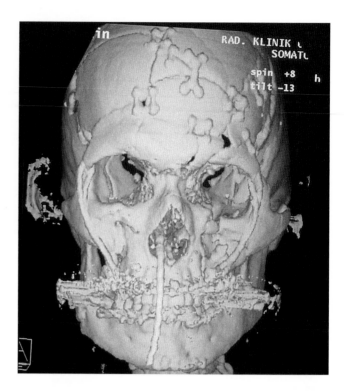

FIGURE 14-2 Three-dimensional reconstructed tomogram after anterior cranial fossa repair and fixation of the midface with internal suspension wires and intermaxillary fixation as an interim measure. Notice the substantial residual malposition of major midface fragments. *(Courtesy of R. Schmelzeisen, Professor and Medical Director, Department of Maxillofacial and Oral Surgery, Albert-Ludwigs-University, Freiburg, Germany.)*

communication, humidification) imply a diverse range of potential problems, making the development of good outcome measures difficult. Nevertheless, just as fracture configurations tend to follow certain patterns, so do adverse outcomes. Advances in the measurement of esthetic results in other areas of facial surgery[13,14] have emerged following the advent of three-dimensional (3-D) and four-dimensional facial imaging modalities. These techniques are applicable to the assessment of esthetic and functional outcomes in trauma cases.

Much of the perceived disfigurement after facial injury is a consequence of asymmetry, which should be quantifiable with digitization of facial form and the use of software algorithms. There are obstacles to the development of such a tool. For example, all individuals have some degree of facial asymmetry, and this cannot be controlled for. It seems probable, however, that asymmetry in some facial subunits has a disproportionate effect in producing perceived disfigurement.

Refinements in technique to produce improved outcomes demand that we look critically and carefully at results and further develop objective outcome measures despite the obstacles that exist.

ASSESSMENT

The initial assessment of the patient presenting with panfacial and maxillary fractures is no different from that for any other trauma patient and should follow principles of Advanced Trauma Life Support. Compared with isolated injuries localized to the craniomaxillofacial region, the greater energy imparted in producing panfacial trauma implies a higher probability of associated injury, particular to the brain and cervical spine.

In the primary survey of a patient with panfacial trauma, the airway may well be compromised by orofacial hemorrhage and require active management, or the patient may be obtunded with a decreased Glasgow Coma Scale (GCS) score. The potential for concomitant cervical spine injury in panfacial trauma should be remembered. Problems with breathing not related to loss of the airway are uncommon but can occur as a result of foreign bodies (e.g., avulsed teeth, fractured dentures).

Hemorrhage from panfacial trauma does not usually result in cardiovascular compromise unless it is very profuse or has been on going for a considerable time. Any orofacial hemorrhage should be arrested and can usually be controlled with the application of direct or indirect pressure. It is always wise to presume that cardiovascular compromise in the patient with panfacial trauma is related to a source other than orofacial blood loss unless other causes have been ruled out. Many patients with panfacial injury have some degree of head injury that requires appropriate management.

When assessing the patient with a panfacial injury after completion of the primary survey, it is prudent for the maxillofacial surgeon to consider the following questions:

1. Is there an actual or potential airway problem?
2. Is there ongoing hemorrhage?
3. What is the nature and likely outcome of any accompanying head injury?
4. Has a cervical spine injury been diagnosed or definitively excluded?
5. Is there an occult life-threatening injury not detected on primary and secondary survey (i.e., is further investigation or consultation required)? A further comprehensive, top-to-toe evaluation is a prudent measure in the 48-hour period after admission and before any major intervention.
6. What is the precise extent, location, and nature of all injuries to the craniomaxillofacial region?
7. Are there non–life-threatening injuries present that require management by other specialties?
8. Is there any comorbidity that will affect treatment and subsequent rehabilitation?

What follows is primarily a discussion of question 6—the extent, location, and nature of injuries to the facial region—but all the questions listed require an answer in the planning of definitive management. Not only the necessity but also the urgency of liaison with additional specialties such as neurosurgery, ophthalmology, vascular surgery, interventional radiology, and orthopedics requires careful consideration based on timely, detailed, and repeated assessment. Early involvement of the required teams and good communication serve to minimize delays and optimize treatment.

The full assessment begins with a detailed history of the injury. This should be taken from the patient, if possible, or from eye witnesses, ambulance personnel, or other emergency team staff. The object of the detailed history taking is to clearly define the mechanism of injury so as to gain an appreciation of the energy involved. This indicates the probable extent of the facial injuries, and highlights probable associated injuries. A past medical history is important with regard to any intervention, and in the multiply injured patient it is often necessary to obtain this history from relatives.

A detailed craniofacial examination should take place as soon as practicable after the patient is admitted. All findings must be described in detail, and diagrams are very useful. A thorough inspection should identify lacerations, incised wounds, abrasions, and contusions. These should all be examined carefully with consideration to underlying structures that may be damaged, particularly the seventh cranial nerve. During inspection, consideration should be given to the possibility of a cerebrosponal fluid (CSF) leak. The bony structures should be palpated for contour, steps, and mobility. The eyes should be examined in detail, including fundoscopy. However, dilatation of the pupils should be carried out only after discussion with the neurosurgical service. The ears should be examined, and blood behind the tympanic membrane, tympanic perforations, and external auditory canal tears should be noted.

The history and clinical examination guide the use of further investigations. Plain radiographs taken under less than ideal circumstances are usually noncontributory. Furthermore, plain film images frequently fail to provide sufficiently detailed information regarding the nature and extent of skull base fractures, orbital wall injuries, pterygoid plate fractures, and sagittal fractures of the maxilla and condylar process of the mandible. Computed tomographic (CT) scanning is the major diagnostic investigation, with multiplanar and 3-D reconstruction and manipulation of the images on the radiology department workstations or on the surgeon's own Picture Archiving and Communication System (PACS) being necessary to get the best detail from the information available.

Interpretation of CT scans is first directed toward determining the presence, extent, and location of skull base involvement, as well as underlying brain parenchymal injury and intracranial hemorrhage. The axial images reveal the posterior wall in frontal sinus fractures. The cribriform plate region is often more clearly seen on coronal images, and the orbital roof region is well visualized in axial, coronal, and sagittal planes. Fractures detected in the ACF are often associated with dural tears that communicate with the upper airway. Meningitis is a short- and longer-term risk, although this is not well quantified. ACF repair is frequently indicated, with varying thresholds across neurosurgical units. However, consultation is always indicated in the presence of such injuries.

The scans of the middle cranial fossa are next scrutinized. Here, we pay particular attention to the greater wing of the sphenoid in the lateral orbit. If facial fractures extend in continuity with the middle cranial fossa, mobilization and reduction of anterior zygomatico-orbital segments risks production or exacerbation of intracranial hemorrhage, dural tears, and direct brain injury (Fig. 14-3). Fractures involving the orbital apex with potential involvement of the optic foramen are occasionally seen. In the presence of a traumatic optic neuropathy accompanying such injuries, high-dose steroids are recommended. Other workers perform optic nerve decompression procedures in addition (see Chapter 10).

FIGURE 14-3   **A** and **B,** Computed tomograpnic (CT) axial scans demonstrate craniofacial fractures involving the right lateral orbit extending to the orbital apex. There is a small associated extradural hemorrhage, and a traumatic optic neuropathy was present. Neurosurgical intervention was not required. The traumatic optic neuropathy was managed with high-dose corticosteroids with subsequent improvement in visual acuity. Associated mandibular fractures were managed operatively. In this circumstance, the displaced zygomatico-orbital complex was not treated as part of the primary management. Because of the risks associated with mobilization of the zygomatico-orbital complex, this is one of the few circumstances in which secondary delayed management with osteotomy and bone grafting is advocated. This case illustrates the importance of CT imaging in delineating the relationships of facial injuries to possible injuries in the skull base.

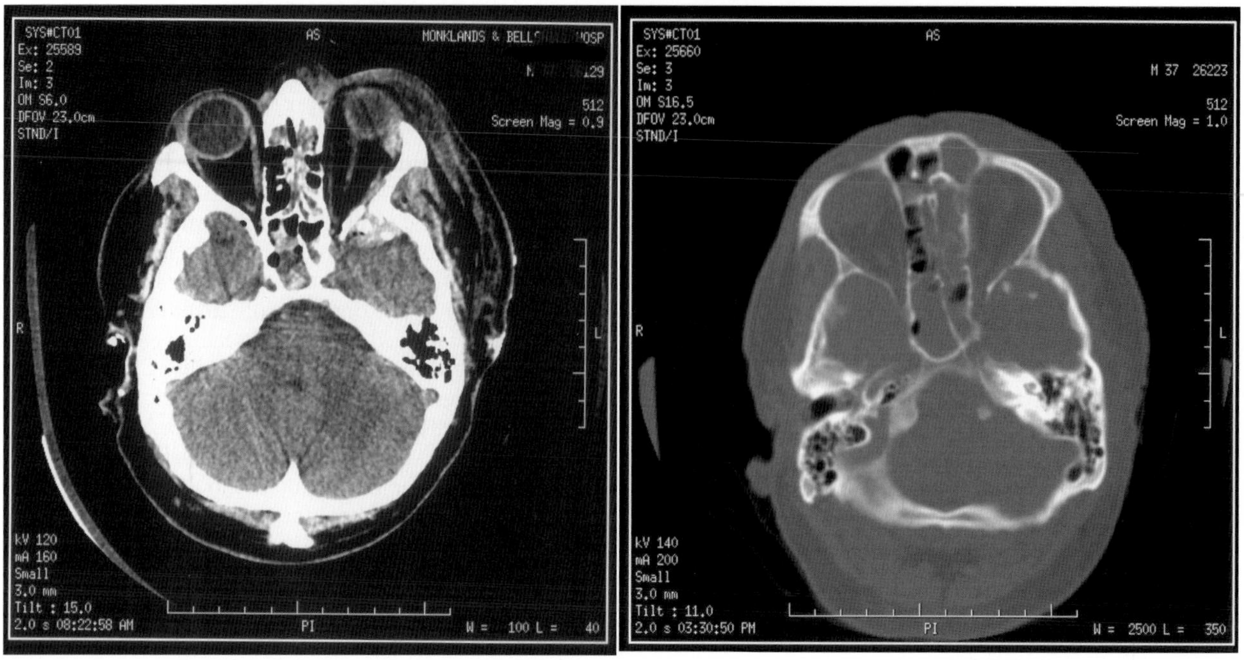

There is little information that cannot be obtained from a careful scrutiny of the axial, coronal, and sagittal images (Fig. 14-4). That said, 3-D CT reconstructions have a role to play in the assessment of facial injuries, because they give a good overview of the injury and make visualization of the relationships of the various fragments easier. However, care needs to be taken in their interpretation, because interpolation of data among images can lead to underestimation of the true extent of injury. Three-dimensional imaging is particularly helpful in the visualization of fracture patterns and displacement of condylar fractures (Fig. 14-5).

Angiography is not often necessary but can be used both diagnostically and therapeutically. Penetrating wounds can cause injury to important vessels, and angiography should be considered (Fig. 14-6). Interventional techniques are used when other measures to arrest hemorrhage have not been, or are not likely to be, successful (Fig. 14-7).

The use of evoked responses, particularly to assess the optic pathway, has been advocated, but at present this type of investigation is a research tool. In the future it may have a greater role in assessment of the optic pathway in the unconscious patient.

A full dental assessment is important and can be undertaken clincally in all cases. If the patient can cooperate, an orthopantomogram (OPG) is helpful. If there are dentoalveolar fractures or other factors that make the establishment of the pre-injury occlusion difficult, the use of dental

models allows assessment of the occlusion and enables the construction of custom-made arch bars and an acrylic interocclusal wafer. It is often necessary to section the models, mimicking the fractures, to allow for an accurate reduction. The inspection of wear facets and the use of pre-injury photographs and orthodontic casts (if available) aid the correct reestablishment of the dental occlusion.

Once the full assessment and targeted investigations have been performed, the following key questions can be answered and, particularly for more complex injuries, a planning meeting for the surgical team convened to formulate an individualized operative strategy. These can be prolonged procedures, and planning optimizes efficiency with respect to both intraoperative decision making and allocation of resources. Treatment planning should considered.

1. What is the current airway, and what sort of airway is required for the planned proceedure?
2. What is the extent of the bony skeletal injury?
   - Is the ACF involved?
   - Is the frontal sinus involved? If so, is there evidence of nasofrontal outflow tract injury and, in particular, obstruction?
   - What is the extent of naso-orbitoethmoidal injuries?
   - What is the extent of malar-orbital injuries, particularly of the medial orbital wall?
   - What is the extent and type of maxillary injuries?

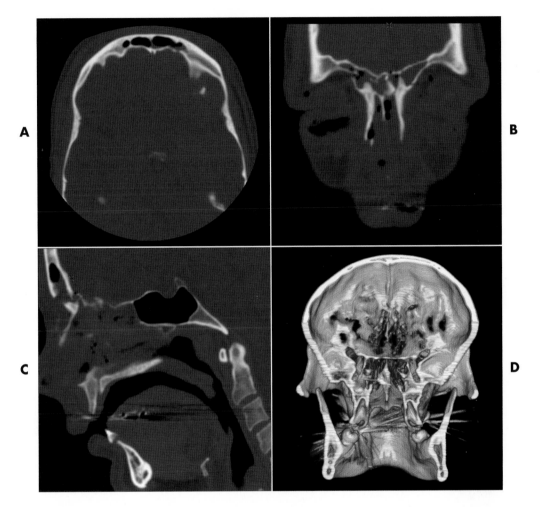

FIGURE 14-4 **A** through **C,** Careful clinical examination and scrutiny of axial, coronal, and saggital computed tomographic images provides as much information as three-dimensional reformatted images, often with more detail (**D**).

- What is the extent and type of mandibular injuries (particularly condylar injuries)?
- Is there any bone loss (either absolute or effective)?
3. What is the extent of any soft tissue injury?
  - What is the extent and type of lacerations?
  - Is there any tissue loss?
  - Is there any injury to cranial nerves?
  - Is there any injury to the globe or optic tract?
4. Is there an actual or potential cervical spine injury?
5. Is there potential for exacerbation of a coexisting head injury?
6. Is there any potential vascular injury?
7. What other injuries exist, and how do plans for their management affect our planning?
8. If injuries are unilateral, can intraoperative navigational techniques be employed to assess the bony reductions?

The main aspects of the formulated management plan should be

- timing of the interventions
- airway management
- surgical access
- sequencing of repair
- bone graft donor sites
- soft tissue repair and reconstruction

The need for any particular equipment (e.g., preformed orbital plates, canthal tendon wires) must be anticipated and access to it assured.

These aspects must be considered in relation to the general state of the patient with particular reference to the current and anticipated respiratory status, cardiovascular status, nutritional state, coexisting injury, and comorbid disease.

OPERATIVE STRATEGY: STATE-OF-THE-ART MANAGEMENT

MANAGEMENT PRINCIPLES

Restoring pre-injury form and function to the facial region requires precise anatomic reconstitution of the craniofacial skeleton and overlying soft tissue drape. The cranial cavity must be sealed off from the upper aerodigestive tract, preventing subsequent infection. Orbital volume

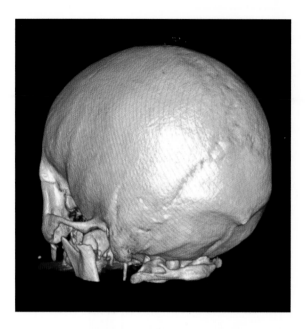

FIGURE 14-5 Subcondylar fractures of the mandible are better visualized in three-dimensional reformatted images compared with axial scans.

and configuration must be restored, providing support and projection to the globes and supporting structures. The form of the external nose is restored, and an unimpeded nasal airway is reestablished. Correct jaw relationships are reestablished and maintained with a precise restoration of the pre-existing dental occlusion. The form of the face is restored in three-dimensional space (i.e., width, anteroposterior projection, and vertical height). The soft tissue drape of the face must be supported in its pre-injury location before scar development and maturation lead to soft tissue shrinkage. It is the secondary alteration in the character of soft tissues that so often frustrates secondary attempts to correct posttraumatic deformity. Primary repair represents the best opportunity to restore form and function.

Achieving these goals requires appropriate surgical access to, and exposure of, the craniofacial skeleton. All fractures are exposed directly, allowing accurate assessment of the degree of bony comminution and displacement. Failure to achieve direct visualization of all fractures and bone segments is a common reason for persistent deformity.[15] This problem particularly applies in the orbital and nasoethmoidal regions, where procedures are performed through small incisions in patients who have a comminuted fracture pattern.

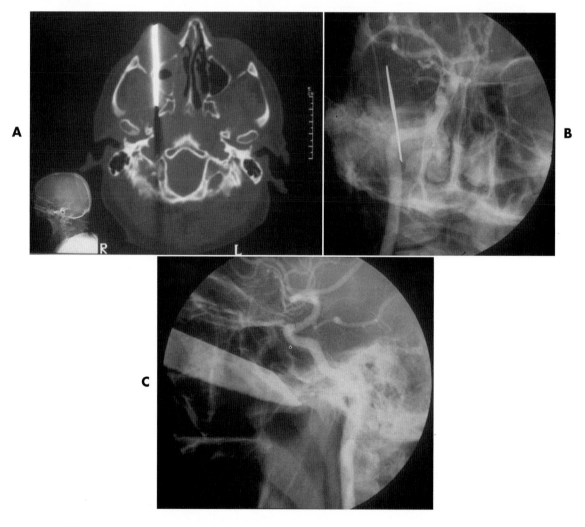

FIGURE 14-6 **A,** Patient with knife in face. It is not possible to see the relationship to vessels from plain views. Angiography helps determine these relationships (**B** and **C**).

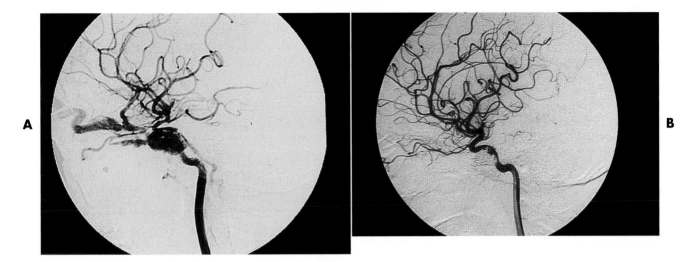

FIGURE 14-7 **A** and **B,** A traumatic caroticocavernous fistula managed with embolization.

Comminuted fractures in this region are an indication for the wider exposure afforded by a coronal flap, usually in combination with a lower eyelid access incision. Once the fracture anatomy is visualized, reduction and internal fixation are performed, linking unstable segments to adjacent stable areas of the craniofacial skeleton. Severely damaged areas with comminution represent areas of effective bone loss and are replaced with primary bone grafting, restoring support and contour. Only in the presence of a heavily contaminated or infected wound is primary bone grafting omitted and recourse made to delayed grafting techniques. The results are not as favorable when there is delay in grafting because of the effects of fibrosis and tissue shrinkage.

If elements of the bony skeleton and soft tissue are absent, primary bone grafting and, on occasion, flap repair are indicated; no attempt should be made to reduce the size of the defects by accepting a less than anatomical reduction. Advancement of local tissues across areas of loss creates secondary deformity that may be irreversible. Skin or mucosal loss should, in general, be managed with grafting, or occasionally with free tissue transfer, in the primary treatment phase.[16] Absolute or effective bone loss is similarly managed with bone-grafting techniques. In the case of composite tissue loss, a composite free flap primary repair may be indicated. The overriding principle is to restore and maintain spatial relationships.

An inevitable consequence of the surgical exposure required to effect precise reduction and stabilization of the facial skeleton is that the overlying soft tissue drape is detached. Often, although good restoration of skeletal form is produced, the results are compromised because of failure to restore the correct relationship of the soft tissues to the underlying facial skeleton.[17] This applies particularly to the orbital region. The medial canthal tendon is an obvious problem area, although complete bone detachment is quite rare. However, wide exposure means that the lateral canthus is also inferiorly displaced on occasion and requires reattachment at its normal location, 2 mm cephalad and posterior to its medial counterpart.

An important superficial muscular aponeurotic system supporting adhesion exists around the orbital rim. In addition, a series of the muscles of facial expression (zygomaticus major, zygomaticus minor, levator labii superioris, levator labii alaeque nasi) arise from the periosteum in the infraorbital region. Detachment of periosteum in this area allows its descent along with the origin of these muscles of facial expression. Unless this is reattached, thinning in the infraorbital region is seen, with a corresponding fullness of the nasolabial fold. This may also contribute to the lower eyelid retraction and scleral show sometimes seen after fixation of fractures of the infraorbital rim via a lower eyelid approach.

In the temporal region, a further system of adhesions exists supporting the superficial musculo-aponeurotic system (SMAS). Loss of support and descent of the SMAS may contribute to, and accentuate, the temporal hollowing seen after coronal flap access to the upper and midface skeleton. It is probable, however, that much of this hollowing is a consequence of ischemic atrophy of the fat pad that lies between the leaves of deep temporal fascia above the zygomatic arch. This fat is perfused by the middle temporal artery, a branch of the superficial temporal artery, which is susceptible to injury during dissection to expose the zygomatic arch.

Management of the soft tissue drape after treatment of facial fractures has received insufficient attention in the literature, with some notable exceptions.[17] We do not have clear answers to all of these soft tissue drape problems but seek here to give them their deserved attention and to describe some practical solutions we have adopted in attempting to restore proper facial soft tissue support.

KEY POINTS
- Restore and maintain spatial relationships
- Replace missing and severely damaged (comminuted) bone segments
- Replace missing soft tissue cover
- Restore the correct relationship of the soft tissue drape to the underlying facial skeleton

TIMING

Procedures performed at admission are confined to those that are life-saving. The maxillofacial surgeon may be called on to provide a surgical airway or to arrest hemorrhage. Thereafter, once the patient is under observation and stable, an individual plan is drawn up.

Patients typically fall into two broad groups: (1) those whose injuries at initial presentation require a definitive airway, usually an orotracheal airway, and who are therefore on an intensive care unit, intubated and ventilated, and (2) those whose facial injuries are such that the airway is not threatened.

In both groups, the upper and middle facial injuries usually result in considerable swelling of the face, and we believe that it is advantageous to allow this swelling to settle before definitive repair of the underlying bony injury is undertaken. This generally involves a planned delay in definitive treatment of 5 to 10 days, mostly determined by the reduction of swelling and the availablity of the required operating room time. Depending on the age of the patient, definitive treatment can be delayed for up to 2 weeks without substantially compromising outcome, but these delayed procedures present greater technical difficulty in achieving adequate reduction and fixation. Beyond 2 weeks, progressive difficulty is encountered, at least in part, because of the accelerated callus formation seen in head-injured patients. Furthermore, beyond 7 days, internal healing and fibrosis, in the setting of malpositioned skeletal support, prevents a natural redraping of the mimetic soft tissues of the face. In our practice, the most common reason for a longer delay is an accompanying brain injury.

In the first group, there are a number of reasons why prolonged intubation may be undesirable. In particular, it may delay the assessment of a head injury or clinical assessment of the cervical spine. In such cases, consideration must be given to whether the orotracheal tube can be safely removed or whether a surgical airway should be secured.

If there is a mandibular fracture, consideration should be given to staging the overall management, with the mandibular fracture being addressed first (within 24-48 hours after injury). If the mandible has condylar fractures, these should also be addressed, and care must be taken not to increase the mandibular width when fixing the fractures. If there is a palatal or maxillary dentoalveolar fracture, a helpful guide to reduction of the mandible is lost. In such instances, one can either decide to address these fractures at the same time to reestablish the maxillary arch width and thereby help with establishing the correct mandibular width when the mandible is reduced and fixed, or one can undertake the best anatomical reduction of the mandible that is possible at this time to stabilize it, being mindful that at the next proceedure (to fix the rest of the fractures) a review of the mandibular reduction may be required.

The use of dental study models (casts) and appropriately segmented and custom-made arch bars, can be invaluable, particularly in establishing the maxillary and mandibular width.

If there is no mandibular injury and no imperative to reduce the sedation early, then procedures undertaken in the first 24 to 48 hours are limited to débridement of wounds with excision of necrotic tissue and closure of wounds that involve no tissue loss. On occasion, the soft tissue injuries provide the obvious means of access to reduce and fix the underlying facial fractures (Fig. 14-8). If this is the case, a balanced decision must be made whether it is best to reduce and fix the midfacial fractures (in the presence of any

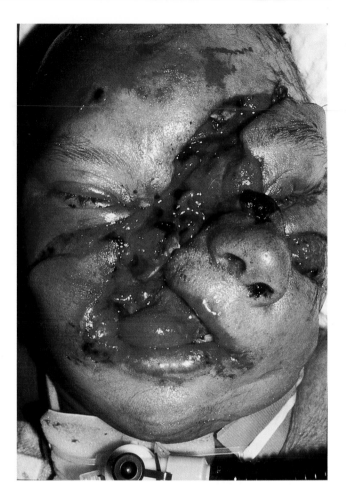

FIGURE 14-8 Soft tissue injuries may provide direct access to management of underlying fractures.

swelling) and close the soft tissue wounds early, accepting the difficulty the swelling may present to accurate fracture reduction, or whether it is better to close the soft tissues injuries early without reducing the fractures and then selectively reopen them for access to underlying fractures when the swelling has resolved.

In all cases, the opportunity is taken to perform a thorough examination with the patient under anesthesia. Impressions for dental models can be obtained. Second- and third-look procedures and appropriate débridement are indicated if there has been massive tissue injury with necrosis and if marginally viable tissue is present.

AIRWAY MANAGEMENT

In panfacial fractures, if unrestricted access is required to the middle and lower face, a surgical airway is our usual practice. Submental intubation provides an alternative route to tracheostomy if the period of ventilatory support is likely to be short[18] (Fig. 14-9). If an ACF repair is to be performed, a surgical airway is usually indicated. This reduces the potential for development of a cranial aerocele associated with coughing in the early postoperative period.

In maxillary fractures with no skull base involvement, we have found that nasotracheal intubation allows adequate access. However, if the upper midface is involved and a

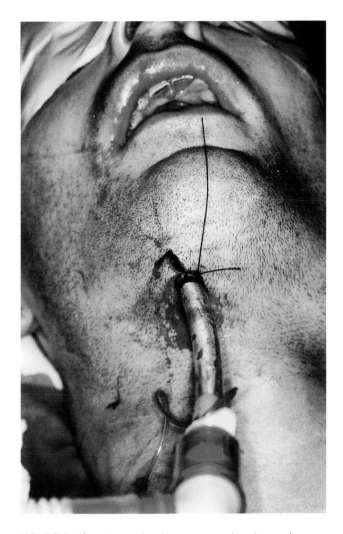

FIGURE 14-9 Submental intubation is a simple technique that gives unimpeded access to the facial region. It is a useful alternative to tracheostomy if it is envisaged that airway support will be required for a short duration.

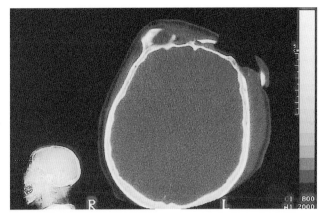

FIGURE 14-10 Despite extensive disruption of the anterior frontal sinus wall, the force transferred in this injury was dissipated in disrupting the well-pneumatized frontal sinus, leaving the posterior wall intact.

However, detachment of the soft tissue drape, particularly the periosteum, from the facial skeleton has secondary consequences, as outlined earlier. Exposure commensurate with visualization and accurate reduction and fixation are required, but no more than that. If the periosteum can be left attached, it should be, maintaining the correct spatial relationship between the facial skeleton and overlying mimetic soft tissues in at least a few points. This is likely to greatly facilitate accurate and secure repositioning of intervening areas of detachment. Our preferred adjective to describe access and exposure is *appropriate* rather than *wide*.

> KEY POINTS
> - Consider degree of comminution as well as site of fractures in planning access
> - Leave soft tissue drape attached to craniofacial skeleton where possible

coronal flap is indicated, either submental intubation or tracheostomy is recommended to ensure a safe and unencumbered procedure.

ACCESS

Some time ago Manson et al.[17] divided the facial skeleton into anterior and posterior areas from the viewpoint of access requirements. Low-level midfacial fractures, pyramidal fractures, and fractures of the horizontal body of the mandible may be approached via the buccal sulcus and small cutaneous incisions, provided there are no more than one or two large fragments. The presence of multiple fractures at a higher level, comminution of facial subunits, or fractures of the condylar process of the mandible necessitate posterior access incisions, usually a coronal flap, the latter is not commonly used these days for condylar access. The essential point is that not only the location but also the severity of the injury must be considered in planning access. Greater fragmentation implies greater difficulty in achieving adequate stability, necessitating better fixation, with or without bone grafting, and therefore wider exposure.

SURGICAL ANATOMY OF THE FACIAL SKELETON

The face may conceptually be divided into three zones or subunits with different purposes. The upper subunit is composed of the frontal bone; its principal purpose is protection of the frontal lobes of the brain, but it also forms the roof of the orbit and encloses the cribriform plate of the ethmoid, subserving the special sense of olfaction. It contains the frontal sinus, whose extent varies from individual to individual, with a trend toward increasing pneumatization with age.

Sufficient force directed over the frontonasal region produces a central fracture with fracture lines that may involve the frontomaxillary and the weak frontoethmoid vomerine buttress. If the frontal sinus is large, it absorbs a large proportion of the force, and the posterior wall may remain intact without dural exposure or injury (Fig. 14-10). With small linear cracks in the posterior wall of the frontal sinus, the dura may remain intact, but with greater disruption dural tears occur, leading to CSF rhinorrhea. The significance of injury to the nasofrontal tract in patients who have sustained frontal sinus trauma has been recognized.[19]

If the frontal sinus is rudimentary or the fracture extends beyond the sinus, large segmental fractures can occur, involving the orbital roof and floor of the ACF (Fig. 14-11). These may extend across the sphenoid ridge and, in so doing, jeopardize the internal carotid arteries and the optic nerve, the latter lying within the confined space of the optic canal (Fig. 14-12). It may be safer to expose the ACF before disimpacting the maxilla under such circumstances. Laterally, extensive fractures involving the frontal bone, greater wing of the sphenoid, and the temporal and parietal bones present the potential for injury to the middle meningeal artery. If there is displacement of bony segments in this region, neurosurgical colleagues must be consulted. Mobilization of depressed fractures of the zygomatic complex under such circumstances should also be performed with direct visualization through a coronal flap and in an institution with neurosurgeons present and available in the event of intracranial complications.

The middle subunit of the face has a very different structure, characterized by areas of lower structural integrity and enclosure within a bony framework of supportive pillars or struts. Gruss and Mackinnon[20] made an important conceptual advance in the mid-1980s when they described the vertical supportive pillars of the midface: the paired frontonasal maxillary pillars anteromedially, the zygomaticomaxillary pillars laterally, and the pterygoid processes posteriorly. In individuals with fully developed sinuses, these pillars are relatively weak in the midface superior to the alveolar process of the maxillae. It is unfortunate for the surgeon undertaking repair of midfacial fractures that the most robust of these supportive pillars, the pterygoid plates, are inaccessible for direct operative repair.

Later authors described horizontal facial buttresses. Superiorly, the frontal bar of the upper facial subunit is included. Inferiorly, the horizontal buttress is described as comprising the maxillary alveolus and palatal processes with a contribution from the horizontal process of the palatine bone. The middle horizontal buttress is composed of the zygomatic arches, the body of the zygomatic bones, and the infraorbital

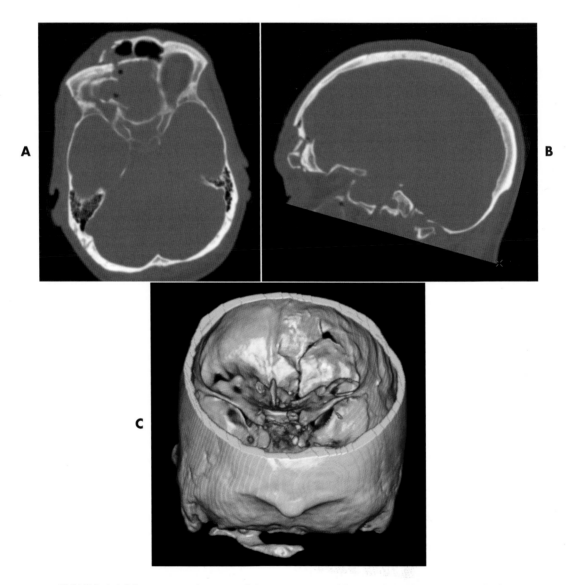

FIGURE 14-11 Extensive disruption of the anterior cranial fossa includes the posterior wall of the frontal sinus. Air is seen within the anterior cranial fossa.

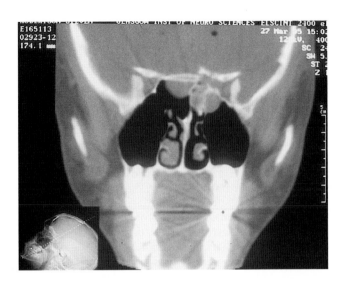

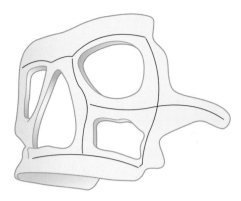

FIGURE 14-14 Model depicts the horizontal and vertical lines of elective osteosynthesis for the midface. The bone is thicker at these sites. *(Courtesy of R. Schmelzeisen, Professor and Medical Director, Department of Maxillofacial and Oral Surgery, Albert-Ludwigs-University, Freiburg, Germany.)*

FIGURE 14-12 Fracture extending across the sphenoid ridge. Such fractures jeopardize the optic nerve and internal carotid artery.

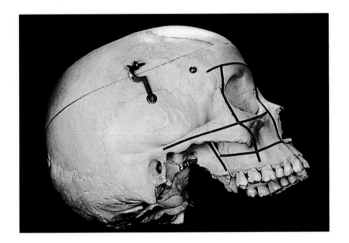

FIGURE 14-13 The vertical and horizontal buttresses of the midface define the lines of elective osteosynthesis. Notice the absence of a sagittal buttress between the palate and the frontal bar in the central midface.

The mandible forms the skeletal structure of the lower face. Its surgical anatomy is described elsewhere in this text. It has good structural integrity as a consequence of its functional role and well-developed associated musculature. The specific problem presented by mandibular fractures in association with midfacial injuries lies with its importance in reestablishing correct facial width. Difficulties commonly arise with fracture patterns that occur in the symphysis and parasymphyseal region, particularly those associated with fractures of the condylar process. Force delivered from an anterior direction produces retrodisplacement of the mandible as it fractures, with widening at the mandibular angles. Displacement is maintained by insertion of the suprahyoid musculature into the symphyseal region of the mandible, which also places torsional forces on the fracture segments[15] (Fig. 14-15).

When there is a corresponding sagittal fracture of the maxilla or an absence of teeth, guides to the reestablishment of facial width are lost, and an operative strategy designed to overcome this difficulty must be planned.

rim. These transversely oriented supportive elements link the zygomaticomaxillary processes and the nasomaxillary processes[17,21] (Fig. 14-13). This conceptual model has value because it marks important horizontal and vertical lines of elective osteosynthesis in repair of the facial skeleton (Fig. 14-14). In reality, surgeons naturally opt for these thicker bony struts for osteosynthesis, because outside of these areas, the bone is too thin for adequate fixation of the plates.

Manson et al. made the point that what is notably absent is a robust sagittal supportive pillar in the central part of the face extending from posterior to anterior.[17] The septovomerine complex is weak. The lateral wall of the nose between the perpendicular processes of the palatine bone and the nasomaxillary processes has very little structural integrity. Central midface collapse is therefore a common consequence of severe midfacial injury and requires specific attention if successful repair is to be achieved.

KEY POINTS AND PITFALLS
- Principle of subunit reconstruction
- Horizontal and vertical buttresses mark sites of elective osteosynthesis in the midface
- Bone grafting may be required in the relatively weak midface
- Lack of a central midface sagittal buttress explains the frequent occurrence midface collapse after severe injury
- Excessive width and corresponding lack of anteroposterior projection are common errors in the repair of midface fractures

SEQUENCE OF OPERATIVE REPAIR IN PANFACIAL INJURIES

Manson et al. described panfacial fractures as comprising two facial halves separated by a fracture at the Le Fort I level. The lower facial half was further divided into an upper occlusal level, comprising the maxillary and mandibular alveolar processes with their associated teeth as well as the palate, and a lower unit comprising the vertical ramus and horizontal basal

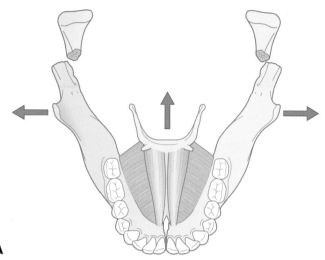

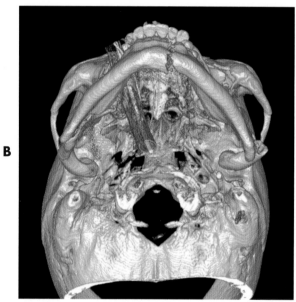

FIGURE 14-15 **A** and **B,** Fractures involving the symphysis and the condylar regions of the mandible frequently result in an increase in facial width with decreased anterior projection. This position is maintained by the pull of the suprahyoid musculature.

mandible. The upper facial half was divided into an upper unit, comprising the frontal bone with its supraorbital ridges and roof of orbits, and a midfacial unit[17] (Fig. 14-16). This model has descriptive utility and is employed here.

Our preferred definitve operative sequence is to commence with management of the lower facial half. (In some cases, a mandibular component to the injury may have already been treated.) The occlusal subunit is first reconstituted. This is an important determinant of lower facial width. Sagittal fractures of the maxilla, in association with mandibular fractures, result in loss of all reference points for reestablishment of the correct width and therefore of anterior projection in the lower face (Fig. 14-17). Standard techniques rely on establishment of a seemingly correct dental occlusion, followed by fixation of mandibular fractures, to which the upper facial repair is related. This approach not infrequently results in decreased anterior projection and increased lower

facial width. Manson's group found that split palate fractures accompany 8% of midface fractures.[22] However, the incidence of sagittal fractures is greater when midface fractures are a consequence of motor vehicle accidents, as high as 20% to 25%.

Rowe and Killey[1] pointed out that gross separation of the maxilla must result in associated fractures of the zygomatico-orbital complex, an observation subsequently demonstrated to be generally correct.[23] Denny and Celik studied the distribution of sagittal fractures of the maxilla in a series of patients and found about 15% to be comprised of dentoalveolar fractures, with the remainder involving the palatal vault.[24] These were equally distributed between true sagittal and parasagittal fractures. Manson et al. stated that, although sagittal fractures occur in younger individuals, parasagittal fractures are preponderant in adults.[25] The palatal suture is structurally akin to the cranial sutures. Persson and Thilender[26] found synostosis of the palatal suture to occur between 15 and 19 years of age, firmly uniting the lateral palatal segments and making parasagittal fracture, in the thinner bone at this site, more probable with advancing years. A lip laceration extending into the gingivobuccal sulcus, accompanied by tooth loss, is strongly suggestive of sagittal fracture of the maxilla. A mucosa tear in the palate is sometimes seen. However, sagittal fractures may be present in the absence of any of these signs. Careful palpation for such injury and scrutiny of axial and coronal CTs is necessary, because this is an important diagnosis to make in correctly reestablishing facial width.[22]

Manson and others have advocated direct exposure of the palatal fracture via a longitudinal incision and limited subperiosteal exposure of the palatal shelves.[22,25] Reduction by the application of lateral arch pressure followed by plate and screw fixation in the palate reestablishes facial width but does not necessarily prevent incorrect angulation of segments. Further plate fixation across the fracture at the anterior alveolus decreases the likelihood of improper angulation or malrotation of segments.

Dentoalveolar segment fractures can greatly complicate treatment and require precise methods of fixation. It is our opinion that the best results are achieved with bony fixation of the dentoalveolar segments, if possible, and use of an acrylic occlusal splint that has sufficient palatal coverage to control angulation of the dentoalveolar segments and yet allow buccal inspection of occlusal relationships. Except with difficult dentoalveolar fractures, we prefer to avoid any intervening wafer and to establish dental intercuspation by direct examination. This allows the identification of small but important occlusal discrepancies that indicate imperfect fracture reduction.

The use of wire intermaxillary fixation using Erich or custom-made arch bars is our standard practice. Before placement in intermaxillary fixation, mobilization of the maxilla should be achieved. However, if a skull base fracture exists and an ACF repair is indicated, mobilization of the maxilla should be deferred until this can be performed with the anterior fossa floor under direct vision. Adequate maxillary mobilization is important. Failure to obtain adequate mobilization and correction of the posterior maxillary lengthening before fixation invites relapse into an anterior open bite on release of intermaxillary fixation.

After the arch width, and therefore the anterior projection at the occlusal level, has been established, fractures of the

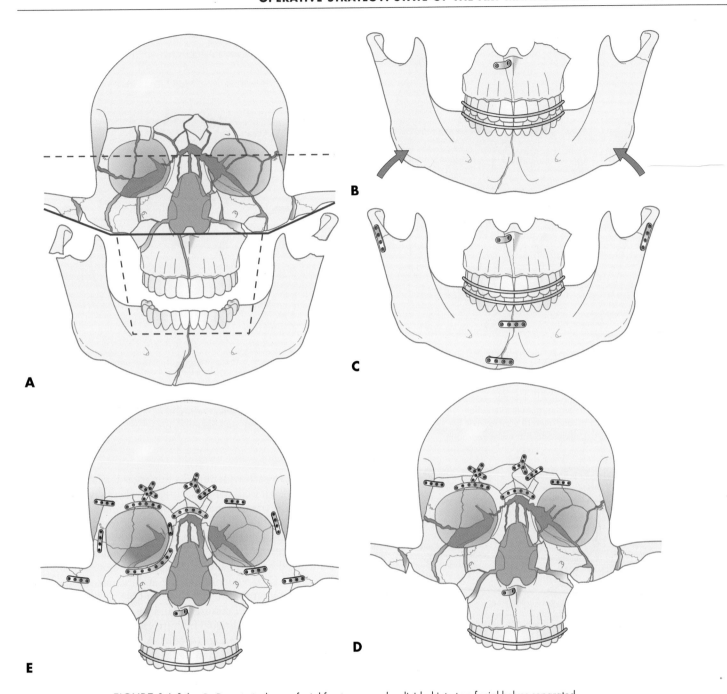

FIGURE 14-16 **A,** Descriptively, panfacial fractures may be divided into two facial halves separated by a fracture at the Le Fort I level. The upper facial half is subdivided into an upper unit comprising the frontal bone and a midfacial unit. The lower facial half is subdivided into an occlusal unit and a lower basal unit. **B,** Establish facial width at the occlusal level. Sagittal fractures of the maxilla and mandibular fractures with splaying of the vertical rami lead to errors with excessive width and deficient anterior projection. Pressure should be applied to the gonial angles to close any lingual gap in the anterior mandible. A useful guide to the correct reduction is the point at which the anterior fracture just starts to open on its labial or buccal surface. At that point, the lingual cortex is acting as a fulcrum. **C,** Fixation of the mandibular condyles, when feasible, helps to prevent excessive width and to restore posterior facial height. **D,** Reassembly of the upper facial subunit precedes midface repair. **E,** Start midface repair at the least injured part of the orbits, and use all visual clues to establish the correct anterior projection.

Continued

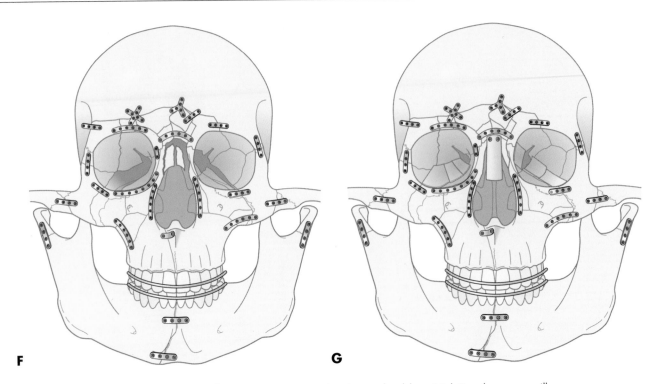

F   **G**

FIGURE 14-16, cont'd   **F,** Buttress reconstruction is completed by miniplating the nasomaxillary and zygomaticomaxillary vertical buttresses. **G,** Volumetric orbital reconstruction, nasal bone grafting, and medial canthopexy are performed, if necessary, before inset of any pericranial or galeofrontalis flap and soft tissue redraping.

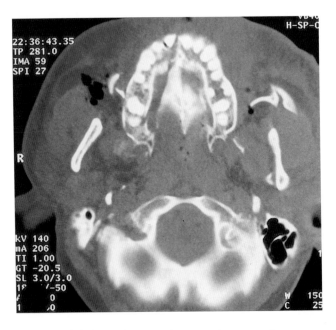

FIGURE 14-17   Axial computed tomographic image of a parasagittal fracture of the palate in a patient with panfacial trauma.

mandible are fixed. The management of mandibular fractures is discussed elsewhere in this text. Here, we confine our comments to the particular problem of low face width and posterior facial height in patients with panfacial trauma. Consideration of the fracture pattern and examination of the mandibular arch form should make it possible to predict any tendency to arch widening. In this regard, a lateral crossbite should be viewed with the greatest skepticism. As stated earlier, the fracture pattern most commonly resulting in increased width is that which involves the symphyseal or parasymphyseal region, especially when fractures of the condylar process are present[27] (Fig. 14-18). Under such circumstances, all fractures should be exposed before any are fixed. If there is clear widening of the arch, it may be helpful to expose the lingual cortex of the mandible via an upper cervical skin incision. Pressure should be applied at the gonial angles to close any lingual fracture gap occurring in the body of the mandible (see Fig. 14-16B). A small lingual gap in the symphyseal region is magnified at the gonial angles and must be closed if the lower facial width is to be reestablished and the correct anterior projection achieved.

Before fixation of fractures of the body, it is prudent to examine any condylar fracture to ensure fragment alignment; it may be that fixation of the condylar fractures is required before fixation of body fractures. However, treatment of condylar fractures is not always feasible. As the energy imparted in fracturing the mandible increases, the location of fractures has a tendency to move from a predominance of subcondylar fractures to more superior locations in the neck and intraarticular region;[28] for this reason, intracapsular fractures are not uncommon in patients with panfacial injuries. The loss of height that occurs with such injuries is usually less than with fracture dislocations occurring in the condylar neck; this injury pattern also occurs in higher-energy trauma but can and should be treated by open reduction and internal fixation. If a coronal flap is indicated for treatment of fractures of the middle and upper face, detachment of the masseter insertion along the zygomatic arch provides good access to

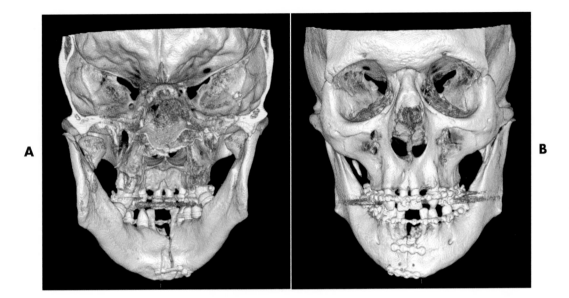

FIGURE 14-18 **A** and **B,** This patient sustained a parasymphyseal fracture as well as high condylar fractures of the mandible. Open reduction and fixation of the mandibular symphysis without due consideration to the condylar injuries resulted in a mandible with excessive width posteriorly, inadequate projection in an anteroposterior plane, and reduced height in the posterior face. This is a common error in fractures of this pattern.

the condylar process of the mandible. In the absence of a coronal flap, our currently preferred approach to the condyle is through a retromandibular incision and transparotid dissection.

Fixation of condylar process fractures is important in reestablishing posterior facial height and preventing subsequent anterior open bite deformity. It indirectly helps establish midfacial height by correctly orienting the occlusal and, therefore, the maxillary plane angle in relation to the skull base (see Fig. 14-16C). In the case of intracapsular condylar fractures with collapse, less precise clues to the correct maxillary and mandibular plane angle must be relied on. The reassembly of midfacial fragments that provides the basis for correct orientation under such circumstances is prone to error in angulation even when there has been no loss of bone segments.

MANAGEMENT OF THE UPPER FACIAL UNIT

Injuries to the frontal bone, the frontal sinus, and the ACF often require, and benefit from, the cooperation of neurosurgical and craniofacial surgeons in a multidisciplinary team. The balance between the neurosurgical concerns of the patient with a brain injury and the need to treat facial injuries often raises issues that can be resolved with close cooperation and communication between the neurosurgical and craniofacial teams. The neurosurgical needs of the patient have to take priority, because the importance of minimizing injury to the brain outweighs the improved outcome that follows early repair of craniofacial fractures. The neurological outcome may be adversely affected by brain retraction in the early stages of an evolving head injury. It is primarily for this reason that we prefer a delayed approach (5-10 days) to the repair of craniofacial injuries.

Anterior fossa fractures are often complex, and they do not follow stereotypical patterns. The anterior fossa floor may be

significantly disrupted with no other fractures more superficial to the area. Imaging should be in three planes (axial, coronal, and sagittal). It is also useful to use multiplanar reconstructions on the CT workstation to view, and fully appreciate, the three-dimensional nature of the fractures. It should also be remembered that, even with the most advanced scanners, all fractures may not be apparent due to the overlapping of thin bone fragments and data interpolation.

If an ACF repair is indicated, access to the ACF through a frontal craniotomy is followed by dural repair. Fractures involving the orbital roof may be impacted and should be reduced under direct vision. If fractures of the ACF extend to the sphenoid ridge, it may be safer to perform an osteotomy and advance the frontal bar into the correct position, leaving posterior fractures unreduced, and to graft resulting defects in the orbital roof with split calvarial bone.

The anterior skull vault is not subjected to muscular forces, and stable fixation is readily achieved with small (1-mm) plating systems. These have the advantage of more readily providing the correct contour when comminution has occurred. Fixation plates should be placed in a transverse plane whenever possible. This orientation facilitates their removal, should it become necessary, via a local incision parallel to the relaxed skin tension lines.

The management of frontal sinus injuries is an important issue and remains the subject of some controversy. The frontal sinus drains via the short frontonasal duct into the anterior end of the hiatus semilunaris of the middle meatus in the lateral wall of the nose or directly into the anterior ethmoid air cells,. This has led to the term frontonasal *outflow tract*, rather than *duct*, to describe the drainage of the frontal sinus. Outflow obstruction is almost always seen in cases in which postoperative complications develop. Obstruction can lead to entrapment of mucus with chronic infection. The frontal sinus mucosa may then develop mucus retention cysts. By an unknown mechanism, mucoceles erode adjacent bone and may extend intracranially or into the orbit. If the mucoid contents of the cyst become infected, a mucopyocele results. Mucopyocele formation may lead to orbital or cranial abscess formation, orbital cellulitis, meningitis, or osteomyelitis of the frontal bone. These complications can occur many years after the initial repair, and it is this long-term risk that makes obtaining satisfactory data so difficult.

Most reports have described this complication in small numbers of trauma cases, and there have been no comparative trials. Stanwix et al.[29] have recently reported 30 years' experience with frontal sinus fractures and highlighted the importance of assessment of the frontonasal outflow tract. In particular, they demonstrated that nasofrontal tract injury, and especially obstruction, is almost always evident in patients who develop complications from frontal sinus fracture. They developed an algorithm for the management of frontal sinus fractures. Treatment modalities include observation, reconstruction, or cranialization and obliteration, depending on the status of the outflow tract.

A number of authors have recommended frontonasal duct and frontal sinus obliteration when fractures involve the frontal sinus. Abdominal fat, temporalis muscle, and bone graft have been recommended for this purpose. The danger of using fat in the presence of comminuted or missing sinus walls was emphasized in an animal experimental model,[30] and there is no reason to believe that nonviable muscle would pose any less risk. Furthermore, before obliteration, all sinus mucosa must be removed by thorough curettage and bur obliteration. This represents a considerable undertaking in a well-pneumatized frontal bone, in which the sinus may extend posteriorly almost to the lesser wing of sphenoid and laterally to the zygomatic processes of the frontal bone. The posterior wall is thin, and dural injury a risk. Filling of the resultant defect with bone graft requires a large amount of what is a valuable commodity in panfacial trauma.

Our experience is in accordance with that of Gruss et al.[31] If ACF repair is required, cranialization of the frontal sinus should be performed. The posterior or cranial wall of the frontal sinus is burred away in its entirety, and the sinus mucosa is curetted and burred, ensuring thorough removal. The frontonasal outflow is identified inferomedially and obliterated with bone graft with subsequent placement of a pericranial or galeofrontalis flap inset to seal the ACF from the nasal cavity below (Fig. 14-19). If injury is limited to the anterior wall of the frontal sinus without dural involvement, no attempt is made at sinus obliteration. Gruss et al.[31] stated that:

> …when bone is securely reduced and grafts rigidly applied … when non delayed debridement is accomplished, the chance of mucocoele formation is minimal. The premise that the naso-frontal duct will resume function in a majority of patients appears legitimate. Early intervention and reconstruction are hallmarks of this approach. The presence of improperly reduced bone segments, comminuted sequestra, foreign bodies, and torn mucosal shreds leave the patient susceptible to the development of mucopyocoele.

If the anterior wall of the sinus and nasoethmoidal region are comminuted, stenting of the nasofrontal ducts for 4 weeks with Silastic tubing (a portion of nasogastric tube is suitable)

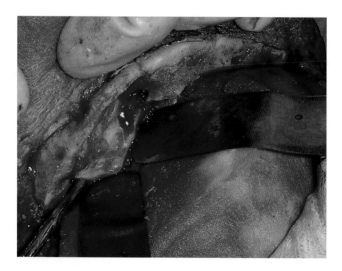

FIGURE 14-19 When an anterior cranial fossa repair is planned, due consideration must be given to the requirement for a pericranial or galeofrontalis flap inset to seal the floor of the anterior fossa. Such thin flaps are readily introduced through the craniotome cut at the inferior edge of the frontal bone flap. This slide shows removal of the posterior wall. *(Courtesy of Robert Bentley, Kings College Hospital, London.)*

seems prudent. These can be inserted through the anterior wall defect before reconstitution and brought out through the external nares, to which they are secured.

After débridement, the anterior wall is reconstructed by reassembly of bone fragments with bone grafting where necessary (see Fig. 14-16D). It is often necessary to map and mark the fragments to allow reassembly (Fig. 14-20). If a map is not used, it is surprisingly difficult and time-consuming to piece the pieces back together correctly, even when there are only a few. On occasion, bone deformation occurs prior to fracture; under such circumstances, a perfect reduction cannot be achieved.

Inadequate reduction in the supraorbital ridge is a potential problem and leads to flattening with inadequate anterior projection (Fig. 14-21). Comminution of the supraorbital ridge may require primary bone grafting to prevent this occurrence, especially when major segments are displaced and ACF repair is not judged to be indicated. Onlay bone grafting is indicated; this allows restoration of an even contour with a symmetrical anterior projection.

Reconstruction of the orbital rim and roof can also be problematic when comminution is present. Exophthalmos and downward displacement of the globe, which is very difficult to safely correct secondarily, may occur. Care must be exercised in contouring the orbital rim and ensuring that the reconstructed roof of the orbit is approximately 3 mm cephalad to the rim where it lies above the globe. This can be satisfactorily achieved only from above with exposure of the ACF. Failure to reconstruct the orbital roof when there is a large bony dehiscence risks development of a pulsating exophthalmos.

If ACF repair is required, insetting of the pericranial or galeofrontalis flap and fixation of the frontal bone flap is deferred until midface repair is complete. This maintains unimpeded access.

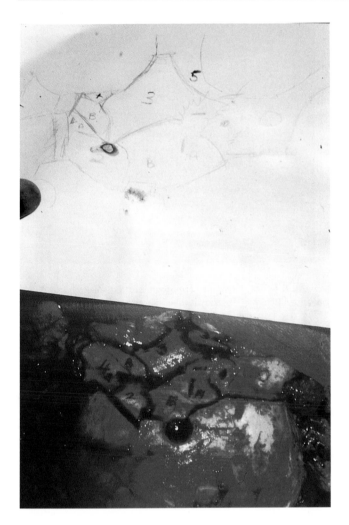

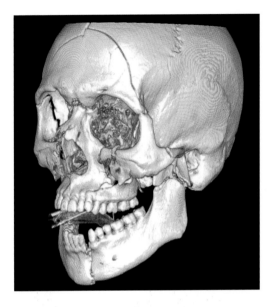

FIGURE 14-22 An intact greater wing of sphenoid can be a guide to correct reduction of the fracture at this level.

FIGURE 14-20 Before removal of frontal bone fragments, a map is constructed of the constituent pieces. This greatly facilitates reassembly.

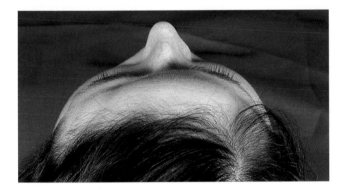

FIGURE 14-21 Posttraumatic recession or flattening of the supraorbital region.

MIDFACE FRACTURES

In the midface, zygomatico-orbital and nasoethmoidal reconstruction that reestablishes the correct width and anterior projection in relation to a stable frontal bar follows from fixation of the upper face (see Fig. 14-16E). Finally, with a stable upper midface, the occlusal unit is fixed in the

anterior vertical buttress regions at the appropriate height (see Fig. 14-16F).

The midface presents several major reconstructive difficulties after severe facial trauma. Comminution of this delicate structure is the rule rather than the exception in panfacial injury. The greater the comminution, the more difficult it becomes to achieve adequate stability, even in the presence of precise reduction and fixation of individual fragments. Furthermore, errors of a few millimeters in restoring orbital volume and configuration, canthal reattachment, and occlusal relationships are noticeable and often difficult to correct with secondary procedures. A wide midface with collapse in an anteroposterior plane, enophthalmos, and traumatic telecanthus were common sequelae of management with closed techniques in a former era and continue to frustrate contemporary efforts. As elsewhere in the facial skeleton, a complete diagnosis and planning of an operative strategy, bearing in mind common errors, maximize the likelihood of a satisfactory outcome.

On the basis of preoperative imaging and intraoperative findings, the least injured part of the orbital region is identified, and repair of the midfacial skeleton commences at that point. A successful approach has been to identify an intact greater wing of sphenoid in the lateral orbit (Fig. 14-22). If not fractured, this robust structure gives a good indication of the correct angulation and therefore the width and anterior projection of the lateral midface. Gruss[15] prefers to rely on the zygomatic arches and to commence reconstruction at that point. Our experience has been more in accordance with that of Manson et al.,[17] who have found few clues to the correct lateral projection of the zygomatic arch. A common error is to overreduce laterally, which results in an increased facial width and inadequate anterior projection.

If the greater wing of sphenoid is fractured and the zygomatic arch is used as the key to the lateral facial reconstruction, it is important to recall that the zygomatic arch has a straight sagittal orientation between the zygomatic process of the temporal bone and the zygomatic prominence. A temporary wire placed at the frontozygomatic suture establishes vertical height in this region and allows manipulation in the transverse and anteroposterior planes. The zygomatic arch is a muscular process that is the origin of the masseter muscle. It is subject to significant functional stress and is not, of itself, robust. Displacement with loss of anterior projection after initial good reduction of fixation has been described. We routinely fix this region with a 1.5-mm plate and screw system in adults, believing that lighter fixation provides insufficient stability.

Fixation of the medial orbital region takes as its reference the nasal process of the frontal bone, reconstituted or uninjured. The frontal process of the maxilla is the key structure in this region, because this forms a substantial part of the important frontonasomaxillary vertical buttress. Establishing the correct transnasal width of this structure, and therefore restoring anterior projection to the nasal pyramid, is problematic. Common errors in the naso-orbitoethmoid region are increased width and collapse in an anteroposterior plane and malposition of medial canthal tendons. Although the height of the fractured frontal process of the maxilla usually can be readily established if it is not comminuted, the orientation of this structure in all other planes is difficult because the nasal bones and inferior orbital rim are frequently fragmented. Therefore, reduction of the frontal process of the maxilla where it meets the frontal bone is frequently associated with significant angular errors. All visual clues must be used to achieve its correct orientation. Fixation of the frontal process of the maxilla at the glabella is followed by reassembly of the inferior orbital rim. Every effort should be made to retrieve fragments that have been displaced posteroinferiorly into the maxillary sinus and to ensure that the jigsaw of fragments is reassembled with plate fixation. Visual assessment of the width at the medial canthal level is important at this stage (see Fig. 14-16F).

After the horizontal and vertical buttresses of the upper midface have been reestablished, fixation of the occlusal unit at the correct vertical height is performed with fixation at the zygomaticomaxillary and nasomaxillary vertical buttresses. It is important to consciously seat the mandibular condyles into the glenoid fossae if an anterior open bite dental relationship is to be avoided. To prevent persistent posterior maxillary lengthening, it may be necessary to remove displaced bone fragments in the posterolateral maxilla at the Le Fort I level. At this point, the vertical and horizontal midfacial buttress reconstruction should be complete.

Although diagrammatic representaions show ideal reductions and perfect alignment, in practice perfect reduction at the zygomaticomaxillary and nasomaxillary vertical buttresses and a perfect occlusion rarely are achieved. Some minor discrepancy is to be expected; if such a discrerpancy does exist, it is better to have correct occlusion with a minor discrepancy in the bony alignment at the Le Fort I level than to have an ideal bony alignment at the expense of the occlusion. That said, any discrpancy should be small. A large discrepancy might indicate a signifcant malalignment of the bony reduction above or below the Fort I level (Fig. 14-23).

Next, reconstruction of the medial, lateral, and inferior walls of the orbits is accomplished with the emphasis on precise volumetric reconstruction. This can be undertaken with titanium plates or mesh of various forms or with bone

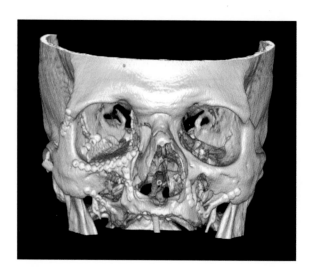

FIGURE 14-23 Computed tomogram of a patient with upper and midfacial fractures. Fixation devices are placed along the midfacial vertical and horizontal buttresses.

grafts. In most cases, the canthus remains attached to a fragment of bone and can be reduced with the use of a small plate via a coronal incision.

Medial canthal tendon reattachment is performed after orbital wall reconstruction. This key soft tissue structure inserts into the anterior lacrimal crest of the frontal process of the maxilla and the posterior lacrimal crest on the lacrimal bone. Treatment is aimed at restoring attachment at the anterior lacrimal crest. Exposure and identification of the medial canthus is required for successful repair of traumatic telecanthus. Attempts to identify and reposition a totally detached medial canthus via a coronal flap have been unsuccessful in correcting telecanthus in our experience and that of others.[17] The medial canthus is readily exposed via a short (4-5 mm) horizontal incision that begins 2 to 3 mm medial to the medial commissure of the palpebral fissure. Dissection through this small wound brings the 2- to 3-mm, white band of fibrous tissue that forms the medial canthal tendon into clear relief. Its attachment to the frontal process of the maxilla, where this is a substantial fragment, should not be disturbed. If comminution exists, however, transnasal canthopexy is indicated.

Common errors in canthal repositioning are twofold: undercorrection in width (which is overcome by direct canthal ligament exposure and wire capture) and fixation of the canthus too far anteriorly, which creates an unnatural appearance of the medial canthus. It is essential to locate the canthus behind the most anterior part of the globe within the orbital rim. This can be achieved by passage of the transnasal canthopexy wire through a cantilevered microplate fixed in the glabellar region. This plate terminates at the desired location for canthal attachment, and the transnasal wire is passed through the vacant screw hole at the end of this plate. The wire then passes across the nasal pyramid and is tied over a toggle (short length of plate) on the contralateral side at the desired canthal width (Fig. 14-24). Subsequent canthal drift is to be anticipated, and overcorrection is desirable. It is probable that this drift is, at least in part, a consequence of delayed bone resorption in the glabellar region. Each canthus is managed independently of its counterpart.

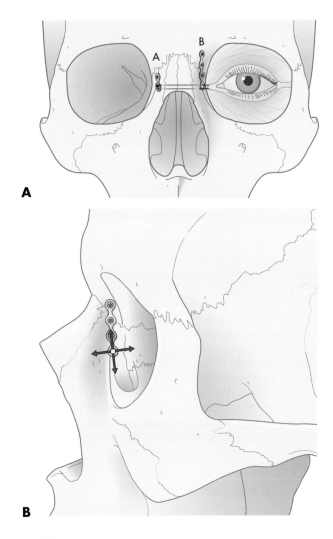

FIGURE 14-24 A, Medial canthopexy. The medial canthus is directly exposed and captured with wire. The wire is passed through the distal hole of a miniplate on the ipsilateral side (positioning plate), passed transnasally, and tied over a toggle plate on the contralateral side of the nasoethmoid complex. A, toggle plate; B, positioning plate. **B,** Medial canthopexy. Once the medial canthus has been captured and the transnasal wire has been placed, the positioning plate is moved into the desired location and fixed with screws in the accessible glabella region. Final tightening over the toggle plate is then performed.

Collapse of the glabellar region is a consequence of two factors. As elsewhere in the face, excessive width leads to inadequate anterior projection; therefore, reducing the width of the bony radix to approximately 20 mm in Caucasians is an important treatment objective. Effective bone loss due to comminution, with subsequent resorption of small fragments, explains both early and delayed inadequate projection of the nasal pyramid when the intercanthal width is satisfactory. Primary bone grafting with split calvaria is indicated if comminution of the nasal bones has occurred. The bone graft is cantilevered with plate or screw fixation to the glabella. Common errors in primary nasal bone grafting are obliteration of the radix, which results in a Greco-Roman nose. Overextension of the bone graft into the nasal tip results

in an unnatural appearance in this region and may lead to graft exposure from ulceration through the skin.

There are difficulties in establishing adequate stability of fixation in the midface. The delicate bone architecture, its fragmentation, and the necessity of using relatively light fixation devices all contribute. As Manson pointed out, the lever principle means that relatively small forces at the occlusal level result in significant deforming influences when the first point of good fixation is the frontal bar.[17]

If significant fragmentation of the midface has occurred, postoperative intermaxillary fixation is a prudent measure during the initial healing phase. Primary bone grafting seems to enhance both initial and subsequent development of midfacial stability after operative repair and is also recommended in the presence of significant bone loss.

It is possible now to assess the bony reduction at this point intraoperatively with the use of mobile CT scanning machines in the operating room. This should not be particularly time-consuming, adding only 10 to 15 minutes to the procedure. Being able to check the position of the bony reconstruction at this point may well improve outcomes and reduce the need for secondary surgery, because any errors that are seen can be corrected immediately.

KEY POINTS AND PITFALLS

- Establish the facial width at the occlusal level.
- Repair of fractured mandibular condyles is important in preventing excessive lower facial width and restoring posterior facial height.
- If the ACF is fractured, defer maxillary mobilization until the anterior fossa has been exposed.
- Cranialize the frontal sinus if ACF repair is performed; otherwise, repair the anterior wall and stent the frontonasal duct.
- Commence midface repair at the least injured part of the orbits.
- The greater wing of sphenoid provides a good guide to zygomatic width and anterior projection if it is uninjured.
- Excessive width and inadequate anterior projection are common errors in naso-orbitoethmoidal repair.
- If there is comminution of the midface, primary bone grafting and intermaxillary fixation enhance stability.

CLOSURE AND SOFT TISSUE DRAPE

Surgical Anatomy

Moss et al.[32] made the point that true ligaments exist in the medial midface (zygomatic and masseteric ligaments) as well as in the lower face (mandibular ligament). These connective tissue condensations comprise a discrete cylindrical attachment of fibrous tissue that arises from either deep fascia or periosteum. They cross the sub-SMAS plane to the undersurface of the SMAS, where they divide into numerous branches and then attach to the dermis through a subcutaneous fascial system. More superior attachments around the orbit and temporal region differ in that they retain the SMAS plane only, allowing considerable mobility to occur at a cutaneous level (Fig. 14-25). Rather than true ligaments, these attachments take the form of fibrous tissue septa and adhesions.

A temporal ligamentous adhesion supports the region immediately superior to the eyebrow at the junction of the middle and lateral thirds. Located at the intersection of the temporal, frontal, and periorbital region, this fibrous

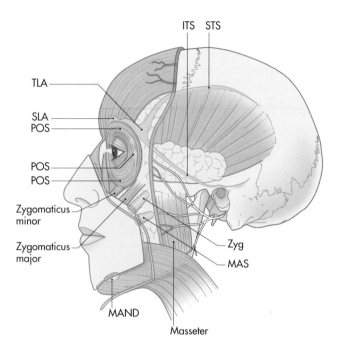

FIGURE 14-25 Schematic diagram of the ligamentous and septal retaining apparatus for the superficial musculo-aponeurotic system and overlying integument. Supraorbital ligamentous adhesion (SLA), temporal ligamentous adhesion (TLA), superior temporal septum (STS), inferior temporal septum (ITS), periorbital septum (POS), zygomaticus major, zygomaticus minor, zygomatic ligament (Zyg), masseteric ligament (MAS), and mandibular ligament (MAND) are shown. Notice that the important attachments around the orbit and temporal region retain the superficial musculo-aponeurotic system (SMAS) only, whereas the ligamentous structures of the cheek region and mandible run from deep structures, traverse the SMAS, and insert into dermis.

adhesion is a well-defined structure from which three further zones of fixation radiate. The temporal ligamentous adhesion inserts onto the deep surface of the frontalis muscle, where it meets the temporoparietal fascia laterally. It is a broad adhesion lying about 1 cm above the superolateral orbital rim. From this adhesion, the superior temporal septum radiates posterosuperiorly, arising from the pericranium along the superior temporal line and inserting into the line of junction between the temporoparietal fascia and galea. The inferior temporal septum takes an oblique course along a line extending from the lateral corner of the temporal ligamentous adhesion toward the root of the zygomatic process. It consists of crisscross fibers that pass from the deep temporal fascia to their insertion into the deepest layer of the temporoparietal fascia.

The division of deep temporal fascia into its deep and superficial leaves, with an intervening fat pad, is above the level of the inferior temporal septum. The most cephalad temporal branches of the facial nerve lie on the deep surface of the temporoparietal fascia, just caudal to this inferior temporal septum. In developing a coronal flap, incision of the outer layer of the deep temporal fascia cephalad to the inferior temporal septum will preserve this supporting structure and facilitate repositioning of the SMAS layer at the time of closure. It also ensures that the temporal branches of the facial nerves are protected.

A periorbital septal adhesion gains origin from three-quarters of the circumference of the orbital rim extending from the corrugator origin around to the inferomedial bony origin of the orbicularis oculi. The septum has two or more broader adhesions, named the lateral brow and lateral orbital ligamentous thickenings. The lateral orbital thickening is located superolaterally to the lateral canthal tendon insertion, and the lateral brow thickening arises from a bony crest on the lateral supraorbital rim. Both of these ligaments insert into and retain the deep surface of orbicularis oculi.[32] Esthetic surgeons recognize the importance of these supporting structures in facial rejuvenation procedures and aim to release and reposition them superiorly and posteriorly.

The zygomaticus major, zygomaticus minor, levator labii superioris, and levator labii alaeque nasi originate in a line across the malar eminence and along the infraorbital region to the frontal process of the maxilla. All originate from periosteum and are important in supporting the soft tissue of the cheek and upper lip. In the lower face, the mandibular ligament is found in the anterolateral region of the mandible adjacent to the origin of the depressor angulioris.[33] The importance of the mentalis muscle in preventing lip and chin ptosis has been emphasized in the esthetic facial literature. In accessing the facial skeleton by means of wide-exposure and subperiosteal dissection, release of many of these supporting structures, particularly around the orbit, will occur. These attachments of the mimetic soft tissues have important esthetic consequences, and accurate periosteal repositioning is an important part of treatment. If this is not feasible, additional measures should be taken to reestablish support for the SMAS layer.

Operative Details

Closure commences with the reestablishment of periosteal continuity across the inferior orbital rim. If periosteal continuity cannot be reestablished, suspension of the periosteum, and therefore the mimetic soft tissue drape, must be provided for. The zygomatic ligament as it lies medial to zygomatic minor directly supports the skin of the midface. Often the cheek prominence is not directly fractured; if possible, periosteum should be left undisturbed at this location to prevent detachment of the zygomatic ligament. If detachment is necessary, non-resorbable sutures should be used to resuspend the cheek tissue. We use two 2-0 nylon sutures from the periosteum of the cheek and infraorbital region to the deep temporal fascia above and lateral to the frontozygomatic suture.

Lateral canthal descent is commonly seen after treatment of orbital trauma requiring extensive periosteal detachment. If a lateral canthotomy has been performed for access, the lower tarsal plate should be directly reattached to the lateral orbital rim. We have observed relatively frequent abnormalities of contour of the palpebral fissure when lateral canthotomy and cantholysis were performed for access. Other workers have reported a similar experience.[34] If a canthotomy is performed, the lateral canthal orbital septum is grasped with a non-resorbable suture and secured to the lateral orbital rim 2 mm cephalad and posterior to the medial canthus. It is prudent to overcorrect.

Closure of the incision in the deep temporal fascia created in raising the coronal flap is important in our opinion. Detachment at the zygomatic arch of the lateral SMAS is often necessary, and any gap in closure of the deep temporal fascia above implies lateral SMAS descent, because an adhesion exists between the two layers, with consequent fullness below and hollowing above. A "skeletonized" lateral orbit is a not uncommon consequence of severe orbital injury and its repair; SMAS descent may be an important contributor (Fig. 14-26).

If an ACF repair has not been necessary, closure of periosteum in the supraorbital region is usually performed continuously with that of the deep temporal fascia. Every effort is made to restore the height of periosteal redraping.

If an ACF repair has been performed, suspension sutures may be employed in the frontal region from supraorbital periosteum to superior bone anchoring points. The highest point of the eyebrow is at the junction of the middle and lateral thirds in the youthful face, and this should be borne in mind when suspension sutures are applied. Closure of the galeal layer at the coronal incision provides further support for the SMAS and is important in preventing subsequent scar widening.

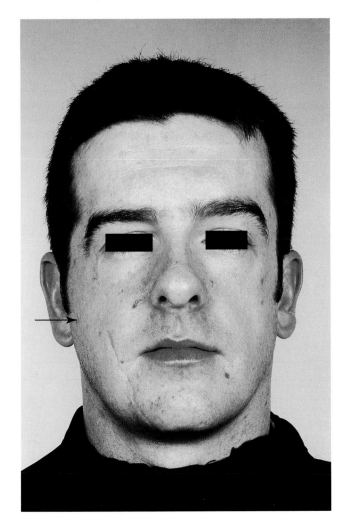

FIGURE 14-26 Lateral canthal descent and a mildly skeletonized lateral orbit with hollowing in the temporal fossa and fullness below (arrow). This patient sustained a right-sided orbital injury. There has been descent of the superficial musculo-aponeurotic system (SMAS) on the right. Notice the comparative vertical positions of the most anterior part of the hairline.

In creating exposure to the anterior mandible, the mentalis muscle is an important structure. Maintenance of an adequate cuff of muscle attached to the labial surface of the mandible to allow layered closure may be helpful in preventing subsequent lower lip and chin ptosis. If muscle reapproximation is not possible, the use of bone-anchoring devices is advisable. The use of chin supportive strapping is recommended while substantial postoperative soft tissue edema is present. Closure of the periosteal layer in buccal sulcus incisions is achievable if exposure is created with this goal in mind. Wherever feasible, an effort should be made to achieve closure of periosteum and muscle origins followed by mucosal closure in a double-layered wound approximation.

MANAGEMENT OF BALLISTIC AND AVULSIVE INJURIES OF THE FACE

Gunshot wounds to the face have recently been reported to be associated with a mortality rate of 14.5% due to injuries other than the facial wound. This relatively high mortality, despite modern trauma resuscitation protocols, emphasizes the need for particular care in the early management of these injuries.[35]

Low-energy ballistic injuries do not differ significantly from blunt trauma in their effects on the damaged parts, and management is the same. High-energy avulsive and ballistic injuries have a different pathophysiology. The zone of tissue injury sustaining direct impact is typically avulsed, pulverized, and destroyed by the impact. This zone typically widens from the surface point of impact as the energy imparted dissipates through the affected tissues and secondary projectiles (bones and teeth) are recruited. Surrounding the resulting zone of tissue necrosis, there is a zone of relative tissue injury, the extent of which varies with the degree of energy transferred. Within this zone, an evolving pattern of tissue loss develops over ensuing days. Previously marginally viable tissues may become necrotic as the massive swelling associated with an acute inflammatory response and bacterial insult combine to adversely affect areas of marginal perfusion. Ultimately, the inflammatory response subsides, macrophage infiltration is seen at the tissue level, and the contused soft tissue components heal with a variable degree of internal fibrosis, depending on the magnitude of the injury sustained. The effects of fibrosis are to render affected areas variably hypovascular, rigid, and contracted.

What previous generations of surgeons have learned is the primacy of an adequate blood supply. At each stage, the surgical team seeks to exert a favorable influence by minimizing the potential for further bacterial insult and avoiding any intervention that could add surgical trauma in the wound evolution stage or otherwise adversely affect tissue perfusion. The essential difference between what is proposed here and more traditional management protocols is the timing. High-energy ballistic and avulsive wounds have largely been managed with a regimen of débridement, sequential dressings, external skeletal fixation, and delayed secondary reconstruction after scar maturation. The problem with this strategy is that fibrosis with contracture fixes soft tissues and displaced bone segments in rigid, hypovascular, collagen-rich scar. Deformity occurring as a consequence is often impossible to correct secondarily. Collapse of the central facial region is frequently seen. The use of external fixators to maintain the spatial relationship of major bony fragments, and therefore the associated soft tissue relationships, is all too frequently frustrated by fibrosis, shrinkage, and inward collapse of intervening bone and soft tissue. Even if tissue perfusion has been maximized by minimal interference, the ultimate functional and esthetic outcome is frequently compromised.

It is for these reasons that treatment protocols that seek to optimize functional and esthetic outcome without compromising safety through serial débridement and a delayed primary reconstruction are gaining increasing acceptance in civilian practice. These are complex injuries with potential loss of mucosal lining, bone, and overlying soft tissue, which will have serious consequences for the affected functional and esthetic subunits of the face. Management of these injuries challenges the resourcefulness of the resuscitation team, the maxillofacial trauma surgical team, and rehabilitation specialties. Care of these patients according to the described protocol also challenges the resources of all but large hospitals.

Once the airway is secured, active external bleeding should be controlled. Truncal, head, and limb injuries take precedence over facial injuries in the early management (day 1). It is frequently possible to perform an initial débridement concurrently with the management of trunk or limb injuries. In emergency treatment of bleeding in the head and neck region, care is taken to preserve vascular pedicles that might be used later in definitive reconstruction. However, an expanding hematoma should be investigated with angiography, and embolization should be performed if indicated.

After resuscitation and treatment of life-threatening problems, a tracheostomy is performed, replacing the orotracheal tube. Even if the airway is patent, massive swelling is to be anticipated over the ensuing 48 hours. Necrotic soft tissue is excised, and fragments of teeth and devitalized detached bone fragments are removed. Significant bone fragments that are attached to viable soft tissue should be left undisturbed. Severed branches of the facial nerve are repaired or tagged for later identification. The wound is copiously lavaged with a warmed normal saline solution, and broad-spectrum antimicrobial agents are administered.

After this initial procedure, an intermediate phase of wound management ensues, the purpose of which is wound stabilization. This phase is necessitated by the evolving pattern of tissue loss that is seen when high levels of energy are imparted to the tissues. The treatment strategy is to minimize loss of marginally viable tissue by doing nothing that would further impair tissue perfusion and by controlling all variables that lead to bacterial growth. Hematomas, persistent dead space, retained foreign bodies, and necrotic tissue are the principal culprits favoring infection. To stabilize the wound, planned serial reexploration is performed every 24 to 36 hours. Any necrotic tissue is débrided, hematomas are evacuated, the wound is lavaged, and an antibiotic-impregnated nonadherent dressing is applied.

Robertson and Manson[36] advocated reduction and fixation of fractures within the first day or so after admission, with primary closure of wounds or advancement of mucosa to skin where tissue loss has occurred. They cited optimal support for soft tissue healing as their reason for early skeletal fixation by wide exposure and direct fixation and minimization of bacterial colonization as the reason for early wound closure.

Until further evidence emerges demonstrating safety, we do not advocate the use of such aggressive intervention during the wound stabilization period. Attempts to advance tissues and achieve closure early in the wound evolution may lead to tension, and therefore ischemia, of already vulnerable wound margins as progressive and gross tissue edema develops. As swelling starts to resolve and the wound stabilizes, typically after 72 hours, primary closure of wounds becomes safe. Serial evaluation in the operating room is repeated until no further débridement is required and the wound is stable and viable.

Definitive management is possible by 5 to 10 days after injury. The principles of definitive management are the same as for blunt trauma or low-velocity ballistic injuries. Precise skeletal fixation is achieved by appropriate exposure and internal fixation of bone segments with primary bone grafting of midfacial defects. Restoration and maintenance of correct spatial relationships to support the soft tissue drape is emphasized. The survival of bone grafts and that of major fragments that have been converted to free grafts by wide exposure, depends on a well-vascularized and complete soft tissue cover. This often presents a considerable challenge in the management of high-energy avulsive and ballistic injuries. Rotation and advancement of tissue within the zone of relative injury requires careful judgment and can be hazardous. If there has been a loss of mucosal lining as well as bone and other soft tissues, composite free flap transfer is usually indicated. If there has been considerable soft tissue loss in the absence of a skeletal defect, we would also give serious consideration to the import of a soft tissue flap. If free tissue transfer is employed, recipient vessels outside the zone of relative injury should be used. Once the definitive reconstruction has stabilized, secondary revision of bulky or color-mismatched tissue can be performed. Serial excision of skin flaps is frequently possible through rotation or advancement of local skin without disturbing the now well-established spatial relationships.

KEY POINTS
- Initial débridement is followed by an evolving pattern of tissue loss.
- Serial débridement is performed during the evolution phase to stabilize the wound.
- Wound stabilization is followed by primary reconstruction.

MANAGEMENT OF FRACTURES OF THE EDENTULOUS MAXILLA

Trauma in the elderly is an increasing phenomenon related to increased longevity. It is reckoned that the geriatric population in the United States will have expanded by 50% in 2050. Approximately 6% of maxillary fractures occur in edentulous patients.[37] As in the dentate, fractures of the edentulous maxilla are less common than mandibular fractures until the age of 65 years, after which the incidence of maxillary fractures equals that of mandibular injuries.[38] The probable explanations are increasing maxillary pneumatization that occurs with age, declining bone resilience, and atrophy of the relatively strong alveolar process. Maxillary fractures in the elderly population tend to be more comminuted than in younger people.

Triage of the elderly patient who has sustained a facial injury is crucial at the outset of treatment. The in-hospital mortality rate for elderly patients with a craniomaxillofacial injury in one review was 11.1%. This reflected the likelihood of a coexistent head injury, and the fact that this age group may have significant comorbid disease. The GCS and trauma scores have a direct relation to eventual outcome. In this group of patients, the significant mortality rate occurred tpredominantly in those with a lower GCS score and a higher trauma score.

Nonunion is extremely rare in the maxilla, and for undisplaced or minimally displaced fractures, if there is no obvious comminution, simple management with a soft diet and appropriate analgesics allows adequate healing. If definitive surgical management of the fractured edentulous maxilla is indicated, the goals are the same as in the dentate population. Facial height, width, and anterior projection must be restored with anatomical reduction of the facial buttresses. Primary bone grafting and augmentation of the anterior and middle facial buttresses may form an integral part of the definitive management.[37]

In our own practice, we have observed a high incidence of malposition of the Le Fort I segment in the open reduction and internal fixation of edentulous fractures. We believe this to be a consequence of the lack of intraoperative visual clues to guide correct positioning of this alveolus-palatal fragment. An overreliance on correct reassembly of comminuted buttresses is the operative strategy we believe to be directly responsible. Errors have occurred in all three dimensions, with the maxilla rotated, canted, and retropositioned. Although some of these errors can be compensated for in denture construction, this is by no means universally the case. Dentures and acrylic splints can provide useful aids to the repositioning of the maxilla when the mandible is intact, and reduction of any mandibular fractures is essential. We advocate the use of some form of prosthesis that allows for intraoperative intermaxillary fixation in all cases in which open reduction and internal fixation are undertaken.

KEY POINTS AND PITFALLS
- Comminution is likely to be present.
- Buttress reconstruction augmented with bone graft is often required.
- Overreliance on reassembly of comminuted fragments frequently results in malposition of the Le Fort I segment.
- Use of dentures or splints and intraoperative intermaxillary fixation is recommended.

REFERENCES

1. Rowe NL, Killey HC: *Fractures of the facial skeleton*, ed 2, Edinburgh, 1968, Churchill Livingstone.
2. Wolfe SA: The influence of Paul Tessier on our current treatment of facial trauma, both in primary care and in the management of late sequelae. *Clin Plast Surg* 24:515-518, 1997.
3. O'Sullivan ST, Snyder BJ, Moore MH et al: Outcome measurement of the treatment of maxillary fractures: a prospective analysis of 100 consecutive cases. *Br J Plast Surg* 52:519-523, 1999.
4. Manson PN, Glassman D, Vanderkolk C et al: Rigid stabilization of sagittal fractures of the maxilla and palate. *Plast Reconstr Surg* 85:711-717, 1990.
5. Gruss JS: Complex nasoethmoid-orbital and midfacial fractures: role of craniofacial surgical techniques and immediate bone grafting. *Ann Plast Surg* 17:377-390, 1986.
6. Jackson IT: Classification and treatment of orbitozygomatic and orbitoethmoid fractures: the place of bone grafting and plate fixation. *Ann Plast Surg* 16:77-81, 1986.
7. Guerrissi JO: Maxillofacial injuries scale. *J Craniofac Surg* 7:130-132, 1996.
8. Bagheri SC, Dierks EJ, Kademani D et al: Application of a facial injury severity scale in craniomaxillofacial trauma. *J Oral Maxillofac Surg* 64:408-414, 2006.
9. Catapano J, Fialkov JA, Binhammer PA et al: A new system for severity scoring of facial fracture: development and validation. *J Crainiofac Surg* 21:1098-1103, 2010.
10. Girotto JA, McKenzie E, Fowler C et al: Long-term physical impairment and functional outcomes after complex facial fractures. *Plast Reconstr Surg* 108:312-327, 2001.
11. Al-Quiranny JA, Stassen LF, Dutton GN et al: Diplopia following midfacial fractures. *Br J Oral Maxillofac Surg* 29:302-309, 1991.
12. Haug RH, Adams JM, Jordan RB: Comparison of the morbidity associated with maxillary fractures treated by maxillomandibular and rigid internal fixation. *Oral Surg Oral Med Oral Pathol Oral Radiol Endodont* 80:629-637, 1995.
13. Devlin MF, Ray A, Raine P et al: Facial symmetry in unilateral cleft lip and palate following alar base augmentation with bone graft: a three demensional assessment. *Cleft Palate Craniofac J* 44:391-395, 2007.
14. Downie J, Mao Z, Rachel Lo TW et al: A double-blind, clinical evaluation of facial augmentation treatments: a comparison of PRI 1, PRI 2, Zyplast and Perlane. *J Plast Reconstr Aesthet Surg* 62:1636-1643, 2009.
15. Gruss JS: Advances in craniofacial fracture repair. *Scand J Plast Reconstr Hand Surg* 27(suppl):67-81, 1995.
16. Foster RD, Anthony JP, Singer MI et al: Reconstruction of complex midfacial defects. *Plast Reconstr Surg* 99:1555-1565, 1997.
17. Manson PN, Clark N, Robertson B et al: Subunit principles in midfacial fractures: the importance of sagittal buttresses, soft tissue reductions, and sequencing treatment of segmental fractures. *Plast Reconstr Surg* 103:1287-1306, 1999.
18. Caron G, Paquin R, Lessard MR et al: Submental endotracheal intubation: an alternative to tracheotomy in patients with midfacial and panfacial fractures. *J Trauma* 48:235-240, 2000.
19. Rohrich RJ, Hollier L: The role of the nasofrontal duct in frontal sinus fracture management. *J Craniomaxillofac Trauma* 2:31-40, 1996.
20. Gruss JS, Mackinnon SE: Complex maxillary fractures: role of buttress reconstruction and immediate bone grafts. *Plast Reconstr Surg* 78:9-22, 1986.
21. Stanley RB: Rigid fixation of fractures of the maxillary complex. *Facial Plast Surg* 7:176-184, 1990.
22. Hendrickson M, Clark N, Manson PN et al: Palatal fractures: classification, patterns, treatment with rigid internal fixation. *Plast Reconstr Surg* 101:319-332, 1998.
23. Rimmell F, Marenette LJ: Injuries of the hard palate and the horizontal buttress of the midface. *Otolaryngol Head Neck Surg* 109:499-505, 1993.
24. Denny AD, Celik N: A management strategy for palatal fractures: a 12 year review. *J Craniofac Surg* 10:49-57, 1999.
25. Manson PN, Glassman D, Vanderkolk C et al: Rigid stabilization of sagittal fractures of the maxilla and palate. *Plast Reconstr Surg* 85:711-717, 1990.
26. Persson M, Thilender B: Palatal suture closure in man from 15 to 35 years of age. *Am J Orthodont* 72:42-51, 1977.
27. Ellis E, Tharanon W: Facial width problems associated with rigid fixation of mandibular fractures. *J Oral Maxillofac Surg* 50:87-94, 1992.
28. Marker P, Nielsen A, Bastian HL: Fractures of the mandibular condyle. Part 1. Patterns of distribution and causes of fracture in 348 patients. *Br J Oral Maxillofac Surg* 38:417-421, 2000.
29. Stanwix MG, Nam AJ, Manson PN et al: Critical computed tomographic diagnostic criteria for frontal sinus fractures. *J Oral Maxillofac Surg* 68:2714-2722, 2010.
30. Donald PJ, Ettin M: The safety of frontal sinus fat obliteration when sinus walls are missing. *Laryngoscope* 92:190-193, 1986.
31. Gruss JS, Pollock RA, Phillips JH et al: Combined injuries to the cranium and the face. *Br J Plast Surg* 42:385-398, 1989.
32. Moss CJ, Mendelson BC, Taylor GI: Surgical anatomy of the ligamentous adhesions in the temple and periorbital regions. *Plast Reconstr Surg* 105:1475-1490, 2000.
33. Furnas DW: The retaining ligaments of the cheek. *Plast Reconstr Surg* 83:11-16, 1989.
34. Yaremchuk MJ: Orbital deformity after craniofacial fracture repair: avoidance and treatment. *J Craniomaxillofac Trauma* 5:7-12, 1999.
35. Demetriades D, Chahwan S, Gomez H et al: Initial evaluation and management of gunshot wounds to the face. *J Trauma* 45:39-41, 1998.
36. Robertson B, Manson PN: High energy ballistic and avulsive injuries. *Surg Clin North Am* 79:1489-1502, 1999.
37. Crawley WA, Azman P, Clark N et al: The edentulous Le Fort fracture. *J Craniofac Surg* 8:298-306, 1997.
38. Farmand M, Bauman A: The treatment of the fractured edentulous maxilla. *J Craniomaxillofac Surg* 20:341-344, 1992.

CHAPTER 15

Mandibular Fractures in Adults

Mike Perry, Risto Kontio

Mandible fractures are among the commonest fractures of the face,[1] and much has been published about their management. Yet despite this wealth of clinical research, debate continues over what is considered to be best practice in some types of fracture. Management has evolved considerably over the past 3 decades, with advances occurring not only in the techniques used to repair fractures but also in our understanding of fracture healing,[2] and the importance of the soft tissues in this process. These developments have resulted in improved outcomes and fewer complications, notably infection and malunion. Consequently patients are now much more likely to be restored to their pre-injury function and occlusion. Transoral, semirigid fixation is commonly undertaken for most "routine" mandibular fractures, thereby avoiding the need for external incisions with their attendant shortcomings. *Wire* intermaxillary fixation (IMF, also known as maxillomandibular fixation—MMF) is now rarely indicated as definitive treatment, although elastic IMF may still be used to "fine tune" the bite and provide additional fracture support with some semirigid techniques. External approaches and rigid fixation are now usually reserved for more complex cases (such as those that involve extensive comminution, infected fractures, continuity defects, or when immediate bone grafting is required).

However, current indications for semirigid and rigid fixation are not absolute and a degree of overlap still exists between the two, the final decision often being based on personal experience and that gained from reported clinical outcomes and prospective studies. Many aspects of management are still controversial and the literature is replete with publications arguing the case for or against various strategies. Surgical access, biomaterials, plate size and design, and specific fracture groups (such as edentulous, comminuted, or pathological fractures) are just a few areas where controversy continues. For the novice this may sometimes be confusing. This lack of consensus suggests that additional confounding factors may play a role in final outcomes. Patient compliance and their biological variation, aftercare and our individual technical skills, to name a few, no doubt contribute variably to our final results. Nevertheless, these developments have resulted in a faster, safer and a more comfortable return to function.[3] Some of these developments and controversies are discussed.

A BRIEF HISTORICAL OVERVIEW

Very early descriptions of mandibular fractures came from the Egyptians in 1650 B.C. and also from Hippocrates who described the treatment of a fractured mandible using circumferential wiring.[4] Later references to fractures and their management include the the Edwin Smith Surgical Papyrus,[5,6] Salicetti in 1275[7,8] and Gilmer in 1887.[9,10]

For much of the 20th century, initial attempts at managing mandibular fractures were limited mostly to maxillomandibular fixation (described later), or Gunning-type splints.[11,12] Direct fixation through an open approach was generally avoided in this preantibiotic era, due to high infection rates. Only on occasion was this was used in selected cases, or in some edentulous patients.[13] Fracture fixation using "bone plates" was later reintroduced, initially into the German-speaking literature by Luhr and Spiessl in 1968 and 1972.[14] Further work has since helped to develop many of the principles now advocated by the Arbeitsgemeinschaft für Osteosynthesefragen (Association for Osteosynthesis/Association for the Study of Internal Fixation [AO/ASIF]).[15]

Initial attempts at fracture fixation were based on the orthopedic principles of the time, in which callus formation was believed to indicate a failure of the healing process, due to movement at the fracture site. This resulted in the development of rigid, but bulky "compression" plates, which by necessity were placed through large skin incisions in an attempt to provide absolutely rigid fixation. However it later became recognized that satisfactory reduction and healing was also possible without requiring this degree of rigidity, using much weaker fixation (i.e., IMF). But some considered it to be potentially dangerous and was certainly unpleasant for the patient. Each of these two approaches (rigid fixation and IMF) had advantages and disadvantages over the other. IMF in some countries required the patient to remain in hospital for the 6 weeks or so of fixation and posed an obvious threat to the airway. On the other hand compression plating had high morbidity, such as unsightly scarring, risks of nerve injury (facial and inferior alveolar), plate infection, and the need for a second procedure to remove the plates. It was also a very unforgiving technique, which could not be used to repair the thinner bones of the upper facial skeleton.

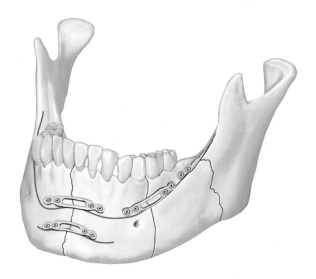

FIGURE 15-1. Champy's lines of osteosynthesis.

In the 1970s, Michelet introduced a new technique for mandible fixation using smaller "miniplates" which could be placed through the mouth. These "monocortical" plates could be secured using much smaller screws which only needed to engage the outer cortical bone. This advance was subsequently modified by Champy and colleagues, whose biomechanical studies resulted in the concept of "ideal lines of osteosynthesis"[16,17] (Fig. 15-1). This concept was analogous to the principle of the suspension bridge. By defining lines of tension across a load-bearing fracture, smaller and thinner plates (and sometimes wires) could provide adequate fixation to enable bone healing. The key development here was that the fracture support, provided by these smaller plates, was considered adequate and did not need to be rigid—hence the term *semirigid*. Consequently the use of monocortical screws allowed greater flexibility in plate positioning over these lines of tension. This use of smaller miniplates was subsequently extended into the rest of the facial skeleton, being miniaturized further for periorbital and cranial non–load-bearing areas and are now in common use today.

Most recently, bone-plating systems made from resorbable polymer have been developed. Material-related complications (such as migration of titanium, thermal paresthesia and the need to remove plates) have all been reported and this has led to the search for more biocompatible materials. These polymers are generally degraded by hydrolysis into water and carbon dioxide and have been reported in some cases to reach mechanical rigidities similar to that of titanium. Resorbable materials were initially designed for use in craniofacial surgery, due to the minimal loading requirements. However as they became stronger, their use was later extended to the treatment of midfacial fractures and then orthognathic surgery. Within the past decade increasing reports have been published of their use in mandibular fractures,[18-20] although it is still unclear whether or not all systems are comparable to the commonly used miniplates. Biodegradable materials have a number of disadvantages (costs, brittleness, difficult handling, inflammation and swelling during degradation). These need to be balanced against those of titanium (cost, infection, possible long-term toxicity and need for removal).[21]

Even more recently the use of adhesives to fix bone fragments has received interest in both orthopedic and maxillofacial surgery. The idea itself is not new[22,23]—the notion of bonding bone using biological materials was proposed by Gluck more than a century ago. Adhesives have several advantages over plating. They can secure small fragments and may therefore be useful in comminuted fractures. It has been suggested that by providing more diffuse fixation, adhesives result in a more uniform distribution of loads across the fracture site, compared to the irregular loading that occurs at screw sites. This may reduce the risk of overloading the plate and subsequent failure. It has also been reported that some adhesives act as "subchondral spacers", smoothing out joint surface irregularities in articular fractures. However, compared to those adhesives used in soft tissue trauma, the biocompatible requirements for bone adhesives need to be stricter, if they are to be safe, easy to use, and effective in load-bearing fractures. Cyanoacrylates, methacrylates, aldehyde-based, and fibrin systems have all been evaluated at some point and research is still ongoing. Adhesives related to polymethylmethacrylate (PMMA), used extensively in dentistry and in hip surgery, show some promise, but this is still a relatively new field of research.[24-28]

EPIDEMIOLOGY

Much has been published on the causes of mandible fractures, which vary from culture to culture, but include assault, motor vehicle collisions, work-related injury, falls, sport-related injury, pathologic fractures, and projectile missiles. A number of large reviews have been published over the years with differences in etiology, varying between different clinical settings.[29-31] In urban populations, the most frequent cause of mandibular fractures is often interpersonal violence, while in more rural areas motor vehicle collisions are a more common cause. Young men are almost universally more commonly injured than women and in many countries alcohol is often a significant contributing factor—hence the (paraphrased) expression "Testosterone and alcohol are a potentially dangerous mix"!

INITIAL ASSESSMENT

"If you leave the patient facing towards heaven, it won't be long before they get there" (paraphrased, original source unknown), underlines the importance of good initial care and assessment.

The immediate care of the traumatized patient is covered elsewhere, but is especially important when complex mandibular fractures exist.[32,33] The American college "ATLS" system of care in the multiply injured patient is commonly regarded as the gold standard and is now taught in over 40 countries worldwide. However its "blind," unthinking, application to patients with coexisting facial injuries can result in a number of complications (notably airway), especially in those patients with associated head injuries, a full stomach, and high blood alcohol. Such patients need close observation and should never be left unattended while immobilized on a spine board.

Crudely speaking, patients can be placed into one of two groups:

1. High-velocity or deceleration injuries, where coexisting torso injuries exist and ATLS principles are required
2. The "walking wounded," where other injuries have been ruled out

In both scenarios assessment always starts with the airway, while simultaneously protecting the cervical spine until injury can be excluded. "Clearing" the neck by clinical examination can usually be done in alert, cooperative patients and many guidelines exist. Where concerns exist about cervical spine injury, imaging is necessary, although how this is best done is more controversial. The best approach is to follow local evidence-based protocols, which usually exist in most trauma units.

With regard to initial assessment (during the primary survey), establishing the presence of those mandibular fractures placing the airway at risk, is a crucial early step. Although an appropriate verbal response is encouraging, direct inspection of the oropharynx must always be undertaken to rule out oral bleeding, mobile and unstable fractures, loose teeth, and foreign bodies, all of which place the airway at risk in supine patients. Correctly fitting rigid collars restrict mouth opening, making assessment difficult (Fig. 15-2), but in all cases of significant facial trauma should be loosened enough to enable thorough examination. During this time manual in-line immobilization of the neck provides continued protection. Precise sizing and placement of collars is important—poorly fitting ones can displace mandibular fractures and aggravate ongoing swelling. Swallowing may be painful and ineffective in mandibular fractures and vomiting is an ever-present risk in all patients, unless the airway has been secured. The use of opiates (recreational or for pain relief) can also compromise the airway in these patients. Airway adjuncts such as the jaw thrust and chin lift can be difficult with comminuted fractures and if unable to sit up, patients who are at high risk of vomiting may require intubation to protect the airway.

However not all patients vomit and the difficulty therefore lays in deciding who should have their airway secured as a precaution. This decision is even more critical if inter-hospital transfer or imaging (notably CT) outside the relative safety of the resuscitation room is necessary. For these reasons senior staff with skills in airway management should be involved at an early stage in such cases.

CLINICAL FEATURES

With all trauma patients, knowledge of the mechanism of injury can give clues to the possibility of unrecognized injuries. For instance, a blow to the forehead can result in blindness, even if there are no fractures present and deceleration injuries to the torso can result in mediastinal bleeding ("bell clanger" effect). Such injuries can easily be overlooked and bear relevance to us if transfers to maxillofacial units are being considered.[34] These, and many others, need to be actively considered and excluded. Similarly, with regard to the mandible, certain mechanisms may also suggest particular injury patterns.[35] The classic "guardsman's fracture" (midline/parasymphyseal fracture associated with bilateral fractures of the condyles, following a faint or fall onto the chin), is an example where both condyles need to be carefully assessed.

The hallmark of a mandible fracture is a change in the patient's occlusion (Fig. 15-3). However a normal occlusion does not rule out a mandible fracture. Clinical features are listed in Box 15-1. If a fracture is felt *not* to be present, "springing" the mandible by manually compressing the angles (much akin to springing the pelvis), should elicit no pain and is a useful test to avoid unnecessary imaging. *Change* in the occlusion is one of the commonest physical findings, but can be easily overlooked or misinterpreted in patients with pre-existing abnormal dental or skeletal relationships, hence *change* in the occlusion. However, occlusal changes may also arise as a result of an effusion in the TMJ, or following fractures of the alveolus, teeth, or the maxilla. Occasionally a

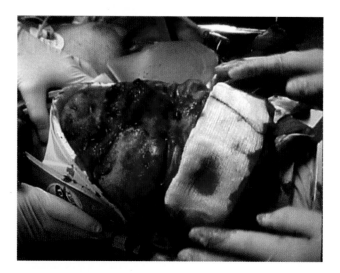

FIGURE 15-2 *Patients with unstable mandibular fractures are at high risk of airway compromise if placed in the supine position, but this may be unavoidable.*

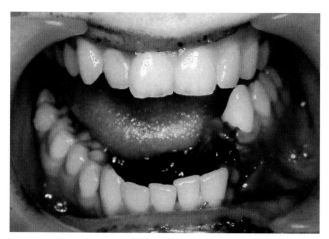

FIGURE 15-3 *Obvious change in bite after fracture. Such displaced fractures are a risk to the airway (see Fig. 15-2) and inferior alveolar and mental nerves, and are very uncomfortable to the patient. This needs to be temporarily reduced as soon as possible.*

displaced fracture of the zygoma can "flex" the ipsilateral maxilla resulting in premature contact with the mandible on the same side and diagnostic confusion. Numbness of the lower lip is also a useful sign. This may signify stretching of the inferior alveolar nerve during fracture displacement at the moment of impact, but it can also occur in the absence of a fracture. Documentation of numbness is important as its persistence is often a source of patient dissatisfaction and litigation. Sublingual hematoma is highly suggestive of a fracture involving the lingual plate of the mandible. It should be watched closely in those patients taking anticoagulant medication, notably warfarin, because continued bleeding can result in airway compromise.

IMAGING

Radiographic studies (usually plain films) are not always necessary to exclude fractures of the mandible, so long as a thorough clinical examination has failed to elicit signs of one. In an alert and cooperative patient, springing the mandible and asking them to forcefully open the mouth against resistance at the symphysis are two useful tests. If neither elicit pain the bone is at least clinically intact. However, when a fracture or fractures are evident or suspected, imaging is required,

usually as plain films in the first instance, although in some cases with computed tomography (CT).

The principle with plain radiography is to obtain at least two films taken at right angles to each other. Often this is thought to be achieved by obtaining an orthopantomogram (OPT or OPG) and a posteroanterior (PA) view of the mandible, to help visualize the condyles. In reality the direction of view at the symphysis is similar in both films and certainly not at ninety degrees, but this practice has become historical in many units and together with clinical examination seems to be reliable. If doubt exists in the symphyseal region a true lower occlusal view is a useful additional view. This is particularly useful in visualizing the lingual plate and the presence of any avulsion fractures. Panoramic films (OPT) (Fig. 15-4) provide a good overview of all regions of the mandible[36] and are also useful in examining the existing dentition, buried teeth, and location of the inferior alveolar canal. Depending on patient positioning, OPTs may also incidentally view the maxilla, zygomatic arch, hyoid bone, and upper cervical spine, although diagnostic accuracy is limited. However, in order to obtain an OPT the patient must be able to stand, a requirement which may not be possible in the multiply injured scenario (and in some alcohol-related ones too). If this is not possible oblique views can often be obtained to view any regions of interest. This is more labor intensive and costly and subjects the patient to a higher dose of radiation, but at least is possible in the supine patient. Alternatively, imaging can be withheld until the patient is in a better condition. This may be possible in those fractures and patients in whom immediate intervention is not required.

Additional periapical or occlusal radiographs are often helpful in viewing specific areas of concern, especially when dental, alveolar, or oblique fractures are suspected. Selective tomograms or transcranial views of the TMJ are occasionally useful if CT facilities are not available, but are now mostly of historical interest only.

Computed tomography (CT) currently offers the most detailed and comprehensive view of the facial skeleton, but is more expensive and time-consuming. Two-mm cuts usually provide enough detail when imaging the entire facial skeleton. CT may be undertaken in clinical situations where the patient is not able to undergo routine radiographic techniques, such as may occur in the presence of torso, cervical spine, or brain injury. With the newer high-speed machines, the extra time required to image the face is now considerably

BOX 15-1	Symptoms and Signs of Mandibular Fractures (Not All May Be Present)

- Pain, especially on talking and swallowing
- Swelling, bruising
- Bleeding from the periodontium
- Sublingual hematoma
- Drooling
- Altered bite, with palpable step in the dental arch
- Mobility of fractured segment, with palpable crepitus
- Numbness of the lower lip
- Trismus and difficulty in moving the jaw
- Loosened teeth
- With medial displacement of the condyle, injury to the trigeminal nerve can result in ipsilateral facial numbness (rare)
- The facial nerve may be damaged by a direct blow over the ramus, resulting in ipsilateral facial weakness (rare)

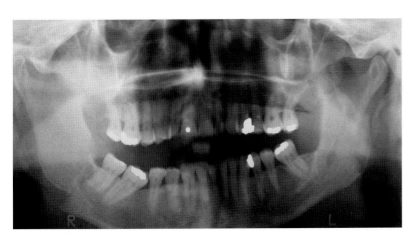

FIGURE 15-4 OPT (OPG). Although technically this particular image is inadequate, it still gives a very good overview of the mandible.

reduced, and the previous arguments against wasting valuable time to image the face no longer apply. Images can now be viewed in any plane (in addition to the standard axial, coronal, and sagittal views), with three-dimensional reconstruction. If necessary (which is rarely required in mandibular fractures), accurate models of the facial skeleton can now be fabricated and used to create custom-made implants or prostheses. More recently the use of cone-beam computed tomography (CBCT) in dentistry has been extensively reported. It is now regarded by some as an accurate and reliable alternative to conventional CT, providing good quality images with less radiation.[37,38] Both CT and CBCT are usually reserved for complex fractures, to help in the planning of fractures of the condyle, or when concomitant midfacial or orbital injuries are present. However, for most "walking wounded" fractures plain films are enough.

Other imaging studies can be helpful in very specific circumstances, but are rarely required. Magnetic resonance imaging (MRI) is of very limited value in evaluating bony injuries, but may be helpful to delineate injuries to the intracapsular disc of the TMJ or associated soft tissues. Ultrasound has occasionally been used to determine condylar position after fractures. Supraselective angiography and embolization can be used when significant bleeding is associated with facial fractures.[39,40]

CLASSIFICATION OF MANDIBULAR FRACTURES

A number of classifications for mandibular fractures now exist, some of which are based on orthopedic experiences. Despite obvious similarities between the long bones and the mandible, some important differences exist. These include differences in development, presence of the dentition, complex muscle attachments, and synergistic bilateral articulations. Fractures of the mandible are often classified and described based on the relationship of the fractured segments, anatomic region, associated muscular anatomy and the involvement of the dentition. Unfortunately these are of limited usefulness when it comes to the "nuts and bolts" of planning treatment. However the influence of the pterygomasseteric muscle sling and its role in displacing angle fractures (favorable and unfavorable fractures) is important when closed management is being considered. The terms *favorable* and *unfavorable* refer to the orientation of the fracture (as viewed in the horizontal or vertical plane) and the likelihood of subsequent impaction or displacement of the bone fragments (Fig. 15-5).

BASIC PRINCIPLES OF FRACTURE MANAGEMENT

Whatever type of treatment is undertaken, the main aims in management are as follows:

- Adequate (or anatomical) reduction of the fractures
- Adequate stability to allow healing
- Restoration of pre-injury occlusion
- Restoration of mandibular function
- Avoidance of complications (notably infection, malunion, nonunion, and nerve injury)

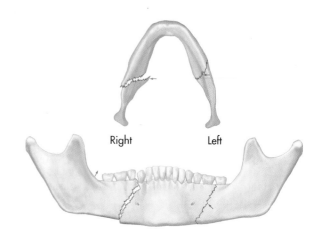

FIGURE 15-5 Favorable and unfavorable fractures of mandible. Unfavorable fracture (Right) resulting in displacement at fracture site caused by pull of masseter muscle. Favorable fracture (Left) in which direction of fracture and angulation of muscle pull resists displacement. *(From Hupp JR, Ellis E, Tucker MR:* Contemporary oral and maxillofacial surgery, *ed 5, St. Louis, 2008, Mosby.)*

Regarding the first two points, what is considered as "adequate" is still not clearly defined in the literature and opinions vary, hence the many alternative treatments which have been successfully used. For example, perfectly acceptable functional outcomes can be achieved in patients without *anatomical* reduction of the fracture. Furthermore, intermaxillary fixation (IMF), semirigid fixation, and rigid fixation are all well know to result in healing, yet the degree of stability each produces across fracture sites varies between them. These points are discussed later.

In orthopedic surgery it is often taught that the success of fracture management depends not only on the condition of the bones and how well they are repaired, but also (and mostly) on the condition of the overlying soft tissues. Consider for example two identical fractures, one of which is closed and covered by healthy, well-vascularized soft tissues, the other being exposed through a mucky (infected), open wound following a crush injury. Whether the fracture is in the leg, arm, or mandible, intuitively outcomes would seem to be better with the first fracture than with the second. This is not the whole story, but does highlight the importance of the soft tissues and in particular the blood supply in the healing process. In this regard the mechanism of injury gives useful clues as to the likelihood of injury to the soft tissues. Comminution in a fracture implies high energy transfer—more energy is also transferred to the soft tissues in the process of sustaining the fracture. Compare, for instance, fractures following a single punch, being kicked by a horse, blast injury, and being shot. Each mechanism carries with it increasing amounts of kinetic energy, potentially compromising the vascularity of the tissues. The worse the blood supply, the greater the chances of infection, non-healing, and /or sequestration.

Excessive movement across the fracture also has an adverse effect in healing by preventing vascularization of the fragments. The judgment here is what do we mean by "excessive"—micromovement has been shown to stimulate bony union.

CLOSED VERSUS OPEN TREATMENTS

In general, treatment is usually composed of the following elements:

1. Reduction (such as closed manipulation or open reduction)
2. Stabilization (for example with IMF, transosseous wires)
3. Fixation (internal or external)
4. Rehabilitation

By and large, these components can be achieved by either "closed" or "open" treatments. In many fractures, *closed* treatment (i.e., the fracture is not exposed) involves analgesia, judicious use of antibiotics if the fracture is contaminated (often via the periodontium), and a soft diet until a firm callus has formed (usually around 4-6 weeks). This may also be termed *conservative* treatment. In some fractures, IMF may be used to provide additional support and/or pain relief. This approach works well in fractures where the mandible appears undisplaced, stable, with no change in occlusion, and the fracture pattern is "favorable", that is, unlikely to displace spontaneously (from muscle activity). Outcomes are usually good in compliant and motivated patients. Some clinicians may prescribe antibiotics if the fracture involves a periodontal socket (making it technically compound, or open). Patients must be kept under regular review for approximately 1 month after which the fracture should have healed sufficiently to allow them to return to a normal diet. However, closed treatment does not reduce fractures *anatomically*—it is wrong to assume that just because the teeth meet, the fractures are in the anatomically correct position.

If the occlusion is deranged or other signs of fracture displacement or mobility are present, then either closed treatment or open reduction can be undertaken. As a temporary first-aid measure, pain relief may be achieved by infiltration of local anesthesia around the fracture site, or if possible by an inferior alveolar nerve block. If the neck is cleared, a soft collar can be used to support the mandible. If the fracture can be reduced manually, a "bridle wire" can be passed around the teeth either side of the fracture and tightened to help reduce it, provide support, and prevent movement (Fig. 15-6). In effect this is the maxillofacial equivalent of an orthopedic backslab used to support limb fractures. By itself, or in conjunction with intermaxillary fixation (IMF), this should be considered when significant delays in repair (i.e., surgery the next day) are anticipated. Any loose dentoalveolar fractures can also be splinted with this technique.

With displaced or mobile fractures a number of treatment options are available. These include:

1. Intermaxillary fixation with wire or elastics (closed techniques)
2. Open reduction and internal fixation via a transoral approach
3. Open reduction and internal fixation via a transcutaneous approach
4. External fixation

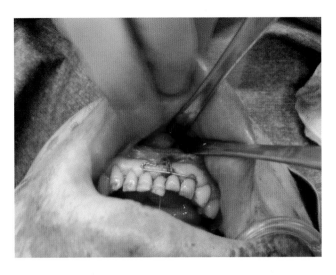

FIGURE 15-6   Two-layer approach to symphyseal fracture. (Notice also the bridle wire.)

Each of these has its own specific set of advantages and disadvantages. The choice of fixation depends on the site and type of fracture, condition of the overlying soft tissues, the patient's general condition and preferences, as well as the personal preference and technical skills of the surgeon. Open treatments tend to be used when closed treatment is inappropriate or has failed. With open treatment, surgical exposure of the fracture site and (hopefully) anatomical reduction and fixation is carried out.

Currently there are two schools of thought when undertaking fixation of mandibular fractures.

1. **Mandibular fractures need rigid fixation.** This can be achieved using dynamic compression osteosynthesis. However, this requires an external approach (with a resulting scar and risks to the mandibular branch of the facial nerve), bicortical screw fixation (with risks of injury to the dental roots and inferior alveolar nerve), and a second procedure to remove the bulky plate once the fracture has healed. The natural curvature of the mandible also makes this a technically demanding procedure, as the plate must fit precisely to avoid distortion of the bone. The thick plates are very difficult to contour, even in experienced hands. Nevertheless, this is a reliable treatment, with a good "track record" and patients can return to normal function quickly. Lag screws also provide rigid fixation and can be placed intraorally (see later). However these are also technically demanding and are only suitable for certain fracture configurations.
2. **Mandibular fractures do not need rigid fixation.** Following fracture, the initial phase of healing is characterized by an inflammatory response within the surrounding hematoma. This is followed by fibrovascular ingrowth and soft callus formation by osteogenic cells. For these processes to occur successfully, the fracture must be adequately stabilized. However, rigid fixation is not essential. Consider for example other land mammals. These may sustain fractures in the wild, which go onto soundly unite, albeit nonanatomically, without any form of artificial stabilization. Furthermore, studies have shown that micromovement, which

can occur following semirigid fixation, encourages callus formation and healing. Callus is no longer regarded as a failure of healing. It is just an indication that there is movement across the fracture. Excessive palpable callus is clearly undesirable but, by and large, bone remodeling reduces this over time.

To achieve semirigid fixation large reconstruction plates are not needed. Instead, smaller miniplates, placed along Champy's lines or zones of tension, produce compression across the fracture. For this to work the periosteum needs to be mostly intact, with good abutment of the fracture ends. Finite element model analysis supports this approach.[41,42] If necessary, fine tuning of the bite is possible with elastic IMF. Routine removal of the miniplates is not necessary. However, compared to rigid fixation, miniplates are reported to be more likely to get infected and patients still require a soft diet for the same period of time as if treated by IMF.

Within the United Kingdom both techniques are used. However the use of miniplates to apply semirigid fixation is usually the first choice for most mandibular fractures. Nevertheless the rigid approach still has a role to play, particularly in comminuted and in some infected fractures, or where bone grafting is required. If semirigid fixation is not going to be successful, rigid fixation or IMF may then be undertaken. The role of fixation in the edentulous mandible is discussed later.

TIMING OF SURGICAL REPAIR

Ideally all fractures should be repaired as soon as possible, but this does not always happen. For all open fractures (i.e., those associated with an overlying laceration, or involvement of the periodontium), it is generally assumed that the longer the delay in repair, the more likely infection will occur. However what is not clear from the literature is how long a delay is possible without significantly increasing the risks of complications or the likelihood of poor outcomes.[43,44] Although some clinicians may feel that a delay of more than a few days may put patients at risk, several studies have failed to demonstrate a direct relationship between delays in repair and any increase in complication rates.[45,46] Excessive fracture mobility, poor oral hygiene, and smoking are probably more likely to result in poor outcomes, and if these can be minimized safe delays may be possible. By and large, it appears that in the absence of airway problems, active bleeding, and excessively mobile (and painful) fragments, most patients can be safely deferred until the next day, or even longer. General anesthesia can be risky and is best avoided late at night. When prolonged delay is anticipated, temporary support using a collar, bridle wire, and/or temporary IMF may be useful interim measures.

SPECIFIC TREATMENTS

CLOSED TECHNIQUES

IMF is commonly used in minimally displaced fractures and in fractures of the condyle (a controversial topic in itself, which is discussed elsewhere). Arch bars (wired or bonded to the teeth),[47] hooks, or eyelets (many types exist) are applied

to the upper and lower dentition using circumdental wires or adhesives. These are then used to hold the teeth into occlusion. This approach is based on the (erroneous) assumption that if the bite is restored, the bones will be anatomically reduced. This is not always the case, although adequate reduction usually occurs, enough to restore a functional occlusion. Many products now exist and the choice between them is often a matter of personal preference. Whatever fixation device is used, it is important to place it carefully so as not to damage the gingiva or periodontal pocket. Plastic circumdental ligatures (rather like bag-ties or the plastic wrist restainers used by some law enforcers), with cleats, are claimed to speed up the process of applying IMF (Fig. 15-7). Arch bar systems which are bonded to the teeth can sometimes be unreliable, since a dry field during bonding may be difficult to achieve.

All these techniques rely heavily on the presence of an intact dentition and are therefore limited in usefulness in the partially dentate/edentulous patient, or when dentoalveolar injuries coexist. Alternatively the use of bicortical bone screws (IMF screws), which allow the passage of wire ligatures, avoids the need for dental anchorage, but care is required in screw placement if teeth exist nearby (Fig. 15-8). An adequate number of opposing teeth is still required in order for the occlusion to be stable while held in IMF.

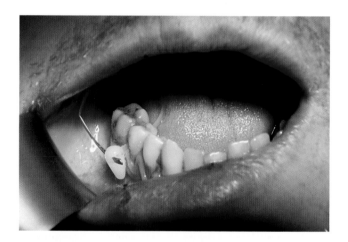

FIGURE 15-7   Rapid intermaxillary fixation (IMF) placement.

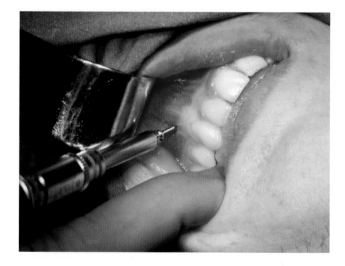

FIGURE 15-8   Intermaxillary fixation (IMF) screw placement.

One potential complication of IMF is that the condyles can be inadvertently distracted out of the glenoid fossae if the fixation is too tight (notably with wires). The fracture then heals in the incorrect position, only to be noticed once the IMF is released. This is particularly important in condylar fractures. For this reason elastics are often used rather than wires, to provide a degree of "give" and allow the condyles to settle in their correct positions (remember that fracture immobilization only has to be adequate and not necessarily rigid).

SPECIFIC TREATMENTS: OPEN REDUCTION AND INTERNAL FIXATION

It is now widely accepted that most displaced craniofacial fractures are best treated by direct exposure, anatomical reduction and internal fixation using miniplates (or microplates), with monocortical screws. This is termed *open reduction and internal fixation,* abbreviated to ORIF. In contrast to closed methods, this approach enables visualization of the fractures), thereby (hopefully) seeing that they are anatomically reduced. Some surgeons now argue that by seeing that the fracture has been reduced and fixed anatomically, postoperative "check X-rays" are no longer required. Fractures involving the mandibular symphysis, parasymphysis, body, and angle can be adequately exposed through a transoral approach, thereby avoiding the need for visible scars. Fortunately the rich blood supply of the maxillofacial skeleton allows wide subperiosteal dissection and exposure of the mandible, without compromising vascularity and healing, in most cases.

Several well-known approaches exist. Whenever possible incisions should be at least 5 mm from the mucogingival junction. This avoids damaging the attached gingiva and periodontal tissues, minimizing the risk of subsequent dehiscence and gingival recession. With anterior fractures, a one- or two-layer approach is possible (see Fig. 15-6). Care is required during exposure and retraction, to avoid damaging (by incision, diathermy, or traction) the mental nerves as they leave the mental foramen. The mentalis muscles are divided prior to incising the periosteum, leaving a small cuff attached to the bone. When closing, it is important to close this incision as a separate layer to avoid a "witch's chin" deformity (chin ptosis) and to ensure the repaired fracture is covered with well vascularized tissue. Some surgeons apply a chin dressing for further support postoperatively.

Further back, the ramus, angle, and body of the mandible can be approached through a one-layer posterior vestibular incision. This starts in proximity to the lower end of the external oblique ridge, passing anteriorly, again maintaining a 5-mm cuff of tissue below the mucogingival junction. Full-thickness mucoperiosteal flaps are then elevated to visualize these areas. Other variants of these approaches exist, but whichever is used, all enable the direct visualization and placement of plates across most mandibular fractures. With the development of the percutaneous trocar, posterior plates can now be placed even "deeper" than before (e.g., condylar neck and lower border of the mandible) via the transoral route, with screw placement via a small skin incision. Rigid plates can also be placed transorally with this technique in some cases.

A number of well-described techniques also exist for approaching the mandible externally. Although the entire mandible can be exposed extraorally, these approaches are usually reserved for condylar fractures, comminution involving the lower border, bone grafting, and in severely atrophic mandibles. While fractures in the anterior region can be approached through a submental incision, in most cases adequate access is possible intraorally.

The submandibular (Risdon) approach places an incision in the submandibular region approximately 1.5 to 2 cm below the inferior border of the mandible. This approach requires careful dissection in order to avoid the mandibular or cervical branches of the facial nerve that run in this region (Fig. 15-9). These are usually found on the undersurface of the deep cervical fascia. Dissection is carried down to the periosteum of the lower border of the mandible, which is then incised and elevated to expose the fractures before fixation. A similar blunt dissection technique in the retromandibular region provides access to the ramus and condylar neck. This can be either behind or through the parotid capsule and gland. Here, care is also required not to damage any of the branches of the facial nerve.

Like parotid surgery, good assistance is required in both approaches. Often facial nerve injury arises not from direct injury to the facial nerve or its branches, but from overzealous traction in an attempt to improve visualization of the fractures through a small skin incision. Finally, preauricular or endaural incisions can be used to expose high condylar neck fractures or to access the joint space.

Choosing the Type of Plate

Miniplates and monocortical screws have without doubt revolutionized the treatment of mandibular fractures. Many systems are now available, providing plates and screws of varying shapes and sizes, and extending the role of semirigid fixation to increasingly more complex fractures. Consequently the need for heavy compression plates at the lower mandibular border (using bicortical screws) has become less. However, some argue that rigid fixation avoids the need for IMF, has less risk of infection[48,49] and allows patients to function much earlier. More precise anatomic reduction and

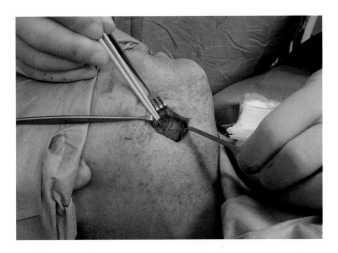

FIGURE 15-9 External approach to the lower border, demonstrating the mandibular branch of cranial nerve VII.

greater stability is also possible. One of the problems commonly reported with miniplates is loosening of screws due to excessive, intermittent loading where they engage the bone. This concept has led to the development of minilocking plates, which arose following the success of the larger locking reconstruction plates used in ablative/ reconstructive surgery.

The Case for Locking Plates
Risto Kontio

Before the introduction of reconstruction plates, surgeons carried out primary reconstruction with osteomyocutaneous regional flaps, external fixators, and bone grafts. Over the past few decades, reconstructive techniques and bone fixation plates have revolutionized the treatment of continuity defects and fractures. Open surgical semirigid or rigid plate fixation is now a standard technique. Various plate designs have improved both intraoperative handling and postsurgical results in the management of facial bone defects and fractures.

Initial reconstruction plates (bridging plates) were nonlocking in nature. When nonlocking screws were tightened, pressure was translated through the plate to the underlying bone. Friction between the plate and the bone surface "locked" the bone-screw-plate combination. Locking technology exploits the benefits of an external fixator. The theory of the locking plate and screw system is based on a solid integration of screw and plate that allows greater rigidity in the plating system. Cordey et al.[50] showed that the friction between the screw head and the plate is the main weak point of the entire fixation. In conventional plating systems, fixation is provided by the screw thread inserted into the bone, which creates a friction lock between the plate and the bone. Torsional forces between the bony fragments lead to a loss of this friction lock and result in reduced primary stability. In newer systems, the locking plate becomes united to the screw through a second set of threads within the head of the screw (Fig. 15-10). As the surgeon completes the tightening, the screw locks itself to the plate, creating a single functional unit and minimizing the transmission of pressure to the underlying bone. The lock of plate to screw prevents screw migration and axial movement of the screw.

In the 1980s, the AO/ASIF introduced the titanium hollow-screw osseointegrated reconstruction plate. This system integrated the concepts of internal and external fixation. At present, there are several types of rigid locking reconstruction plates and semirigid locking plates (1.5-2.0 mm) on the market.

Several benefits exist with the locking plate system. Poor adaptation of conventional bone plates causes displacement of the mobile bony fragments when the screws are tightened. This often leads to inexact repositioning and impairment in primary stability. With locking plates, in contrast, the fixator principle keeps the bony fragments (and fracture lines) in the planned, reduced position even if the plate is not precisely adapted (Fig. 15-11). Therefore, exact plate adaptation is not necessary.[51,52] Axial movement of the screw is also reduced by this locking mechanism. In a locking plate system, the forces generated between the threaded portion of the plate and the screw itself reduce compressive forces between the surface of the plate and the bony cortex, allowing better periosteal function and less risk of surface necrosis. Locking plate systems therefore have the following advantages over conventional plates and screws: (1) less precision required in plate adaptation, (2) less alteration in the osseous relationship after screw tightening, (3) greater stability across the fracture site, and (4) less screw loosening.

The main disadvantage of locking plate systems is the need for precise positioning of the screw in relation to the plate. Locking systems require perpendicular placement of the plate-screw interface, and a drill guide is often required. In intraoral surgery, this is not always practical. The other drawback is the cost. At the time of this writing, six-hole 2.0-mm locking plates are more than one-third more expensive than nonlocking 2.0-mm conventional plates, and the cost of locking screws is almost double of that of nonlocking screws.

Chiodo and Ziccardi and their co-workers designed an experimental study to try to incorporate some of the patient variability factors regarding plate fixation.[53] Fresh bovine bone was used. They concluded that locking systems have an advantage over conventional plates in areas where access is difficult, plate adaptation is less than ideal, or small continuity defects exist. Haug et al. showed that better results were

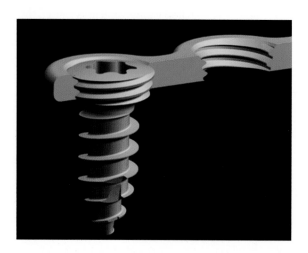

FIGURE 15-10   Plate and screw design of a locking system.

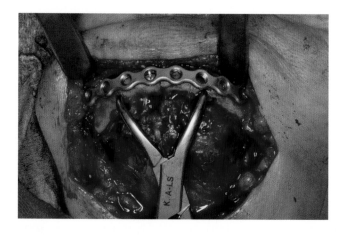

FIGURE 15-11   Application of locking plate to anterior edentulous mandible.

achieved with a locking system than with conventional plates in a study of polyurethane mandibles.[54] They concluded that the locking plate system does not need a friction lock between plate and bone for stability; as a result, there is decreased pressure and, in theory, less disturbance of periosteal perfusion and less bone necrosis. Gellrich et al. retrospectively compared two rigid locking plate systems (THORP and UniLock) in patients with mandible reconstruction after tumor-ablative surgery. A total of 107 patients had mandible defects reconstructed by the plate bridging technique. The UniLock 2.4 system was shown to be slightly superior to the THORP system. This may be explained by the less bulky design of the UniLock 2.4 system.[55] However, this clinical situation is not directly comparable with routine trauma fractures.

Kirkpatrick et al. examined the incidence of infection when a locking reconstruction bone plate system was used.[56] Fifty-six locking bone plates were placed in 42 patients. Two patients with three fracture sites (6%) developed postoperative infection that required further therapy. The authors found an incidence of postoperative infection with locking reconstruction plates similar to that stated by other research groups. They concluded that the use of locking reconstruction plates can facilitate the management of complicated fractures but does not eliminate all complications.

The primary goal of mandible osteosynthesis is to achieve the pre-injury occlusion. Studies of the UniLock 2.0 system have shown that 5% to 10% of patients can have minor postoperative occlusal discrepancies.[52] Similar studies on conventional miniplates showed postoperative malocclusions in approximately 5% of patients.[57,58] However, Chiodo et al. did not show any statistically significant differences between locking and nonlocking plate designs when they were placed in an identical manner.[53]

Another prospective, randomized clinical trial was conducted in 90 consecutive patients with 122 mandibular fractures.[59] Patients were randomly assigned to receive locking 2.0-mm or nonlocking 2.0-mm plates. Short-term complication rates were similar. This study did not consider other factors such as the costs of the two systems. Locking plates in most countries are significantly more expensive.

Loosening of screws and plates is considered to be one of the main risk factors for increased rates of infection and complications. Sauerbier et al. showed that the UniLock 2.0 system had a major complication rate of only 2%, with loosening of only one screw.[60] Provided that the UniLock 2.0 plates are inserted correctly, the risk of screw loosening seems to be minimal. This fact, combined with decreased pressure and stress to the underlying bone, may allow increased bony healing and regeneration.

Both laboratory and animal models have shown locking-type systems to function as well as, or better than, conventional plates, with less critical plate adaptation when bridging continuity defects. The conventional plating system is inherently weaker when bone quality or quantity is compromised. If bone quantity or quality is poor, decreased strength and increased failure of nonlocking plating are likely. Locking plating may be beneficial in such circumstances.

However, the use of rigid locking plates in the treatment of mandible continuity defects still has a high rate of complications (30%-40%), including plate fracture, screw loosening, plate exposure, wound infection, and malocclusion.[61]

Continuity defects are particularly relevant in oncology but also are occasionally seen in trauma cases. The average time until hardware fails is 1.5 years. Plate exposure is closely associated with radiation therapy and with reconstruction of lateral defects using a plate only or a plate and soft tissue flap. Because of these high rates of complications with mandible reconstruction plates, definitive bridging reconstruction should be used only for older patients and those with rapidly progressing disease. Primary bridging osteosynthesis of mandibular defects is regarded as efficient temporary reconstruction to support and keep the facial contours intact on a temporary basis, allowing for a delayed secondary bony reconstruction.

Alternative Strategies in Repair

As materials have become stronger, fixation devices have become smaller. The use of microplates for internal fixation of mandibular fractures has now been reported, although this is not routinely undertaken in many units.[62]

Part of the reason for this diversity of opinion (rigid versus semirigid fixation) and the wide range of fixation kits currently available is due to the still unanswered question, "How rigid does fixation need to be?" IMF certainly does not immobilize fractures rigidly, yet it clearly works and they heal even if not anatomically. Those surgeons who advocate the use of two or more plates across a fracture, or the use of larger (2.3- and 2.7-mm) plates, argue that this is necessary in order to neutralize all forces across the fracture and adequately stabilize it. On the other hand, others argue that this is unnecessary and that smaller plates provide sufficient fixation, requiring less soft tissue dissection and fewer complications.[63]

A further technique originally developed in orthopedics is that of the lag screw.[64,65] This is sometimes a useful compromise between the rigid and semirigid techniques, especially in the anterior mandible. Here, a screw hole is drilled perpendicular to the fracture, essentially "kebabing" (passing through) both bone fragments. The screw is then passed while the fracture is anatomically reduced. Either by design of the screw, or by overdrilling the proximal hole (in the fragment closest to the screw head), only the distal fragment is engaged by the end of the screw. This allows the fragments to be compressed on tightening. Varying combinations of this technique are possible, using multiple screws or plates and lag screws (Fig. 15-12). Whatever arrangement is chosen the aim is always the same: to attain at least adequate fixation of the fracture while minimizing the amount of soft tissue/periosteal dissection.

When used effectively, lag screws offer excellent reduction and near-rigid fixation. Lag screw fixation of fractures involving the posterior mandible and ramus regions is also possible, but is more technically demanding. Often, a percutaneous trocar is necessary to place the screw without damaging the inferior alveolar nerve or teeth. This technique offers a quick and precise method of reduction in selected cases.

How Many Plates Are Required?

In the anterior mandible (symphysis/parasymphysis) it is generally accepted that a minimum of two plates is required in order to resist the torsional forces produced by the attached muscles (Fig. 15-13). The upper plate should ideally be placed 5 mm or more below the apices of the teeth to minimize risks

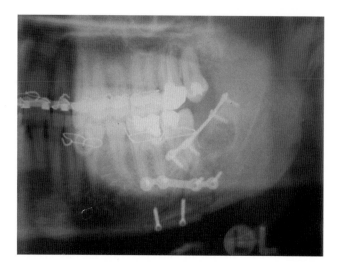

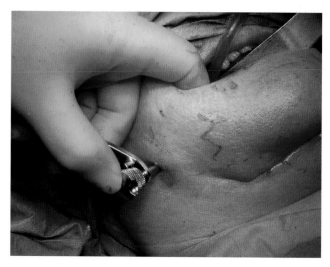

FIGURE 15-12   Repair of comminuted fracture with a combination of plates and lag screws.

FIGURE 15-14   Transbuccal access for screw placement.

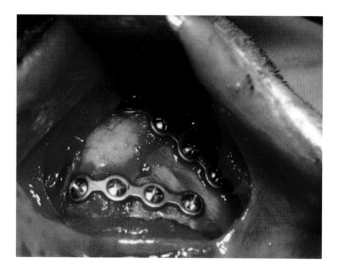

FIGURE 15-13   Two-plate fixation for parasymphyseal fracture.

to the apical blood supply. The lower plate is ideally placed as low as possible (i.e., along the lower border) for maximal stability. Two plates next to each other is not the best arrangement. In reality, what is needed is two remote points of fixation, rather than two plates. On this basis some fractures can be successfully managed using a single plate as one point and the lower teeth as the other, by splinting them with a short arch bar or circumdental wire. In essence the teeth and arch bar acts like a little external fixator. This technique works well with most simple fractures but depends on healthy lower teeth and supporting structures. If either are damaged, diseased, or loose it is not recommended to try this. In selected cases of incomplete anterior fractures where the lower mandibular border has not been completely split, but the upper end of the fracture is separated, a small arch bar by itself can often suffice to close and support the fracture. IMF is not needed. These techniques are only of use in selected cases where there has been incomplete splitting or minimal separation of the bones and good interlocking of the fragments. In all other cases, two or more plates are usually required.

Posteriorly, some surgeons have looked at the role of two miniplates in angle fractures. This has been done in an attempt to enhance stability, yet avoid the external incisions required for larger plates. Different treatment strategies have been reported, all with good success rates. According to AO/ASIF principles, two bone plates should be used.[66] Here the upper plate should be positioned high, while the other is ideally placed on the lower border. However, this has been challenged, and many believe that one plate is enough.[67] If only one bone plate is used, it should be positioned high, along "Champy's line" at the external oblique ridge. Unfortunately this requires contouring a "propeller" twist in it, which can sometimes be difficult. This site may also result in the plate being placed directly under the mucosal incision, with an increased risk of exposure. For these reasons some surgeons now prefer a "transbuccal" approach, whereby one or two plates are secured more buccally. This requires a percutaneous trocar technique to drill the holes and place the screws (Fig. 15-14). For body fractures, fixation with one plate or two plates gives equally good clinical results.

At present, it is not entirely clear whether one bone plate or two plates are required for treatment of simple mandibular fractures. Two miniplates do not seem to confer any significant extra clinical benefit in angle fractures.[63] On the other hand, Champy's original recommendation was for two plates in the anterior mandible. With comminuted fractures (discussed later), stability between all the fragments is considerably less. There are also more "pieces" to put together. Consequently, plates will have to carry increased loads and more may be required.

EXTERNAL FIXATION

External fixation is a technique which can provide rapid fixation (in critically ill patients), with minimal soft tissue disruption. As such its benefits lay in temporary fixation (in patients being transferred, or too sick to undergo lengthy surgery), or when there is extensive comminution of the mandible and/or significant soft tissue injury. It is also particularly useful in maintaining space and orientation in continuity defects. External fixation is especially useful in mandibular fractures associated with high energy transfer such as gunshot wounds, where additional and unpredictable tissue necrosis needs to be anticipated for up to several weeks following initial injury. Following blast or ballistic injuries it can "buy time" allowing devitalized tissue to declare itself, while maintaining fragment orientation. These concerns also apply when the surrounding soft tissues have been compromised by other causes, such as previous radiotherapy. As with other closed treatments this is essentially a "blind" technique (in that the fractures are not visualized). However, combinations of closed techniques may be useful in grossly comminuted fractures with multiple small fragments. This avoids wide periosteal stripping which can further compromise vascular supply, and risk subsequent necrosis and/or infection of the smaller bone fragments.

In order to obtain effective stability two pins are required on each side of the fracture. In orthopedics as healing progresses, the degree of rigidity can be modified (dynamization), thereby reducing the potential effects of stress shielding. This can also be done in the mandible although it is not as essential. The position of the bones can also be adjusted (often without general anesthesia) if postoperative radiographs show inadequate reduction. Many types of devices exist, some specifically designed for the mandible, others fabricated from general external fixation kits. If a kit is unavailable acrylic cross bars can be easily fabricated with the aid of an endotracheal tube/chest drain and acrylic resin (Fig. 15-15). During the hardening phase the reaction is exothermic, so care should be taken to avoid burning the patient's skin.

Unfortunately the bulky apparatus is often disliked by patients. Care is required not to injure themselves, a particular problem in alcoholics, children, and uncontrolled epileptics. Even modern miniature devices are still relatively obtrusive. Placement normally involves skin punctures which can leave unsightly scars. More recently, the external fixator has had a new lease on life as a means of callus distraction, and although a very successful technique, scarring and awkwardness still remain significant problems. Pin sites can also become infected. After 6 to 8 weeks, loosening of the bone pins commonly occurs. Some surgeons argue that external

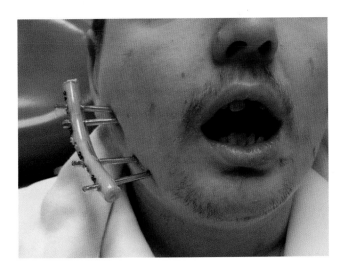

FIGURE 15-15 "Poor man's external fixator", using endotracheal tube and acrylic resin.

fixation may also have a role in the management of pediatric mandibular fractures (in cooperative patients) by minimizing risks to the developing tooth buds.[68]

AFTERCARE AND FOLLOW-UP

Relatively little has been published about the follow-up process of patients and protocols vary considerably, often without any evidence base. Anecdotally, patients may be discharged from care as soon as 1 month following treatment, or they may be kept under review for well over a year. Within the United Kingdom financial and other constraints undoubtedly play a part in the decision to discharge patients, as well as other factors, such as the surgeon's "specialists interest", and the high rates of nonattendances commonly seen. In the postoperative management phase a number of decisions must be made, many of which are based on personal experience and opinion:

1. **Oral Hygiene.** This needs to emphasised to patients, especially when intraoral incisions or lacerations have occurred, or IMF is used. Many regimens exist, from regular hot salt water mouthwashes, to a variety of antiseptically based ones. The ideal frequency is not known, but some antiseptics, such as chlorhexidine, can stain enamel if overused. Tooth brushing should be advised as soon as the oral environment will allow.

2. **Postoperative imaging.** In various areas of maxillofacial trauma, including the mandible, there appears to be a growing trend towards not taking "postop views", in all but the complex cases. This is an interesting point. On the one hand it is argued that this is not necessary, since the surgeon should know if his repair has been adequate or not. It reduces the need for unnecessary irradiation and in the vast majority of cases it does not alter what we do—the decision to re-operate is based on clinical assessment, not on an "X-ray." On the other hand, it is argued that without postoperative views we cannot evaluate our results, improve our care, or train the next generation of surgeons. There are also medicolegal issues as well if the patient returns with loose hardware—is this a surgical failure, or did they just get thumped (assaulted) again? Although, a small number of publications have challenged the need for postoperative views, at the moment this is not widespread established practice.

3. **Antibiotics.** This area has been well published on, but regimens still vary. If antibiotics are to be administered they should certainly be given at the time of surgery (or on admission), rather than commenced postoperatively. Concerns about bacterial resistance are always present and these need to be weighed against the risks of infection developing, such as in comminuted fractures, debilitated patients, and if there have been delays. Ideally all infections should be reviewed every 48 hours and the need for antibiotics reassessed, but this is not practical for the vast majority of cases. Discussion with your local microbiologist may be of value and local audits help define local policies.

4. **Postoperative elastics.** The use of these (or not) following semirigid fixation, and how tight they are applied varies considerably, depending on a number of factors. For single

and simple fractures they may not be used at all. The rationale for elastics is to help support the mandible (and fractures) while "fine tuning" the occlusion if the fracture has not been anatomically reduced. This appears to work, presumably by allowing the dentition to readjust, although very little has been published about this aspect of management. How long elastics should be used for is also poorly discussed in the scientific literature and in clinical practice is often based on personal experience.

5. **Return to normal diet.** 4 to 6 weeks seems to be an approximate time length for most fractures, depending on their complexity. Considering the significant amount of force a healthy mandible can generate on biting, this is an interestingly short time frame when one considers the limbs, which can take 3 to 4 months of immobilization before weight bearing.

6. **Plate removal.** The literature is not clear on this. Several reports have been published on the migration of titanium particles into the neck and further afield, questioning how inert titanium really is. As yet, the very long-term effects of titanium are still unknown. Some units routinely remove the fixation plates, although the evidence indicating that this is necessary is currently weak. Most units do not remove plates unless there have been significant complications.

7. **Rehabilitation.** Once the fracture has healed, patients should be encouraged to mobilize the jaw. Prolonged IMF restricts mouth opening by capsular contraction at the TMJs. The surrounding soft tissues also should not be forgotten. High-energy injuries may result in fibrosis, both in the skin and in the deeper tissues and these often need vigorous massage and other exercises to facilitate neuromuscular recovery. Many protocols and devices exist. Chewing gum and lollipop sticks are a cheap alternative. The most important element however is patient compliance to a long-term regimen.

8. **Length of follow-up.** This varies considerably and is influenced by many factors. While early discharge may "free up" time to see more patients it is only with long-term follow-up that long-term outcomes can be known. However, what is meant by "long term"? Some complications (for instance condylar resorption) may take years to occur and some injuries (notably scars and nerve injuries) years to recover. Conversely, untreated infections can rapidly progress over a matter of days in high-risk patients and may need very close follow-up initially. Follow-up—whether it be weekly, monthly, or annually—is generally not based on biology, but rather on our astronomical calenders! A pragmatic biological approach is ideally required on a case by base basis. Prolonged dental follow-up (usually by the patient's dentist) is also recommended. In the long term, teeth can devitalize and stain in the absence of obvious injury, either as a result of the initial impact or subsequent screw placement.

COMPLICATIONS IN MANDIBULAR FRACTURE MANAGEMENT

Complications following treatment may arise as a result of the effects of the original injury, the treatment itself, inadequate aftercare, or patient non-compliance postoperatively. These may be considered as anatomical (i.e., cosmetic deformity) or functional in nature. Fortunately complication rates have improved since the early days of wire fixation, but even the most sound fixation techniques can have problems.

MALUNION AND NONUNION

If fractures are assessed critically, malunion (i.e., nonanatomical union) is a relatively common outcome. However, most cases do not result in any clinical difficulties and these minor discrepancies are usually accepted by both patients and clinicians. Low-grade infection can result in delayed union, nonunion, or loosening of the screws and plates enough to result in malunion. With nonunion, a number of risk factors are associated, notably smoking and infection. Other risks include poor reduction of the fractures (resulting in soft tissue interposition), inadequate immobilization, the presence of foreign bodies, devitalized teeth or bony fragments, malnutrition, and debilitation.

Arch deformity following fracture repair is often the result of inadequate reduction. This is more common when the mandible has sustained fractures at multiple sites, or when associated with an unrecognized palatal split in the maxilla. Here the upper dental arch no longer acts as a reference point in reduction. Failure to anatomically reduce the fractures results in occlusal discrepancies, compromising the patient's ability to bite and chew. It can also result in poor esthetics. Bone is a plastic material and can undergo deformation as well as fracturing (especially in children). Consequently, minor residual deformity may still occur, even in those fractures which appear to be anatomically reduced. Familiarity in dental anatomy and functional occlusion (and their variants) certainly helps during treatment. Preoperative study models (with or without model surgery) and splint fabrication may also aid fracture reduction in complex cases.

If malalignment is noticed early in the postoperative phase it may be corrected by returning the patient to the operating room for repeated reduction. When this is not recognized the fractures will go on to heal in a nonanatomical position (malunion). Minor malunions do not usually cause major clinical problems, because the dentition often readjusts to a new bite. Alternatively, judicious selective grinding can balance the "neo-occlusion" satisfactorily. However, significant malunions of the mandible can produce facial asymmetry and/ or functional disturbances, which can only be resolved by carefully planned osteotomies. For this reason close follow-up during the healing process is necessary.

The commonest cause of nonunion is excessive mobility across the fracture site. Movement of the bone ends disrupts fibrovascular ingrowth, thereby reducing osteoblast migration. Instead of bony healing, fibrosis at the fracture occurs—fibrous union. Other contributing factors to nonunion include impaired healing capacity secondary to illness or self-neglect, smoking, and infection. In some cases (atrophic edentulous mandibles in frail patients), nonunion may be accepted if movement at the fracture site is not significant. But in most other cases further treatment is required. The management of nonunion requires excision of scar tissue within the fracture gap, together with bone fixation. Bone grafting may also be required although treatment strategies may vary from patient to patient.

INFECTION

Infected fractures are often seen in clinical practice, with rates varying from less than 1% to 32%.[69-71] They can be very difficult to manage. These are commonly seen in those patients who either neglect themselves, are poorly compliant, or present late with infection. Of all the facial bones, the mandible is the one most likely to become infected following injury. This is probably due to a combination of continued movement of the fractures from muscular pull, associated poor oral hygiene, and relatively less vascularization compared to the other bones of the face. Infection is especially a concern when there is a communication externally, or with the oral cavity via the periodontium in patients with poor oral hygiene. Alcohol, smoking, and excessive movement across the fracture site are the main contributing factors to the development of infection. Other risk factors include immunocompromise (notably diabetes and alcoholism), substance abuse, gross contamination, and preexisting periodontal disease.[72,73]

Most infections are usually mild, with intraoral swelling and discomfort. However these can progress to cellulitis, abscess formation, fistula, osteomyelitis, and, rarely, necrotizing fasciitis. A number of treatment options are available, based on the patient (general health, compliance, and wishes), the jaws (number of teeth, periodontal status), the fracture (its site and complexity), the infection (acute or chronic, presence of suppuration), and the associated soft tissues (healing potential). No one treatment has been shown to be the most appropriate for all case scenarios and various options and protocols are available.

Depending on the general condition of the patient, severity of the infection, time since repair, and adequacy of reduction, treatment may include:

- oral or intravenous antibiotics with our without incision and drainage of any pus.
- antibiotics and IMF.
- antibiotics and immediate removal of plates with or without IMF or external fixation if fracture is mobile.
- antibiotics and immediate removal of plates with or without rigid fixation if fracture is mobile.[74]
- for minor infections, treat with antibiotics and leave the plates in situ, or remove them later.

The principles of management are therefore to control the infection (incision and drainage, and antibiotics), remove any focus of infection (dental roots, third molars, sequestra, or plates and screws), optimize the healing environment (patient's health, oral health) and immobilize the fracture. This latter principle is where opinions vary and a number of strategies have been reported. IMF is the traditional method, keeping the fixation device remote from the infection, but has drawbacks as previously outlined. External fixation is a useful alternative. Rigid internal fixation may seem inappropriate, but in fact has a well-published success rate if properly undertaken. The key here is that fixation is rigid. Review of the literature shows that this approach is biologically sound and clinically effective so long as the fixation is rigid.

Most infections are polymicrobial. A member of the penicillin family is a good choice for treatment of early infections (if the patient is not allergic), whereas clindamycin may be used for chronic infections. If the infection fails to respond quickly, underlying causes should be considered and discussion with your local microbiologist is recommended. Laboratory studies (e.g., complete blood count, erythrocyte sedimentation rate, C-reactive protein) can be useful if there is systemic involvement, or immunosuppression is suspected, but in most cases management can be guided by regular clinical follow-up. CT and MRI may be required in severe infection or those which fail to respond to treatment. This helps to assess the degree of bony involvement, identify sequestra, and look for soft tissue collections or swelling. Specimens for bacterial culture and sensitivity should be sent as early as possible.

Osteomyelitis is rare in non-immunocompromised patients. Clinically, low-grade osteomyelitis can be confused with simple nonunion. Plain radiographs, CT, and MRI may be required to define the site of infection and delineate the region of the mandible affected. Radionuclide scans have been helpful, but lack specificity. Treatment includes surgical débridement, copious irrigation, and long-term antibiotics. If bone loss is extensive, the area should be immobilized and allowed to heal for several weeks prior to any definitive attempts at reconstruction with bone grafts or other methods.

NERVE INJURY

Fractures that involve the mandibular parasymphysis, body, or angle may result in injury to the inferior alveolar or mental nerves. The degree of deficit often depends on the amount of fracture displacement at the moment of impact and the type of nerve injury that results from this. Numbness can also be iatrogenic in origin. This is a common cause of litigation and therefore numbness *prior* to any treatments should always be recorded. Ideally patients with paresthesia following fracture should be observed during the postoperative period and the level of neurosensory return documented. As a "rule of thumb" sensory recovery can take up to 2 years to occur. Dysesthesia may be an encouraging sign in some cases as the nerve begins to regenerate, although it can also be a long-term troublesome symptom. Rubbing the affected area is said to induce "collateral macrosprouting" and encourage nerve ingrowth from adjacent regions. Rarely surgical exploration, decompression, and, if necessary, repair may be considered between 3 and 6 months.[75] Immediate management of inferior alveolar nerve injury at the time of mandibular fracture repair has also been reported where there has been significant fracture displacement, anesthesia, and an obviously injured nerve.[76] It is perhaps worth noting that in orthognathic surgery the lowest incidence of nerve injury occurs with wire fixation, with higher rates following most rigid fixation techniques. This would suggest that trauma itself is not the only cause of nerve injury.

SPECIAL CONSIDERATIONS

MANAGEMENT OF THE TOOTH IN LINE OF THE FRACTURE

Teeth are often involved in fractures of the mandible. The canine and third molars especially provide points of weakness in the bone, hence fractures at these sites are relatively common. The concern with retained devitalized or periodontally involved teeth is that they may encourage infection in the fracture and ultimately nonunion or abscess formation. However this is not likely in every case. Vital, functional or unerupted teeth with surrounding healthy periodontal tissues can be safely left in situ in most instances and, if problems develop, removed once the fracture has healed. Indications for removal of the tooth therefore include:

- Root fractures (devitalized roots can act as a nidus for infection).
- The tooth interferes with fracture reduction. This is often the case in underdeveloped third molars.
- The presence of obvious pericoronal or periodontal infection.
- The presence of associated pathology (e.g., cysts).

If a tooth needs to be removed it is sometimes better to plate the fracture first, then remove the plate before elevating the tooth. Removing bone to get a tooth out should be avoided as much as possible. This decision is particularly relevant for wisdom teeth, which sometimes help to stabilize the fracture. Once they have been elevated, precise reduction and stabilization of fractures can often become tricky.

CORONOID FRACTURES

This is an uncommon fracture, comprising around 0.5% to 1% of all mandibular fractures. Often it arises as an avulsion-type fracture, due to the pull of the attached temporalis muscle tendon.[77] However, impacts directly onto the side of the face can also result in these fractures. In such scenarios the zygomatic arch may also be fractured. Management of isolated coronoid fractures is usually nonsurgical. When the zygomatic arch has been fractured it is commonly taught that there is a risk of ankylosis between the two healing sites and that surgical treatment is necessary. Being such a rare fracture the evidence for this is more anecdotal, although it seems logical. Coronoidectomy of the fracture fragment is a relatively easy procedure if the fractured tip hasn't retracted upward. If no surgery is undertaken, aggressive jaw exercises (chewing gum is useful for this) may prevent ankylosis.

PATHOLOGICAL FRACTURES

These are rare fractures, comprising around 1% or 2% of all mandibular fractures. Their management can be extremely difficult, time consuming, and outcomes are often unsatisfactory. Definitions vary and include "fractures that result from normal function or minimal trauma in a bone weakened by pathology", and "a fracture which occurs through a preexisting lesion or in a diseased part of the bone". These definitions include a diverse group, but do not include the severely atrophic mandible, which can be argued not to be pathological, but rather a consequence of aging. Nevertheless both groups are difficult to treat and are considered together in some studies. The atrophic mandible is discussed separately later. Although a significant number of pathological fractures are due to osteoradionecrosis (ORN), newer etiologies such as bisphosphonate-induced osteonecrosis and fractures following implant placement are now becoming more frequent.

Only a few large series have been published, making sound evidence-based management difficult and controversial.[78] This is complicated by the fact that these fractures have a number of different predisposing causes which may affect bone healing in different ways. Patients may be immunocompromised, and present with grossly infected and nonviable bone. Treatment of the pathology usually takes priority, with fracture management depending on the resulting bony defect. Benign pathologies such as cysts have been successfully managed by marsupialization/enucleation together with external fixation, reconstruction plates, and bone grafts. In those cases where there is good bone-to-bone contact across the fracture, miniplate fixation has been reported to be reliable.[79] However in cases where healing is compromised, bone may need to be excised, and the resulting defect temporarily reconstructed using large reconstruction plates. Treatment of the defect will then depend on how much viable bone remains following this. Preoperative magnetic resonance imaging (MRI) may be useful in delineating the extent of marrow involvement, as an aid in deciding how much bone will need to be resected. Resecting back to bleeding bone may not be adequate and some reports recommend resection up to 1 cm past clinically "normal" looking bone. Some surgeons have attempted to preserve the inferior alveolar nerve, although results have been disappointing.

Options for reconstruction include primary free bone graft, delayed secondary bone graft, and primary microvascular reconstruction. This last choice provides the best outcomes with large defects (over 6 cm), as well as the ability to supply healthy soft tissues to the pathologic site. This has been used successfully in cases of ORN, bisphosphonate osteonecrosis, and osteomyelitis.

At the other end of the treatment spectrum, nonsurgical measures are sometimes successful. These are highly case dependent but may be considered in minimally displaced fractures, secondary to benign pathology, in patients too frail for surgery or who refuse treatment. Successful management has been reported with simple measures such as a soft diet and leaving out the dentures. The aim here is to achieve a fibrous pain-free union with intact overlying mucosa.

COMMINUTED FRACTURES

These are technically difficult to repair and commonly associated with complications.[80] Comminution implies high energy transfer at the moment of impact, a significant proportion of which is transferred to and damages the surrounding soft tissues. Often the overlying skin is split and so many of these fractures are open and contaminated. Not only is the vascularity compromised but multiple fragments, some small, are difficult to stabilize without using an excessive number of plates, all of which are foreign bodies. These small fragments are often difficult to manipulate and secure, while maintaining their soft tissue attachments, and are therefore at risk of becoming devitalized later on. All this results in a high risk for fragment necrosis, sequestration, nonunion, infection, and in some cases continuity defect. The key to successful management is therefore maintaining adequate immobilization of the fragments and sufficient vascularity, while minimizing contamination and preventing subsequent infection.

Traditionally, management of these fractures used closed techniques, thereby avoiding periosteal stripping and further devitalizing the bone. However, these techniques cannot guarantee adequate immobilization of all the fragments, although they do work well in selected cases. A number of techniques are available and have been previously discussed, notably IMF and/or external fixation. More recently, a more aggressive approach of open reduction and rigid internal fixation has been advocated. A number of reports have argued that maintaining the periosteal attachment, and therefore blood supply, is not as critical as providing stabilization of the bony fragments, so long as the fixation is rigid. Two elements are essential—the fixation needs to be fully load-bearing and there must be absolute stability across the fracture. Under these circumstances small bone fragments can then be replaced and fixed as free bone grafts, with a good chance for rapid bone healing and a low rate of infection.

The choice therefore lays between maximizing the soft tissue attachments and vascularity (using IMF / external fixation) and maximizing stability across the fragments (by load-bearing osteosynthesis).[81] Unfortunately the application of both is mutually exclusive, although some surgeons compromise by using smaller miniplates, with less periosteal dissection, supplemented with IMF. Whichever approach is undertaken there will always be a risk of infection, nonunion, or malunion. With very high impact energies, such as blast injuries, some surgeons recommend delaying treatment at least several days or longer. This enables nonvital tissue to demarcate itself, which can then be excised as part of the definitive repair. Once the airway is secure and hemorrhage controlled, these injuries are not life-threatening and can wait while further imaging (notably CT) helps define the extent of the fracture. Temporary IMF or external fixation can be used in the interim.[82]

THE ATROPHIC MANDIBLE

Fractures of the severely atrophic edentulous mandible are a difficult challenge. Once teeth are removed, progressive resorption of the alveolar crest and basal bone occurs, especially when the overlying mucosa is loaded with a dental prosthesis. With a depleted or absent dentition to dissipate the energy of impact and stabilize the segments, many fractures are significantly displaced due to impact and subsequent pull of the attached muscles. Greater understanding in fixation techniques and bone healing has now resulted in better outcomes. It is often stated that with increasing age there is decreased vascularity in the mandible, secondary to decreased flow in the inferior alveolar artery.[83] This study was based on angiograms carried out for vascular problems, so it may not be a "normal" situation. Consequently, the edentulous mandible depends more on the surrounding periosteum for its nutrition. In addition, the elderly mandible is often sclerotic and has decreased osteoblastic activity. With this loss of bone volume and vascularity the mandible becomes more susceptible to fracture. To add to these difficulties many patients are elderly, in whom general health and ability to heal is reduced. Not surprisingly therefore there is a significant rate of nonunion, malunion, and infection. A direct relationship between the height of the bone in the fractured area and the incidence of complications has been shown and this forms the basis of a simple classification system. Atrophic edentulous mandibles can be classified as class 1 (16-20 mm), class 2 (11-15 mm), or class 3 (10 mm or less). Fixation failure more often occurs with fibrous union or nonunion, when the height of the mandible is less than 10 mm. At heights above 20 mm conventional miniplate fixation is usually effective and mandibles with 30 mm or more vertical height are considered as nonatrophic.[84]

A number of treatment options are available; each has advantages and disadvantages compared to the others. These include nonintervention, the use of existing dentures wired to the jaw (with or without IMF), external fixators, miniplating (both sub- and supraperiosteal), and heavier reconstruction plates. Elective bone grafting has also been shown to be a useful adjunct, although this does carry the risk of additional morbidity at the donor site.

In minimally displaced fractures, a very soft diet and close observation may allow fibrous union to occur. Although not an anatomical result, this avoids surgery in often very frail patients, whose dentures can be realigned to fit, once the fracture is firm. Close observation is essential to ensure that the bone fragments do not erode through the overlying mucosa. Closed reduction may also be effective although immobilizing the fracture with the patient's denture is often difficult, even if it fits well. Nevertheless this is a useful option in patients unwilling or unable to undergo general anesthesia. Alternatively, occlusal splints (Gunning) may be fabricated to reestablish arch relationships. Longer periods of maxillomandibular fixation are recommended in elderly patients to allow for healing. External fixation can be used in patients where there are major concerns about healing, or where the bone is comminuted.

Open reduction in the atrophic mandible may be undertaken in many cases and is considered by some to give superior results. This approach is based partly on the orthopedic literature, which has shown a good relationship between stability and healing in poorly vascularized bone. It is also well reported that small avascular bone fragments or bone grafts, if adequately stabilized, will become incorporated and promote healing. Different philosophies exist and fixation varies from the use of large rigid reconstruction plates to the less aggressive use of semirigid miniplates.[85] Current areas of controversy in the literature include:

- open versus closed treatment.
- intraoral versus extraoral approach.
- subperiosteal versus supraperiosteal dissection.
- type of internal fixation hardware (miniplates versus rigid plates, locking versus nonlocking systems).
- simultaneous bone grafting.[86]

Fixation with transosseous wiring is often associated with a relatively high incidence of complications due to the amount of soft tissue stripping required and the lack of rigidity achieved. This can also occur when small miniplates are used. Near-rigid internal fixation is therefore recommended by some surgeons. This usually requires the use of at least 2.0-mm plating kits, with at least three screws on each side of the fracture. Larger reconstruction plates (2.7 mm) have also been recommended, but carry the risk of nerve injury and devascularization of the bone. The larger screws themselves can fracture the severely atrophic mandible during placement. Smaller kits (2.3 mm) require less periosteal stripping. In some cases, simultaneous bone grafting may be undertaken, although there is little in the literature to demonstrate that this provides major benefit. However, bone grafts may be useful in patients presenting late with non-united fractures. These are believed to increase the osteogenic potential of the fracture site. Grafting has to be balanced against the risks of potential morbidity at the donor site (rib, iliac crest, and tibia have all been used).

To date, the best way to manage these difficult fractures has not been clearly identified. The literature can be somewhat confusing if taken on face value. However it is worth noting that a 2007 Cochrane database review on the management of fractured edentulous atrophic mandibles found that there was inadequate evidence for the superior effectiveness of any single approach over the other alternatives.[87] Until a high level of evidence is available, treatment decisions should continue to be based on the clinician's prior experience and must always be considered on a case by case basis. Close follow-up is advised.

CONCLUSION

The successful management of fractures of the mandible requires a sound understanding of its complex anatomy, pathophysiology, articulations, dental occlusion, and related structures and biomechanical forces. Modern fracture repair is based on anatomic reduction, stabilization and (semi) rigid internal fixation techniques. Yet these are unlikely to work if either the patient or soft tissue environment are significantly compromised. It is not just a case of fixing the bones with big plates. Continued research in materials and techniques will further refine our treatments. Good aftercare is important in all trauma—just because the operation went well, it does not mean that the outcome will be good.

REFERENCES

 1. Vetter JD, Topazian RG, Goldberg MH, et al: Facial fractures occurring in a medium-sized metropolitan area: recent trends. *Int J Oral Maxillofac Surg* 20:214-216, 1991.
 2. Sakou T: Bone morphogenetic proteins: from basic studies to clinical approaches. *Bone* 22:591-603, 1998.
 3. Ellis E: Advances in maxillofacial trauma surgery. In Fonseca RJ, Walker RV, Betts NJ et al., editors: *Oral and maxillofacial trauma*, Philadelphia, 1997, Saunders, pp 308-363.
 4. Hippocrates: Oeuvres completes, trans. E.T. Withington, London, 1928, Loeb Classical Library.
 5. The Edwin Smith surgical papyrus, trans. Breasted JH. Chicago, 1930, University of Chicago Press.
 6. Lipton JS: Oral surgery in ancient Egypt as reflected in the Edwin Smith papyrus. *Bull Hist Dent* 30:108, 1982.
 7. Salicetti G: *Cyrurgia*, 1275, first printed at Piacenza, c. 1475-1476.
 8. Prevost N: *Translation of Salicetti's* Cyrurgia. Lyons, 1492.
 9. Gilmer TL: A case of fracture of the lower jaw with remarks on the treatment. *Arch Dent* 4:388, 1887.
10. Dorrance GM, Bransfield JW: *The history of treatment of fractured jaws*, Washington, DC, 1941, Army Medical Museum.
11. Ivy RH: Fracture of condyloid process of the mandible. *Ann Surg* 61:502, 1915.
12. Cole PP: Dental surgery and injuries of the jaw. *Br J Dent Sci* 60:77, 1917.
13. Heslop IH, Clarke PB, Becker R, et al: Mandibular fractures: treatment by open reduction and direct skeletal fixation. In Rowe NL, Willams JL, editors: *Maxillofacial injuries*, Edinburgh, 1985, Churchill Livingstone, pp 293-336.
14. Luhr HG: Stable osteosynthesis in fractures of the lower jaw. *Dtsch Zahnaertz* 23:754, 1968.
15. Spiessl B: *New concepts in maxillofacial bone surgery*, Berlin, 1976, Springer-Verlag.
16. Michelet FX, Deymes J, Dessus B: Osteosynthesis with miniaturized screwed plates in maxillofacial surgery. *J Maxillofac Surg* 1:79, 1973.
17. Champy M, Lodde JP, Schmitt R, et al: Mandibular osteosynthesis by miniature screwed plates via a buccal approach. *J Maxillofac Surg* 6:14, 1978.
18. Turvey TA, Bell RB, Tejera TJ, et al: The use of self-reinforced biodegradable bone plates and screws in orthognathic surgery. *J Oral Maxillofac Surg* 60:59-65, 2001.
19. Suuronen R: Biodegradable fracture fixation devices in maxillofacial surgery. *Int J Oral Maxillofac Surg* 22:50, 1993.
20. Eppley BL, Prevel CD, Sarver D: Resorbable bone fixation: its potential role in craniomaxillofacial trauma. *J Craniomaxillofac Trauma* 2:56, 1996.
21. Suuronen R, Kallela I, Lindqvist C: Bioabsorbable plates and screws: current state of the art in facial fracture repair. *J Craniomaxillofac Trauma* 6:19-27; discussion 28-30, 2000.
22. Bloch B: Bonding of fractures by plastic adhesives: preliminary report. *J Bone Joint Surg Br* 40B:804-812, 1958.
23. Weber SC, Chapman MW: Adhesives in orthopaedic surgery: a review of the literature and in vitro bonding strengths of bone-bonding agents. *Clin Orthop Relat Res* 191:249-261, 1984.
24. Perry MJ, Youngson CC: In vitro fracture fixation: adhesive systems compared with a conventional technique. *Br J Oral Maxillofac Surg* 33:224-227, 1995.
25. Donkerwolcke M, Burny F, Muster D: Tissues and bone adhesives—historical aspects. *Biomaterials* 19:1461-1466, 1998.
26. Shermak MA, Wong L, Inoue N, et al: Fixation of the craniofacial skeleton with butyl-2-cyanoacrylate and its effects on histotoxicity and healing. *Plast Reconstr Surg* 102:309-318, 1998.
27. Yilmaz C, Kuyurtar F: Fixation of a talar osteochondral fracture with cyanoacrylate glue. *Arthroscopy* 21:1009.e1-1009.e3, 2005.
28. Ruiz AJO, Vicente A, Alonso FC, et al: A new use for self-etching resin adhesives: cementing bone fragments. *J Dent* 38:496-502, 2010.
29. Haug RH, Prather J, Indresano AT: An epidemiologic survey of facial fractures and concomitant injuries. *J Oral Maxillofac Surg* 48:926-932, 1990.
30. Ellis E, Moos KF, El-Attar A: Ten years of mandibular fractures: an analysis of 2137 cases. *Oral Surg Oral Med Oral Pathol* 59:120, 1985.
31. Olson RA, Fonseca RJ, Zeitler DR, et al: Fractures of the mandible: a review of 580 cases. *J Oral Maxillofac Surg* 40:23, 1982.
32. Perry M: Advanced Trauma Life Support (ATLS) and facial trauma: can one size fit all? Part 1. Dilemmas in the management of the multiply injured patient with coexisting facial injuries. *Int J Oral Maxillofac Surg* 37:209-214, 2008.
33. Perry M, Morris C: Advanced Trauma Life Support (ATLS) and facial trauma: can one size fit all? Part 2. ATLS, maxillofacial injuries and airway management dilemmas. *Int J Oral Maxillofac Surg* 37:309-320, 2008.
34. Sansevere JJ, Badwal RS, Najjar TA: Cervical and mediastinal emphysema secondary to mandible fracture: case report and review of the literature. *Int J Oral Maxillofac Surg* 22:278-281, 1993.
35. Shuker ST: The effect of a blast on the mandible and teeth: transverse fractures and their management. *Br J Oral Maxillofac Surg* 46:547-551, 2008.
36. Chayra GA, Meador LR, Laskin DM: Comparison of panoramic and standard radiographs for the diagnosis of mandibular fractures. *J Oral Maxillofac Surg* 44:677-679, 1985.
37. White SC: Cone-beam imaging in dentistry. *Health Phys* 95:628-637, 2008.
38. Ilgüy D, Ilgüy M, Fisekcioglu E, et al: Detection of jaw and root fractures using cone beam computed tomography: a case report. *Dentomaxillofac Radiol* 38:169-173, 2009.
39. Mokoena T, Abdool-Carrim AT: Haemostasis by angiographic embolization in exsanguinating haemorrhage from facial arteries: a report of two cases. *South Afr Med J* 80:595-597, 1991.
40. Cannell H, Silvester PC, O'Regan MB: Early management of multiply injured patients with maxillofacial injuries transported to hospital by helicopter. *Br J Oral Maxillofac Surg* 31:207-212, 1993.
41. Fernandez JR, Gallas M, Burguera M, et al: A three-dimensional numerical simulation of mandible fracture reduction with screwed miniplates. *J Biomech* 36:329-337, 2003.
42. Arbag H, Korkmaz HH, Ozturk K, et al: Comparative evaluation of different miniplates for internal fixation of mandible fractures using finite element analysis. *J Oral Maxillofac Surg* 66:1225-1232, 2008.
43. Moulton-Barrett R, Rubinstein AJ, Salzhauer MA, et al: Complications of mandibular fractures. *Ann Plast Surg* 41:258-263, 1998.
44. Biller JA, Pletcher SD, Goldberg AN, et al: Complications and the time to repair of mandible fractures. *Laryngoscope* 115:769-772, 2005.
45. Koulocheris P, Sakkas N, Otten JE: Maxillomandibular fixation with Otten mini-hooks. *Br J Oral Maxillofac Surg* 45:679-680, 2007.
46. Hermund NU, Hillerup S, Kofod T, et al: Effect of early or delayed treatment upon healing of mandibular fractures: a systematic literature review. *Dent Traumatol* 24:22-26, 2008.
47. Baurmash D: Closed reduction, an effective alternative for comminuted mandible fractures. *J Oral Maxillofac Surg* 62:115-118, 2004 (letter).
48. Ellis E, Sinn DP: Treatment of mandibular angle fractures using two 2.4 mm dynamic compression plates. *J Oral Maxillofac Surg* 51:969-973, 1993.

49. Luhr HG: Compression plate osteosynthesis through the Luhr system. In Kruger E, Schilli W, editors: *Oral and maxillofacial traumatology*, Chicago, 1982, Quintessence, pp 319.

50. Cordey J, Borgeaud M, Perren SM: Force transfer between the plate and the bone: relative importance of the bending stiffness of the screw friction between plate and bone. *Injury* 31(suppl 3):C21-C28, 2000.

51. Gutwald R, Büscher P, Schramm A, et al: Biomechanical stability of an internal mini-fixation-system in maxillofacial osteosynthesis. *Med Biol Eng Comp* 37:280, 1999.

52. Ellis E 3rd, Graham J: Use of a 2.0-mm locking plate/screw system for mandibular fracture surgery. *J Oral Maxillofac Surg* 60:642-646, 2002.

53. Chiodo TA, Ziccardi VB, Janal M, et al: Failure strength of 2.0 locking versus 2.0 conventional Synthes mandibular plates: a laboratory model. *J Oral Maxillofac Surg* 64:1475-1479, 2006.

54. Haug RH, Street CC, Goltz M: Does plate adaptation affect stability? A biomechanical comparison of locking and nonlocking plates. *J Oral Maxillofac Surg* 60:1319-1326, 2002.

55. Gellrich NC, Suarez-Cunqueiro MM, Otero-Cepeda XL, et al: Comparative study of locking plates in mandibular reconstruction after ablative tumor surgery: THORP versus UniLOCK system. *J Oral Maxillofac Surg* 62:186-193, 2004.

56. Kirkpatrick D, Gandhi R, Sickels JE: Infections associated with locking reconstruction plates: a retrospective review. *J Oral Maxillofac Surg* 61:462-466, 2003.

57. Nakamura S, Takenoshita Y, Oka M: Complication of miniplate osteosynthesis for mandibular fractures. *J Oral Maxillofac Surg* 52:233-238; discussion 238-239, 1994.

58. Choi BH, Kim KN, Kang HS: Clinical and in vitro evaluation of mandibular angle fracture fixation with the two-miniplate system. *Oral Surg Oral Med Oral Pathol Oral Radiol Endod* 79:692-695, 1995.

59. Collins CP, Pirinjian-Leonard G, Tolas A, et al: A prospective randomized clinical trial comparing 2.0-mm locking plates to 2.0-mm standard plates in treatment of mandible fractures. *J Oral Maxillofac Surg* 62:1392-1395, 2004.

60. Sauerbier S, Kuenz J, Hauptman S, et al: Clinical aspects of a 2.0-mm locking plate system for mandibular fracture surgery. *J Craniomaxillofacial Surg* 38:501-504, 2010.

61. Coletti DP, Ord R, Liu X: Mandibular reconstruction and second generation locking reconstruction plates: outcome of 110 patients. *Int J Oral Maxillofac Surg* 38:960-963, 2009.

62. Burm JS, Hansen JE: The use of microplates for internal fixation of mandibular fractures. *Plast Reconstr Surg* 125:1485-1492, 2010.

63. Ellis E, Walker WR: Treatment of mandibular angle fractures using one noncompression miniplate. *J Oral Maxillofac Surg* 54:864-871, 1996.

64. Terheyden H, Springer I, Warnke P, et al: Internal fixation of median or paramedian fractures of the mandible with a novel lag screw system. *Int J Oral Maxillofac Surg* 34(1 suppl):66, 2005.

65. Ellis E 3rd: Lag screw fixation of mandibular fractures. *J Craniomaxillofacial Trauma* 3:16-26, 1997.

66. Kroon F, Mathisson M, Cordey JR, et al: The use of miniplates in mandibular fractures: an in-vitro study. *J Craniomaxillofacial Surg* 19:199-204, 1991.

67. Siddiqui A, Markose G, Moss KF, et al: One miniplate versus two in management of mandibular angle fractures: a prospective randomised study. *Br J Oral Maxillofac Surg* 45:223-225, 2007.

68. Blakey GB, Ruiz RL, Turvey TA: Management of facial fractures in the growing patient. In Fonseca RJ, Walker RV, Betts NJ, et al, editors: *Oral and maxillofacial trauma*, Philadelphia, 1997, Saunders, pp 1003-1043.

69. Bochlogyros PN: A retrospective study of 1521 mandibular fractures. *J Oral Maxillofac Surg* 43:597-599, 1985.

70. Busuito MJ, Smith DJ Jr, Robson MC: Mandibular fractures in an urban trauma center. *J Trauma* 26:826-839, 1986.

71. James RB, Kent JN: Prospective study of mandibular fractures. *J Oral Surg* 39:275-281, 1981.

72. Passeri LA, Ellis E, Sinn DP: Relationship of substance abuse to complications with mandibular fractures. *J Oral Maxillofac Surg* 51:22-25, 1993.

73. Moulton-Barrett R, Rubinstein AJ, Salzhauer MA, et al: Complications of mandibular fractures. *Ann Plast Surg* 41:258-263, 1998.

74. Koury M, Ellis E 3rd: Rigid internal fixation for the treatment of infected mandibular fractures. *J Oral Maxillofac Surg* 50:434-443; discussion 443-444, 1992.

75. Zuniga JR: Advances in microsurgical nerve repair. *J Oral Maxillofac Surg* 51(suppl 1):62-68, 1993.

76. Thurmuller P, Dodson TB, Kaban LB: Nerve injuries associated with facial trauma: natural history, management, and outcomes of repair. *Oral Maxillofac Surg Clin North Am* 13:283-293, 2001.

77. Philip M, Sivarajasingam V, Shepherd P: Bilateral reflex fracture of the coronoid process of the mandible: a case report. *Int J Oral Maxillofac Surg* 28:195-196, 1999.

78. Gerhards F, Kuffner HD, Wagner W: Pathological fractures of the mandible: a review of the etiology and treatment. *Int J Oral Maxillofac Surg* 27:186-190, 1998.

79. Coletti D, Ord R: Treatment rationale for pathological fractures of the mandible: a series of 44 fractures. *Int J Oral Maxillofac Surg* 37:215-222, 2008.

80. Ellis E 3rd, Muniz O, Anand K: Treatment considerations for comminuted mandibular fractures. *J Oral Maxillofac Surg* 61:861-870, 2003.

81. Abreu ME, Viegas VN, Ibrahim D, et al: Treatment of comminuted mandibular fractures: a critical review. *Med Oral Patol Oral Cir Bucal* 14:E247-E251, 2009.

82. Futran ND: Management of comminuted mandible fractures. *Oper Tech Otolaryngol* 19:113-116, 2008.

83. Bradley JC: Age changes in the vascular supply of the mandible. *Br Dent J* 132:142-144, 1972.

84. Luhr HG, Reidick T, Merten HA: Results of treatment of fractures of the atrophic edentulous mandible by compression plating. *J Oral Maxillofac Surg* 54:250-254, 1996.

85. Ellis E III, Price C: Treatment protocol for fractures of the atrophic mandible. *J Oral Maxillofac Surg* 66:421-435, 2008.

86. Van Sickels JE, Cunningham LL: Management of atrophic mandible fractures: are bone grafts necessary? *J Oral Maxillofac Surg* 68:1392-1395, 2010.

87. Nasser M, Fedorowicz Z, Ebadifar A: Management of the fractured edentulous atrophic mandible. *Cochrane Database Syst Rev* 24:CD006087, 2007.

CHAPTER 16

Condylar Fractures

Richard A. Loukota, Khalid Abdel-Galil

According to most large series reported in the literature, fractures of the mandibular condyle account for 26% to 57% of all mandibular fractures. The male-to-female sex ratio ranges from 3:1 to 2:1 depending on which population is studied. Between 48% and 66% of patients with condylar fractures also have a fracture of the mandible body or angle.

Approximately 84% of condylar fractures are unilateral, and the most common causes are interpersonal violence, sports injury, falls, and road traffic accidents. According to Silvennoinen et al.,[1] approximately 14% are intracapsular, 24% condylar neck, 62% subcondylar, and 16% associated with severe displacement. The highest incidence of fractures is seen in patients between 20 and 39 years of age.

Fractures may be classified according to their location: intracapsular or condylar head, condylar neck, and subcondylar. Further subdivision may be made according to deviation, displacement, and dislocation of fragments in relation to the glenoid fossa. The importance of any classification is to be able to identify a subgroup so that outcomes can be meaningfully compared.

To avoid confusion, it should be noted that in the literature from continental Europe, the term "dislocation" may be used to indicate *displacement,* as it would be called in the United Kingdom and in the United States. Likewise, the European term "luxation" may be used instead of *dislocation* (UK/USA). In this chapter, the UK/USA nomenclature is used.

Classifications include that of Spiessel and Schroll[2]:

Type I:	Undisplaced condylar neck fracture
Type II:	Displaced low condylar neck fracture
Type III:	Displaced high condylar neck fracture
Type IV:	Fracture-dislocation — low neck
Type V:	Fracture-dislocation — high neck
Type VI:	Head or intracapsular fracture

Other classifications include those of MacLennan[3] and Lindahl and Hollender.[4]

The classification adopted by the Strasbourg Osteosynthesis Research Group (SORG)[5] in their pan-European prospective, randomized, controlled trial[6] was as follows (Fig. 16-1):

1. Diacapitular fracture (through the head of the condyle): The fracture line starts in the articular surface and may extend outside the capsule.

2. Fracture of the condylar neck: The fracture line starts somewhere above line A, the perpendicular line through the sigmoid notch to the tangent of the ramus; in more than half of cases, it runs above the line A in the lateral view.

3. Fracture of the condylar base: The fracture line runs behind the mandibular foramen and, in more than half of cases, below line A.

There has been a change in the evolving nomenclature of fractures of the condylar head. Previously, these fractures were known as *intracapsular* fractures, but it was found that in large numbers of cases, the condylar head fracture extends outside and inferior to the capsule on the medial aspect. This name was therefore abandoned because it is anatomically incorrect. The more accurate name, *diacapitular* fracture, was then adopted.

Subsequently, a more anatomical nomenclature was proposed,[7] in which condylar head fractures were divided into three types (Fig. 16-2). More recently, the importance of associated ramus shortening with these injuries was highlighted as an indicator for open intervention.[8] Almost any direction of fracture propagation is possible, and in general, the greater the displacement of fragments, the less favorable the outcome.

Condylar fractures are complicated by their intimate relationship with the temporomandibular joint (TMJ). Direct fracture involvement of the joint or prolonged immobilization during treatment can lead to problems with deranged occlusion, internal derangement of the joint, ankylosis, and reduced mandibular growth. Symptomatically, these conditions manifest with long-term pain, limitation of jaw movement and function, asymmetrical growth, and malocclusion. TMJ ankylosis due to trauma is thought to account for only 0.4% of ankylosis cases.

In contrast to mandibular body fractures, which are now almost universally treated with osteosynthesis plates, there exists considerable variation in the management of condylar fractures in patients older than 12 years of age. Protagonists of conservative (closed) treatment methods cite evidence in the literature of satisfactory outcome with closed fracture management. They believe that the risks of scar formation, seventh nerve injury, and vascular compromise to the condylar head usually are not justified in simple condyle fractures.

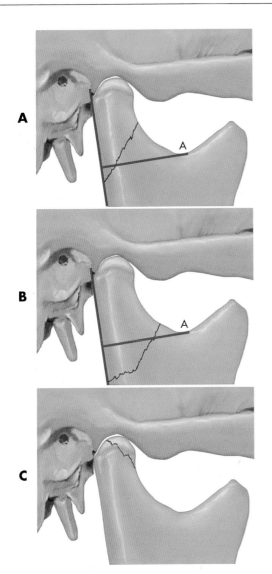

FIGURE 16-1 Strasbourg Osteosynthesis Research Group (SORG) classification of condylar fractures: **(A)** high or condylar neck fracture; **(B)** low or condylar base fracture; **(C)** diacapitular fracture.

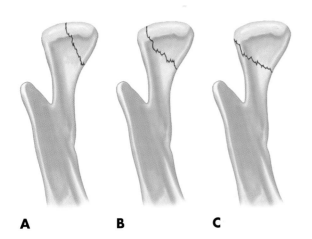

FIGURE 16-2 Types of condylar head fracture: type A, through the medial part of the condylar head; type B, through the lateral part; type C, near the attachment of the lateral capsule.

In this chapter, we attempt to draw on the published literature, consensus practice, and our own unit's policies to guide the reader in practical decision making when managing these fractures.

CLINICAL FINDINGS AND INVESTIGATIONS

Most condylar fractures are a result of blunt trauma to the anterior mandible. Forces are transmitted to the condylar region, where posterior movement of the mandible is limited by the glenoid fossa, the TMJ capsule, and insertion of the lateral pterygoid muscles. When the force is sufficient to overcome the strength of the condylar region, fracture follows. Trauma involving the open mouth leads to flexion fractures of the condyle. Symmetrical impact is said to cause bilateral fractures. Unilateral impact causes contralateral condylar fractures, and shearing forces are thought to produce intracapsular fractures. Closed-mouth fractures tend to distribute some of the energy to the occlusal surface of the teeth, and cuspal fractures are common.

Under the influence of the masticatory muscles, the mandibular ramus may shorten vertically and produce premature occlusal contacts distally (Fig. 16-3). The condylar fragment can dislocate out of the fossa, usually in an anterior direction; however, it may displace laterally, medially, or centrally into the middle cranial fossa. Any combination of fractures is possible, and joint maceration poses considerable surgical and healing difficulties.

Direct trauma to the TMJ area is unusual but may be associated with fractures of the zygomatic complex.

The derangement of the occlusion may give an indication of the fracture pattern. A unilateral fracture with sufficient fragment overlap or dislocation results in premature posterior contact and midline deviation on the affected side. Bilateral condylar fractures with overlap or dislocation produces bilateral posterior premature contact and anterior open bite with little or no chin deviation.

Comminuted mandibular fractures with bilateral condyle fractures produce crossbites and tend to increase the interangular distance, making accurate reduction challenging. Failure to recognize and correct this increased interangular distance leads to fixation of the body with a malocclusion (Fig. 16-4). Accurate reduction with the use of temporary intermaxillary fixation (IMF) avoids this problem and is

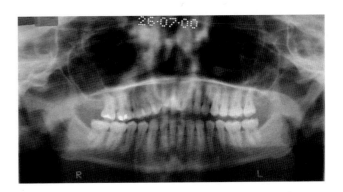

FIGURE 16-3 Orthopantomogram demonstrating right condylar fracture with anterior and left-sided open bites.

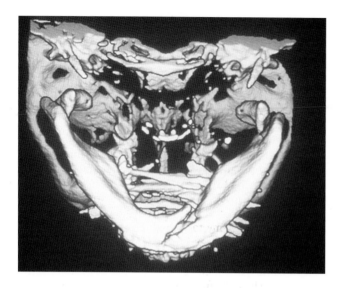

FIGURE 16-4 Three-dimensional computed tomogram demonstrates symphyseal and bilateral condylar (Guardsman's) fractures in which the fixation of the symphyseal fracture has been inadequate with splaying of the lingual cortex and increase in the interangular distance.

worth the time and effort before fixation of the mandibular body with miniplates.

Radiological imaging in two planes is required. An orthopantomogram (OPG) and posteroanterior (PA) mandible films are commonly used. Other projections include reverse Towne's, lateral oblique, and basic tomographic views.

If surgery is being considered, computed tomography is recommended and may identify previously undiagnosed sagittal (diacapitular) or comminuted fractures. If meniscus and capsular disruption are suspected, magnetic resonance imaging is also advisable.

MANAGEMENT STRATEGIES

The aims of condyle fracture treatment are to achieve:

- pain-free mouth opening with interincisal distance >40 mm.
- good movement of the jaw in all excursions.
- restoration of the pre-injury occlusion.
- stable TMJs.
- good facial and jaw symmetry.

Much of the debate is based on the fact that not all of these goals have an equal impact on the patient's quality of life and outcome. For example, a jaw that deviates on opening is less of a problem than a severe anterior open bite.

INDICATIONS FOR OPEN REDUCTION AND INTERNAL FIXATION

Absolute indications for open reduction and internal fixation (ORIF) in adult patients are:

- displacement into the middle cranial fossa or external auditory meatus.

- inability to obtain adequate occlusion by nonsurgical treatment.
- invasion by foreign body or gross contamination.
- lateral extracapsular displacement.

Relative indications are:

- bilateral fractures in edentulous jaws.
- IMF contraindicated for medical reasons.
- bilateral condyle fractures associated with comminuted midface fractures.

INDICATIONS FOR NONSURGICAL TREATMENT

Nonsurgical treatment may be the appropriate management strategy in cases of:

- condylar neck fractures in children <12 years of age.
- high condylar neck fractures without displacement.
- intracapsular (diacapitular) condylar fractures without loss of ramus height.
- poor anesthetic risk.

CONSERVATIVE CLOSED FUNCTIONAL TREATMENT

Definition of Closed Treatment

Closed treatment is treatment of condylar fractures by means other than surgical exploration, reduction, and fixation of the fracture line (i.e., not involving an open surgical exposure of the fracture). Traditionally, this has been achieved by arch bars, splints fitted over the remaining dentition, IMF, screws, or bonded brackets. Once reduction of the occlusion has been achieved, a period of immobilization may be required to encourage bony healing. Early mobilization is advised to minimize the risk of fibrous and bony TMJ ankylosis. This method of treatment is based on the principle that condylar nonunion is unlikely despite mobilization.

Definition of Closed Functional Treatment

Closed functional treatment involves the principles of closed treatment but is followed by at least 3 months of rehabilitation, including guiding elastics and mobilization regimens. It was found that when a full range of jaw movement is attained, normal jaw growth is not hindered. Adult muscles are more powerful than children's and commonly cause jaw shift, leading to malocclusion. The application of elastics to guide the occlusion allows some degree of remodeling and articulation in its new position. Early mobilization reduces the development of soft tissue scarring and promotes increased mobility. Use of intermittent maxillomandibular elastic traction each night, followed by release in the morning for full daytime use, results in daily stretching of the soft tissues. The motion enables linear and circumarticular healing of these tissues sufficient to allow a full range of joint and jaw movement. Scarring and tethering are inevitable, but this treatment may allow full jaw mobility. Repeated holding of the jaw in occlusion at night results in a balance between remodeling of the condylar fracture and firm extension of the soft tissue healing. These are the principles of closed functional treatment.

To encourage mobilization, mechanical devices have been developed to provide continuous passive motion. However, they are cumbersome and expensive. An alternative is the use of wooden spatulas to achieve 40 mm of interincisal opening. The number of spatulas placed between the upper and lower molar and premolar teeth is gradually increased until the desired opening is achieved. They are then taped together to allow use four to five times per day during the 3 months of rehabilitation. Protrusive and excursive movements are equally important during this period.

The literature is inconclusive regarding the success of conservative treatment, because series are often contradictory. Original work carried out by the Chalmers J. Lyon Club[9] provided the basis for the conservative approach, with good results reported in 120 cases treated conservatively. MacLennan[3] and Blevins and Gores[10] also published results supporting conservative treatment.

Based on research showing that bony union occurs in condylar fractures whether IMF is applied or not, the restoration of occlusion in a unilateral or bilateral condylar fracture through the use of IMF for 7 to 10 days and nonrigid immobilization for 3 to 4 weeks has provided a satisfactory functional outcome in many reported series. If there is gross displacement of the condylar fragment, IMF can achieve function through bony union of the fracture ends followed by pseudoarthrosis and re-education of the TMJ system over a 2- to 6-month period.

These early studies have been criticized heavily. In the case of the Chalmers J. Lyon Club, only 60 of the 120 patients were examined; the remainder were surveyed by mail. In MacLennan's study, only 67 of the 120 patients were examined, and Blevins and Gore used a postal questionnaire. Furthermore, there was no stratification of severity of injury, and the caseloads spanned all ages. Subsequently, it was found that bony remodeling and restoration of function vary with age, raising questions about the interpretation of these series.

EVIDENCE SUPPORTING CLOSED TREATMENT OF UNILATERAL CONDYLAR FRACTURES IN ADULT PATIENTS

Over a 12-year period, Marker et al.[11] reviewed 348 patients who had closed treatment of mandibular condyle fractures. IMF was applied for 4 weeks in patients with condylar fractures alone and for 6 weeks in those with combined fractures of the mandible body. Patients were assessed for complaints, mouth opening, malocclusion, and deviation after treatment and again after 1 year. In this series, 72% of patients had unilateral fractures, and 28% had bilateral condylar fractures. After 1 year, 13% of patients stated that they had one or more physical complaints, including reduction in mouth opening, deviation on opening, malocclusion, clicking, and limited chewing ability. In these 13%, there was no difference in severity or frequency of symptoms according to whether a unilateral or bilateral fracture pattern was present. However, there was an association between cause of fracture and complaint. Unilateral fractures caused by sporting accidents and bilateral condylar fractures caused by road traffic accidents produced the greatest number of subjective complaints, although this difference was not statistically significant. Only 3% of the 348 patients complained of pain in the TMJ or muscles.

Mouth opening was recorded as abnormal immediately after treatment in 55% of cases; after 1 year, this had fallen to only 10%. In these patients, there was an almost equal distribution between unilateral and bilateral fracture pattern. Among patients with persistent limitation of movement at 1 year, 69% were treated by IMF and the remainder had soft diet alone. Malocclusion was detected in only 2% of the 348 patients assessed. On review of the degree of displacement and malocclusion, it was found that 31% of patients with bilateral displacement but only 5% of those with unilateral displacement developed malocclusion. Of the overall 2% with malocclusion, most could be treated with simple occlusal grinding; the remainder of patients were not concerned and did not wish further treatment. Only one patient required a sagittal split osteotomy to correct the malocclusion. Deviation on opening was recorded in 10% of cases and was more frequently associated with high forces at impact. The results were amalgamated to conclude that there were more complaints in the bilateral fracture group compared with the unilateral fracture group when measured objectively.

There was no record of the degree of angulation or overlap at presentation in Marker's publication, but Silvennoinen et al.[1] estimated that 50% of condylar fractures would fall into the operative category, and that estimate suggests that there should be more dissatisfied patients. However, complaints were few. Marker's group therefore concluded that such rules are by no means a definite criterion for surgery. They advocated closed treatment but were cautious in applying this method to dislocations of the condylar head and bilateral fractures.

Joos and Kleinheinz[12] published a prospective study of 122 adult patients with 138 condylar fractures. Fracture types were limited to Spiessel type II and type IV low condylar neck fractures. The patients were allowed to choose between closed and open treatment. Assessment included clinical examination, three-dimensional axiography, radiographic assessment, and ultrasound TMJ evaluation. The results showed no significant differences in outcome. The authors also tried to predict mathematically the potential for vertical repair and angulation repair in the nonoperated condyle. They concluded that 6 degrees of angulation can resolve and 4 mm of height can be regained. However, angles greater than 37 degrees can remodel little and lead to clinical problems.

Hidding et al.[13] retrospectively analyzed 34 patients with unilateral displaced fractures of the condylar neck; 20 were treated surgically by ORIF and 14 by closed treatment. Outcome was assessed subjectively and analytically by axiography, radiography, and clinical and functional examination. Although some significant differences in measurement parameters were found, they could not conclude from the patients' own mastication ability that one group recovered better than the other. One possible limitation to this paper is that results were measured only 5 years after treatment, and possible long-term sequelae are not predictable. However, Dahlstrom et al.[14] suggested that there was little long-term change in their series. The authors concluded that ORIF of the displaced condylar fracture should be undertaken on the grounds of better measurement criteria rather than subjective outcome.

Konstantinovic and Dimitrijevic[15] compared surgical versus nonsurgical treatment of unilateral condylar process fractures. By computer-simulated graphic presentations of PA radiographs of the mandible, actual posttreatment condylar reduction was compared with ideal reduction as determined by the computer. Based on standardized clinical evaluation (maximal mouth opening, deviation, and protrusion), no statistical difference was found between the open treatment (n = 26) and closed treatment (n = 54) groups. However, the radiographic examination showed a statistically better position of the surgically reduced condyle process fracture. This study would seem to discourage open surgery on the grounds of overtreatment. However, the patients' treatment methods were not randomized, and there were many more patients with severe condylar displacement in the surgical group, as stated in the article. Therefore, if one assumes that the likelihood of problems after trauma becomes greater as the degree of condylar displacement increases, then this study also tends to support open treatment, because the two groups had similar treatment results.

Dahlstrom et al.[14] reported on a 15-year follow-up of conservatively treated condylar fractures in 36 patients. This series provides the best data available on the long-term outlook of closed treatment. Those patients who had sustained their injury in childhood had excellent results, with no growth restriction. Adults had some degree of restriction, as did the teenage group (12-19 years). Twice as many patients in the older group experienced symptoms of dysfunction compared with the younger group. Radiologically, the younger group showed better ability to restore condylar morphology. Interestingly, the symptoms and signs at 6 months were similar to those at 15-year follow-up, suggesting that long-term gradual improvement cannot necessarily be expected. Also, it may be concluded that future study design may not need to be protracted.

In a prospective evaluation of 26 class VI fractures randomized to ORIF or conservative treatment, Landes et al.[16] failed to demonstrate a benefit of the former treatment modality. Based on their results, the authors advocated closed treatment of these injuries. However, this study was based on a small cohort of patients, some of whom were not randomly allocated in order to achieve a balanced distribution between the two groups, thus deviating from the original protocol.

A study by Ellis et al.[17] looked at the position of the condylar fragment when closed treatment was deemed appropriate and found that the condylar position was different after IMF than at the outset of treatment. This brings up the question: If the condyle position in an individual meets operative criteria after IMF, should conservative treatment be abandoned for ORIF? In this study, 65 patients were treated by closed treatment. Coronal and sagittal displacement was assessed before, immediately after, and 6 weeks after IMF, and a statistically significant difference (mean, ↕5.5 degrees) in the coronal position of the condylar process before and after arch bars was found. The change in a sagittal plane was not statistically significant. Other planes of movement were noticed but did not reach significance. Further changes were noted at 6 weeks' follow-up. The authors concluded that care must be taken in basing treatment decisions on the degree of displacement or dislocation of the condylar process observed on presurgical radiographs.

In a more recent study by Ellis,[18] all unilateral extracapsular fractures treated over a 10-year period (1998-2008) were reviewed retrospectively. Ellis concluded that the determination of which patients would not benefit from ORIF can be made clinically during surgery more reliably than with preoperative imaging studies. This conclusion was based on intraoperative assessment of mandibular deviation and "dropback." If these are not found at operation, then open treatment is not necessary. However, closed functional treatment can also be used successfully in patients displaying deviation and the dropback phenomenon.

EVIDENCE SUPPORTING OPEN TREATMENT OF UNILATERAL FRACTURES IN ADULT PATIENTS

Palmieri et al.[19] studied 136 patients with fractures of the condylar process; 74 were treated by closed methods and 62 by open methods. The patients were assessed for mandibular and condylar mobility at 6 weeks, 6 months, and 1, 2, and 3 years after surgery. A jaw-tracking device was used to assess mandibular motion. Radiographs were traced and digitized to assess condylar displacement and condylar mobility. It was accepted that patients treated by open reduction had significantly greater initial displacement of their condylar fractures compared with the closed-treatment group. As expected, condylar malposition persisted after closed treatment compared with open treatment. At 6 weeks, some measures of mobility were significantly greater in patients treated by the closed method compared to ORIF. However, after 6 weeks, there were minimal differences between the two groups, and subsequently there was significant improvement in mobility in the ORIF group. No measure of presurgical displacement correlated with mobility measures in patients treated by ORIF. However, several measures of condylar displacement correlated with measures of mobility in patients treated by the closed method, indicating that the more displaced the condylar process, the more limited the mobility. The authors concluded that patients treated by ORIF had somewhat greater condylar mobility than those treated by the closed method, even though the former group had more severely displaced fractures before surgery, and that ORIF can produce functional benefits in patients with severely displaced condylar process fractures.

Worsaae and Thorn[20] published a series in which they evaluated 52 patients (24 with dislocated fractures) who were randomly assigned to receive either ORIF (24 patients) or closed treatment (28 patients). All fractures were unilateral, and the condyles were displaced from the fossa or overlapped at the fracture site (or both). All patients were 18 years of age or older and dentate. High condylar neck fractures were excluded from the study. The open treatment consisted of a submandibular incision and wire osteosynthesis followed by 6 weeks of IMF. The nonsurgical (closed) treatment consisted of an average of 30 days of IMF (range, 0 to 47 days). Both treatment groups had a median of 7 days of interarch training elastics after release of IMF. The mean follow-up period was 21 months for the ORIF group and 30 months for the closed treatment group, with each group having the same range, 6 to 64 months. The complication rate was 39% (11/28) in the nonsurgical group and only 4% (1/24) in the surgical group. The one patient with a problem in the surgical group had a collapse of the repositioned condyle and developed a malocclusion and muscle pain. In the nonsurgical group, there were three patients with mandibular asymmetry, eight with malocclusions, three with reduced mouth opening (<35 mm), two with persistent headaches, and six with muscle pain and impaired masticatory function. The median mouth opening for both groups was 45 mm, despite the relatively long periods in IMF; therefore, the extent of mouth opening alone did not separate the two groups. This study could have produced better results if more rigid fixation had been used instead of wire osteosynthesis. Also, IMF was used in both treatment groups.

Eckelt[21] published a series of 103 patients treated by ORIF, 26 of whom had bilateral fractures. The results were far more superior than those achieved with closed treatment. He reported normal anatomical alignment in 84% and limitation of protrusion in only 6% of cases.

Hidding et al.[13] investigated 34 patients with displaced fractures of the condylar neck, of whom 20 had been treated by open reduction and 14 by closed functional treatment. Assessment was by clinical, radiographic, and axiographic means. The clinical results were almost equal in both groups, but instrumental registration and radiographic findings showed considerable deviation in joint physiology in the closed-treatment group. Nineteen of the 20 patients who underwent surgery showed near-anatomical reconstruction with good functional results. It might reasonably be assumed that these patients would do better functionally in the long term as well.

Takenoshita et al.[22] reported a comparison of open and closed reduction in 36 cases of condylar fracture with a 2-year follow-up. Sixteen patients underwent ORIF via preauricular and short Risdon incision, followed by 3 weeks of IMF. The other 20 patients were treated by only 3 weeks of IMF. The two groups were not randomly selected. The ORIF group was selected for surgery because they had dislocated or severely displaced condylar processes. The authors' comparison showed that both groups had a similar result. If one assumes that severe condylar displacement is more likely to result in compromised jaw function, for which there is some evidence, then ORIF was beneficial for this surgical group. Again, IMF was used in both groups studied.

In a prospective investigation spanning 7 years, Ellis et al.[23] studied occlusal results after open and closed treatment of unilateral condylar fractures. Treatment was decided according to patient choice after explanation of the two treatment modalities. Assessment of occlusion was made by examination of posttreatment standardized occlusal photographs by an orthodontist (blinded condition) and by surgeon (unblinded). Patients treated by ORIF had significantly more pretreatment condylar displacement than those treated by the closed technique. Patients treated by the closed technique had a significantly greater percentage of malocclusion than those treated by ORIF.

Hlawitschka et al.[24] compared the results of open and closed treatment of diacapitular fractures of the mandible. Fifteen such fractures, associated with ramus shortening, were treated by ORIF. Outcomes were compared with those of 34 similar fractures treated with the use of a closed-technique. After ORIF, patients showed better radiological results with regard to mandibular ramus height, resorption, and pathological changes to the condyle. In both groups, some signs of dysfunction persisted, although there were slightly better results in the ORIF group. In 30% of the closed treatment group, lateral deviation during mouth opening, crepitus, and occlusal disturbances were noted. No cases of occlusal disturbance were observed in the ORIF group.

Axiographic examinations revealed significant limitation of movement of the fractured condyle in both groups. However, after open treatment, the TMJ displayed significantly fewer irregularities in the condylar paths.

More recently, several clinical trials have attempted to address the clinical controversy surrounding decision making in relation to condylar fracture treatment.[6,25,26] The data provided by these randomized, prospective studies indicate that better functional results can be expected by open reduction and internal fixation for moderately displaced condylar fractures with ramus shortening compared with closed treatment.

The SORG prospective, randomized trial involved seven international centers and compared operative and conservative treatment of displaced condylar fractures.[6] The results were clearly in favor of the operative approach. The trial reported on 66 patients treated for 79 fractures and followed up for 6 months. Evaluation included radiographic assessment and clinical, functional, and subjective parameters including visual analogue scales for pain and the Mandibular Function Impairment Questionnaire index for dysfunction. Operative treatment was found to be superior in terms of all of the objective and all but one of the subjective functional parameters.

In another prospective, randomized trial, conducted between 2007 and 2009, both treatment options for condylar fractures yielded acceptable results. However, operative treatment was superior in terms of all objective and subjective functional parameters except occlusion.[25]

BILATERAL CONDYLAR FRACTURES IN ADULTS

In the consensus study by Baker et al.,[27] bilateral undisplaced fractures of the condyle were managed similarly by surgeons throughout the world. However, the introduction of condylar displacement, dislocation, and intracapsular fracture patterns revealed great variation in treatment preference when dealing with bilateral condylar fractures.

The Gronigen Consensus Group[28] determined that there was good evidence that displaced bilateral condylar fractures benefit from treatment of at least one side by ORIF. It was accepted that this may cause an increased risk of even further displacement on the other side. It was noted that some displaced bilateral fractures can be treated successfully by the closed method but that predicting a favorable outcome is difficult.

Newman[29] published a series of 61 patients with bilateral condylar fractures; 51% of patients had bilateral condylar fractures alone, and the remainder also had other fractures, mainly parasymphyseal. Almost half of the condylar fractures (46%) were undisplaced. In 39 patients (21%), the condylar fractures were managed by the closed method with wire rigid IMF for a mean of 37 days; 13 patients had conservative management (no intervention), and 9 patients (15%) with 10 fractured condyles underwent ORIF. The most common complaint after treatment was persistent limitation in mouth opening, which was significantly less in the ORIF group compared with the IMF group (mean opening ± standard deviation, 44 ± 2 mm versus 28 ± 2 mm; $P < .01$). More importantly, 10% of the patients treated by IMF required orthognathic surgery to correct a persistent anterior open bite, despite the long periods in rigid IMF. The authors also commented that most of those requiring orthognathic surgery had minimal angulation at presentation. They concluded that the risk of complications from ORIF were minimal and that, in the case of bilateral condylar fractures, ORIF should be undertaken on at least on one side if displacement or angulation is present.

Our unit policy involves the use of interarch elastic traction for a period of 1 week, followed by further assessment. If the occlusion is found to be satisfactory and the condylar fragments are undisplaced on OPG and PA views, we treat the fracture by the closed method. If the fragments are seen on one side to be overlapped by more than 2 mm or if the angulation is greater than 10 degrees, we select ORIF of the displaced fracture. If both sides show significant displacement and measurement of angulation and overlap are greater than the values stated, we advise ORIF on both sides (Fig. 16-5), with each side being assessed on its own merits.

Particular care is needed to achieve very accurate reduction of the fragments before fixation. It may not be possible to hold the teeth in occlusion during the fixation procedure, because a downward distraction of the angle may be the only way to retrieve and reduce the condylar fragment. Once satisfactory fixation is achieved, the patient can be mobilized immediately postoperatively. To date, we have not experienced any seventh nerve injury that would change this policy.

The benefits of ORIF are:

- direct visualization of the fragments for accurate reduction and fixation.
- early mobilization of the mandible.
- early restoration of normal mouth and jaw activity.

Reported complications of open treatment include:

- poor esthetic result from the skin incision (particularly relevant if keloid scarring is likely).
- neural damage, especially to the facial nerve.
- intraoperative bleeding from the maxillary artery.
- loss of blood supply to the condylar head, leading to avascular necrosis.

MANAGEMENT OF CONDYLAR FRACTURES IN PANFACIAL INJURY

Panfacial injuries pose considerable challenges to the maxillofacial surgeon. Reduction and fixation of the facial skeleton must restore the correct anteroposterior (AP), lateral (width), and vertical dimensions. In the case of severe comminution of the midface and mandible, the only point of reference from which to start reconstruction is the stable posterior area (temporal bone and proximal zygomatic arch). One works sequentially to restore the AP projection, followed by reduction in width and restoration of the nasoethmoidal and orbital complex. Attention is then applied to accurate restoration of posterior vertical height by repositioning and fixation of the condylar ramus fracture. Access to the condylar fragment can be gained by extending the coronal incision that was used to access the zygomatic arch. Once posterior vertical height is restored, the anterior mandible can be fixed with accurate reduction in intercondylar width. Finally, occlusion is attended to, with fixation being applied lastly at the Le Fort I level, although some surgeons prefer to fix the occlusion at an earlier stage.

SURGICAL APPROACHES

SUBMANDIBULAR APPROACH (RISDON APPROACH)

The Risdon approach (Fig. 16-6) is best suited for low fractures of the condylar neck and ramus.

Anatomical Points of Importance

The marginal mandibular branch of the facial nerve runs on the deep surface of the platysma and is most likely to be no more than 1.5 cm below the lower border of the mandible. The facial artery runs vertically at the anterior border of the masseter muscle. The facial vein runs with the facial artery but posterior to it.

Preparation and Draping

Conventional draping is done to allow exposure of the surgical field with the ear visible posteriorly and the corner of the mouth and lower lip anteriorly.

Incision Marking and Vasoconstriction

The proposed skin incision is marked before a vasoconstrictor (normal saline with 1:200,000 adrenaline) is infiltrated. The incision should be 1.5 to 2 cm below the lower border of the mandible (if possible), employing the natural skin creases. These do not parallel the lower border but do provide ease of extension, if required, with good cosmesis.

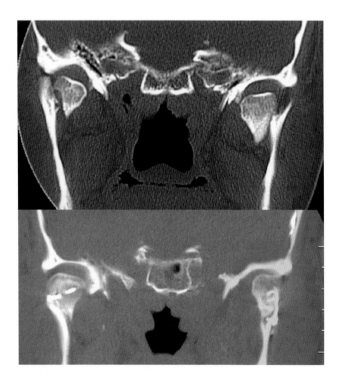

FIGURE 16-5 Composite computed tomographic scan showing preoperative and postoperative position after bilateral condylar fractures.

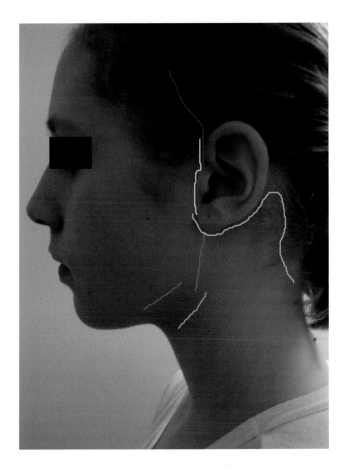

FIGURE 16-6   Position of the various incisions for surgical management of condylar fractures. *Blue*, Bramley-Al Khayat; *yellow*, preauricular; *turquoise*, rhytidectomy; *red*, retromandibular; *green*, submandibular; *purple*, submandibular (continental).

If there is shortening of the posterior mandibular height by telescoping of fragments, this should be taken into account when the site of the incision is planned.

Dissection

The skin and platysma are incised, exposing the superficial layer of deep cervical fascia. Care must be taken to avoid cutting the facial artery and vein. If they limit access, they can be tied and ligated or retracted. The marginal mandibular branch of the facial nerve lies superiorly and should be retracted gently with Langenback retractors. The dissection continues to the pterygomasseteric sling, which is incised with a scalpel along the inferior border, its most avascular area. With the aid of a periosteal stripper, the masseter is lifted off the lateral ramus. The dissection is continued superiorly, the entire lateral surface of the ascending ramus of the mandible is exposed to the TMJ and the coronoid process. The fractured end of the proximal fragment is frequently embedded in the masseter and needs to be dissected free. Care must be taken not to shred the muscle or perforate the oral mucosa anteriorly.

Closure

It is possible to repair the pterygomasseteric sling with resorbable sutures. The insertion of a vacuum drain helps to reduce hematoma formation. Platysma can be closed by a running

resorbable suture followed by interrupted subcuticular stitches. Finally, the skin is closed with nylon.

SUBMANDIBULAR APPROACH—CONTINENTAL

The continental submandibular incision is at the level of the lower mandibular border. Dissection is carried out above the masseter, identifying the seventh nerve branches. Medial dissection, splitting the masseter muscle to the ascending ramus, gives good exposure.

RETROMANDIBULAR APPROACH

The retromandibular approach is more suitable for low condylar fractures (Fig. 16-7). There are a number of approaches that surgeons call "retromandibular." The most common type is described first.

Anatomical Points of Importance

The main trunk of the facial nerve divides into the temporofacial and cervicofacial divisions. The marginal mandibular branch courses obliquely, inferiorly and anteriorly. It often arises from the main trunk behind the posterior border of the mandible, crossing the ramus at its lower border. This allows good access with relative safety between the buccal branch and the marginal mandibular nerve. The retromandibular vein courses through the parotid gland superficial to the external carotid artery.

Preparation and Draping

Draping should expose the entire earlobe and the angle of the mandible. The mouth should also be visible.

Incision Marking and Vasoconstriction

The incision line begins 0.5 cm below the earlobe and continues inferiorly for 3 to 3.5 cm. It is located behind the ascending ramus of the mandible and may be extended inferiorly. Normal saline with 1:200,000 adrenaline is injected into the operative field.

Dissection

The skin and subcutaneous tissue are incised, revealing the parotid capsule. Before the capsule is incised, the skin is undermined to allow retraction. The superficial musculoaponeurotic system (SMAS) and parotid capsule are then incised, and blunt dissection directly onto the posterior edge of the mandible is undertaken with a hemostat. The hemostat should be opened parallel to the anticipated direction of the nerve. The marginal mandibular branch may be directly encountered, or it can be sought with the aid of an electric nerve stimulator. Once the nerve has been identified, retraction can be performed in a superior or inferior direction. A flat instrument placed behind the ascending ramus holds the mandible steady to allow sharp dissection with a blade through the pterygomasseteric sling, subperiosteally. Blunt dissection superiorly, stripping periosteum, exposes the fracture ends. Care must be taken when disimpacting the condylar fragment from the masseter muscle.

Closure

It is possible to repair the pterygomasseteric sling with resorbable sutures. The insertion of a vacuum drain helps reduce

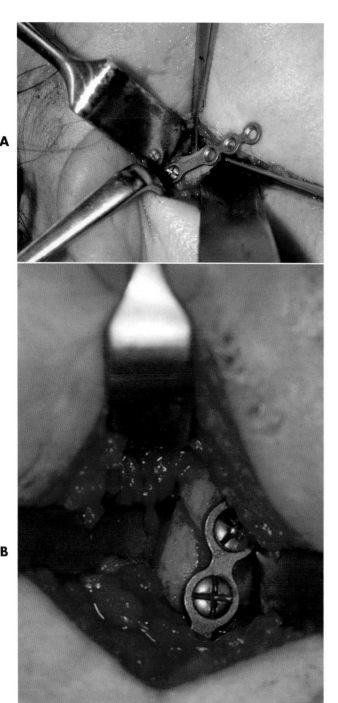

FIGURE 16-7 Retromandibular approach demonstrating placement of fixation plate before (**A**) and after (**B**) reduction of the proximal fragment.

hematoma formation. Closure of the parotid capsule and SMAS layer must be meticulous to reduce the chance of formation of a salivary fistula. Platysma, once defined, can be closed by a running resorbable suture followed by interrupted subcuticular stitches. Finally, the skin is closed with nylon.

RETROMANDIBULAR APPROACH—DEEP

Some surgeons dissect down to the sternocleidomastoid muscle, then deep to the superficial lobe of the parotid gland, and approach the posterior ramus from a deep angle, with the branches of the seventh nerve superficial to the dissection.

RETROMANDIBULAR APPROACH—HORIZONTAL THROUGH PAROTID

Some surgeons have advocated dissection above the parotid gland and incision horizontally through the parotid gland and masseter muscle, between the buccal and marginal mandibular branches of the seventh nerve, to gain access to the ascending ramus.

MODIFIED BLAIR INCISION APPROACH

The modified Blair approach is suitable for both low and high condylar fractures. It combines the preauricular and retromandibular approaches and offers increased exposure. It is particularly good for demonstrating the upper TMJ and the meniscus. It is used for repositioning and fixing intracapsular and very high TMJ fractures.

PREAURICULAR AND AURICULAR APPROACH

This approach gives good access to the TMJ, allowing repair of capsular disruption, and is suitable for high condylar fractures. The facial nerve is preserved in the modification by Al Khayat and Bramley (Fig. 16-8). The incision is started superiorly through the scalp, and the temporalis fascia is identified. Development of the flap in this plane is carried out anteroinferiorly to a point at which the fat is visible through the superficial layer of temporalis fascia, about 2 cm above the zygomatic arch. The skin is dissected off the tragus and the cartilaginous external acoustic meatus. This plane is avascular, and dissection ends with exposure of the postglenoid tubercle. The superficial layer of the temporalis fascia is incised at 45 degrees anterosuperiorly to avoid the facial nerve. The periosteum of the arch is incised and raised as one flap with the outer layer of the temporalis fascia. Periosteum may be incised as far forward as is necessary to gain good exposure to the TMJ capsule. Ligation of the superficial temporal vessels is often required during this approach. The sharp condylar neck fragment often tears laterally through the capsule as it telescopes superiorly. Dissection of the condylar neck is performed by lateral capsular incision and periosteal stripping down the condylar neck to expose sufficient fixation surface.

The condylar head is usually deep and anteriorly sited and requires mobilization to deliver it laterally and upward into accurate reduction. Kocher's bone-holding forceps or artery clips can be used to grasp the condylar head fragment while the neck and ramus are pulled inferiorly by the assistant's fingers pushing intraorally on the molar region. A bone hook

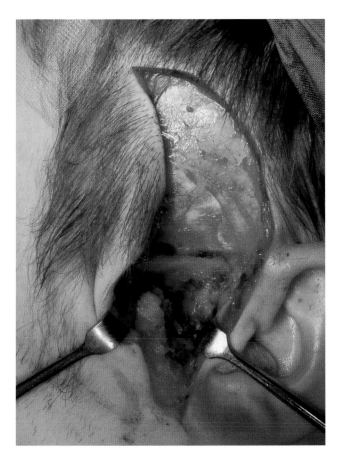

FIGURE 16-8   Bramley-Al Khayat approach.

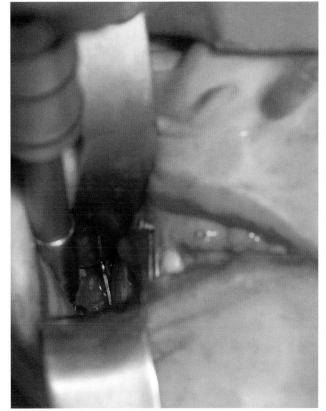

FIGURE 16-9   Intraoral approach demonstrating use of the right-angled drill.

can help in moving the condylar neck but may risk splitting it if pulled too forcefully; we prefer the intraoral pressure method. Closure in layers is required to restore anatomy, and a small vacuum drain prevents hematoma formation.

RHYTIDECTOMY APPROACH

Anatomical Points of Importance

In addition to the other structures mentioned previously, the great auricular nerve courses at 45 degrees to the sterno-cleidomastoid, anterosuperiorly, just deep to the SMAS.

Preparation and Draping

Draping should allow direct visualization of the corner of the eye and the mouth. The ear should be fully exposed along with the descending hairline and 2 to 3 cm of hair behind the ear.

Skin Marking and Vasoconstriction

The incision begins 1.5 to 2 cm superior to the zygomatic arch, just behind the hairline and in front of the ear. The incision then curves inferiorly under the earlobe and for about 3 mm onto the posterior surface of the auricle; this allows scarring to be less noticeable.

Incision and Dissection

The incision is through the skin and subcutaneous tissue only. Wide blunt dissection deep to the subcutaneous tissue is

performed, and the anterior surface is undermined widely. Once the lateral surface has been exposed, the dissection continues as in the standard retromandibular approach.

Closure

It is possible to repair the masseter and medial pterygoids with resorbable sutures. Closure of the parotid capsule and SMAS layer must be meticulous to reduce the chance of formation of a salivary fistula. Platysma can be closed by a running resorbable suture followed by interrupted subcuticular stitches. The insertion of a vacuum drain helps reduce hematoma formation. Finally, the skin is closed with nylon.

TRANSORAL APPROACH

The transoral technique has the advantage of avoiding facial scarring and risk of injury to the facial nerve. However, facial nerve injury has been reported during this approach, and warnings should be included when obtaining patient consent.

The major disadvantage is limited access, which makes fragment control difficult and the procedure surgically more challenging. The introduction of right-angled instruments with illumination has expanded the use of this approach (Fig. 16-9). It should be reserved for fractures that involve the low condylar region. It may not be possible to align the posterior border perfectly, and slight errors of reduction are inevitable.

An incision is made over the anterior border of the vertical ramus, extending into the lower buccal sulcus. The temporalis muscle is stripped from the anterior ascending ramus, and the masseter is stripped by subperiosteal dissection. It is important to do this extensively, because it allows easier retraction and visibility. A Bauer retractor placed in the sigmoid notch can sometimes aid reduction. A Merrill-Levassier fiberoptic retractor can be used to aid reduction while applying fixation.

A transbuccal trocar is introduced and drilling occurs transbuccally; the plate is introduced transorally. It may be difficult to maintain fixation in the posterior thick cortical bone, and the drill may enter the fracture line or the weaker subsigmoid area.

Mokros and Erle[30] reported a series of 34 patients with low subcondylar fractures approached transorally. They employed a 90-degree drill and screwdriver, a special reduction hook, and retractors.

Undt et al.[31] retrospectively reviewed 55 patients who had 57 condylar neck fractures treated with transoral miniplate osteosynthesis. They concluded that satisfactory reduction and fixation can be achieved with avoidance of facial scarring.

ENDOSCOPIC APPROACH

Endoscopically assisted reduction and fixation of fractures of the condyle has been used for more than a decade and is gaining increased interest worldwide. It enables transoral access to the condylar neck region of the mandible, allowing treatment of fractures in that region with minimal or no facial scarring while also minimizing the risk of facial nerve injury.

Schoen et al.[32] assessed the functional results of endoscope-assisted transoral reduction and fixation of displaced bilateral condylar fractures in 13 patients. After 6 and 12 months, all patients demonstrated a pre-injury range of TMJ motion, including those with comminution at the fracture site. These and other authors have reported a steep learning curve during use of this technique.

In a prospective, randomized, controlled trial involving centers from North America, Europe, and Asia, patients with condylar neck fractures were randomized to receive either ORIF with an extraoral (submandibular, preauricular, or retromandibular) approach or a transoral endoscopic procedure. The investigators measured primary functional outcome using the asymmetrical Helkimo dysfunction score at 8 to 12 weeks and 1 year after surgery.[33] This showed that comparable functional results were achieved after reduction and internal fixation by either technique. A marginally better early cosmetic outcome and fewer complications were the associated advantages of the transoral approach. A reduced occurrence of facial nerve damage was also associated, but this was not supported by comparative statistical analyses.

RETROAURICULAR APPROACH

The retroauricular approach requires transection of the external auditory canal. It is favored by some surgeons and is thought to be particularly useful for access to condylar head fractures. A further benefit is the cosmesis of the scar, which is hidden behind the pinna. Potential risks of the

approach are stenosis of the external meatus and, if the meatus is sectioned at a deep level, damage to the tympanic membrane.

TECHNIQUES OF REDUCTION

Reduction of the fractured condyle can be very difficult, especially when the condylar head is medially dislocated. In these cases, surgical instruments must be employed to try to reposition the condyle (Fig. 16-10). The use of the curved elevator, Howarth's elevator, and the tracheostomy hook have all been advocated. Some surgeons have drilled rigid fixation wires into the fragment to gain control. Kocher's bone-holding forceps may be used to grasp and reduce fragments but can crush and split the condylar head and therefore must be used with caution. In cases of severe and difficult reduction, the lateral pterygoid insertion may be cut to give greater mobility and reducibility, but preservation of the periosteal attachment to the condylar head is mandatory to preserve a blood supply to the proximal fragment. We do not agree with the idea of temporarily removing the condyle and replacing it as a free graft, because the risk of avascular necrosis is high. Gross comminution in the noncompound, noncontaminated fracture of the condylar head should not be excised, because doing so results in loss of vertical height. We believe that leaving the fragments in situ offers the potential for repair with nonrigid IMF. As in all fracture management, accurate

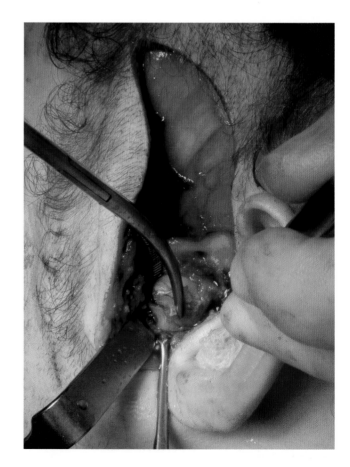

FIGURE 16-10 Kocher's forceps being used to reduce the proximal fragment.

reduction is mandatory, and care must be taken in orienting the condyle, because the correct orientation is not always obvious from the fracture ends.

Downward traction on the mandible can be achieved by double-gloved intraoral pressure in the molar region, temporary wiring, or screw and wire traction on the lower border if surgical exposure allows. There is no substitute for practice to gain competence at reduction, and surgeons will adopt instrumentation according to their own preference. We prefer the presence of two assistants during condylar surgery to ensure optimal exposure and reduction.

In cases of condylar fracture requiring ORIF with simultaneous fixation of body or symphyseal/parasymphyseal fracture, we fix the condyle first, to provide greater mobility and easier reduction of the condyle. As mentioned earlier, bilateral fractures with body or symphyseal/parasymphyseal fracture require particular attention to intercondylar distance when plating the noncondylar area. The tendency to open posteriorly can result in crossbite and malocclusion; external palm pressure applied simultaneously at the angles of the mandible reduces this splaying before the plating and corrects the crossbite.

FIXATION

Historical methods of fixation include transosseous wire fixation, external fixation, and Kirschner wire (K-wire) fixation. Current methods are discussed in the following paragraphs.

Miniplate Osteosynthesis

Condylar plate and screw systems are designed to withstand and overcome any biomechanical deforming forces that may arise, thereby minimizing micromotion of the bone ends. Under conditions of stability and perfect fracture reduction, the primary bone healing will occur. In this situation, new bone forms along the surface of the fracture without fibrous tissue intervening. High condylar fractures may accommodate only one plate due to bony limitations (Fig. 16-11). A 2-mm plate with two screws above and below the fracture parallel to the posterior border provides adequate stability in most cases, in our opinion.

Hammer et al.[34] reported inadequate stability leading to plate failure or screw loosening in more than one third (35%) of cases treated with single adaptational plating. They questioned whether a period of maxillomandibular fixation was needed in combination with plating. Other authors have also reported fractures of plates used in condylar neck fractures and suggested that condylar plates should be stronger and thicker than the thinner adaptational plates.

Byung-Ho et al.[35] studied the strengths of condylar plates in cadaver mandibles. They loaded the condyle to simulate functional loading, and fixation included a miniplate (four screws), a mini dynamic compression plate (four screws), a 2.4-mm plate (four screws), and a double miniplate. They found that the only system able to withstand normal forces of loading was the double miniplate. This mechanical advantage stems from the neutralizing effect of the plates on the functional stresses in the condylar neck. In vitro strain measurements of the condylar process showed that the highest level of tensile strain occurred on the anterior and lateral surfaces and the highest compressive strain on the posterior surface. The two miniplates applied at the posterior

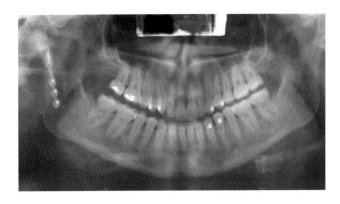

FIGURE 16-11   Postoperative orthopantomogram after open reduction and internal fixation of a right condylar fracture using a single osteosynthesis plate.

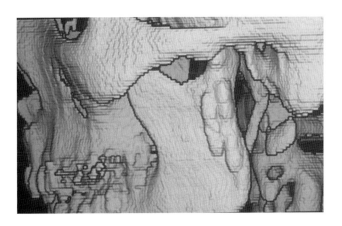

FIGURE 16-12   Postoperative three-dimensional computed tomogram shows left condylar fracture after open reduction and internal fixation by two osteosynthesis plates.

and anterior border of the condylar neck seem to have the advantage of restoring the tension and compression trajectories.

In the case of low condylar fracture, two plates may be required to achieve stability (Fig. 16-12). At least two screws should be placed in the condylar fragment and at least two in the main mandibular segment. The posterior plate should parallel the posterior ascending ramus, and the anterior plate can be angulated across the fracture line.

Eckelt and Hlawitschka[36] commented that a disadvantage of miniplating is the occasional need to remove the plates. This necessitates reexploration of the wound, which entails a much greater risk of injury to the facial nerve due to its tethering and anatomical distortion. This has led to the development of alternative minimal access techniques, which are discussed later.

Dynamic Compression Plating

Because the fractures are generally oblique, any compression effect during plating could lead to overlap of the fragment ends and loss of ramus height. A review of current practice indicates that dynamic compression plating has little place in condylar fractures; treatment is adequate with miniplates placed in the neutral mode.

Lag Screw Osteosynthesis

A true lag screw has threads only on the distal end; when these threads engage the far cortex, the screw head seats against the near cortex and, on tightening, provides compression. This method is biomechanically advantageous because of the central location of the lag screw. The screw is placed in the interior of the condyle, so there is no need to open the joint capsule to place the fixation device. This permits a less traumatic operation than with miniplates, which may require the joint to be opened if the proximal fragment is short.

Lag screw osteosynthesis was first described in condylar fractures by Wackerbauer in 1962. Advantages of lag screws include rapid application of rigid fixation and close approximation of the fractured parts because of the large amount of compression generated. Contraindications to lag screw use are loss of bone in the fracture gap and comminution that would cause displacement and overriding of segments when compression is applied.

Many designs of lag screw are available, but the more simple designs rely on the spherical head of the screw to act as a wedge. Combining the screw with a washer or angled plate (e.g., Wurzburg lag screw plate) eliminates localized high stresses and transforms them into pressure, which is better tolerated than crushing forces under the screw head. This prevents the screw head from penetrating the cortical bone. Lag screws with washers can be turned twice as tightly as those without washers before the surface bone begins to crack.[37] Authors have reported problems with lag screw systems, commenting that there is a tendency toward lateralization and rotation of the condylar head if the screw is not placed centrally. There is also a steep learning curve to this technique.

The Eckelt screw is one of the most popular lag screws in use today (Fig. 16-13). Its use requires an open approach with preparation of a gliding canal between the buccal and lingual cortex of the larger fragment. This has a butt area at the lower border of the mandible that retains the device during tightening. The condylar head is reduced in one of three ways. First, by means of a thin elevator placed medially to the posterior border of the mandible and moved cranially, it is possible to

push the fragment laterally and reduce it. Second, the reduction can be achieved by the use of specifically designed forceps to hold the condylar head on its dorsal aspect. Third is the use of a reduction pin that is screwed into the condylar fragment and is manipulated to achieve reduction.

A gliding channel is drilled in the ramus of the mandible, parallel to the posterior border between the inner and outer cortices. The condylar fragment is then drilled with a narrow drill, and a measuring gauge allows the correct screw length to be chosen. The lag screw is then inserted through the gliding channel into the condylar head and tightened with a nut. This provides good apposition of fragments and allows early mobilization. The screw can be removed with the use of local anesthesia and a simple stab incision.

Eckelt and Hlawitschka[36] published a series of 230 patients who had undergone lag screw fixation over a 16-year period, showing an overall success rate of 90%. Fragment reduction and healing were present in 93.4% of cases. In 6.6% of cases healing occurred in a displaced position, and incomplete reduction occurred in 3.5% of cases. Screw fracture or twisting after return to function occurred in 4.2% of cases. Stability of fixation allowing early mobilization was present in 91.1% of patients. In 5.8%, there was instability attributed to extreme anatomical features and complicated fracture patterns. These cases were recognized preoperatively, and additional methods of fixation were used in conjunction with the lag screw. Surgical errors were reported: the screw was too short to engage the condylar fragment in 3.1%, the screw was too long in 1.5%, and there was anterior/medial malplacement of the screw in 4.2%. Once these errors were discovered, IMF was used postoperatively for 2 to 3 weeks, and the lag screw was removed prematurely. Only three cases of screw fracture were encountered at the proximal end of the thread, and screw bending occurred in only two cases. Screw migration may be caused by insufficient cooling of the drill, remodeling processes in the fracture gap, or disturbed blood supply to the condylar fragment. Twenty-one percent of patients reported transient facial nerve weakness limited to the marginal mandibular branch, and only one patient reported long-term problems with this nerve. The authors advocated supraplatysmal dissection to improve nerve protection.

Krenkel[37] described placement of a lag screw halfway up the ascending ramus. Welk[38] reported a 3.5% rate of contraindication to lag screws due to an extremely narrow or distorted ascending ramus and thin condylar neck. In another 9.3%, reduced loading capacity was observed in the case of lateral bending forces due to considerable perforations of the lateral cortex after difficult screw placement. Teranobu et al.[39] reported that certain racial differences of mandibular form may preclude lag screw use. Because of these potential problems, Hibi et al.[40] recommended a modified osteosynthesis method that combines the miniplate and lag screw in atrophic mandibles. Kitayama[41] described lag screw insertion via an intraoral approach, but positioning in the condylar fragment can be eccentric, leading to displacement on tightening.

Pin Fixation

Pin fixation uses 1.3-mm K-wires placed into the condyle under direct vision. This technique requires an open approach to the condylar head and traction applied to the lower border of the mandible. It is beneficial if the dorsal surface of the

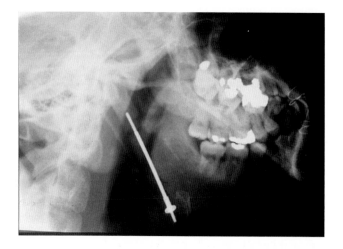

FIGURE 16-13 Postoperative lateral oblique radiograph taken after open reduction and internal fixation of condylar fracture using the Eckelt screw.

head can be seen, to enable assessment of the reduction of the fracture before fixation. Not all K-wires need to be passed through the surgical access site; a transbuccal approach may be used, but this must be protected by a trephine. The direction of wire placement varies depending on the fracture configuration. Usually, a minimum of three convergent K-wires is needed to ensure stability.

Bioresorbable Plates and Pins

The use of resorbable fixation devices is now well established in orthognathic and craniofacial practice. Authors cite good healing results with financial and psychological benefits. However, plate resorption may take more than 2 years. Materials used include self-reinforced poly-L-lactide screws (SR-PLLA), polyglycolide pins, and absorbable α-hydroxy polyesters.

Rasse[42,43] reported that the replacement of wires with resorbable polydioxanone pins gave good stability and avoided the need for a second-stage removal procedure. Nehse and Maerker[44] also recommended polydioxanone, polylactide, or autologous bone pins for temporary stabilization of subcondylar fractures but admitted that shortened IMF and functional therapy were mandatory with these fixation methods. They concluded that, at that time, resorbable materials could not replace miniplate or traction screw, but did enhance the armamentarium available to the surgeon in the management of subcondylar fractures.

Eppley[45] reported their experience of using polylactic-polyglycolic copolymer plates in maxillofacial trauma; the results were encouraging, but to date no large series has been reported with regard to the mandibular condyle fracture.

CONDYLAR FRACTURES IN CHILDREN

Fractures of the facial skeleton in children account for only 5% of all facial fractures in a given population and are seen most commonly between the ages of 6 and 12 years. In most pediatric cohorts, the most common maxillofacial fracture sites are the nose and the dentoalveolar complex, followed by the mandible, orbit, and midface. The male-to-female ratio is between 2.4:1.0 and 2.9:1.0. Among the mandibular fractures, involvement of the condyle occurs in 43.3% to 72%.

In a retrospective analysis of 101 children younger than 16 years of age with condylar fractures, Thoren et al.[46] found that 22% were intracapsular and 78% extracapsular. There was only a preponderance of intracapsular fractures (58%) among patients younger than 6 years of age. In the older children, 78% of fractures were confined to the condylar neck. Subcondylar fractures accounted for only 4% of cases. They found displacement to be present in only 6% of cases but commented that dislocation of the condyle from the glenoid fossa was common at all ages. The sex of patient and the cause of the injury had no bearing on the fracture site.

In 1992, Thoren et al.[47] reported on a series of 220 mandibular fractures in children. They found that condylar fractures were prevalent in those patients younger than 10 years of age, but children older than 10 years showed fracture patterns similar to those observed in the adult population, with body and angle fractures being more common than condylar fractures.

As with adult patients, the management of childhood condylar fractures is controversial but consensus is now emerging that conservative treatment is the preferred method, especially in the younger patient. In older pediatric patients with severely displaced fractures, the debate continues. It is now accepted that the condylar cartilage and its condylar growth center, which traditionally was thought to provide the dominant growth impetus, is not as important as previously claimed. Traditionally, the mandible was likened to a long bone with the cartilage acting as an epiphyseal growth plate. Along with this growth center, appositional bone formation occurred at the sites of insertion of masseter at the angle of the mandible and temporalis at the coronoid, leading to the development of the mandible in combination with alveolar margin stimulation.

Moss[48,49] proposed the functional matrix theory, which states that the mandible develops in conjunction with the morphogenetic demands of the enveloping soft tissues, particularly muscle and ligaments, acting through their periosteal attachments. In this theory, the mandibular condyle is not the site of primary growth but has a secondary adaptive response, allowing the condylar head to stay in the fossa as the mandible develops. The predominant growth is downward and forward in response to the demand of the functional matrix.

However, the condyle does have an important role in growth, because condylectomy leads to reduced anteroposterior growth, and trauma to the condylar region can result in unilateral or bilateral underdevelopment of the mandible. If the condyle has lost its lead role in mandibular growth, how are these findings to be explained? It is postulated that in these cases the matrix has been damaged in some way, possibly secondary to soft tissue trauma. The presence of ankylosis may also be significant in that it limits movement. Patients with juvenile arthritis (Still's disease) have been shown to have impaired anterior movement of the mandible by fibrous ankylosis. In these patients, the condyle has lost its potential to remodel into the glenoid fossa.

As a result of this theoretical model, it was commonly believed that ankylosis and maldevelopment would occur in children younger than 10 years of age, in fracture-dislocations and intracapsular fractures of the condylar head, and in compound fractures with comminution of the condylar head.

The treatment of condylar fractures in children is complicated by poor patient compliance, difficulty in applying IMF, and crowded mandible and maxillae with developing teeth. The methods employed to provide temporary immobilization include arch bars, acrylic splints, IMF screws, and bonded brackets with heavy elastics. The period of immobilization need only be 1 to 2 weeks to allow early bone healing, followed by aggressive active mobilization of the mandible to prevent ankylosis. In addition, the use of guided elastics for up to 6 to 8 weeks normally restores occlusion.

The 1999 Gronigen Consensus[28] and a consensus study by Baker et al.[27] corroborated the practice of most units in stating that ORIF has little or no role in the treatment of childhood condylar fractures. Numerous studies looking at the outcome of conservative fracture management in children have confirmed that closed functional treatment gives excellent results based on the growing patient's potential to remodel the condylar head and restore function.

Hovinga et al.[50] studied 25 patients with childhood condylar fractures treated by the closed method over a 15-year period. They treated only 5 patients with IMF, the remainder being treated by early mobilization. The results were excellent with regard to masticatory function and patient satisfaction. High condylar fractures showed better regenerative tendency than intracapsular and low condylar fractures. Asymmetry was observed in only 4 patients by the trained observer and was not noticed by the patients. All deviations were distributed over all fracture types. The measurement of ascending ramus height did show some variation in 63.6% of cases but was usually not clinically significant. Only one case of intracapsular fracture exhibited considerable growth disturbance. Only 1 patient with persistent malocclusion required corrective osteotomy, and in that case, the fracture was of a low condylar type. The findings of this series are in keeping with those of others who have assessed conservative closed functional treatment in children.

Other authors have assessed condylar repair by different methods, including electronic computer-assisted recording of condylar movement, spiral computed tomography, nuclear magnetic resonance, plain radiographic assessment, and OPG. Subtle findings including bony spurs, neoarthrosis, bifid condyle, altered condylar angle, asymmetry, and shorter condylar height are seen, but these findings appear not to cause functional problems and support the adaptive remodeling theory (see Fig. 16-10). This further confirms the role of conservative treatment in children.

SPECIFIC TREATMENT STRATEGIES

Young Patients with Maximum Remodeling Potential

In patients younger than 12 years of age, the adaptive mechanisms should restore function without a period of immobilization. We therefore advocate analgesia and early mobilization in all planes of mandibular movement.

Two patient groups need particular caution: those with major disruption of occlusion and those at risk for ankylosis or defective development.

Significant occlusal disharmony, consisting of open bite and possible retropositioning of the mandible, may be seen after bilateral fracture-dislocation. In these cases, the potential for spontaneous correction by overeruption of teeth is limited. Treatment in these instances should be by a conservative immobilization regimen, as for an adult. If there is a unilateral condyle fracture with major occlusal disruption, a period of immobilization for 10 to 14 days should be undertaken. Bilateral fractures may require immobilization for 3 weeks.

Young patients at risk for ankylosis or defective development, or both, include those with close proximity of the fractured condylar neck to the glenoid fossa (i.e., intracapsular fractures and fracture-dislocation with telescoping) and those who have compound fractures with associated coronoid and zygomatic fractures. In these cases, it must be assumed that there is damage to the meniscus and capsule. A conservative, nonimmobilization regimen may be used if the patient has minimal symptoms. However, in the presence of severe pain, a period of IMF (for no longer than 14 days) is recommended, followed by active mobilization.

Adolescent Patients

Similar principles apply to 12- to 17-year-old age group as to the younger group, with slight modification. If a malocclusion is present, the capacity for spontaneous correction is less than in the younger age group. A malocclusion is therefore an indication for IMF for 2 to 3 weeks. The dentition at this stage tolerates simple eyelet wires or arch bars. Failure of conservative treatment would lead the clinician to apply adult principles of treatment to the older members of this group.

INDICATIONS FOR OPEN REDUCTION AND INTERNAL FIXATION

In pediatric patients, the indications for ORIF are rare. They include:

- failed conservative functional treatment.
- a fractured condyle that directly interferes with jaw opening or movement.
- a fracture that causes severe loss of ramus height with severe anterior open bite.
- a condylar fragment that is dislocated into the middle cranial fossa.

The best chance for full and functional recovery is obtained by causing as little trauma as possible to the surrounding tissues during the surgery. The use of bioresorbable fixation may be beneficial in this setting. We advise that only experienced surgeons undertake this procedure in the young patient.

COMPOUND FRACTURES

Early operation with copious irrigation is indicated in both pediatric and adult patients with compound fractures. In severe compound cases with gross comminution, removal of nonviable bone fragments is indicated at the time of exploration and closure. A swab for culture and sensitivity should be taken, followed by at least 5 days of broad-spectrum antibiotic therapy. Early mobilization should be encouraged.

In the young patient, cephalometric assessment should be performed postoperatively and repeated at follow-up to ensure adequate mandibular growth.

COMPLICATIONS

MALOCCLUSION

Fractures close to the TMJ have a surprisingly favorable outcome. The bilateral condylar fracture causes the most malocclusions. Ellis[51] commented that, despite accurate occlusion in these cases with rigid IMF and elastics, some patients drift into anterior open bite after the elastics have been removed for 12 to 24 hours. This is not a uniform finding. He postulated that the more displaced the condyles, the more adaptation is needed to maintain the normal occlusal relationship.

Most investigators conclude that the mandible functions as a class 3 lever system during biting. This means that the mean force vector of the elevator muscles is located between the fulcrum (TMJ) and the load (bite point). Loss of the fulcrum or its displacement would significantly alter this relationship. In such cases, the normal function of the elevators tends to raise the gonial angle farther than normal, resulting in premature contact of the posterior dentition.

In Ellis' experience, some patients can achieve normal occlusion despite displacement. He postulated that somehow the elevator muscles stay minimally active and do not contribute to the foreshortening. If they selectively activate the posterior temporalis muscle, the coronoid process is pulled posteriorly, allowing rotational closure of the mandible into occlusion with the maxilla. This results in inefficiency of the biting force but allows for the establishment of a new temporomandibular articulation by skeletal and dentoalveolar adaptations. Most patients cannot achieve this on their own and need IMF elastic traction as a guide. After nonsurgical treatment, a new temporomandibular articulation is established, resulting in restoration of the class 3 lever. As the mandibular plane becomes steeper, the condylar stump approaches the skull base, and once the remodeling is complete, the posterior vertical dimension stabilizes. Reestablishment is age related, and younger patients may show normal TMJ morphology. Older patients show altered morphology, with the new articulation being more inferior at the base of the articular eminence. The extrusion of anterior teeth and intrusion of posterior teeth restores the occlusion.

Persistent malocclusion can be corrected only by orthognathic surgery once the new articulation is stable. An asymmetrical anterior open bite can be corrected by a Le Fort I osteotomy. An asymmetrical open bite or deviation of the mandible can be corrected by ascending ramus surgery.

MANDIBULAR HYPOMOBILITY

An interincisal opening of less than 40 mm is regarded as mandibular hypomobility. It is accepted that trauma is a cause of ankylosis. However, it is rare after condylar fractures and has been estimated to occur in only 0.2% to 0.4% of cases. Hypomobility has been reported to persist in 8% and 10% of condylar fractures. Some patients function well at this reduced level of opening, but some authors have found that masticatory dysfunction is higher in those patients who never regained a normal range of motion. Ellis recommended physiotherapy during recovery in the acute phase. Reducing the period of IMF can also help reduce hypomobility.

ASYMMETRY

Ellis commented that asymmetry in function is very common. Deviation toward the side of the fracture has been reported in 50% of patients studied. It is presumed to be caused by reduced lateral pterygoid function or by pseudarthrosis on the side of the fracture, or both. The greater the condylar displacement, the greater the deviation. Asymmetry in mandibular growth has been shown to occur in approximately 25% of patients with fractures during the growing years. It is not always undergrowth; overgrowth also has been reported to occur. From studies of patients with ankylosis, it is known that encouraging mobility leads to less growth disturbance. This principle should be applied to condylar fracture management.

DYSFUNCTION AND DEGENERATION

Dysfunction and condylar degeneration have been shown to occur not only on the fractured side but also on the contralateral side. It is believed that fracture-dislocation is most likely to lead to late problems. Ellis admitted that it is difficult to determine the level of dysfunction, but after a literature review, he estimated that it occurs in between 9% and 85% of condylar fractures. Dysfunction has also been linked to long periods of fixation and to increasing age. Condylar degeneration is not limited to closed treatment but occurs in open cases too. Ellis estimated that 65% of patients are completely symptom free, but the clinician may detect subtle symptoms and signs of dysfunction, such as deviation on opening, a long centric slide, TMJ clicking, popping, and locking. The difficulty is that these are prevalent in the population and may have existed before injury.

IATROGENIC INJURY

Cause, of iatrogenic injury include:

- deterioration in oral hygiene secondary to IMF or elastics that may lead to decay of dentition.
- injury to dentition by fixation methods.
- malnutrition and weight loss due to use of IMF or elastics.
- airway risk from fixation methods.
- scars.
- seventh nerve injury (reported incidence: permanent injury, 1%; transient injury, 10%-15%).
- salivary fistulae.
- Frey's syndrome.
- altered sensation of the ear or temple.

ESTHETIC ASPECTS

Mandibular asymmetry after trauma can be corrected by ramus osteotomy. This is not frequently a major complaint of the patient. Minor, subtle deviations may go unnoticed and can be treated expectantly.

ASSESSMENT SCORES AND OUTCOMES

Several methods, both objective and subjective, have been described for the assessment of outcome after surgery on the TMJ complex. The Helkimo dysfunction score consists of three indices evaluating anamnestic and clinical dysfunction, occlusion, and articulation disturbance. It is an accepted, valid, and reliable tool that is used to determine the functional outcome after surgery of mandibular and TMJ disorders and after orthognathic surgery.[52-54]

As in most surgical disciplines, clinicians managing condylar injuries are responsible for monitoring and recording the outcomes of treatment. This should include functional assessments of jaw mobility and excursions (opening, lateral excursion, and protrusion), occlusal changes, and subjective pain and discomfort. Such monitoring facilitates future clinical decision making and assists in the standardized dissemination of treatment results.

CONCLUSION

In recent years, an increased number of fractures of the condylar region of the mandible have been surgically treated, and the indications for this approach seem to be supported by the literature.[6,21,23-25] The potential benefit appears to be present regardless of the anatomical position of the condylar fracture; it depends more on the extent of the displacement of the proximal fragment.[55] The benefits of fixation of condylar head fractures have also been identified.[56]

Accumulating Level I evidence supports ORIF of condylar fractures if the following clinical conditions are met: adult unilateral fractured condyle with fragment override of greater than 2 mm or angulation of greater than 10 degrees with occlusal disturbance (or both). With less displacement, a trial of nonrigid IMF should be given, with clinical and radiological reassessment after 1 week and surgery still being an option. Endoscopic assistance, performed with a transoral approach, may provide an alternative means for treating a subset of these injuries, reducing visible scar formation and possibly facial nerve damage.

There now seems to be a sufficient body of evidence and consensus that the fracture type that gives most long-term functional problems is bilateral condylar fractures with displacement. The risks of surgical approaches are less than initially thought and should not preclude ORIF. Restoration of condylar height with adequate stabilization and restoration of the occlusion, followed by early mobilization, are the goals.

Bilateral condylar fractures should be treated on their own merit (i.e., according to the guidance given earlier for each of the fractures). Aggressive mobilization should help to restore jaw mobility. Children younger than 12 years rarely need ORIF, and the surgeon must have clear justification to undertake it in that age group.

REFERENCES

1. Silvennoinen U, Lizyka T, Lindqvist C, et al: Different patterns of condyle fractures: an analysis of 382 patients in a 3-year period. J Oral Maxillofac Surg 50:1032-1037, 1992.
2. Spiessel B, Schroll K: Gelenkfortsatzund gelenkkopfchenfrakturen. In Higst H, editor: Spezielle frakturen-and luxationslehre BD.I/I, Stuttgart, 1972, Thieme.
3. MacLennan DW: Consideration of 180 cases of typical fractures of the mandibular condylar process. Br J Plast Surg 5:122-128, 1952.
4. Lindahl L, Hollender L: Condylar fractures of the mandible: a radiographic study of remodelling processes in the temporomandibular joint. Int J Oral Surg 6:153-165, 1977.
5. Loukota RA, Eckelt U, De Bont L, et al: Subclassification of fractures of the condylar process of the mandible. Br J Oral Maxillofac Surg 43:72-73, 2005.
6. Eckelt U, Schneider M, Erasmus F, et al: Open versus closed treatment of fractures of the mandibular condylar process: a prospective randomized multi-centre study. J Craniomaxillofac Surg 34:306-314, 2006.
7. Neff A, Mühlberger G, Karoglan M, et al: Stabilität der Osteosynthese bei Gelenkwalzenfrakturen in Klinik und biomechanischer Simulation [Stability of osteosyntheses for condylar head fractures in the clinic and biomechanical simulation]. Mund Kiefer Gesichtschir 8:63-74, 2004.
8. Loukota RA, Neff A, Rasse M: Nomenclature/classification of fractures of the mandibular condylar head. Br J Oral Maxillofac Surg 48:477-478, 2009.
9. Members of the Chalmers J Lyon Club: Fractures of the mandibular condyle: a post-treatment survey of 120 cases. J Oral Surg 5:45-73, 1947.
10. Blevins C, Gores RJ: Fractures of the mandibular condyloid process: results of conservative treatment in 140 patients. J Oral Surg 19:392-406, 1961.
11. Marker P, Nielson A, Bastian HL: Fractures of the mandibular condyle. Part 2. Results of treatment of 348 patients. Br J Oral Maxillofac Surg 38:422-426, 2000.
12. Joos U, Kleinheinz J: Therapy of condylar neck fractures. Int J Oral Maxillofac Surg 27:247-254, 1998.
13. Hidding J, Wolf R, Pingle D: Surgical versus non surgical treatment of fractures of the articular process of the mandible. J Craniomaxillofac Surg 20:345-347, 1992.
14. Dahlstrom L, Kalmberg KE, Lindhall L: 15 Years follow-up of condylar fractures. Int J Oral Maxillofac Surg 18:18-23, 1989.
15. Konstantinovic V, Dimitrijevic B: Surgical versus conservative treatment of unilateral condylar process fractures: clinical and radiographic evaluation of patients. J Oral Maxillofac Surg 50:349-352, 1992.
16. Landes CA, Day K, Lipphardt R, et al: Closed versus open operative treatment of nondisplaced diacapitular (class VI) fractures. J Oral Maxillofac Surg 66:1586-1594, 2008.
17. Ellis E, Palmieri C, Throckmorton G: Further displacement of condylar process fractures after closed treatment. J Oral Maxillofac Surg 57:1307-1316, 1999.
18. Ellis E 3rd: Method to determine when open treatment of condylar process fractures is not necessary. J Oral Maxillofac Surg 67:1685-1690, 2009.
19. Palmieri C, Ellis E, Throckmorton G: Mandibular motion after closed and open treatment of unilateral mandibular condylar process fractures. J Oral Maxillofac Surg 57:764-775, 1999.
20. Worsaae N, Thorn J: Surgical versus non surgical treatment of unilateral dislocated low subcondylar fractures: a clinical study of 52 cases. J Oral Maxillofac Surg 52:353-360, 1994.
21. Eckelt U: Zugschraubenosteosynthesebei unterkiefergelenkfortsatzfrakturen. Dtsch Zeitschrift Mund Kiefer Gesichtschir 15:51-57, 1991.
22. Takenoshita Y, Ishibashi H, Oka M: Comparison of functional recovery after nonsurgical and surgical treatment of condylar fractures. J Oral Maxillofac Surg 48:1191-1195, 1990.
23. Ellis E 3rd, Simon P, Throckmorton GS: Occlusal results after open or closed treatment of fractures of the mandibular condylar process. J Oral Maxillofac Surg 58:260-268, 2000.
24. Hlawitschka M, Loukota R, Eckelt U: Functional and radiological results of open and closed treatment of intracapsular (diacapitular) condylar fractures of the mandible. Int J Oral Maxillofac Surg 34:597-604, 2005.
25. Singh V, Bhagol A, Goel M, et al: Outcomes of open versus closed treatment of mandibular subcondylar fractures: a prospective randomized study. J Oral Maxillofac Surg 68:1304-1309, 2010.
26. Danda AK, Muthusekhar MR, Narayanan V, et al: Open versus closed treatment of unilateral subcondylar and condylar neck fractures: a prospective, randomized clinical study. J Oral Maxillofac Surg 68:1238-1241, 2010.
27. Baker AW, McMahon J, Moos KF: Current consensus on the management of fracture of the mandibular condyle: a method by questionnaire. Int J Oral Maxillofac Surg 27:258-266, 1998.
28. Bos R, Ward Booth P, de Bont L: Mandibular condyle fractures: a consensus (editorial). Br J Oral Maxillofac Surg 37:87-89, 1999.
29. Newman L: A clinical evaluation of the long-term outcome of patients treated for bilateral fractures of the mandibular condyles. Br J Oral Maxillofac Surg 36:176-179, 1998.
30. Mokros S, Erle A: Transoral miniplate osteosynthesis of mandibular condyle fractures: optimising the surgical method. Fortschr Kiefer Gesichtschir 41:136-138, 1996.
31. Undt G, Kermer C, Rasse M, et al: Transoral miniplate osteosynthesis of condylar neck fractures. Oral Surg Oral Med Oral Pathol Oral Radiol Endodont 88:534-543, 1999.
32. Schoen R, Fakler O, Metzger MC, et al: Preliminary functional results of endoscope-assisted transoral treatment of displaced bilateral condylar mandible fractures. Int J Oral Maxillofac Surg 37:111-116, 2008.
33. Schmelzeisen R, Cienfuegos-Monroy R, Schön R, et al: Patient benefit from endoscopically assisted fixation of condylar neck fractures: a randomized controlled trial. J Oral Maxillofac Surg 67:147-158, 2009.
34. Hammer B, Schier P, Prein J: Osteosynthesis of condylar neck fractures: a review of 30 patients. Br J Oral Maxillofac Surg 35:288-291, 1997.
35. Byung-Ho C, Kyung-nam K, Moon-Key K: Evaluation of condylar neck fracture plating techniques. J Craniomaxillofac Surg 27:109-112, 1999.
36. Eckelt U, Hlawitschka M: Clinical and radiological evaluation following surgical treatment of condylar neck fractures with lag screws. J Craniomaxillofac Surg 27:235-242, 1999.
37. Krenkel C: Axial anchor screw (lag screw with biconcave washer) or slanted screw plate for osteosynthesis of fractures of the mandibular condylar process. J Craniomaxillofac Surg 20:348-353, 1992.
38. Welk A: Morphologische undtersuchungen zur indikation der zugschraubenosteosynthese nach eckelt bei kiefergelenkfortsatzfrakturen [medical dissertation], Geifswald, Germany, 1997.
39. Teranobu O, Yamada K, Eida K: Evaluation of lag screw osteosynthesis for condylar process fractures of the mandible. Int J Oral Maxillofac Surg 26(suppl):239, 1997.
40. Hibi H, Sawaki Y, Ueda M: Modified osteosynthesis for condylar neck fractures in atrophic mandibles. Int J Oral Maxillofac Surg 26:348-350, 1997.

41. Kitayama S: A new method of intra-oral open reduction using a screw applied through the mandibular crest of condylar fractures. *J Maxillofac Surg* 17:16-21, 1989.

42. Rasse M: Diakapituläre Frakturen der Mandibula. *Die operative versorgung: tierexperiment und klinik*, Vienna, 1993, Habilitationsschrift Med Fakultat Universitat Wien.

43. Rasse M: Diakapituläre Frakturen der Mandibula: Eine neue Operationsmethode und erste Ergebnisse. *Zeitschrift fur Stomatologie* 90:413-428, 1993.

44. Nehse G, Maerker R: Indications for various reconstruction and osteosynthesis methods in surgical management of subcondylar fractures of the mandible. *Fortschr Kiefer Gesichtschir* 41:120-123, 1996.

45. Eppley BL: A resorbable and rapid method for maxillomandibular fixation in pediatric mandible fractures. *J Craniofac Surg* 11:236-238, 2000.

46. Thoren H, Ilzuka T, Hallikainen D, et al: An epidemiological study of patterns of condylar fractures in children. *Br J Oral Maxillofac Surg* 35:306-311, 1997.

47. Thoren H, Ilzuka T, Hallikainen D, et al: Different patterns of mandibular fractures in children: an analysis of 220 fractures in 157 patients. *J Craniomaxillofac Surg* 20:292-296, 1992.

48. Moss M: The primacy of functional matrices in orofacial growth. *Dental Practitioner* 19:65-73, 1968.

49. Moss M, Salentijn L: The capsular matrix. *Am J Orthodont* 56:474-491, 1969.

50. Hovinga J, Boering G, Stegenga B: Long-term results of nonsurgical management of condylar fractures in children. *Int J Oral Maxillofac Surg* 28:429-440, 1999.

51. Ellis E: Complications of mandibular condyle fractures. *Int J Oral Maxillofac Surg* 27:255-257, 1998.

52. Helkimo M: Studies on function and dysfunction of the masticatory system. II. Index for anamnestic and clinical dysfunction and occlusal state. *Sven Tandlak Tidskr* 67:101-121, 1974.

53. Helkimo M: Studies on function and dysfunction of the masticatory system. I. An epidemiological investigation of symptoms of dysfunction in Lapps in the north of Finlandc *Proc Finn Dent Soc* 70:37-49, 1974.

54. Helkimo M: Studies on function and dysfunction of the masticatory system. 3. Analyses of anamnestic and clinical recordings of dysfunction with the aid of indices. *Sven Tandlak Tidskr* 67:165-181, 1974.

55. Schneider M, Erasmus F, Gerlach KL, et al: Open reduction and internal fixation versus closed treatment and mandibulomaxillary fixation of fractures of the mandibular condylar process: a randomized, prospective, multicenter study with special evaluation of fracture level. *J Oral Maxillofac Surg* 66:2537-2544, 2008.

56. Hlawitschka M, Loukota R, Eckelt U: Functional and radiological results of open and closed treatment of intracapsular (diacapitular) condylar fractures of the mandible. *Int J Oral Maxillofac Surg* 34:597-604, 2005.

CHAPTER 17

Dentoalveolar Injuries

Richard R. Welbury

Dental trauma in childhood and adolescence is common. By 5 years of age, 31% to 40% of boys and 16% to 30% of girls have suffered some dental trauma; by 12 years, these figures are 12% to 33% and 4% to 19%, respectively. Boys are affected almost twice as often as girls in both the primary and permanent dentitions.

Most dental injuries involve the anterior teeth, especially the maxillary central incisors. The mandibular central incisors and maxillary lateral incisors are less frequently involved. Concussion, subluxation, and luxation are the most common injuries in the primary dentition, whereas uncomplicated crown fractures are most common in the permanent teeth.

The most accident-prone ages are between 2 and 4 years for the primary dentition and between 7 and 10 years for the permanent dentition. Coordination and judgment are incompletely developed in young children, and most injuries in the primary dentition are the result of falls in and around the home. In the permanent dentition, most injuries are caused by falls and collisions associated with playing and running, although bicycles are a common accessory. The place of injury varies in different countries according to local customs, but accidents in the schoolyard remain common. Sports injuries usually occur in the teenage years and are commonly associated with contact sports such as soccer, rugby, ice hockey, and basketball. Injuries due to road traffic accidents and assaults are most commonly associated with the late teenage years and adulthood and are often closely related to alcohol abuse. One form of injury in childhood that must never be forgotten is child physical abuse or nonaccidental injury; more than 50% of affected children have orofacial injuries.

The exact mechanisms of dental injuries are largely unknown, and experimental evidence is lacking, but injuries can result from either direct or indirect trauma. Direct trauma occurs when the tooth itself is struck. Indirect trauma is seen when the lower dental arch is forcefully closed against the upper (e.g., by a blow to the chin). Direct trauma implies injury to the anterior region, whereas indirect trauma favors crown or crown-root fractures of the premolars and molars with the possibility of jaw fractures in the condylar regions and in the symphysis. The factors that influence the outcome or type of injury are energy impact, resilience of the impacting object, shape of the impacting object, and angle of direction of the impacting force.

Increased overjet with protrusion of upper incisors and insufficient lip closure are significant predisposing factors to traumatic dental injuries. Injuries are almost twice as frequent among children with protruding incisors, and the number of teeth affected in a particular incident is also greater. The second major group of children with predisposition to traumatic injuries are the accident prone. They sustain repeated trauma to their teeth, with reported frequencies ranging from 4% to 30%.

CLASSIFICATION OF DENTOALVEOLAR INJURIES

Correct and appropriate treatment demands accurate diagnosis. Table 17-1 summarizes the classification of dento-alveolar injuries based on the World Health Organization (WHO) system.

HISTORY AND EXAMINATION

HISTORY SPECIFIC TO DENTOALVEOLAR INJURIES

The exact nature of the accident gives information on the type and severity of dentoalveolar injury to be expected. In a minor, a discrepancy between the history and the clinical findings should raise suspicion of child physical abuse or nonaccidental injury.

Lost teeth or fragments should be accounted for. If there is a history of loss of consciousness and teeth or teeth fragments cannot be found, a chest radiograph is essential. Similarly, if there is a soft tissue laceration of the upper or lower lip, anteroposterior and lateral soft tissue views of the lips should be obtained.

The time interval between injury and treatment significantly affects the prognosis for both the pulp and the periodontal ligament (PDL).

A history of previous dentoalveolar trauma can affect pulpal sensibility tests and the recuperative capacity of the pulp and periodontium.

In a minor, a history of previous dentoalveolar trauma could raise suspicion about the possibility of child physical abuse or whether the minor is just accident prone.

TABLE 17-1	Classification of Dentoalveolar Injuries
Type of Injury	**Description**
Injuries to the Hard Dental Tissues and the Pulp	
Enamel infraction	Incomplete (crack) of enamel without loss of tooth substance
Enamel fracture	Loss of tooth substance confined to enamel
Enamel-dentine fracture	Loss of tooth surface confined to enamel and dentine not involving the pulp
Complicated crown fracture	Fracture of enamel and dentine exposing the pulp
Uncomplicated crown-root fracture	Fracture of enamel, dentine, and cementum but not involving the pulp
Complicated crown-root fracture	Fracture of enamel, dentine, and cementum and exposing the pulp
Root fracture	Fracture involving dentine, cementum, and pulp. Can be subclassified into apical, middle, and coronal third
Injuries to the Periodontal Tissues	
Concussion	No abnormal loosening or displacement but marked reaction to percussion
Subluxation (loosening)	Abnormal loosening but no displacement
Extrusive luxation (partial avulsion)	Partial displacement of tooth from socket
Lateral luxation	Displacement other than axially with comminution or fracture of alveolar socket
Intrusive luxation	Displacement into alveolar bone with comminution or fracture of alveolar socket
Avulsion	Complete displacement of tooth from socket
Injuries to Supporting Bone	
Comminution of mandibular or maxillary alveolar socket wall	Crushing and compression of alveolar socket; found in intrusive and lateral luxation injuries
Fracture of mandibular or maxillary alveolar socket wall	Fracture confined to facial or lingual/palatal socket wall
Fracture of mandibular or maxillary alveolar process	Fracture of the alveolar process that may or may not involve the tooth sockets
Fracture of the mandible or maxilla	May or may not involve the alveolar socket
Injuries to Gingiva or Oral Mucosa	
Laceration of gingiva or oral mucosa	Wound in the mucosa resulting from a tear
Contusion of gingiva or oral mucosa	Bruise not accompanied by a break in the mucosa, usually causing submucosal hemorrhage
Abrasion of gingiva or oral mucosa	Superficial wound produced by rubbing or scraping of the mucosal surface

MEDICAL HISTORY SPECIFIC TO DENTOALVEOLAR INJURIES

Features of the medical history that are relevant to dentoalveolar injuries include the following:

- *Bleeding disorders:* Close liaison with hematologists is crucial if soft tissues are lacerated or teeth are to be removed.
- *Allergies:* Alternative antibiotics need to be prescribed.
- *Congenital heart disease or rheumatic fever:* These are not necessarily contraindications to reimplantation of teeth; however, the advice of the physician should be sought. If endodontic treatment is likely to be difficult or may involve a persistent necrotic focus, then the risk of bacterial endocarditis is significant, and reimplantation may be contraindicated after a risk-versus-benefit analysis.
- *Severe immunosuppression:* This is a contraindication to any procedure that is likely to require prolonged endodontic treatment with a persistent necrotic focus.
- *Tetanus prophylaxis:* This should be checked with the physician. Usually, a tetanus toxoid booster is required if there is soil contamination of a wound and the patient has not been given a tetanus booster in the previous 5 to 10 years.

EXTRAORAL EXAMINATION

Severe facial swelling and bruising may indicate underlying bony injury. Lacerations require careful débridement to remove all foreign material before suturing (Fig. 17-1). Antibiotics or tetanus toxoid or both may be required if wounds are contaminated. Limitation of mandibular movement or mandibular deviation on opening or closing of the mouth may indicate a jaw fracture or dislocation.

INTRAORAL EXAMINATION

The intraoral examination must be systematic and should include recording of any laceration, hemorrhage, or swelling of the oral mucosa or gingiva. All lacerations should be

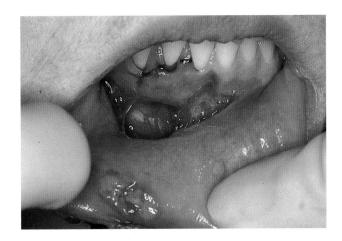

FIGURE 17-1 Soft tissue injuries of the lip and gingiva require thorough débridement.

cleaned to remove any foreign bodies (see Fig. 17-1). Lacerations of the lips or tongue must be sutured, but those of the oral mucosa heal very quickly and may not need suturing. Orofacial signs of child physical abuse may be present (see later discussion). Any abnormalities of occlusion, tooth displacement, fractured crowns, or cracks in the enamel must also be noted.

The following signs and reactions to tests are particularly helpful:

- *Mobility:* Degree of mobility is estimated in a horizontal and a vertical direction. If several teeth move together en bloc, a fracture of the alveolar process should be suspected. Excessive mobility may also suggest root fracture or tooth displacement.
- *Reaction to percussion:* This is tested in a horizontal and a vertical direction and compared against a contralateral uninjured tooth. A duller note may indicate root fracture.
- *Color of tooth:* Early color change is visible on the palatal surface of the gingival third of the crown.
- *Reaction to sensibility tests:* Thermal tests with warm gutta percha or ethyl chloride are widely used. However, an electrical pulp tester in the hands of an experienced operator is more reliable. Nevertheless, vitality testing, especially in children, is notoriously unreliable and should never be assessed in isolation from the other clinical and radiographic data. Neither negative nor positive responses should be trusted immediately after trauma. A positive response does not rule out later pulpal necrosis, and although a negative response suggests pulpal damage, it does not necessarily indicate a necrotic pulp. The negative reaction is often caused by a shockwave effect that has damaged the apical nerve supply. The pulp in such cases may have a normal blood supply. In all vitality testing, the reaction of uninjured contralateral teeth should be included and documented for comparison. In addition, all teeth adjacent to the obviously injured teeth should be regularly assessed, because they have probably suffered concussion injury. In the future, advances in Doppler technology will allow the clinician to measure whether the vascular supply to individual teeth is intact. Doppler probes are currently too expensive for the general dental practitioner, but research has shown them to be a reliable tool.

RADIOGRAPHIC EXAMINATION

Three types of radiograph allow the clinician to accurately diagnose and treat all dentoalveolar injuries:

- *Periapical:* Reproducible periapical projections made with the long cone technique are best for accurate diagnosis and clinical audit. Two radiographs at different angles may be essential to detect a root fracture. However, if access and cooperation are difficult, one anterior occlusal radiograph rarely misses a root fracture. A small periapical film placed inside the upper or lower lip will detect tooth fragments or foreign bodies in the vertical plane.
- *Occlusal:* This projection can detect root fractures and displacements when the mouth cannot open enough to accommodate a periapical film. An occlusal film held by

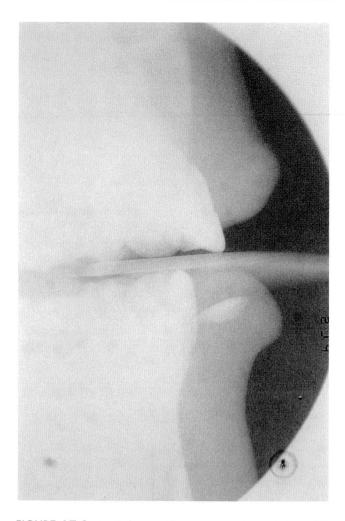

FIGURE 17-2   Tooth fragment from an upper incisor is lodged in the lower lip.

the patient or by a helper at the side of the mouth can be used to detect tooth fragments or foreign bodies in the lateral plane (Fig. 17-2).
- *Dental panoramic tomograph:* This is essential in all dentoalveolar trauma cases and may detect an unsuspected underlying bony injury.

PHOTOGRAPHIC EXAMINATION

Good clinical photographs are useful to assess treatment outcomes and for medicolegal purposes.

STATE-OF-THE-ART MANAGEMENT OF INJURIES TO THE PRIMARY DENTITION

During its early development, the permanent incisor is located palatally to the apex of the primary incisor and in close proximity to it. With any injury to a primary tooth, there is a risk of damage to the underlying permanent successor (Fig. 17-3). Parents should be advised that in all cases of trauma involving the primary dentition, there is a 50%

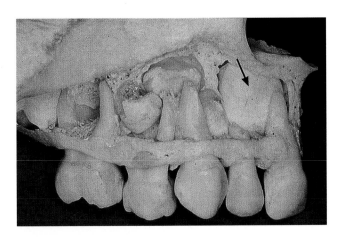

FIGURE 17-3 *The close proximity of developing permanent tooth germs to the roots of the primary dentition. The* arrow *indicates permanent central incisor germ.*

chance of developmental disturbances to the permanent successor teeth.

Children aged 2 to 4 years are most likely to injure their primary dentition. Realistically, this means that few restorative procedures are possible; in most cases, the decision is between extraction or maintenance without extensive treatment. A primary incisor should always be removed if its maintenance would jeopardize the developing tooth bud.

A traumatized primary tooth that is retained should be assessed regularly for clinical and radiographic signs of pulpal or periodontal complications. Radiographs may even detect damage to the permanent successor. Soft tissue injuries in children should be assessed weekly until healed. Tooth injuries should be reviewed every 3 to 4 months for the first year and then annually until the primary tooth exfoliates and the permanent successor is in place.

UNCOMPLICATED CROWN FRACTURE

In cases of uncomplicated crown fracture, the sharp edges should be smoothed or the crown morphology restored with a bonded restoration if cooperation allows.

COMPLICATED CROWN FRACTURE

In complicated crown fracture, pulp extirpation, root canal obturation with resorbable zinc oxide cement, and a bonded restoration to restore crown morphology can be achieved with reasonable cooperation. However, in many cases, extraction of the tooth is the only realistic option.

CROWN-ROOT FRACTURE

In crown-root fractures, the pulp is invariably exposed and the fracture line extends well below the gingival margin. Restorative treatment is extremely difficult, and the tooth is best extracted.

ROOT FRACTURE

In cases of root fracture without displacement and with only a small amount of mobility, the tooth should be kept under observation. If the coronal fragment becomes nonvital and symptomatic, it should be removed. The apical portion usually remains vital and undergoes resorption. If there is marked displacement and mobility, only the coronal portion should be removed. Unnecessary searching for small apical root fragments runs the risk of iatrogenic damage to the permanent successor tooth.

CONCUSSION, SUBLUXATION, AND LUXATION INJURIES

In all instances, associated soft tissue damage should be cleaned by the parent twice daily with 0.2% chlorhexidine solution using cotton buds or gauze swabs until healing occurs.

- *Concussion*: These injuries require periodic review with close observation for signs of nonvitality.
- *Subluxation*: If there is slight mobility, parents should be advised to keep the traumatized area as clean as possible and to give the child a soft diet for 1 to 2 weeks.
- *Extrusive luxation*: These teeth are usually very mobile and require extraction.
- *Lateral luxation*: If the crown is displaced palatally, the apex moves buccally, away from the permanent teeth germ. If the occlusion is not gagged, conservative treatment to await some spontaneous realignment is possible. If the crown is displaced buccally, the apex will be displaced toward the permanent tooth bud, and extraction is indicated to minimize further damage to the permanent successor.
- *Intrusive luxation*: This is a common injury. The aim of investigation is to establish the direction of displacement by thorough radiographic examination. If the root is displaced palatally toward the permanent successor, the primary tooth should be extracted to minimize possible damage to the developing permanent successor. If the root is displaced buccally, periodic review to monitor spontaneous reeruption should be undertaken. Review should be weekly for 1 month, then monthly for a maximum of 6 months. Most reeruption occurs between 1 and 6 months. If reeruption does not occur, ankylosis is likely, and extraction is necessary to prevent ectopic eruption of the permanent successor.
- *Exarticulation (avulsion)*: Replantation of avulsed primary incisors is not recommended because of the risk of damage to the permanent tooth germs. Space maintenance is not necessary after loss of a primary incisor, because only minor drifting of adjacent teeth occurs. The eruption of the permanent successor may be delayed for about 1 year as a result of abnormal thickening of connective tissue overlying the tooth germ.

INJURIES TO SUPPORTING BONE

Most fractures of the alveolar socket in primary dentition do not require splinting, because bony healing is rapid in small children. Jaw fractures are treated in the conventional manner, although stabilization after reduction may be difficult due to lack of sufficient teeth.

STATE-OF-THE-ART MANAGEMENT OF SEQUELAE OF INJURIES TO THE PRIMARY DENTITION

PULPAL NECROSIS

Necrosis is the most common complication of primary trauma. Evaluation is based on tooth color and radiographic findings. Vitality testing is unreliable and of no clinical benefit in primary teeth. Teeth of a normal color rarely develop periapical inflammation, and mildly discolored teeth also may be vital. A mild gray color occurring soon after trauma may represent intrapulpal bleeding with a pulp that is still vital. This color may recede, but if it persists, necrosis should be suspected. Radiographic examination should be scheduled every 3 months to check for periapical inflammation. Failure of the pulp cavity to reduce in size is an indicator of pulp death. Teeth should be extracted whenever there is evidence of periapical inflammation, to prevent possible damage to the permanent successor.

PULPAL OBLITERATION

Obliteration of the pulp chamber and canal is a common reaction to trauma. Clinically, the tooth becomes yellow or opaque. Normal exfoliation is usual, but occasionally periapical inflammation develops and extraction is required. Annual periapical radiography is advisable to detect infection and to check physiological root resorption. If resorption does not occur, the permanent successor will erupt in an ectopic position.

ROOT RESORPTION

Internal resorption may be seen with concussion, subluxation, and luxation injuries and in external inflammatory resorption with intrusive injuries. Extraction is usually the preferred treatment for these types of root resorption.

INJURIES TO DEVELOPING PERMANENT TEETH

Injury to the permanent successor tooth can be expected in 12% to 69% of cases of primary tooth trauma and in 19% to 68% of jaw fracture. Intrusive luxation causes most disturbances. Avulsion of a primary incisor also causes damage if the apex moved toward the permanent tooth bud before the avulsion. Most damage to the permanent tooth bud occurs before 3 years of age, during its developmental stage. However, the type and severity of disturbance are closely related to the age at the time of injury. Changes in the morphology and mineralization of the crown of the permanent incisor are most common, but later injuries can cause radicular anomalies.

Injuries to developing teeth can be classified as follows:

- White or yellow-brown discoloration of enamel—injury at 2 to 7 years of age
- White or yellow-brown discoloration of enamel with circular enamel hypoplasia—injury at 2 to 7 years of age
- Crown dilacerations (Fig. 17-4)—injury at about 2 years of age

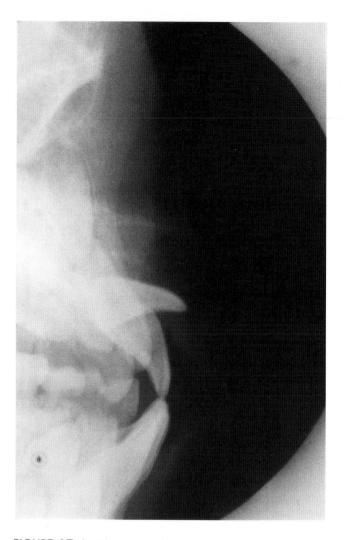

FIGURE 17-4   Dilaceration of an upper permanent central incisor resulting from an intrusion injury to the primary incisor at the age of 2 years.

- Odontoma-like malformation—injury before 1 to 3 years of age
- Root duplication—injury at 2 to 5 years of age
- Vestibular or lateral root angulation and dilaceration—injury at 2 to 5 years of age
- Partial or complete arrest of root formation—injury at 5 to 7 years of age
- Sequestration of permanent tooth germs
- Disturbance in eruption

The term *dilaceration* describes an abrupt deviation of the long axis of the crown or root portion of the tooth. This deviation results from a traumatic nonaxial displacement of already formed hard tissue in relation to developing soft tissue.

The term *angulation* describes a curvature of the root that results from gradual change in the direction of root development without evidence of abrupt displacement of the tooth germ during odontogenesis. This may be vestibular (i.e., labiopalatal) or lateral (i.e., mesiodistal). Evaluation of the full extent of complications after injuries must await complete eruption of all permanent teeth involved. However, most serious sequelae (disturbances in tooth morphology) can be diagnosed radiographically within the first year after the trauma.

Injuries to the infant alveolus, even before the eruption of primary teeth, can cause disturbances in tooth morphology of the primary teeth and, more rarely, of very early-developing permanent teeth.[1]

Eruption disturbances of the permanent teeth may involve the following:

- Delayed eruption due to connective tissue thickening over a permanent tooth germ as a result of early primary predecessor loss
- Ectopic eruption due to lack of eruptive guidance as a result of premature loss of the primary predecessor or failure of physiological resorption of the primary predecessor
- Impaction and failure of eruption in teeth with malformations of crown or root

TREATMENT OF INJURIES TO THE PERMANENT DENTITION

Yellow-brown discoloration of enamel with or without hypoplasia is treated with (1) acid-pumice microabrasion, (2) composite resin restoration (localized, veneer, or crown), and (3) porcelain restoration (veneer or crown in the anterior, fused to metal crown in the posterior).

Crown dilaceration is treated with (1) surgical exposure with or without orthodontic alignment, (2) placement of a temporary crown until root formation is complete, (3) removal of the dilacerated part of the crown with or without one-stage root canal obturation, and (4) coronal restoration.

Vestibular root angulation is treated with combined surgical and orthodontic realignment. For other malformations, extraction is usually the treatment of choice. Disturbance in eruption is treated by surgical exposure with or without orthodontic realignment.

STATE-OF-THE-ART MANAGEMENT OF INJURIES TO THE PERMANENT DENTITION

Most traumatized permanent teeth can be treated successfully. Prompt and appropriate treatment instituted after correct diagnosis improves the prognosis.

The aims and principles of treatment can be broadly categorized into three parts.

1. Emergency treatment
   - Retain vitality of fractured or displaced teeth
   - Cover exposed dentine with a bonded restoration
   - Treat exposed pulp tissue
   - Reduce and immobilize displaced teeth
   - Antibacterial mouthwash, antibiotics, and tetanus prophylaxis
2. Intermediate treatment
   - May require pulp treatment
   - Minimally invasive coronal restoration
3. Permanent treatment
   - Stimulated root end closure
   - Root filling with or without root extrusion

- May require gingival and alveolar collar modification
- Semipermanent or permanent coronal restoration

Trauma cases require painstaking follow-up to disclose any complications and institute the correct treatment. The intervals between examinations depend on the severity of the trauma, but the following schedule is a guide: 1 week, 3 weeks, 6 weeks, 3 months, 6 months, 12 months, and then annually for 4 to 5 years. At these times, color, mobility, percussion, and sensibility are routinely noted, and radiographs are examined for periradicular conditions and changes within the pulp cavity.

INJURIES TO THE HARD DENTAL TISSUES AND THE PULP

The various types of injury to the hard dental tissues and the pulp are summarized in Table 17-1.

Enamel Infraction

Enamel infractions are incomplete fractures without loss of tooth substance. Without proper illumination, they are easily overlooked. Periodic follow-up is necessary, because the energy of the blow may have been transmitted to the periodontal tissues or the pulp.

Enamel Fracture

With enamel fractures, no restoration is needed, and treatment is limited to smoothing of any rough edges and splinting if there is associated mobility. Periodic review is undertaken as for enamel infractions.

Enamel-Dentine Fracture

Immediate treatment of enamel-dentine fractures is necessary because of the involvement of dentine. The pulp requires protection against thermal irritation and against bacteria via the dentinal tubules. Restoration of crown morphology also stabilizes the position of the tooth in the arch.

Emergency protection of the exposed dentine can be achieved in two ways. A bonded composite resin or compomer bandage may be used. (Conventional glass ionomer cement alone will not be retained because of its poorer physical properties and bond strength.) Alternatively, glass ionomer cement supported within an orthodontic band or the incisal end of a celluloid crown former or stainless steel crown may be used. These serve as temporary retainers until further eruption occurs.

Intermediate restoration of most enamel-dentine fractures can be achieved by two methods. Acid-etched composite may be applied freehand or with the use of a celluloid crown former. With recent improvements in composite technology, most of these restorations can be regarded as semipermanent or permanent. With larger fractures, more enamel surface area should be used for bonding; a complete celluloid crown former is used to construct a "direct" composite crown. At a later age, this can be reduced to form the core of a porcelain jacket crown preparation. Alternatively, the crown fragment can be reattached (Figs. 17-5 and 17-6). This method of restoration has become feasible since the development of dentine bonding agents. However, few long-term studies have been reported, and the longevity of this type of restoration is largely unknown.[2] In addition, there is a tendency for the distal

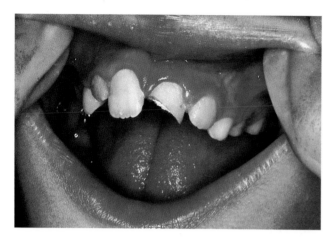

FIGURE 17-5 An enamel-dentine fracture of the upper left central incisor.

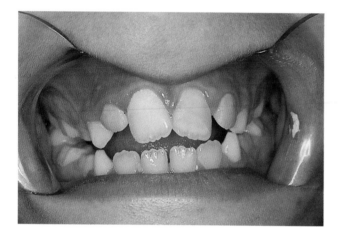

FIGURE 17-6 Same patient as in Figure 17-5, after reattachment of the coronal fragment.

fragment to become opaque or to require further restorative intervention in the form of a veneer or jacket crown.

If the fracture line through dentine is not very close to the pulp, the fragment may be reattached immediately. If it runs close to the pulp, it is advisable to place a suitably protected calcium hydroxide dressing over the exposed dentine for at least 1 month while storing the fragment in saline, which should be renewed weekly. The procedure is as follows:

- Check the fit of the fragment and the vitality of the tooth.
- Clean the fragment and the tooth with pumice-water slurry.
- Isolate the tooth with a rubber dam.
- Attach the fragment to a piece of gutta percha to facilitate handling.
- Etch the enamel for 30 seconds on both fracture surfaces, extending for 2 mm from the fracture line on the tooth and the fragment. Wash for 15 seconds and dry for 15 seconds.
- Apply dentine primer to both surfaces and then dry for 15 to 30 seconds.

- Apply enamel-dentine bonding agent to both surfaces and then lightly blow away any excess. Light-cure for 10 seconds.
- Place the appropriate shade of composite resin over both surfaces, and position the fragment. Remove the gross excess and cure for 60 seconds labially and palatally.
- Remove any excess composite resin with sandpaper discs.
- Remove a 1-mm gutter of enamel on each side of the fracture line, both labially and palatally, to a depth of 0.5 mm using a small round or pear-shaped bur. The finishing line should be irregular in outline.
- Etch the newly prepared enamel, wash, dry, apply composite, cure, and finish.

Enamel-Dentine Pulp Fracture (Complicated Crown Fracture)

In a tooth with an immature apex, the major concern is preservation of pulp vitality to allow continued root growth. The injured pulp must be sealed from bacteria so that it does not become infected during the period of repair. Pulpotomy or partial pulpotomy is the treatment of choice to retain vital radicular pulp. However, for the best chance of success, treatment should be initiated within 24 hours after the injury. If radicular pulp vitality is not maintained or the pulpal exposure is wide, total pulp extirpation (pulpectomy) is the only treatment choice. Nonsetting calcium hydroxide is spun into the root canal and changed every 3 months to stimulate root end closure so that a permanent root canal filling can be obturated against a closed apex. The average time for stimulated root end closure to occur with nonsetting calcium hydroxide is between 9 and 12 months.[3,4] Mineral trioxide aggregate (MTA) is being used increasingly to create an apical stop at an open apex, before backfilling of the canal with gutta percha. This reduces the number of treatment visits required.

In a tooth with a mature apex and a complicated crown fracture, the treatment of choice is either pulpotomy or extirpation and obturation. However, if the exposure is very small and recent, direct pulp capping can be attempted.

Uncomplicated Crown-Root Fracture

After removal of the fractured piece of tooth, crown-root fractures commonly extend vertically a few millimeters incisal to the gingival margin on the labial surface but down to the cementoenamel junction palatally. Before placement of a restoration, the fracture margin must be brought supragingival by gingivoplasty or by extrusion (orthodontically or surgically) of the root portion.

Complicated Crown-Root Fracture

Complicated crown-root fractures are treated similarly to uncomplicated ones with the addition of endodontic requirements. If extrusion is planned, the final root length must be no shorter than the final crown length; otherwise, the result will be unstable. Root extrusion can be successful in a motivated patient and leads to a stable periodontal condition.

Root Fracture

Root fractures occur most frequently in the middle or apical third of the root. The coronal fragment may be extruded or luxated. Luxation is usually in a lingual or palatal direction.

If displacement has occurred, the coronal fragment should be repositioned as soon as possible by gentle digital manipulation, and the position should then be checked radiographically. Mobile root fractures need to be functionally splinted to encourage repair of the fracture. Apical-third fractures, in the absence of concomitant PDL injury, are often firm and do not require splinting; however, they need to be regularly reviewed to check pulpal status, and they should be treated endodontically if necessary.

Apical-, middle-, and coronal-third fractures must be splinted functionally. A functional splint is one that includes one abutment tooth on either side of the fractured tooth. Apical-third and middle-third fractures should be splinted for 4 weeks and coronal-third fractures for a longer period, up to 4 months.[5] The splint should allow color observations and sensitivity testing, as well as access to the root canal if endodontic treatment is required. Splint design and placement techniques are discussed later.

In about 80% of all root-fractured teeth, the pulp remains viable and repair occurs in the fracture area. Three main categories of repair are recognized:

1. Repair with calcified tissue if the fracture line is invisible or hardly discernible
2. Repair with connective tissue if there is a narrow, radiolucent fracture line with peripheral rounding of the fracture edges
3. Repair with bone and connective tissue if a bony bridge separates the two fragments

In addition to these changes in the fracture area, pulp canal obliteration is commonly seen. Fractures in the coronal third of the root can be repaired as well as those in the middle or apical thirds as long as no communication exists between the fracture line and the gingival crevice. If such a communication exists, splinting is not recommended, and a decision must be made to extract the coronal fragment and retain the remaining root, extract the two fragments, or internally splint the root fracture. The last option is unlikely to achieve long-term success.

If the coronal fragment is extracted and the root is retained, the remaining radicular pulp should be removed and the canal temporarily dressed before obturation with gutta percha. Three options are now available for the radicular portion:

1. Post, core, and crown restoration if access is adequate.
2. Extrusion of the root, either surgically or orthodontically, if the fracture extends too far subgingivally for adequate access. Rapid orthodontic extrusion over 4 to 6 weeks aiming to move the root a maximum of 4 mm is the best option. This is achieved by cementing a J hook made from 0.7-mm stainless steel wire into the canal and using elastic traction applied over an arch wire cemented to one tooth on either side of the injured tooth. Retention for 1 month after the end of movement is advised to prevent relapse. If esthetics is a particular concern, an orthodontic bracket can be bonded to a temporary crown made over the J hook. The temporary crown length will need to be reduced as extrusion occurs.
3. Use of a mucoperiosteal flap to cover the root. This maintains the height and width of the arch and facilitates later placement of a single tooth implant.

Pulpal necrosis occurs in about 20% of root fractures and is the main obstacle to adequate repair. The amount of displacement of the coronal portion is important for pulpal prognosis and hard tissue union. Most cases of necrosis are diagnosed within 3 months after a root fracture. A persistent negative response to electrical stimulation is usually confirmed on radiography by radiolucencies adjacent to the fracture line.

The apical fragment almost always contains viable pulp tissue. In apical- and middle-third fractures, any endodontic treatment is usually confined to the coronal fragment. After completion of endodontic treatment, repair and union between the two fragments with connective tissue is a consistent finding. In coronal-third fractures that develop necrosis, the radicular portion can be retained, both portions can be extracted, or the fracture can be internally splinted (see earlier discussions).

INJURIES TO THE PERIODONTAL TISSUES

As the severity of periodontal injury increases, there is a decrease in pulpal prognosis for the teeth involved (Table 17-2) and an increase in the amount of expected root resorption (Table 17-3). Table 17-2 demonstrates clearly that pulpal prognosis is superior for all categories of injury in teeth with open or immature apices. In these immature teeth, the neurovascular bundle can survive some edema and movement around the open apices, whereas in the mature tooth, any mobility and edema within the narrow confines of the small apical foramen often leads to pulpal necrosis. Correct

TABLE 17-2	5-Year Pulpal Survival Data for Injuries Involving the Periodontal Ligament	
Type of Injury	Open Apex (%)	Closed Apex (%)
Concussion	100	96
Subluxation	100	85
Extrusive luxation	95	45
Lateral luxation	95	25
Intrusive luxation	40	0
Replantation	30	0

TABLE 17-3	Prevalence of Resorption after Periodontal Ligament Injury	
Type of Injury	Open Apex (%)	Closed Apex (%)
Concussion	1	3
Subluxation	1	3
Extrusive luxation	5	7
Lateral luxation	3	38
Intrusive luxation	67	100
Replantation	Frequent	Frequent

diagnosis and treatment of all periodontal tissue injuries aims to improve pulpal prognosis and decrease future resorption sequelae.[6]

Concussion

In concussion injury, the impact force causes edema and hemorrhage in the PDL fibers, and the tooth is firm in the socket. The treatment is:

- occlusal relief.
- soft diet for 7 days.
- immobilization with a functional splint for 2 weeks if tenderness to percussion (TTP) is significant or the apex is closed.
- chlorhexidine 0.2% mouthwash twice daily.

Subluxation

In subluxation, in addition to the concussion injury, there is rupture of some PDL fibers, and the tooth is mobile in the socket, although not displaced. The treatment is the same as for concussion injuries.

In subluxation injuries, the immature apex tooth may not require splinting. However, the mature apex tooth should always be splinted to rest the periodontal tissues and protect the neurovascular bundle as it enters the small apical foramen.

Extrusive Luxation

In extrusive luxation, there is rupture of the PDL and pulp. Treatment for extrusive luxation should include:

- local anesthetic.
- atraumatic repositioning with gentle but firm digital pressure.
- nonrigid functional splint for 2 weeks.
- antibiotic therapy (e.g., amoxicillin 250 mg three times daily (if <6 years old, 125 mg three times daily) for 5 days.
- chlorhexidine 0.2% mouthwash twice daily while splint is in position.
- soft diet for 2 weeks.

Extrusive luxation is discussed further in the next section.

Lateral Luxation

In lateral luxation, there is rupture of the PDL and pulp and damage to the alveolar plate or plates (Figs. 17-7 and 17-8). Treatment for lateral luxation should include:

- local anesthetic.
- atraumatic repositioning with gentle but firm digital pressure.
- nonrigid functional splinting for 4 weeks.
- antibiotic therapy (e.g., amoxicillin 250 mg three times daily (if <6 years old, 125 mg three times daily) for 5 days.
- chlorhexidine 0.2% mouthwash twice daily while splint is in position.
- soft diet for 4 weeks.

Antibiotics may have a beneficial effect in promoting repair of the PDL. They do not appear to affect pulpal prognosis.

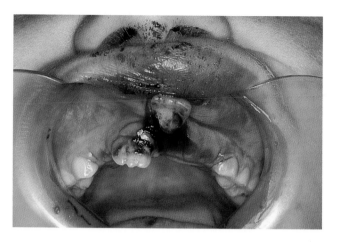

FIGURE 17-7   Labial lateral luxation of upper left central incisor at age 8 years.

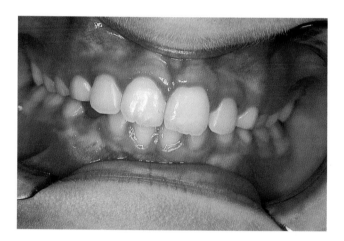

FIGURE 17-8   Same tooth as in Figure 17-7 at age 18 years, after correct treatment.

After the splinting period for extrusion (2 weeks) or for lateral luxation (4 weeks), radiographic images of the teeth are obtained. If there is no evidence of marginal breakdown, the splint can be removed. If marginal breakdown is present, the splint should be retained for a further 2 to 3 weeks.

For extrusion and lateral luxation injuries, the decision whether to progress to endodontic treatment depends on the combination of clinical and radiographic signs (see later discussion). Five-year pulpal survival figures (see Table 17-2) show that prognosis is significantly better for open apex teeth, but nevertheless a proportion of mature teeth involved in luxation injuries exhibit on radiographs a natural healing phenomenon known as transient apical breakdown (TAB), which can mimic apical infection. Ambivalent clinical and radiographic signs should be given the benefit of the doubt until the next review.

With more significant damage to the PDL in both extrusive and lateral luxation injuries, there is an increased risk of root resorption (see Table 17-3). Thirty-five percent of mature teeth that have undergone lateral luxation show subsequent evidence of surface resorption. This is because the PDL has been irreversibly damaged by crushing against the alveolar

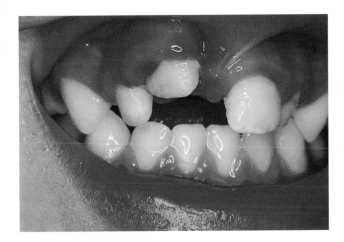

FIGURE 17-9 Intrusive injury to the upper right permanent central incisor.

plates, as opposed to the tearing that occurs in extrusive luxation injury.

In cases of lateral luxation with late presentation (>2 days after the injury), the displacement cannot be reduced with gentle finger pressure. It is not advisable to use more force, because this could further damage the PDL. Orthodontic appliances, either a removable type or a sectional fixed appliance, can be used to reduce the displacement over a period of a few weeks.

Intrusive Luxation

Intrusive luxation injuries result from an axial, apical impact, and there is extensive damage to PDL, pulp, and alveolar plates (Fig. 17-9).

Two distinct treatment categories exist, for open and closed apex.[5] If the apex is open, the displacement can be disimpacted (with forceps if necessary) and allowed to erupt spontaneously. If there is no spontaneous movement within 3 weeks, rapid orthodontic repositioning is started. Alternatively, disimpaction and surgical repositioning can be performed, followed by functional splinting for 4 weeks. The pulpal status is monitored clinically and radiographically at 1, 3, and 6 months, and endodontic therapy is started if necessary. The use of nonsetting calcium hydroxide in the root canal does not preclude orthodontic movement. Once apexification has occurred, the canal is obturated with gutta percha.

Intrusive luxation with a closed apex is treated with elective orthodontic or surgical extrusion immediately, followed by functional splinting for 4 weeks. Elective pulp extirpation is performed before splint removal. Obturation with gutta percha is performed after initial calcium hydroxide dressing.

If endodontic treatment is commenced within 2 weeks after an injury to the PDL, some authors suggest that the initial intracanal dressing should be a polyantibiotic or antibiotic/steroid paste. The reason is that if nonsetting calcium hydroxide is inadvertently spun through the apex before the PDL fibers have healed, it can cause replacement resorption. Sixty percent of PDL fibers are healed 2 weeks after an injury.

At the outset, all patients with intrusive luxation injuries should receive antibiotics, chlorhexidine mouthwash, and a soft diet. The risk of pulpal necrosis in these injuries is high, especially in the closed apex (see Table 17-2). The incidence of resorption and ankylosis sequelae is also high (see Table 17-3).[7,8]

Avulsion and Replantation

Replantation of avulsed teeth should always be attempted, although it may offer only a temporary solution due to the frequent occurrence of external inflammatory resorption (EIR).[9-13] Even if resorption occurs, the tooth may be retained for years, acting as a natural space maintainer and preserving the height and width of the alveolus to facilitate later implant placement.

Successful healing after replantation can occur only if there is minimal damage to the pulp and the PDL. The type of extra-alveolar storage medium and the extra-alveolar time (EAT)—the time the tooth has been out of the mouth—are critical factors. The suggested protocol for replantation can be divided into advice on the telephone, immediate treatment in surgery, and review.

The following advice should be given to patients and families over the telephone:

- Do not touch root; hold the tooth by its crown.
- Wash the tooth gently under cold tapwater for 10 seconds.
- Replace the tooth into the socket or transport it in a suitable medium to the hospital.
- If the tooth is replaced, bite gently on a handkerchief to retain the tooth until arrival at the hospital.

The best transport medium is the tooth's own socket. Nondentists may be reluctant to replant a tooth, and milk is an effective iso-osmolar medium. Saliva, the patient's buccal sulcus, specific tooth transport media, and normal saline are alternatives.

The following points are important in the immediate treatment:

- Do not handle root; if the tooth has been replanted, remove it from the socket.
- Rinse the tooth with normal saline. Note the state of root development. Store the tooth in saline.
- Apply local analgesia.
- Irrigate the socket with saline, and remove clot and any foreign material.
- Push the tooth gently but firmly into the socket.
- Apply a nonrigid functional splint (which will remain in place for 2 weeks).
- Check the occlusion.
- Obtain baseline radiographs (periapical or anterior occlusal). Determine whether any other teeth have been injured.
- Prescribe antibiotics, chlorhexidine mouthwash, and soft diet as described previously.
- Check the patient's tetanus immunization status.

Before splint removal at 2 weeks, radiographs are obtained. If there is an open apex and EAT was less than 45 minutes, observation is appropriate. Otherwise, endodontic therapy is commenced before splint removal, as follows:

1. Open apex and EAT >45 minutes
   a. Initial intracanal dressing: polyantibiotic or antibiotic/steroid paste
   b. Subsequent intracanal dressings: nonsetting calcium hydroxide
   c. Replace calcium hydroxide every 3 months until an apical barrier forms or form an apical stop with MTA
   d. Obturate the canal with gutta percha
2. Closed apex
   a. Initial intracanal dressing: polyantibiotic or antibiotic/steroid paste
   b. Subsequent intracanal dressing: nonsetting calcium hydroxide
   c. Obturate with gutta percha

Radiographic review is performed at 1, 3, 6, 12, 18, and 24 months, then annually. If resorption is progressing unhalted, nonsetting calcium hydroxide is kept in the tooth until exfoliation, changing it every 6 months.

The immature tooth with an EAT of less than 45 minutes may undergo pulp revascularization (see Table 17-2). However, these teeth require regular clinical and radiographic review, because once EIR occurs, it progresses rapidly.

Replantation of Teeth with a Dry Storage Time of Greater Than 1 Hour

If a mature tooth has a dry storage time of greater than 1 hour, the PDL will be nonvital. The PDL and the pulp should be removed at chairside and the tooth placed in 2.4% sodium fluoride solution acidulated to pH 5.5 for 20 minutes. The root canal is then obturated with gutta percha, and the tooth is replanted and splinted with a nonrigid functional splint for 4 weeks. The aim of this treatment is to produce ankylosis, which allows the tooth to be maintained as a natural space maintainer, perhaps for a limited period only. The sodium fluoride is believed to slow down the resorptive process.

Pulpal and Periodontal Status

Pulpal necrosis, the most common complication, is related to the severity of the periodontal injury (see Table 17-2). Immature teeth have a better prognosis than mature teeth due to their wide apical opening Slight movements can occur without disruption of the apical neurovascular bundle.

Necrosis usually can be diagnosed within 3 months after the injury, but in some cases, it may not be evident for 2 years or longer. Both clinical and radiological signs are often required to diagnose necrosis.

Sensitivity Testing

Most injured teeth respond negatively to electrical pulp testing immediately after the trauma. Most pulps that recover test positively within months, but responses have been reported as late as 2 years after injury. Therefore, a negative test by itself should not be regarded as proof of necrosis. Endodontics should be postponed until at least one other clinical or radiographic sign is present.

Tooth Discoloration

Initial pinkish discoloration may be caused by subtotal severance of apical vessels that leads to penetration of hemoglobin from such ruptures into the dentine tubules. If the vascular system repairs itself, most of this discoloration will disappear.

If the tooth becomes progressively gray, necrosis should be suspected. A gray color that appears for the first time several weeks or months after trauma signifies decomposition of necrotic pulp tissue and is a decisive sign of necrosis. Color changes are usually most apparent on the palatal surface of the injured teeth.

Tenderness to Percussion

TTP may be the most reliable isolated indicator of pulpal necrosis.

Periapical Inflammation

Radiological periapical involvement secondary to necrosis can be seen as early as 3 weeks after trauma. In mature teeth, TAB may be mistaken for periapical inflammation.

Arrest of Root Development

If necrosis involves the epithelial root sheath before root development is complete, no further root growth will occur. In an injured pulp, necrosis may progress from the coronal to the apical portion; residual apical vitality may result in formation of a calcific barrier across a wide apical foramen.

Failure of the pulp chamber and root canal to mature and reduce in size on successive radiographs compared with contralateral uninjured teeth is also a reliable indicator of necrosis.

Root Resorption
Inflammatory Root Resorption (External)

External inflammatory root resorption is a pathognomic sign of necrosis and requires immediate endodontic treatment. Resorptive areas are usually evident within 3 weeks to 4 months after injury. External inflammatory resorption is most frequently associated with intrusive luxation and replantation. It is initiated by PDL damage resulting in resorption cavities in cementum but is propagated and potentiated by infected necrotic pulpal products that stimulate an increase in inflammatory response in the PDL via the dentinal tubules. "Punched-out" areas of resorption on the external root surface are associated with adjacent bony radiolucencies. If EIR is not present within 1 year after injury, it is unlikely to occur. Left untreated, inflammatory root resorption will destroy the tooth completely within months. Treatment consisting of extirpation, débridement, and nonsetting calcium hydroxide is necessary. In most cases, arrest and cemental repair will occur.

Inflammatory Root Resorption (Internal)

Internal inflammatory root resorption is an infrequent complication caused by chronic pulpal inflammation. It is often without clinical symptoms and is seen radiographically as a ballooning of the near-parallel walls of the root canal. It progresses rapidly to perforation of the root surface. Early endodontic treatment with extirpation, mechanical and chemical débridement, and nonsetting calcium hydroxide has a good chance of success.

Pulp Canal Obliteration

In up to 35% of injured teeth, there is progressive hard tissue formation within the pulpal cavity leading to a gradual narrowing of the pulp chamber and root canal and partial or total obliteration. There is a reduced response to vitality testing, and the crown appears slightly yellow or opaque. The exact initiating factor that produces this response from the odontoblasts is unknown. It is more common in immature teeth and in luxation injuries than in concussion and subluxation injuries. Although radiographs may suggest complete calcification, there is usually a minute strand of pulpal tissue remaining. Up to 13% of these teeth can give rise to periapical inflammation as long as 5 to 15 years after the initial injury. Instrumentation of these canals can be difficult and prolonged and may result in perforation. Current clinical opinion would support allowing pulp canal obliteration to occur rather than initiating prophylactic endodontic treatment.

Replacement Resorption (Ankylosis)

Ankylosis is the most severe type of external root resorption; it is significantly related to replantation of avulsed incisors that had an extended extra-alveolar dry period. It is caused by extensive damage to the PDL and the cementum, which results in the establishment of bony union (ankylosis) between the alveolar socket and the root surface. The tooth then becomes essentially part of the bone, and as such, it is constantly remodeled, resulting in continuous resorption of cementum and dentine. Radiographically, the periodontal space disappears and tooth substance is gradually replaced by bone. Most resorption is evident within 2 months to 1 year after injury; it can be detected clinically by a high, metallic percussion note.

There is no effective treatment for ankylosis, but because the rate of progression is relatively slow, the tooth can be maintained for up to 10 years. However, such teeth can be a problem in a growing child, because they may cease to move or grow with the rest of the jaw and cannot be moved orthodontically. Nonsetting calcium hydroxide can increase replacement resorption if it is extruded through the apex of an injured tooth before PDL healing has occurred. For this reason, the initial intracanal dressing should be polyantibiotic or antibiotic/steroid for the first 2 weeks after injury to the PDL.

Conclusion

The initial treatment of PDL injuries is often the easiest part of the management. All injuries should be seen by a specialist in pediatric dentistry or restorative dentistry within days after the initial injury so that appropriate endodontic and periodontal management can be undertaken. Why go to the trouble of replanting a tooth in the middle of the night only to lose it 6 months later through external inflammatory resorption as a result of inadequate endodontic management?

INJURIES TO THE SUPPORTING BONE

The extent of the alveolar fracture should be verified clinically and radiographically (Figs. 17-10 and 17-11). If there is displacement of the teeth such that their apices have risen up and are positioned over the labial or lingual/palatal alveolar plates (apical lock), they require extrusion first, to free the apices before repositioning.

The segment of alveolus with teeth requires only 4 weeks of rigid splintage (composite-wire type), using two abutment teeth on either side of the fracture (Fig. 17-12), together with

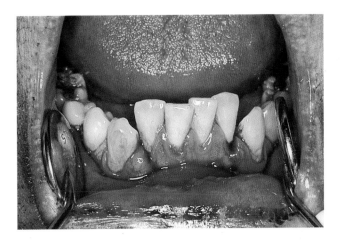

FIGURE 17-10 Dentoalveolar fracture "carrying" all lower incisors.

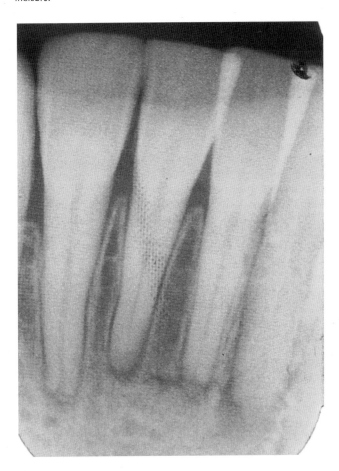

FIGURE 17-11 Periapical radiograph of the same dentoalveolar fracture as in Figure 17-10.

antibiotics, chlorhexidine, soft diet, and tetanus prophylaxis check.

Pulpal survival is more likely if repositioning occurs within 1 hour after the injury. Root resorption is rare.

SPLINTING

Trauma may loosen a tooth either by damaging the PDL or by fracturing the root. Splinting immobilizes the tooth in the

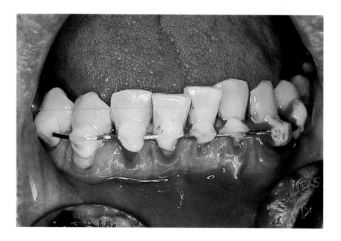

FIGURE 17-12   *Same dentoalveolar fracture as in Figures 17-10 and 17-11 after reduction, showing rigid composite-wire splint.*

correct anatomical position so that further trauma is prevented and healing can occur. Different injuries require different splinting regimens.[5,13] A functional splint involves one, and a rigid splint two, abutment teeth on either side of the injured tooth.

Splinting Regimens
Periodontal Ligament Injuries
Sixty percent of PDL healing occurs within 10 days, and healing is complete within 1 month. The splinting period should be as short as possible, and the splint should allow some functional movement to prevent replacement root resorption (ankylosis). As a general rule, exarticulation (avulsion) injuries require 2 weeks and lateral and extrusive luxation injuries require 4 weeks of functional splinting.

Root Fractures
Apical-third and middle-third injuries require 4 weeks of functional splinting to encourage a repair with either calcified tissue or connective tissue. Coronal third injuries require longer stabilization time, up to 4 months. If there is a lot of mobility, the fracture site becomes filled with granulation tissue and the tooth remains mobile.

Dentoalveolar Fractures
Dentoalveolar fractures require 4 weeks of rigid splinting.

Types and Methods of Constructing Splints
Acrylic Resin
In the acrylic resin method, temporary crown material is formed into a thin sausage shape and applied to the incisal half of the labial surfaces of the crowns after acid etching. It is the ideal splint for a single operator to apply (e.g., in after-hours accident and emergency work).

Resin-Wire Splint
The resin and wire splint method uses a temporary crown material made of either a composite resin or an acrylic resin. The composite resin is easier to place, but the acrylic resin is easier to remove.

The technique for a functional resin-wire splint is as follows:

- Bend a flexible orthodontic wire to fit the middle third of the labial surface of the injured tooth and one abutment tooth on either side.
- Stabilize the injured tooth in the correct position with soft red wax palatally.
- Clean the labial surfaces. Isolate, dry, and etch middle crown of the teeth with 37% phosphoric acid for 30 seconds; wash and dry the teeth.
- Apply to the center of the crowns a 3-mm diameter circle of unfilled and then filled composite resin or of acrylic resin.
- Position the wire into the filling material, and then apply more composite or acrylic resin.
- Use a brush lubricated with unfilled composite resin to mold and smooth the composite. Acrylic resin is more difficult to handle; smoothing and excess removal can be done with a flat plastic instrument.
- Cure the composite for 60 seconds, or wait for the acrylic resin to cure.
- Smooth any sharp edges with sandpaper discs.

For a rigid splint, use the same technique but incorporate two abutment teeth on either side of the injured tooth. These splints should not impinge on the gingiva and should allow assessment of color change and sensitivity testing.

Orthodontic Brackets and Wire
For displacement injuries and exarticulations, orthodontic bracket and wire splints have the advantage of allowing a more accurate reduction of the injury by gentle forces.

Interdental Wiring
Interdental figure-of-eight wiring on an arch wire ligated to the teeth with ligature wire should not be used except as a temporary measure, because it compromises gingival health.

Foil and Cement Splint
A temporary splint made of soft metal (cooking foil or a milk bottle top) and cemented with quick-setting zinc oxide–eugenol cement is an effective measure that can be used by a single operator or while awaiting construction of a laboratory-made splint.

The technique is as follows:

- Cut foil to size: long enough to extend over two or three teeth on each side of the injured tooth and wide enough to extend over the incisal edges and 3 to 4 mm over the labial and palatal gingiva.
- Place foil over teeth and mold it over labial and palatal surfaces. Remove any excess.
- Cement the foil to the teeth with quick-drying zinc oxide–eugenol cement.

Laboratory Splints
Thermoplastic and acrylic splints are used if it is not possible to make a satisfactory splint by the direct method, such as in a 7-year-old patient with traumatized maxillary incisors, unerupted lateral incisors, and carious or absent primary canines. There are two methods, both of which require alginate impressions. Very loose teeth may need to be supported by wax, metal foil, or wire ligature so that they are not removed with the impression.

- *Acrylic splints*: There is full palatal coverage, and the acrylic is extended over the incisal edges for 2 to 3 mm on the labial surfaces of the anterior teeth. The occlusal surfaces of the posterior teeth should be covered to prevent any occlusal contact in the anterior region. This also aids retention, and Adams cribs may not be required. The splint should be removed for cleaning after meals and at bedtime.
- *Thermoplastic splints*: The splint is constructed from polyvinylacetate-polyethylene (PVAC-PE) copolymer, in the same way as a mouthguard, with extension onto the mucosa. It is usually removed after meals and at bedtime, but with more severely loosened teeth, it can be retained at night.

Both forms of laboratory splint allow functional movement and therefore promote normal periodontal healing. However, they may compromise general gingival health if oral hygiene is not maintained.

CHILD ABUSE

A child is considered to be abused if he or she is treated in a way that is unacceptable in a given culture at a given time. Child abuse is now recognized as an international issue and has been reported in many countries.[14] Each week, at least 4 children in Britain and 80 children in the United States die as a result of abuse or neglect. At least 1 of every 1000 children in Britain suffers severe physical abuse, such as fractures, brain hemorrhage, severe internal injuries, or mutilation, and in the United States more than 95% of serious intracranial injuries during the first year of life are the result of abuse. Although some reports do prove to be unfounded, the common experience is that proven cases of child abuse are four to five times as common as they were 2 decades ago. In the United States, a national emergency was declared in 1990 by the U.S. Advisory Board on Child Abuse and Neglect because there were 2.4 million cases of child maltreatment in the previous year.

The significant scientific paper in this area was published in 1962.[15] In "The Battered Child Syndrome," pediatrician Henry Kempe and his co-workers proposed that previously unexplained fractures and head injuries seen in children must have been caused nonaccidentally. The paper was a watershed, and subsequently many health workers realized that children under their care had similar nonaccidental injuries.

In the United Kingdom, the Children Act of 1989 defined four categories of abuse that could result in a child's being placed on an "at-risk" registry: physical abuse, sexual abuse, emotional abuse, neglect. Currently, approximately 34,000 children are listed on such registries or subject to a child protection plan in England and Wales. However, each category of abuse is not a diagnosis on its own but merely a symptom of disordered parenting. The aim of intervention and placement of a child on an at-risk registry is to diagnose and cure the disordered parenting. Fewer than 4% of children who come to the attention of Child Welfare Services are actually removed from the family environment because of significant risk; most families receive help and guidance so that they can function better. There is evidence that children do significantly better with their own parents rather than parental substitutes. Of those children who are severely abused in

TABLE 17-4 — Incidence of Orofacial Injuries in Child Physical Abuse

Type of Injury	Incidence (%)
Extraoral	
Contusions and ecchymoses	66
Abrasions and lacerations	28
Burns and bites	4
Fractures	2
Intraoral	
Contusions and ecchymoses	43
Abrasions and lacerations (including frenal tears)	29
Dental trauma	29

the United States, an estimated 35% to 50% [16] will suffer additional serious injury, and 50% could die if returned to their home environment without intervention.

At least 50% of children diagnosed as having suffered physical abuse have signs on the head, neck, face, and mouth that are visible to the dental practitioner.[17-22] Indeed, the dental practitioner may be the first professional to see or suspect the abuse. Injuries may take the form of contusions and ecchymoses, abrasions and lacerations, burns, bites, dental trauma, or fractures. The incidences of common orofacial injuries seen in child physical abuse are presented in Table 17-4. However, orofacial injuries are not limited to physical abuse alone. Signs on the head, neck, face, and mouth may be seen in up to 16% of cases of sexual abuse and up to 33% of neglect cases.[21] Therefore, a dental practitioner's awareness of the possibility of physical abuse may provide an opportunity for intervention. If this opportunity is missed, there may not be a further opportunity for many years.

The following points should be considered whenever doubts or suspicions are raised.

1. Could the injury have been caused accidentally, and if so, how?
2. Does the explanation for the injury fit the child's age and the clinical findings?
3. If the explanation of cause is consistent with the injury, is the cause itself within normally acceptable limits of behavior?
4. If there has been any delay seeking advice, were there good reasons for the delay?
5. Does the story of the accident vary?
6. What is the nature of the relationship between parent and child?
7. What is the child's reaction to other people?
8. What is the child's reaction to any medical or dental examinations?
9. What is the general demeanor of the child?
10. Have any comments made by the child or the parent/ caregiver given concern about the child's upbringing or lifestyle?
11. What is the child's history of previous injury?

Dental practitioners should be aware of any established system in their locality that is designed to cope with cases of child abuse. In the United Kingdom, each Local Authority Social Services Department is required to set up an Area Child Protection Committee. Dental practitioners are advised how to refer, and to whom, if they are concerned about a patient.

Awareness of child protection issues among dental practitioners varies.[18,19,23-26] This is directly related to undergraduate and postgraduate training programs, with younger practitioners tending to have greater knowledge. In addition, specialist training programs in pediatric dentistry now include child protection issues. In board examinations in the United States and membership examinations in the United Kingdom, such knowledge is now essential for certification and recertification.

Since 1989, it has been mandatory for dental practitioners in the United States to report cases of child abuse. In the United Kingdom in 2003, a high-profile enquiry by Lord Laming into the death of an 8-year-old girl in London led to recommendations about procedures and training for all agencies in regular contact with children.[27] Despite these legislative advances, there is underreporting of suspected cases by dental practitioners. This problem appears to be related both to practitioners' level of knowledge of the signs of a child in need and, probably more significantly, to their lack of understanding of how Child Welfare Services works and what happens to a child and family after a referral is made. These defects can be addressed only by participation in interagency training with all professionals involved in child protection.

Dental neglect is now recognized as often being part of more generalized neglect. Child neglect is a form of child maltreatment and is defined as "the persistent failure to meet a child's basic physical and/or psychological needs, likely to result in the serious impairment of the child's health or development."[28] Similarly, dental neglect can be defined as "failure by a parent or guardian to seek treatment for visually untreated caries, orofacial infections and pain; or failure to follow through with treatment once informed that the above condition(s) exist, to ensure a level of oral health essential for adequate function and freedom from pain and care."[29] However, for police to implement this definition adequately would be very difficult, because there are significant barriers including poverty, ignorance, and lack of access to adequate dental care.

Forty-five percent of all child protection plans in England and Wales are filed for neglect. This number is likely to rise as the poverty gap increases in developed countries.

KEY POINTS

- Boys experience dental trauma almost twice as often as girls.
- Maxillary central incisors are the most commonly involved teeth.
- Regular clinical and radiographic review is necessary to limit unwanted sequelae, institute appropriate treatment, and improve prognosis.
- Injuries to the developing permanent dentition occur in half of all instances of trauma to the primary dentition.
- Splinting for avulsion, luxation, and root fractures should be functional to allow physiological movement and promote healing of the PDL and should not exceed 2 to 3 weeks.
- Splinting for dentoalveolar fractures should be rigid and should extend for 3 to 4 weeks.
- Endodontic management of some PDL injuries must start within 7 to 10 days after the injury. Referral to pedodontic and restorative specialists is mandatory.
- In all luxation injuries, the prognosis for pulpal healing is better with an immature apex.
- Root resorption increases with the severity of damage to the PDL.
- The prognosis for replantation of avulsed teeth is best if it is undertaken within 1 hour after the injury, with a hydrated PDL.
- Orofacial injuries are found in at least 50% of cases of child physical abuse.

REFERENCES

1. Cole BOI, Welbury RR: Malformation in the primary and permanent dentitions following trauma prior to tooth eruption. *Endodont Dent Traumatol* 15:294-296, 1999.
2. Andreasen FM, Noren JG, Andreasen JO et al: Long-term survival of fragment bonding in the treatment of fractured crowns: a multicenter clinical study. *Quintessence Int* 26:669-681, 1995.
3. Mackie IC, Bentley EM, Worthington HV: The closure of open apices in non-vital immature incisor teeth. *Br Dent J* 165:169-173, 1988.
4. Kinirons MJ, Srinivasan V, Welbury RR et al: A study in two centres of variations in the time of apical barrier detection and barrier position in nonvital immature permanent incisors. *Int J Paediatr Dent* 11:447-451, 2001.
5. Flores MT, Andersson L, Andreasen JO et al: Guidelines for the management of traumatic dental injuries. 1. Fractures and luxations of permanent teeth. *Dent Traumatol* 23:66-71, 2007.
6. Andreasen JO, Andreasen FM: *Textbook and colour atlas of traumatic injuries to the teeth*, ed 3, Copenhagen, 1994, Munksgaard.
7. Kinirons MJ, Sutcliffe J: Traumatically intruded permanent incisors: a study of treatment and outcome. *Br Dent J* 170:144-146, 1991.
8. Al-Badri S, Kinirons MJ, Cole BOI et al: Factors affecting resorption in traumatically intruded permanent incisors in children. *Dent Traumatol* 18:73-76, 2002.
9. Mackie IC, Worthington HV: An investigation of replantation of traumatically avulsed permanent incisor teeth. *Br Dent J* 172:17-20, 1992.
10. Andreasen JO, Borum MK, Jacobsen HL et al: Replantation of 400 avulsed permanent incisors: papers 1, 2, 3, 4. *Endodont Dent Traumatol* 11:51-89, 1995.
11. Barrett EJ, Kenny DJ: Survival of avulsed permanent maxillary incisors in children following delayed replantation. *Endodont Dent Traumatol* 13:269-275, 1997.
12. Kinirons MJ, Gregg TA, Welbury RR et al: Variations in the presenting and treatment features in reimplanted permanent incisors in children and their effect on the prevalence of root resorption. *Br Dent J* 189:263-266, 2000.
13. Flores MT, Andersson L, Andreasen JO et al: Guidelines for the management of traumatic dental injuries. II. Avulsion of permanent teeth. *Dent Traumatol* 23:130-136, 2007.
14. Welbury RR: Child physical abuse (nonaccidental injury). In Andreasen JO, Andreasen FM, editors: *Textbook and colour atlas of traumatic injuries to the teeth*, ed 3, Copenhagen, 1994, Munksgaard.
15. Kempe CH, Silverman FN, Steele BF et al: The battered child syndrome. *JAMA* 181:17-24, 1962.
16. Kittle PE, Richardson DS, Parker JW: Examining for child abuse and neglect. *Pediatric Dentistry* 8:80-83, 2003.
17. Cairns AM, Moq JYQ, Welbury RR: Injuries to the head, face, mouth and neck in physically abused children in a community setting. *Int J Paediatr Dent* 15:310-318, 2005.
18. Cairns AM, Moq JYQ, Welbury RR: The dental practitioner and child protection in Scotland. *Br Dent J* 199:517-520, 2005.

19. Uldum B, Christensen HN, Welbury RR et al: Danish dentists' and dental hygienists knowledge of and experience with suspicion of child abuse or neglect. *Int J Paediatr Dent* 20:361-365, 2010.

20. Becker DB, Needleman HL, Kotelchuck M: Child abuse and dentistry: orofacial trauma and its recognition by dentists. *J Am Dent Assoc* 97:24-28, 1978.

21. Da Fonseca MA, Feigal RJ, Ten Bensel RW: Dental aspects of 1248 cases of child maltreatment on file at a major county hospital. *Paediatr Dent* 14:152-157, 1992.

22. Jessee SA: Physical manifestations of child abuse to the head, face and mouth: a hospital survey. *J Dent Child* 62:245-249, 1995.

23. Needleman HL, MacGregor SS, Lynch LM: Effectiveness of a statewide child abuse and neglect educational program for dental professionals. *Paediatr Dent* 17:41-45, 1995.

24. Adair SM, Wray IA, Hanes CM et al: Perceptions associated with dentists' decisions to report hypothetical cases of child maltreatment. *Paediatr Dent* 19:461-465, 1997.

25. Adair SM, Wray IA, Hanes CM et al: Demographic, educational, and experimental factors associated with dentists' decisions to report hypothetical cases of child maltreatment. *Paediatr Dent* 19:466-470, 1997.

26. Welbury RR, Macaskill SJ, Murphy JM et al: General dental practitioners perception of their role within child protection: a qualitative study. *Eur J Paediatr Dent* 2:89-95 2003.

27. The Victoria Climbie Inquiry Report: Department for Education. www.publications.gov.uk   http://news.bbc.co.uk/2/hi/in_depth/uk/2002/victoria_climbie_inquiry/default.stm

28. Child Protection and the Dental Team: *Department of Health England.* www.cpdt.org.uk

29. Definition of Dental Neglect: American Academy of Pediatric Dentistry. *Pediatric Dentistry Reference Manual* 32:13, 2010/2011.

CHAPTER 18

Eyelid and Lacrimal Injuries

Anthony G. Tyers

The eyelids protect the eyes. Spontaneous blinking sweeps away microscopic debris and moistens the eyes with tears. A dust fragment or bright light stimulates reflex blinking, and during sleep, the eyes are protected by continuous eyelid closure. Without adequate eyelids, the combined effects of desiccation and repeated minor trauma would soon lead to painful blindness. Neglected eyelid trauma can have the same disastrous result.

The distress that inevitably accompanies facial trauma can be reduced considerably by a cosmetic and functional outcome that restores normality as far as possible, especially to the midface. This is achieved by careful assessment in the hours after trauma and appropriate early management with later adjustment if necessary. A multidisciplinary approach is appropriate for all but the most superficial injuries. Photographs add to the written record, aid in planning late adjustments, and provide an accurate graphical record for medicolegal purposes.

ANATOMY

Thorough knowledge of the anatomy of the periorbital region is essential for an accurate assessment and repair of eyelid and canthal trauma.

SURFACE ANATOMY

The upper and lower lids enclose the palpebral aperture, and they join at the medial and lateral canthi (Fig. 18-1). The average size of the palpebral aperture in an adult is 30 mm horizontally and 10 mm vertically between the centers of the lids. In the upper lid, the delicate preseptal skin (inferior to the brow) and the pretarsal skin (superior to the lashes) meet at the upper lid skin crease, 6 to 10 mm from the lash line in an adult and lower in a child. The skin crease in the upper lid is formed by the insertion of the levator aponeurosis into the orbicularis muscle at this level. There is often redundant skin superior to the skin crease in the upper lid so that a skin fold is created that covers the skin crease when the eye is open. Superior to the skin crease, the fullness in the upper lid is caused by orbital fat. A less obvious skin crease may be visible in the lower lid 4 to 5 mm from the lash line. Fullness in the lower lid also is caused by orbital fat. The lateral canthus lies

at a slightly higher position than the medial canthus, and it rises further in upgaze.

EYELID STRUCTURE

An eyelid is conveniently divided into two anatomical lamellae (Figs. 18-2 and 18-3). The anterior lamella includes the skin and the orbicularis muscle. The posterior lamella is formed by the tarsal plate and the conjunctiva. Any reconstruction of the eyelid must restore the anterior covering lamella (skin) and the posterior lining lamella (mucosa) for the lid to function normally.

The skin of the eyelids is the thinnest in the body. It is attached loosely to the orbicularis muscle and more firmly attached in the region of the canthal tendons.

The orbicularis oculi muscle is the main protractor of the eyelids (Fig. 18-4). It is a flat sheet of concentric fibers encircling the palpebral aperture and spreading out beyond the orbital rims. It is divided into concentric zones: palpebral and orbital. The palpebral part overlies the eyelids. It is subdivided into a pretarsal part overlying the tarsal plates and a preseptal part anterior to the orbital septum in the upper and lower lids. The orbital part of the orbicularis muscle lies peripheral to the palpebral part. Because the orbicularis muscle is supplied by the facial nerve, lacerations that damage the nerve may compromise eyelid closure.

The anatomy of the lymphatic drainage of the lids is important in facial trauma. Lacerations or surgical incisions that cut the lymphatic drainage may result in prolonged edema of the eyelid tissues. The lateral two thirds of the upper lid and the lateral one third of the lower lid drain to the preauricular and parotid lymph nodes. The medial one third of the upper lid and the medial two thirds of the lower lid drain to the submandibular nodes.

LATERAL CANTHAL TENDON

The pretarsal muscles join laterally and insert by a common tendon into Whitnall's tubercle, a bony prominence in the lateral orbital wall 5 mm posterior to the lateral orbital rim. The preseptal muscles join laterally to form a lateral raphe, which is connected to the underlying tendon. Deep to the muscle insertions, a Y-shaped fibrous thickening in the orbital septum joins the lateral ends of the tarsal plates to

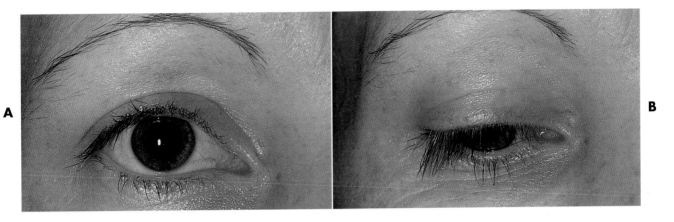

FIGURE 18-1   Surface anatomy of the eyelids in the primary position (**A**) and downgaze (**B**).

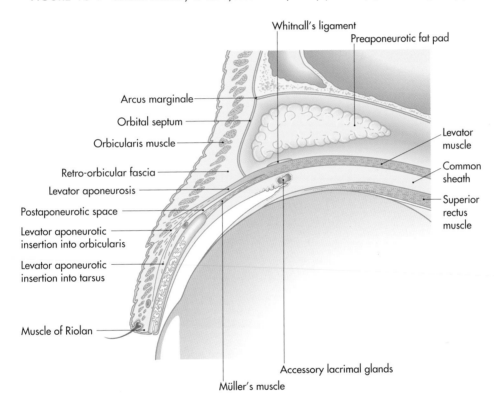

FIGURE 18-2   Section through the upper eyelid.

Whitnall's tubercle. These structures together form the lateral canthal tendon.

MEDIAL CANTHAL TENDON

The medial canthal tendon is complex anatomically, and some controversy surrounds the details of the anatomy. It has a fibrous and a muscular component. The muscular component is the insertions of the preseptal and pretarsal muscles (Fig. 18-5). The fibrous component is attached laterally to the medial ends of the tarsal plates as two limbs of a Y. The stem of the Y inserts medially, and it has an anterior and posterior component. The anterior component inserts on the frontal process of the maxilla just anterior to the anterior lacrimal crest level with the upper part of the lacrimal sac. The

posterior part leaves the deep surface of the anterior part just lateral to the anterior lacrimal crest. It passes medially and posteriorly, lateral to the lacrimal sac, and inserts on the posterior lacrimal crest. The muscle insertions are divided into superficial and deep heads, which also insert into the anterior and posterior lacrimal crests. Contraction of the preseptal orbicularis muscle during blinking activates the lacrimal pump mechanism, which facilitates the passage of tears from the palpebral aperture through the canaliculi into the lacrimal sac.

In practice, the detailed anatomy of the medial canthal tendon is not evident at surgery. The fibrous part is clearly visible, especially the anterior component. The posterior components of the medial canthal tendon are the main anchor for the medial ends of the lids. It is important to

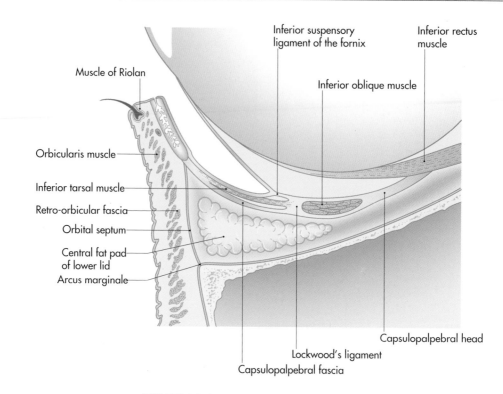

FIGURE 18-3   Section through the lower eyelid.

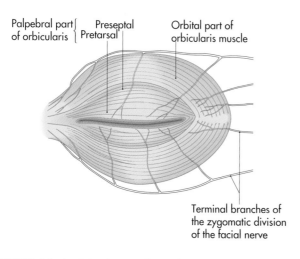

FIGURE 18-4   Orbicularis oculi muscle and terminal branches of the facial nerve.

reconstruct the posterior component by reattaching the canthal tissues to the posterior lacrimal crest if it has been divided by medial canthal trauma.

UPPER AND LOWER LID RETRACTORS

The levator palpebrae and Müller's muscles working together maintain the normal position of the upper lid when the eye is open (see Fig. 18-2). The levator muscle arises from the roof of the orbit immediately anterior to the optic foramen. It passes forward above the superior rectus muscle to end just posterior to the orbital septum as an aponeurosis. The aponeurosis passes forward into the lid and is inserted into the orbicularis muscle at the level of the upper lid skin crease and

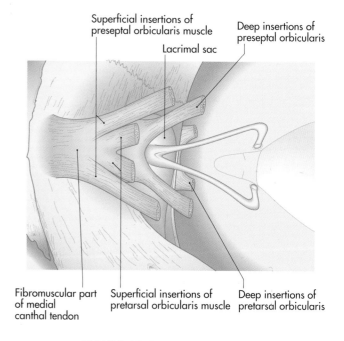

FIGURE 18-5   The medial canthus.

into the lower one third of the anterior surface of the tarsal plate. The orbital septum inserts into the anterior surface of the aponeurosis soon after its origin from the levator muscle. The aponeurosis expands medially and laterally to insert into the region of the medial and lateral canthal tendons as the medial and lateral horns of the aponeurosis (Fig. 18-6).

Müller's muscle lies deep to the levator aponeurosis, between it and the conjunctiva. It arises from the deep surface of the levator muscle at the point of origin of the levator

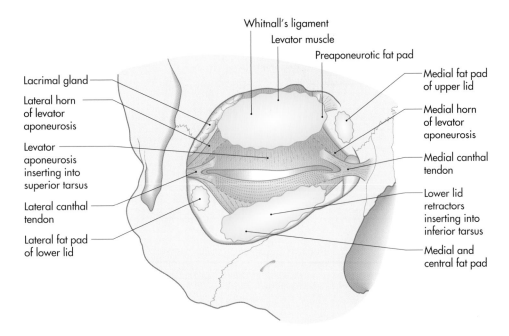

FIGURE 18-6   Extraconal fat pads and insertions of the upper and lower lid retractors.

aponeurosis. It descends to insert into the superior border of the tarsal plate. The preaponeurotic fat pad lies posterior to the septum and superior to the levator muscle. This fat gives the upper lid its fullness, and it is an important surgical landmark.

The structure of the lower lid is similar. The lower lid retractors are vestigial but important in maintaining lower lid position. The central fat pad in the lower lid is similar anatomically to the preaponeurotic fat in the upper lid.

THE LACRIMAL SYSTEM

Tears are produced by the lacrimal gland, which lies between the globe and the superior temporal quadrant of the anterior orbit, just within the orbital rim (Fig. 18-7). As it becomes the lateral horn, the lateral edge of the levator aponeurosis creates a deep cleft in the lacrimal gland, dividing it into two lobes, a larger orbital lobe above the lateral horn and a smaller palpebral lobe below the lateral horn. The palpebral lobe is just visible in the lateral end of the superior conjunctival fornix if the lateral end of the upper lid is lifted. Fine secretory ductules pass from the palpebral lobe to penetrate the conjunctiva of the superior fornix laterally.

Blinking spreads tears across the cornea, and they usually move in a medial direction toward the lacrimal puncta in the upper and lower lids approximately 6 mm from the medial canthus. The puncta normally lie within the tear film, and eversion of the puncta hinders the collection of tears. Canaliculi pass from the puncta medially to the lacrimal sac. The initial 2 mm of each canaliculus passes vertically into the lid before turning medially. At the medial canthal angle, the canaliculi pass posterior to the anterior limb of the medial canthal tendon and usually join to form a common canaliculus 3 to 5 mm lateral to the lacrimal sac. The common canaliculus opens into the sac 2 to 3 mm behind the anterior limb of the medial canthal tendon. The lacrimal sac is situated within the fossa and is bounded by the anterior and posterior lacrimal crests. The sac empties inferiorly into the nasolacrimal duct that passes down through the bony nasolacrimal canal, which is about 12 mm long, to open into the lateral wall of the nose under the inferior turbinate, which is approximately 15 mm from its tip and 30 to 35 mm from the external nares.

ASSESSMENT

HISTORY

An accurate account of the cause of the trauma allows a preliminary estimate of the depth and extent of the injury. Blunt trauma frequently leads to diffuse contusion with irregular wound edges, whereas sharp objects cause wounds with smoother edges that are often deeper.

EXAMINATION

Tissue swelling or a reduced level of consciousness may prevent a full assessment. A stepwise approach to the examination of the periocular soft tissues is helpful.

Gross Pathology

The examination assesses edema, ecchymosis, crepitus, and hematoma. It is important to differentiate an orbital hematoma from preseptal hemorrhage. An orbital hematoma has a sharply limited edge (Fig. 18-8). The globe may be proptosed and eye movements reduced. In contrast, preseptal hemorrhage (Fig. 18-9) may be extensive, causing considerable local swelling but without proptosis of the globe or limitation of eye movements. A subconjunctival hemorrhage arising from an orbital hemorrhage (Fig. 18-10) has no posterior edge but disappears posteriorly around the equator of

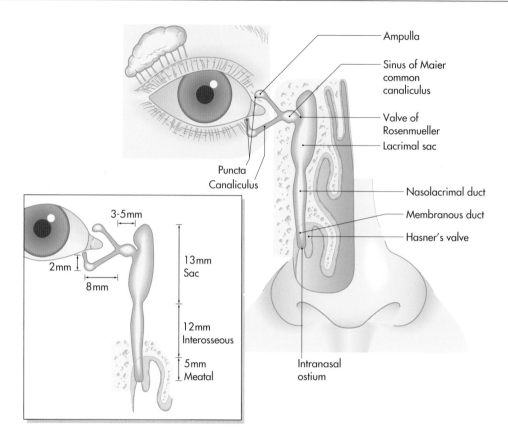

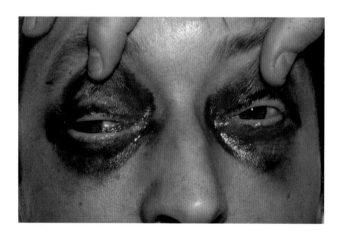

FIGURE 18-7   Lacrimal drainage system.

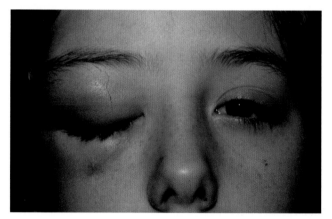

FIGURE 18-8   Bilateral orbital hematomas.

FIGURE 18-9   Periorbital hematoma.

the globe. Subconjunctival hemorrhages due to direct trauma (Fig. 18-11) may be localized with the whole edge visible, although the posterior edge is often well posterior and may not be visible.

Record entry wounds, estimate the depth of wounds, and document any possible loss of tissue. Record whether the lid margins are involved in any laceration. Notice lacerations involving the medial canthus, the presence of telecanthus, and aponeurosis or lacerations in the upper lid that may have damaged the levator muscle.

Exclude blunt or penetrating trauma to the eye, particularly penetrating injury of the globes if the eyelids are

lacerated (Fig. 18-12). Check the visual acuity. Examine the pupils for their size at rest and their reaction to light.

The swinging flashlight test (Fig. 18-13) is valuable for identifying optic nerve trauma. To perform this test, dim the lights in the examination room, and if the patient is able to cooperate, indicate a distant target to look at. With a bright light, illuminate first one eye for 2 seconds and then the other for 2 seconds. Swing the light backward and forward in this fashion, and observe the pupil reactions. In the absence of optic nerve trauma (or disease) or widespread retinal trauma, the pupils remain small in both eyes, apart from momentary dilatation during the transit of the light from one eye to the

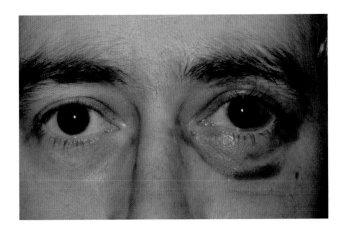

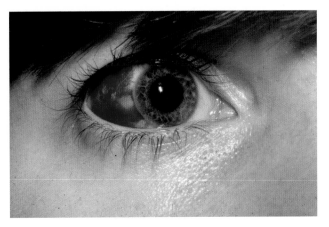

FIGURE 18-10   Subconjunctival and orbital hemorrhage and a fracture of the zygoma.

FIGURE 18-11   Spontaneous subconjunctival hemorrhage.

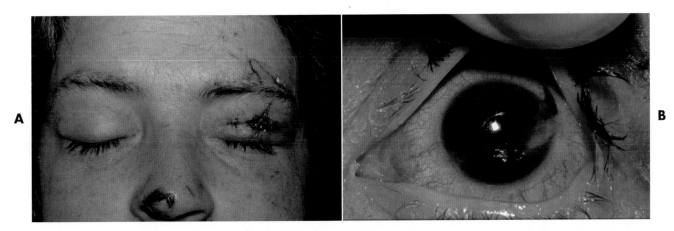

FIGURE 18-12   Upper lid laceration (**A**) with an underlying penetrating eye injury (**B**).

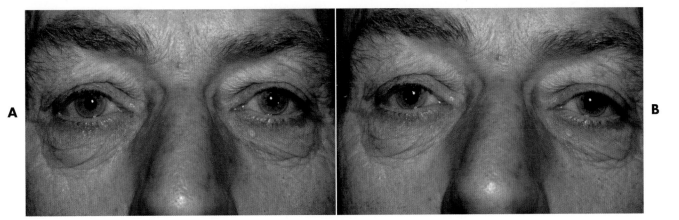

FIGURE 18-13   Right relative afferent pupil defect (RAPD). **A,** Light in front of normal left eye; both pupils constrict. **B,** Light in front of abnormal right eye; both pupils dilate.

other. In the presence of unilateral trauma to the optic nerve or with widespread retinal trauma, the pupil on that side dilates instead of remaining constricted as the light is moved from the normal eye to illuminate that eye. If the patient is mobile, a slit-lamp examination with measurement of the intraocular pressures is important at this stage.

Eyelid Position

The examination evaluates the vertical position of the eyelids and the shape and position of the canthi. Although the vertical distance between the center of the upper and lower lids varies, the palpebral aperture is commonly used as a measure of the position of the lids. It has the disadvantage that the lower lid is used as the reference point for the position of the upper lid. In trauma and often in lid disease, the lower lids are not level (Fig. 18-14), and a false impression of the lid positions is given. A better measure is the margin reflex distance (MRD). The patient is asked to look at a flashlight (Fig. 18-15). The distance from the corneal light reflex to each upper lid and each lower lid is recorded. This gives an accurate record of the position of all four lids. It remains reasonably accurate even if one eye is displaced by hemorrhage, swelling, or an underlying squint. The MRD is recorded in the following manner:

$$
\begin{array}{cc}
3 & 1 \\
\text{MRD} & \\
5 & 5
\end{array}
$$

In this case, the right upper lid is 3 mm and the left upper lid 1 mm above the corneal light reflexes. Both lower lids measure 5 mm from the light reflexes.

The distance between the medial canthi should be approximately one half of the distance between the centers of the pupils with the eyes in the primary position. Telecanthus and any displacement of the lateral canthi should be documented. Disruption of the canthal tendons frequently leads to rounding of the angle of the canthi.

Eyelid Movement

To estimate the function of the levator muscle of each upper lid, stabilize the brow with a thumb, and hold a ruler directly in front of the eyelids. Ask the patient to look up and down, and measure the excursion of the upper lid in millimeters (Fig. 18-16). The normal upper lid moves 12 to 15 mm from upgaze to downgaze. If there is no measurable levator function because of swelling or hemorrhage, look for any evidence of muscle action. The levator may cause only the slightest movement of the lid or dimpling of the upper lid skin. Bruising alone without transection of the levator can lead to a marked decrease in levator function (Fig. 18-17). Surgical emphysema causes a mechanical ptosis that resolves over several days as the emphysema disappears (Fig. 18-18).

Eye Position

Measure the position of each globe in all three planes. A ruler is used to measure the vertical and horizontal position

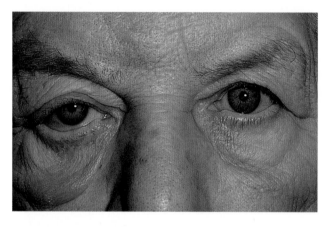

FIGURE 18-14 The value of margin reflex distance (MRD). The asymmetrical lower lids provide poor reference points for measuring the relative positions of the upper lids.

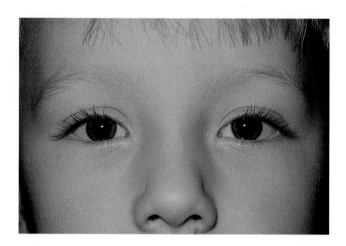

FIGURE 18-15 Corneal light reflexes as reference points for measuring the position of the lids.

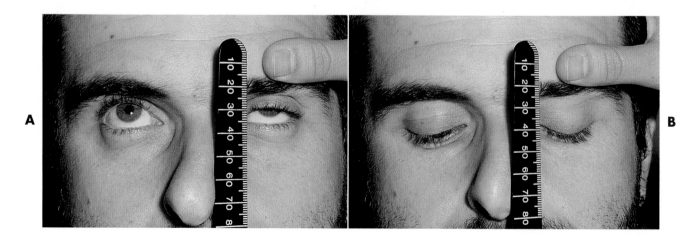

FIGURE 18-16 With the brow fixed, measure the upper lid excursion in upgaze (**A**) and downgaze (**B**).

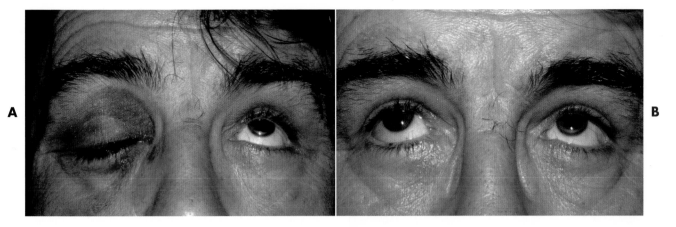

FIGURE 18-17 **A,** Orbital and periorbital hematoma with bruising of the levator muscle. **B,** Full recovery after 2 months.

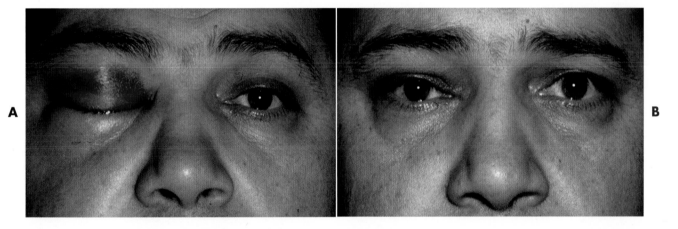

FIGURE 18-18 **A,** Extensive surgical emphysema. **B,** Full recovery after 1 week.

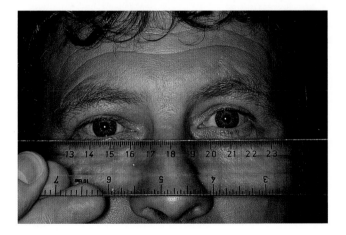

FIGURE 18-19 Measuring vertical and horizontal displacement of the eye.

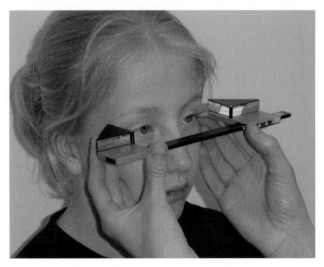

FIGURE 18-20 Measuring proptosis with a Hertel exophthalmometer.

of the globes (Fig. 18-19). The center of the pupil and the medial limbus are useful reference points. A Hertel exophthalmometer is used to measure anteroposterior position (Fig. 18-20). Because the Hertel exophthalmometer rests on the lateral orbital rims, it is not accurate in the presence of displacement of the zygoma. In this case, a rough estimate of anteroposterior displacement of the eyes can be made by looking over the patient's forehead from behind (Fig. 18-21). The relative positions of the eyes can be assessed easily.

Eye Movement

Check that the eyes move together in horizontal and vertical directions. Record the presence of diplopia and the direction of gaze in which the images are most widely separated.

Lacrimal System

Inspect the medial canthal areas and the nose. A fine probe (size 00) may be passed into the lacrimal puncta and along the canaliculi to assess continuity. Alternatively, saline stained with fluorescein may be gently syringed through the canaliculi (Fig. 18-22). As a result of nasoethmoidal fractures that have damaged the walls of the nasolacrimal duct or sac, the fluid may leak through a defect into the tissues and give the false impression of a patient's nasolacrimal system. Patency of the lacrimal system is confirmed if fluid can be seen beneath the inferior turbinate. Fluid stained with fluorescein fluoresces green with a cobalt blue light.

Special Studies

It is important to exclude retained foreign bodies within the periocular tissues or globes. They are easily visible with plain radiography or computed tomography.

A photographic record of the extent of the injuries at presentation is useful for medicolegal purposes and for planning future treatment. The photographic department may not be available, and it is helpful to have access to an alternative camera in the department. The most useful magnifications are for one eye (1:1), both eyes (1:3, 1:4), and full face (1:10). A suitable standard film (nondigital) camera should have a lens with an approximately 100-mm focal length, a suitable flash, and 100 ISO film speed. A digital camera should be capable of the same range of magnifications and a resolving power in excess of 3 megapixels.

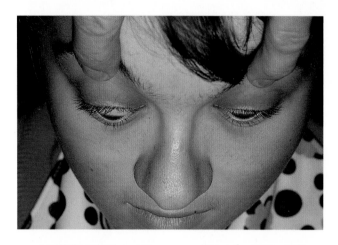

FIGURE 18-21 Estimating proptosis by viewing from above.

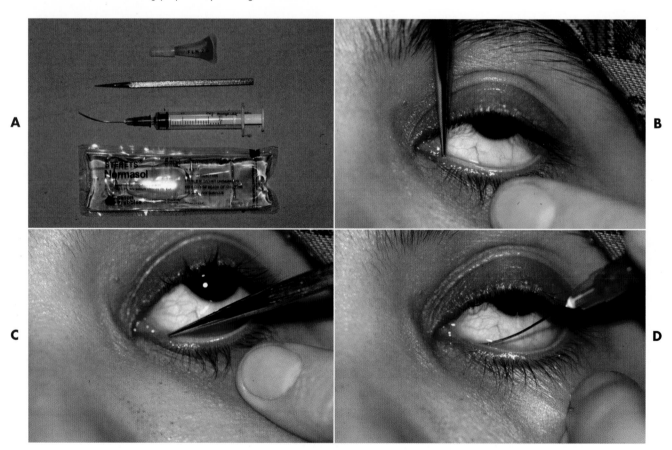

FIGURE 18-22 **A,** Equipment for syringing the lacrimal system. **B,** After local anesthetic drops have been instilled, gently dilate the punctum, first vertically and then horizontally (**C**) a short distance along the canaliculus. **D,** Pull the lid laterally to straighten the canaliculus, and pass the lacrimal cannula along the canaliculus until the medial wall of the lacrimal sac can be felt as a hard stop. Inject saline gently. In a patent system, the patient feels the fluid in the throat.

MANAGEMENT PRIORITIES AND ANESTHESIA

Complex periorbital trauma should be approached systematically. The order of priority in addressing injuries in the emergency examination room and the operating room is as follows:

- Life-threatening injuries
- Decision on timing of any fracture stabilization
- Sight-threatening injuries, including corneal exposure
- Lacrimal drainage system
- Medial canthal tendon
- Lid margins
- Lateral canthal tendon
- Levator muscle and aponeurosis
- Penetrating trauma of eyelids and periocular region

General anesthesia is appropriate for children and most adults. However, local anesthesia may be particularly helpful in repairing the levator muscle or aponeurosis. In an adult patient with limited local swelling for whom general anesthesia is not required for other reasons, local anesthesia allows the levator to be identified more easily by asking the patient to look up and down during surgery. The lid level is also set more accurately if the patient is awake. A 2% solution of lidocaine with 1 : 100,000 epinephrine provides a good level of anesthesia and hemostasis. If local anesthesia is indicated because the patient is unfit for general anesthesia but local infiltration is difficult because of wide local contusion, a regional block (e.g., frontal block, infratrochlear block, infraorbital block) avoids the injection of large volumes of local anesthetic.

ACUTE MANAGEMENT OF EYELID AND LACRIMAL TRAUMA

SIGHT-THREATENING TRAUMA

Management of fractures affecting the optic canal and of penetrating ocular injury is considered elsewhere. Exposure of the cornea due to an inability to close the lids requires immediate treatment. If the lids are intact, chloramphenicol ointment should be put into the eye and the lids taped closed. If there is loss of lid tissue, the cornea should be protected by creating a moist chamber; eye pads are best avoided, but a plastic cartella shield can be placed over the eye and the gaps sealed with tape. Alternatively, a thin sheet of plastic food wrap or cling film can be placed directly over the eye and lids and taped around the edges to the forehead and cheek to create a sealed, moist space. If there is enough lid tissue to close the lids, a temporary tarsorrhaphy suture of 4-0 Prolene placed over bolsters is an effective way of providing temporary protection of the cornea. If the loss of tissue does not allow a suture to be used, early reconstruction of the defect is required (see "Reconstruction of Full-Thickness Eyelid Defects").

LACRIMAL DRAINAGE SYSTEM

Lacerations of the inner canthus commonly damage the canaliculi. The lacrimal sac is damaged less often, but

nasoethmoidal fractures can cause complex medial canthal disruption. Bony nasolacrimal canal fractures can obstruct the nasolacrimal duct. The management of trauma to the lacrimal drainage system depends on the site of the trauma.

Canaliculus Laceration within 8 mm of the Punctum

There is controversy about the need to repair a single, divided canaliculus, especially the upper canaliculus. A single, intact canaliculus is probably adequate in most patients to avoid watering, and the risk of iatrogenic injury to the normal canaliculus, especially with a pigtail probe, is significant. However, most lacrimal surgeons advise careful repair of any lacerated canaliculus when possible. The surgery is best undertaken within 24 hours of the injury; late repairs are less successful. A microscope is necessary for accurate repair.

The cut canaliculus can normally be identified easily and is situated posteriorly within the lid close to the lid margin. If one canaliculus is damaged, a monocanalicular stent, such as a Mini-Monoka stent (FCI Ophthalmics, Novamed Ltd., Dundee, Scotland), is easy to place, and it has an advantage over the Veirs rod because it is not easily dislodged during the healing period. If both canaliculi are damaged, a single canalicular stent can be used in each canaliculus, but a better alternative is bicanalicular silicone tubes, such as Ritleng tubes (FCI Ophthalmics). They are convenient and can be left in situ for 6 months or longer. However, they can be difficult to insert. Most systems using silicone lacrimal intubation tubes have probes attached to the tubes that are passed through the canaliculus in each lid and down the nasolacrimal duct to emerge below the inferior turbinate. Retrieving the probes can be difficult. The Ritleng tubes have a different system of intubation that is easier to insert.

After the tubes are in place, the lower ends within the nose are knotted together or joined with a suture or a Watzke sleeve and may be sutured within the ala of the nose with a 6-0 monofilament suture. However, the suture collects mucus and may gradually detach from the tissues. Silicone tubes can erode like a cheese wire through the puncta and canaliculi if they are too tight or abrade the cornea if they are too loose.

Insertion of a Monocanalicular Stent

Technique The Mini-Monoka stent is a silicone tube that is self-retaining within the canaliculus (Fig. 18-23). Its shape does not allow it to migrate down the canaliculus into the lacrimal sac. To insert it, pass the tube through the canaliculus and across the laceration into the distal canaliculus and lacrimal sac (Fig. 18-24). Locate the angle of the stent within the proximal canaliculus, where it will be retained for 3 months or longer without attention.

An alternative material is thin silicone tubing. It must be passed through both canaliculi because it does not have the angled, self-retaining end for single canaliculus intubation.

Complications The stent may fall out and can usually be replaced under local anesthesia. After removal of the stent, it is common for the canaliculus to narrow or stenose and to become nonfunctional. Little can be done to overcome this, but a watering eye is not inevitable if the other canaliculus is patent.

Insertion of Bicanalicular Tubes

Technique There are several systems for bicanalicular intubation. The commonly used Crawford tubes are more difficult to insert than the Ritleng system. The principle is the same: Fine silicone tubing is passed through the upper and lower canaliculi, and the ends are passed down the nasolacrimal duct and retrieved from the exit of the duct beneath the inferior turbinate (Fig. 18-25).

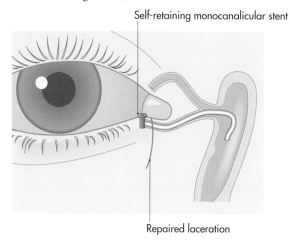

Self-retaining monocanalicular stent

Repaired laceration

FIGURE 18-23 Position of the monocanalicular stent in lower canaliculus repair.

Complications The loop of tubing may ride up within the nose and appear as a large loop within the palpebral aperture, abrading the cornea. It can be pulled down within the nose with the aid of a nasal endoscope and fine forceps. Alternatively, if it is too tight, the loop in the inner canthus may cheese-wire through the canaliculi. It should be loosened within the nose if this occurs.

Repair of the Canaliculus

Technique Pass a silicone stent through the lacrimal punctum and across the laceration in the canaliculus. Place two or three fine sutures, such as 8-0 to 10-0 Vicryl or nylon, in the submucosal tissue surrounding the canalicular lumen to approximate the edges. Repair the lid tissues in layers (Fig. 18-26).

Complications Stenosis of the repair is common despite adequate stenting. Providing the other canaliculus is patent, watering of the eye is not inevitable. The traditional alternative of a pigtail probe passed between the canaliculi through the common canaliculus is considered unsuitable because of the risk of iatrogenic damage, and it is best avoided.

Canaliculus Laceration More Than 8 mm from the Punctum or in the Common Canaliculus

It is usually impossible to repair the distal canaliculus or common canaliculus directly. If the cut end of the canaliculus

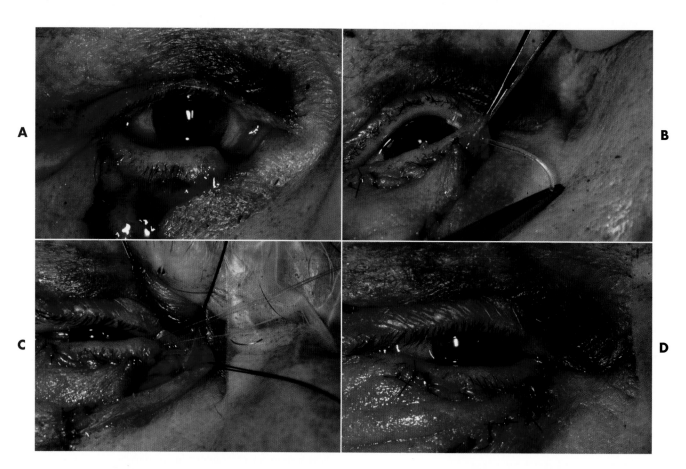

FIGURE 18-24 **A** to **D,** Insertion of a Mini-Monoka tube through the punctum, across the laceration, and into the medial cut end of the canaliculus before the lacerations in the canaliculus and the lid are sutured.

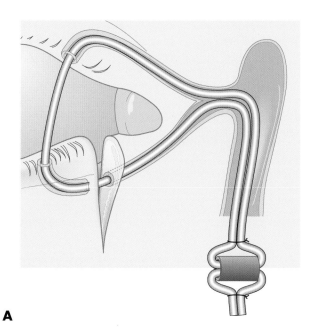

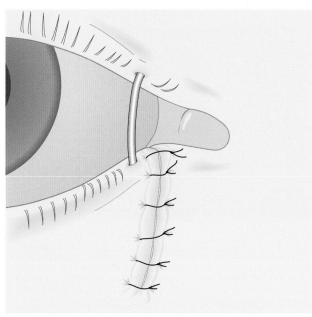

A

B

FIGURE 18-25 **A,** Bicanalicular intubation for single or double canalicular lacerations. **B,** The wound is sutured in layers.

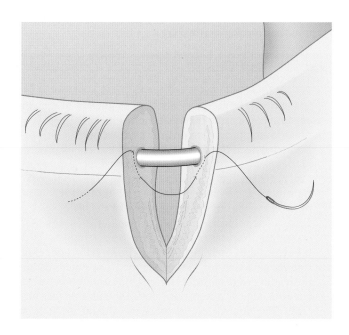

FIGURE 18-26   Repair of a cut canaliculus.

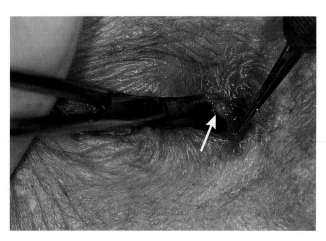

FIGURE 18-27   The canaliculus is identified medially.

is visible, the options are to marsupialize the canaliculus into the conjunctival sac or to place a silicone stent. Lacerations occurring more medially, through the common canaliculus, cannot be repaired, and a Lester Jones tube may be required if watering is significant.

Marsupialization of the Canaliculus
Technique
1. Identify the lower canaliculus in the medial cut edge (Fig. 18-27).
2. Cut the canaliculus longitudinally for about 5 mm (Fig. 18-28).

3. Separate the cut edges of the opened canaliculus (Fig. 18-29), and place two 7-0 absorbable sutures between the corners of the cut canaliculus and the adjacent conjunctiva. This helps to hold the canaliculus open (see Fig. 18-40).

Complications The marsupialized canaliculus may not drain tears. Silicone tubes introduced through the canaliculi and down the nasolacrimal duct as described previously give the best chance of restoring patency. The medial canthal tendon is often damaged at the same time. If the posterior part of the tendon has been disrupted, it must be repaired.

Lacrimal Sac

If the lacrimal sac has been damaged but the canaliculi and common canaliculus are intact, a dacryocystorhinostomy with the insertion of silicone tubes is usually required. It may

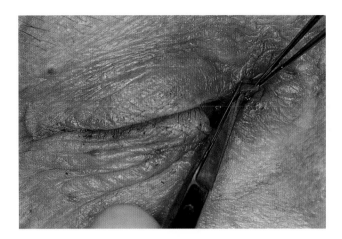

FIGURE 18-28   Cut along the posterior wall to open the canaliculus for 5 mm.

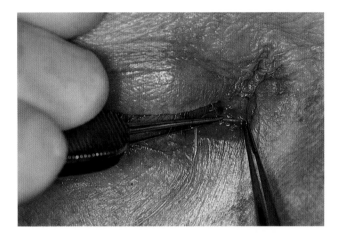

FIGURE 18-29   The corners of the marsupialized canaliculus can be secured open with fine absorbable sutures.

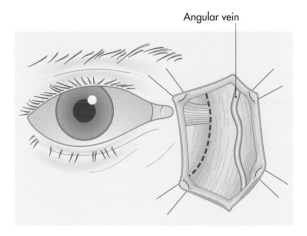

FIGURE 18-30   Position of the incision into the periosteum of the anterior lacrimal crest. The medial canthal tendon is seen laterally and the angular vein medially.

be appropriate to undertake this surgery at the time of the primary repair. However, if there is complex disruption in the region of the medial canthus, it is preferable to defer definitive lacrimal surgery for several months until the tissues have healed. If the canaliculi and sac are severely damaged, it is unlikely that a patent lacrimal system can be achieved with any surgery. The tissues should be allowed to heal, and a Lester Jones bypass tube should be inserted at a later date if watering is a problem.

Dacryocystorhinostomy

Technique The principle of dacryocystorhinostomy is that the bone between the lacrimal sac fossa and the middle meatus of the nose (see Fig. 18-31, circled area) is removed. The mucosa of the lacrimal sac and the mucosa of the nose are incised, and anterior and posterior flaps, respectively, are anastomosed to create a direct connection between the lacrimal sac and the middle meatus.

1. Pack the nose and especially the region of the middle meatus with a nasal decongestant, such as a 4% solution of cocaine.

2. Make a straight incision about 15 mm long and 8 mm medial to the inner canthus. One third should be superior to the medial canthal tendon and two thirds inferior. Deepen it through the orbicularis muscle to identify the anterior limb of the medial canthal tendon as it inserts into the anterior lacrimal crest.

3. Using a periosteal elevator, such as Rollet's rougine, cut through or disinsert the medial canthal tendon and the adjacent periosteum along the anterior lacrimal crest. Reflect it laterally to expose the lacrimal sac fossa as far as the posterior lacrimal crest. The angular vein may be encountered during this dissection (Fig. 18-30).

4. Using a small, right-angled elevator, create a gap in the suture between the lacrimal bone and the frontal process of the maxilla in the floor of the lacrimal sac fossa. Fracture out a small piece of bone, and then reintroduce the right-angled elevator to push the underlying nasal mucosa away from the deep surface of the bone.

5. Using bone nibblers, enlarge the hole in the lacrimal sac fossa until the floor of the fossa has been removed. After the removal of each small piece of bone, reintroduce the right-angled elevator to separate the nasal mucosa from the leading edge of the enlarging rhinostomy. Extend the anterior edge of the ostium onto the anterior lacrimal crest. The final defect in the bone should be at least 15 mm in diameter (Fig. 18-31).

6. Pass a lacrimal probe through the lower canaliculus into the lacrimal sac to tent up its medial wall (Fig. 18-32). Make a vertical incision in the medial wall of the lacrimal sac to expose the tip of the lacrimal probe. Enlarge this vertically to the fundus of the sac superiorly and the nasolacrimal duct inferiorly.

7. Make a vertical cut in the nasal mucosa about one third of the distance from the posterior edge of the bony defect. From the ends of this incision, make transverse incisions to improve the mobility of the flaps (Fig. 18-33).

8. Suture the posterior flap of the lacrimal sac to the posterior flap of nasal mucosa with three or four interrupted, 6-0, absorbable sutures (Fig. 18-34). Introduce tubes at this point if necessary. To do this, pass the metal introducers along the superior and inferior canaliculi into the

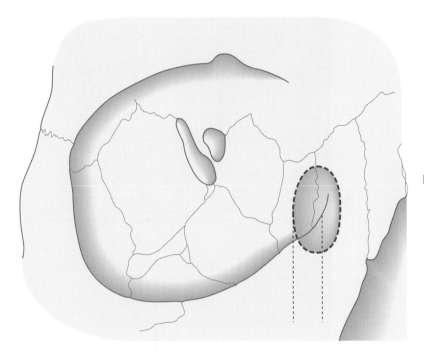

FIGURE 18-31   Area of bone removal.

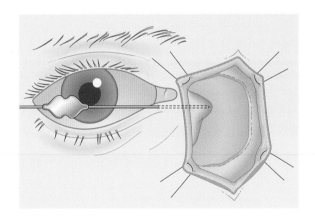

FIGURE 18-32   Probe tenting the medial sac wall before opening it.

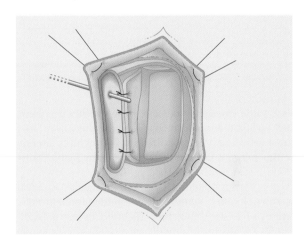

FIGURE 18-34   Posterior flaps of the lacrimal sac and nose sutured.

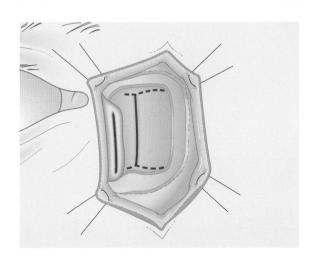

FIGURE 18-33   Vertical cut into the lacrimal sac laterally and H-shaped cut into the nasal mucosa medially.

lacrimal sac. Cut off the metal introducers. Tie a knot 5 to 10 mm from the point where the tubes enter the lacrimal sac or pass the tubes through a fine sleeve (e.g., Watzke's sleeve) located at the same point. Pass fine, curved artery forceps up the nose into the dacryocystorhinostomy site, and draw the ends of the tubes down the nose. Another knot or sleeve can be used to secure the lower ends of the tubes. Cut the tubes to leave their ends just within the nose.

9. Close the anterior flaps with three or four 6-0 absorbable sutures. Close the muscle and skin in two layers.

10. If tubes have been used, they should be removed at 3 months.

Complications Dacryocystorhinostomy is successful in about 85% of patients, although more than this achieve patency of the lacrimal drainage system but with residual

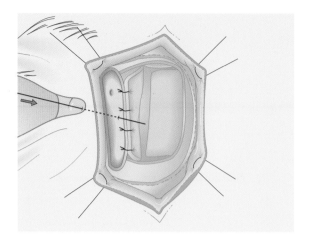

FIGURE 18-35   Guidewire from the inner canthus to the ostium.

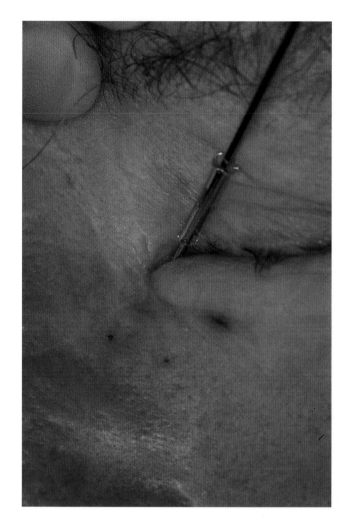

FIGURE 18-36   Lester Jones tube over a guidewire at the inner canthus.

watering of the eye. Repeat surgery can be difficult, and the results are often disappointing.

Insertion of Lester Jones Bypass Tube

Technique A Lester Jones tube is passed from the medial canthus behind the medial end of the lower lid through the soft tissues and the bony rhinostomy of a dacryocystorhinostomy into the middle meatus of the nose.

1. Follow steps 1 to 8 as for a standard dacryocystorhinostomy.
2. Pass a fine, pointed, guidewire from the junction between the caruncle and the medial end of the lower lid in a downward and posterior direction through the lateral wall of the lacrimal sac and through the bony ostium into the middle meatus of the nose (Fig. 18-35).
3. Pass a 2-mm trephine over the guidewire to create a narrow channel. Remove the trephine, and estimate the length of Lester Jones tube required to reach from the inner canthus to the middle meatus. Pass a Lester Jones tube of the correct length along the guidewire (Fig. 18-36). Check its position; the medial end should be 2 to 3 mm from the nasal septum (Fig. 18-37), and the lateral end should lie close to the lower fornix behind the medial end of the lower lid (Fig. 18-38; see also Fig. 18-41) so that tears can enter it easily. A 6-0 Prolene suture may be wound around the neck of the tube and through the adjacent lid to anchor it for the first week.
4. Close the lacrimal sac and the wound as for a dacryocystorhinostomy.
5. The tube should be irrigated twice daily by sucking saline drops through it.

Complications The tubes may become blocked or fall out. Regular cleaning by inhaling saline drops through the tube maintains patency in most patients. If the tube becomes blocked and cannot be cleared with syringing or if it falls out, it must be replaced, usually under general anesthesia.

Nasolacrimal Duct

If the nasolacrimal duct has been damaged by a fracture through the nasolacrimal canal but the lacrimal sac and

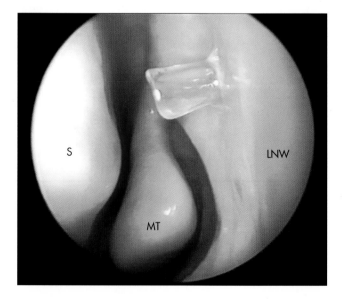

FIGURE 18-37   Good tube position. LNW, lateral nasal wall; MT, middle turbinate; S, septum.

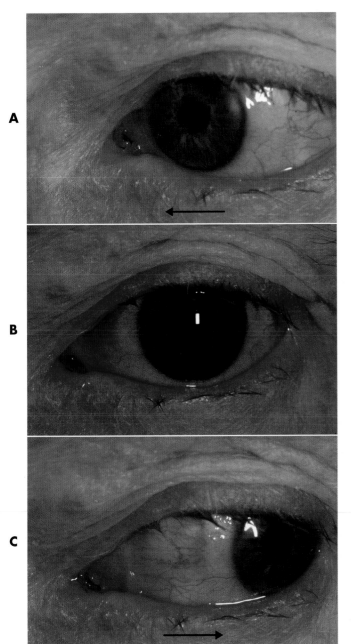

FIGURE 18-38 **A,** Proximal end of the tube. There is no tube-eye touch (**B**) or displacement (**C**) with eye movement.

canaliculi are intact, a dacryocystorhinostomy is appropriate. This is usually deferred until the tissues have healed.

Extensive Trauma with No Reconstruction Possible

Extensive damage to the lacrimal drainage system cannot be repaired with any significant chance of patency. The tissues are allowed to heal, and if watering becomes a problem, a Lester Jones bypass tube is inserted at a later date.

MEDIAL CANTHAL TENDON

Disinsertion or disruption of the medial canthal tendon may occur with nasoethmoidal and Le Fort II fractures or with local penetrating injuries. The anterior limb of the medial

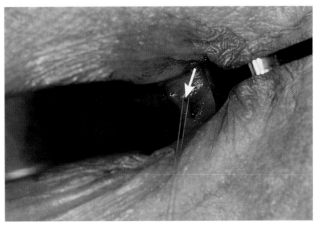

FIGURE 18-39 Suture placed in the periosteum of the posterior lacrimal crest and right inner canthus.

canthal tendon can be ignored. The posterior limb, however, should be identified and reattached to the posterior lacrimal crest. The periosteum over the posterior lacrimal crest is slightly thickened and offers a good anchor point for a double-armed, 5-0, nonabsorbable suture, which then passes forward to the severed tissues at the medial canthal angle. This repair is performed after any canalicular repair, and care must be taken to avoid further damage or distortion of the canaliculi.

If it is not possible to achieve adequate fixation to the posterior lacrimal crest, alternative anchorage in the region of the posterior crest must be provided. This is achieved with local wiring or a transnasal wire anchored to the medial canthal tendon of the opposite side. A miniplate or microplate attached to the anterior lacrimal crest and angled back toward the posterior lacrimal crest can provide adequate posterior fixation. If there have been fractures in the region of the lacrimal fossa with loss of fixation points, a transnasal wire may be preferred to attempted direct refixation of the medial canthal tendon to the periosteum. A transnasal wire is also required for bilateral medial canthal tendon disruption, especially if there is disruption of the normal bone anchor points. The wire must be passed through the floor of the lacrimal sac fossa as far posteriorly as possible. Care must be taken preoperatively to establish the position of the cribriform plate to avoid injury at surgery.

Suture Reattachment of the Medial Canthal Tendon to the Posterior Lacrimal Crest
Technique

1. Using blunt dissection with scissors directed posteriorly and medially lateral to the lacrimal sac, expose the posterior lacrimal crest at or just above the level of the medial canthus.
2. Place a malleable retractor gently against the globe to improve the exposure, and insert both needles of a double-armed, 5-0, nonabsorbable suture, directed posteriorly through the periosteum of the posterior lacrimal crest (Fig. 18-39).
3. Pass one needle of the 5-0 suture through the edge of the tarsal plate in the lateral wound edge close to the lid

margin, adjusting its position as necessary so that when the suture is tightened, the lid is drawn medially and posteriorly to lie against the eye. Pass the second needle through the tarsal plate 2 to 3 mm inferior to the first (Fig. 18-40). Tie the 5-0 suture with a single throw to draw the lateral wound edge medially.

4. Close the conjunctiva to ensure that the 5-0 fixation suture is well covered. Tighten the 5-0 fixation suture further, and tie it. Close the skin with 6-0 sutures.

Complications

The suture holding the medial canthus attached to the posterior lacrimal crest may become detached, resulting in migration of the canthus. It will need to be replaced.

Transnasal Wire Insertion to Fix the Canthi

Guidelines for inserting a transnasal wire were provided earlier (see "Insertion of a Monocanalicular Stent"). A traumatic telecanthus treated with this technique is shown in Figure 18-41.

LID MARGINS

Lid margin lacerations are common. Accurate repair, avoiding distortion or a notch, ensures comfort, corneal protection, and good function with regard to the spread of tears. If the lid margin cannot be approximated because of limited local loss of tissue, it may be necessary to release tissue in the region of the lateral canthus to allow direct closure. If tissue loss is more extensive, larger flaps and reconstruction of both eyelid lamellae may be required (see "Reconstruction of Full-Thickness Eyelid Defects").

Direct Closure
Technique

The technique is identical for upper and lower lids (Fig. 18-42).

1. Place a 6-0 or 7-0 absorbable suture through the cut edges of the tarsal plate close to the lid margin, but avoid including the conjunctiva (Fig. 18-43). Tie the knot on the anterior surface of the tarsal plate.

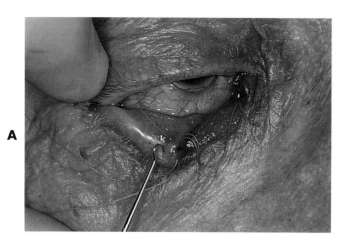
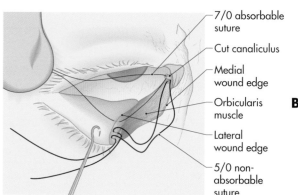

FIGURE 18-40 **A** and **B,** Posterior lacrimal crest suture passed through the cut medial edge of the tarsal plate. Notice the 7-0 absorbable suture anchoring the marsupialized canaliculus.

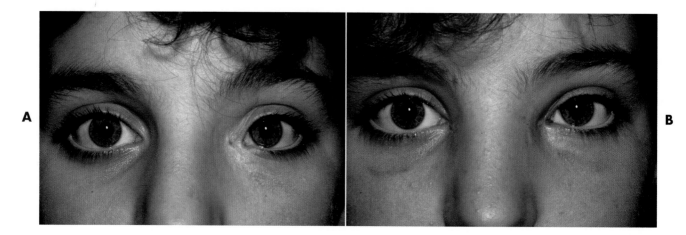

FIGURE 18-41 **A** and **B,** Traumatic telecanthus treated with a transnasal wire. A Lester Jones tube has been inserted at the same time.

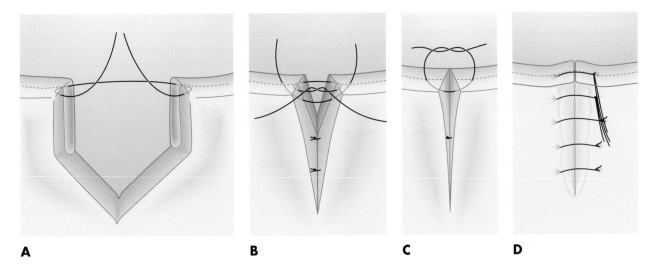

A   B   C   D

FIGURE 18-42 **A** to **D,** Principles of direct lid margin closure.

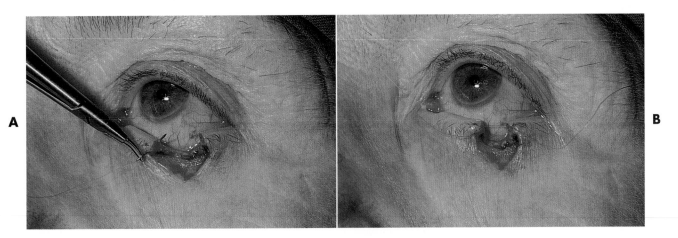

A   B

FIGURE 18-43 **A** and **B,** The first suture is placed through the tarsal plate at the posterior lid margin on either side of the wound.

2. Place two more absorbable sutures through the edges of the tarsal plate in the same way to close the posterior lamella of the lid. Place a 6-0 suture through the gray line (squamous-mucosal junction) at the lid margin. Pass it across the wound and out through the gray line on the opposite side (Fig. 18-44). Tie the suture to support closure of the margin. Leave the suture ends long.

3. Close the orbicularis muscle within the wound with two or three 6-0 or 7-0 absorbable sutures. Close the skin with 6-0 or 7-0 sutures. Pass the long end of the lid margin suture beneath the skin closure sutures to prevent it damaging the cornea (Fig. 18-45). The lid margin and skin sutures can be removed after 1 week (Fig. 18-46).

Complications

A small notch may appear at the lid margin despite every effort to prevent it. It is best left alone. If an obvious notch or distortion of the lid margin is present (Fig. 18-47), allow the lid to heal for several months, excise the notch, and resuture the lid. Occasionally, the lid repair breaks down. Remove the sutures, and allow the lid to heal without further attempt to suture it. The result is usually surprisingly good, but if there

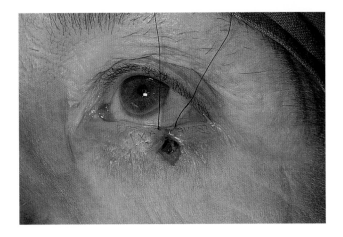

FIGURE 18-44 The tarsal plate is closed with the lid margin suture in situ through the gray line.

is local distortion, this area of the lid margin should be excised and the lid resutured.

LATERAL CANTHAL TENDON

Disruption of the lateral canthal tendon leads to a rounded lateral canthal angle and displacement of the canthus

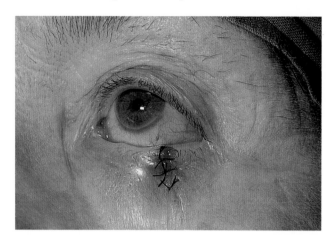

FIGURE 18-45   The eyelid wound is closed.

medially and forward. The lateral canthal tendon should be reattached to Whitnall's tubercle. This is sometimes possible with a simple suture through the periosteum overlying Whitnall's tubercle. If this is not possible, a periosteal flap fashioned from the periosteum overlying the lateral orbital rim and based medially within the orbit provides adequate anchorage. Alternatively, a wire passed through the lateral canthal tissues and through holes drilled in the lateral orbital rim provides secure fixation.

Periosteal Flap
Technique
A periosteal flap is used to support the upper or lower lid, or both, laterally when the lateral canthal tendon is inadequate (Fig. 18-48). It is useful in lid reconstruction when lateral fixation of the posterior lamella is required or when the tendon is lax or absent and the lateral canthus has moved medially.

1. Make a horizontal incision from the lateral canthus to expose the lateral orbital rim. At the level of the proposed new lateral canthal tendon, mark two horizontal lines on the periosteum, 8 to 10 mm apart, extending from the medial border of the lateral orbital rim to the temporalis

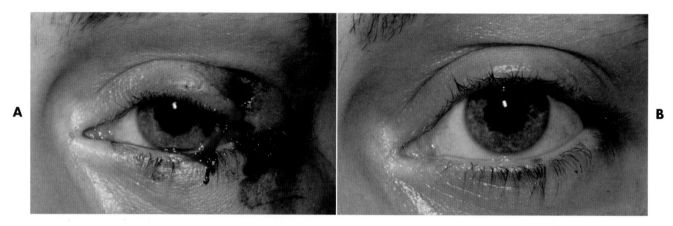

FIGURE 18-46   **A,** Upper lid lacerations with potential tattooing. **B,** Repair after careful removal of debris from the skin and wounds.

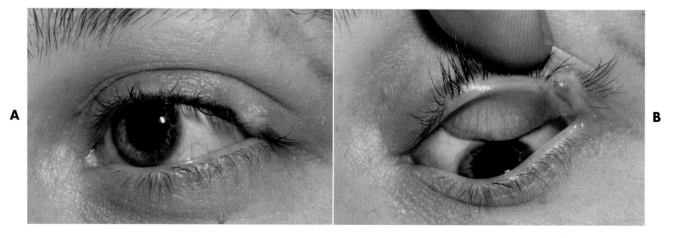

FIGURE 18-47   **A** and **B,** Upper lid margin distortion and tattooing due to inaccurate closure and incomplete removal of debris during the original operation.

fascia laterally. If support for both lids is required, cut a broader strip of periosteum to allow it to be split later. Mark the lateral extent of the flap with a vertical line (Fig. 18-49).

2. Incise the edges of the flap, leaving the periosteum intact medially, and lift the flap of periosteum with a periosteal elevator. Leave the base of the flap attached to the periosteum within the lateral rim of the orbit (Fig. 18-50).

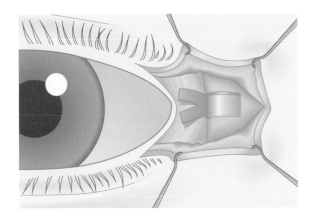

FIGURE 18-48 Principle of a periosteal flap.

3. To attach the canthal tissues or the reconstructed posterior lamella to the periosteal flap, pass one or two double-armed, 5-0 nonabsorbable sutures through the lid tissues, and then pass both needles through the periosteal flap.
4. Tie the sutures to support the lid tissues. There should be minimal horizontal lid laxity. If a broader strip of periosteum has been cut for the support of both lids, split it into an upper and a lower limb, and attach them to the posterior lamellae of the upper and lower lids in the same way.
5. Close the incision in two layers (Fig. 18-51).

Complications

The canthus can drift medially over several months. Resuture to the periosteal flap usually corrects this. Granuloma may form within the wound. Excise it, and resuture the wound, taking care to cover the periosteal flap and sutures with orbicularis muscle during closure.

LEVATOR MUSCLE AND APONEUROSIS

Laceration of the levator apparatus manifests with ptosis. However, severe bruising and local swelling or surgical emphysema may also present with poor levator function and ptosis (see Figs. 18-17 and 18-18). Wounds in the upper lid must be explored to their depths and any damage to the

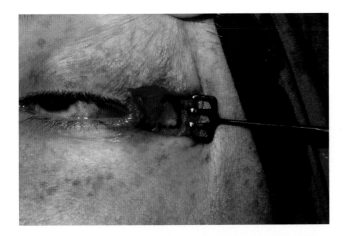

FIGURE 18-49 Periosteum of the lateral orbital rim is exposed.

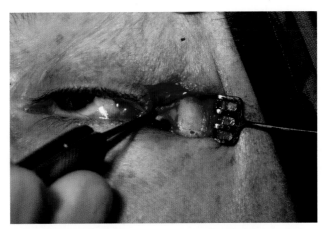

FIGURE 18-50 Cut for a periosteal flap.

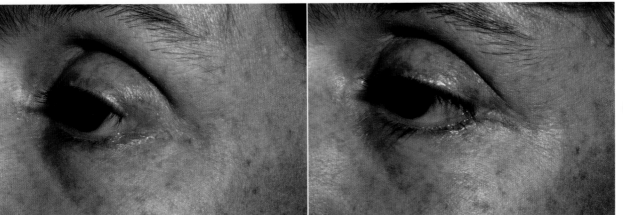

A

B

FIGURE 18-51 **A,** Rounded canthus due to detachment of the lateral canthal tendon. **B,** Repaired with a periosteal flap.

levator identified. Fat visible within the wound in the upper lid is usually preaponeurotic fat, and it indicates that the septum has been cut. Brow fat that extends down from the brow on the anterior surface of the septum may also be visible. Preaponeurotic fat is lighter and more mobile than brow fat.

A tear in the levator aponeurosis or muscle should be repaired with 6-0 absorbable sutures. The septum should not be repaired. The levator can be repaired through the main wound in the upper lid if it is large. If it is not or if there is doubt about the adequacy of exposure, it is preferable to close the primary wound and make a second, formal incision within the upper lid skin crease to expose the levator and aponeurosis and repair it formally (Fig. 18-52).

If no damage to the levator is identified, the cause of the ptosis may be local bruising. Levator function and ptosis will improve as the bruising subsides.

PENETRATING EYELID AND PERIOCULAR TRAUMA WITHOUT TISSUE LOSS

Early repair of skin and orbicularis wounds within the first 8 hours is preferable. The repair may be delayed for 24 to 48 hours if circumstances demand, although it becomes progressively more difficult due to edema. It may also be more difficult to decontaminate the wounds adequately. The wound must be cleaned and irrigated and all visible foreign bodies removed. The skin must be cleaned meticulously of all embedded foreign material, with firm scrubbing with a brush if necessary to avoid tattooing (Figs. 18-53 and 18-54). Dead tissue is excised, but tissue removal should be kept to a minimum.

The wounds should be explored carefully to determine the depth and nature of any damage. Fat visible within a wound may indicate laceration of the septum. This does not present a problem. The fat should be pushed back into position and the septum left open.

Close the wounds with absorbable sutures to the orbicularis muscle and 6-0 monofilament sutures to the skin. Closure of lid margin lacerations is described previously.

PENETRATING EYELID AND PERIOCULAR TRAUMA WITH TISSUE LOSS

Tissue loss should be assessed. Distortion of the tissues due to edema or hemorrhage may give the impression of actual loss of tissue. However, loss often is not confirmed during surgery (Fig. 18-55).

The principles of reconstruction of defects in the lids and periocular tissues are the same as for reconstruction after tumor removal. A reconstructed eyelid must have an anterior covering layer (skin) and a posterior lining layer (mucosa). One of these layers must have a blood supply. There must also be adequate support for the lids medially and laterally. In planning the method of reconstruction, excess tension or distortion should be avoided. The skin graft color should be matched accurately with careful choice of the donor site. Definitive repair in the hours after an injury should be

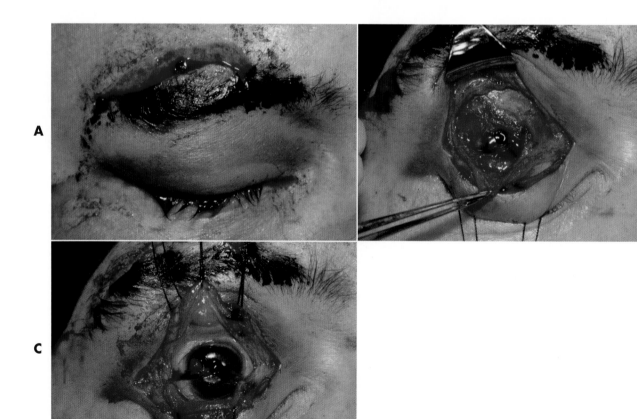

FIGURE 18-52 **A** to **C,** An oblique laceration above the brow transects the levator aponeurosis (exposed through a second incision at the upper lid skin crease) and penetrates the cornea.

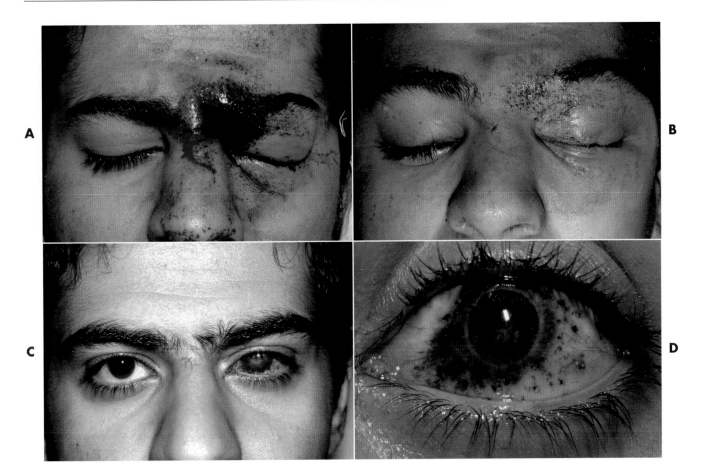

FIGURE 18-53 **A,** Embedded debris after a close-range gunshot with a blank. **B,** Careful scrubbing removed as much foreign material as possible. **C,** The appearance 1 year later shows that tattooing of the cornea and conjunctiva could not be avoided. **D,** Notice the corneal graft to restore clarity to the central cornea.

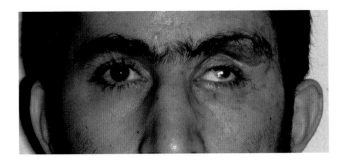

FIGURE 18-54 Marked tattooing was caused by failure to remove debris during the original operation.

considered only if adequate cleansing of the wounds has been possible and the viability of the tissues is certain.

Reconstruction of Partial-Thickness Eyelid and Periocular Defects

Partial-thickness defects of the lids or periocular region may be closed directly or may require reconstruction of the anterior covering layer with a skin graft or a skin flap. Direct closure of wounds must be performed in a direction that does not cause distortion of the lid margin, such as ectropion or local retraction. In the lower lid, this usually means a closure wound placed at right angles to the lid margin (Fig. 18-56).

Closure with a skin flap or graft is indicated if the defect is too large for direct closure. Many different configurations of skin flap may be used in the periocular region. Local sliding or transposed flaps are common (Fig. 18-57).

Skin grafts may be partial or full thickness. Partial-thickness (split-thickness) grafts are usually reserved for large defects or those in the upper lid above the skin crease when skin from the opposite upper lid is not available. Full-thickness grafts are best taken from the upper eyelid; they give an excellent color match and good mobility. The graft is taken from the skin superior to the skin crease (Fig. 18-58). Alternative donor sites include the postauricular region and the supraclavicular fossa.

Reconstruction of Full-Thickness Eyelid Defects

Full-thickness defects of up to one fourth of the lid length may be closed directly as described previously. Defects up to about one third of the lid require release of the upper or lower limb of the lateral canthal tendon—a lateral cantholysis—before they can be closed directly.

Full-thickness eyelid defects larger than about one third of the lid length (or up to one half in the elderly) require the reconstruction of the posterior lining layer and the anterior

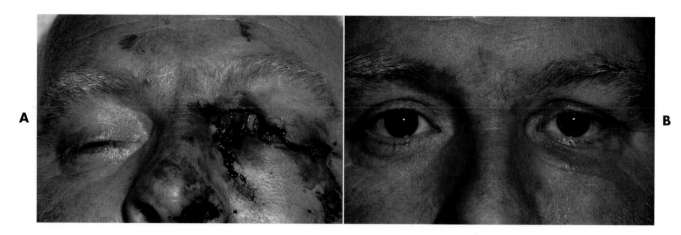

FIGURE 18-55 **A,** Apparent loss of tissue, which was not confirmed during the operation. **B,** The final result after a simple repair with careful attention to restoration of the anatomy.

FIGURE 18-56 **A** and **B,** Direction of closure of small lower lid wounds to avoid vertical traction.

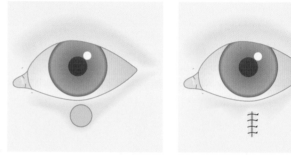

covering layer. When both layers have to be reconstructed, at least one of them must have a blood supply. This means combining an anterior skin flap with a posterior graft or an anterior skin graft with a posterior flap. Alternatively, both may be flaps.

Lateral Cantholysis

Lateral cantholysis is a technique used almost exclusively in the lower lid. In the upper lid, great care is needed when releasing the septum to avoid damage to the lacrimal gland. Up to one third of the lid length can be reconstructed with the extra tissue made available by a cantholysis.

Technique

1. Make a horizontal cut from the lateral canthus to the orbital rim. Take care not to cut obliquely downward or upward through either limb of the lateral canthal tendon (Figs. 18-59 and 18-60).
2. Pull the lid medially to put the lateral canthal tendon on stretch. It can be felt as a tight band just posterior to the orbicularis muscle and between the muscle and the conjunctiva. Expose this limb of the tendon by spreading scissors either side of it (Fig. 18-61).
3. Cut this limb of the tendon laterally (Fig. 18-62).
4. Close the lid defect in the standard way. Close the lateral wound in layers with 6-0 sutures (Fig. 18-63).

If the defect cannot be closed without undue tension, the orbital septum between the lateral tarsal fragment and the

inferior orbital rim must be cut to allow the lateral tissues to move further medially. To do this, grasp the medial cut end of the tendon, and pull it laterally and slightly upward to put the septum on stretch. Gently introduce scissors between the orbicularis muscle and the conjunctiva along the superior or inferior orbital rim, and cut the septum as far medially as necessary to allow closure of the lid. With each cut into the septum, the lid can be felt to "give" and become more mobile.

Complications

Slight notching of the lid margin at the outer canthus may occur if there has been excessive dissection to expose the lateral canthal tendon. It is best left alone, but if extensive, local resuturing can improve the profile of the lid margin.

Posterior Graft with an Anterior Flap

If the posterior layer is reconstructed with a graft, the anterior layer must be reconstructed with a skin flap. Grafts for the posterior (lining) layer can come from oral mucosa, tarsal plate, or hard palate. Tarsal plate grafts usually are taken from the upper lid. Other grafts, such as donor sclera or ear cartilage, are less satisfactory because they do not have a mucosal lining, and their use typically is restricted to the lower lid.

Tarsal Plate Grafts

Technique A full-thickness tarsal plate from the upper lid is an excellent posterior lamellar graft with a mucosal lining when only a small area is required. It may be taken from the ipsilateral or contralateral side.

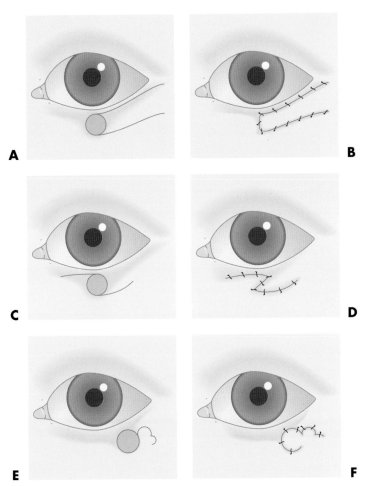

FIGURE 18-57   Principles of sliding (**A** and **B**), O-Z (**C** and **D**), and bilobed (**E** and **F**) flaps for reconstruction of lower lid defects.

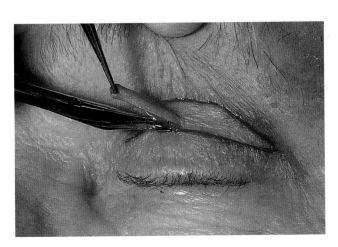

FIGURE 18-58   Taking a full-thickness skin graft from the upper lid.

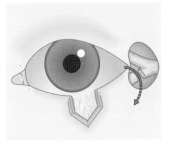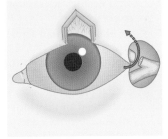

FIGURE 18-59   **A** and **B**, Principle of lateral cantholysis.

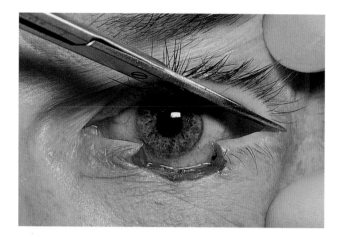

FIGURE 18-60   Horizontal cut at the lateral canthus.

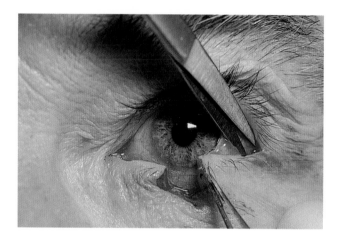

FIGURE 18-61   Exposing the lower limb of the lateral canthal tendon. Notice the traction on the lid to put the tendon on stretch.

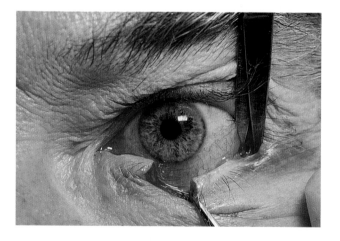

FIGURE 18-62   Cutting the lower limb of the lateral canthal tendon.

1. Evert the upper lid over a Desmarres retractor, and insert a stay suture close to the lid margin. Measure on the tarsal plate 4 mm from the lid margin at several points, and mark off along this line the length of graft required (Fig. 18-64).

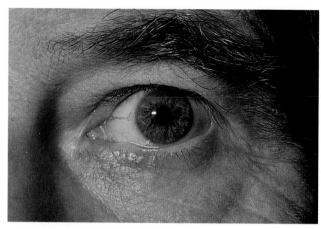

FIGURE 18-63   The result 2 months after routine closure of the central defect with a cantholysis.

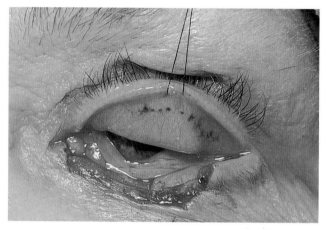

FIGURE 18-64   Incision in the tarsal plate is marked 4 mm from the lid margin.

2. Incise the full thickness of the tarsal plate along the mark. Make vertical cuts from each end of the first incision to the superior border of the tarsal plate and extend them superiorly for 2 mm into the conjunctiva. Undermine and excise the graft with about 2 mm of conjunctiva attached (Fig. 18-65). Allow the donor site to granulate.

Complications   If the incision in the tarsal plate was made less than 4 mm from the lid margin, buckling of the lid may occur during healing. Once healed, the distorted area should be excised and resutured. Occasionally, lid retraction occurs with healing. Release of the upper lid retractors is necessary to correct this.

Many different flaps are used for the anterior (covering) layer. The small Tenzel flap and the larger McGregor flap are useful for defects up to about half the lid. A nasojugal flap medially or a transposed cheek flap laterally are commonly used for larger defects. These flaps are best for defects that do not extend far inferiorly into the cheek. Larger defects involving cheek skin often require a larger flap, such as the Mustarde cheek rotation flap.

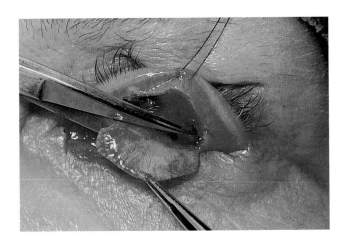

FIGURE 18-65   Tarsal plate graft is excised with 2 mm of conjunctiva superiorly.

Tenzel Flap

Technique   The Tenzel flap technique allows direct closure of upper or lower lid defects up to about one half of the lid length (Fig. 18-66).

1. Mark the semicircular flap approximately 22 mm in the vertical and 18 mm in the horizontal direction. Begin the mark as a lateral continuation of the line of the lid to be reconstructed. Continue more steeply upward (for reconstruction of the lower lid) or downward (for reconstruction of the upper lid), curving the line to achieve the correct dimensions. Finish level with the canthus and no further lateral than the end of the eyebrow (Fig. 18-67).
2. Make an incision along the mark, and undermine the flap in the plane just deep to orbicularis muscle. Reflect the flap to expose the lateral canthus. Cut the appropriate limb of the lateral canthal tendon (Fig. 18-68).
3. For closure of a lower lid defect, free the septum. Close the eyelid defect in the usual way. Pull the lid gently laterally

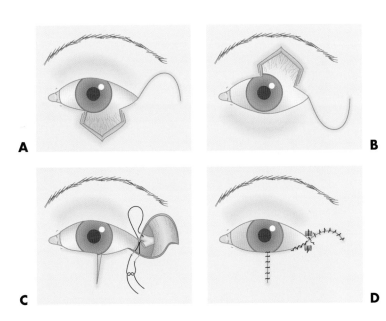

A

B

C

D

FIGURE 18-66   **A** to **D,** Principle of a Tenzel semicircular flap.

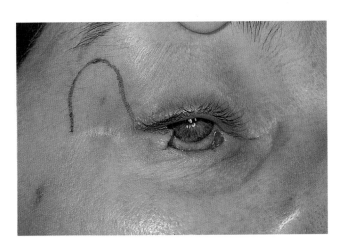

FIGURE 18-67   The incision is marked for a Tenzel flap.

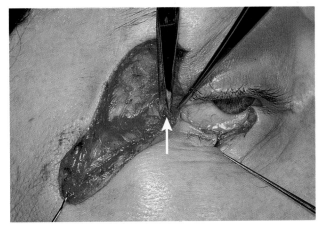

FIGURE 18-68   The flap is reflected, and the lower limb of the lateral canthal tendon is cut.

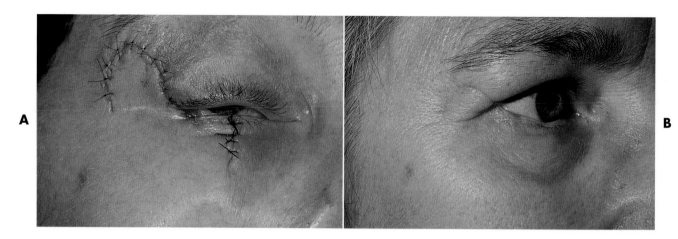

FIGURE 18-69   **A,** End of the operation. **B,** Six months later.

to remove any horizontal lid laxity. Support the flap with a 4-0 nonabsorbable suture to the deep tissues. Where the flap edge crosses the lateral canthus, fix it to the opposite limb of the lateral canthal tendon with a 4-0, long-acting, absorbable suture to create a new canthus.
4. Close the edge of the flap in two layers with 6-0 catgut and a 6-0 nonabsorbable suture to the skin. Remove the surface sutures after 5 days (Fig. 18-69).

Complications Shallow notching of the lid margin at the outer canthus may occur. If marked, resuture the affected lid to correct the notch.

McGregor Flap

Technique The McGregor flap uses a Z-plasty, which helps to avoid a dog ear in the superior edge of the wound and partly hides the scar by breaking the line.

1. Mark an incision from the lateral canthus toward the ear with a gentle, convex curve upward (for the lower lid) or downward (for the upper lid). Mark a Z with the stem along the main incision, placing the more lateral limb of the Z on the same side of the main incision as the lid to be reconstructed (Fig. 18-70).
2. Reflect the flaps, keeping deep to the orbicularis muscle and medial to the orbital rim but superficial to orbicularis, within the subcutaneous fat and lateral to the orbital rim. Undermine beyond the flaps. Cut the appropriate limb of the lateral canthal tendon, and mobilize the lateral part of the lid.
3. Close the defect in the lid. Transpose the flaps in the usual way, and close the skin (Figs. 18-71 and 18-72).

Complications Shallow notching of the lid margin at the outer canthus may occur. If marked, resuture the affected lid to correct the notch.

Nasojugal Flap

Technique The nasojugal flap is used for medial lower lid defects (Fig. 18-73).

1. Reconstruct the posterior lamella with a suitable graft. The flap should be almost vertical in the nasojugal area, with

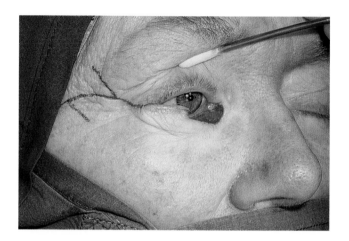

FIGURE 18-70   The McGregor cheek flap is marked.

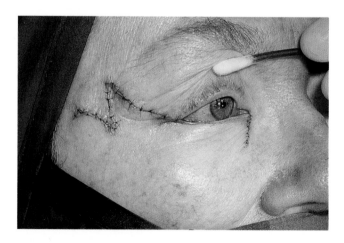

FIGURE 18-71   The defect is closed. Flaps are transposed, and the skin is closed.

its base just inferior to the medial canthus. Care is needed in the design of the flap to ensure that it is long enough to fill the defect (Fig. 18-74).
2. Raise the flap, staying superficial to the facial muscles and within the fat layer.

3. Close the cheek wound first. Transpose the flap into the defect, and trim it to fit. Close the skin with interrupted 6-0 sutures (Fig. 18-75).
4. Close the lid margin with a continuous 6-0 suture, which unites the skin and the mucosa of the posterior lamellar reconstruction.

Complications Nasojugal skin is thicker than eyelid skin, and the reconstruction may be rather bulky. Later debulking is possible if necessary (Fig. 18-76). Necrosis of the tip of the

flap is unusual. If it occurs, wait to see how much of the flap survives, and then reconstruct the defect that remains if necessary.

Transposed Cheek Flap
Technique Large lower lid defects that extend to the lateral canthus can be reconstructed with a transposed flap based near the outer canthus and extending down into the cheek (Fig. 18-77). Take care to design the flap with sufficient length and width to fill the defect. It must be lined, usually with oral mucosa. To close the secondary defect, undermine the edges of the wound.

Complications Cheek skin is thicker than eyelid skin, and the reconstruction may be rather bulky. Later debulking is possible if necessary. Necrosis of the tip of the flap is unusual. If it occurs, wait to see how much of the flap survives, and then reconstruct the defect that remains if necessary.

Posterior Flap with an Anterior Graft
If the posterior layer is reconstructed with a flap of tarsus and conjunctiva with its blood supply intact (i.e., Hughes procedure), a skin graft typically is used to fill the anterior defect, although a flap may be used.

Hughes Procedure
Technique The Hughes procedure is a two-stage technique to reconstruct full-thickness defects in the lower eyelid (Fig. 18-78). A broad strip of upper tarsal plate on a pedicle of

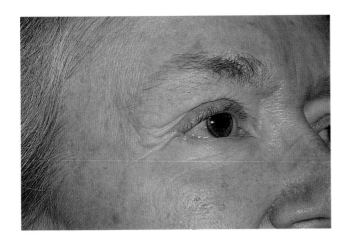

FIGURE 18-72   Four months after a McGregor cheek flap.

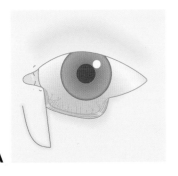

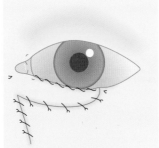

FIGURE 18-73   **A** and **B,** Principle of a nasojugal flap.

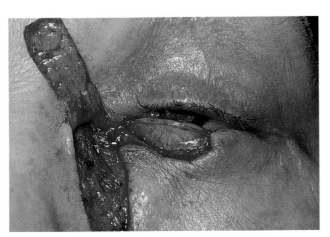

FIGURE 18-74   For a nasojugal flap, the posterior lamella is reconstructed with a tarsal plate graft.

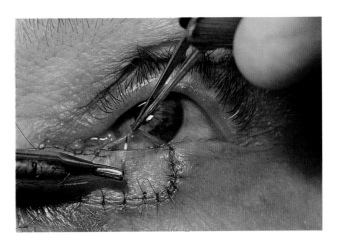

FIGURE 18-75   Nasojugal flap at the end of the operation.

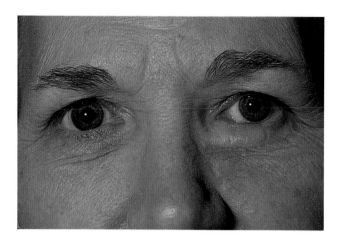

FIGURE 18-76 Nasojugal flap 6 months after surgery.

conjunctiva is used to reconstruct the posterior lamella of the lid. It may be covered with a skin graft or flap. The pedicle is divided after a few weeks. The use of the Hughes flap is restricted to relatively shallow lower lid defects that do not extend much beyond the inferior border of the tarsal plate.

1. Insert a stay suture of 4-0 silk through the tarsal plate close to the lid margin, and evert the lid over a Desmarres retractor. Mark a line 4 mm from and parallel to the lid margin. Mark on this line the horizontal length of tarsal plate required. From these marks, draw vertical lines to the superior tarsal border to delineate the flap. Incise the tarsal plate through its full thickness along the marks. Raise the flap of tarsus by dissection in the pretarsal space as far as the superior border of the tarsal plate (Fig. 18-79).

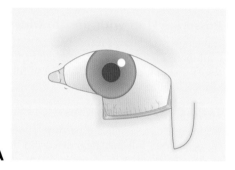

A

B

FIGURE 18-77 **A** and **B,** Principle of a transposed cheek flap.

FIGURE 18-78 **A,** Principle of a Hughes reconstruction of a central lower lid defect. **B,** Posterior lamella is reconstructed with a flap of tarsoconjunctiva from the upper lid. **C,** Anterior lamella is reconstructed with a full-thickness skin graft.

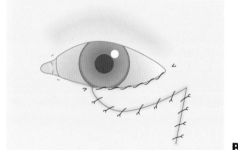

A

B

C

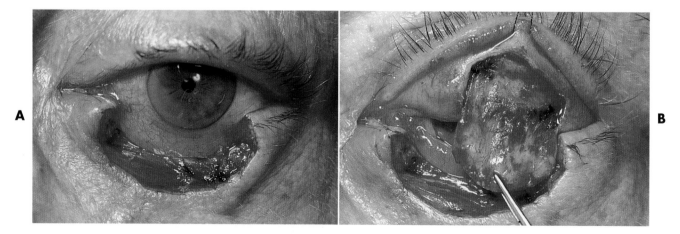

A

B

FIGURE 18-79 **A,** Large lower lid defect. **B,** Tarsoconjunctival flap is cut for reconstruction of the posterior lamella.

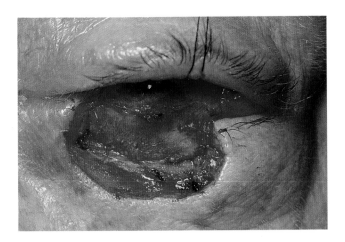

FIGURE 18-80   The tarsoconjunctival flap is sutured into the defect.

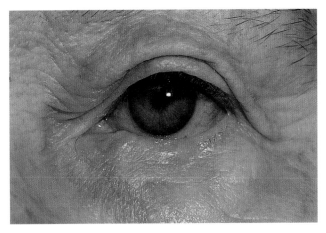

FIGURE 18-82   Three months after division of the bridge of conjunctiva.

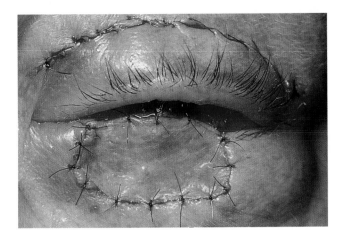

FIGURE 18-81   Skin graft from an upper lid.

2. Suture the flap into the defect with 6-0 catgut sutures. Begin by suturing the ends of the superior border of the upper tarsal plate to the lower lid margins at the edges of the defect. Suture the remaining edges of the tarsus to the conjunctiva (Fig. 18-80).
3. Reconstruct the anterior lamella with a full-thickness skin graft or a local flap of skin and muscle (Fig. 18-81).
4. After about 3 weeks, divide the pedicle 2 to 3 mm superior to the tarsal plate and the skin graft (Fig. 18-82). Suture the free edge of the conjunctiva to the skin with a continuous, 6-0, monofilament suture. Remove this suture at 5 days. The upper lid retractors are advanced by the procedure and must be recessed to prevent upper lid retraction. To do this, dissect between the conjunctiva and the retractors until the lid is at a satisfactory level. Allow the proximal conjunctiva to retract. A downward traction suture on the upper lid may be needed for 24 hours.

Complications Retraction of the upper lid may follow the second stage if the upper lid tissues have not been freed sufficiently. Dissect further between the conjunctiva and the upper lid retractors until the lid is at the correct level.

Closure with Flaps for Both Lamellae

Both anterior and posterior lamellae may be reconstructed with flaps (i.e., a tarso-conjunctival flap posteriorly and a local skin flap anteriorly.) Composite flaps (e.g., Cutler-Beard bridge flap), which include all layers of the lower lid inferior to the tarsal plate, are useful for larger central upper lid defects.

Cutler-Beard Bridge Flap

Technique The Cutler-Beard bridge flap is a two-stage technique for reconstruction of large, full-thickness defects in the upper lid (Fig. 18-83).

1. Draw a horizontal line 5 mm inferior and parallel to the lash line of the lower lid. On this line, mark the width of flap required to fill the defect in the upper lid, and draw two vertical lines as far as the inferior orbital rim (Fig. 18-84).
2. Incise along the lines. Perforate the full thickness of the lid at the corners of the flap, and with a pair of scissors inserted between the stab incisions, complete the horizontal full-thickness incision. Extend this inferiorly along the vertical lines to the inferior conjunctival fornix to create an inverted U-shaped flap. Pull the flap up posterior to the lower lid margin (Fig. 18-85).
3. Suture it into the upper lid defect in three layers, including conjunctiva to conjunctiva and orbicularis muscle of the lower lid to the levator aponeurosis and orbicularis muscle of the upper lid, with interrupted, 6-0, absorbable sutures. Then close skin to skin with interrupted, 6-0, nonabsorbable sutures. Remove the sutures after 5 days (Fig. 18-86).
4. After 6 weeks, estimate whether the flap has stretched enough to reduce the tension. If it is still tight, leave it in place for another 3 weeks. If it has stretched and feels less tight, divide the bridge to restore the upper lid margin. To do this, pass a squint hook posterior to the flap, and carefully incise the layers of the flap, making the initial incision convex downward to allow for retraction. Leave an excess of conjunctiva (Fig. 18-87).
5. Suture the conjunctiva to skin over the new lid margin with a continuous, 6-0, monofilament suture. Remove this on day 5. Replace the pedicle of the bridge into the lower

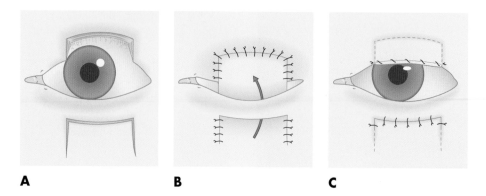

FIGURE 18-83   **A,** Principle of a Cutler-Beard reconstruction of an upper lid defect. **B,** A full-thickness flap from the lower lid is sutured into the defect. **C,** The bridge is divided after 6 weeks.

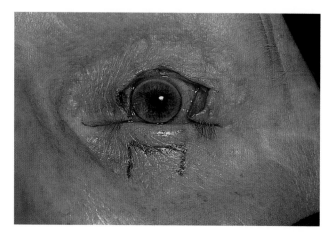

FIGURE 18-84   Defect in the upper lid. The Cutler-Beard bridge flap is marked.

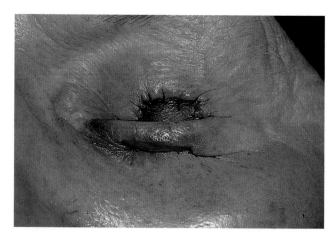

FIGURE 18-86   The flap is sutured into the defect in layers.

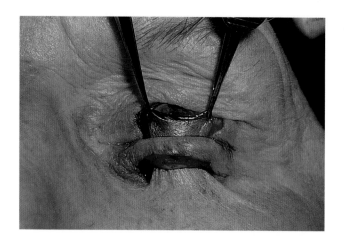

FIGURE 18-85   The flap is cut and placed into the defect.

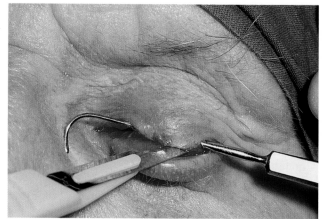

FIGURE 18-87   The bridge is divided at 6 weeks.

lid defect, and repair it in layers to avoid a fistula through the lid (Fig. 18-88).

Complications   The reconstructed upper lid margin is relatively unstable and may develop entropion. If this occurs, a graft of donor sclera or ear cartilage may need to be inserted between the lamellae of the reconstructed lid. The margin may be irregular at the edges of the bridge flap. Allow the lid

to heal, and excise the notches if necessary. Skin hairs may cause irritation, and they can be treated with cryotherapy.

Reconstruction of Full-Thickness Periocular Defects

Small defects can be closed directly or with small, local skin flaps. It is important to avoid vertical tension in the upper or lower lids. It is better to allow a scar to cross the relaxed skin

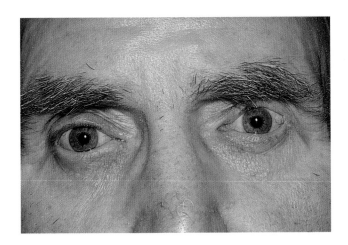

FIGURE 18-88 Six months after left upper lid reconstruction with a Cutler-Beard flap.

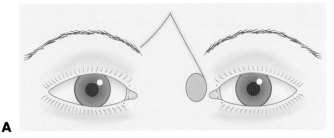

A

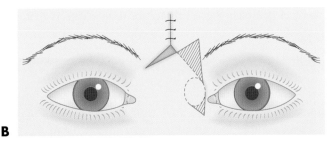

B

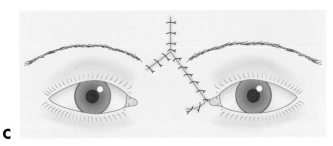

C

FIGURE 18-89 **A** to **C,** Principle of a glabellar flap. A V-shaped flap in the glabella is converted to a Y to allow the flap to slide into a medial canthal defect.

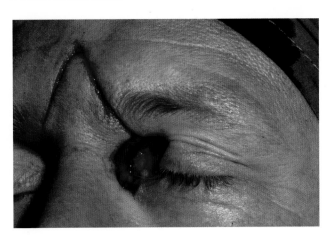

FIGURE 18-90 The glabellar flap is marked.

tension lines than to close with vertical tension. Larger defects require a local flap or skin graft.

Medial Canthus Reconstruction

A medial canthal defect that cannot easily be closed directly is usually reconstructed with a skin flap, such as a glabellar flap, if it is mainly above the medial canthal tendon and especially if it is relatively deep, or with a skin graft below the medial canthal tendon. A deep defect below the canthal tendon also may be closed with a local flap. Vertical tension spanning the tissues above and below the canthus and within 8 mm medial to the canthus has a tendency to form a web. It is then preferable to use a small skin graft.

In reconstruction of the medial canthus, it is important to perform lacrimal drainage system repair first, reconstruct the medial canthal tendon, and then remedy the overlying soft tissue defect.

Technique A full-thickness skin graft may be used for superficial defects at the inner canthus (Fig. 18-89). If the defect is deep, a glabellar flap is preferred, and it does not require a posterior lamellar reconstruction. An inverted V is created in the glabellar region and converted to a Y to allow the flap to be transferred to the inner canthus. If the defect is small, the flap is used as a sliding flap, and the excess is trimmed off. If the defect is large, the flap may be used as a transposed flap with little trimming necessary. If the defect extends into the upper or lower eyelid, supplementary procedures may be needed to reconstruct the residual lid defect.

1. Mark an inverted V, centered in the midline of the forehead. One limb of the V is drawn to the lateral border of the canthal defect; the other is drawn to the medial end of the opposite brow (Fig. 18-90). Undermine the flap, dissecting in the layer of subcutaneous fat. Extend the dissection beyond the boundaries of the flap to allow it to be placed without tension into the canthal defect.
2. After the position is satisfactory, insert one or two 4-0 nonabsorbable sutures between the deep surface of the flap and the tissues of the canthus to anchor the flap. Undermine either side of the forehead defect to allow closure

with minimal tension. Close the forehead in two layers to just above the brows.
3. Trim the excess tissue from the glabellar flap. Suture the flap into the canthal defect with 6-0 absorbable sutures to the subcutaneous tissues and 6-0 nonabsorbable sutures to the skin. Complete the closure of the forehead (Fig. 18-91). Remove all skin sutures after 1 week (Fig. 18-92).

Complications A fold or dog ear commonly occurs on the bridge of the nose, especially if the defect is large. Leave it for

6 weeks, and then trim it if necessary. Poor application of the flap to the hollow at the inner canthus and the appearance of telecanthus can be avoided by careful placement and suturing of the flap at operation.

Larger Upper or Lower Lid Defects Extending into the Medial Canthus

Occasionally, an upper or lower lid defect extends into the inner canthal area, and a more complex combination of reconstructive techniques is needed. In the canthus, a glabellar flap is usually a good choice for deeper defects that are mainly superior to the medial canthal tendon; other local flaps are used for deep defects below the medial canthal tendon. Skin grafts are appropriate for shallow defects. The residual defect in the lid is closed with one of the techniques described in "Reconstruction of Full-Thickness Defects of the Eyelids" (Figs. 18-93 and 18-94).

Medial and Lateral Support

A reconstructed lid must have adequate medial and lateral support to prevent the lid drooping. This is especially important in the lower lid. A defect that includes the medial or

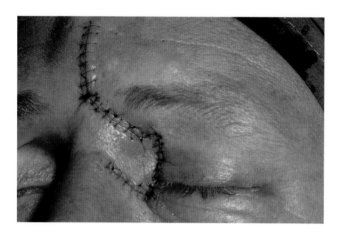

FIGURE 18-91   The glabellar flap is sutured into the defect.

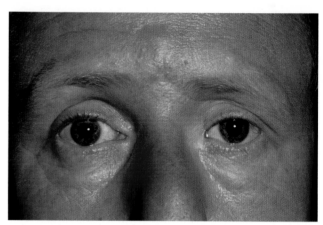

FIGURE 18-92   One year after repair of a large medial canthal defect with a glabellar flap.

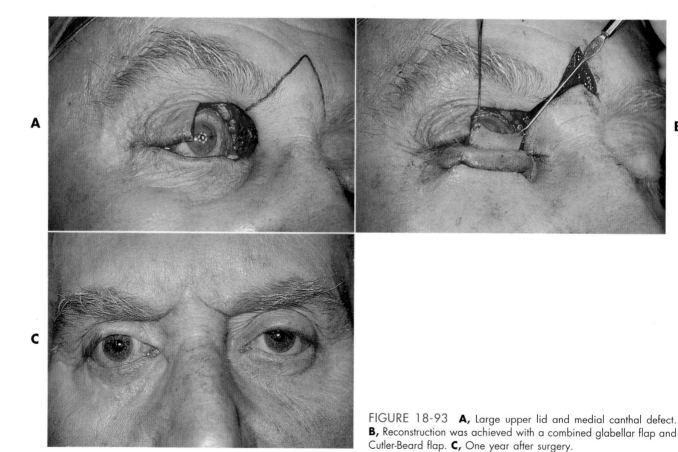

FIGURE 18-93   **A,** Large upper lid and medial canthal defect. **B,** Reconstruction was achieved with a combined glabellar flap and Cutler-Beard flap. **C,** One year after surgery.

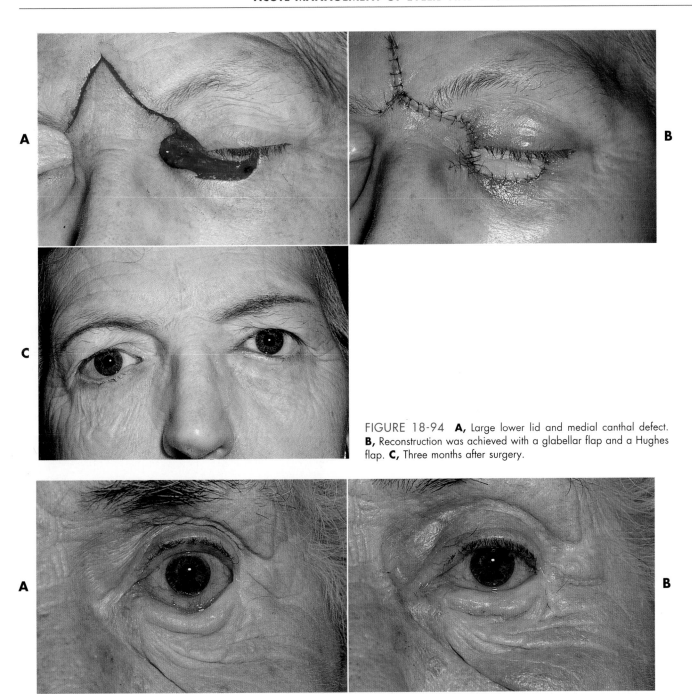

FIGURE 18-94 **A,** Large lower lid and medial canthal defect. **B,** Reconstruction was achieved with a glabellar flap and a Hughes flap. **C,** Three months after surgery.

FIGURE 18-95 **A,** Lax lower lid after multiple reconstructions. **B,** Support is provided with a sling of autogenous fascia lata.

lateral canthal tendon must be reconstructed in such a way that the support is restored. Medially, the tissues of the reconstructed lid should be attached to the posterior lacrimal crest; this ensures that the lid is pulled posteriorly and medially and that it is well applied to the globe.

Laterally, there should be an attachment in the region of Whitnall's tubercle directly to the periosteum or with a periosteal flap or with a wire. If the lid droops despite all attempts to support it, a sling of autogenous fascia lata may be needed. This is attached to the medial canthal tendon, and after traversing the lid close to the lid margin, it is passed through holes in the lateral orbital rim (Fig. 18-95).

Lateral Canthus

After correcting any disruption of the lateral canthal tendon, defects of the lateral canthus are closed directly, if small, or with a local flap.

Cheek or Temple

Assess facial nerve function. Close small defects directly, avoiding vertical tension, especially in the lower lid. Local flaps are used to close larger defects. The O-Z plasty is particularly useful in these areas. Alternatively, a full-thickness skin graft may be needed.

LATE REPAIR OF EYELID AND LACRIMAL TRAUMA

If the initial repair of an eyelid injury is unsatisfactory but the eye is adequately protected, revision can be deferred for 6 months to allow the scars to mature. In planning a revision, ophthalmic plastic surgeons usually collaborate with maxillofacial colleagues in case revision of the fractures is required at the same time. It is easier to make appropriate adjustments if the initial repair is anatomically correct. If it is not, the tissues should be dissected to reconstruct the injury and display the anatomy. The lid is then reconstructed and the appropriate adjustment made.

LIDS

Common late deformities of the lids include cicatricial ectropion or entropion, lid retraction, distortion or notching of the lid margins, and ptosis.

Cicatricial ectropion is caused by a shortage of skin in the lower lid. If it is caused by a contracted linear scar, it is corrected with a Z-plasty. If there is a more diffuse shortage of scarred skin, a full-thickness skin graft is used.

Cicatricial entropion is caused by shortening of the posterior lining lamella of the lid. Choice of the appropriate operation for the degree of scarring is important, and the surgery can be difficult. In the lower lid, entropion is corrected by fracturing the tarsal plate and inserting everting sutures or by inserting a graft of oral mucosa to release the contraction. In the upper lid, the operation used depends on the degree of scarring and amount of associated upper lid retraction. The principle is that the anterior lamella of the lid is moved up in relation to the posterior lamella, everting the lid margin. In more severe scarring, it may be necessary to divide the tarsal plate to evert the scarred lid margin.

Retraction of the upper or lower lid is usually caused by shortening of the upper or lower lid retractors, possibly combined with scarring in the anterior or posterior lamella. The retracted lid is explored and the retractors released. The operation can be difficult. If it is necessary to release the anterior or posterior lamella at the same time to achieve a satisfactory lid position, the defect is reconstructed as outlined for cicatricial ectropion and entropion.

Notching and distortion of the lid margin are usually caused by inaccurate initial closure (see Fig. 18-47). It is usually easiest to excise the initial repair scar and close the lid margin accurately.

Ptosis may result from trauma to the levator apparatus or adhesion within the lid between the upper lid retractors and adjacent structures, such as the orbital rim periosteum. Brain injury can result in bilateral ptosis with reduced levator function (Fig. 18-96). Ptosis is assessed as previously described by measuring the degree of ptosis (i.e., margin reflex distance), the function in the levator muscle, and the adequacy of eye movements.

The surgery can be complex and the anatomy difficult in severe lid injuries (Fig. 18-97). The upper lid is explored through a skin crease incision and the anatomy displayed. Adhesions are divided. The preaponeurotic fat can conveniently be used to provide a barrier to prevent readhesion of the tissues. If the levator function is good, the levator

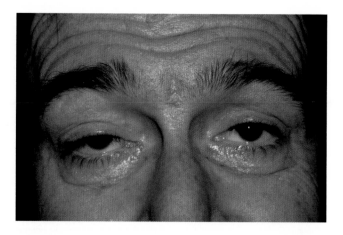

FIGURE 18-96 Bilateral ptosis with poor levator function after severe head injury.

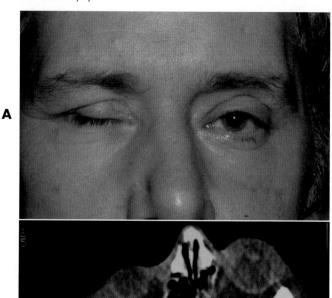

A

B

FIGURE 18-97 **A** and **B,** Severe injury to the right orbit with complex ptosis.

aponeurosis is shortened and advanced to the tarsal plate to correct the ptosis (Fig. 18-98). If the levator function is poor despite the division of any adhesions, it may be necessary to consider a brow suspension procedure. Care is needed to avoid corneal exposure postoperatively.

MEDIAL CANTHUS

Persistent telecanthus requires reattachment of the medial canthal tendon to the posterior lacrimal crest or adjustment to a unilateral or transnasal wire if it was inserted during the

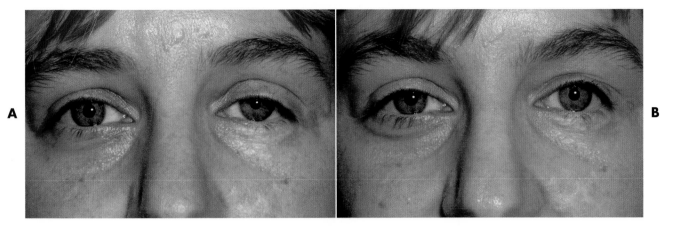

FIGURE 18-98   **A,** Simple traumatic ptosis with moderate levator function. **B,** Correction is achieved with a skin approach to levator resection.

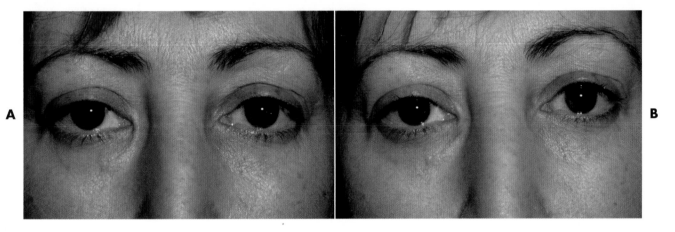

FIGURE 18-99   **A** and **B,** Web at the inner canthus is corrected with a Z-plasty.

original operation. Webbing of the skin at the medial canthus should be corrected with a Z-plasty or possibly a skin graft (Fig. 18-99). If the canthus has been displaced vertically, a Z-plasty may be required to correct the position (Fig. 18-100). Care should be taken to preserve the lacrimal drainage apparatus if it is patent and functioning. It is better to leave the medial canthus with slight distortion than risk damage to the lacrimal apparatus.

LATERAL CANTHUS

Displacement with rounding of the canthus requires reestablishment of the attachment to the region of Whitnall's tubercle with a periosteal flap or a wire. Displacement of the canthus in a vertical direction may require a Z-plasty to correct the position.

LACRIMAL DRAINAGE SYSTEM

Narrowing of the punctum can be improved with a "one-snip" procedure that opens the vertical 2 mm of proximal canaliculus. Eversion of the punctum can be corrected

with retropunctal cautery if slight or with the excision of a diamond of tarsoconjunctiva inferior to the punctum and closure with 7-0 absorbable sutures. More severe degrees of eversion may be associated with shortage of skin or an ectropion and require a full-thickness skin graft.

Blockage in the canaliculi is difficult to treat. If a block is found in both canaliculi within 8 mm of the puncta, it is not possible to reconstruct the connection with the lacrimal sac. A Lester Jones bypass tube is indicated if watering is significant.

Distal block in both canaliculi more than 8 mm from the puncta can be reconstructed by excision of the scarred canaliculi and anastomosis of the patent proximal canaliculi directly to the lacrimal sac. Usually, a dacryocystorhinostomy is also performed. This canaliculodacryocystorhinostomy is not always functional, even if the system is patent on syringing.

Scarring at the distal end of the common canaliculus at its entry into the lacrimal sac can be excised. A dacryocystorhinostomy is performed, and silicone tubes are inserted for 3 months. If the lacrimal sac and adjacent tissues are disrupted,

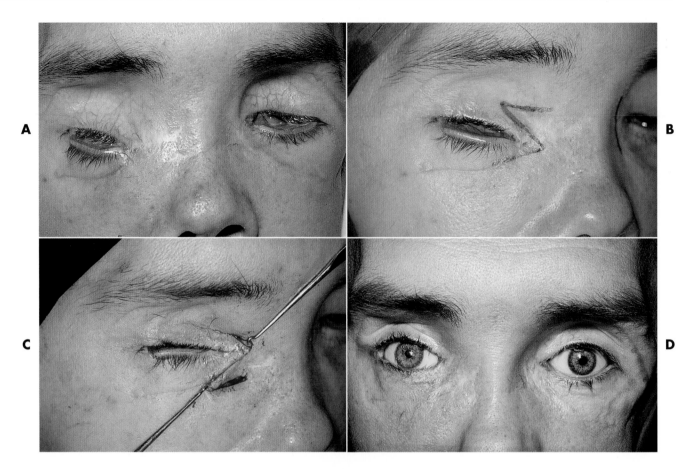

FIGURE 18-100   **A,** Severe midface trauma with loss of both eyes. Z-plasty (**B**) and transnasal wire (**C**) placement to correct the position of the medial canthi. **D,** Result, with artificial eyes.

it may not be possible to reestablish patent drainage. A Lester Jones bypass tube is then required.

RECOMMENDED READING

Bartley GB: Acquired lacrimal drainage obstruction: an etiologic classification system, case reports, and review of the literature. *Ophthal Plast Reconstr Surg* 8:237, 1992.

Bartley GB: Acquired lacrimal drainage obstruction: an etiologic classification system, case reports, and a review of the literature. Part 3. *Ophthal Plast Reconstr Surg* 9:11, 1993.

Beyer RW, Levine M: A method for repositioning or extraction of lacrimal system tubes. *Ophthal Surg* 17:496, 1986.

Borges AF: Relaxed skin tension lines (RSTL) versus other skin lines. *Plast Reconstr Surg* 73:144, 1984.

Bosniak S: *Principles and practice of ophthalmic plastic and reconstructive surgery*, Philadelphia, 1996, WB Saunders.

Collin JRO: Immediate management of lid lacerations. *Trans Ophthalmol Soc U K* 102:214, 1982.

Collin JRO, editor: *A manual of systematic eyelid surgery*, ed 2, Edinburgh, 1989, Churchill Livingstone.

Crawford JS: Intubation of obstruction in the lacrimal system. *Can J Ophthalmol* 12:289, 1977.

Cutler NL, Beard C: A method for partial and total upper lid reconstruction. *Am J Ophthalmol* 39:1, 1955.

Guzek JP, Ching AS, Hoang TA, et al: Clinical and radiologic lacrimal testing in patients with epiphora. *Ophthalmology* 104:1875, 1997.

Harrington JN: Reconstruction of the medial canthus by spontaneous granulation (laissez faire): a review. *Ann Ophthalmol* 14:956, 1982.

Harvey JT, Anderson RL: Transcanalicular removal of prolapsed Silastic tubing after nasolacrimal intubation. *J Ocular Ther Surg* 2:294, 1982.

Hawes MJ, Segrest DR: Effectiveness of bicanalicular silicone intubation in the repair of canalicular lacerations. *Ophthalmic Plast Reconstr Surg* 1:185, 1985.

Jones LT: An anatomical approach to problems of the eyelids and lacrimal apparatus. *Arch Ophthalmol* 66:111, 1961.

Jones LT: The cure of epiphora due to canalicular disorders, trauma and surgical failures on the lacrimal passages. *Trans Am Acad Ophthalmol Otolaryngol* 66:506, 1962.

Levine MR: *Manual of oculoplastic surgery*, Boston, 1966, Butterworth-Heinemann.

Linberg JV: *Contemporary issues in ophthalmology: lacrimal surgery*, vol 5, Edinburgh, 1988, Churchill Livingstone.

Maurice DM: The dynamic drainage of tears. *Int Ophthalmol Clin* 13:103, 1973.

McGregor IA: *Fundamental techniques of plastic surgery*, ed 8, Edinburgh, 1989, Churchill Livingstone.

McNab AA: *Manual of orbital and lacrimal surgery*, Edinburgh, 1994, Churchill Livingstone.

Moss ALH: Medial canthal tendon reconstruction. *J Maxillofac Surg* 12:131, 1984.

Mustarde JC: *Repair and reconstruction in the orbital region*, ed 3, Edinburgh, 1991, Churchill Livingstone.

Olver J: *Colour atlas of lacrimal surgery*, Oxford, 2002, Butterworth-Heinemann.

Patrinely JR, Anderson RL: A review of lacrimal drainage surgery. *Ophthalmic Plast Reconstr Surg* 2:97, 1986.

Rodriguez RL, Zide BM: Reconstruction of the medial canthus. *Clin Plast Surg* 15:255, 1988.

Salasche SJ, Grabski WJ: *Flaps for the central face*, Edinburgh, 1990, Churchill Livingstone.

Shore JW, Rubin PAD, Bilyk J: Repair of telecanthus by anterior fixation of cantilevered miniplates. *Ophthalmology* 99:1133, 1992.

Smit TJ, Mourits M: Monocanalicular lesions: to reconstruct or not. *Ophthalmology* 106:1310, 1999.

Spoor TC, Nesi FA: *Management of ocular, orbital and adnexal trauma*, New York, 1988, Raven Press.

Stranc MF: The pattern of lacrimal injuries in nasoethmoid fractures. *Br J Plast Surg* 23:339, 1970.

Tenzel RR: Reconstruction of the central one half of an eyelid. *Arch Ophthalmol* 93:125, 1975.

Tyers AG, Collin JRO: *Colour atlas of ophthalmic plastic surgery*, ed 3, Oxford, 2008, Butterworth-Heinemann.

Veirs ER: Malleable rods for the immediate repair of traumatically severed canaliculus. *Trans Am Acad Ophthalmol Otolaryngol* 66:262, 1962.

Welham RAN: Immediate management of injuries of the lacrimal drainage apparatus. *Trans Ophthalmol Soc U K* 102:216, 1982.

Welham RAN, Henderson PH: Results of dacryocystorhinostomy: analysis of the causes of failure. *Trans Ophthalmol Soc U K* 93:601, 1973.

CHAPTER 19

Primary Repair of Facial Soft Tissue Injuries

Barry L. Eppley

The complex and specialized anatomical regions of the face merit consideration because they have significant influence on facial appearance. The need for many secondary soft tissue procedures in these areas can be obviated by skillful primary surgery.[1] In this chapter, special attention is given to injuries of the scalp, forehead, brow, eyelid, nose, lips, ear, and important deeper structures such as the facial nerve, the lacrimal gland, and the parotid duct.

Initial care of soft tissue injuries should be undertaken as described in Chapter 6, and the following discussion assumes that these principles have been followed:

- Primary Advanced Trauma Life Support (ATLS) care
- Control of hemorrhage
- Early intervention for soft tissue injuries
- Careful evaluation of damage to nerves, ducts, and blood vessels
- Careful evaluation of any ocular injuries
- Identification of foreign bodies
- Clinical and radiological examinations to exclude bone fractures

SCALP AND FOREHEAD

The scalp, with its well-defined five layers, represents a single anatomical unit that, including the forehead, extends from the supraorbital margins anteriorly to the superior nuchal line posteriorly. The musculoaponeurotic galea provides a source of vascular perforators to the skin, and its fibrous composition makes it a good anchor for deep sutures. The galea is readily mobilized, facilitating wound closure and the development of local flaps. The subgaleal fascia is the plane in which scalp avulsions almost exclusively occur (Fig. 19-1).

Scalp injuries, particularly avulsions, often bleed profusely, and patients presenting with hemorrhagic shock require aggressive fluid resuscitation and blood replacement. Blood loss can be minimized with the application of pressure dressings or ligation of the galeal vessels and temporary suturing or stapling of the wounds. The vigorous blood supply of the scalp enhances the viability of tissue fragments that would not survive elsewhere. Near-complete avulsions of scalp segments may survive on small bridges of tissue or even as isolated islands. Only obviously devitalized tissue should be débrided. Scalp tissue that appears to have even a tenuous blood supply should be given the benefit of the doubt and retained, because the hair that it contains is a valuable resource. Any nonviable tissue can be readily removed and usually is not a source of infection. The robust blood supply serves as an adjunct in the prevention of infection. Scalp infections are uncommon even in contaminated wounds, and the resistance to infection makes it unnecessary to clip or shave hair from wound edges, unless doing so aids the alignment of the tissues.

Primary closure is the method of choice when there is no significant tissue loss (<3 cm). The wound edges tend to contract, and what initially appears to be a large defect may be relatively easily closed with subgaleal undermining (Fig. 19-2). Wounds on the vertex of the scalp are usually more difficult to close because of the decreased tissue mobility in that region. Scoring of the galea on its deep surface is a well-described procedure to facilitate closure. It consists of transverse incisions made perpendicular to the axis of advancement. Care should be taken not to damage the more superficial subcutaneous vessels.

A layered primary closure is carried out if the galea has been lacerated. The galea adheres tightly to the overlying skin, and its approximation facilitates skin closure. Failure to repair this layer may result in cosmetic deformity, ranging from a depressed scar to asymmetrical brow contraction. Closure of the galea also prevents the spread of wound contaminants to the intracranial cavity through the emissary veins, which connect the skin to the venous sinuses. Satisfactory galeal closure prevents the development of most potential problems, including osteomyelitis and meningitis. The galea is approximated with interrupted, 2-0 or 3-0, slowly resorbable sutures.

Because a noticeable scalp scar is determined primarily by the presence of alopecia, great care should be paid to follicular viability. Dermal sutures are used sparingly, or not at all, to reduce the possibility of hair follicular damage. Restoring the continuity of the galea obviates the need in most cases for dermal sutures, relieving tension on the skin sutures so they may be removed early. Closure of the skin is carried out using non-interlocking, continuous sutures of 3-0 nylon or Prolene in adults and 4-0 sutures in children (Fig. 19-3). Metallic staples may also be used, but their removal is painful.

SPLIT-THICKNESS SKIN GRAFTING

Placement of a split-thickness skin graft is the treatment of choice for most larger scalp defects that are not amenable to

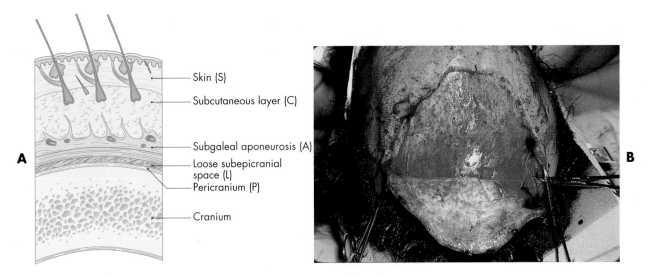

FIGURE 19-1 **A,** The five layers of the scalp include the skin (S), subcutaneous tissue (C), subgaleal aponeurosis (A), loose subepicranial space (L), and pericranium (P). **B,** Scalp avulsions commonly occur in the subgaleal plane.

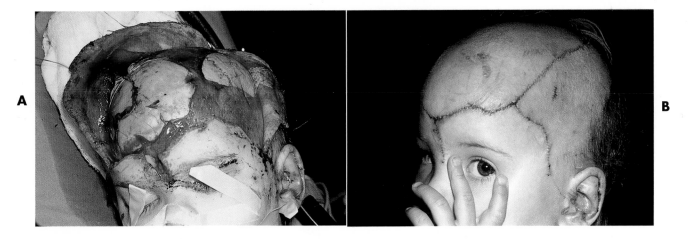

FIGURE 19-2 Extensive scalp lacerations with degloving in a 4-year-old (unrestrained passenger) who was involved in a motor vehicle accident. **A,** Intraoperative view. **B,** View 7 days postoperatively.

primary closure. The pericranium must be intact, because grafts cannot succeed on denuded bone. Split-thickness skin grafts provide a rapid and reliable method for wound coverage in the acute setting (Fig. 19-4). The 0.14- to 0.20-inch-thick grafts are harvested with a dermatome, usually from the lateral thigh. They can be placed as sheet grafts if encroaching on the forehead, but they typically are meshed in a 1.5:1 ratio and placed with minimal expansion. Meshing the graft has two purposes: It engrafts better without bolstering by allowing fluid egress, and it results in greater wound contracture, which is subsequently beneficial. Because scalp skin grafts are ultimately esthetically undesirable due to contour depression and alopecia, they are usually serially excised about 6 months after placement. Because split-thickness skin grafts contract by 20% to 40%, the reduction in size of the defect aids secondary excision and closure. In grossly contaminated wounds and those in which the viability of the pericranium is questionable, a homograft (cadaveric) or xenograft (porcine) may be used as a temporary biological dressing until the placement of an autograft is considered appropriate.

The lack of a pericranium obviates the success of a skin graft. In the absence of a pericranium, the outer table of the cranium typically is removed, exposing the well-vascularized diploë, which is an excellent bed for grafting. This can be done by burring away the outer table or drilling multiple holes through the outer table; either method allows granulation tissue to cover the exposed bone. After about 3 weeks, there should be a satisfactory covering of healthy granulation tissue on which the graft can be placed. Although this is an effective method to achieve epithelial coverage, it does require a considerable delay between bone removal and placement of the graft, and it is likely to leave a poorly contoured defect.

FLAPS

Unless there are contraindications, a flap procedure provides a more expedient solution than grafting or removal of the

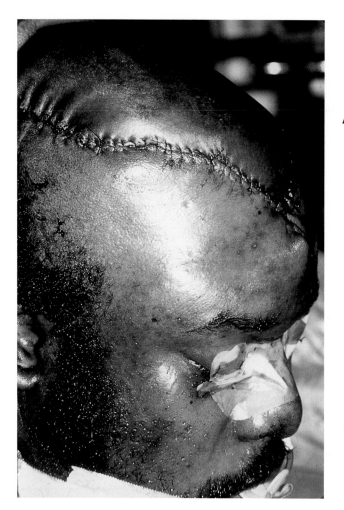

FIGURE 19-3 Scalp skin closure can be done expeditiously with a running suture or staples.

outer bone plate. A locally based pericranial flap is used if the defect is small, or a free tissue transfer is employed for larger defects. Pericranial flaps enable the transfer of a thin, vascularized cover onto which a skin graft can be placed. Although originally thought to be random in nature, much of the blood supply of flaps is derived from the overlying subgaleal fascia, which usually is elevated with the flap. To be effective and reliable, the pericranial flap should be centered on a major vascular territory with minimal dissection close to the pedicle (Fig. 19-5). The blood supply is extremely sensitive, and postoperative graft dressings should be very lightly applied.

Use of Local Flaps

Flaps using local scalp tissue are appropriate for relatively small, partial- or full-thickness defects (3-5 cm wide). Local flaps permit closure of the defect with hair-bearing skin of similar thickness. Their use is appropriate for the cover of clean, sharply defined lacerations when surrounding tissue viability is not compromised. Many traumatic scalp wounds are the result of crush or avulsion injuries in which adjacent tissue damage is inevitable. Flap elevation may further compromise an already tenuous blood supply, and local flaps that must be raised and rotated have only limited use in these circumstances (Fig. 19-6).

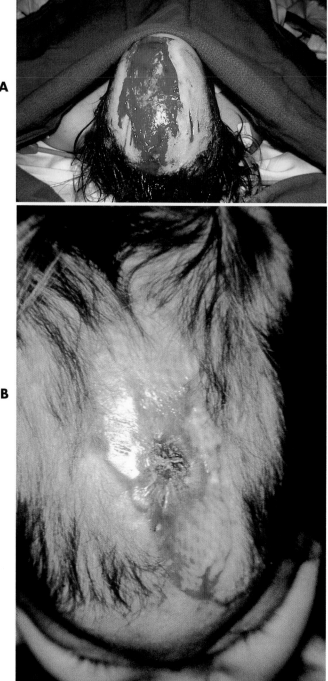

FIGURE 19-4 Split-thickness skin grafting on the scalp. **A,** Partial scalp avulsion in a 3-year-old boy due to a dog bite with the underlying pericranium intact. **B,** Ten days after split-thickness skin grafting with approximately 90% success. A small, central eschar represents the only area of unsuccessful grafting, which will heal secondarily.

Use of Free Tissue Transfer

The transfer of free, vascularized flaps is a long and potentially demanding procedure, and the timing must be considered with care. It is not a procedure to start late at night with tired or inexperienced surgeons and anesthetists; it should be a planned, semi-elective procedure. Wet-dry dressings may be applied to large, denuded defects until free, vascularized tissue transfer can be arranged. Flaps should be muscular for bulk and should have maximal vascularity. The flap of choice usually is the latissimus dorsi because of its large surface area,

relatively long pedicle, and ease of harvest (Fig. 19-7). Other options include the rectus abdominis muscle, scapular or parascapular flaps, and the omental fat flap.[2] Most of these options require a simultaneously placed split-thickness skin graft for outer coverage of the flap.

REPLANTATION

Microsurgical scalp replantation is the treatment of choice for total or near-total scalp avulsion. These uncommon injuries have a classic presentation and are usually caused by entanglement of long hair in rotating machinery. Separation occurs in the subgaleal, loose areolar plane at the peripheral margins of the scalp, where the galea is less resistant to applied force. Partial-avulsion injuries are rare, and the scalp and forehead typically are removed as a single anatomical unit (Fig. 19-8). The upper eyelids and portions of the ears may be included in the avulsed segment because of the intimate relationship between the muscular segments of the galea and these structures.[3]

Microsurgical replantation, if successful, is esthetically and functionally superior to any other method of wound closure or coverage. It restores normal hair growth in unscarred areas, and a large amount of the avulsed segment, such as eyelids and ears, can be expected to survive (see Fig.

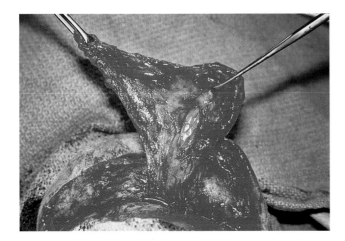

FIGURE 19-5   Pericranial flaps usually must have a defined vessel to ensure viability. A frontal pericranial flap based on the supraorbital-supratrochlear vessels is one option.

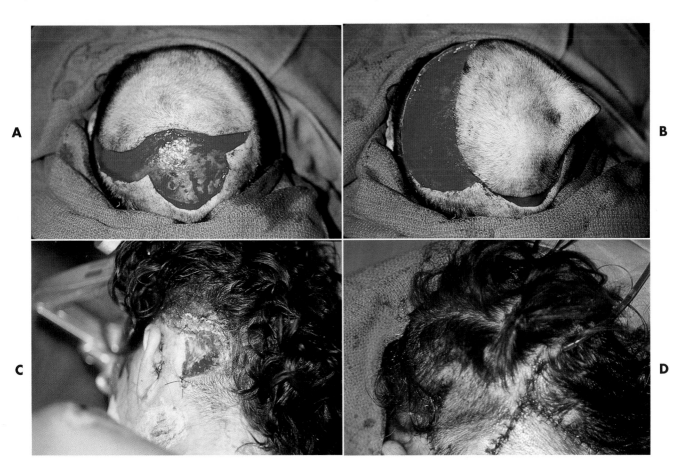

A **B** **C** **D**

FIGURE 19-6   Coverage of avulsed scalp defects with rotational flaps. **A,** Débrided scalp avulsion defect from dog bite in 4-year-old boy. **B,** Rotational flap coverage, with the wake of the flap to be covered with a skin graft. The flap was needed because of the exposed bone underneath the avulsion. **C,** Small occipital scalp defect seen 8 days after avulsive injury from a rollover motor vehicle accident in 21-year-old woman. **D,** Coverage of exposed bone with a scalp transpositional flap.

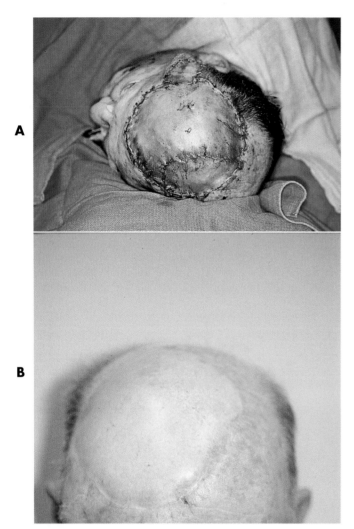

FIGURE 19-7 Coverage of a large scalp wound with a free latissimus muscle flap covered with a skin graft. **A,** Intraoperative view with the free muscular flap sewn into the defect. The microvascular anastomoses are in the right neck, and the muscle is covered with unmeshed, split-thickness skin grafts. **B,** View 6 months postoperatively of the healed flap and no contour deformity.

19-8C). Provided that the avulsed segment is not severely crushed and mutilated and the period of warm ischemia was not greater than 12 hours, every effort should be made for replantation.[4]

Successful replantation depends on emergency access to the operating room, finding suitable recipient vessels in the surrounding temporal scalp or neck (which is always possible), and finding suitable vessels in the avulsed segment (which is not always possible). Vein grafts may be needed to move the microvascular repair out of the zone of injury and reduce tension along the vessels and across the anastomoses. Although the scalp can survive with only one arterial anastomosis, it is preferable to identify at least two vessels suitable for repair. It is possible (although rare) to identify and repair bilateral superficial temporal and occipital arteries. Because venous congestion is the predominant cause of most postoperative flap failures, it is essential to ensure adequate venous outflow. If no suitable veins are available, venous outflow can be achieved by anastomosis of a scalp artery directly to a recipient vein. The use of medicinal leeches is an option, but a large scalp replant requires four to six leeches concurrently, and the patient needs extensive transfusions until venous outflow is reestablished. Most established scalp replants require secondary revision of the scars, eyelids, ears, and any large remaining areas of alopecia.[5] If it is not possible to replant the scalp, coverage may be obtained using one of the methods previously described (Fig. 19-9).

If avulsion occurs in the forehead region, primary closure can be a problem because of the difficulty in recruiting local tissue to cover the defect. Extensive mobilization and release of the galea can help, but only for closure of defects of several centimeters. Reduction of the width of the forehead causes problems with medial or superior eyebrow transposition and frontal hairline disturbances, neither of which is easy to restore secondarily without recreating the original defect. Initial repair is usually best managed by coverage with a split- or full-thickness skin graft. If the avulsion is only of partial thickness, with preservation of some or all of the frontalis muscle, a full-thickness graft or unmeshed, thick, split-thickness graft may produce a reasonable result without significant contour deformity (Fig. 19-10A and B). If only pericranium is left, a split-thickness skin graft produces a healed but depressed wound that will require secondary reconstruction through tissue expansion or local flaps, or both (see Fig. 19-10C and D).

The eyebrow is the most valuable esthetic structure of the forehead. Preservation of hair-bearing skin and accurate realignment of the eyebrow unit is essential (Fig. 19-11). Eyebrow hair should not be shaved because it may not fully regrow, and the likelihood of secondary eyebrow deformities is increased even if it does regrow. After a portion of the eyebrow is lost, the remaining portion should be put back together along its preinjury arc, even if this creates a larger forehead defect. Closure of the wound with the eyebrow canted up or down can make secondary reconstruction more difficult, although a Z-plasty often can provide an effective solution. Significant eyebrow loss ultimately requires free scalp grafts or micrograft hair transplants for reconstruction (see Figs. 19-10D and 19-11D).

EYELIDS

In the management of eyelid injury, associated trauma to the underlying globe must be excluded. If the cornea has been exposed, care should be taken that the cornea remains moist by regular saline irrigation or placement of a saline-soaked dressing. At the time of repair, it is good practice to protect the cornea with a soft lens or shield. If injury is not seen or suspected, an ophthalmologist's opinion is not immediately necessary, and visual acuity can be assessed by simple tests. If an injury is suspected, an expert evaluation is mandatory. A common error is to miss a foreign body. Lifting the lids away and carefully inspecting the depths of the fornices is a simple but important procedure. Corneal abrasions are common in facial trauma, and pain and irritation of the injured eye are typical findings. Definitive diagnosis requires ophthalmological assessment with fluorescein dye and slit-lamp examination.

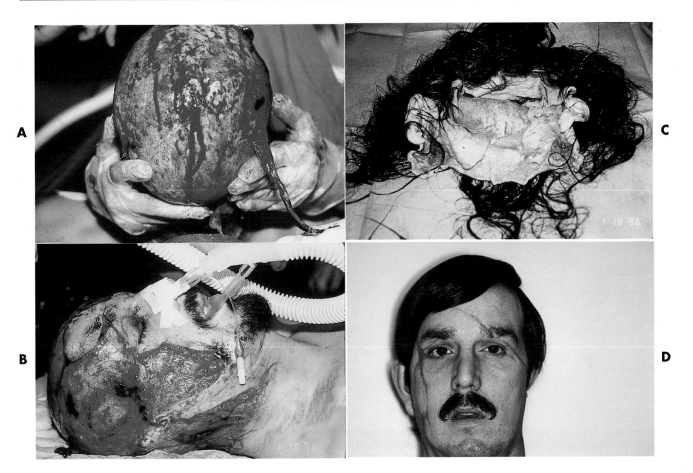

FIGURE 19-8 Microsurgical scalp replantation. **A,** A 33-year-old man sustained a complete scalp avulsion when his hair became entangled in machinery. **B** and **C,** Total scalp avulsion, including the ears and eyebrows. **D,** Successful scalp replantation with survival of the eyebrows and most of both ears. *(Courtesy of A. Michael Sadove, MD, Indianapolis, In.)*

With appropriate treatment, healing is usually rapid and uncomplicated. In rare cases, devastating infection can occur with *Pseudomonas,* which warrants an immediate ophthalmological intervention.

For practical purposes, the eyelid has two layers: an inner layer comprising the tarsal plate and conjunctiva and an outer layer of skin and orbicularis muscle (Fig. 19-12A). Apposition of skin, muscle, and tarsal plate is important, because conjunctival lacerations frequently heal adequately on their own. Lacerations in the upper eyelid may disrupt the levator aponeurosis and, if not properly repaired, result in postoperative downward positioning of the upper eyelid (i.e., ptosis). Downward positioning of the lower eyelid (i.e., ectropion) is usually the result of lacerations that run perpendicular to the lid margin; it is caused by poor anatomical realignment, tissue loss, or canthal disruption.

Full-thickness eyelid lacerations should have the lid margin approximated first by lining up the gray line (i.e., squamous-mucosal junction) or the meibomian gland orifices with 7-0 Vicryl suture, with the tail of the suture left long so it can be sewn down by the adjacent sutures. The remainder of the laceration is repaired in layers with 6-0 Vicryl for the tarsus and muscle; 6-0 plain or chromic gut, with the knots inverted to prevent corneal irritation, for the conjunctiva; and 6-0 or 7-0 nylon or Prolene for the skin (see Fig. 19-12B and C). Approximating the tarsus and the ciliary margin are the crucial steps provided there is no significant tissue loss.[5] For partial-thickness injuries with skin loss, full-thickness skin grafts from the avulsed segment (if available) or from the opposite upper eyelid or postauricular area can be used. For small, full-thickness defects involving less than one third of the lid, primary closure can be carried out. Many defects involving up to one half of the lid can be primarily closed with release of the lateral canthus (Fig. 19-13). Defects larger than one half of the lid require a cheek advancement (i.e., Mustarde rotation flap) or an upper lid switch procedure. Use of these more extensive flap procedures, which are often only one-time use techniques, is not advised in the acute trauma setting. In some cases with more superficial loss, a full-thickness graft from the other upper eyelid is desirable.

LACRIMAL APPARATUS

Any injury to the medial aspect of the eyelids, particularly the lower lid, may involve the lacrimal system (Fig. 19-14). Inspection and cannulation of the punctum with probes can confirm the injury (see Fig. 19-14A to C). Repair is usually carried out by loop intubation with the puncta initially

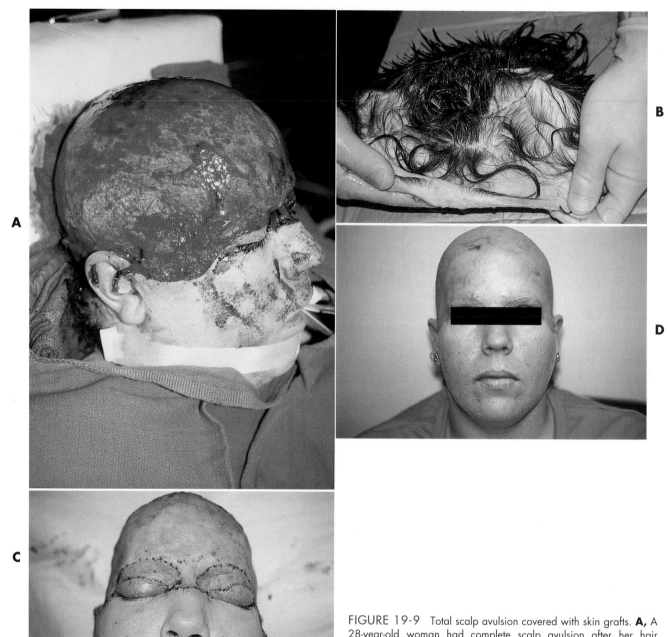

FIGURE 19-9   Total scalp avulsion covered with skin grafts. **A,** A 28-year-old woman had complete scalp avulsion after her hair became entangled in machinery. **B,** Avulsed scalp segment. **C,** Because the scalp was not replantable due to poor vessel quality, immediate coverage was achieved with meshed and unmeshed (fore-head and upper eyelid), split-thickness skin grafts. **D,** Almost 100% of the graft was successful 3 weeks after the initial surgery.

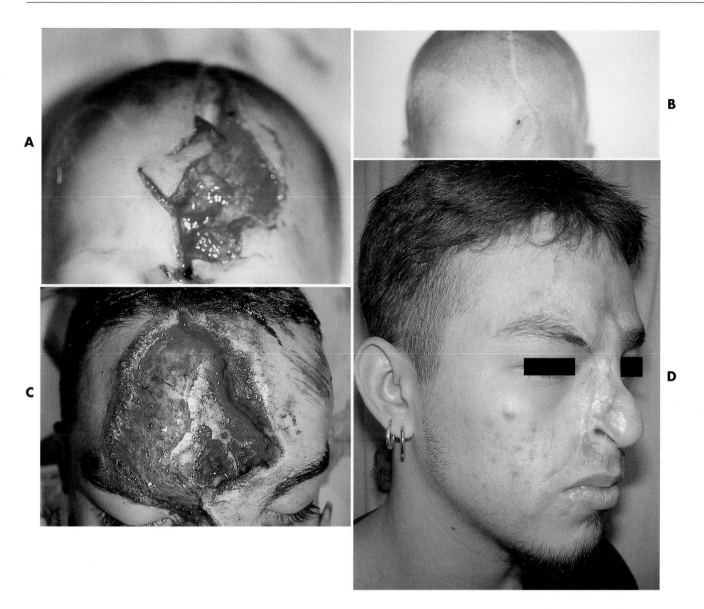

FIGURE 19-10 Forehead avulsion with skin graft coverage. **A,** Because of a dog bite, a 4-year-old boy had avulsion of the central forehead that left the pericranium and galea intact. **B,** Three months postoperatively, an unmeshed, split-thickness skin graft provides coverage with minimal contour deformity. **C,** After a motorcycle accident, a 24-year-old man had a large forehead and eyebrow (partial) avulsion with only the pericranium left intact. **D,** The postoperative result at 1 year shows that multiple revisions of the forehead, eyebrow, and nose will be needed.

cannulated with Silastic stents that pass into and through the lacrimal duct into the nose, where they are tied[6] (see Fig. 19-14D and E). Repair of the canaliculi, sac, or duct can then be done with 9-0 nylon, but this approach is often more theoretical than practical. Completion of the lid repair and keeping the stents in place for at least 3 months often results in adequate tear drainage. Injury to the upper canaliculus alone rarely causes epiphora.

Retrograde probing is an alternative to loop intubation. The specialized probes are passed through the uninjured punctum into the common canaliculus and then into the proximal end of the cut canaliculus. This can be useful when the punctum proximal to the laceration cannot be entered.

CANTHAL LIGAMENTS

Disruption of the canthal ligaments is uncommon, but an attempt should be made to reattach disrupted ligaments to the orbital walls. Untreated, this injury produces a very ugly deformity. As long as a small fragment of bone remains attached to the ligament, the result is reasonably predictable. Small microplates can be used to hold the bone fragment and canthus in the correct position. If the canthus is completely free, it is difficult to restore its original position. Wires passed through these small canthal stumps look fine in diagrams, but they frequently cut through the fine tissues, especially if the wound is treated late and more force is needed. A useful way

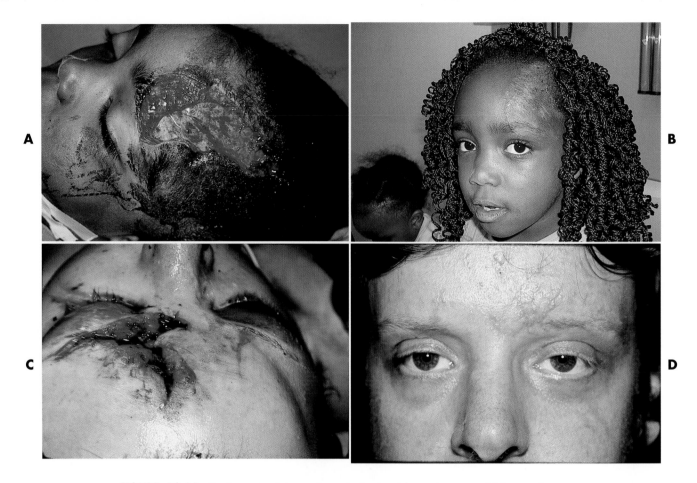

FIGURE 19-11   Realignment of the eyebrow in forehead lacerations reestablishes an important esthetic landmark. **A,** A 4-year-old girl had an extended scalp-to-eyelid laceration due to a motor vehicle accident. **B,** Postoperative result at 6 weeks. Despite healing scars, the alignment of the eyebrow produces a good early result. **C,** A 31-year-old man had deep forehead lacerations and partial eyebrow loss after a motor vehicle accident. **D,** Proper alignment of the eyebrow, even if deficient, has been achieved and the area can be secondarily grafted without the need for additional skin surgery.

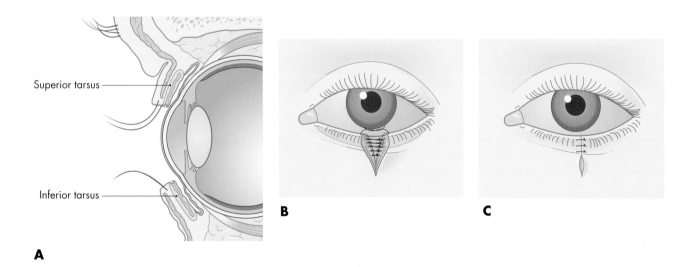

FIGURE 19-12   **A,** The eyelid consists essentialy of two layers: an inner lamella of conjunctiva and tarsus and an outer lamella of skin and orbicularis muscle. **B,** Closure of the inner lamella. **C,** Closure of the outer lamella.

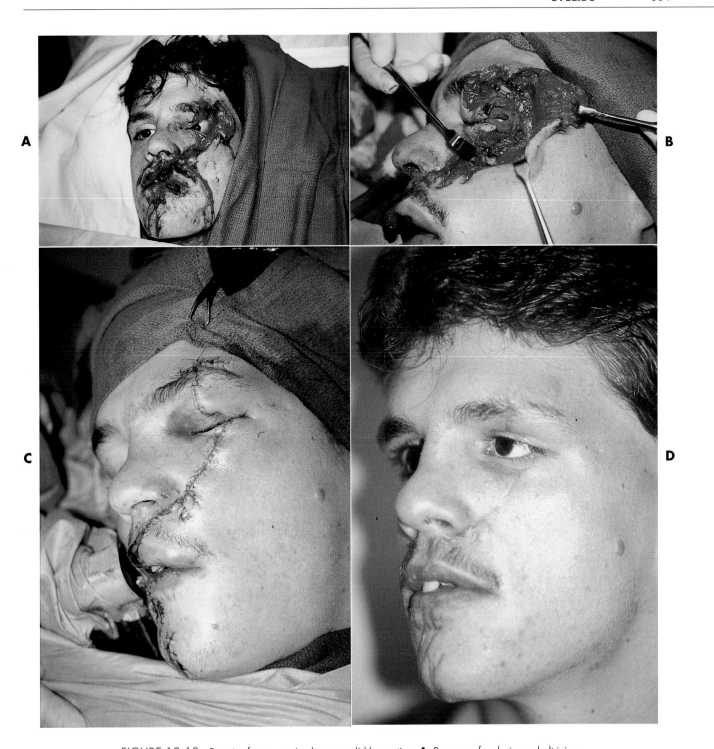

FIGURE 19-13   Repair of an extensive lower eyelid laceration. **A,** Because of a chainsaw belt injury, a 26-year-old man had a severe laceration with loss of about one fifth of the lower eyelid. **B,** Bony repair of the periorbital skeleton before eyelid reconstruction. **C,** Immediate postoperative result shows that a lateral canthotomy is required for lower eyelid closure. **D,** The 3-month postoperative result shows no lower eyelid notching.

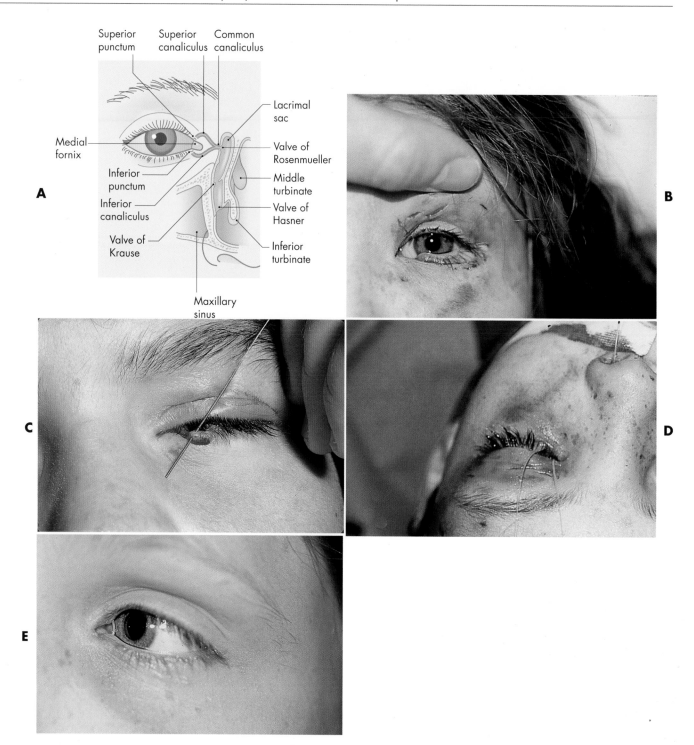

FIGURE 19-14   Repair of lacrimal duct injuries. **A,** Anatomy of the nasolacrimal system. **B,** Medial laceration of the lower eyelid in a 9-year-old girl was caused by a dog bite. **C,** Cannulation with a probe confirms the lacrimal transection in a different patient. **D,** Anterograde cannulation of nasolacrimal system through the upper and lower eyelid puncta with Crawford tubes. **E,** The tubes are kept in place for 3 months after repair of the laceration. The Silastic loop can be seen in the medial aspect of the eye between the puncta.

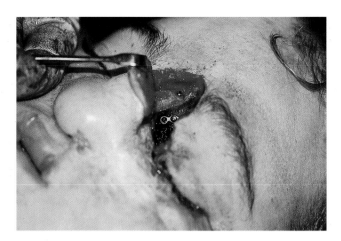

FIGURE 19-15 A metallic plate is placed on the inner orbital wall for medial canthal reattachment during orbital repair. A 15-year-old girl sustained these injuries in a motor vehicle accident.

to prevent this problem is to place a clear acrylic button (allowing skin necrosis to be detected) over the canthal skin and run the wire through the button and the ligament. With this method, the acanthus is "pulled" and "pushed" into position. The wire canthopexy has to be fixed to an artificial anchorage, which in the medial canthal area can be provided by placement of a small miniplate (Fig. 19-15). In the lateral canthal area, a small hole placed through the lateral orbital wall works well. If the soft tissue injury is associated with underlying skeletal injury, it is common to find comminution of the bone, and transnasal fixation may be required.

NOSE

Lacerations to the nose are usually uncomplicated, but they may involve the underlying cartilaginous or bony structures, and unsuspected injuries may be overlooked (Fig. 19-16). The rich vascular supply of the nose through the septum and enveloping skin makes it difficult for any portion of the nose not to survive, providing some pedicle remains. Full-thickness lacerations should be closed in three layers: the mucous membrane (4-0 chromic), torn cartilages (5-0 or 6-0 polydioxanone [PDS] or clear nylon), and the overlying skin (6-0 nylon). After the cartilaginous and bony framework is anatomically aligned, the nasal skin usually approximates if there has been no significant tissue loss. Dermal sutures often are unnecessary, which is fortuitous, because the thick sebaceous skin with its high bacterial content is prone to suture abscesses. If there has been cartilaginous loss, consideration should be given to the placement of a primary cartilage graft to resist postoperative contracture and depression of the scar, although this technique is not frequently needed.

ABRASION OR AVULSION INJURY

Abrasion and avulsion injuries are common, and the nose is frequently exposed to abrasive tangential forces. Partial-thickness avulsions are best left alone and treated topically, because they have a remarkable ability to heal. With deeper

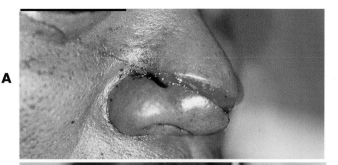

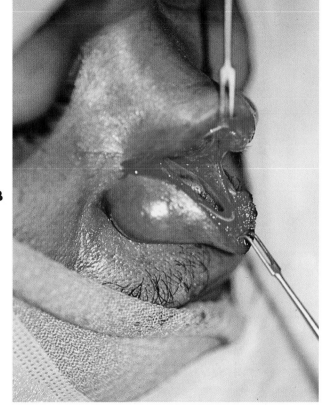

FIGURE 19-16 Nasal laceration caused by a knife. **A,** A 47-year-old man has a superficial laceration across the distal nose. **B,** Intraoperative evaluation of the laceration shows its complete transection through the alar cartilages and septum.

lesions that penetrate the dermis, full-thickness skin grafts from the preauricular or postauricular area provide the best color match and prevent significant depression of the healed wound. Split-thickness grafts produce a translucent, contracted appearance and should be considered only for partial-thickness avulsions when some dermis remains. Full-thickness grafts should be secured with a tie-over dressing for at least 5 to 7 days, because revascularization may not be complete for at least 1 week after placement. The timing of graft placement may be delayed from the acute setting to allow for an improved recipient bed if the risk of contamination is high or there is exposed cartilage (Fig. 19-17). Survival of the nasal skin can be remarkable even with very large avulsive injuries attached by a narrow pedicle. As long as there is bleeding from the dermal edges of the cut tissue, the nasal flap should be replaced and can be expected to survive (Fig. 19-18).

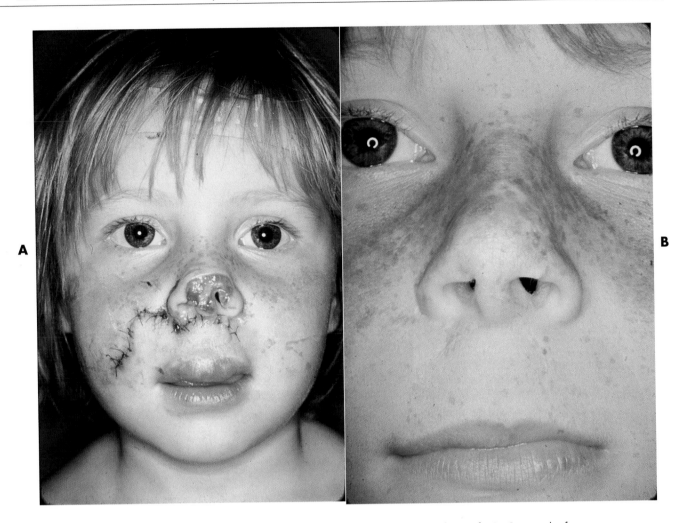

FIGURE 19-17   Reconstruction of the nasal tip with a full-thickness skin graft. **A,** One week after nasal tip avulsion caused by a dog bite in a 4-year-old boy. **B,** Results 1 year after secondary reconstruction with a full-thickness skin graft and secondary cartilage grafting.

AMPUTATION INJURY

Amputation injuries are dramatic, and management depends on the size of the separated part. For nasal segments 2.5 cm long or smaller, replacement with a composite graft may be successful (Fig. 19-19). Complete revascularization through existing vascular channels may occur, and although it may initially appear that the segment is not viable, it may "pink up" 10 to 14 days later. Patience and reassurance of the patient are necessary before deciding that it has not survived. Systemic anticoagulants do not improve the success of the composite replacement, although topical vasodilators (e.g., nitroglycerin paste) have been helpful. If the amputated part is not available, consideration should be given, especially for small, clean defects of the nostril margin, to composite grafting; the ear is a suitable donor site. Success rates vary, but this approach may avoid prominent disfigurement.

For larger nasal amputations, nonvascularized replantation cannot succeed, and the segment should be discarded. In children, the size limitation of the replanted nasal segment may be increased because composite grafts are more forgiving and the difficulty in reconstructing a growing nose justifies

the risk. In a few instances, the amputated nose has been successfully replanted using microvascular techniques, but this requires a very clean amputation of the part and a short period of warm ischemia.[7]

SEPTAL HEMATOMAS AND HEMORRHAGE

A septal hematoma usually manifests as an anterior nasal swelling that is obstructive and tender. Drainage should be performed without delay to prevent abscess formation and avascular necrosis of the septal cartilage. Treatment is best carried out using a hemitransfixion incision and mucosal approximation with transseptal, 4-0, plain gut sutures. Plastic septal stents can be used and secured with large, transseptal, Prolene sutures.

Most nasal bleeding stops spontaneously, but it occasionally persists and requires active management. Underlying skeletal injury may be the cause of bleeding and should be suspected in such instances. If the bleeding arises from the anterior aspect, simple packing may suffice. If the bleeding arises from the posterior aspect, postnasal and anterior packing may be required. Several adjuncts, including balloon

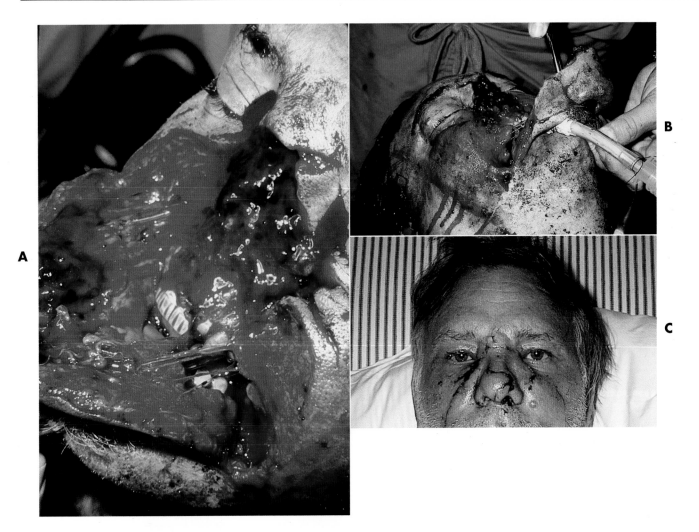

FIGURE 19-18 A 53-year-old man sustained a large nasal avulsion in a motor vehicle accident. **A** and **B,** The entire nose and midfacial tissue are avulsed, remaining attached only by the upper lip. **C,** Reattachment of the pedicled nasal flap, with complete survival 1 week after the injury.

catheters, are commercially available (Fig. 19-20). Occasionally, operative intervention is required to establish the source of bleeding and tie off the regional vessels. The blood supply to the nasal cavity below the middle turbinate arises from the external carotid and that above the turbinate from the internal carotid system. Exploration of the medial orbital wall to identify the anterior and posterior ethmoidal arteries may be necessary.

LIPS

The key to successful repair of the lips is ensuring correct approximation and alignment of the orbicularis oris muscle and the vermilion border. The orbicularis muscle should be repaired with 4-0 or 5-0 Vicryl or Dexon, and enough sutures should be placed to prevent dehiscence of the muscle. If not properly repaired, loss of lip height, notching, and an incompetent sphincter may result. It is helpful at this stage to accurately align the vermilion border using 5-0 nylon or Prolene

before proceeding to closure of the mucosal or skin surface (Fig. 19-21). The intraoral mucous membrane is then closed with 4-0 chromic or plain gut. The skin is closed using 5-0 chromic for the dermis and 6-0 nylon or Prolene for the skin. Ideally, the laceration should cross the vermilion border at 90 degrees to facilitate correct alignment, but most lacerations do not, and removal of tissue to make this conversion is of uncertain merit in the acute setting.[8]

Management of avulsion injuries depends on the size of the defect. In rare cases of very little vermilion loss, the recovered piece may be successfully replaced as a free composite graft (Fig. 19-22). Usually, however, it is best to complete a wedge excision, because it can be performed, with up to one fourth of the lip lost or removed, without any functional or esthetic defect other than the scar (Fig. 19-23). In larger defects with loss of up to 50% of the lip, primary closure can still be carried out, but some degree of microstomia will result. Postoperative lip-stretching exercises help, but the total circumoral surface area will be decreased. With defects greater than 50% of the lip, primary closure is not possible.

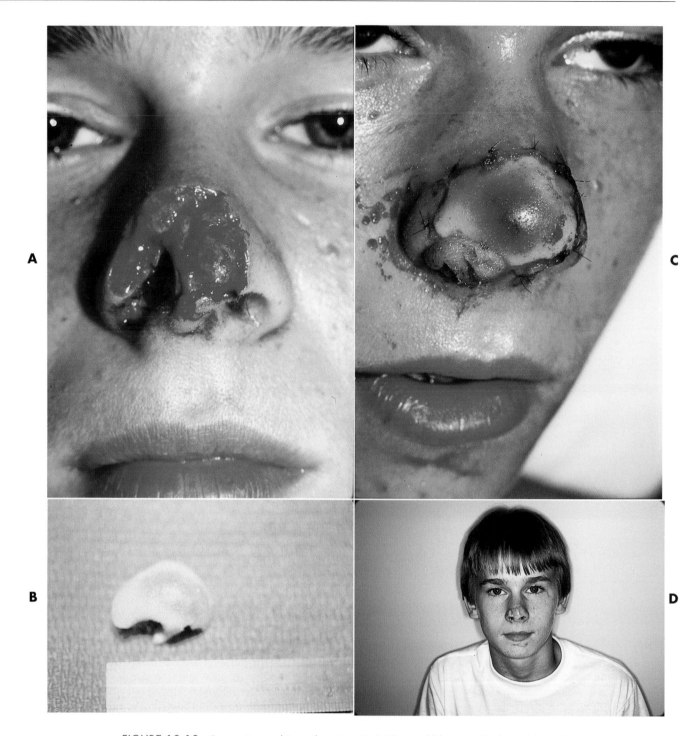

FIGURE 19-19   Composite nasal tip replantation. **A,** A 12-year-old boy sustained nasal tip avulsion after a dog bite. **B,** Avulsed nasal tip segment. **C,** Replantation of a composite piece. **D,** One year after surgery, much of the replanted skin survives. *(Courtesy of A. Michael Sadove, MD, Indianapolis, In.)*

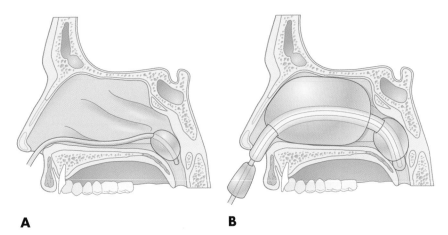

FIGURE 19-20 Treatment of nasal epistaxis by silicone catheters. **A,** A Foley catheter is a simple and effective device for management of posterior epistaxis. While inflated posteriorly, Vaseline gauze is packed anteriorly. **B,** More sophisticated, double-balloon designs obviate the need for anterior gauze packing.

A   **B**

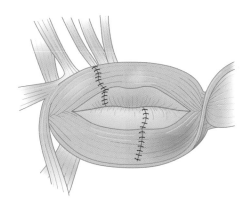

FIGURE 19-21 Layered lip anatomy and closure. The circumoral musculature puts a near-circumferential pull on lip wounds. The key points are muscle reapproximation and alignment of the vermilion-cutaneous junction.

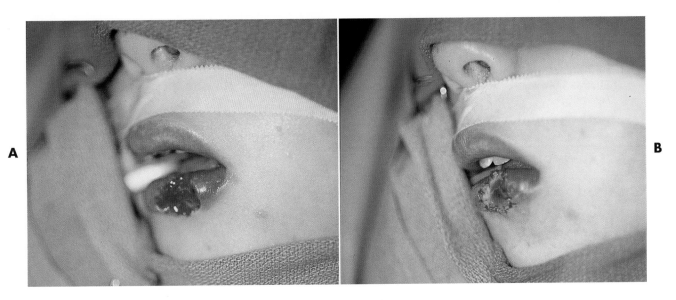

FIGURE 19-22 Vermilion avulsion of the lower lip. **A,** A 4-year-old girl sustained a small vermilion avulsion because of a dog bite. Primary closure requires extending a wedge excision into the skin. **B,** Preservation and replantation of the avulsed vermilion segment was ultimately successful.

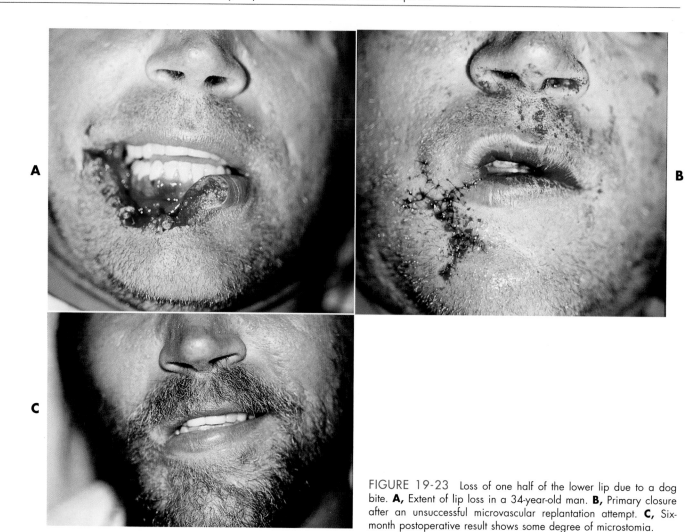

FIGURE 19-23   Loss of one half of the lower lip due to a dog bite. **A,** Extent of lip loss in a 34-year-old man. **B,** Primary closure after an unsuccessful microvascular replantation attempt. **C,** Six-month postoperative result shows some degree of microstomia.

In such circumstances, a skin-to-mucosal closure is the treatment of choice, with secondary surgery to re-create the oral aperture. Some form of rotational flap is required.

Rarely, an amputated lip segment can be replanted because the labial vessels in the remaining and avulsed lip are fairly easy to locate due to their predictable position.[9] However, the avulsed nature of most lip amputations makes it very difficult to reestablish flow in stretched vessels with significant intimal damage (Fig. 19-24).

INTRAORAL WOUNDS

Mucosal lacerations of the cheek, vestibules, floor of the mouth, tongue, and palate commonly occur. They most often result from compression or shearing of the mucosa against the dentition (natural or otherwise) or underlying bone, but they can result from a penetrating injury or be associated with mandibular or maxillary fractures.

PALATE

Injuries to the palatal mucosa most commonly occur in children as a result of a fall while sucking a foreign body (e.g.,

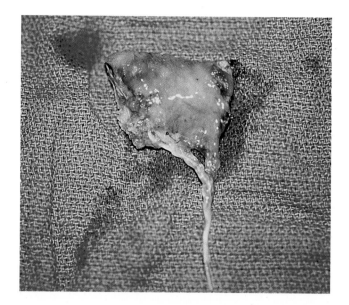

FIGURE 19-24   Avulsed lower lip segment from the patient described in Figure 19-23. These avulsions severely injure the labial vessels, making reestablishing vascular flow very difficult. The strand of tissue coming from the lip segment is a branch of the mental nerve.

toothbrush, pencil). The injury tends to be toward the posterior aspect, crescentic with the convexity anterior, and likely to involve the soft palate; or it may occur with maxillary fracture, most likely associated with a split palate and lying in the sagittal plane. In the former scenario, care should be taken to ensure that no foreign bodies are retained and, depending on the extent of the laceration, the wound may be tacked closed or not. Occasionally, a through-and-through wound results along the posterior edge of the maxilla, separating the soft palate from its anterior attachment. In this case, the nasopharyngeal and oral surfaces should be repaired if practical. With an underlying maxillary fracture, the initial requirement is to stabilize and fix the fracture and repair the soft tissues of the nasal floor (if required) and palate to avoid development of an oronasal fistula.

CHEEKS AND LIPS

Lacerations to the cheek or mucosa along the inner lip surface should be closed with 4-0 chromic or plain sutures and, depending on the depth of injury, with dermal sutures as required. Care should be taken in the cheek to ensure that the parotid papilla or duct is not compromised.

FLOOR OF MOUTH

In most instances, lacerations in the floor of the mouth can remain unsutured. Inexperienced suturing in this area may result in damage to the submandibular or sublingual salivary ducts or the lingual nerve. Through-and-through wounds require exploration and suturing in layers to avoid fistula formation.

TONGUE

To prevent notching and marginal deformities, significant tongue lacerations should be closed in layers with loosely tied, 3-0 chromic or Vicryl sutures in anticipation of muscular edema. Although rare, profuse bleeding can obstruct the airway, and early intubation is recommended in these cases.

DEGLOVING INJURY

Degloving injuries in the anterior mandibular region occur when significant compression and downward shearing forces are applied to the lower lip and chin. The mental nerves and vessels often remain intact, and some degree of the alveolar mucosa is stripped from the anterior mandible, commonly exposing the outer table from the alveolus to the chin point as far back as the mental foramina. The injury frequently results from hitting the chin and lower lip against the ground after a fall from a bicycle or skateboard. The wound typically is contaminated with particulate debris and requires thorough cleaning before the mucosa is fastened back in its original position. It often is not possible to approximate the original positions of the tissues, and exposed areas subsequently heal by secondary intention. External strapping or bandaging is recommended for the first 48 hours after repair.

Mucosal injury may be the first indication of child abuse, and this should be considered if the explanation appears incompatible with the injury.

EAR

The ear is similar to the nose in that there is a potential for disruption of a complex cartilaginous framework. Only the lobule, consisting of skin and adipose tissue, is devoid of cartilage. The large area of perichondrium and cartilage predisposes to hematoma formation after blunt injury. An enlargement of the ear with loss of definition usually indicates a hematoma and warrants immediate incision and drainage to prevent cartilaginous and fibrous disfigurement, the so-called cauliflower ear. After incision and drainage, bolsters should be placed and tied through and through onto the anterior and posterior surfaces of the ear to prevent reaccumulation of the hematoma; this is a more reliable and comfortable method than circumferential, tight pressure dressings (Fig. 19-25).

The unique structures of the ear warrant conservative débridement, because their replacement can be difficult. The blood supply is extensive, and many large ear segments can survive on narrow skin flaps. The cartilage must be approximated before closure of the overlying skin. The elastic cartilage of the ear does not heal by cartilaginous ingrowth but by the development of a fibrous scar between the cut edges, and it should be sutured with an undyed, slowly resorbing or clear, permanent suture for a more secure closure.[10] Because the shape and position of the ear are determined primarily by the support provided by the outline of the helical rim and antihelix, repair of the cartilaginous components is critical. Repair of the cartilage within the concave hollows of the ear, such as the concha and triangular fossa, is less critical because unsupported soft tissue healing alone can maintain

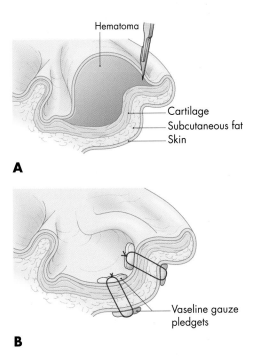

A

B

FIGURE 19-25 Auricular hematoma. **A,** An incision is made over the hematoma, and the clot is evacuated. **B,** After evaluation, pressure is applied by through-and-through chromic sutures tied over a bolster placed on the side of the hematoma to prevent reaccumulation.

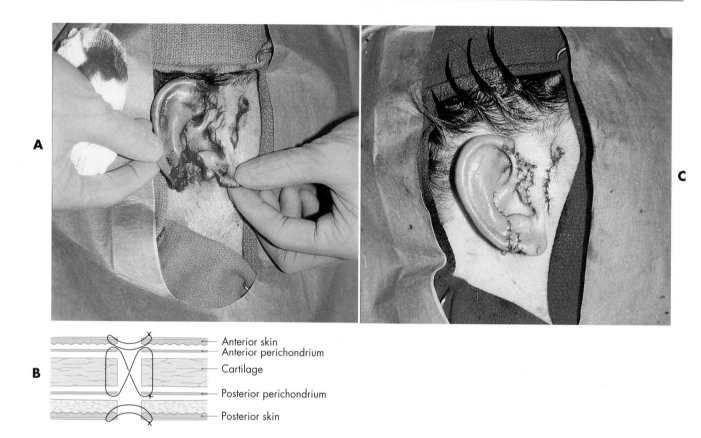

FIGURE 19-26 Closure of ear lacerations requires careful attention to cartilage repair. **A,** Partial ear transection. **B,** Figure-of-eight sutures through the cartilage prevent the edges from overriding each other. The skin is closed with simple sutures or everting mattress sutures. **C,** Closure of a partial ear transection.

the concavity. Notching of the helical rim is common after transection and repair and is particularly noticeable. Attention should be paid to cartilage realignment and skin closure in this area, with the use of vertical mattress sutures to evert the skin if necessary. Suturing of the dermis is rarely necessary, because the cartilaginous repair typically relieves any likely tension across the skin closure and the dermis is usually quite thin (Fig. 19-26).

Avulsion injuries vary greatly, but most involve some degree of tearing and crushing. Replacement of small avulsions as composite grafts may be considered, and there is usually little risk other than that of secondary removal and reductive closure with delayed reconstruction. Only the smallest segments (<1.0-1.5 cm) are likely to survive, and depending on the components involved, it may be more expedient and with less risk to complete a wedge excision and close primarily. For injury involving segmental avulsions of the upper two thirds of the helix, the retained cartilage may be denuded of skin and buried in the postauricular area with the torn or cut skin edges of the ear sutured into the same area, facilitating the subsequent use of a postauricular flap for secondary reconstruction and avoiding an operative stage and a donor site.

Most large, incomplete avulsions, even if attached by a very narrow pedicle, can survive with simple reattachment. However, although the skin pedicle usually offers adequate vascular inflow, the venous outflow may not be sufficient. This situation becomes evident in the immediate postoperative period by the presence of bluish discoloration and sluggish to nonexistent capillary refill, which are classic signs of venous congestion. Leeches used for several days often salvage the situation. One or two leeches, changed twice daily, combined with the typical ooze after removal allow the venous system rapidly to reestablish itself. There can be surprisingly significant blood loss with this technique, and the hematocrit should be monitored daily. A broad-spectrum antibiotic active against *Aeromonas*, a common gram-negative bacterium found in the gut of the leech, should be prescribed. Despite the nursing care needed and its unappealing nature, the salvage of tissue from venous congestion with leech therapy can be remarkable (Fig. 19-27).

If the ear avulsion is complete, a microvascular repair provides the best hope for successful replantation (Fig. 19-28). The success rate is low because of the very small size of the vessels (≤0.5 mm), difficulty in finding recipient vessels in the remaining wound bed and donor vessels in the amputated segment, and the intimal damage to the vessels that occurs with the more common avulsive injury. However, the arterial inflow from a single arterial anastomosis combined with postoperative leech therapy for venous outflow makes success possible, particularly in children.[11] For every large avulsed ear segment with a limited period of warm ischemia, microvascular replantation should be attempted. If microvascular replantation is not possible, placing the cartilage in a

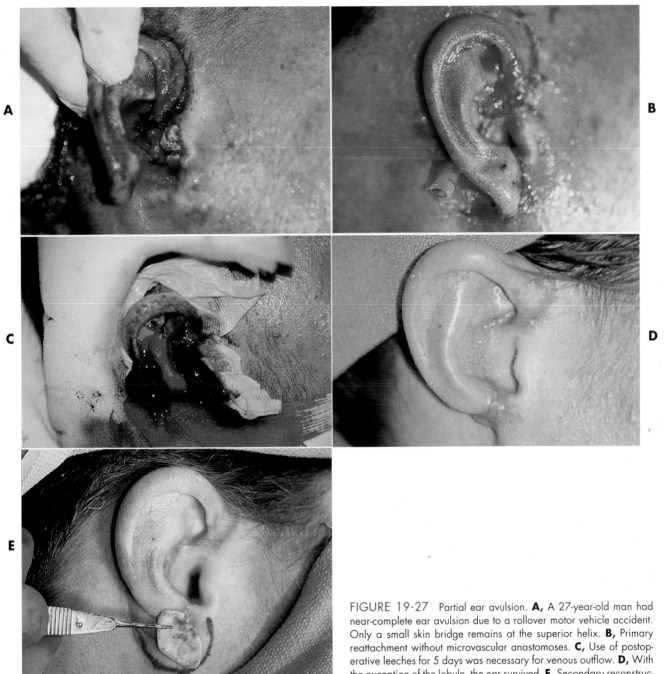

FIGURE 19-27   Partial ear avulsion. **A,** A 27-year-old man had near-complete ear avulsion due to a rollover motor vehicle accident. Only a small skin bridge remains at the superior helix. **B,** Primary reattachment without microvascular anastomoses. **C,** Use of postoperative leeches for 5 days was necessary for venous outflow. **D,** With the exception of the lobule, the ear survived. **E,** Secondary reconstruction was done with a cartilage graft and release.

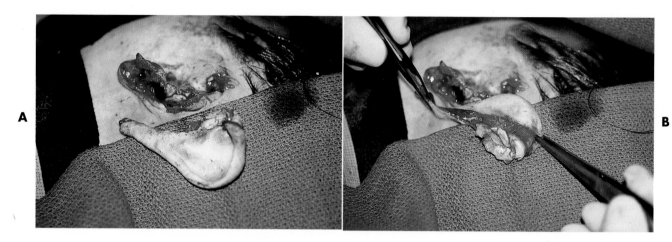

FIGURE 19-28 An 18-year-old girl (unrestrained passenger) sustained a total ear amputation during a rollover motor vehicle accident. **A,** Complete transection through the concha. **B,** The severe crush mechanism of the avulsion made the small (0.25-mm) vessels unusable for a microvascular replantation attempt.

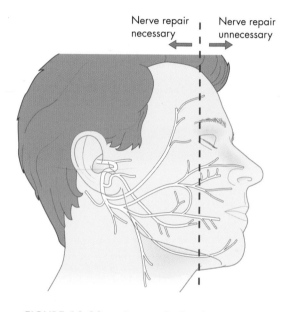

FIGURE 19-29 Indications for facial nerve repair.

postauricular subcutaneous pocket (i.e., pocket principle) should be considered.[12] It is uncovered weeks later and used as part of the secondary reconstruction.

FACIAL NERVE

Because lacerations of the lateral face, involving an area from the temporal region to the neck, may involve branches of the facial nerve, facial nerve function must be assessed as part of the examination. Injuries to the nerve anterior to a vertical line from the lateral canthus or the midpupillary line do not require repair and do not cause permanent loss of muscle function because the superficial facial muscles are innervated through their posterior aspects (Fig. 19-29). Posterior to these vertical lines, severed branches of the facial nerve should be repaired under microscopic guidance

within the first 24 hours of injury, if possible. In this early period, the distal nerve ends can be stimulated and identified.[13,14]

With either an epineural or a fascicular repair, surgery should be done using appropriate magnification with loupes or the operating microscope. If large branches are involved, an epineural repair may be adequate if a reasonable alignment and orientation of the fascicles within the sheath can be achieved. After cleaning and trimming of the nerve ends, simple interrupted sutures are placed using 10-0 nylon or Prolene on a 75- to 100-µm needle. Three to five sutures usually are needed (Fig. 19-30). In the smaller, more distal branches, the fascicles may be directly repaired with 11-0 suture material. There is some dispute about which method of repair—epineural alone or fascicular—produces the better functional outcome.[15] This argument often becomes moot, because the size of the nerve and its number of fascicles usually dictate the repair technique used.

If there has been loss of nerve tissue and continuity cannot be restored without unacceptable tension across the anastomosis, a primary nerve graft using the sural nerve should be considered (Fig. 19-31). The nerve graft can be harvested quickly and is associated with minimal morbidity (i.e., lateral plantar anesthesia) at the donor site.

Severe functional deficits arise from transections of the peripheral, single nerve branches, the frontal and marginal mandibular nerves. They have no cross-innervation with other branches, and motor function therefore never recovers without their anastomosis. However, they tend to be the hardest nerves to find and the least forgiving of a poor repair (Fig. 19-32).

Transection of the main nerve trunk as it exits from the stylomastoid foramen poses a difficult problem. Although the nerve trunk at this level is large, a sufficient proximal segment may not be available to facilitate a repair. Mastoid bone can be removed, and this may expose enough of the proximal segment to complete the repair. In rare circumstances, a proximal segment may not be available, and consideration should be given to a primary crossfacial nerve graft. The sural nerve graft, usually about 16 to 20 cm long, is anastomosed to the

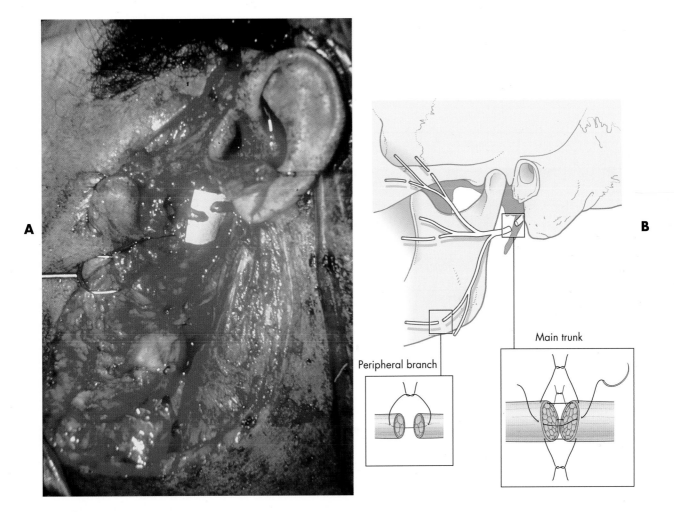

FIGURE 19-30 Primary repair of facial nerve transection. **A,** Typical location of nerve branch transections on the lateral face. **B,** Suture technique of epineural repair of facial nerve transections.

distal branches of the normal nerve on the opposite side of the face and then tunneled across the upper lip to the site of injury (Fig. 19-33). There is no advantage in delaying the repair under these circumstances unless the wounds are severely contaminated. Primary crossfacial nerve grafting offers the best hope for return of spontaneous and symmetrical facial expression. If the graft does not restore function to the remaining distal nerve branches, it can be used for a gracilis muscle transfer for smile reanimation.

PAROTID DUCT

Because the parotid duct runs parallel to the buccal branch of the facial nerve, traversing the middle third of a line drawn from the tragus to the midpoint of a line drawn between the alar of the nose and the vermilion border of the upper lip, lacerations in this area may sever the duct and the nerve branch. Saliva is rarely present in the wound after transection, and the injury easily can be missed (Fig. 19-34A).

Retrograde cannulation of Stensen's duct can confirm or refute transection of the duct (see Fig. 19-34B). The duct is large, usually 4 to 5 mm in diameter, which makes finding the proximal portion a simple procedure under loupe

magnification. The injection of colored dyes from the distal end is often recommended, but this seems unnecessary because it only colors and obscures the operative field. The proximal portion can be found by expressing saliva from the parotid gland.

The repair is carried out with 6-0 or 7-0 nylon or Prolene over a plastic stent; the Silastic tubing from an angiocatheter of a similar size to that of the duct can suffice. The stent is allowed to extend from the papilla for about 1 cm and is sutured to the mucosa with a 4-0 chromic suture. The stent is retained for about 2 weeks and then removed if it has not already become dislodged.[16]

If a section of the duct is missing and there is not enough residual duct to satisfactorily reconstitute the lumen, there are three practical options: to reconstruct the duct with a vein graft, to create a new oral opening by diverting the proximal stump through the oropharyngeal wall, and to ligate the duct and hope for eventual atrophy without creating a source of chronic infection.

Lacerations to the parotid gland itself should be repaired in layers (i.e., capsule, subcutaneous tissue, dermis, and skin) to avoid fistula formation. Lacerations involving the substance of the gland usually do not pose a problem unless adequate drainage of saliva is obstructed. If saliva collects

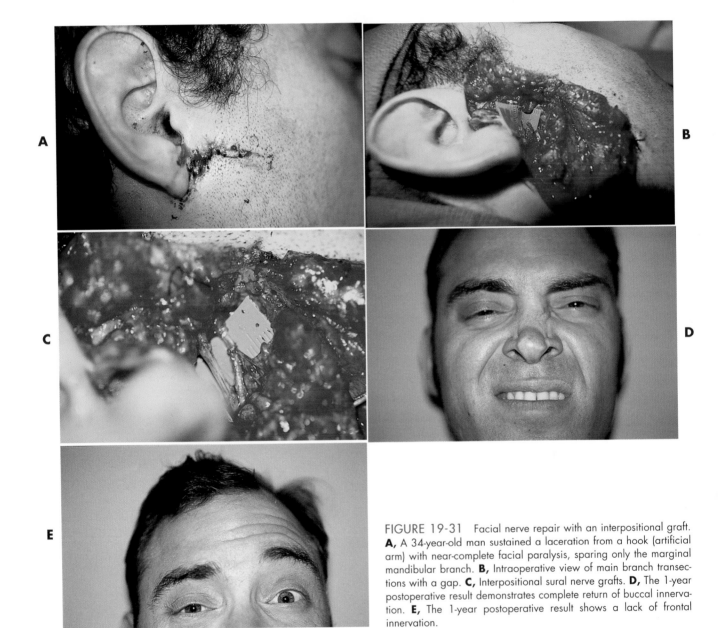

FIGURE 19-31   Facial nerve repair with an interpositional graft. **A,** A 34-year-old man sustained a laceration from a hook (artificial arm) with near-complete facial paralysis, sparing only the marginal mandibular branch. **B,** Intraoperative view of main branch transections with a gap. **C,** Interpositional sural nerve grafts. **D,** The 1-year postoperative result demonstrates complete return of buccal innervation. **E,** The 1-year postoperative result shows a lack of frontal innervation.

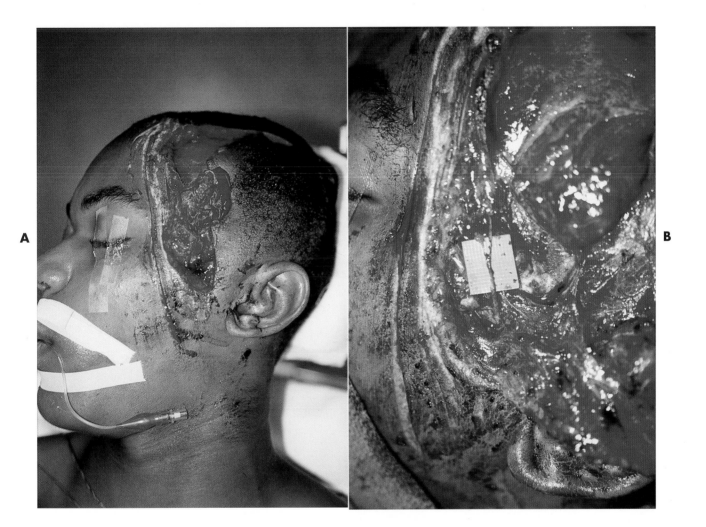

FIGURE 19-32 Transection of the terminal frontal branch of the facial nerve. **A,** A 16-year-old boy sustained severe left temporal lacerations in a motorcycle accident. **B,** Identification and repair of the frontal nerve branch transection. These facial nerve branches usually consist of only one or two fascicles.

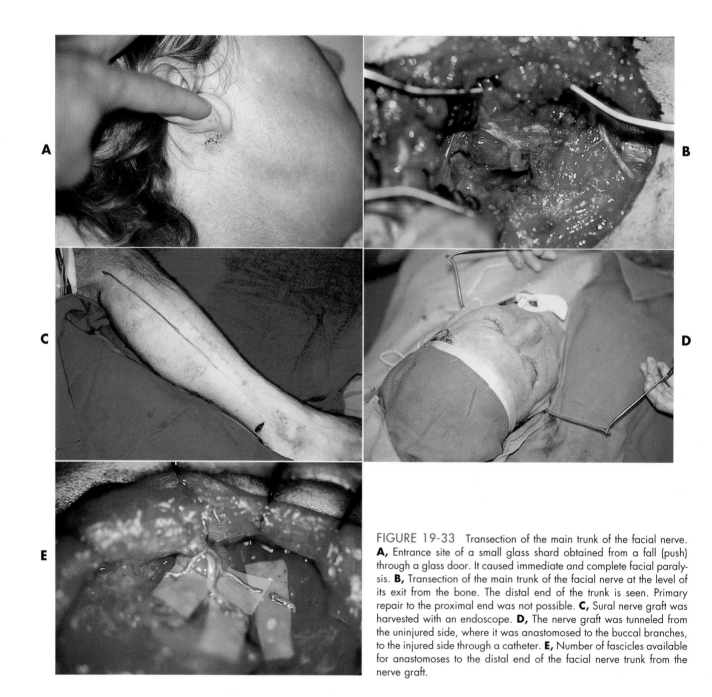

FIGURE 19-33 Transection of the main trunk of the facial nerve. **A,** Entrance site of a small glass shard obtained from a fall (push) through a glass door. It caused immediate and complete facial paralysis. **B,** Transection of the main trunk of the facial nerve at the level of its exit from the bone. The distal end of the trunk is seen. Primary repair to the proximal end was not possible. **C,** Sural nerve graft was harvested with an endoscope. **D,** The nerve graft was tunneled from the uninjured side, where it was anastomosed to the buccal branches, to the injured side through a catheter. **E,** Number of fascicles available for anastomoses to the distal end of the facial nerve trunk from the nerve graft.

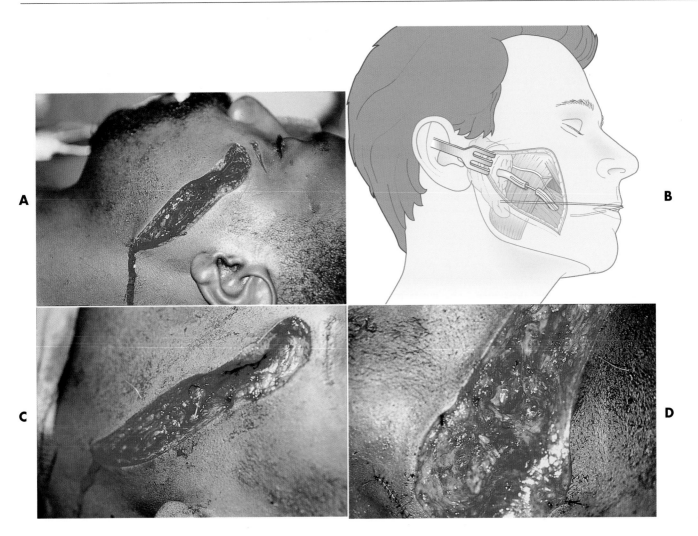

FIGURE 19-34 Parotid duct repair. **A,** A 27-year-old man sustained transfacial laceration by a knife, and parotid duct laceration was suspected. **B,** Diagram of probing of the parotid duct laceration. **C,** Intraoperative probing of the parotid duct laceration. No facial nerve branches were injured. **D,** Repair of the parotid duct laceration over a stent.

within the wound and persists after multiple aspirations, the wound needs to be further explored to ensure that no transection has been missed and the repair has not failed. Persistent collection of saliva in the presence of a restored duct may benefit from the use of botulinum toxin to block the parasympathetic innervation.[17]

REFERENCES

1. Holt GR: Concepts of soft tissue trauma repair. *Otolaryngol Clin North Am* 23:1019-1030, 1990.
2. Sadove AM, Eppley BL: Major craniomaxillofacial reconstruction aided by microsurgical transfer. *J Craniofac Surg* 1:77-87, 1990.
3. Sadove AM, Moore TS, Eppley BL: Total scalp, ear, and eyebrow avulsion: aesthetic adjustment of the replanted tissue. *J Reconstr Microsurg* 6:323-328, 1990.
4. Thomas A: Total face and scalp replantation. *Plast Reconstr Surg* 102:2085-2087, 1998.
5. Schultz RC: Treatment of soft tissue injuries to the face. In Smith JW, Aston SJ, editors: *Plastic surgery*, Boston, 1991, Little, Brown, pp 325-345.
6. Osguthorpe JD, Hoang G: Nasolacrimal injuries: evaluation and management. *Otolaryngol Clin North Am* 24:59-73, 1991.
7. Hammond DC, Bouwese CL, Hankins T, et al: Microsurgical replantation of the amputated nose. *Plast Reconstr Surg* 105:2133-2136, 2000.
8. Zide BM: Deformities of the lips and cheeks. In McCarthy JG, editor: *Plastic surgery*, vol 3, part 2, Philadelphia, 1990, WB Saunders, p 2014.
9. Wong SS: Successful replantation of a bitten-off lower lip: case report. *J Trauma* 47:602-604, 1999.
10. Templer J, Renner GT: Injuries of the external ear. *Otolaryngol Clin North Am* 23:1003-1018, 1990.
11. Concannon MJ, Puckett CL: Microsurgical replantation of an ear in a child without venous repair. *Plast Reconstr Surg* 102:2088-2093, 1999.
12. Pribaz JJ, Crespo CD, Orgill DP, et al: Ear replantation without microsurgery. *Plast Reconstr Surg* 99:1868-1872, 1997.
13. Zuker RM, Eppley BL: Facial reanimation. In Coleman JJ III, editor: *Plastic surgery: indications, operations, and outcomes*, vol III, St Louis, 2000, Mosby, pp 1611-1623.
14. Kelly KJ: Soft-tissue injury to the face. *Oper Tech Plast Reconstr Surg* 5:246-256, 1998.
15. Baker DC: Facial paralysis. In McCarthy JG, editor: *Plastic surgery*, vol 3, part 2, Philadelphia, 1990, WB Saunders, p 2258.
16. Dumpis J, Feldmane L: Experimental microsurgery of salivary ducts in dogs. *J Craniomaxillofac Surg* 29:56-62, 2001.
17. Marchese RR: Management of parotid sialocele with botulinum toxin. *Laryngoscope* 109:344-346, 1999.

CHAPTER 20

Reconstruction of Large Hard and Soft Tissue Loss of the Face

Barry L. Eppley

The distinctive features of the human face and its visibility to other people pose major challenges in facial reconstruction. When large or massive defects of the face are present, these challenges become truly great. Situations that induce extensive injury with such large losses of facial tissue are infrequent outside of wartime, the most common cause being gunshot wounds—either accidental, self-inflicted, or of criminal origin. Gunshots often produce unpredictable patterns of facial injury with large composite defects that may severely compromise multiple orofacial functions including breathing, eating, speaking, and seeing. Rarely, severe motor vehicle, industrial, or home accidents cause extensive damage, but this is usually of a more blunt nature, with crushing and comminution of facial structures rather than large tissue loss. Glass or metal shards may produce long and deep lacerations with underlying bone fractures, but this is usually a less complicated problem than the tissue loss that occurs with high-energy penetrating missiles and the blast effect from discharge of a gun close to the face.

When presented with a patient who has sustained a severe injury with loss of facial tissues, it can be bewildering to know where to begin after the initial resuscitation, control of bleeding, and systemic stabilization. The successful reconstruction of these facial defects involves replacement of much of the missing tissue before significant scarring and contracture have occurred. Such an approach demands early surgical intervention and the knowledge and application of every known reconstructive procedure and often new, creative designs.

GUNSHOT PATHOPHYSIOLOGY

Although large composite facial defects can occur from numerous causes, they are most consistently produced by firearms. This problem is most significant in the United States, where the continued upward trend in firearm injuries will soon eclipse motor vehicles as the leading cause of traumatic death.[1] As more of these facial insults occur, their management benefits from a basic understanding of ballistics and the mechanisms of tissue injury.

Scientific investigation of the interaction of penetrating projectiles with body tissues has a significant history but is often misunderstood in the medical literature. Although a large number of gun and bullet types exist, the mechanisms by which the projectile disrupts tissue are quite basic and are purely mechanical in nature. Initially, the bullet crushes sufficient tissue to make a hole (entrance), through which it penetrates the underlying tissue (permanent cavity). Depending on the caliber and the speed at which the bullet is traveling, the walls of the permanent cavity radiate outward to form a temporary cavity (Fig. 20-1). The permanent cavity exhibits obvious tissue destruction, but the damaging effect in the temporary cavity is variable. A third mechanism, powder gases that follow the bullet out of the barrel and are forced into the tissues, occurs only in wounds in which the gun is in close contact with the skin at the time of firing.[2]

The tissue damage produced by a projectile depends on numerous factors including its shape, construction, and mass, not just its velocity alone. This is best illustrated by comparing three well-known types of bullets, all of which travel at about the same projectile velocity. From a distance of 15 feet, the tissue damage caused by a .22 caliber bullet is less significant than that caused by a .44 Magnum hollow-point bullet. The increased size and deformation of the .44 Magnum bullet on impact account for the greater tissue damage. Both of these pale, however, when compared with the tissue disruption caused by a load of 00 buckshot from a 12-gauge shotgun. The pellets from a shotgun hit so close together that they shred tissue for a diameter of up to 10 cm, causing the greatest harm of any small firearm[2] (Fig. 20-2).

What makes the face unique in most gunshot injuries is that an unimpeded, through-and-through bullet wound occurs in only a minority of cases. The facial bones make up much of the volume of the face, and bone is almost always struck within 1 to 2 cm of the entry point in any facial area. This anatomical difference from the trunk and extremities accounts for two distinct considerations in evaluating and treating gunshot wounds to the face. First, the damage caused by projectiles is a function of tissue density (decreased elasticity). Facial bones, when hit, suffer significant damage, because they have the second highest specific gravity of any body tissue (exceeded only by the enamel of the teeth). Second, when bullets entering the face hit bone, they deform or yaw. Yaw causes them to change direction, altering their original straight path. Yawing of deformed bullets results in an unpredictable path, producing a large temporary cavity and damaging more tissue (Fig. 20-3). Such behavior demands a thorough search for potential injury in all craniofacial areas, not just the structures between the entrance wound and the exit site, if an exit site exists at all (Fig. 20-4).

WOUND CLASSIFICATION

Certain patterns of facial injury caused by penetrating missiles have been reported in the literature. These are based on either the path of the missile (entrance and exit wound) or the pattern of tissue injury or loss that occurs. The four general patterns of involvement for gunshot wounds are the frontal cranium, the orbit, the lower midface, and the mandible (Fig. 20-5). The location of the exit wound provides a rough guide to the pattern, which is most accurately predicted by the locations of the entrance and exit wounds. In general, skin and bone complications are less severe in the upper face and cranial area. In the lower face, there is greater comminution of fractures and damage to the intraoral lining.[3]

More clinically useful is an appreciation of the zones of facial tissue injury and tissue loss based on the patterns of gunshot wounds. These include the central face, the lateral mandible, the lateral midface and orbit, and the lateral cranium and orbit (Fig. 20-6). In each case, a wide zone of

FIGURE 20-1 Characteristic wound profile of a bullet traveling through tissue. Notice the large amount of tissue destruction (detached muscle) and the size of the temporary cavity compared with the permanent cavity. The false belief that a bullet damages tissue in direct proportion to its velocity is widespread. Tissue destruction is based as much on bullet shape and construction as on its velocity.

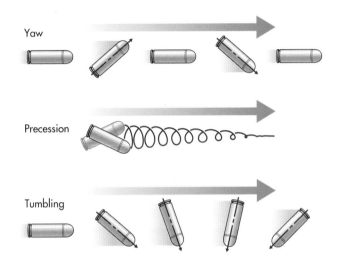

FIGURE 20-3 Variations in the motion of bullets that lead to greater tissue damage. These variations are usually caused by the bullet's striking facial bones after entering the skin and can radically change its straight-line course through the face.

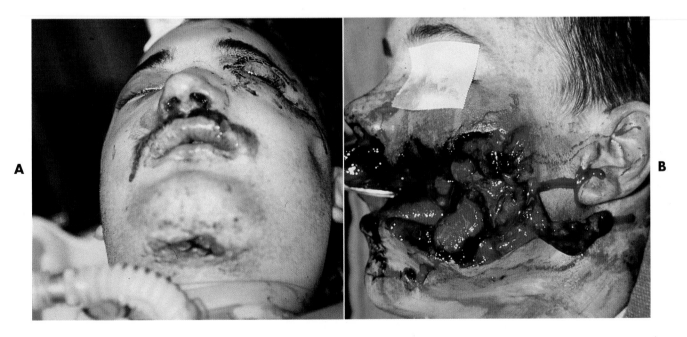

FIGURE 20-2 Differences in facial damage caused by two different bullet types that travel at roughly the same velocity and were fired at roughly the same distance from the face. **A,** A .38 caliber handgun. **B,** A 20-gauge shotgun.

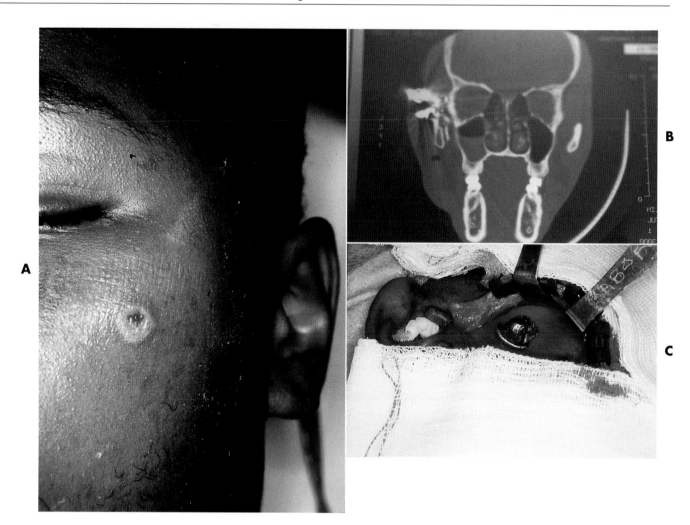

FIGURE 20-4 Dramatic change of bullet path caused by striking facial bone. Patient was shot on one side of the face (malar area), and the bullet ended up on same side of the face (temporal area). **A,** Left malar entrance site. **B,** Axial computed tomographic image of left temporal location of bullet. **C,** Location of bullet in left temporal area. The bullet was removed due to masticatory pain.

hard and soft tissue injury surrounds a smaller zone of actual hard and soft tissue loss. The important point is to appreciate that the zone of injury is more expansive than that of tissue loss and must be factored into the plan of reconstruction.

STATE-OF-THE-ART MANAGEMENT: BASIC PRINCIPLES

The historical approach to early management of ballistic injuries to the face included multiple débridements, daily dressing changes, and delayed reconstruction. This was fostered and appeared rational based on the rate of complications that developed when early reconstruction was undertaken, which included infection, wound breakdown with necrosis, and ultimate collapse of the reconstructed facial segments. The application of craniofacial surgical and diagnostic techniques has revolutionized the management of blunt facial injuries but still frequently fails in cases of gunshot facial wounds if the fundamental differences between these two types of facial

injuries are not appreciated. Recognition of the absence of tissue and the devascularized, compromised quality of some of the remaining hard and soft facial tissues is paramount in choosing the appropriate reconstructive techniques and the timing of their application.

The facial gunshot wound, first and foremost, must be controlled by débridement of necrotic, nonviable tissue; elimination or evacuation of hematoma and infection; obliteration of dead space with vascularized tissue; and re-creation of adequate skin and mucosal lining.[1] In addition to understanding this most important conceptual approach, the initial management of facial gunshot wounds should take into account several basic principles derived from the unique anatomy of the face and the behavior of penetrating missiles.

TREAT THE WOUND, NOT THE WEAPON

The exact gun type and circumstances that caused the facial wound, while of interest, do not guide or alter the subsequent

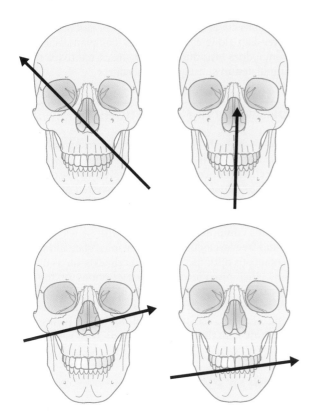

FIGURE 20-5   General patterns of facial gunshot wounds: frontal cranium, orbit, midface, and mandible. The locations of the entrance and exit wounds are a rough guide to the type of pattern. *(Adapted from Clark N, Birely B, Robertson B et al: High-energy ballistic and avulsive facial injuries: classification, patterns, and an algorithm for primary reconstruction. Plast Reconstr Surg 98:583-601, 1996.)*

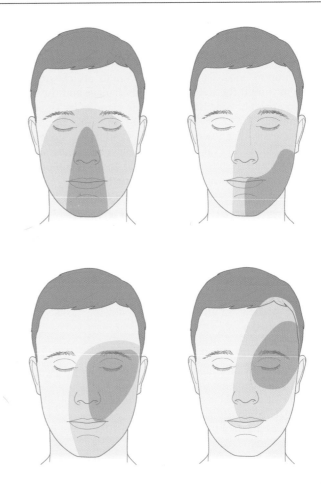

FIGURE 20-6   Zones of facial involvement based on the pattern of the facial gunshot wound: central face (*upper left*), lateral face and mandible (*upper right*), midface and orbit (*lower left*), and orbit and skull (*lower right*). Zones of tissue loss (entrance and exit wounds) are blacked out, and the surrounding zones of tissue injury are indicated by diagonal lines. *(Adapted from Clark N, Birely B, Robertson B et al: High-energy ballistic and avulsive facial injuries: classification, patterns, and an algorithm for primary reconstruction. Plast Reconstr Surg 98:583-601, 1996.)*

surgical management. Victims and observers of gunshot wounds are unreliable and frequently misrepresent many of the events of the shooting, particularly the type of weapon and the distance of fire. Focus on the facial damage present, and do not concern yourself with the details of the gun. The only gun-specific information that really matters is whether it was a single-bullet or a multiple-pellet firearm. However, the facial wound itself usually makes this obvious. Much is made of whether the penetrating missile is of high or low velocity, but this does not usually change the required treatment.

PROVIDE PRIMARY CARE AFTER BASIC TRAUMA RESUSCITATION

In patients with significant injuries and severe facial tissue damage, management of the airway is of supreme importance. Intubation, or preferably tracheostomy, should be liberally done. In addition to solving issues of early airway patency and obstructive bleeding, this facilitates the numerous subsequent reconstructive procedures. Oral or nasal intubation often hinders proper access for the reconstruction, even many months later. It is not uncommon to keep a tracheostomy or feeding tube in place for up to 1 year after the injury in cases of severe facial tissue loss. Patients tolerate

airway and feeding tubes well, and they do not preclude breathing around the tracheostomy tube or oral feeding between reconstructive surgeries.

PROVIDE ADEQUATE ANTIBIOTIC COVERAGE IN THE IMMEDIATE INJURY STATE

A bullet is not sterilized by being fired. Penetrating projectiles carry bacteria into the wound. When combined with the presence of devitalized tissues and open wounds, a near-ideal bacterial culture medium may exist that can overcome even the superior blood supply of the face. Group A β-hemolytic streptococci and clostridia were historically reported from battlefield gunshot wounds but have been almost eliminated since the development of antibiotics during World War II. A broad-spectrum cephalosporin or penicillinase-resistant antibiotic should be given. Subsequent surgeries are covered as for any other facial reconstructive procedure.

MAINTAIN A HIGH LEVEL OF SUSPICION FOR VASCULAR INJURY

By definition, most facial gunshot wounds are classified as being in zone II (between the cricoid cartilage and the mandibular angle) or zone III (between the mandibular angle and the skull base). Vascular injury in these zones may be obscure and not easily diagnosed by clinical examination. Computed tomographic (CT) evaluation is especially helpful for assessment of major vessels and the cranial and orbital contents. When in doubt, consider carotid angiography.

PROVIDE INITIAL SURGICAL TREATMENT WITH MINIMAL DÉBRIDEMENT AND PRIMARY CLOSURE

After stabilization, the patient should be taken to the operating room as soon as possible. This permits a thorough wound exploration and determination of what type of reconstruction will be needed. At this time, the following tasks can be accomplished:

- Remove loose teeth and bone.
- Remove obvious bullet fragments, but do not dissect and retrieve fragments that lie deep.
- Débride only obviously nonviable tissue.
- Irrigate copiously with saline.
- Close as much of the soft tissue as possible, going from the inside out.
- Stabilize facial bones by direct plate and screw and maxillomandibular fixation if enough teeth and jaw structures are present, or use an external mandibular or cranial halo (midface) fixator if large bone segments lack continuity and flail segments are present.

PLAN FOR EARLY RECONSTRUCTION WITH TISSUE REPLACEMENT

Early reconstruction with tissue replacement is the cornerstone of contemporary reconstruction of large facial defects. Early replacement of hard and soft tissue deficits provides the best long-term results. Until recently, treatment consisted of initial wound débridement, packing of extensive defects, and serial dressing changes followed by surgical débridement procedures until soft tissue closure could be achieved. Concerns about contamination and lack of reliability of local tissues were overriding themes. It is now clear that there is no facial advantage to allowing the wound to heal by secondary intention or skin grafting of open wounds before reconstruction is initiated. The historical approach allowed a tremendous amount of scar formation and contracture to occur, making the formal reconstruction attempts much more difficult and often leading to partial or patchwork results. Facial tissue should be replaced as soon as the patient is stable and the margins of wound viability are clear.[4] Neurological and ophthalmological injuries frequently cause the initial reconstruction to be delayed, but often it can still be performed within the first weeks after injury. A pre-reconstruction CT scan, preferably three-dimensional, can be very informative as to the extent of missing bone.[5]

The contemporary approach employs liberal use of microvascular tissue transfers to replace missing bone, oral lining, and cutaneous cover, often in a single operation. Although a single free flap alone cannot provide complete facial reconstruction, it does introduce healthy, unscarred tissue that can be manipulated in subsequent procedures.

RECONSTRUCTIVE FLAP OPTIONS

The concept of early tissue replacement in extensive traumatic facial wounds is very similar to the reconstruction of facial defects after oncologic resection. Knowledge of a variety of tissue flaps, some that must be transferred as free tissue and others pedicled in design, provides powerful reconstructive options that permit early facial intervention. These include flaps composed of free bone with or without a skin paddle and free fasciocutaneous, free muscular, and pedicled fasciocutaneous options. Several superb texts are available on this topic that provide detailed descriptions of the entire scope of tissue flap anatomy, and the reader is referred to these for descriptive detail and operative guidance.[6] The following sections are not meant to be all-inclusive but describe those flaps that are commonly used for facial gunshot wounds.

FREE FIBULAR FLAP

The fibula is the longest bone that can be transferred by microsurgical techniques. It is often described as an ideal mandibular replacement in terms of bony stock, but this is not entirely accurate. It has very similar cross-sectional thickness but inadequate vertical height—usually less than half that of a normal dentate mandible. Its available length, up to 24 cm, does allow it to be used for long bone defects. The pedicle is large and very reliable, and septocutaneous branches make formation of a significant skin paddle possible. It is a truly expendable long bone with little donor morbidity other than an external scar if properly harvested.

Fibular transfer depends on the endosteal and periosteal blood supplies from the peroneal artery. The endosteal circulation is supplied through a nutrient artery that typically enters the middle third of the fibula. The pedicle of the peroneal artery is rather short, usually about 6 to 8 cm at best. A single central artery with a diameter of 2 to 3 mm is surrounded by two venae comitantes. In addition to the nutrient and periosteal vessels to the fibula, the peroneal artery gives off multiple branches to all of the surrounding muscles of the leg and to the lateral leg skin. There are two to six cutaneous perforating branches of the peroneal artery which travel along the posterior crural septum and through the soleus and flexor hallucis longus muscles. They supply a longitudinally oriented area of skin that can be raised as a septofasciocutaneous flap with the central axis along the posterior crural septum (Fig. 20-7A).

The fibular free flap is most commonly used for mandibular reconstruction, particularly of the symphysis and angle, where osteotomies may be required to provide a three-dimensional reconstruction. When used with a skin paddle, it offers replacement of the external skin, lip, or lining of the buccal mucosa or floor of the mouth[7,8] (see Fig. 20-7B,C). If only a small amount of bone is needed, such as in reconstruction of the anterior maxilla, a long vascular pedicle can be created by use of the more distal end of the bone.

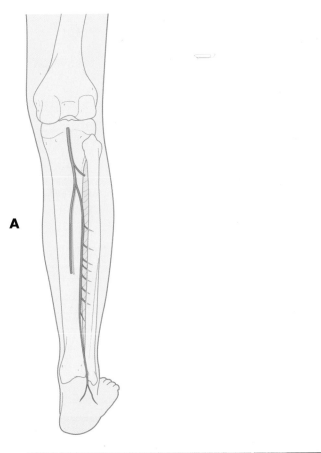

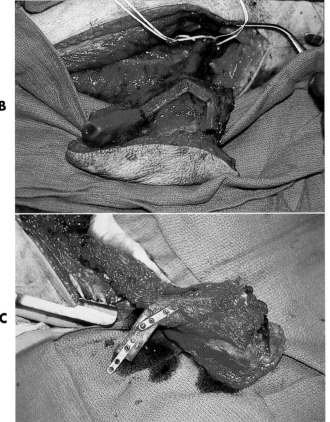

FIGURE 20-7   Fibular free flap. **A,** Peroneal blood supply. **B,** Large segments of mandible can be replaced; this requires multiple osteotomies and shaping of the fibula. **C,** The need for shorter bone lengths creates a longer vascular pedicle by using the distal end.

FREE SCAPULAR FLAP

The scapular flap has gained utility because it provides good bone stock with a large pedicle that is long and relatively easy to find. The circumflex scapular pedicle is a branch of the subscapular system, with a pedicle length of 5 to 6 cm and vessel diameters up to 2.5 mm. The direct vascular connection between the circumflex scapular artery and the periosteum of the scapula makes osseous transfer possible. The lateral border of the scapula provides a 10- to 14-cm segment of straight bone located between the glenoid fossa and the tip of the scapula.[9] The lateral inferior axillary border of the scapula also receives a periosteal pedicle (angular) from a branch of the thoracodorsal artery and associated venae comitantes. If the thoracodorsal branch is included with the circumflex scapular pedicle, a second vascularized bone segment may be designed with the scapular flap.[10] The overlying soft tissue can be harvested with the bone transfer, either with or without the overlying skin. The skin is thick and hairless and has only a thin layer of subcutaneous fat, which is usually advantageous in the face. The donor site can be closed primarily, even when a skin paddle is used, and the back scar is often wide but acceptable. One of its most significant advantages is the wide arc of movement between the skin paddle and the osseous portion of the flap, which is related to the differing transverse (skin paddle) and descending (bone) branches of the circumflex scapular pedicle (Fig. 20-8).

The scapular region also provides an excellent source of vascularized fasciocutaneous tissue, which was used long before its potential for bone transfer was recognized. The soft tissue is based on the horizontal or descending branch of the circumflex scapular artery in either a horizontal (scapular) or vertically oriented (parascapular) design. This provides thin, pliable tissue, up to 10 cm in width with skin attached, or larger if only the fascial component is required.

The one disadvantage to the scapular flap is the necessity for significant arm rotation to properly visualize and dissect the pedicle through the triangular space. This precludes a two-team approach with simultaneous flap elevation and facial recipient site preparation.

Use of the scapular free flap has been described for both mandibular and maxillary bone reconstruction. It is a good choice when a straight piece of bone is required. The use of a skin paddle with bone makes it useful for a variety of composite defects about the orofacial and orbitomaxillary regions. The fascial or fasciocutaneous component alone provides an excellent source of vascularized soft tissue fill.

FREE RADIAL FLAP

The radial forearm provides a potentially large, thin fasciocutaneous free flap on the ventral surface. It was historically described as a useful osteocutaneous flap, but the radius is a poor source of good bone stock and places the donor bone at a significant risk of postoperative fracture. If bone is needed, other free flap options (e.g., fibula, scapula) are usually better. The forearm should be used as a source of thin soft tissue only.

Almost all or any part of the skin and fascia extending from the antecubital fossa to the wrist may be elevated based on the radial artery and its septocutaneous branches. The more distal the skin flap is designed, the longer the pedicle

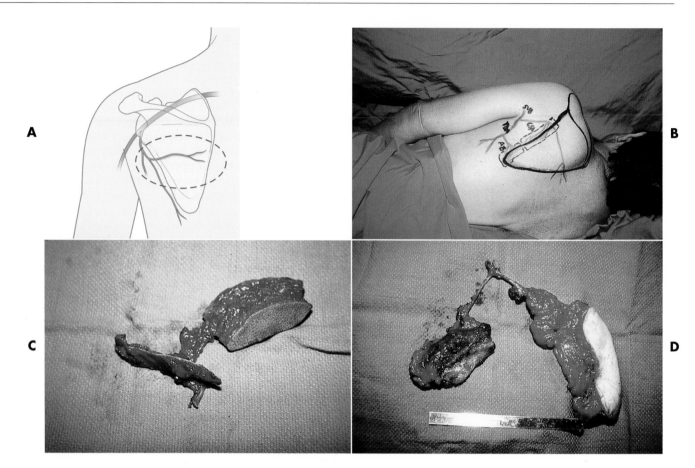

FIGURE 20-8   Scapular free flap. **A** and **B,** Subscapular blood supply with two distinct branches to the lateral border of the scapula. **C,** Lateral scapular bone graft with skin island (common scapular artery). **D,** Bipedicled design with the inferior edge of the scapula based on the ascending branch.

will be. The radial artery is of good size (2.5 mm) and has a very consistent anatomy; it courses between the bellies of the brachioradialis and pronator teres in the upper forearm and between the tendons of the brachioradialis and flexor carpi radialis in the lower forearm. Most of the septocutaneous-fasciocutaneous branches are in the distal half of the radial artery and are easily identified emerging from the intermuscular septum, which must be preserved during harvest, at the radial border of the flexor carpi radialis muscle[11] (Fig. 20-9).

The radial forearm flap has numerous advantages as a soft tissue source, including a large amount of thin tissue, a long and large pedicle, and ease of harvest. These qualities make it particularly well suited for lining intraoral defects or as an external skin cover.[12] However, the harvest of a flap from an extremity requires several precautions to avoid significant donor site complications. It is essential that the inflow to the hand be preoperatively evaluated with an Allen test to confirm that circulation through the ulnar artery is sufficient for survival of the hand. This should be reconfirmed during flap dissection by placement of a microvascular clamp distally and release of the tourniquet before division of the radial artery. The peritenon covering the tendons of the flexor carpi radialis, brachioradialis, and finger flexors must be preserved to avoid skin graft failure and possible loss of the tendons postoperatively.

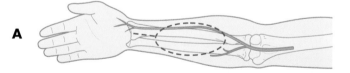

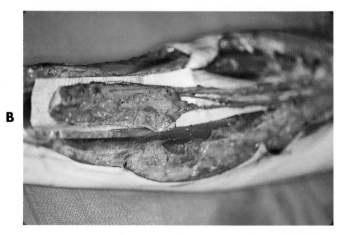

FIGURE 20-9   Radial forearm flap. **A,** Radial blood supply. **B,** Thin fasciocutaneous components of the flap (turned over).

FREE LATISSIMUS FLAP

The latissimus dorsi is a large, flat, triangular muscle that offers the largest source of well-vascularized soft tissue in the body, measuring up to 25×35 cm in size. Its tendon attaches to the humerus proximally with broad attachments to the lower thoracic and sacral vertebrae, the posterior iliac crest, and the external abdominal muscles. Although it is responsible for adduction, extension, and rotation of the humerus, it is a completely expendable muscle in most patients as long as they have intact synergistic shoulder girdle musculature. Its dominant pedicle is the thoracodorsal artery and venae comitantes, which is a major branch off the subscapular artery. The thoracodorsal pedicle (2.5 mm in vessel size) offers reasonable length, approximately 8 cm, but this can be significantly extended if the distal portion of the muscle is the only tissue required. A reliable, large skin paddle can also be obtained, because there are extensive vascular communications to the overlying back skin.[13] When a skin paddle is taken, the donor site can almost always be primarily closed. Whereas rotation of the muscle into the head and neck area can be done around the axilla with tunneling on top of the pectoralis muscle, it will extend only to the lower face and may potentially be compromised by compression of the overlying tissues. It is of far greater utility when transferred as a free microvascular flap (Fig. 20-10).

The latissimus dorsi free flap has numerous applications in reconstruction of the face. Over the past 20 years, it has been equally applied to the midface and the mandible with great reliability.[14] Its wide muscular expanse makes it uniquely suited for extensive scalp replacement and calvarial coverage when combined with skin grafting. The reliability of its skin paddle can provide for reconstruction of large defects of the external skin cover, particularly in the lateral face. The patient position necessary for harvest does make it difficult for a simultaneous two-team approach, but the speed at which the flap can be raised makes this of little significance.

FREE RECTUS FLAP

The paired, vertically oriented rectus muscles of the abdomen provide another reliable donor source for vascularized tissue. This long, flat muscle, measuring about 6 cm in width and 25 cm in length, is easy to harvest because of its constant anatomy, and this can be done simultaneously with facial work in a two-team approach. It lies within an anterior and posterior fascial sheath, and its dissection is complicated only by the release of the tenacious attachments of three sets of horizontal inscriptions. Although there are dual dominant pedicles, the inferior epigastric is always used because of its larger size, longer length, and easier dissection. Entering at the underside of the lateral surface of the muscle, the inferior epigastric is about 2.5 mm in diameter with a fairly short pedicle length of 4 to 5 cm.[15] The length of the muscle typically makes the usable pedicle length longer than that of the actual vessels. A vertical or horizontally oriented skin paddle can be taken, but this is rarely done in facial reconstruction. The donor site, even if a skin paddle is taken, can always be primarily closed. Previous abdominal surgery with any horizontal scar across the rectus territory precludes its use.

The musculocutaneous territories supplied by the inferior epigastric have their greatest use in breast reconstruction, but

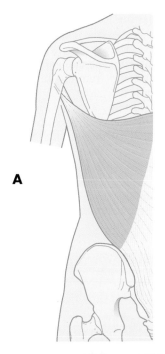

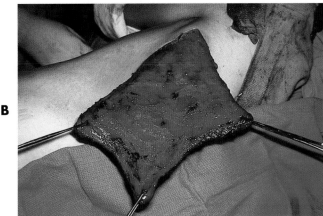

FIGURE 20-10 Latissimus dorsi flap. **A,** Muscle location. **B,** Size of muscle harvested through a lateral thoracic incision.

they also have significant value in a variety of head and neck sites. When combined with a skin graft, they can be used for outer coverage of scalp and skull defects[16] and as vascularized fill for a wide variety of lower facial wounds. The long length of the muscle rarely makes its short pedicle length a problem (Fig. 20-11). However, extending the pedicle into the neck for anastomosis requires a very wide subcutaneous tunnel to avoid postoperative venous congestion of the flap.

FREE SERRATUS FLAP

The free serratus flap provides a very long pedicled musculofascial flap that has excellent utility for facial applications.[17] Its long pedicle (15-20 cm) combined with the length of muscle and fascia can easily reach the midface when anastomosed into the neck. It can be raised with both skin and muscle, but the amount of rib obtained is not sufficient for most facial reconstructive needs. The serratus is a thin, broad muscle that originates from the outer surface of ribs 8 and 9 and inserts on the ventral surface of the scapula. It has a dual blood supply from the lateral thoracic artery and branches of the thoracodorsal artery. Most commonly, the flap is based on the thoracodorsal branch as it emanates from the under-surface of the latissimus dorsi, because it is easier to elevate. The serratus has very predictable anatomy and is easy to identify and dissect out between the lateral borders of the latissimus and the pectoralis, tracing the pedicle up into the axilla (Fig. 20-12).

PEDICLED FOREHEAD FLAP

The median forehead flap is primarily used for nasal coverage and reconstruction. The forehead is the single best source of

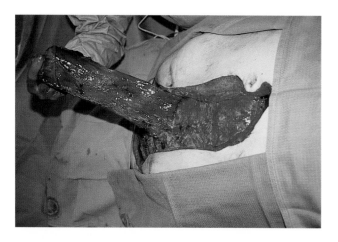

FIGURE 20-11   Rectus muscle flap. This is the muscle raised on the superior pedicle that is not used for free tissue transfer (inferior pedicle). The length and width of the muscle can be appreciated, however.

external nasal skin replacement; its color and thickness are similar to those of the nose. The supratrochlear vessels are the dominant pedicle and supply the entire central forehead skin, including the frontalis, corrugator, and procerus. These vessels are a terminal branch of the ophthalmic artery; they are 1 mm in diameter and have a short (1-2 cm) pedicle length. Because this a rotational flap, these dimensions are of no significance other than to appreciate that the vessels emerge over the supraorbital rim deep to the frontalis and may easily be injured during dissection of the flap. The supra-orbital vessels are a minor pedicle but should be preserved if possible. The base of the flap can be fairly narrow compared with the distal end and may be skeletonized down to the vessels to aid the 180 degrees of flap rotation that is usually required. The flap length is determined by the height of the frontal hairline; usually, at least 7 to 8 cm is necessary to cover the most distal nasal defects. With low hairlines, an oblique flap orientation improves flap length.

In extensive defects involving the nasal tip, columella, and upper lip, a "gull-wing" design at the distal end of the flap design is often used.[18] In large nasal defects, tissue expansion of the flap itself should be avoided due to unfavorable post-operative contraction. However, preoperative tissue expansion lateral to the flap can aid greatly in donor site closure[19] (Fig. 20-13).

REGIONAL CONSIDERATIONS

CENTRAL FACE

Lower Face and Mandible

The lower face and mandible is the facial area most frequently affected in severe gunshot wounds, which are usually

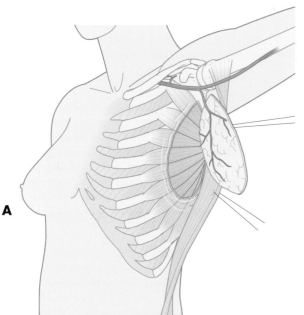

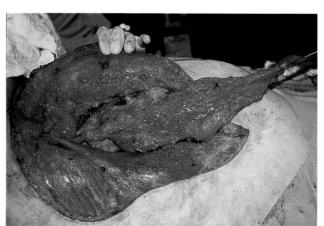

FIGURE 20-12   Serratus muscle flap. **A,** Thoracodorsal blood supply of the serratus muscle. **B,** The muscle can be long and narrow with a very long vascular pedicle.

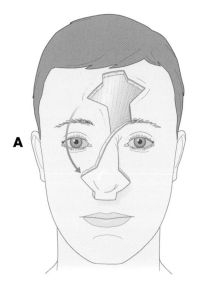

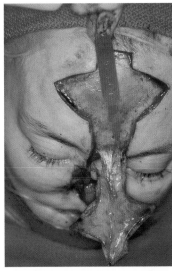

FIGURE 20-13   Median forehead flap. **A,** Maximal flap design of forehead flap. **B,** Raising of the flap design based on the supratrochlear vessels (*red arrow*).

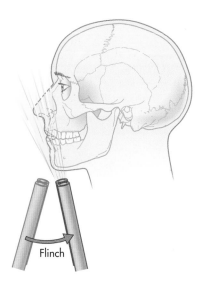

FIGURE 20-14   Classic angle of gunshot impact from a self-inflicted injury. The flinch makes it a nonlethal wound but often eliminates much of the anterior facial structures.

self-inflicted. This typical injury is produced when the patient fires under the chin with the neck hyperextended (Fig. 20-14). Usually, only the anterior lower and midface is blown off, resulting in a nonlethal injury. The lateral mandible with attached masseter and temporalis muscles are sufficiently posterior and internal that they often are spared and continue to provide excursion to the lower jaw. Loss of the anterior mandible and lip and their importance in breathing, speech, and mastication make destruction of this orofacial region a serious functional handicap. The functional abnormalities may be further aggravated if significant damage has occurred to the tongue and surrounding muscles that are attached to the anterior mandible. Bony reconstruction of the anterior mandible helps provide a stable suspension of the hyocervical musculature, whereas soft tissue reconstruction of the lip and chin allows oral continence to be restored. If significant tongue muscle is lost or severe scarring has occurred on the

floor of the mouth, this dynamic soft tissue complex will sorely be missed and can only poorly, if at all, be replaced or reconstructed. At best, we can only replace the lining defect and possibly provide a mechanical dam that can aid in speech and deglutition.

The reconstruction of this submental injury includes restoring the continuity of the three major components that are usually lost: the lining, bony structures, and external cover. During the first procedure after the initial injury, obvious devitalized soft tissue should be débrided and bony stabilization of the flailed lateral mandibular segments carried out. This can be done with a reconstruction plate (preferably) or with an external fixator. It is perfectly acceptable to have the reconstruction plate exposed in the immediate postoperative period, because the chin tissues may be missing. This poses no significant increase in the risk of infection, and its exposure will shortly be remedied by a free flap reconstruction. We prefer use of the reconstruction plate to an external fixator, which creates additional scarring in the uninjured lateral facial skin and is usually in the way for placement of the free flap and neck microvascular anastomoses.

Almost always, the use of free vascularized bone for anterior mandibular reconstruction is desired as the second stage of reconstruction. This may follow the initial débridement and stabilization as soon as the patient is able, often within the first 10 to 14 days of hospital admission. Even in small segmental bone loss (<6 cm), vascularized bone offers numerous advantages over any other method. Reconstruction can be performed immediately and regardless of the amount of soft tissue present; it does not rely on surrounding tissue vascularity for survival; it does not disturb other local anatomy and can offer a single-stage solution to the tissue loss problem. Bone donor options are essentially three: radius, scapula, and fibula. The fibula is preferred because it has ample bone and a long pedicle of good vessel caliber (particularly if only the distal portion is used). It can be shaped to some degree by selective osteotomies and is fairly easy to harvest because its anatomy is consistent with no significant postoperative morbidity.

The radius has much thinner bone of more limited quality and creates a very noticeable donor site. The scapula is an excellent source of vascularized bone, but it can be more difficult to harvest and precludes simultaneous work on the face and back because of positioning needs (Fig. 20-15).

Repair of the lining deficit is often ignored or not considered important, but such deficits frequently cause late functional disturbances. The loss of lining is usually greatest between the lip and anterior mandible. This poses great problems for the long-term stability of any reconstructed vertical lip height and for a pliable separation from the alveolus if dental restoration must be done and hygienically maintained. In theory, elevation and rotation of surrounding oral and buccal mucosa can provide some coverage. In reality, these flaps look good in drawings but cannot reach the midline and often do not survive after transfer. The use of tongue flaps is appealing, because they can easily be drawn up over a reconstruction plate or anterior bony reconstruction. However, they should be avoided, because they lead to speech and deglutition problems and induce the potential for future restriction in tongue mobility. For these reasons, the skin paddle of a vascularized bone transfer offers a versatile and robust fascial and skin composite reconstruction. All of the commonly used free bone flaps previously described can be used as composite flaps with fascia and skin if desired.

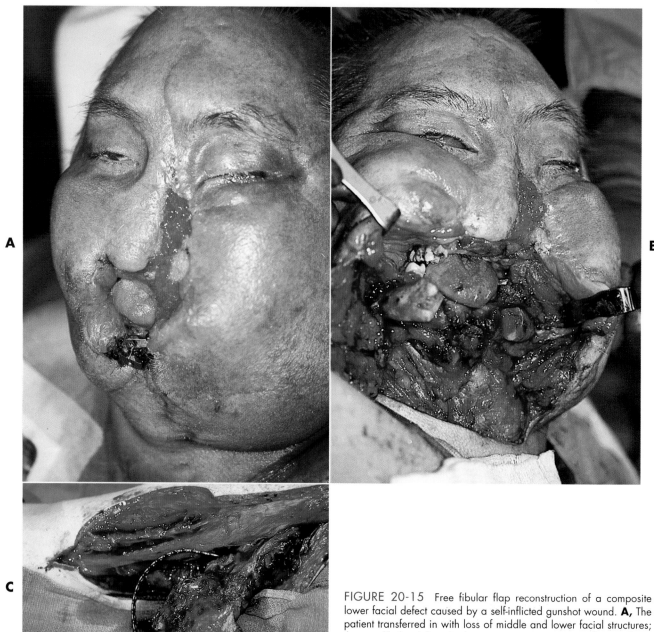

FIGURE 20-15 Free fibular flap reconstruction of a composite lower facial defect caused by a self-inflicted gunshot wound. **A,** The patient transferred in with loss of middle and lower facial structures; the mandibular defects had a spanning reconstruction plate in place. **B,** The lower facial defect is exposed, and the old reconstruction plate is removed. **C,** Fibular donor site with composite flap. The bone has been osteotomized and shaped according to a template from a new reconstruction plate.

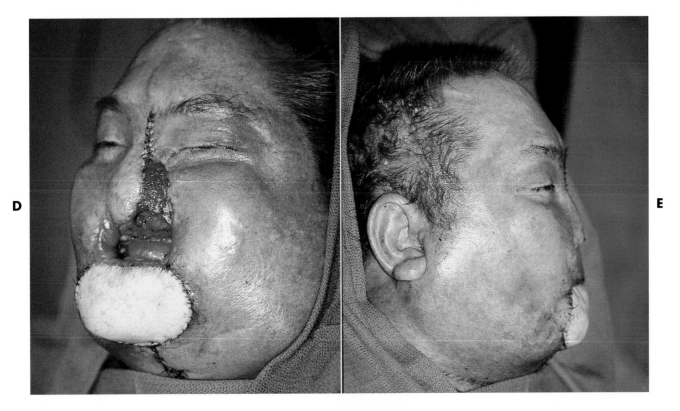

D

E

FIGURE 20-15, cont'd **D,** Frontal view of free fibular flap in position with leg skin used for chin and submental skin replacement. The skin color and texture never match, and this has to be accepted. **E,** Lateral view of reconstruction.

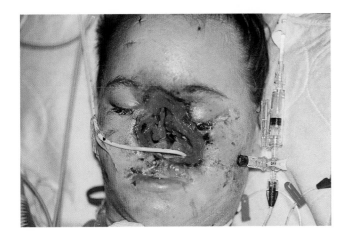

FIGURE 20-16 Midfacial avulsion caused by the patient's being struck by a flying tire cleat from a racecar that struck the wall. Such a nonlethal but composite midfacial avulsion injury is very rare.

Midface

The midface is often impacted obliquely from an inferior angle due to a submentally directed gunshot. A direct midface impact is seldom seen, because this is usually a lethal injury (Fig. 20-16). Midface wounds are frequently part of a concomitant pattern of tissue loss that includes the anterior mandible, lip, and chin as well as the upper lip, anterior maxilla, and nose.

Such injuries to the midface are the most difficult of all facial injuries to reconstruct because of the shape and contour of the component parts. Many small and delicate bone and soft tissue elements are present, as are a labyrinth of air spaces, cavities, and canals. Reconstruction of the lining of these delicate structures can, at times, be an impossible task. Whereas the lining of the upper aerodigestive tract can fill in rather quickly with granulation tissue from neighboring areas, the ultimate result is collapse of the overlying soft tissue and complete obliteration of nasal breathing and sinus drainage. The presence of these air-filled cavities throughout the midface also imposes an increased risk of postoperative infection and makes it very difficult to build anatomical structures on top of such cavities. Reconstructive efforts are also complicated by the prominent position of the midface with the protruding and individualized nose, which is such an important element in the recognition of one's face.

The typical gunshot wound creates a cone of injury which, after cautious débridement, leaves a large central facial defect without support. With smaller defects and limited soft tissue loss, immediate reconstruction with free bone grafts and local coverage can be done. However, this is the exceptional case. Most of these defects involve significant tissue loss, making this approach impractical. Even those midfacial defects that appear small are almost always missing important lining of the mouth or nose that is certain to ultimately compromise any limited approach. The absence of lining and the presence of the sinuses and open communication with the mouth and nose make it mandatory to both control the wound and replace lining and bone. This is best done, simultaneously or through various stages, with vascularized tissue.

In smaller facial gunshot wounds, the entrance wound is usually more diminutive than the amount of internal hard and soft tissue loss. In these cases, the nose is often spared, and the defect is primarily intraoral. The thin bone of the maxilla and the tight tissue of the alveolus and vestibule make transfer of any local tissue difficult. Vascularized fibula works well for replacement of missing maxilla (Fig. 20-17). It offers a long pedicle that is ideal for reaching the neck vessels by tunneling subcutaneously from the facial wound into the neck. A skin paddle usually is not necessary, because the

muscle cuff on the fibular bone rapidly becomes covered with mucosa (see Fig. 20-17D). If more lining is needed, a skin paddle of more than adequate dimensions can be carried with the bone, although this is often quite bulky in the limited confines of the midface and mouth. This bone also provides excellent bone stock into which endosseous implants can be eventually placed (see Fig. 20-17F).

With moderate tissue loss from midfacial gunshot wounds, some portion of the upper or lower lips is usually involved or missing. This is far more common than a midfacial injury without lip involvement. Reconstruction of this composite midfacial wound must provide not only bone and lip

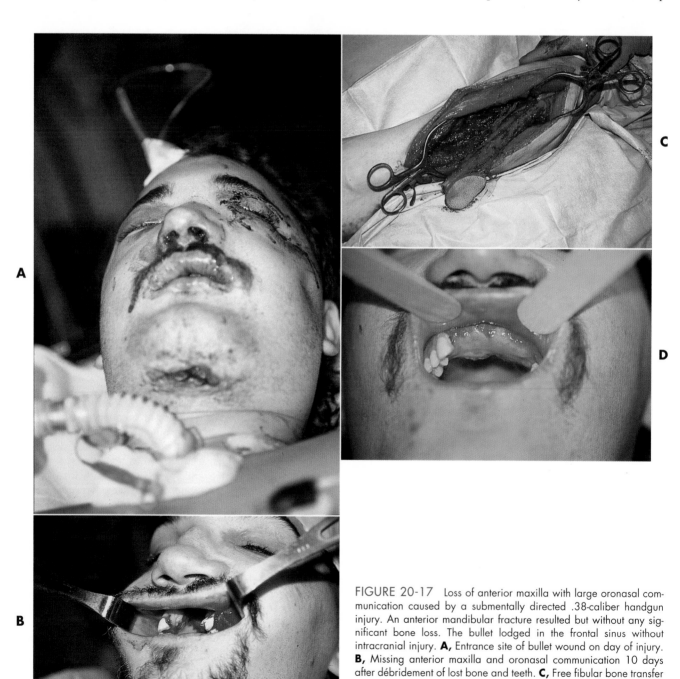

FIGURE 20-17   Loss of anterior maxilla with large oronasal communication caused by a submentally directed .38-caliber handgun injury. An anterior mandibular fracture resulted but without any significant bone loss. The bullet lodged in the frontal sinus without intracranial injury. **A,** Entrance site of bullet wound on day of injury. **B,** Missing anterior maxilla and oronasal communication 10 days after débridement of lost bone and teeth. **C,** Free fibular bone transfer using the very distal end of the bone and discarding the skin paddle, thus creating a very long vascular pedicle. **D,** Three months after reconstruction, the muscle over the bone is completely covered with mucosa.

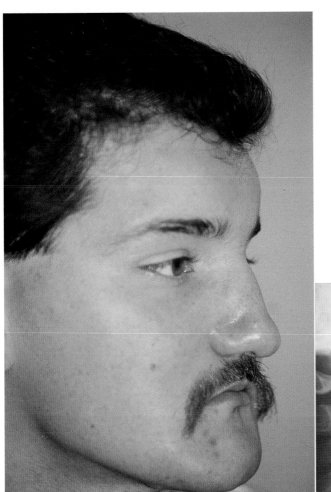

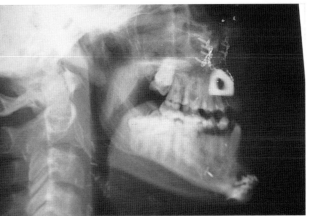

E   F

FIGURE 20-17, cont'd   **E,** Lateral facial view with reasonable horizontal projection taken 3 months after surgery. **F,** Two-year postoperative radiograph showing cross-section of fibular bone in the anterior maxilla.

replacement but also a vestibule. In some instances, one lip is left relatively unaffected (ideally, the lower lip), allowing an eventual cross-lip transfer, which is the best solution to any upper lip and vestibule problem. Reconstruction takes place in two major stages: an initial microvascular bone flap for replacement of the missing maxilla, followed by a regional cross-lip transfer (Fig. 20-18). If the amount of missing upper lip is significant (50% or more) or the lower lip is concomitantly damaged, lip reconstruction may have to be done by incorporating the lip replacement from the skin paddle of the microvascular transfer.

In larger midfacial defects, particularly if some or all of the nose is missing, the provision of lining can present a tremendous challenge in reconstruction. Failure to provide adequate lining may leave areas of bone exposed, increasing the chance of infection and loss of tissue; it can increase the scarring and resorption of normal cavities and overlying tissue; and it can produce unwanted retraction and contraction of the midface, which may later prove difficult to resolve. Local flaps and skin grafts may be effective in more limited cases, but the amount of lining required usually makes these a poor option.

In these cases of severe midfacial tissue loss, one should think about either vascularized obliteration of the base of the midfacial defect or extensive vascularized replacement of missing bone and soft tissue. In vascularized obliteration, the sinuses and nasal airway are replaced with vascularized muscle or fat to initially control the wound and allow it to heal (Fig. 20-19). The previous placement of a tracheostomy tube obviates any need for a patent nasal airway, at least in the short term. This also allows bones to heal after the fixation of fractures or the placement of bone grafts across the maxilla, zygoma, or orbital floors or rim.

The latissimus dorsi or rectus muscle provides excellent fill of the midface, but the sheer bulk of muscle mass requires that the facial skin be split for passage of the muscle and its pedicle into the neck (see Fig. 20-19C, and D). The length of pedicle needed to traverse the midface to the neck limits the number of free flap tissue options. The omentum is also an excellent choice for fill, and its very pliable, amorphous form allows it to fill all midfacial cavities. Its slender pedicle permits creation of a subcutaneous tunnel into the neck without a facial split. With these flaps, the risk of infection is dramatically reduced, and a vascularized base is established onto which the anterior maxilla, upper lip, or nasal reconstruction can be based. This does not mean that a future free or pedicled flap reconstruction will not be needed; it simply provides

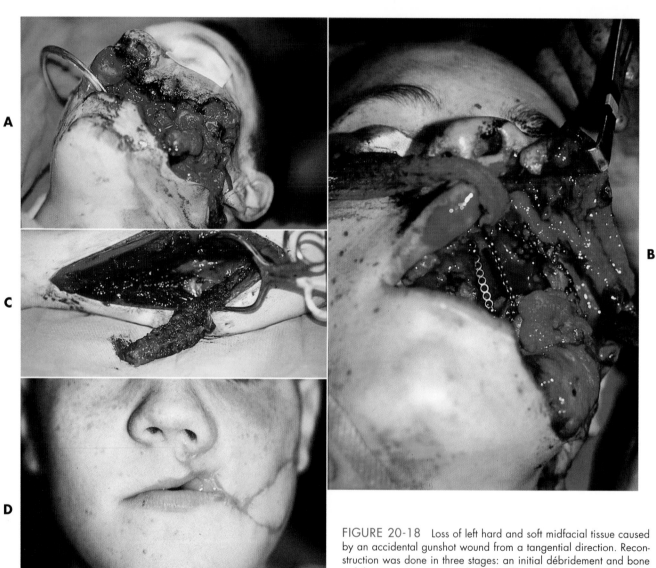

FIGURE 20-18   Loss of left hard and soft midfacial tissue caused by an accidental gunshot wound from a tangential direction. Reconstruction was done in three stages: an initial débridement and bone stabilization, a microvascular bone flap, and a cross-lip transfer. **A,** Facial injury as seen in the emergency room. **B,** First-stage débridement and stabilization of remaining maxillary segments. **C,** Second-stage (7 days later) free fibular bone flap using only the distal end with no skin paddle. **D,** Frontal facial view obtained 6 months after surgery.

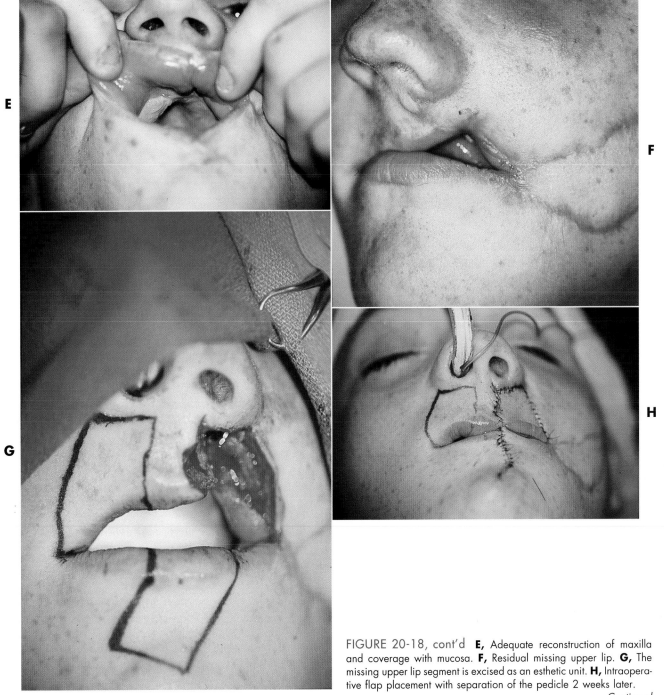

FIGURE 20-18, cont'd **E,** Adequate reconstruction of maxilla and coverage with mucosa. **F,** Residual missing upper lip. **G,** The missing upper lip segment is excised as an esthetic unit. **H,** Intraoperative flap placement with separation of the pedicle 2 weeks later.

Continued

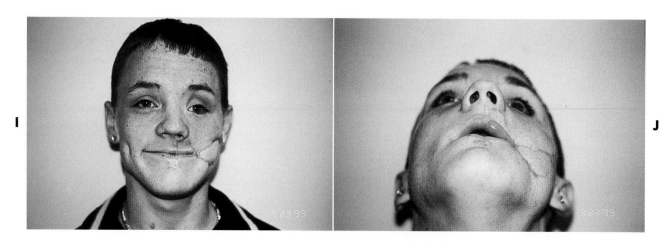

FIGURE 20-18, cont'd   **I,** Facial view 1 year after injury. **J,** Submental view 1 year after reconstruction demonstrates midfacial projection and restoration of lip contours. Further orbital and scar revision work is planned.

early control of the open facial wound until secondary facial reconstruction can be carried out (Fig. 20-20). This is particularly useful in patients with very large facial wounds and in those whose mental status is not yet clear. Attempts to reestablish a nasal airway can be done secondarily, as the final midfacial reconstructive procedure, through the use of a nasal stent or trumpet around which a skin graft is wrapped and passed through the vascularized muscle or fat to the posterior choana.

In other patients, a more anatomically based free flap reconstruction of the midface can be done early. This works best when the midfacial defects are not massive, the facial wounds are clean, the viability of adjacent tissue margins is clear, and the mental status of the patient is more defined. Free flap reconstruction of midfacial defects often involves very clever flap designs and well planned patterns for tissue replacement[20-22] (Fig. 20-21). Much of this technique has been learned from oncological resection of the midface, where one flap does not fit all defects. The composite creation of palatal-maxillary-orbital bone and soft tissue fill or lining, or both, requires preoperative design of the flap components, which must then be properly traced out for the flap harvest. This design must be done with the location and orientation of the vascular pedicle in mind to avoid a major surprise when the tissue is transferred to the face. Although no one flap can be universally applied, scapular and fibular osteocutaneous composite flaps are most commonly used.[20] They offer adequate bone and attached soft tissue, which can have a different arc of rotation from that of the bone. This is a particular asset in the scapular flap, because a bipedicled flap design can be created.

The reestablishment of a nose depends on recreating a support framework of cartilage and bone and an external skin cover. With severe loss of lining, the placement of these structures is highly dependent on having a vascularized base onto which they can be placed. The rebuilding of the nasal framework is fairly straightforward, and either bone or cartilage may be used to make an L-strut with lateral support (Fig. 20-22). Lateral alar support is important to prevent the eventual skin coverage from contracting completely around the

tip of the framework. Because of decreased resorption potential, we prefer cartilage rather than bone for the majority of the framework whenever possible. This requires rib harvests from the free-floating ninth and eighth ribs, which are easy to harvest. It is important to recruit or wrap any surrounding vascularized tissue around the framework to eliminate nonvascularized dead space underneath the graft reconstruction.

The more difficult challenge is in the reconstruction of the nasal skin cover, which frequently includes part or all of the upper lip also. For smaller defects of nasal cover, the pedicled forehead flap remains the most ideal option. It has the best color match, is fairly similar in skin texture and thickness (albeit slightly thicker in most patients), and is easy to harvest, with a very predictable survival. Its use frequently involves a three-stage procedure: transfer, separation of the pedicle weeks later, and eventual revision of the transferred tissue or donor site or both (Fig. 20-23). This method is almost always available in facial gunshot wounds, because the forehead is usually spared from the blast. The donor site is left with a vertical scar, which initially seems undesirable given that it may be one of the few esthetic facial units that has not been violated by the initial injury. However, with eventual fading and blending, the scar usually looks surprisingly good, even if the forehead donor wound cannot be completely closed after harvest.

One helpful maneuver is the use of tissue expansion before forehead flap transfer. This is done not to create more tissue for transfer but to help close the midline forehead defect. Preexpansion of the forehead flap itself intuitively seems helpful but will only result in a nasal skin reconstruction that ultimately undergoes significant contraction. Tissue expanders should be placed outside the outline of the flap to expand the residual forehead tissue. This allows a very large flap to be taken and still permits primary closure of the forehead. This is particularly useful in total nasal reconstruction. It is important also not to forget the importance of nasal lining and coverage of the framework from an intranasal standpoint. Failure to do so results in eventual extrusion, infection, and loss of the framework.

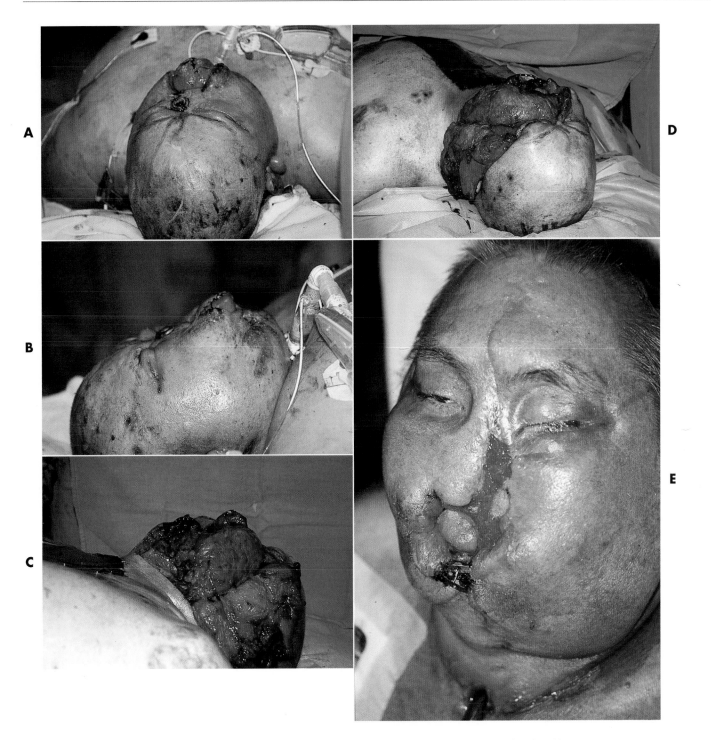

FIGURE 20-19   Self-inflicted gunshot wound to the face with loss of all central midfacial and lower facial structures. The patient was transferred in with a nasal trumpet in place and the skin closed around it. First-stage reconstruction was done with a vascularized muscle fill of the entire midface. **A,** Preoperative frontal facial view. **B,** Preoperative lateral facial view. **C,** Facial split with latissimus muscle flap in place and vascular anastomoses in the neck. **D,** Superior view of vascularized muscle fill of the midface. **E,** Healed midfacial wound is now ready for more definitive reconstruction of the middle and lower face.

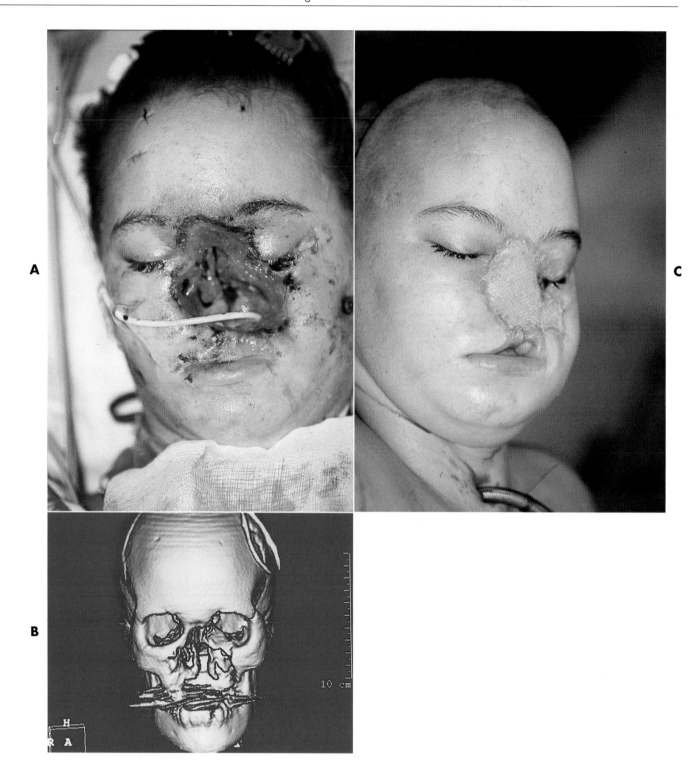

FIGURE 20-20 Vascularized obliteration of midfacial avulsive defect. **A,** Preoperative frontal facial view of the same patient as in Figure 20-16. **B,** Three-dimensional computed tomographic scan demonstrates the extent of midfacial bone loss. **C,** One month after surgery, facial view shows well-healed skin graft overlying the muscle flap.

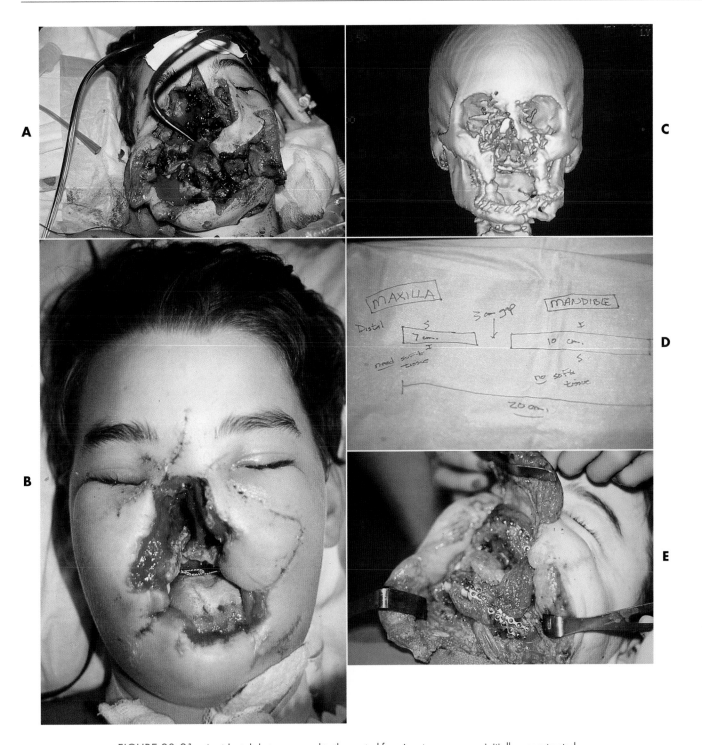

FIGURE 20-21   Accidental shotgun wound to the central face in a teenager was initially reconstructed with a composite free flap for concomitant maxillary and mandibular reconstruction. **A,** Appearance in the emergency room. **B,** Appearance after initial débridement and bone stabilization. **C,** Three-dimensional computed tomographic scan demonstrates extent of midfacial bone loss. **D,** Design of first-stage free flap reconstruction using a long fibular flap. A bone gap is created in the middle so that the flap can be turned to fill both the maxillary and mandibular defects, with the skin paddle covering the external nasal skin defect. **E,** Intraoperative flap positioning with vessels anastomosed in the neck.

Continued

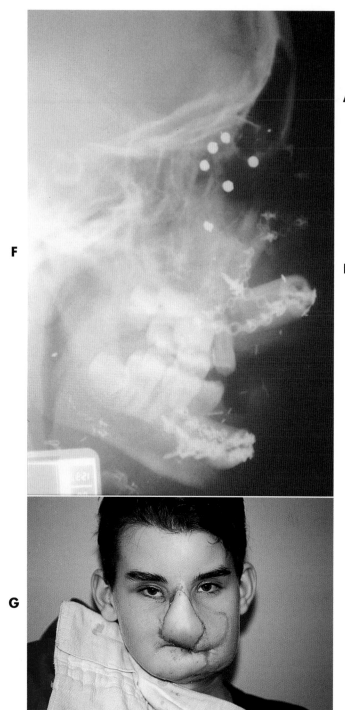

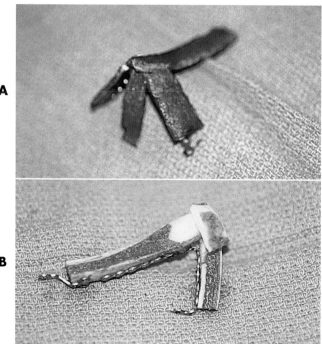

FIGURE 20-22 Nasal framework reconstruction using cranial bone (**A**) or rib cartilage (**B**).

FIGURE 20-21, cont'd **F,** Radiographic appearance of bone placement 1 month after surgery. **G,** Facial view 3 months after surgery. The patient still requires nasal framework placement, skin shaping, and upper and lower lip reconstruction.

If total nasal reconstruction is needed, particularly if portions of the upper lip are also missing, the amount of tissue from the forehead can be inadequate. In these circumstances, coverage of a nasal framework with a free tissue transfer is often the only option. Donor requirements are a thin fasciocutaneous or muscle flap (which requires a skin graft) and a

long vascular pedicle, which must reach into the neck. Minimum pedicle lengths of 12 to 15 cm are needed. The radial forearm fasciocutaneous free flap is probably the first choice, because it best fulfills these requirements. Despite the color and texture differences, it produces good coverage of nasal frameworks (Fig. 20-24). Multiple revisions will ultimately be necessary for shaping, contouring, and the placement of nostrils. Other available free flap options exist, such as serratus muscle and scapular fascial flaps, but these require skin grafts because their cutaneous components are too large and bulky to be useful for nasal cover.

With orbital involvement, the typical reconstructive problems are re-creation of the orbital lining after enucleation due to a penetrating injury to the globe and secondary correction of vertical dystopia resulting from the loss of bony support due to missing floor or walls. In most gunshot wounds involving loss of the globe, the eyelids are still present, and the issue is to provide some vascularized fill of the intraorbital space that will eventually accommodate a prosthesis. If the intraorbital defect is fairly isolated, options include a pedicled temporalis musculofascial flap (Fig. 20-25) and a small free tissue transfer such as a radial forearm flap (see Fig. 20-24). The temporalis flap is appealing because of its proximity and ease of harvest; however, it provides a limited amount of tissue fill, because the very distal end of the flap consists of fascia alone and is often sufficient only for creating lateral orbital lining. In many cases, however, this flap provides enough vascularized lining to line the orbital floor, cover bone grafts, and allow placement of a skin or mucosal graft, and it may provide enough to allow an orbital prosthesis to be made. Donor site morbidity is minimal other than the temporal scar from the

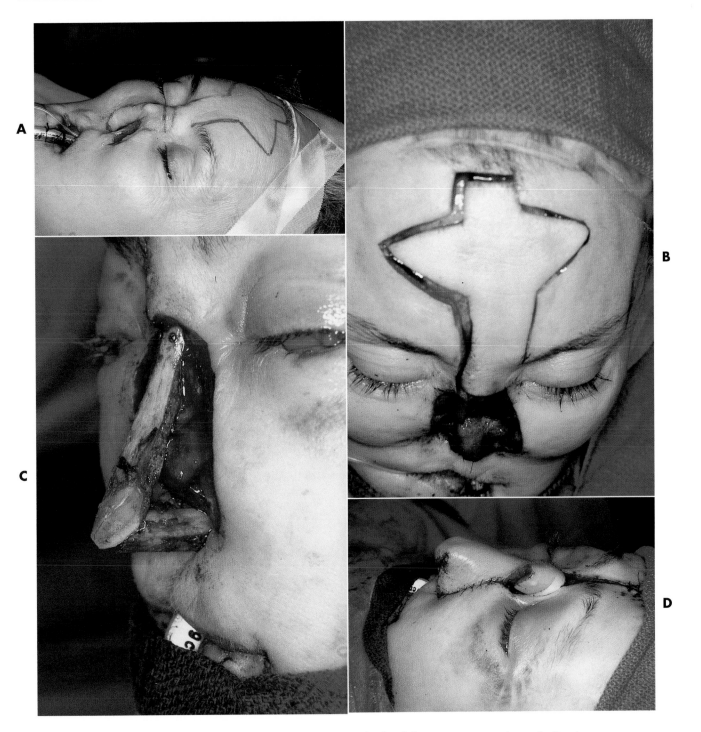

FIGURE 20-23 Total nasal reconstruction with a forehead flap in a patient with a self-inflicted gunshot wound. **A,** Preoperative appearance 6 months after the initial injury. **B,** Forehead flap design. **C,** Rib graft nasal framework reconstruction. **D,** Flap coverage of the nasal framework with the pedicle turned 180 degrees.

Continued

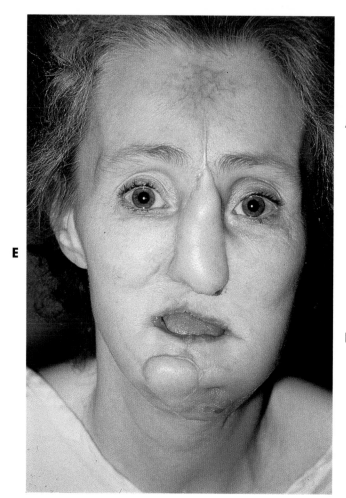

E

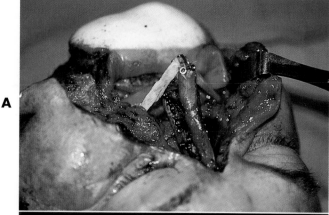

A

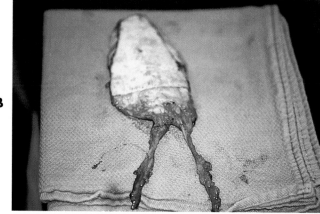

B

FIGURE 20-23, cont'd **E,** Three months after surgery, there is secondary healing of the central forehead defect. Further revisions still are needed.

FIGURE 20-24   Total nasal reconstruction using vascularized fasciocutaneous cover. **A,** Nasal framework fabricated from rib cartilage. **B,** Radial fasciocutaneous free flap harvested with a vascular pedicle located at the inferior end.

coronal incision and the potential for temporal hollowing if a large amount of muscle is taken with the fascia. For larger defects or if the ipsilateral temporal region is also damaged, free vascularized tissue is needed. The radial forearm flap can provide more than adequate soft tissue and skin for the orbit and is the preferred choice in many of these more complex orbital cases (Fig. 20-26).

In cases of vertical dystopia, repositioning and reconstruction of the bony box is the main method of correction. This is usually accomplished by completely rebuilding the orbital floor and rim, which is best done with autologous cranial bone or alloplastic materials. Proponents exist for each method, but the patient's anatomy and problem must be carefully considered. If there is good vascularized tissue around the orbit and the sinus is obliterated, any autologous or alloplastic method can work with a low risk of infection. Titanium mesh is commonly used, because it is easily adapted and can be secured to the surrounding bone. Autologous cranial bone may or may not be combined with it, although the need for bone grafting with a rigid titanium mesh that reestablishes and secures the intraorbital volume is not

completely obvious. Bone grafting is another viable method, but the amount of graft needed can often be deceiving, and some form of graft fixation is still required. For orbital defects of poor tissue quality with an underlying open sinus exposure, titanium mesh is probably best, because it is very well tolerated even when exposed and predictably maintains the elevation of the globe. In certain cases in which the bullet has passed through the maxilla and obliterated the pillars, the entire orbital box shifts down as a result of orbitomalar displacement. In these patients, an osteotomy and repositioning, with or without bone grafting, may be done (Fig. 20-27). This approach is superior to globe elevation by floor reconstruction alone, because it more effectively addresses the lack of malar projection and lower eyelid support.

One specific issue with orbital reconstruction in facial gunshot wounds is the frequent need for eyelid repositioning and reconstruction. As the globe elevates, the eyelid often does not follow because of scar contracture or actual loss of lid tissue. The liberal use of canthal reconstructions and release and full-thickness skin grafting on the lower lid are often needed. One should resist the temptation to simply pull up the lower eyelid through the medial or lateral canthus, particularly if the amount of movement is significant. This would result in postoperative ectropion. Most significant

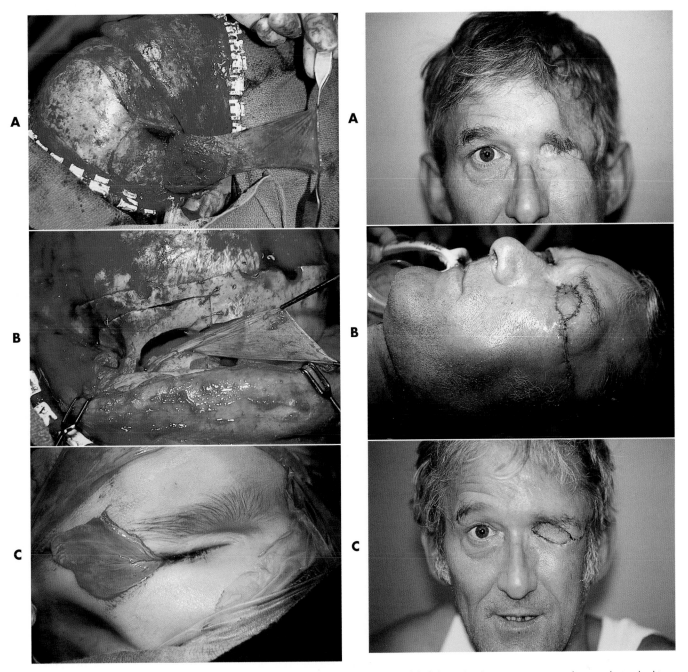

FIGURE 20-25 Pedicled temporalis fascial flap for orbital lining. **A,** Harvest of the temporalis fascial flap. **B,** Extent of fascial reach through the orbit. **C,** Amount of thin fascial tissue that can be gained for intraorbital lining.

FIGURE 20-26 Orbital reconstruction with vascularized skin. **A,** Preoperative appearance of healed temporo-orbital gunshot wound with significant loss of hard and soft tissues. **B,** Intraoperative placement of small radial fasciocutaneous flap into orbit after frontotemporal cranioplasty. **C,** Result 3 months after surgery.

movements require more lower eyelid tissue, which is obtained by full-thickness skin grafting or interposition of more tissue through a temporalis fascial flap.

LATERAL FACE

The side of the face provides a less complicated array of anatomical structures and contours, and the tissue loss is somewhat simpler to reconstruct. Many single-bullet injuries to the face do not result in large hard or soft tissue loss. Shortly after skin entrance, the bullet strikes bone, causing a comminuted fracture and changing the path of the bullet. Reconstruction in these cases focuses on bony reduction and stabilization, because the entrance and exit sites are small (Fig. 20-28). Small amounts of tissue loss, either intraoral lining or external skin cover, can be tolerated, because local tissue rearrangement can be done and may permit the placement of free bone grafts (Fig. 20-29). Loss of intraoral lining is less well tolerated than loss of external skin cover. Oral

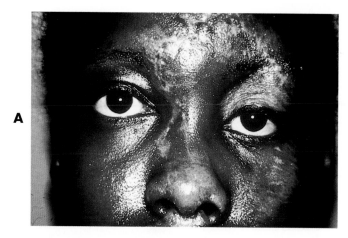

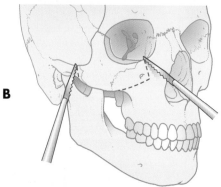

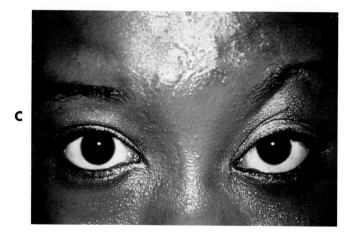

FIGURE 20-27   Repositioning of the orbital box through osteotomies. **A,** Preoperative facial view of severe orbital dystopia caused by loss of left maxillary support from a gunshot wound. **B,** Osteotomy design, cranial bone grafting, and plate and screw fixation. **C,** Result 6 months after surgery.

lining loss results in scar contracture, decreased oral opening, and difficulty with subsequent dental rehabilitation. External skin loss results in undesirable visible scarring but does not usually cause serious functional handicaps.

The ratio of bone mass to soft tissue is greater on the side of the face, and for this reason bullets do not often traverse the entire width of the face, particularly in the lower third, due to the presence of the mandible. Shotgun wounds, however, spare little in their path. Because almost all of these

firearm discharges occur at close range, the amount of composite destruction is significant. Even if large soft tissue loss has not occurred, the blast effect from the bullet frequently damages surrounding bones, including the maxilla and zygomatico-orbital complex (see Figs. 20-29A and 20-31B).

Many lateral facial defects involve through-and-through wounds with moderate to large mandibular bone defects. The loss of inner and outer lining obviates any successful efforts at free bone grafting. The use of free fibular or scapular flaps with a skin paddle oriented to the side with the greatest lining loss is the most common method of immediate reconstruction in these cases. Although the skin paddle does not produce a good color match with the surrounding facial skin, it provides ample coverage for most defects (Fig. 20-30). The relatively flat contour of the lateral face makes shaping and positioning of the flap almost two-dimensional, rather than a three-dimensional effort. In very large composite defects, the amount of internal and external lining needed may make even these free flaps inadequate (Fig. 20-31). In such cases, a large soft tissue flap can be placed initially to establish external coverage, which usually involves the greater amount of surface area loss. Once the wound has been controlled, a second free flap can be placed to reconstruct the lost bone and internal lining.

Many lateral facial wounds result in direct injury to facial nerve branches. This typically involves the buccal and marginal mandibular branches, sparing innervation to the frontal and orbital areas. Primary nerve repair is usually impossible due to the blast injury, and early nerve grafting is difficult without adequate soft tissue coverage and an ability to find the distal ends of the nerve. Secondary nerve or muscular reconstruction is rarely done, because restoration of facial movement in the injured area is prohibited by the transplantation of reconstructed tissue and the resultant surrounding scar.

PROSTHETIC RECONSTRUCTION

The severity of tissue loss and the complexity of facial structures, particularly in the midfacial area, make reconstruction of extensive defects an almost overwhelming challenge. The practicalities of access to experienced and expert surgical care, the economics and physical stamina required to undergo a large number of surgical procedures, and the age and medical and mental status of the patient raise certain philosophical questions. Most pertinently, how far should one go in providing autogenous reconstruction? Autogenous tissue has limitations in the formation and detail that can be obtained in certain facial features. Prostheses, when fabricated by skilled anaplastologists, provide an unparalleled artistic replication of the patient's lost facial features. The development and refinement of osseo-integrated implant techniques have enabled prosthetic replacement to be a viable alternative or, more commonly, an adjunct to the reconstruction of complex facial loss. Osseo-integrated prosthetic reconstruction has certain advantages, such as a more limited surgical burden on the patient, but is not without its own level of demand for a good outcome. Most importantly, there must be an adequate amount of bone volume and density at key locations to allow implants of proper length and orientation to be placed so that the prosthesis is stable and does not

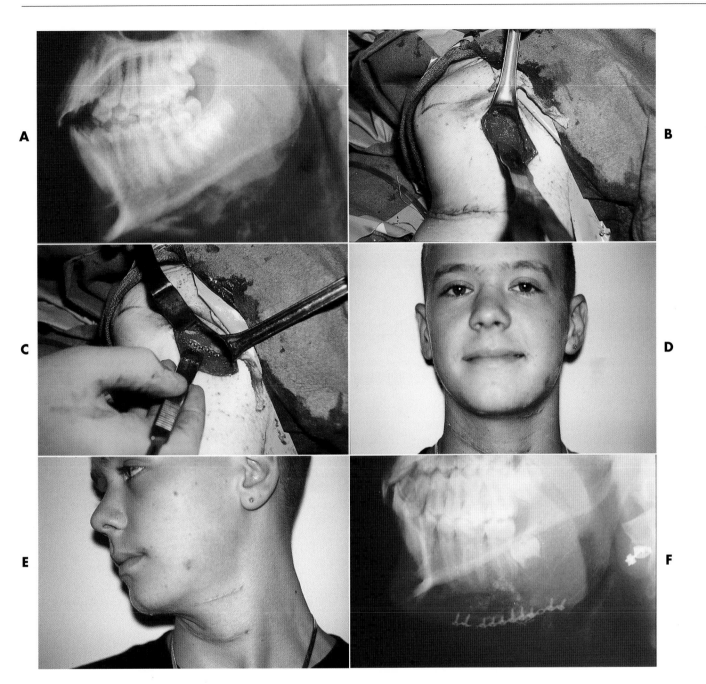

FIGURE 20-28 Gunshot wound to the lateral face that struck the mandible with no soft tissue deficit. **A,** Preoperative lateral facial film. **B,** Comminution and loss of inferior bone of the mandible body. **C,** Because there was good soft tissue cover, immediate reconstruction with bone fragments and iliac marrow was performed. **D,** Facial view 3 months after surgery. **E,** Lateral facial view 3 months after surgery. **F,** Radiographic appearance 3 months after surgery.

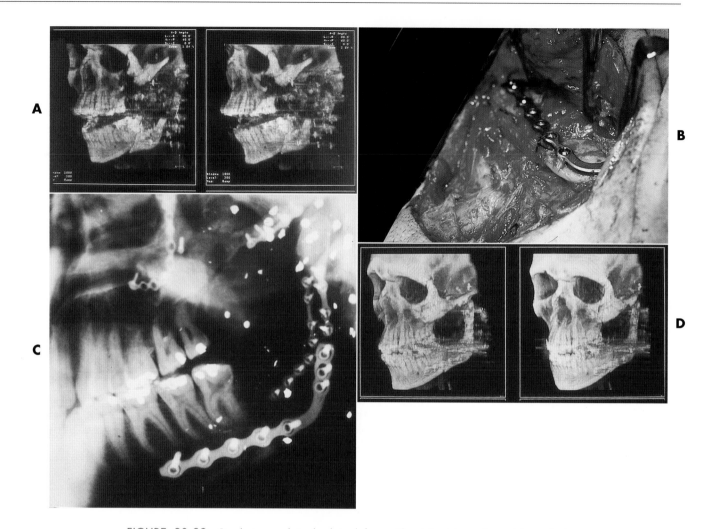

FIGURE 20-29   Gunshot wound to the lateral face with minimal loss of overlying soft tissue. **A,** Three-dimensional computed tomographic (3-D CT) scan shows obliteration of the left ramus of the mandible. **B,** Reconstruction with plate and iliac marrow. **C,** Postoperative panoramic tomographic view. **D,** Postoperative 3-D CT scan shows good alignment of the condyle and ramus. *(Courtesy of Dr. Anders Westermark, Stockholm, Sweden.)*

produce any significant amount of rocking or torque on the bone fixtures. Adequately thin attached tissue around the abutments and adequate access for maintenance are also required.

In most cases, prosthetic reconstruction of severe facial defects is not a simple choice between reconstruction with autogenous tissue or a prosthesis supported by osseo-integrated implants. Although each of these approaches has advantages and disadvantages, both are frequently needed and can be combined in stages. The defect is usually reconstructed initially with a vascularized osseous or osseocutaneous flap, followed secondarily by implant placement.[23,24]

CONTROVERSIES

The concept of reconstruction of severe facial wounds involving large tissue loss with vascularized tissue is well accepted and commonly used today; there is no other satisfactory method of reconstruction in these cases. However, some controversy exists regarding the timing of this reconstructive procedure. Should the procedure be done early (e.g., within the first few days to weeks), or should it be delayed for several weeks to months? Given the risk of a large operation and the limited available flap options in the body, an argument can be made for delaying vascularized reconstruction until a more ideal time, but this time is not often defined. Given that most of these facial injuries occur in healthy patients with noncompromised necks (i.e., no previous surgery and no irradiation), the initial vascularized reconstructive procedure should probably be done after the patient is stable, the viability of the tissue margins is fairly obvious, and the status of vital functions within the field (brain function and vision) is fairly well defined. In some cases, these issues are known within the first few days after the injury.

For patients with large composite tissue loss in the face, little controversy exists regarding the use of microsurgical techniques, given the lack of other viable treatment options. With smaller defects, particularly those that involve small

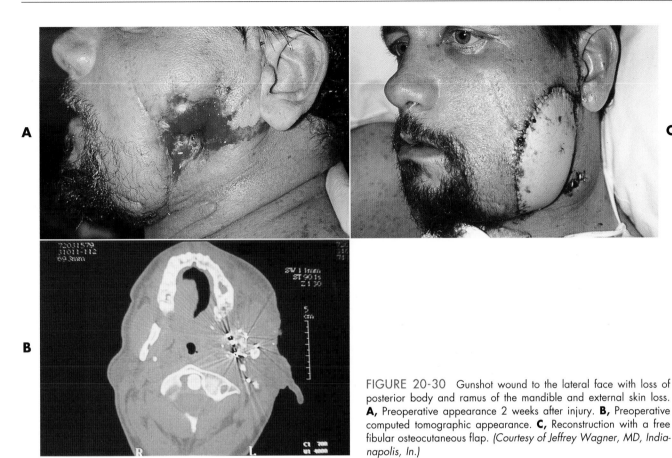

FIGURE 20-30 Gunshot wound to the lateral face with loss of posterior body and ramus of the mandible and external skin loss. **A,** Preoperative appearance 2 weeks after injury. **B,** Preoperative computed tomographic appearance. **C,** Reconstruction with a free fibular osteocutaneous flap. *(Courtesy of Jeffrey Wagner, MD, Indianapolis, In.)*

mandibular segments, the issue of nonvascularized versus vascularized reconstructive techniques is often encountered. In most patients with large traumatic facial wounds, the tissues were noncompromised before the injury, so the use of bone grafts should have the potential for near-normal healing. The type of bone graft required is usually determined by the amount of soft tissue loss. Without an adequate soft tissue cover, free bone grafts often become exposed, leading to partial or complete graft loss. The soft tissue concern has principally to do with the intraoral lining. With small losses of mucosal lining, it may be possible to recruit enough local tissue to obtain reconstructive cover. Even if this results in loss of vestibular depth, secondary correction through release and skin grafting can be done after the free graft has revascularized and undergone osseous healing. This approach becomes increasingly inadequate as the amount of missing lining increases.

The concept of prefabrication of a flap transfer is based on the use of delay procedures and interposition of specialized vascularized tissue in certain areas of the body, from which a frame or pattern can be made that will simulate the complete tissue needed in another region of the body. This is best illustrated by nasal replacement, in which the nose, complete with lining, bone, and skin, can be initially constructed on the forehead, forearm, back, or abdomen. After maturity, the nose is harvested on a vascularized pedicle that has been relocated into the area and is then transplanted to the face by microvascular surgery. This concept has obvious appeal,

because the complex anatomy of the nose can be put together in pieces at a distant site first, before being transferred to the face, where such manipulations are more difficult. This concept has also been used clinically for other complex facial areas, such as extensive midfacial defects.[25] Despite its theoretical advantages and reported successes in selected clinical cases, the actual use of prefabrication is more difficult and often less satisfactory than one would envision. It is a concept that clearly has merit but is not yet ready for universal application. Many composite tissue free flaps, if properly designed, can achieve the desired reconstructive goals in one operation rather than two. Furthermore, the reverse of prefabrication can be done very successfully—that is, placement of vascularized soft tissue first, followed by free bone grafting secondarily.

The role of prosthetic (alloplastic) as opposed to autogenous reconstruction must be considered in both primary and secondary efforts. The tremendous surgical effort and expertise, patient endurance and tolerance of numerous operations over a prolonged period, the economic and resource costs, and the esthetic quality of the final facial result make a prosthetic replacement a viable option in selected patients. The use of endosseous implants for attaching oral and facial prostheses overcomes the traditional problems associated with glues and dental anchorage methods. Which patients with large facial defects should receive this therapy is open to debate, and numerous factors must be considered in addition to defect size and location.

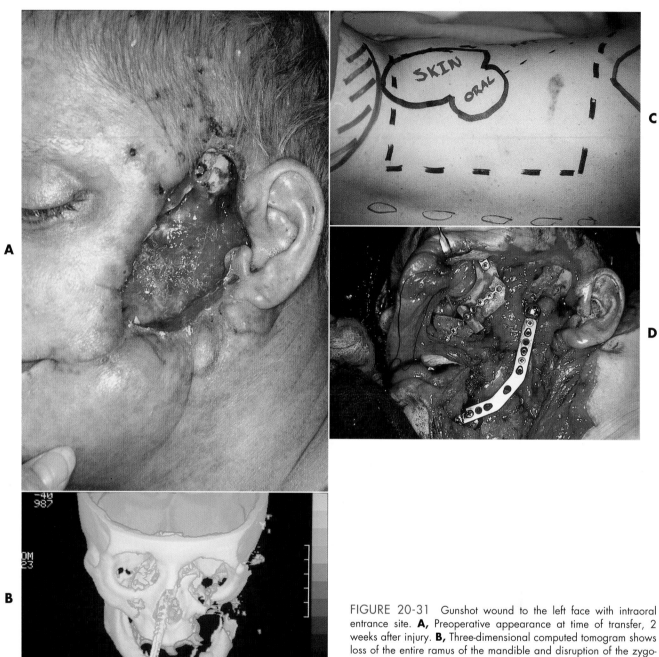

FIGURE 20-31   Gunshot wound to the left face with intraoral entrance site. **A,** Preoperative appearance at time of transfer, 2 weeks after injury. **B,** Three-dimensional computed tomogram shows loss of the entire ramus of the mandible and disruption of the zygomatic complex. **C,** First-stage reconstruction with a free latissimus musculocutaneous flap (design on back). **D,** Plate fixation of fractures and temporary alloplastic (metal) reconstruction of mandibular segment before flap inset.

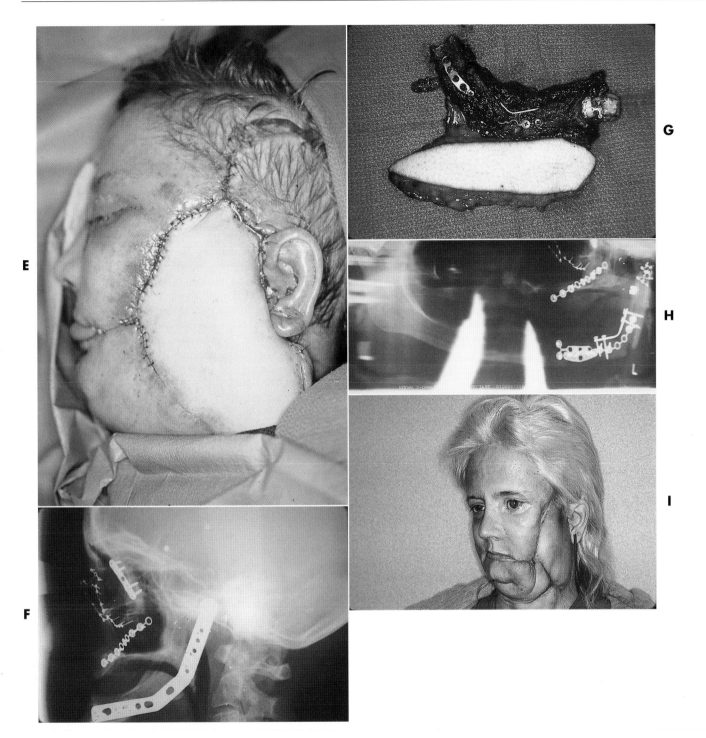

FIGURE 20-31, cont'd   **E,** Latissimus flap inset over bony reconstruction. **F,** Immediate postoperative radiographic appearance. **G,** Second-stage mandibular reconstruction was performed 6 months later with a free fibular osteocutaneous flap. Skin was used for intraoral lining. **H,** Postoperative panoramic tomogram. **I,** Nine months after a second free flap reconstruction, scar revisions and skin flap adjustments are needed, but good, well-vascularized tissue is present.

FACE TRANSPLANTATION

BERNARD DEVAUCHELLE

One of the most exciting developments in facial reconstruction is that of face transplantation. Free tissue transplantation was once used only for simple bone and soft tissue injuries; the idea of transferring part or almost a whole face is a relatively new concept in maxillofacial surgery. Use of tissue transplantation in functional organs such as kidney and heart is well established, and the ongoing evolution of microsurgical tissue transfer has made face transplantation a reality.

Clearly, face transplantation is an extension of free tissue transfer procedures. The important additional complications are the need to ensure motor and sensory innervation and to prevent rejection. Prevention of rejection consists of a highly specialized treatment regimen undertaken by internal medicine physicians who specialize in transplantation; it will not be discussed further in this surgical text.

Composite facial replacement is currently limited to patients with the most severely traumatized faces, those disfigurements in which tissue loss is so great that conventional facial reconstructive methods fall far short of the mark. These "facial cripples" have historically been relegated to numerous and ongoing inadequate reconstructive attempts and usually live at the outer margins of society. Nothing short of a face transplant will suffice in some cases.

Face transplants are allotransplants, coming from other humans, and should be considered a facial reconstruction only if there is restoration of motor and sensory function. The first aim of such surgery is functional rehabilitation of the face, taking it beyond just restoration of facial shape. Esthetic reconstruction should be considered only in its broad meaning, including normal facial expression.

ANATOMICAL CONDITIONS FOR FACE TRANSPLANTATION

Anatomical consideration in terms of the vascular independence of each esthetic zone is the first condition of the procedure, as it is with other flaps. The facial vascular supply is from the external carotid artery. The vascular territory anastomoses with the internal carotid artery; less known is the vascular anastomosis network of the facial artery with the internal maxillary artery.

The very rare reported cases of face transplantation confirm the main role of the facial artery. This supply is thoroughly assessed for the middle and lower face without any consideration for skeletal structures. Techniques are completely different according to the necessity to re-anastomose the facial vessels, the temporal vessels, or the whole external carotid artery system. The anatomy of these allografts can be described by their topographical division into five types.

The *lower central facial allograft (type I)* includes harvesting the donor's nose, lips, and chin from the cutaneous surface to the deep mucosa. The graft is vascularized by the two facial pedicles, which are dissected down to their emergence from the large vessels of the neck and contain all the of oral cleft muscles harvested by subperiosteal elevation, from the zygomatic and maxillary bones to the mandibular rim. These muscles are reinnervated by zygomatic, buccal, and mandibular branches of the facial nerve (cranial nerve VII), which are dissected as separate segmental rami or traced more proximally up to their common origin on the trunk of the facial nerve. The sensory nerves of the allograft are the mental (V3) and infraorbital (V2) branches of cranial nerve V, which are exposed at the corresponding bony foramina and lengthened on their proximal course by intraosseous dissection.

The standard allograft just described (referred to as type IA) concerns only the soft tissues of the face. It may be extended laterally to the cheeks and up to the preauricular areas. In the latter case, it also contains the parotids. It is raised on the external carotid and jugular axes and on the proximal trunk of the two facial nerves. If necessary, it can

also extend deeper to include the middle part of the mandibular arch, which is used to restore the bone support to the chin; this is the type IB allograft (B = bone). The mandibular bone segment is vascularized by the periosteal network of the two submental arteries, which are connected in the area of the mental foramina with the inferior alveolar arteries. The submental vessels must therefore be included and left undamaged when the type IB graft is harvested. Consequently, this graft contains an additional skin surface corresponding to the submandibular region next to the hyoid bone.

The *midfacial allograft (type II)* contains the nose, upper lip, cheeks, and muscles elevating the oral cavity; it is raised equally on the right and left facial pedicles. Although it can consist of soft tissues only (type IIA), it usually includes the anterior part of the maxillae and zygomatic arches and a variable segment of the anterior palate (type IIB). Its sensitivity is restored by the infraorbital nerves (V2), and its motor reinnervation relies on restored continuity of the zygomatic and buccal rami of the facial nerve (VII), if possible, along with that of the buccal nerves (V3) if tonicity to the buccinator muscles is to be restored. Depending on the extent of the defect to be reconstructed, the allograft may be very wide, extending on both sides of the midline, or it may be unilateral. In some cases, it can be more or less extended downward, toward the lower portion of the cheek (Fig. 20-32).

The *upper facial allograft (type III)* includes the superficial planes of the forehead, eyelids, and root of the nose and the deeper planes of the frontalis, glabellar, and orbicularis oculi muscles. It is raised on the two superficial temporal pedicles and on the supraorbital sensory nerves (V1). Deep dissection of the allograft around the palpebral sulci must include the preseptal and periosteal anastomotic vascular circle around the orbital rim in order to incorporate the shunts connecting the intracranial and extracranial vascular networks. Restoration of palpebral blink activity is delicate but may be mediated by restoring the continuity of the frontal and zygomatic branches of the facial nerves (VII). To date, this segmental transplantation model remains theoretical, because it has never been implemented clinically.

Unlike the three composite transplants just discussed, which are segmental and are linked to large functional neurovascular territories of the face, the *total facial skin allograft (type IV)* is a purely segmental transplant that is designed to restore, in a single segment, the cutaneous cover of the whole facial mask and a variable portion of scalp, according to its laboratory description. It is vascularized by the two facial and superficial temporal pedicles, which are harvested separately or in a continuous fashion along the external carotid and jugular axes. It is pierced by three artificial orifices for the nostrils, lips, and eyelids and can be likened to a carnival mask placed over a face in which all of the deeper functional structures are supposed to be intact and able to adhere to the deep surface of the facial allograft. It does not, therefore, have any intrinsic motor activity, and was not initially described as sensate. However, it now seems technically possible to reinnervate the cutaneous surface of a type IV allograft by using a deeper dissection plane to include the three segmental terminal branches of the left and right trigeminal nerves. The name *full face allograft,* often suggested to describe this transplant, is therefore somewhat erroneous and inaccurate. Although it covers a wider area than segmental allograft types

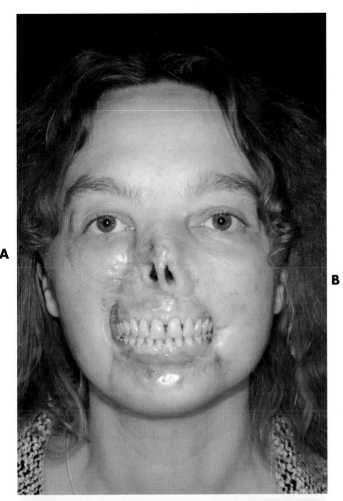

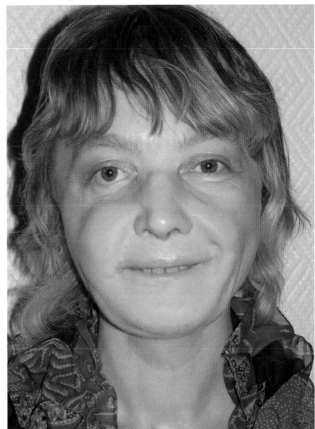

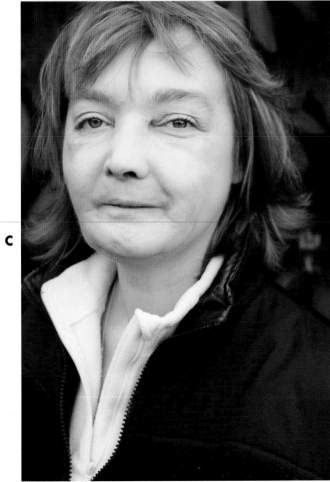

FIGURE 20-32 **A,** Type II facial transplant candidate. **B, C,** Appearance after face transplantation. *(Courtesy of Dr. Bernard Devauchelle.)*

I, II, or III, this theoretical transplant was devised to resurface extensive burns to the face. Even devoid of any functional purpose, it does constitute a partial facial allograft and could therefore be applicable to either a hemiface or the whole facial cutaneous cover. To avoid any ambiguities with regard to nomenclature, this allograft should be referred to as a *partial* (type IVp) or a *full* (type IVf) composite tissue allograft of the facial mask.

Strictly speaking, a true *full facial allograft (type V)* ought to be performed as a multisegmental or composite transplant combining the partial allograft types I, II, and III in a single block of uniform thickness. This would have to be harvested on the entire external carotid axis with the confluent jugular veins on both sides of the donor's head. It would contain all of the muscles of expression, the common trunks of both facial nerves, and the three segmental branches (V1, V2, and V3) of the two trigeminal nerves. In the deeper planes, it could involve soft tissues only, including the superficial musculo-aponeurotic system (SMAS), with or without the periosteal plane; this is called a *full soft tissue facial allograft (type VA)*. Alternatively, it could include the maxillary and mandibular arches, if necessary; this is a *full hard and soft tissue facial allograft (type VB)*. Although theoretically conceivable, these allografts correspond to such extensive tissue defects that they are hardly ever encountered clinically. They belong more to the realm of virtual or conceptual surgery rather than practical reality.

To date, clinical experience has focused on allograft types I and II. In the four documented cases, the composite allografts survived entirely successfully after microsurgical transplantation. Three were harvested from a heart-beating donor with a facial morphology comparable to the recipient's, and one was obtained from a cadaveric donor. In none of these cases was partial necrosis of any tissue transplant component reported, and preoperative hemodynamic observation of the allografts showed at all times that the entire transplant was fully vascularized on unilateral arterial and venous anastomoses. Moreover, wound healing along the lines of the cutaneous and mucosal sutures was satisfactory in every case. These results can be explained by the intense anastomotic collateral blood supply of the facial vessels. They were achieved by four different teams, providing the first evidence of the vascular reliability of face transplants when the fundamental rules of microsurgery are observed. Vascular anastomoses must always be performed on large-caliber vessels and should be bilateral, even when the entire transplant could survive on a single vascular axis. This rule prevents the harmful consequences of thrombosis of one of the two arterial or venous axes supplying the transplant. However, if the allograft predominantly concerns a single hemiface, this precaution is not necessary. Only by a larger series of operated patients can these preliminary conclusions be confirmed with regard to the reliability and primary survival of composite facial allografts.

INDICATIONS FOR FACE TRANSPLANTATION ACCORDING TO TOPOGRAPHY

There is no mandatory link between large composite defects and anatomical studies on the feasibility of the transplantation. Each patient is a unique case. However, it is possible to define different topographical types in relation to indications

for face transplantation, and in some cases the severity of the defect demands face transplantation as an ideal solution.

Middle Face (Lips-Chin-Nose Triangle)

The middle face is without doubt the best area for a face transplant because of the impossibility of reconstructing both function and esthetics of the lips with traditional procedures. Face transplantation for this esthetic and functional unit, even extending onto the nasolabial area, over the nose, or down under the chin, provides the double advantage of perfect esthetic restoration of the face and vascular independence. Restoration of sensation is very achievable. Motor function is ensured by musculo-muscular sutures except for the orbicularis oris muscles. The skin margins are also easy to match with the recipient skin. The possibility of including skeletal structures (nasal bone and cartilage, premaxillary region, mandibular arch) can be envisaged. Beyond that, there remains the question of the quality of the vascular supply from the internal maxillary artery and the necessity to adapt the initial dissection to the transplant and the vascular anatomosis.

Upper Face (Fronto-Orbito-Eyelid Region)

Large upper facial injuries are very rare. For many reasons, disfigurement of this area is not a good indication for face transplantation. From a vascular standpoint, this region depends on several terminal branches (internal frontal artery, facial artery, superficial temporal artery). The restoration of eyelid function, which is the essential point of the reconstruction, is currently not achievable because of the complexity of both the anatomical and the physiological aspects. The large disfigurement is usually associated with blindness, which raises other ethical considerations. Some defects of this region are more frequently associated with an extended defect in the orbitofrontal and nasomaxillary regions and could suggest transplantation of an upper face.

Lateral Face

Some severe lateral defects (e.g., after a large benign tumor resection) could be an indication for face transplantation. Anatomically there is no problem, and, paradoxically, the defect in this area leads to very few functional problems. Hearing will not be important. Facial palsy could be solved by other procedures. The question is more about the esthetic result. Would profile surgery (by comparison with the other side) have a less good result than frontal facial surgery?

Full Face

The first paper on face transplantation, reported in early 2000, expressed the idea that there is only one indication for complete transplantation: a patient with severe burns. From an anatomical and vascular point of view, harvesting of the whole cutaneous face is possible, with the vascular supply from the bilateral external carotid arteries and external jugular veins from the donor and anastomosis on the same pedicles for the recipient, except on one side with a lateral anastomosis on the carotid axis. There is also no problem with including some skeletal structures such as the mandibular arch and the anterior part of the maxilla. Skin extension could also include the ears and the main part of skin hair.

Even if it is obvious that the SMAS is part of the transplant, the difficulties are always from a functional point of view. What is the prognosis in terms of facial movement with simple facial nerve anastomosis? How can the complexity of eyelid movement be solved? As far as sensation is concerned, it is very important to ensure continuity of the different branches of the trigeminal nerve and those of the cervical plexus. It is too early to answer these questions, because the follow-up of face transplantation cases done to date is too short.

The demand for full or partial face transplantation will always be very rare indeed, but it may occur more frequently for burn patients. This surgery demands a dedicated team, and I would like to acknowledge my co-workers, Stephanie Dakpe and Sylvie Testelin (CMF, Amiens, France) and Benoit Lengelé (Plastic Surgeon, Brussels, Belgium).

CURRENT STATE OF THE ART

Composite facial allotransplantation is an efficient and accessible surgical procedure in which the rejection phenomena can be prevented and treated with basic immunosuppressive drugs, just as with immunosuppressive treatment after organ transplantation. It can be argued that face transplantation is an extensive surgical procedure with immunosuppressive treatment that carries health risks (e.g., infections, skin cancers) and treats a problem with severe psychological but no health risks.[26] This keeps the use of face transplantation limited to only those patients with the greatest of facial tissue loss.

CONCLUSION

Large defects of the midface and lower face result in loss of many specialized tissues. As initially described in 1965, "massive compound facial injuries create a sense of dismay, which may lead to therapeutic inertia."[27] Successful reconstruction of these defects entails early action involving replacement of the tissues before significant scarring and contracture have occurred. There are no specific algorithms of reconstruction that can be applied to all patients; each facial gunshot wound creates a unique set of tissue requirements. Thorough evaluation of the facial wound, including radiographic assessment, preferably with three-dimensional CT scanning, delineates the extent of the missing tissue. Lining, bony structures, and soft tissue cover are the three basic elements that need to be replaced in almost all of these injuries. Immediate or early repair, usually with the aid of microsurgical tissue transfer, not only provides for quicker healing of the facial wound but maintains the relationships among the remaining key landmarks that serve as the scaffold for future facial revision and reconstruction. For large defects, more than one free tissue transfer may be necessary to provide enough tissue to restore some semblance of facial form.

Realistic counseling with the patient who has sustained a large facial tissue loss and the patient's family is paramount. This brings in psychological evaluation and support and also helps the patient and family to understand that a large number of reconstructive procedures (commonly 10-15) will be necessary, over an extended period (1-2 years), for the maximal benefit of reconstructive facial surgery to be obtained. Complete pre-injury restoration of facial form and function is almost never achieved in patients with large composite facial defects, but reasonable function and facial proportions can be attained. In selected patients, oral and facial prostheses in conjunction with osseo-integrated implants for anchorage provide an alloplastic alternative or an adjunct to autogenous reconstructions. Most recently, the use of allograft face transplantation is offering hope for those rare traumatized faces in which the tissue defects are beyond any other method of tissue reconstruction.

REFERENCES

1. Centers for Disease Control and Prevention: Deaths resulting from firearm and motor vehicle-related injuries—United States, 1986-1991. *JAMA* 271:495-496, 1994.
2. Fackler ML: Civilian gunshot wounds and ballistics: dispelling the myths. *Emerg Med Clin North Am* 16:17-28, 1998.
3. Robertson B, Manson PN: The importance of serial débridement and "second-look" procedures in high-energy ballistic and avulsive facial injuries. *Oper Tech Plast Reconstr Surg* 20:236-245, 1998.
4. Vasconez HC: Management of massive bone and soft tissue defects of the midface and lower face. *Probl Plast Reconstr Surg* 1:466-481, 1991.
5. Manson PN: Dimensional analysis of the facial skeleton: avoiding complications in the management of facial fractures by improved organization of treatment based on CT scans. *Probl Plast Reconstr Surg* 1:213-237, 1991.
6. Mathes SJ, Nahai F, editors: *Reconstructive surgery: principles, anatomy and techniques,* New York, 1997, Churchill Livingstone.
7. Hidalgo DA: Aesthetic improvement in free flap mandible reconstruction. *Plast Reconstr Surg* 88:574-589, 1991.
8. Schusterman MA, Rees GP, Miller MJ et al: The osteocutaneous free fibula flap: is the skin paddle reliable? *Plast Reconstr Surg* 90:787-798, 1992.
9. Swartz WM, Banis JC, Newton ED et al: The osteocutaneous scapula flap for mandibular and maxillary reconstruction. *Plast Reconstr Surg* 77:530-538, 1986.
10. Coleman JJ III, Sultan MR: The bipedicled osteocutaneous scapula flap: a new subscapular system free flap. *Plast Reconstr Surg* 84:71-79, 1989.
11. Timmons MJ: The vascular basis of the radial forearm flap. *Plast Reconstr Surg* 77:80-87, 1986.
12. Soutar DS, McGregor IA: The radial forearm flap in intraoral reconstruction: the experience of 60 consecutive cases. *Plast Reconstr Surg* 78:1-10, 1986.
13. Bartlett SP, May JW Jr, Yaremchuk MJ: The latissimus dorsi muscle: a fresh cadaver study of the primary neurovascular pedicle. *Plast Reconstr Surg* 67:631-639, 1981.
14. Yamamoto K, Takagi N, Miyashita Y et al: Facial reconstruction with latissimus dorsi myocutaneous island flap following total maxillectomy. *J Craniomaxillofac Surg* 15:288-295, 1987.
15. Taylor GI, Corlett RJ, Boyd JB: The versatile deep inferior epigastric (inferior rectus abdominis) flap. *Br J Plast Surg* 37:330-338, 1984.
16. Miyamoto Y, Harada K, Kodama Y et al: Cranial coverage involving scalp, bone and dura using free inferior epigastric flap. *Br J Plast Surg* 39:483-489, 1986.
17. Inoue T, Ueda K, Hatoko M et al: The pedicled serratus anterior myocutaneous flap for head and neck reconstruction. *Br J Plast Surg* 44:259-267, 1991.
18. McCarthy JG, Lorenc ZP, Cutting C et al: Median forehead flap revisited: the blood supply. *Plast Reconstr Surg* 76:866-893, 1985.
19. Burget GC, Menick FJ: Nasal reconstruction: seeking a fourth dimension. *Plast Reconstr Surg* 77:824-833, 1986.
20. Foster RD, Anthony JP, Singer MI et al: Reconstruction of complex midfacial defects. *Plast Reconstr Surg* 99:1555-1565, 1997.
21. Holle J, Vinzenz K, Wuringer E et al: The prefabricated combined scapula flap bony and soft-tissue reconstruction in maxillofacial defects: a new method. *Plast Reconstr Surg* 98:542-552, 1996.
22. Thomas WO, Harris CN: Subtotal midfacial/total nasal reconstruction following shotgun blast to the face employing composite microvascular serratus, anterior rib, muscle, and scapula tip. *Ann Plast Surg* 38:291-295, 1997.
23. Stevens MR, Heit JM, Kline SN et al: The use of osseointegrated implants in craniofacial trauma. *J Craniomaxillofac Trauma* 4:27-34, 1998.
24. Harris L, Wilkes GH, Wolfaardt JF: Autogenous soft-tissue procedures and osseo-integrated alloplastic reconstruction: their role in the treatment of complex craniofacial defects. *Plast Reconstr Surg* 98:387-392, 1996.
25. Keller K, Vasconez HC: Customized composite reconstruction of extensive midfacial defects. *Ann Plast Surg* 40:291-296, 1998.
26. Lengelé BG: Current concepts and future challenges in facial transplantation. *Clin Plast Surg* 36:507-521, 2009.
27. Moore AM, Winslow P: Initial care of shotgun wounds of the face: report of 2 cases. *Am Surgeon* 31:321-328, 1965.

21

Facial Nerve Injuries

Henning Schliephake, Jarg-Erich Hausamen

Traumatic injuries of the facial nerve are uncommon compared with other causes of facial nerve dysfunction, such as tumors, cerebral ischemia, and idiopathic nerve palsy. Facial nerve damage caused by head or neck trauma may be associated with life-threatening injuries, and therapy focuses on life-saving measures and stabilization of the patient's general condition. Although a traumatic lesion of the facial nerve may not appear to be of primary importance in the emergency room, permanent facial paralysis caused by traumatic injury can severely affect the patient's life thereafter. Loss of facial movement and insufficient eye closure are burdensome, and the social consequences of disfigurement and loss of facial expression are particularly distressing. The sequelae are likely to impair the patient's personal relationships and social life in a profound manner.

Adequate management of the traumatic injuries of the facial nerve requires a thorough knowledge of the complex anatomy of the nerve, sophisticated diagnostic means, and advanced surgical skills in microsurgical nerve repair. The surgeons must provide the conditions for successful recovery or repair of traumatic nerve damage. This chapter discusses initial presentation, diagnostic measures, and timing and techniques of nerve repair.

EPIDEMIOLOGY

Traumatic damage to the facial nerve can be indirect or direct. Indirect damage may be encountered after intracerebral bleeding. Because intracerebral lesions of the facial nerve nucleus or its fascicles are unlikely to be directly repaired surgically, they are not considered in this chapter.

Direct trauma to the nerve can occur along its intratemporal and extratemporal routes. The most common site of direct traumatic lesions is the intratemporal route, and trauma usually is caused by temporal bone fractures (86%).[1] However, only 7% of temporal fractures involve facial nerve damage,[2] which indicates that direct facial nerve injuries in head and neck trauma are uncommon. The second most frequent cause of traumatic damage to the facial nerve is gunshot wounds to the temporal bone,[3] although only 8% of all gunshot wounds in the head and neck are associated with facial nerve injury.[4] Damage to the nerve on the extratemporal route occurs even less frequently. Blunt injuries, stab wounds, severely dislocated mandibular fractures, gunshot wounds, and birth trauma can account for facial paralysis. In gunshot wounds, traumatic damage may occur through blast injury, even if the trunk or the large branches have not been directly severed.[5]

Obstetrical reasons for facial nerve lesions are rare, occurring in approximately 0.07% of deliveries, but facial nerve damage is nevertheless the second or third most common injury caused by obstetrical trauma.[6,7] Only 6.3% of facial nerve disorders result from direct traumatic injuries.[1] Occasionally, late damage to the facial nerve may be associated with posttraumatic vascular malformations.[8,9]

STATE-OF-THE-ART MANAGEMENT

Diagnosis of acute facial nerve damage due to trauma is commonly impaired by the general anaesthetic administered in the emergency room. Facial nerve damage often must be assumed from the location and extent of soft tissue wounds. However, even if direct damage to parts of the facial nerve appears to be very likely from clinical inspection, not every traumatic lesion of the facial nerve is inevitably followed by complete paralysis of the facial muscles. Even in extensive lacerations of facial soft tissues, nerve function may not be damaged, or after initial weakness, a level of adequate function may be recovered (Fig. 21-1).

Several factors influence treatment outcomes. The nerve is completely embedded in soft tissue and has considerable longitudinal elasticity, which accounts for its amazing resistance against mechanical damage, even during direct impact. An extensive system of anastomosis between the trunks of the nerve supplies every region of the facial muscles except the mandibular branch. Multiple nerve supplies, with mutual exchange between fibers of different branches, usually exist between the zygomatic and buccal branches. Isolated damage to one of these branches commonly does not result in a paresis of the corresponding facial muscles. However, clinical evidence of nerve dysfunction based on weakness of the facial muscles is not necessarily associated with severing of, or irreversible damage to, the corresponding nerve fibers.

Nerve damage has been classified into three categories: neurapraxia, axonotmesis, and neurotmesis. Although these categories refer to structural alterations of the nerve at a microscopic level, they are directly related to the patient's prognosis and clinical outcome.

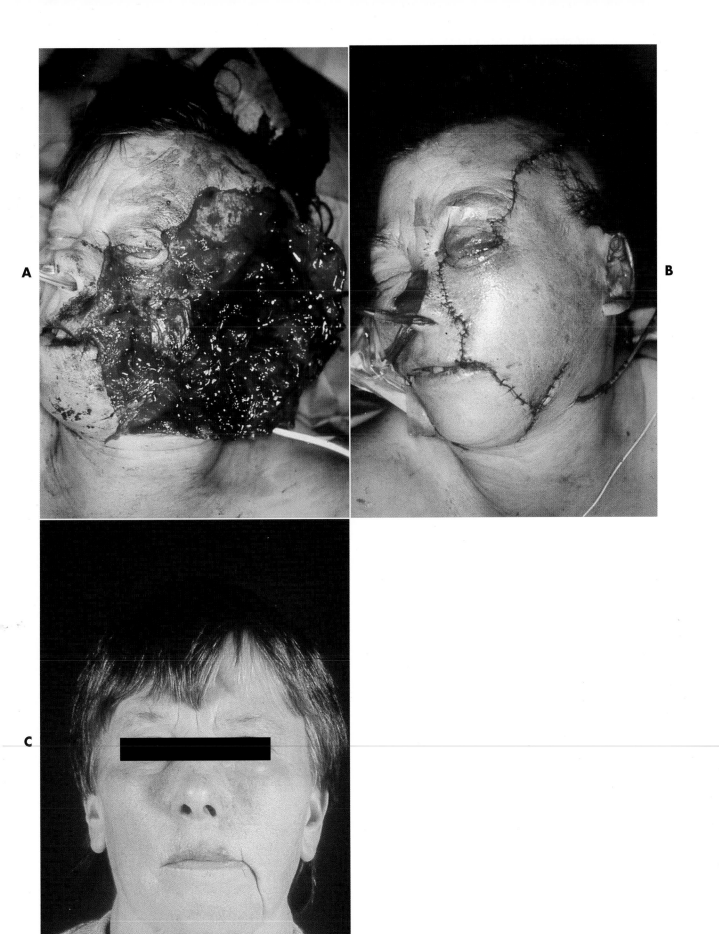

FIGURE 21-1 **A,** Extreme soft tissue laceration of the left cheek. **B,** Status immediately after wound closure. **C,** Facial appearance approximately 6 months later.

Neurapraxia is the simplest type of injury to the nerve, and its clinical manifestation is only temporary. The axons of the nerve remain undamaged, but the myelin sheath sustains injury, such as from compression or hyperextension of the nerve. Resulting edema of the myelin sheath causes temporary dysfunction, from which the nerve recovers within days to weeks.

In axonotmesis, continuity of the nerve is preserved, but damage is more severe due to prolonged compression or a localized ischemic lesion of the nerve. The myelin sheath and the axons are affected. Both components degenerate, but regeneration of axons is guided by the fibrous structures of the nerve, which remain intact. In electromyographic recordings, axonotmesis is characterized by degenerative reactions, retardation of muscle twitching, and complete interruption of nerve conduction. However, because the continuity of the fibrous framework of the nerve has been maintained along the entire length of the nerve, regeneration can proceed to the distal end of the nerve. The axons and the myelin sheath undergo wallerian degeneration, after which their debris is digested by Schwann cells and invading macrophages. Concurrently, Schwann cells proliferate within the basal membrane and arrange themselves into chains known as Hanken-Büngner bands. Regeneration of axons then commences proximal to the site of damage and follows the Hanken-Büngner bands to the periphery. Regeneration of the normal nerve fiber pattern is possible, resulting in more or less complete functional restoration.

In neurotmesis, the nerve is completely severed, and its ends are separated by retraction due to the longitudinal elasticity of the nerve. Clinically and electromyographically, axonotmesis and neurotmesis are identical. The morphological alterations during degeneration of axons and myelin sheath are likewise the same. However, spontaneous regeneration in the peripheral nerve segment is impossible because it depends on bridging the gap between the two retracted nerve ends. Surgical intervention is required to establish continuity of the nerve by direct suturing or grafting.

DIAGNOSIS AND TIMING OF TREATMENT

In conscious and cooperative patients, function of the facial muscles is easily tested by asking the patient to sequentially activate the frontal, periorbital, buccal, and perioral muscles. However, clinical signs of facial nerve palsy also can manifest with some delay in mastoid bone fractures.[10]

In injuries with suspected intratemporal damage to the nerve, diagnostic imaging is required. In temporal bone fractures, computed tomography is preferable to plain radiography, because only 20% to 30% of temporal fractures can be visualized by the latter technique.[11] Magnetic resonance imaging (MRI) provides additional information about facial nerve damage by showing abnormal nerve enhancement, particularly in distal intrameatal nerve segments.[12] MRI enhancement by gadolinium-diethyl-triamine-pentaacetic acid (Gd-DTPA) produces more informative studies for the evaluation of facial nerve pathology and can help to define nerve lesions more accurately.[13-16] Contrast-enhanced scans can identify clinically silent traumatic damage in the temporal bone.[15] Electrodiagnostic tests such as evoked electromyography or electroneuronography play an important role in the objective assessment of facial nerve damage and provide indications for decision making with respect to surgical intervention.[17-19] However, most electrodiagnostic tests are focused on examination of the nerve distal to the stylomastoid foramen and cannot evaluate the nerve across the injury site in intratemporal lesions.[19,20] Pathological findings are obtained on electrodiagnostic nerve testing only if wallerian degeneration of the axons distal to the damaged site has occurred. These diagnostic tools are useful only for late assessment of posttraumatic facial nerve damage.

To provide earlier information about the severity of facial nerve lesions, transcranial magnetic stimulation of the facial nerve after nontraumatic damage has been used to evaluate patients with Bell's palsy.[21,22] This technique has also been applied successfully in the immediate examination of traumatic facial nerve lesions in an experimental setting.[19] However, contradictory results in clinical and experimental studies preclude recommendation of its routine clinical use at this time.

If deep lacerations of facial soft tissues in the buccal and particularly the preauricular area indicate damage on the extratemporal route of the nerve and there is clinical evidence of paresis, meticulous inspection and identification of severed nerve ends is often the only way to positively establish the presence of nerve damage. The functional sequelae of evident damage to individual nerve branches are difficult to predict because of the reasons mentioned earlier, and primary nerve reconstruction after identification of nerve ends is not always indicated. From the experience with crossfacial nerve grafts for facial reanimation, it is known that 50% of facial nerve fibers are sufficient to provide satisfactory muscle tonus at rest and symmetrical movement under voluntary function. Primary repair is recommended only if there is morphological proof that the trunk of the facial nerve itself has been severed. Only in this case should further dissection of the nerve segments be performed. However, if primary repair is not possible because of soft tissue swelling, bleeding, lack of operation time, or serious injury, repair can be delayed. Reconstruction after 3 to 4 weeks may be preferable in many cases because the patient's condition has become stable and soft tissue swelling has gone down. For the severed nerve ends to be identified in the secondary approach, they must be marked during primary care with non-resorbable atraumatic marker sutures that are fixed to the skin.

If the patient has an extratemporal traumatic facial nerve lesion and the surgeon is uncertain whether the injury is only minor (i.e., neurapraxia) or the nerve has been completely severed, no more than 3 months should elapse before possible repair. During this time, the nerve function must be monitored electromyographically, and a decision about whether to perform a reconstruction must be made. If no signs of regeneration are seen during this period, revision and reconstruction should no longer be delayed. Physical therapy such as electrostimulation of the facial muscles and massage should be administered in the meantime.

The interval before secondary nerve repair is limited by the progressive atrophy of the facial muscles on the paretic side of the face. If reconstruction of the nerve is considered, it must be performed at least within the first year postoperatively, because after this period, muscle function, even with reinnervated facial nerve fibers, will be insufficient to accomplish satisfactory movement of the face on the paretic side.

Beyond this interval, reanimation of the paralyzed face must be performed by revascularized transfer of neuromuscular segments. In such procedures, a vascularized segment from the gracilis muscle or the latissimus dorsi muscle with a branch of the supplying nerve is transferred to the face to augment the atrophic facial muscles and allow for innervated function of the transferred muscle.[23-28]

SURGICAL REPAIR

Surgical intervention for repair of traumatic damage to the facial nerve depends on the location of the nerve injury. For intratemporal lesions, decompression surgery of the nerve in the osseous canal through the temporal bone must be considered. For extratemporal lesions, a decision must be made about microsurgical repair of the nerve. Although the former procedure is more a domain of otolaryngology or neurosurgery, the maxillofacial surgeon is involved in the latter.

Microsurgical repair of the extratemporal portion of the facial nerve requires a high standard of technical equipment and surgical training. A surgical microscope with continuously adjustable magnification between 2× and 40× and foot control should be available. Suture material with a 25 μm diameter (10-0) is recommended, and forceps with smooth, nonserrated ends are preferable to avoid trauma to the delicate perineural tissue.

NERVE SUTURING

Basic surgical techniques for repair of the extratemporal part of the facial nerve have been contributed by Conley[29] and Miehlke.[30] Before the use of the microscope for surgical nerve repair, nerve suturing was commonly performed by suturing the epineurium. This was often unsuccessful, mainly because of inadequate preparation of the cross-sectional surface of the nerve ends and insufficient adaptation of the individual fascicles. Surgery has dramatically improved since the introduction of microscopic techniques, which enabled atraumatic handling and precise adaptation of the nerve ends and individual fascicles.[31,32] The poor results obtained with epineural suturing in the earlier era were initially attributed to the epineural location of the suture, and new concepts of perineural suturing with adaptation of individual fascicles were developed. Numerous studies have now shown that both techniques can achieve similar results as long as they are performed with the same accuracy and atraumatic handling of the nerve ends and fascicles.

The differential indication for epineural versus perineural suturing depends on the fascicular structure of the nerve. The three patterns of fascicles are monofascicular, oligofascicular (fewer than five fascicles), and polyfascicular structure[33] (Fig. 21-2). Epineural suturing is considered to be appropriate in monofascicular and oligofascicular nerve ends, and perineural sutures are required only in polyfascicular nerves. Because the facial nerve has a monofascicular or oligofascicular structure at the nerve trunk and its first divisions into peripheral branches, epineural suturing is adequate in most areas of the nerve.

The aim and strategy of microsurgical intervention are defined by the timing of the surgery and the degree of damage to the nerve. In primary repair and any other microsurgical

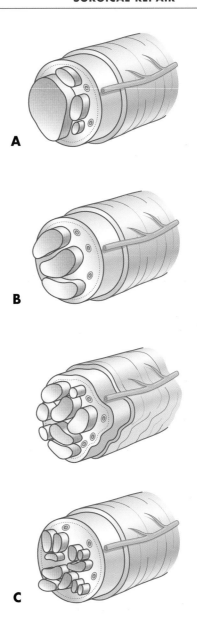

FIGURE 21-2 **A,** Cross-section of a monofascicular nerve. **B,** Cross-section of an oligofascicular nerve. **C,** Cross-sections of polyfascicular nerves.

repair procedure, the nerve ends are dissected free of epineural connective tissue (Fig. 21-3A), because the greatest hazard for axon proliferation from the central nerve end into the peripheral segment is the proliferation of connective tissue at the site of suturing. Intervening connective tissue can prevent axons from further elongation into the distal segment or can turn down already regenerated axons. Possible factors that account for this fibrosis are traumatic dissection of the nerve during preparation for suturing and suturing of the nerve ends while they are under longitudinal tension. Tension-free suturing of the nerve ends and atraumatic dissection are mandatory.

Because the epineural fibroblasts proliferate more rapidly than the fibroblasts and Schwann cells of the endoneural space, the epineural tissue should be removed from the nerve ends to reduce the proportion of connective tissue in nerve cross-section and to allow for more precise adaptation of the

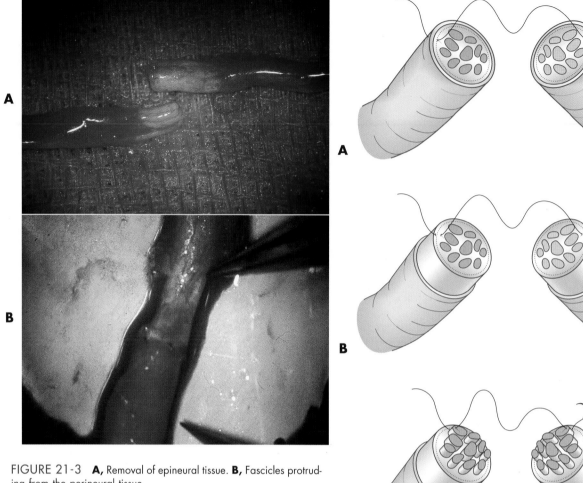

FIGURE 21-3　**A,** Removal of epineural tissue. **B,** Fascicles protruding from the perineural tissue.

fascicles (see Fig. 21-3B). However, removal of the epineurium in facial nerve repair is feasible only at the trunk, because the epineurium becomes very thin on the more peripheral branches and is hardly discernible from the remaining parts.

Before the nerve ends are sutured in primary repair after trauma, they are dissected free of their surrounding tissue and trimmed with serrated scissors until the cut ends look completely undamaged. Subsequently, the epineurium is opened and removed on both ends for a length of 5 to 10 mm with the scissors at a microscopic magnification of 10×. This reveals the location and structure of fascicles at the cross-section of the nerve. After trimming, axons tend to prolapse due to endoneural pressure and longitudinal retraction of the perineural tissue. These protruding axons should be removed to gain a smooth cross-sectional area that facilitates adaptation and suturing of the nerve ends. Protruding axons are grasped with the forceps, pulled forward, and cut with serrated scissors at the level of the epineural or perineural annulus. Suturing can be performed by epineural, perineural, or interfascicular suturing (Fig. 21-4).

The choice of technique is not as important as the precise adaptation of the nerve ends and their fascicles. To ensure mechanically stable and reliable adaptation, three to four sutures are recommended around the complete circumference of the nerve. When microsurgical repair is performed at

FIGURE 21-4　**A,** Microsurgical suturing of the epineurium. **B,** Microsurgical suturing of the perineurium. **C,** Interfascicular microsurgical suturing.

the nerve trunk, it is important to correctly reorient the fascicles in the distal nerve ends to the corresponding proximal ends to ensure restoration of the functional organization of the nerve plexus.

In late secondary repair of lacerated nerves, the nerve ends commonly must be identified in the scar tissue of the former injury. In many cases, the scar tissue serves as a landmark of dissection and orientation to identify the nerve ends. If the nerve ends were marked with sutures during primary care, it is often useful to excise the scar completely and locate the nerve ends distally and proximally from this area along the suture marks. If no marking was performed, dissection and identification of the severed nerve ends is much more difficult using the scar tissue as a starting point. In such cases, it is often preferable to start with exposure of the nerve trunk at the stylomastoid foramen and to proceed along its main branches until the scar area is reached. In the same way, the peripheral branches are identified distal to the scar area and followed proximally (Fig. 21-5).

If the severity of injury to the nerve is unclear, microsurgical neurolysis should be considered first by isolating the nerve from scar tissue and removing the epineurium to examine the fascicles for intact or severed continuity under the microscope. For this purpose, the nerve is located outside the area of former injury and dissected free of scar tissue at magnifications of 10× to 25×. Frequently, a neuroma is encountered that may hide interruption of nerve continuity, but occasionally only increased intraneural scar formation of the fibrous sheath is found, with underlying individual fascicles exhibiting undisturbed continuity. In any case, the epineurium must be removed to examine the intraneural situation. If an endoneural neuroma is found, it is removed, and the nerve ends are treated as described previously for primary nerve repair. If intraneural fibrosis is encountered, an interfascicular neurolysis is required with careful removal of the compromising scar tissue between the fascicles to free the intact nerve components.

CABLE GRAFTING

Direct end-to-end repair of traumatic facial nerve damage is possible only when the nerve has had a straight cut in the area of the trunk or larger peripheral branches without crushing or tearing trauma. Even in primary nerve repair, trauma to the nerve often requires removal of the damaged nerve tissue during trimming. This precludes tensionless suturing of the nerve ends. In primary repair of traumatic nerve damage and in secondary reconstructions if scar formation has separated the nerve ends, a cable graft is necessary to bridge the continuity defect of the nerve. Autogenous nerve grafts usually are the method of choice, although allogeneic nerve grafts also have proved to be functional. However, low-dose immunosuppression is necessary with the use of allogeneic grafts, and the hazard of transmitting infectious diseases is much more serious than the hazard of donor site morbidity from harvesting of autogenous grafts. These risks have precluded allogeneic grafts from clinical use.[34] The possibility of vascularized nerve transfer using the saphenous nerve or the sural nerve has inspired several clinical and experimental approaches. No clear advantage of the increased surgery of such vascularized nerve transfer has been shown compared to nonvascularized nerve grafting with respect to axonal morphology or postoperative nerve function.

Suitable donor sites for nonvascularized nerve grafts include the branches of the cervical plexus in the neck and the sural nerve from the calf. The great auricular nerve from the cervical plexus has been used for cable grafting because its anatomy provides a suitable number of branches that can be connected to the peripheral branches of the facial nerve plexus, and its thicker proximal end is sutured to the central stump of the facial nerve. The sural nerve has a similar morphology of branches.

The branches of the cervical plexus are easily identified on the outer surface of the sternocleidomastoid muscle vertically below the auricle. For exposure, an incision parallel to the course of the muscle or an extended submandibular incision is used. The great auricular nerve and the transverse cervical nerve appear at the lower border of the sternocleidomastoid muscle at the so-called punctum nervosum. The

great auricular nerve courses upward to the auricle, and the transverse cervical nerve runs medially and branches off shortly after the punctum nervosum.

The sural nerve is often preferred if longer or multiple grafts are required. This cutaneous nerve can been conveniently exposed through a horizontal incision behind the lateral malleolus (Fig. 21-6A). During dissection, the lateral saphenous vein may be encountered; it overlies the sural nerve and is commonly preserved. After isolation of the nerve, its proximal course can be identified by gently pulling the nerve and palpating approximately 6 to 8 cm upward from the first incision. At that point, a second horizontal incision is performed, and the nerve is exposed. The nerve runs from the ankle joint to the back of the calf, and the more proximal incisions should be placed further back. The nerve can be followed up to the knee joint, where it joins the lateral sural cutaneous nerve. From the knee to the ankle joint, the sural nerve is 30 cm long. It is important for the reconstruction of the facial nerve that the sural nerve sends off branches in the distal part that allow for reconstruction of large parts of the facial plexus and are easily accessible (see Fig. 21-6B). Preference is often given to the sural nerve over the cervical nerve branches because the former provides longer and stronger grafts.

If there is a discrepancy between the cross-sectional area of the facial nerve and the procured nerve graft, two or more grafts can be connected to the thickest nerve ends (see Fig. 21-6C). In the periphery of the plexus, it is very often the reverse, with thin and tiny branches of the facial nerve sutured with much thicker grafts.

The aims of suturing of nerve grafts to the facial nerve are the same as in primary repair. Suturing must be absolutely tensionless, and atraumatic preparation and handling of the nerve graft are mandatory. The cable nerve grafts must be longer than the length of the nerve defect.

NERVE CROSSOVERS

Indications for crossover anastomoses in facial nerve repair have been considerably reduced by the great advances in extracranial and intracranial treatment of these lesions. However, if the proximal part of the trunk of the facial nerve has been destroyed during trauma, direct suturing or cable grafting will be unsuccessful for nerve repair. Innervation of the facial muscles then must be provided by connecting another cranial motor nerve, such as the hypoglossal, glossopharyngeal, or accessory nerve, to the peripheral facial nerve supply or by providing nerve supply from the opposite, uninjured side by means of a crossfacial nerve graft.

Nerve crossovers using cranial motor nerves have been employed for many years.[35-39] In particular, the hypoglossal nerve and the accessory nerve have been used for this procedure. The nerves that lend their supply to the facial nerve are exposed and cut at a convenient length to reach the facial nerve, and they are anastomosed with the distal end of the facial nerve trunk. Axonal regeneration and neurotization of the previously denervated facial nerve then occurs quickly, originating from the hypoglossal or accessory nerve. However, this method occasionally has resulted in uncoordinated movements through the contralateral nerve and is always associated with functional loss of muscles of the donor nerve supply. Hypoglossal-facial crossover now is the only

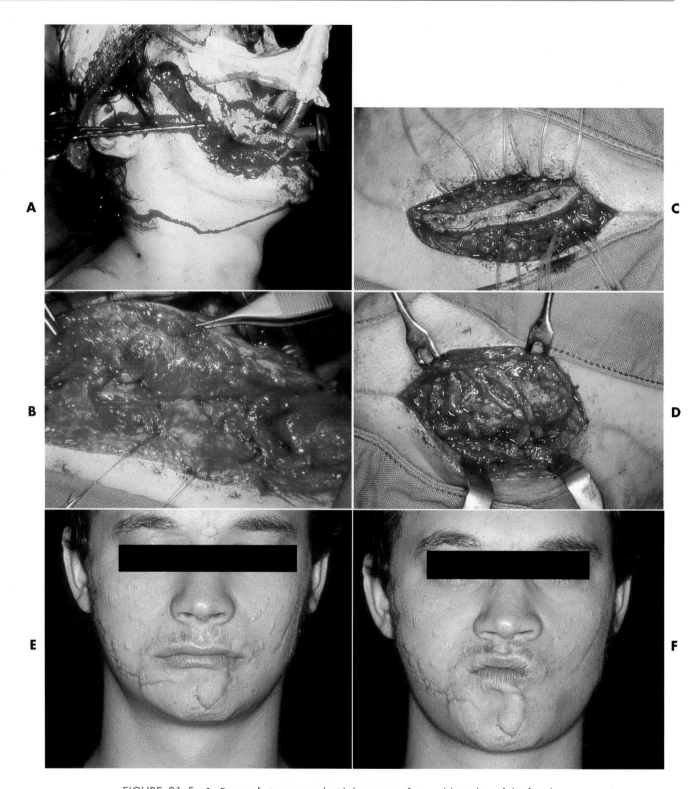

FIGURE 21-5 **A,** Deep soft tissue wound with laceration of several branches of the facial nerve. **B,** Marking of the nerve ends with non-resorbable, atraumatic sutures. **C,** Removal of scar tissue and identification of the individual branches with rubber bands. **D,** Bridging of the defect by cable grafts. **E** and **F,** Postoperative function of the facial nerve.

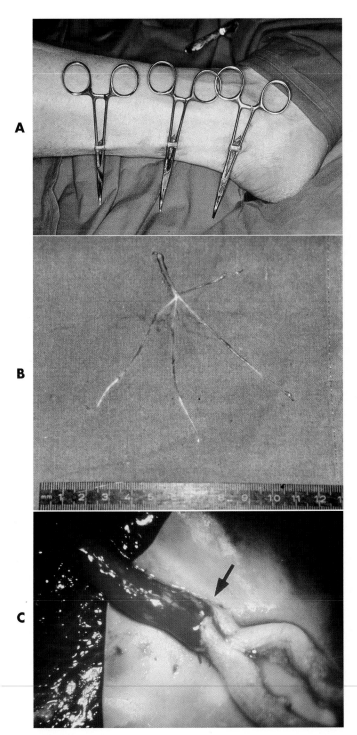

FIGURE 21-6 **A,** Identification of the sural nerve. **B,** Procured sural nerve. **C,** Suturing of two nerve ends from the sural nerve to fit a larger cross-section of the recipient nerve.

crossover anastomosis that is performed using other cranial motor nerves. Usually, the unilateral functional loss of tongue muscles is more easily compensated for by the patient than unilateral limitation of shoulder function in an accessory-facial nerve crossover procedure.

The hypoglossal-facial crossover is a relatively simple operation that can achieve restoration of very good function with regard to both muscular tone of the facial muscles and soft tissue symmetry at rest. It also improves lagophthalmos and permits voluntary movement of the facial muscles to a limited extent. Patients with hypoglossal-facial crossover require a high degree of postoperative muscular training to learn to activate the facial muscles without concurrently activating the tongue muscles. Although voluntary contraction of facial muscles can be accomplished on command, symmetrical affective or emotional expression of the face is not restored fully. Occasionally, moderate intraoral dysfunction, mass movement, and hypertonia of the face can occur. However, these untoward effects are uncommon and usually are well accepted by the patients.

If a hypoglossal-facial crossover is intended after loss of the central part of the facial nerve due to trauma, the distal part of the facial nerve trunk is located in a secondary procedure in the retromandibular fossa, as is done during removal of parotid tumors. From a preauricular incision, the dissection proceeds medially and inferiorly along the outer surface of the cartilage of the external auditory canal. This cartilage forms a triangular prominence before it links with the osseous part of the canal. Approximately 7 to 10 mm medially and inferiorly to that point, the nerve trunk can be located and exposed (Fig. 21-7A). Electrostimulators are indispensable during the final stage of dissection for identification of the nerve. The preauricular incision is then extended into the submandibular region, and the hypoglossal nerve is located beneath the intermediate tendon and the posterior belly of the digastric muscle. From this point, the hypoglossal nerve is followed proximally until it passes over the bifurcation of the carotid arteries. The nerve is then cut distal to the exit of the descending branch on the level of the digastric tendon and transposed cranially over the digastric muscle, where it is sutured to the facial nerve (see Fig. 21-7B to D).

Another type of crossover anastomosis is the faciofacial crossover or crossfacial anastomosis, which was developed in 1971. The principle of this procedure is ingenious: Specific facial nerve fibers reanimate the paretic facial muscles without loss of function of one of the other cranial nerves, providing symmetrical facial movement in emotional expression. The concept is based on the knowledge that approximately 50% of the facial nerve fibers are sufficient for undisturbed function of the facial muscles, so that almost 50% of the neural fibers can be used to reinnervate the paretic side.

To connect the paretic side with the uninjured side, a nerve graft 10 to 15 cm long is required, and it is passed through a subcutaneous tunnel in the upper lip to reach the contralateral side (Fig. 21-8B). The zygomatic branch of the healthy side is commonly selected as the source for innervation of the contralateral side because it contains 40% of the total number of facial nerve fibers and has an intimate exchange of fibers with the buccal branch (see Fig. 21-8C). Because of this extensive system of anastomoses, transection of the zygomatic branch on the uninjured side does not result in paralysis of the periorbital muscles on the healthy side. Stimulation of the contralateral side through the nerve graft to the paretic side enables satisfactory contraction of the orbicularis oculi and the orbicularis oris muscles if it is connected to the zygomatic branch of the severed facial nerve.

The zygomatic branch of the facial nerve is exposed on both sides through a vertical preauricular incision that is located centrally over the parotid gland. For suturing of the

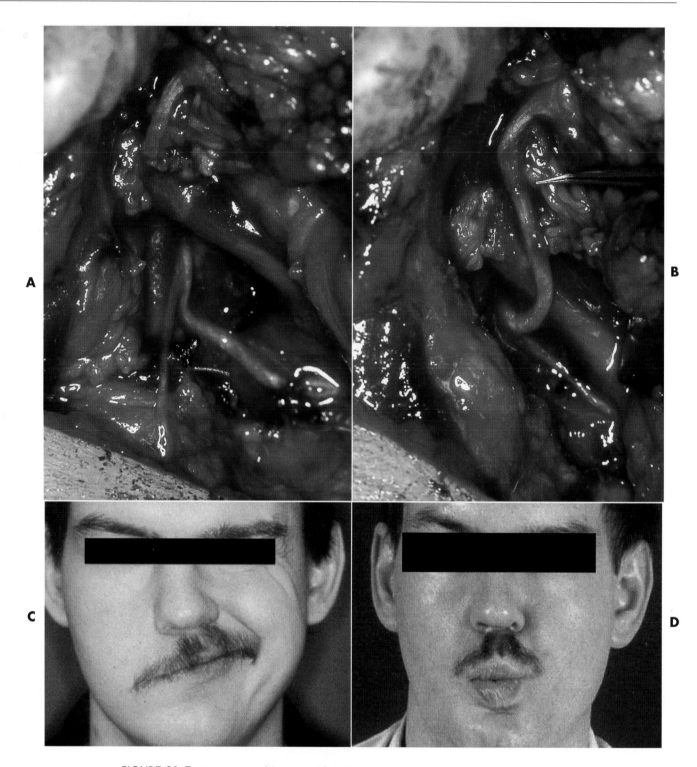

FIGURE 21-7 **A,** Exposure of the severed facial nerve at the stylomastoid foramen and the hypoglossal nerve. **B,** Transposition of the hypoglossal nerve and crossover with the peripheral end of the facial nerve trunk. **C,** Preoperative facial nerve function. **D,** Postoperative facial nerve function.

zygomatic branch on the paretic side, the distal end of the nerve must be reversed by 180 degrees (see Fig. 21-8C to E).

The schedule for crossfacial nerve grafting varies considerably according to the result required. If crossfacial grafting is intended for repair of the contralateral facial nerve, it can be performed as a one-stage or two-stage procedure. In the latter case, the graft is connected to the zygomatic branch on the

healthy side and led through the subcutaneous tunnel. Suturing with the zygomatic arch on the paretic side is done 3 to 4 months later, after proliferation of axons from the nonparetic side into the grafted nerve has commenced. If the crossfacial nerve graft is intended to reinnervate a revascularized muscle segment for facial reanimation after long-standing facial paralysis, the second procedure is performed 10 to 12

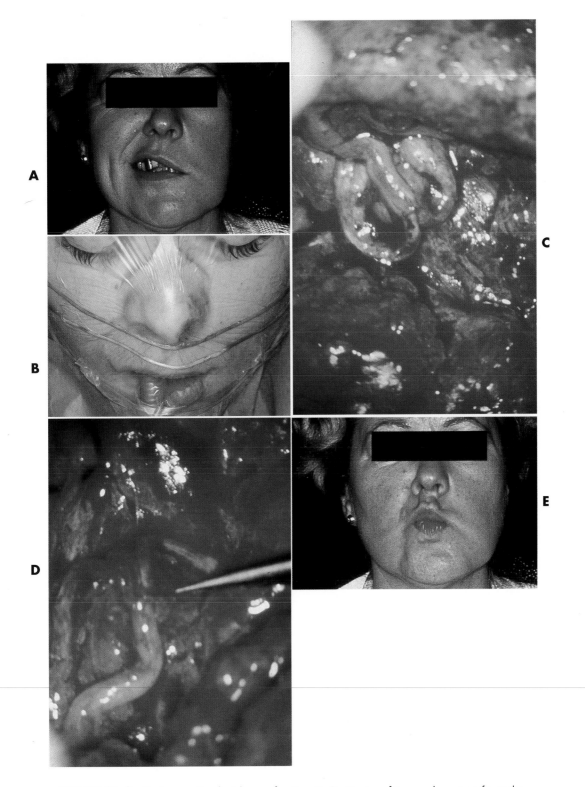

FIGURE 21-8   **A,** Preoperative facial nerve function. **B,** Positioning of two sural nerve grafts on the upper lip on their crossfacial route. **C,** Suturing of the grafts to the zygomatic branch on the healthy side. **D,** Suturing of the graft ends to the zygomatic branch on the paretic side. **E,** Postoperative facial nerve function.

months later, at which time the regenerating axons should have reached the contralateral end of the nerve graft.

NERVE CONDUITS

A newer technique of nerve repair uses the regenerative capacity of the nerve and its inherent growth potential to restore its original morphology. As in many other fields of reconstructive surgery, the use of tissue barriers has been introduced into nerve reconstruction, employing tubes of synthetic, organic, and biologic material that serve as conduits for regenerating axons across a gap of up to several centimeters. The aim of this concept is to avoid sacrifice of autogenous donor nerves in nerve reconstructions across a gap.

Many studies on this topic in clinical and experimental settings have been published.[40-45] The range of results reported is as wide as the experimental approaches used. Some investigators describe positive experiences with the experimental use of collagen or fibronectin nerve guides,[46] but others report no or few advantages for the use of conduits.[47,48] Biologic conduits such as amnion tubes, veins, or avascular muscle grafts demonstrated regeneration in experimental settings across a gap of up to 10 mm that was comparable to that of autogenous nerve grafts.[43,44,49] However, clinical results for gaps of 40 to 58 mm in nerve reconstruction of the upper extremity were poor.[50] When veins are used as nerve conduits, an inside-out vein graft appears to be preferable to a standard autogenous graft.[51]

The application of synthetic conduits appears to be the most widely researched approach, and numerous types of resorbable and non-resorbable polymers are in use.[52-54] However, polymeric conduits have not shown an advantage in nerve regeneration compared with nerve grafts or epineural suturing of nerve ends.[55,56] Healing of nerve gaps of up to 10 mm was worse or did not occur.[48,54,55] Experimental bridging of large gaps of 80 mm by polyglycolic acid tubes resulted in some degree of regeneration but obvious functional deficits.[42] The conduit material does not seem to have a profound effect on outcome,[45] but advances in biologic approaches with the additional application of nerve growth factors or cultivated Schwann cells in these conduits may extend the gap that can be regenerated by the nerve on its own.[41,57,58] Few studies have elucidated the complex effects of conduits in a randomized clinical setting. Weber et al.[40] showed that when a polyglycolic acid conduit is used for repair of nerve gaps of 4 mm or less, improved sensation resulted 1 year postoperatively compared with end-to-end repair of digital nerves. Repair of larger gaps also produced results superior to those obtained with nerve grafts in this area, and clinical use of expanded polytetrafluoroethylene (ePTFE) tubes for repair of trigeminal nerve damage has been successful.[59,60] More research is needed to identify the role of synthetic conduits in clinical nerve repair.

PROBLEMS AND PITFALLS

An unresolved problem in facial nerve reconstruction is the occurrence of uncontrolled or spontaneous (synkinetic) mass movement of the facial muscles. These disturbing effects are prevalent during nerve healing and can affect the facial movements permanently. One of the most frequent synkinetic movements is synchronous elevation of the oral commissure, which is associated with considerable loss of emotional expression. Mass movements can result from poor regeneration of fascicles and from the difficulty in accurately readapting individual fascicles with high precision, even under microscopic control. Several ways to solve this problem have been suggested.

Miehlke and Stennert[38] divided the facial muscles into two functional units: the upper face and the lower face. They concluded that synkinetic movements of the upper and lower functional units could be eliminated by separate reinnervation. They advocated two sources of the reinnervation of the facial muscles. For the repair of the part of the facial nerve plexus that supplies the upper facial muscles, autogenous nerve grafts that connected the peripheral ends with the trunk of the facial nerve were used. The facial nerve supply to the lower face was accomplished through suturing of the hypoglossal nerve to the peripheral nerve ends of this part of the plexus.

Another solution was suggested by Millesi,[61] who used a sophisticated system of interfascicular anastomoses based on anatomic studies of the topographical orientation of certain sectors of the facial nerve cross-section to different groups of facial muscles. To avoid misinnervation in short defects of the trunk of the facial nerve, the use of three to four small nerve grafts is recommended to connect corresponding groups of fascicles in the proximal and peripheral cross-section of the trunk. Bridging of defects between the trunk and peripheral nerve ends can be accomplished by eight nerve grafts that connect these groups of fascicles with the peripheral supply. However, misinnervations can occur even with this technique because of variations in the course of the individual fascicles. Experimental studies also indicate that regenerating fibers may become aberrant at the site of repair and throughout the length of the nerve.[62]

POSTOPERATIVE CARE

Postoperative treatment should commence as early as possible and should be continued until normal facial motion is gained. Three treatment modes are available: neurotrophic vitamins, physical therapy, and electrotherapy.

So-called neurotrophic vitamins have frequently been recommended for enhancement of neural regeneration after nerve trauma. However, apart from severe general metabolic disorders resulting from alcohol abuse or malabsorption, neurotrophic vitamins have no reliable or reproducible effect on nerve regeneration.

Physical therapy is administered to the paretic face to reduce the atrophy of the facial muscles. Massage increases the local perfusion, and percutaneously applied electrical current can enhance this effect. Electrotherapy cannot accelerate reinnervation and does not completely prevent muscular atrophy of the paretic muscle. It is useful in cases of complete paresis and should be continued after reconstruction until the first signs of reinnervation occur. The use of so-called exponential currents has proved to be effective by inducing distinct contraction of paretic muscles.

After onset of visible voluntary contractions, active cooperation of the patient is essential. Electrotherapy is replaced by active muscular exercises. The patient is instructed to voluntarily contract all facial muscles several times per day in front of a mirror. Facial massage should be continued at this stage.

Pulsatile electric currents can be applied in case of residual, chronic facial nerve damage, using battery-powered stimulators at the submotor level for several months. This approach has resulted in decreased motor latencies and has improved House-Brackmann scores.[63]

OUTCOMES OF NERVE RECONSTRUCTION

The results of facial nerve reconstruction are commonly assessed by a mixture of subjective patient criteria and observer-rated criteria.[23,68] Although most observer-rated scales are semiquantitative or provide a summated score of subjective ratings,[26,64] electromyograms provide objective data about voluntary muscle contraction.

Reports on the results of facial nerve reconstruction after trauma are scarce. The prognosis of intratemporal lesions strongly depends on the severity and the delay in the onset of palsy. Incomplete and delayed-onset palsies show good recovery, but patients with immediate onset of complete paralysis have a poor prognosis.[2] Decompression surgery is considered to be beneficial only during the first 24 days in patients with 95% or more degeneration demonstrated on electroneurograms. Blunt injuries to the extratemporal route have been associated with a good prognosis without surgical intervention, which contrasts with injuries to the intratemporal course.[65,66] Results of reconstruction of the facial nerve in the extratemporal part vary considerably according to the techniques used and the time elapsed between trauma and repair. The most favorable results are obtained from direct nerve suturing used in a primary procedure. However, this is not always possible, and the second-best results are achieved by the use of cable grafts that are interposed between the severed nerve ends.

The results of nerve crossover procedures are controversial. Some surgeons prefer crossfacial nerve grafts,[67] but others advocate the hypoglossal-facial nerve crossover.[69] However, the results of nerve crossover procedures are clearly inferior to those of direct facial nerve reconstruction. In all cases, an attempt should be made to perform suturing of severed nerve ends directly or by means of an interposed nerve graft.

The period of reinnervation varies after a completely severed nerve is reconstructed. Depending on the extent of the damage, return of function can be expected in 6 to 12 months. The function of the facial muscles continues to improve thereafter for another year, and usually this is the final result. In cases of long-standing facial palsy with atrophy of the muscles, neurovascular reanastomosed muscle grafts (i.e., gracilis muscle) should be considered (see Chapter 28).

REFERENCES

1. May M: *The facial nerve*, New York, 1986, Thieme, pp 181-216.
2. Brodie HA, Thompson TC: Management of complications from 820 temporal bone fractures. *Am J Otol* 18:188-197, 1997.
3. Qiu WW, Yin SS, Pate WE et al: Neurotologic evaluation of facial nerve paralysis caused by gunshot wounds. *Ear Nose Throat J* 78:270-272, 1999.
4. Stack BC, Farrior JB: Missile injuries to the temporal bone. *South Med J* 88:72-78, 1995.
5. Telischi FF, Patete ML: Blast injuries to the facial nerve. *Arch Otolaryngol Head Neck Surg* 111:446-449, 1994.
6. Bhat V, Ravikumara M, Oumachigui A: Nerve injuries due to obstetric trauma. *Indian J Pediatr* 65:207-212, 1995.
7. Hughes CA, Harley EH, Milmoe G, et al: Birth trauma in the head and neck. *Arch Otolaryngol Head Neck Surg* 125:193-199, 1999.
8. Lalak NJ, Farmer E: Traumatic pseudoaneurysm of the superficial temporal artery associated with facial nerve palsy. *J Cardiovasc Surg* 37:119-123, 1996.
9. Hsu KC, Wang AC, Chen SJ: Mastoid bone fracture presenting as unusual delayed onset of facial nerve palsy. *Am J Emerg Med* 26:386, e1-e2, 2008.
10. Roland JT, Hammerschlag PE, Lewis WS, et al: Management of traumatic facial nerve paralysis with carotid artery cavernosus sinus fistula. *Eur Arch Otorhinolaryngol* 251:57-60, 1994.
11. Turetschek K, Czerny C, Wunderbaldinger P, Steiner E: Temporal bone trauma and imaging. *Radiologe* 37:977-982, 1997.
12. Sartoretti-Schefer S, Scherler M, Wichmann W, Valavanis A: Contrast-enhanced MR of the facial nerve in patients with posttraumatic peripheral facial nerve palsy. *Am J Neuroradiol* 18:1115-1125, 1997.
13. Koike Y, Tojima H, Maeyama H, Aoyagi M: Contrast-enhanced MRI of the facial nerve in patients with Bell's palsy. *Eur Arch Otorhinolaryngol* Dec(suppl):S346-348, 1994.
14. Orloff LA, Duckert LG: Magnetic resonance imaging of intratemporal facial nerve lesions in the animal model. *Laryngoscope* 105:465-471, 1995.
15. Kinoshita T, Ishii K, Okitsu T, et al: Facial nerve palsy: evaluation by contrast enhanced MR imaging. *Clin Radiol* 56:926-932, 2001.
16. Kumar A, Mafee MF, Mason T: Value of imaging on disorders of the facial nerve. *Top Magn Reson Imaging* 11:38-51, 2000.
17. Nosan DK, Benecke JE, Murr AH: Current perspective on temporal bone trauma. *Arch Otolaryngol Head Neck Surg* 117:67-71, 1997.
18. Chang CY, Cass SP: Management of facial nerve injury due to temporal bone trauma. *Am J Otol* 20:96-114, 1999.
19. Har-El G, McPhee JRL: Transcranial magnetic stimulation in acute facial nerve injury. *Laryngoscope* 110:1105-1111, 2000.
20. Metson R, Rebeiz E, West C, Thornton A: Magnetic stimulation of the facial nerve. *Laryngoscope* 101:25-30, 1991.
21. Schriefer TN, Mills KR, Murray NMF, Hess CW: Evaluation of proximal facial nerve conduction by transcranial magnetic stimulation. *J Neurol Neurosurg Psychiatry* 51:60-66, 1988.
22. Parisi L, Coiro P, Valente G, et al: Neurophysiological evaluation of Bell's palsy: electroneurography and transcranial magnetic stimulation. *Eur Arch Otorhinolaryngol* Dec(suppl):253-257, 1994.
23. Schliephake H, Schmelzeisen R: Free revascularized muscle transfer for facial reanimation after long standing facial paralysis. *Int J Oral Maxillofac Surg* 29:243-249, 2000.
24. Harii K, Ohmori K, Torii S: Free gracilis muscle transplantation with microneurovascular anastomoses for the treatment of facial palsy: a preliminary report. *Plast Reconstr Surg* 57:133-156, 1976.
25. Kärcher H: Die Reanimation der langbestehenden Facialisparese. *Fortschr Kiefer Gesichtschir* 35:144-147, 1990.
26. Harii K, Asato H, Yoshimura K, et al: One-stage transfer of the latissimus dorsi muscle for reanimation of a paralyzed face: a new alternative. *Plast Reconstr Surg* 102:941-951, 1998.
27. Terzis JK, Noah ME: Analysis of 100 cases of free muscle transplantation for facial paralysis. *Plast Reconstr Surg* 99:1905-1921, 1997.
28. Ueda K, Harii K, Yamada A: Free neurovascular muscle transplantation for the treatment of facial paralysis using the hypoglossal nerve as a recipient motor source. *Plast Reconstr Surg* 94:808-817, 1994.
29. Conley J: Surgical treatment of tumors of the parotid gland with emphasis on immediate nerve grafting. *West J Surg Obstet Gynecol* 63:534-537, 1955.
30. Miehlke A: *Die Chirurgie des Nervus facialis*, Munich, 1960, Urban & Schwarzenberg.
31. Millesi H: Die operative Wiederherstellung verletzter Nerven. *Langenbecks Arch Chir* 332:347-355, 1972.
32. Samii M: Modern aspects of peripheral and cranial nerve surgery. In Krayenbühl H, editor: *Advances and technical standards in neurosurgery*, vol 2, Vienna, 1975, Springer.
33. Millesi H: Looking back on nerve surgery. *Int J Microsurg* 2:143-155, 1980.
34. Lassner F, Becker MH, Fuhrer S, et al: Time limited immunosuppression in allogenic nerve transplant in the rat. *Handchir Mikrochir Plast Chir* 28:176-180, 1996.
35. Stennert E: Hypoglossal facial anastomosis: its significance for modern facial surgery. *Clin Plast Surg* 6:471-482, 1979.
36. Conley JJ, Baker DC: Hypoglossal-facial nerve anastomosis for re-innervation of the paralyzed face. *Plast Reconstr Surg* 63:63-72, 1979.

37. Evans DM: Hypoglossal-facial anastomosis in the treatment of facial palsy. *Br J Plast Surg* 27:251-260, 1974.

38. Miehlke A, Stennert E: New techniques for optimum reconstruction of facial nerve in its extratemporal course. *Acta Otolaryngol* 91:497-505, 1981.

39. Hausamen JE: Principles and clinical application of micronerve surgery and nerve transplantation in the maxillofacial area. *Ann Plast Surg* 7:428-437, 1981.

40. Weber RA, Breidenbach WC, Brown RE, et al: A randomized prospective study of polyglycolic acid conduits for digital nerve reconstruction in humans. *Plast Reconstr Surg* 106:1036-1045, 2000.

41. Hadlock T, Sundback C, Hunter D, et al: A polymer foam conduit seeded with Schwann cell promotes guided peripheral nerve regeneration. *Tissue Eng* 6:119-127, 2000.

42. Matsumoto K, Ohnishi K, Sekine T, et al: Use of newly developed artificial nerve conduit to assist peripheral nerve regeneration across a long gap in dogs. *ASAIO J* 46:415-420, 2000.

43. Fansa H, Keilhoff G, Forster G, et al: Acellular muscle with Schwann-cell implantation: an alternative biologic nerve conduit. *J Reconstr Microsurg* 15:531-537, 1999.

44. Mohammad J, Shenaq J, Rabinovsky E, Shenaq S: Modulation of peripheral nerve regeneration: a tissue-engineering approach. *Plast Reconstr Surg* 105:660-666, 2000.

45. Strauch B: Use of nerve conduits in peripheral nerve repair. *Hand Clin* 16:123-130, 2000.

46. Kitahara AK, Nishimura Y, Shimizu Y, Endo K: Facial nerve repair accomplished by the interposition of a collagen nerve guide. *J Neurosurg* 93:113-120, 2000.

47. Whitworth IH, Brown RA, Dore C, et al: Orientated mats of fibronectin as a conduit material for use in peripheral nerve repair. *J Hand Surg* 20:429-436, 1995.

48. Vasconelos BC, Gay-Escoda C: Facial nerve repair with expanded polytetrafluoro-ethylene and collagen conduits: an experimental study in the rabbit. *J Oral Maxillofac Surg* 58:1257-1262, 2000.

49. Di Benedetto G, Zura G, Mazzucchelli R, et al: Nerve regeneration through a combined autologous conduit (vein plus acellular muscle). *Biomaterials* 19:173-181, 1998.

50. Tang JB, Shi D, Zhou H: Vein conduits for repair of nerves with a prolonged gap or in unfavourable conditions: an analysis of three failed cases. *Microsurgery* 16:133-137, 1995.

51. Tang J, Wang XM, Hu J, et al: Autogenous standard versus inside-out vein graft to repair facial nerve in rabbits. *Clin J Traumatol* 11:104-109, 2008.

52. Nicoli Aldini P, Perego G, Cella GD, et al: Effectiveness of a bioresorbable conduit in the repair of peripheral nerves. *Biomaterials* 17:959-962, 1996.

53. Giardino R, Nicoli Aldini P, Perego G, et al: Biological and synthetic conduits in peripheral nerve repair: a comparative study. *Int J Artif Organs* 18:225-230, 1995.

54. Evans GR, Brandt K, Widmer MS, et al: In vivo evaluation of poly(L-lactic acid) porous conduits for peripheral nerve repair. *Biomaterials* 20:1109-1115, 1999.

55. Francel PC, Francel TJ, Mackinnon SE, Hertl C: Enhancing nerve regeneration across a silicone tube conduit by using interposed short-segment nerve grafts. *J Neurosurg* 87:887-892, 1997.

56. Ljungberg C, Johansson-Ruden G, Bostrom KJ, et al: Neuronal survival using resorbable synthetic conduit as an alternative to primary nerve repair. *Microsurgery* 19:259-264, 1999.

57. Whitworth IH, Terenghi G, Green CJ, et al: Targeted delivery of nerve growth factor via fibronectin conduits assists nerve regeneration in control and diabetic rats. *Eur J Neurosci* 7:2220-2225, 1995.

58. Mohammad JA, Warnke PH, Pan YC, Shenaq S: Increased axonal regeneration through a biodegradable amnionic tube nerve conduit: effect of local delivery and incorporation of nerve growth factor/hyaluronic acid media. *Ann Plast Surg* 44:59-64, 2000.

59. Pitta MC, Wolford LM, Mehra P, Hopkin J: Use of Gore-Tex tubing as a conduit for inferior and lingual nerve repair: experience with 6 cases. *J Oral Maxillofac Surg* 59:493-496, 2001.

60. Pogrel MA, McDonald AR, Kaban LB: Gore Tex tubing as a conduit for repair of lingual and inferior alveolar nerve continuity defects: a preliminary report. *J Oral Maxillofac Surg* 56:319-321, 1998.

61. Millesi H: Nerve suture and grafting to restore the extratemporal facial nerve. *Clin Plast Surg* 6:333-341, 1979.

62. Choi D, Raisman G: After facial nerve damage, regenerating axons become aberrant throughout the length of the nerve and not only at the site of the lesion: an experimental study. *Br J Neurosurg* 18:45-48,2004.

63. Targan RS, Alon G, Kay SL: Effect of long-term electrical stimulation on motor recovery and improvement of clinical residuals in patients with unresolved facial nerve palsy. *Otolaryngol Head Neck Surg* 122:246-252, 2000.

64. Fisch U, Rouleau M: Facial nerve reconstruction. *J Otolaryngol* 9:487-492, 1980.

65. Simo R, Jones NS: Extratemporal facial nerve paralysis after blunt trauma. *J Trauma* 40:306-307, 1996.

66. Guerrissi JO: Facial nerve paralysis after intratemporal and extratemporal blunt trauma. *J Craniofac Surg* 8:431-437, 1997.

67. Samii M: Zur Indikation, Technik und zu den Ergebnissen der facio-facialen. *Anast Neurochir* 24:90-104, 1981.

68. Hausamen JE, Schmelzeisen R: Current principles in microsurgical nerve repair. *Br J Oral Maxillofac Surg* 34:143-157, 1996.

69. Hausamen JE: Microsurgery of the facial nerve trauma. In Stark RB, editor: *Plastic surgery of the head and neck*, New York, 1987, Churchill Livingstone.

CHAPTER 22

Facial Burns

Barry L. Eppley

Almost one half of the patients who are admitted to a burn unit have some degree of facial burns. Most facial burns are superficial injuries typically caused by flash or splatter mechanisms. Extensive facial burns are uncommon and are usually the result of engulfing flame injuries from large explosions or house fires or scald injuries in children. In either case, the treatment of facial burns is different from that of burns in other locations. Facial tissue that is burned affects esthetic appearance and can negatively affect surrounding orifices such as the eyes, nose, mouth, and ears. Skin grafts are often a poor substitute for native facial skin, and specialized structures such as the eyelids or lips can never be completely restored to their original state.

The primary management of facial burns has a major effect on their outcome and is the subject of this chapter. Secondary burn reconstruction is a much larger topic that is not within the scope of this review.

CAUSES AND CLASSIFICATION OF BURNS

The head, face, and neck are the anatomical sites most likely to sustain thermal injury. The most common cause of facial thermal injury is flash burns, and the least common cause is exposure to hot surfaces.[1] The severity of facial burns depends on the duration of exposure to and the intensity of the burning agent (i.e., heat source). Time and temperature are the prime determinants of the severity of thermal injury; at temperatures between 44° C (110° F) and 51° C (124° F), the rate of cellular destruction doubles with each degree of increase in temperature. At temperatures higher than 51° C (124° F), exposure for 3 minutes or less can result in a full-thickness burn, and above 70° C (158° F), exposure for less than 2 seconds can lead to complete epidermal necrosis.[2]

The specific heat source has an effect on the extent of the facial burn. Noncombustible hot liquids, such as water, are frequently encountered but usually at less than 70° C (158° F), and the duration of exposure is usually very short (<2 seconds) because the liquid runs off quickly from the body surface. Scald burns therefore typically result in only partial-thickness facial burns. Combustible hot liquids, such as grease, are usually heated to much higher temperatures (>100° C), and because of their viscous nature, the duration of exposure is much longer. This often creates contact areas of full-thickness burns. Flash burns to the face cause only a brief exposure to the heat source, resulting in a superficial or partial-thickness burn. The singed eyebrow or nasal hairs from flash burns may make the examiner suspect an inhalation injury, but the absence of carbonaceous soot or difficulty in breathing and the location of the injury make it unlikely that an inhalation injury has occurred. All of these patients should undergo bronchoscopic examination. Flame burns, particularly with ignition of clothing, lengthen exposure to intense heat and make a full-thickness injury more likely.[1]

Burns are traditionally classified as first-, second-, or third-degree injuries, depending on the depth and completeness of dermal involvement. A better anatomical classification is that of superficial, partial-thickness (superficial and deep), and full-thickness burn injuries. All superficial and most partial-thickness burns maintain some dermal circulation, and they are usually capable of healing without excision or grafting. This can be clinically confirmed by the appearance of blisters, pain, and capillary refill. This is the most common type of facial burn because the face is often exposed to heat sources such as flash explosions rather than direct contact with flames (Fig. 22-1). Withdrawal or turning away is a natural protective reaction that frequently spares the face from more severe thermal damage.

Full-thickness burns irreversibly damage the epidermis, papillary dermis, and reticular dermis and result in thrombosis of the subdermal plexus. Clinically, the skin appears pale, with minimal or no capillary refill. Hair shafts are removed easily. This degree of facial burn commonly results from prolonged contact with flames from bed or house fires when the victim is disabled by smoke, alcohol, or drugs (Fig. 22-2). In extensive full-thickness burns, often called fourth-degree injuries, tissues and structures beneath the skin are involved. The skin is usually charred and insensitive. Causes include exposure to more than 1000 volts of electricity or to molten metal or prolonged contact with hot metal or flames. This degree of burn injury is rare in the face.

Describing facial burns as partial or full thickness provides a physiologically based classification system that also designates the approach to management. Although classifying the location and perceived depth of the initial burn is important, understanding the evolving nature of thermal injuries also is essential. It may take several days before the full extent and depth of a burn become apparent. Any early thoughts about surgical excision should be delayed until the burn depth and

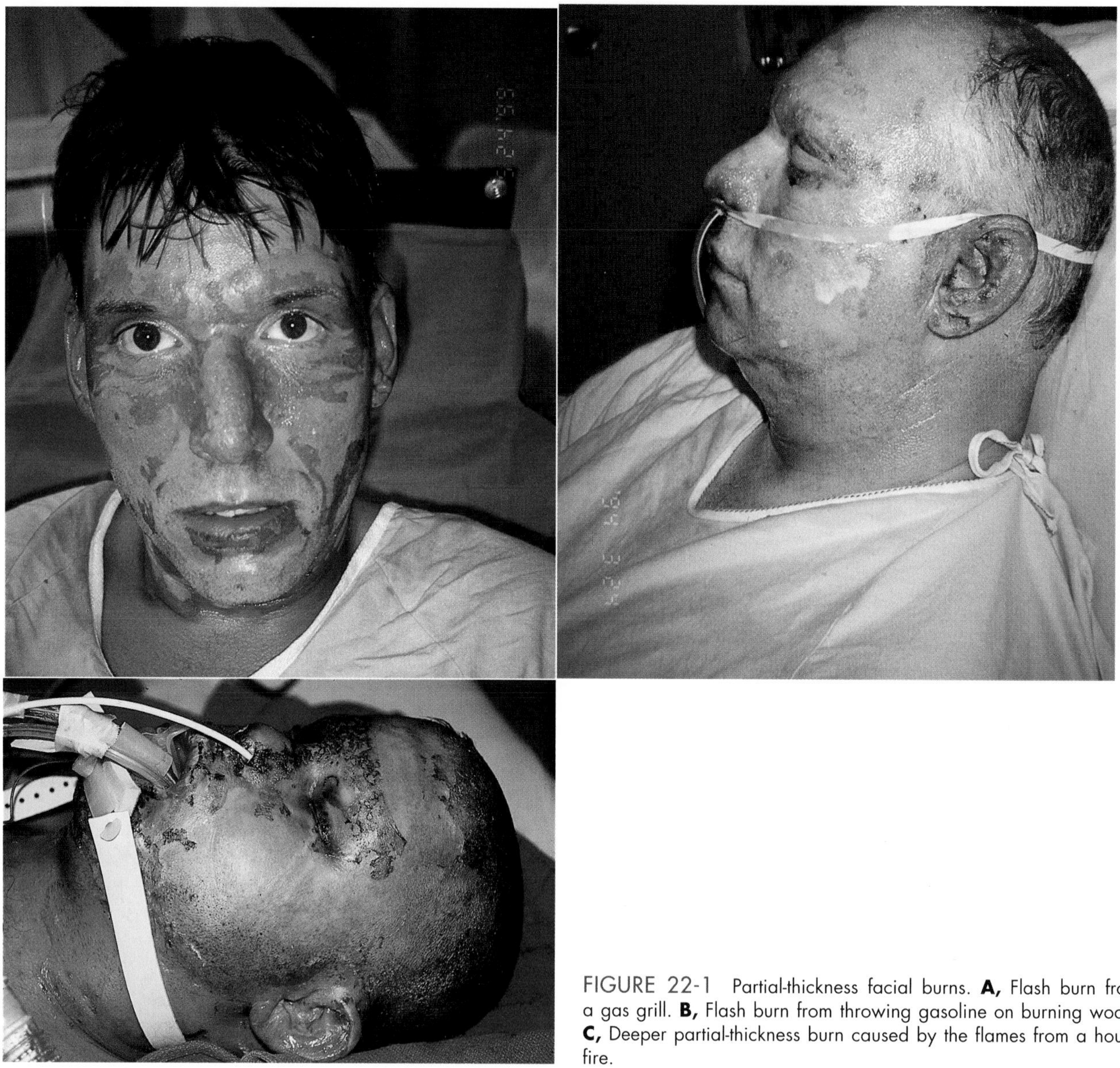

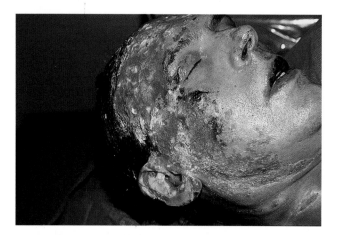

FIGURE 22-1   Partial-thickness facial burns. **A,** Flash burn from a gas grill. **B,** Flash burn from throwing gasoline on burning wood. **C,** Deeper partial-thickness burn caused by the flames from a house fire.

FIGURE 22-2   Full-thickness facial burn from a house fire involving the forehead, cheek, and ear.

margins are clear. Interventions directed toward burn care, such as fluid resuscitation, antibiotics, and topical therapies, may help to prevent conversion of the burn to deeper levels.

ROLE OF TOPICAL ANTIMICROBIALS

The necrotic, nonviable tissue that covers the surface of a burn wound is a fertile medium for bacterial growth. Although excision of the burned tissue is the ultimate treatment for this problem, it is not done until demarcation of the burn is evident and the patient is adequately resuscitated and stabilized. In the interim, the use of topical antimicrobials is the mainstay of infection prevention. Although numerous bacteria, fungi, and viruses have been associated with primary infection of burn wounds, the most devastating are the gram-negative bacteria, particularly *Pseudomonas*. Infected burn wounds may easily progress in depth and extent. Intravenous antibiotics are often of little value because they cannot reach the site of inoculation due to vascular thrombosis.

The most commonly used topical agents are bacitracin, silver sulfadiazine, mafenide acetate, and collagenase (Fig. 22-3). For superficial burns to the face, regular or ophthalmic bacitracin (Bacitracin, E. Fougera and Co., Melville, NY) is the preferred mode of treatment. It contains 500 mg/g of active agent and is a well-tolerated topical antimicrobial agent that causes minimal tissue reactivity. However, it offers no penetration of burn eschar, which is why its use is limited to superficial burns. In deeper partial-thickness and full-thickness burns, 1% silver sulfadiazine (Silvadene or Thermazene, Kendall Company, Marsfield, MA) is commonly used because it has the advantages of good penetration of burn eschar and painless application. It combines the antimicrobial action of silver ions with sulfadiazine. However, Silvadene tends to produce a pseudoeschar if not used appropriately, and this may confuse assessment of the depth of the burn. Mafenide acetate (Sulfamylon, Butek Pharmaceuticals, Morgantown, WV) at a concentration of 85 mg/g is a potent antimicrobial and has the best eschar penetration, but it is associated with pain after application. Silvadene and Sulfamylon must be kept away from the periorbital region because corneal ulceration, conjunctival edema and chemosis, and visual damage may result. In facial burns, all three antimicrobial agents are used in selective applications. In the periorbital area, bacitracin ophthalmic ointment is preferred, regardless of the depth of the burn, because it poses no risk to the eye. In the remainder of the face and scalp, 1% silver sulfadiazine may be liberally applied. Because of the known risk of cartilage exposure and suppurative chondritis from burns, Sulfamylon is used almost exclusively on the ear.

The use of an enzymatic débriding agent such as collagenase (Santyl Ointment, Knoll Pharmaceutical, Whippany, NJ) is helpful for superficial to deep partial-thickness burns. Santyl is a product of the bacterium *Clostridium histolyticum*. It can digest native and denatured collagen in devitalized tissue. In prospective studies, it improved healing and re-epithelialization times in partial-thickness burns compared with Silvadene.[3] Because most of the dry weight of necrotic and viable tissue consists of collagen, a débriding collagenolytic enzyme seems to be an appropriate choice. It can chemically discriminate between viable and nonviable tissue, thereby preserving more viable tissue. This has particular value in the face, where every square millimeter of tissue has esthetic value. Antibiotic powders may be mixed with the ointment. Other débriding ointments include Accuzyme (Healthpoint Medical, San Antonio, TX), a papain-urea preparation (1,100,000 units of papain and 100 mg/g of urea). This débriding ointment is stronger than collagenase and produces significant pain on application. For this reason, I do not use it on the face.

STATE-OF-THE-ART MANAGEMENT

In the acute phase of facial burn management, it is important to rule out heat injury to the upper aerodigestive passages and lungs. The etiology of the burn injury is the single greatest determinant of inhalational injuries. Burns that have occurred outdoors or in open environments are unlikely to cause internal heat injuries. In closed environments, particularly house fires, internal injury should be suspected (Fig. 22-4). Inhaled hot air can directly damage mucous membranes and cause edema. Swelling occurs within the first 24 to 48 hours and, if severe, may lead to airway obstruction and pulmonary insufficiency. In these cases, early endotracheal intubation should be performed. Nasotracheal intubation is preferred to the oral route because it can be easier to perform, is more comfortable when used for longer periods, and can be firmly secured. Fixation of the nasal tube is best done by transseptal suturing (2-3 or 3-0 silk), which provides good security and eliminates the need for tape on the face. When orally placed, the tube can be secured with interdental wires or sutures. If respiratory insufficiency is caused by heat injury, it is usually possible to extubate the patient after several days.

On admission, facial burns are débrided of all loose blisters and eschar. Although there is debate about whether to open blisters, leaving fluid-filled blisters on the face may be an impediment to wound evaluation and healing. In very superficial burns, particularly those involving the periorbital area, bacitracin ophthalmic ointment is used without dressings. Deeper burns may require more aggressive treatment, which is influenced by the anatomical location of the facial burn.

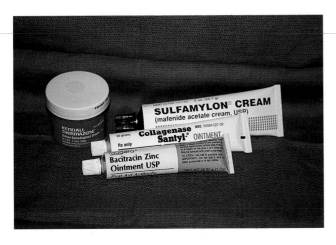

FIGURE 22-3 Commonly used topical agents for facial burns: Bacitracin, Silvadene, Sulfamylon, and collagenase.

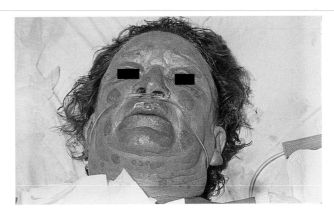

FIGURE 22-4 Patient with a likely inhalation injury with perinasal and perioral burns from a house fire. Bronchoscopy is mandatory.

Tetanus prophylaxis is given to all burn patients unless a booster has been received in the past 5 years. Because routine administration of antibiotics does not protect against burn wound cellulitis or sepsis, their use in the acute setting is not recommended. Unless specifically indicated by obvious wound infection or positive culture results, liberal use of antibiotics contributes to the development of resistant organisms, a common problem in hospital burn units.

SCALP

The scalp is protected from burn injury by a covering of hair, a thick dermis, and an extensive network of subdermal vessels. Most scalp burns can be treated conservatively. The dermal appendages of hair and sweat glands, from which much epithelial regeneration emanates, extend very deeply and allow most burns of the head to heal. They usually do so with minimal hypertrophic scarring because they are stretched out over a tight skull and a maximum number of hair follicles can be preserved (Fig. 22-5). If the scalp burn is likely to heal within 2 weeks, conservative management is warranted. For deeper scalp burns, easy removal of hair follicles is one indicator of a completely irreversible dermal injury. If early excision is needed—usually indicated by an unmistakable white, leathery appearance—the underlying galea, pericranium, or developing granulation tissue makes an excellent bed for skin graft acceptance (Fig. 22-6). Tangential excision in the scalp can result in rapid and significant blood loss, even if its surface area is relatively small. It may be helpful to tumesce the scalp with a dilute solution of epinephrine (1 : 1,000,000) before excision to control the blood loss and reduce the tendency for excessive electrocoagulation of bleeding vessels, which adds another thermal insult.

In occipital scalp burns, the skin is burned and is also exposed to continuous pressure when the patient is in the supine position on the bed. This combination increases the risk of full-thickness tissue necrosis down to the galea and bone. Soft head support and frequent changes in position help to control progression of the burn injury in this area. Pressure-relief mattresses and beds are often used for the more severely burned patients.

In very deep scalp burns, the calvaria can become exposed, posing a difficult problem. Small areas heal by the enveloping development of granulation tissue, which may take several weeks. Management may occasionally require mechanical burring of the outer table of the calvaria to induce the formation of granulation tissue. If larger areas of the calvaria are exposed, local or free vascularized flaps may be necessary for coverage (Fig. 22-7). However, this does not need to be done immediately, because the exposed calvaria does not add any significant risk to the recovering burn patient, and it may be covered with moist dressings until the metabolic status has improved enough for the patient to undergo a major surgical procedure.

EYELIDS AND EYEBROWS

Any patient with periorbital burns must be assumed to have corneal injury until proven otherwise. Corneal injury may result directly from the burn injury or from the presence of a foreign body. Patients with flame burns usually do not have a corneal injury, but those exposed to explosions or chemical burns often do. Chemicals are particularly destructive to the cornea, especially alkaline fluids such as sodium hydroxide. The alkali combines with protein and fat to form soluble soaps, which penetrate and then irreversibly damage the epithelial and stromal cells of the cornea. Acid burns are better tolerated in the eye than alkali burns because of the natural acid-buffering capacity of living tissue. Initial emergency treatment consists of copious, continuous irrigation with water or saline. Low-pressure (<1 psi) application of 0.9% saline with the lids retracted helps to ensure complete flushing of the entire conjunctival sac.

It is important for an ophthalmologist to perform a fluorescein dye examination within the first hours after injury to detect a corneal injury. Because the eyelids swell very quickly, an examination may not be possible the next day. Many corneal injuries heal with topical therapy, which usually includes antibiotic ointments and 1% atropine drops to prevent ciliary and iris sphincter spasm.

If the cornea is exposed, it must be kept lubricated to prevent desiccation. If the surrounding tissue has only minor burns, ophthalmic lubricating ointment with an overlying occlusive film may be adequate. If this is not possible in more severe burns, a scleral lens may be placed. In clinical practice, corneal coverage during the first few days after eyelid burns is not a problem because of the resultant edema, which provides a natural patching mechanism for 48 to 72 hours. The issue of corneal protection becomes relevant as the edema subsides and the globe is again visible. Historically, tarsorrhaphy was often used as a temporary method of eyelid closure, but contemporary burn care has moved away from this treatment because it is often ineffective at lid closure, is prone to separation, and can damage the lid margin, making future reconstruction difficult. I do not advocate its use. If some lid apposition is desirable, it is preferable to use a temporary suture of 4-0 or 5-0 nylon placed between the gray lines of the lid margin off the corneal axis. In more severe cases of exposure, a conjunctival flap (i.e., Gunderson procedure) can help to preserve the integrity of the globe (Fig. 22-8).[4]

Most burns of the eyelids are partial thickness and heal spontaneously without significant scarring. For deep

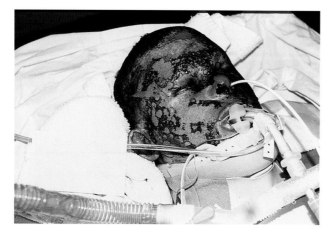

FIGURE 22-5 Superficial scalp burn from house fire will heal on its own.

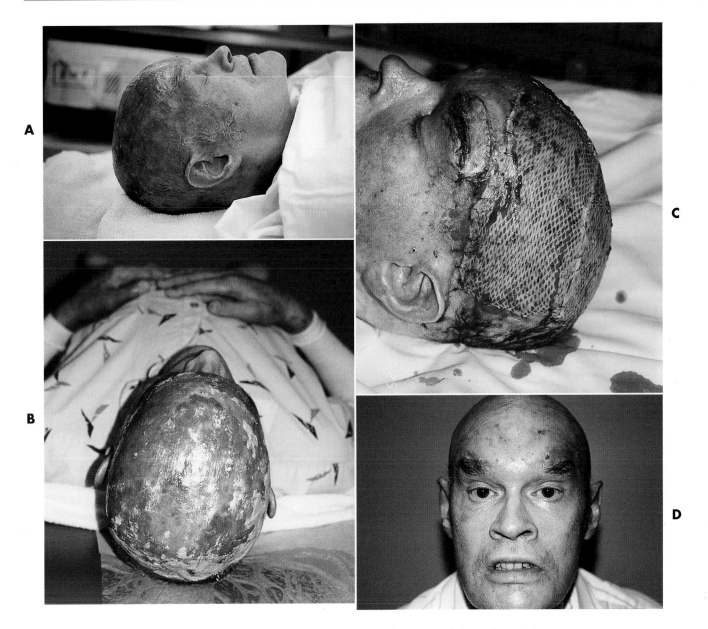

FIGURE 22-6   Deep, partial-thickness scalp burn required excision and skin grafting. **A,** Appearance of the scalp on admission. **B,** Nonhealing scalp burn 10 days later after treatment with topical Silvadene. **C,** Tangential excision and meshed split-thickness skin grafting. **D,** Healing result 10 days later.

partial-thickness or full-thickness burns involving extensive skin loss on the eyelids, skin grafting is necessary as soon as the eschar separates and a healthy bed of granulation tissue develops. Unlike the approach to other facial areas, eyelid burn excision is more theoretical than practical. It is too easy to remove the underlying orbicularis and levator muscles, rendering the eyelid immobile if it is not already so from the depth of the burn. Direct excision of the burn wound is rarely performed. If skin grafting is necessary, I prefer to use full-thickness facial or neck skin on a delayed basis for reconstruction. A full-thickness skin graft of upper eyelid skin is ideal, but in most cases both eyelids are burned, eliminating this option. After application of the autograft, maximal immobilization of the graft to the eyelids must be obtained. The grafts are best secured by tie-over bolster dressings, which remain in place for 5 to 7 days.

Although postponement of eyelid grafting permits it to be done under more favorable wound-healing conditions, corneal exposure or significant lid deformity may develop in cases of severe burns. For these patients, early skin grafting can be performed, with the realization that subsequent contraction and development of ectropion may require further graft reconstruction. Complete loss of significant eyelid tissue (i.e., lid margins and large amounts of upper and lower eyelid tissues) is rare. These cases can be treated with an early masquerade technique, in which the upper and lower eyelid conjunctivae are sewn together and overlaid with a skin graft.[4]

Development of burn ectropion of the eyelids, particularly the lower lid, is a common sequela of significant periorbital burns, whether they are primarily grafted or not. Ectropion may result from an intrinsic mechanism of eyelid contracture or an extrinsic mechanism of surrounding periorbital tissue

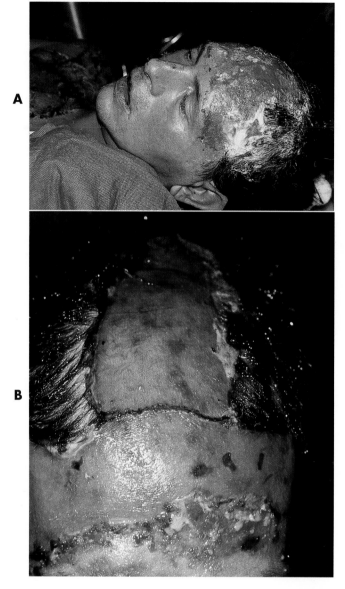

FIGURE 22-7   Full-thickness burn of the anterior scalp and forehead. **A,** Three days after admission. **B,** Ten days after sheet grafting with split-thickness skin.

contracture, or both. In all cases, secondary reconstruction with release and skin grafting is necessary, and this potential need must be appreciated from the outset of management. The dynamic nature of the eyelids combined with their thin tissue quality makes their function very unforgiving of deep partial-thickness and full-thickness burns.

Eyebrows are frequently singed in flash burns and explosive-type injuries. In these circumstances, regrowth almost always occurs. Significant full-thickness injury to the eyebrows may occur with severe burns of the eyelids. Although most follicles lie within the subdermal level, a full-thickness skin injury usually irreversibly damages them. Even if a few follicles survive, they are of no value because the overlying skin must be completely débrided and grafted. Secondary eyebrow reconstruction is delayed until the patient has recovered, and it is often one of the last reconstructive procedures performed.

NOSE

Burns to the nose are common because of its prominent position on the face, and the nose is affected in most facial burns. The thick dermis of the nose, particularly in men, and its rich blood supply account for the high incidence of partial-thickness injuries (Fig. 22-9). In contrast to eyelid injury, burns of the nose usually do not impose the risk of significant functional deformity because the underlying structural framework of cartilage, bone, and mucosal lining is spared. However, the nose has a profound effect on the patient's self-image, and a well-healed, nondeformed nose is desirable.

The main goals of primary nasal burn treatment are to conserve as much tissue as possible and to prevent further injury by iatrogenic means. The initial treatment is to apply bacitracin ophthalmic ointment for more superficial burns and 1% Silvadene for deeper burns. Débridement should be minimal, and excision of the burn can be delayed for 2 to 3 weeks to allow maximal time for demarcation and skin survival. In severe burns with more extensive systemic involvement for which pulmonary management is necessary, endotracheal and nasogastric tubes must be secured so that they do not cause further skin injury through pressure necrosis or adhesive tape tension. This may be accomplished by transseptal suturing of nasal tubes or by use of the oral route if tube placements are likely to be brief. If it appears that the patient is at risk for nostril stenosis due to significant alar involvement, splints can be fabricated and placed early.[5]

EAR

Most facial burns involve the ear. The skin overlying the auricular cartilage is very thin and is susceptible to full-thickness thermal injuries. Even if the ear is not severely burned, suppurative chondritis may develop weeks after the initial injury and may complicate management. Pressure from pillows and circumferential dressings may further damage the ear.

Initial treatment of burned ears has changed significantly over the past 30 years. The original approaches employed early débridement and grafting. Although this technique was effective, significant ear deformities were common. Because 75% of burned ears heal without grafting, less radical excision of only obviously necrotic skin and exposed cartilage is now performed (Fig. 22-10).[5] A regimen of minimal débridement and twice-daily application of Sulfamylon (because of its better penetration of relatively avascular cartilage) is used in most centers. Sulfamylon is applied thickly and often enough to prevent desiccation of the ear. If the cartilage is exposed, time is allowed first for granulation tissue to develop from the normal skin edges, which may take weeks. This produces a better recipient bed for later skin grafting. If the cartilage remains exposed, skin grafting is ultimately performed over its cut edges after débridement back to bleeding tissue. Rarely, the cartilage from an isolated, severely burned ear can be covered by a temporal fascial flap based on the temporal vessels.

Some burn centers employ a topical treatment of antibiotic iontophoresis in place of or in addition to Sulfamylon topical cream for the burned ear. Iontophoresis involves the application of gentamicin sulfate antibiotic (5-10 mg/mL) as a cream or soaked on gauze to the ear, with subsequent application of

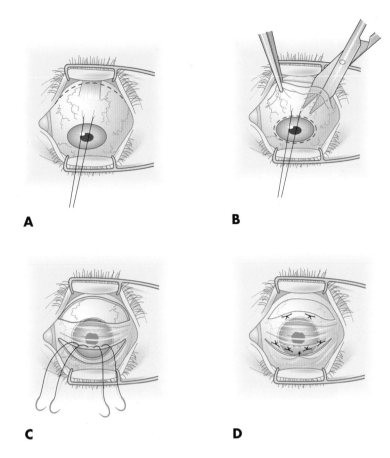

A **B**

FIGURE 22-8 In severe, full-thickness eyelid burns, the globe can be protected by raising and closure of upper and lower conjunctival flaps, which are covered by a skin graft. **A,** Outline of conjunctival flaps. **B,** Sharp elevation of conjunctival flaps. **C,** Suturing upper and lower conjunctival flaps together for corneal coverage. **D,** Vascularized conjunctival bed for skin graft placement.

C **D**

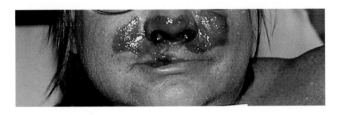

FIGURE 22-9 Partial-thickness perinasal burn will heal on its own with topical therapy.

a direct electrical current (positive electrode of 10-15 mA for gentamicin). A ground (negative pole) is placed somewhere else on the body. There is good experimental evidence for antibiotic penetration into cartilage with this technique, and clinical reports support its effectiveness.[6,7] However, it is not clear that it prevents suppurative chondritis, and it is more cumbersome than Sulfamylon cream alone. Its greatest benefit may be as an adjunctive treatment in established chondritis, because it may minimize the need for significant amounts of cartilage resection.

Avoiding pressure on the ear is another important aspect of primary management. The patients should not be allowed to use pillows, which are an unappreciated source of pressure. If necessary, foam can be placed around the pinna to prevent further pressure, but this method is rarely used. No external wound dressings are needed for ear coverage, because antibiotic cream is sufficient.

All burned ears have the potential for suppurative chondritis, which is often not seen until weeks after the initial injury. The symptoms of infectious chondritis are a red, hot,

tender, swollen ear. Purulence is uniformly present, is often green, and is usually found by culture to be *Pseudomonas aeruginosa* (in most cases) or *Staphylococcus aureus*. The burn may be healed by that time, and cartilage might never have been exposed. Prompt treatment is necessary to prevent loss of all ear cartilage. The abscess is opened through a limited bivalving incision, and cartilage is débrided as necessary. Systemic antibiotics are given in conjunction with topical Sulfamylon. Because of the cartilage débridement and subsequent wound contracture, the esthetic outcome is usually poor, and some patients lose most of the ear. Prevention is paramount, and aggressive early treatment is essential, including antibiotic iontophoresis if it is available.[8,9]

LIPS AND MOUTH

The constant motion of the lips and exposure to contaminated salivary fluids make care of burn injuries in this area different from that for other parts of the face. This area commonly develops hypertrophic scarring and contracture after being burned. Because the mouth provides access for eating, hygiene, and intubation, early treatment often focuses on prevention of microstomia. The risk of microstomia usually results from a severe burn in the perioral area, which causes narrowing of the mouth, or from an electrical burn of the oral commissure. In either case, the use of splinting devices is the mainstay of primary treatment.

Oral splinting devices should be fabricated and inserted as soon after the burn as possible. Except for the most severe injuries, tangential excision or excision of lip burns is rarely done. Lip burns typically are allowed to demarcate

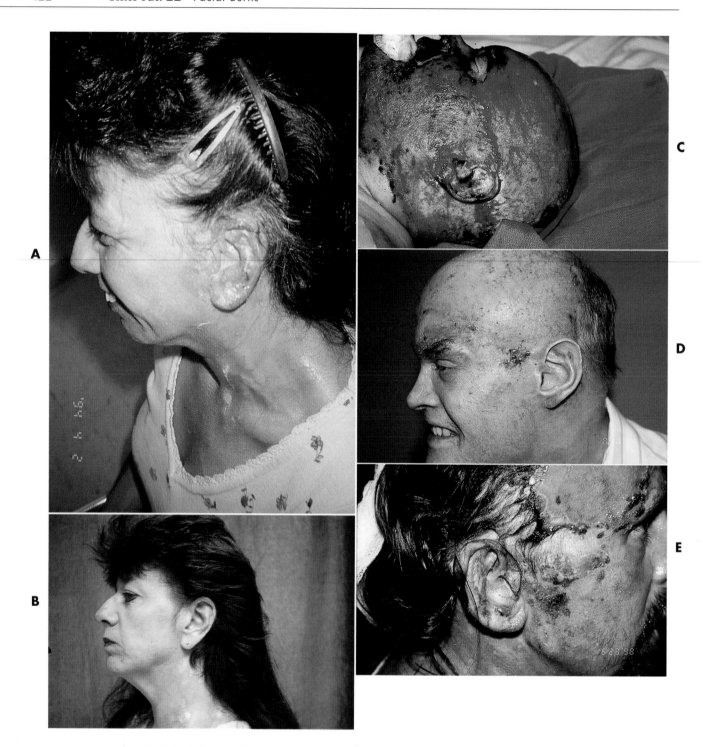

FIGURE 22-10 Partial-thickness ear burns. **A,** Superficial partial-thickness ear burn 3 days after injury. **B,** Spontaneous healing 3 months after injury. **C,** Deeper partial-thickness ear burn on admission. **D,** Complete healing 1 month after injury. **E,** Combination partial- and full-thickness ear burn 3 days after admission.

and heal on their own. Early and continual resistance of contracture for months is usually the best treatment approach, because successful reconstruction of microstomia can be difficult.

Splints are categorized according to their point of anchorage: external (e.g., head and neck straps), self-retaining lip splints; and dental or orthodontic appliances (Fig. 22-11). A dental-based splint is preferred because it attaches to the maxillary teeth and palate intraorally and is less obtrusive than other devices. However, it requires adequate intraoral access for dental impressions, which frequently is difficult, even in the operating room. The other types of microstomia splints do not have to be custom made and are easier to apply, although they are more visible.

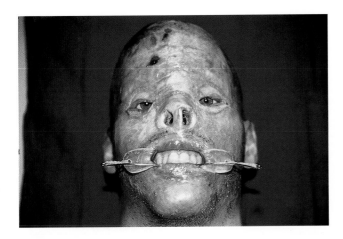

FIGURE 22-11 Splinting of the oral commissure is important in treatment of a perioral burn. The splints are applied early after grafting, when the wound is stable. They may be used for months to counteract sphincteric contractures. In this case, the splint is an extraorally based device with a circumferential strap.

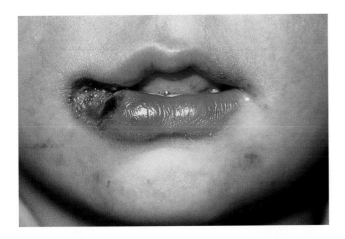

FIGURE 22-12 The classic electrical oral commissure burn is a full-thickness injury with a well-demarcated eschar.

Oral commissure burns are common and are easily treated. This injury typically occurs in toddlers younger than 5 years of age, often a small child who places an electric cord in the mouth. After chewing violates the cord's plastic cover, saliva creates an electrical short circuit, and an arc is created. This produces high heat, up to 3000° C, and chars the portion of the mouth that is in contact with the arc.[10] This energy causes extensive local tissue destruction at the commissure, including a zone of full-thickness burn (Fig. 22-12). No treatment is needed immediately other than the application of bacitracin ointment and warning to the parents that bleeding from the labial artery may occur as the eschar separates several weeks after the injury. Although initially frightening, the bleeding is easily controlled by manual compression. Provided that the child can take fluids and nourishment, there is no need for immediate hospitalization. After allowing several weeks for eschar separation and healing, a palatal splint is fabricated and worn for up to 6 months after the injury on an almost continual basis. With good compliance, subsequent surgical correction usually is unnecessary (Fig. 22-13).[11]

NECK

The neck is frequently involved when the face is burned, although it is unusual to have extensive involvement if there are not also significant upper trunk burns. The neck is often spared in flash burns due to protective clothing, but it can be deeply burned in flame injuries when clothes are ignited. Significant deep neck burns signify greater systemic involvement, and these patients often require fluid resuscitation and intubation. The neck is the rotational mechanism for the head, and deep burns can lead to contracture and a functional deformity that restricts movement.

Superficial and partial-thickness burns of the neck are liberally covered with Silvadene until the demarcation of the wound is clear. Partial-thickness wounds, particularly in men because of the re-epithelialization capabilities of hair-bearing skin, are allowed to heal on their own. In patients with full-thickness neck burns, early excision of the wound is accompanied by the application of a homograft (if the wound bed is uncertain) or large sheets of relatively thick (0.018- to 0.020-inch) split-thickness skin grafts. Not meshing and expanding the skin graft helps to prevent postoperative contracture and gives a better esthetic result, but graft failure is more likely because of the inevitable postoperative movements of the neck that occur and the build-up of subgraft fluid. A good compromise is to use meshed split-thickness skin but with no minimal expansion (Fig. 22-14). An overlying compression dressing or bolster is preferred, but this is not practical in most burned patients with significant skin involvement.

Early excision and coverage of deep neck burns are particularly important in patients who have an inhalation injury requiring extended mechanical ventilatory support (>2-3 weeks). After the neck is successfully grafted and healed, a tracheostomy can be placed through healthy surrounding skin or an intact skin graft.

REMAINDER OF THE FACE

Treatment of burns to areas other than the eyelids, ears, nose, and lips differs somewhat from the approach to those regions. The remaining areas of the face have high esthetic significance but a more favorable geometry, being flatter and covering greater surface areas. They do not impinge significantly on most of the important facial functions. As in all reconstructive facial surgery, the esthetic unit principle applies to the management of burns in these areas (Fig. 22-15).

Facial burns are initially treated, as previously described, by débridement of loose blisters, daily cleaning, and coverage with topical antibacterials. The critical management difference is that if the burns are not healed or expected to heal within 3 weeks of the injury on their own, primary excision and grafting is done. This more aggressive approach to burns in these facial areas yields a better appearance and function than that obtained by allowing spontaneous healing over more than 3 weeks or grafting on granulation tissue. The magnitude and number of subsequent reconstructions are decreased with this technique.[12] The esthetic facial units judged to be incapable of healing within 3 weeks are excised; occasionally, small unburned or healed areas must be included in the excision to preserve the esthetic unit (Fig. 22-16).

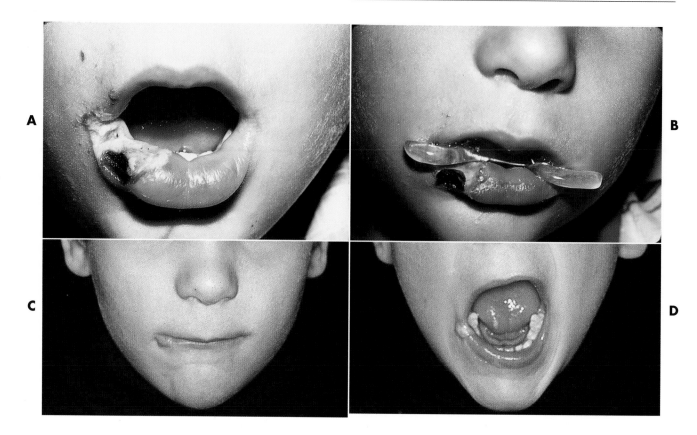

FIGURE 22-13   An electrical burn of the oral commissure was managed without surgery. **A,** Extent of injury. **B,** Use of a splint appliance for 3 months. **C,** Healed result after 1 year. **D,** Oral opening after 1 year.

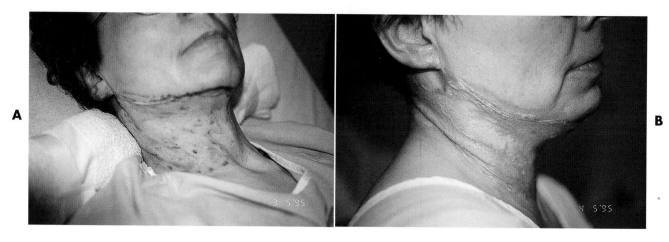

FIGURE 22-14   Skin grafting to the neck is usually done as sheet grafts (unmeshed, split thickness) to decrease the risk of contractures and to improve the esthetic result. **A,** One week after grafting. **B,** One month after grafting.

Excised areas are initially covered with homograft for 48 hours, allowing the egress of serum and blood. Thereafter, thick split-thickness grafts (0.018-0.025 inch) are harvested and placed in an unmeshed fashion according to the esthetic unit guidelines (see Fig. 22-16).[13] In burns of smaller surface area, a better color match can be obtained from scalp, neck, or inner upper arm skin. If the entire face is to be grafted, color match becomes an irrelevant issue.

Some form of postoperative compression of the grafts (e.g., foam, compression garments) is important, and the grafts must be carefully inspected postoperatively several times daily to check for subgraft fluid. Any hematomas or seromas are removed through small graft incisions placed in the relaxed skin tension lines. Once healing has occurred, pressure garments or masks must be worn to lessen the incidence of hypertrophic scarring.

Early excision and grafting of facial burns produces better results than delayed excision or spontaneous healing. Subsequent reconstruction is often limited to junctures, seams, and smaller areas. However, patients who require therapy usually have extensive or deep facial burns and therefore rarely have a normal appearance of the burned areas (see Fig. 22-16). This approach should be reserved only for these more difficult facial burn problems. If the facial burn can heal spontaneously within 3 weeks, it is better left alone.

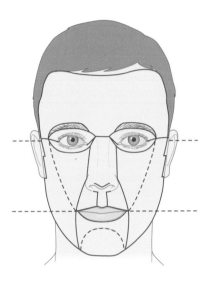

FIGURE 22-15   Esthetic facial units.

CONTROVERSIES

Many aspects of facial burn management are controversial. Contentious areas include the choice of topical agents, early versus late excision and closure of the wound, options for limited versus full facial coverage, and the timing of reconstruction.

For topical agents, most burn centers no longer use Silvadene routinely and are more aggressively using enzymatic débriding ointments. The current approach focuses on prevention of pseudoeschar formation, which is critical in preventing a subeschar proliferation of bacteria, a known mechanism for making burn wounds deeper. Prevention of eschar formation can improve the speed of healing, leading to earlier closure of the wound and decreased likelihood of hypertrophic scarring. Without eschar formation, the physician is better able to assess whether the wound can heal. For the face, this usually translates to a mid-to-late execution of tangential excision. Typically, at least 5 to 7 days should pass before tangential excision of the face is carried out. At that point, the potential for the wound to heal on its own should be evident.

Controversy still exists regarding the choice of options for limited facial burns. It is traditionally better to excise and cover esthetic facial units as a whole. However, this is often impractical, such as in a hemi-forehead burn that would require the sacrifice of much normal tissue. In this circumstance, it is better to think of how primary grafting could be improved by secondary reconstruction. Primary excision and

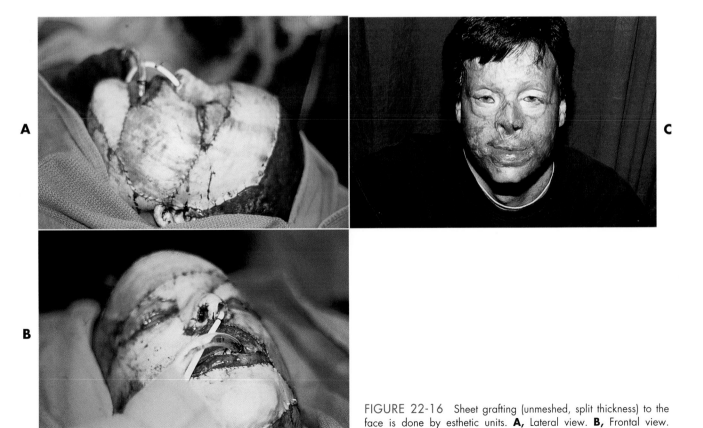

FIGURE 22-16   Sheet grafting (unmeshed, split thickness) to the face is done by esthetic units. **A,** Lateral view. **B,** Frontal view. **C,** One year after grafting.

grafting of a subesthetic unit may be eliminated or improved by secondary reconstruction through the use of tissue expansion or other local flap techniques. The esthetic unit concept is not valid in all cases. If only a small amount of normal skin exists as part of the esthetic unit, it is probably better to remove these areas.

The best donor match for facial burns is the neck, but this is a limited source. Other options must be considered, including upper arm and upper chest skin. For larger burns in which full facial coverage may be needed, a large, thick (0.0015- to 0.0018-inch) sheet graft from the upper back is useful. The color and texture may not be ideal, but it will be homogenous throughout the grafted skin.

The timing of contracture or hypertrophic scar releases is being revised. Historically, contracture releases were not carried out until scar maturation had occurred, which could take 18 to 24 months. In contractures of the eyelid or neck, this is not ideal because of the functional restrictions imposed. Current preference is for earlier releases and coverage to shorten the period of functional impairment. This is particularly useful for eyelid and oral burn scar restrictions.

REFERENCES

1. Morgan RF, Nichter LS, Haines PC, et al: Management of head and neck burns. *J Burn Care Rehabil* 6:20, 1985.
2. Moritz AR, Henriques FC Jr: Studies of thermal injury. II. The influence of time and surface temperature in the causation of cutaneous burns. *Am J Pathol* 23:695, 1947.
3. Hansbrough J: Wound healing: special considerations in the burn patient. *Wounds* 7(suppl A):78A, 1995.
4. Achauer BM, Adair SR: Acute and reconstructive management of the burned eyelid. *Clin Plast Surg* 27:87, 2000.
5. Bernard SL: Reconstruction of the burned nose and ear. *Clin Plast Surg* 27:97, 2000.
6. Purdue GF, Hunt JL: Chondritis of the burned ear: a preventable complication. *Am J Surg* 152:257, 1986.
7. Kaweski S, Baldwin RC, Wong RK, et al: Diffusion versus iontophoresis in the transport of gentamicin in the burned rabbit ear model. *Plast Reconstr Surg* 92:1342, 1993.
8. Rigano W, Yanik M, Barone FA, et al: Antibiotic iontophoresis in the management of burned ears. *J Burn Care Rehabil* 13:407, 1992.
9. Mills DC, Roberts LW, Manson AD, et al: Suppurative chondritis: its incidence, prevention, and treatment in burned patients. *Plast Reconstr Surg* 82:267, 1988.
10. Luce EA: Electrical burns. *Clin Plast Surg* 27:133, 2000.
11. Niazi ZBM, Salzberg CA: Thermal, electrical, and chemical injury to the face and neck in children. *Facial Plast Surg Clin North Am* 7:185, 1999.
12. Engrav LH, Heimbach DM, Walkinshaw MD, Marvin JA: Excision of burns of the face. *Plast Reconstr Surg* 77:744, 1986.
13. Warden GD, Saffle JR, Schnebly A, Kravitz M: Excisional therapy of facial burns. *J Burn Care Rehabil* 7:24, 1986.

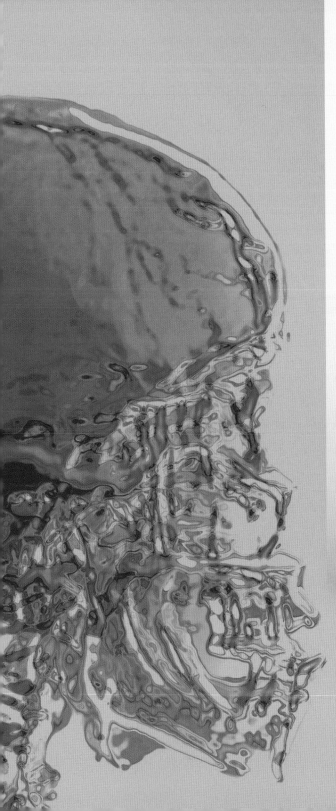

SECTION **III**

Secondary Surgery

CHAPTER 23

Facial Scar Management

Edward Wai-Hei To, Man Kwon Tung, Chi Wang Peter Pang

The face is essential for the expression of emotion and physical state. Scars on the face, in particular, are a stigma in human society and can isolate a person from social contacts. Facial wounds are commonly the result of road traffic accidents, windshield injuries, assaults, animal and human bites, and war injuries. Facial wounds should be aggressively treated to avoid the consequence of an unsightly scar. The presence of separate esthetic units and combined injuries to bone, skin, and vital structures require special attention in the assessment and treatment of facial wounds and subsequent scars.

Although facial scar management is an elective procedure, the appropriate management of acute facial wounds dramatically affects the quality and quantity of scar tissue formation, thus affecting the need for and results of secondary scar revision procedures. It is therefore essential to understand and make use of the principles of wound healing.[1-3]

PRINCIPLES OF WOUND HEALING

Acute Inflammation

As soon as tissue is damaged, the wound is filled by a coagulum. Nerve impulses are generated at the injured site, and the substances released by the damaged cells cause local hyperemia and increased permeability of the vessel wall. This acute inflammatory reaction is the initial step and cornerstone of the healing process. Platelet degranulation and activation of the complement and clotting cascade form a fibrin clot for hemostasis. Chemotactic agents including epidermal growth factor (EGF), insulin-like growth factor 1 (IGF-1), platelet-derived growth factor (PDGF) and transforming growth factor-β (TGF-β) are released during platelet degranulation. Recruitment of neutrophils, macrophages, epithelial cells, mast cells, endothelial cells, and fibroblasts follows. Inflammatory cells proliferate and differentiate for phagocytosis, with further release of cytokines, and form granulating tissue.

The second phase, known as the proliferative phase, spans days 5 to 14 after injury. Capillaries and fibroblasts invade the coagulum in the wound. This new tissue is known as granulation tissue. Blood supply to the area remains high, but permeability of the vessel walls is restored to normal and edema resolves. However, prolongation of the inflammatory process as a result of infection, presence of foreign bodies, and delay in treatment increases the activity of fibrogenic cytokines such as TGF-β and IGF-1, thereby increasing the chance of hypertrophic scar development.

During the maturation phase of wound healing, the collagen scaffold is being remodeled, resulting in increased tensile strength. This process continues for about 1 year under normal conditions.

Scar Formation

In a scar, type I collagen is laid down by fibroblasts. Its appearance ranges from an inconspicuous line to keloid that overgrows the original wound. This process begins on day 4 of wound healing, when the fibroblasts start synthesizing extracellular collagen. The activity of the fibroblasts is increased by fibroblast activation factor, which is liberated by macrophages. Capillaries develop from the vascular endothelium and form a dense vascular network within the newly formed connective tissue. Myofibroblasts differentiate into fibroblasts and produce type I collagen, giving the scar stability. Capillaries are then obliterated, and the original multitude of cells is reduced to a few cell types.

Various factors cause persisting stimulation of the wound, resulting in enhanced cicatrization. Therefore, care is needed to remove all foreign bodies and prevent infection. Adequate débridement should remove all necrotic tissue, and further trauma should be avoided by use of an atraumatic suturing technique.

FACTORS AFFECTING WOUND HEALING

GENERAL FACTORS

The process of healing is more rapid in young patients. Patients with protein, vitamin, or trace element deficiency heal more slowly. Chronic illnesses such as anemia, uremia, uncontrolled diabetes, or immunosuppressive states decrease wound-healing capacity. The long-term use of steroids or immunosuppressive agents for treatment of other medical illnesses could change the inflammatory phase of the wound and lead to delayed formation of new tissue.

LOCAL FACTORS

Blood Supply

A healing wound needs energy and building materials such as oxygen, glucose, amino acids, vitamins, and trace elements. The blood supply to the wound affects the availability of oxygen to the tissue. Blood supply is decreased in the state of shock and in patients with arteriosclerosis or diabetes. Hematoma underneath the wound raises the skin flap, resulting in an impaired blood supply to the tip of the flap via the reticular dermal plexus and causing necrosis of the wound edge and secondary infection. Although the face is rich in blood supply, necrosis of wound edges leads to undesirable scars.

Necrotic Tissue

The facial skin has a rich blood supply, and débridement should be minimal, because most of the tissue will survive and heal.

However, necrotic tissue at the wound edges, caused by direct trauma to the skin, can harbor bacteria. It should be trimmed off before suturing, because devitalized tissue provides an anaerobic medium for the multiplication of anaerobic microbes as well as other microorganisms.

Foreign Bodies

Depending on the mechanism of injury, foreign bodies are common in certain trauma scenarios. Organic foreign bodies (e.g., wooden splinters, soil) and inorganic foreign bodies (e.g., glass or metal shards) should be removed thoroughly during the acute treatment of wounds. These materials not only provide a nidus for bacteria but prolong the inflammatory response of the wound, causing scarring, recurrent infection, and traumatic tattooing.

Previous Irradiation

The patient's head and neck area may have been irradiated for the treatment of cancer or other clinical conditions. The radiation effect to the skin is permanent if the radiation exceeded 15 to 20 Gy over a relatively short period. Radiation-induced atrophy is usually noticed weeks to months after the initial exposure, although further atrophic changes may evolve over 1 or 2 years. The skin is thinned, dry, and hyperkeratotic. Telangiectasia and hyperpigmentation or hypopigmentation are usually prominent features. In the upper dermis, capillaries are reduced in number, and the capillaries, venules, and lymphatics are often widely dilated. Wound healing of irradiated skin is usually slower than that of normal skin, and complications such as infection and dehiscence are more common. Irradiated skin wounds are usually inelastic, and the edges are difficult to approximate in the usual manner.

Infection

Infection of the wound causes an inflammatory reaction and edema. There is an increased number of inflammatory cells, as well as fibrinolysis and breaking down of collagen; hence, the tensile strength of the wound is affected.

Common bacteria causing skin infection are commensals such as *Staphylococcus* and *Streptococcus* species. Wounds that communicate with the nasal or oral cavities may be contaminated with anaerobes. Antibiotics usually are not necessary if there is adequate débridement and cleaning of the wound. Booster tetanus immunization is mandatory in appropriate cases.

TYPES OF WOUND

The nature of the wound is the most important determining factor for the final result of wound healing. The orientation of the wound in relation to the resting skin tension lines (RSTLs), its location and pattern, the degree of tissue trauma, presence of foreign bodies, degree of contamination, and individual tissue response determine the final scar appearance.

Every wound that involves the dermal papilla produces a scar. The most important prognostic factor for the final appearance of the scar is how the wound was inflicted rather than how it was sutured. Surgical technique is important in alleviating the damage caused by the injury but cannot totally reverse it.

LACERATED WOUND

Laceration causes minimal tissue loss. Contamination is usually limited. However, the deep structures such as nerves and underlying organs should be examined for any injury.

CRUSH WOUND

Crush injury is caused by blunt trauma. The wound edges are often irregular, and tissue is lost (Fig. 23-1). All obviously devitalized tissue should be débrided. Traumatized tissue may be left behind, because the blood supply of the facial skin is rich and the chance of recovery is high. Unjustified débridement of facial skin leads to disfigurement, deformity, loss of function, and creation of a bigger scar.

CONTAMINATED WOUND

Contaminated wounds must be cleansed thoroughly. Deep-seated debris encourages inflammation, allergic reactions, and infection, whereas debris embedded within the superficial dermis becomes an unsightly "traumatic tattoo" if left unattended. Thorough scrubbing with a brush while the patient is under general anesthesia is necessary in the acute

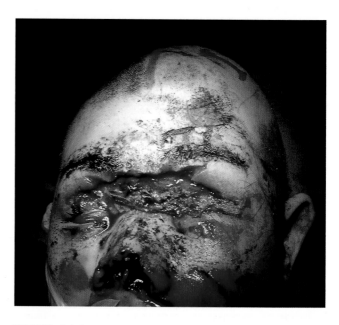

FIGURE 23-1 Badly crushed open facial fracture after a traffic accident.

stage of wound treatment. This can avoid further treatment after the wound has healed.

POTENTIALLY CONTAMINATED WOUND

Wounds that communicate with the nasal or oral mucosa are potentially contaminated by the presence of normal flora, secretions, and anaerobes. They should be closed as soon as possible (i.e., within 6 hours), and patients should be prescribed antibiotics for gram-positive cocci and anaerobic bacteria.

PENETRATING WOUND

Care should be taken in treating penetrating wounds and deep lacerations, because important structures can be damaged. A thorough examination should be carried out and a plan for wound exploration prepared if necessary.

MANAGEMENT OF ACUTE WOUNDS

TIMING

Treatment should be undertaken as early as possible and preferably with the patient under general anesthesia to reduce discomfort and speed up healing. Delay in wound closure increases the risk of infection. For wounds with a low risk of infection, the "golden period" is within 12 to 24 hours after injury. With contaminated wounds or immunocompromised patients, primary closure should be achieved within 6 hours. If the wound carries a high risk of infection, delayed primary closure should be used. However, poor cosmetic outcome, prolonged patient discomfort, and inconvenience are negative factors of this approach and should be thoroughly discussed with the patient.

DÉBRIDEMENT WITH SCRUBBING

Particles of dark color (e.g., dirt, sand, gunpowder) will result in a traumatic tattoo if they remain in the wound. Such discoloration tends to be permanent. This can be easily dealt with by débridement or scrubbing in the acute stage, and these preventive measures cannot be overemphasized (Figs. 23-2 and 23-3).

THOROUGH IRRIGATION TO REMOVE FOREIGN BODIES

It has been said, "The solution to pollution is dilution." Normal saline irrigation remains the best, most economical, and most readily available solution to the problem of contamination. Other antiseptics such as povidone-iodine or hydrogen peroxide are sometimes used; however, these agents can induce tissue reaction, inflammation, and possibly toxicity and should be avoided.

Pressurized irrigation is used in contaminated wounds to remove soil or small foreign bodies. The optimal pressure for irrigation remains debatable, but too high a pressure increases tissue trauma. The recommended pressure of 5 to 8 lb per square inch can be achieved by use of a 16- or 19-gauge needle.

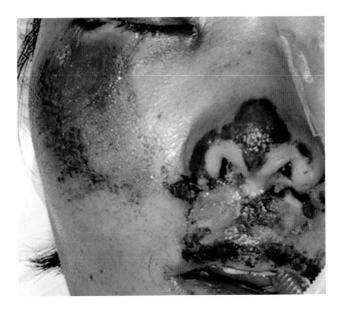

FIGURE 23-2 Fine foreign bodies embedded in an abraded wound.

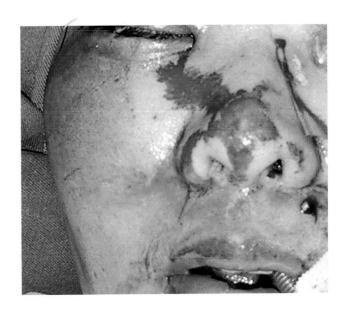

FIGURE 23-3 Clean abraded wound after scrubbing.

TRIMMING OF NECROTIC TISSUE

The potential for skin recovery in blunt facial trauma is great because the blood supply of the face is abundant. Trimming should therefore be limited to obviously dead tissue. The trimming of other tissue such as muscle and nerve should be minimal because it leads to depressed scars and loss of function.

FUNCTIONAL AND ANATOMICAL REPAIR IN LAYERS

Facial appearance and expression depend on the integrity and function of the underlying musculature. Failure of functional and anatomical repair leads to depressed scars, tethering of the overlying skin, or facial asymmetry.

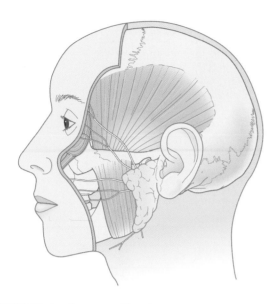

FIGURE 23-4   The course of facial nerve branches and the maximal extent of dissection deep to the superficial musculo-aponeurotic system.

DAMAGE TO FACIAL STRUCTURES

Deep laceration is likely to damage underlying or adjacent organs or structures. Early identification and surgical repair are necessary to avoid unnecessary complications.[4]

The facial nerve emerges from the skull base via the stylomastoid foramen. It emerges into the parotid gland from the posteromedial surface and divides into two main trunks, the temporozygomatic and cervicofacial branches. They are further divided into five branches: temporal, zygomatic, buccal, marginal mandibular, and cervical. They remain under the superficial musculo-aponeurotic system (SMAS) until the line shown in Figure 23-4. The function of the facial nerve should be tested if the clinical situation allows. Wounds superficial to the SMAS behind the line are unlikely to have injured the facial nerve and need not be explored.

Parotid duct injury should be suspected if the wound is situated at the anterior border of the parotid gland or if there is salivary leak. The duct should be repaired with absorbable sutures. Untreated parotid injury leads to fistula formation.

The nasolacrimal duct connects the lacrimal sac at the medial canthus, slopes downward and laterally, and drains to an opening in the inferior meatus. Its injury should be suspected if there is a wound or previous suturing at or below the medial canthus. Cannulation of the duct with a fine probe is necessary before the wound is explored or sutured at that area.

APPROPRIATE USE OF ANTIBIOTICS AND SUTURING MATERIALS

Routine systemic antibiotics are not necessary. The use of antibiotics should be tailored based on host defense status, degree of contamination, mechanism of injury, and likelihood of wound infection. Débridement is the most important step in cleaning up the wound, and antibiotics should not be a substitute.

Prophylactic antibiotics are necessary if the wound is expected to be contaminated, such as animal bites or wounds that communicate with the oral cavity.[5] In medical conditions such as rheumatic heart disease or when host resistance is compromised, as in patients with uncontrolled diabetes and those taking steroids or immunosuppressive agents, antibiotics should also be commenced systemically and early. Commonly encountered organisms are streptococci, staphylococci, and gram-positive bacteria. Penicillin and cloxacillin are the drugs of choice. Patients who are sensitive to the penicillin group should be given erythromycin.

Topical antibiotics (e.g., chloramphenicol ointment) are definitely beneficial. (Very rarely, significant side effects of chloramphenicol have been reported, even when used topically, and in some hospitals its use is prohibited.) Elimination of local infection can reduce the chance of keloid and hypertrophic scar formation.

It is best not to leave any foreign bodies, even stitches, in the wound. If stitches are required at the subcuticular level, the first choice is plain catgut. Synthetic absorbable sutures such as Vicryl are now commonly used to avoid the potential problem of Creutzfeldt-Jakob disease. Stitches that are dissolved by hydrolysis rather than by inflammation have a lower chance of causing keloid and hypertrophic scars. The best result comes from using nonabsorbable monofilament stitches that are removed on day 3 to 7.

Tetanus passive immunization should be given if necessary. A booster dose should be given if the patient's previous immunization was more than 10 years ago. Active immunization should be given if the wound is heavily contaminated.

ASSESSMENT OF EXISTING SCAR

TYPES OF SCAR

Good Scar

A desirable scar should be inconspicuous with the face at rest as well as in the dynamic situation. It should be flat, the same color as the surrounding skin, soft, narrow, and oriented in the same direction as the RSTL.

Bad Scar

A bad scar causes disfigurement and catches the observer's eye. It is usually raised or depressed, hyperpigmented or hypopigmented, wide, and crossing the RSTL. However, the disfigurement may also be exaggerated in the patient's mind. This largely depends on the patient's gender, cultural background, profession, and attitudes. Therefore, before deciding the best method of revision of a scar deformity, it is important to communicate clearly with the patient and forestall any disappointment. It should be emphasized to the patient that a scar can only be improved or reduced and not completely erased.

Depressed Scar

A depressed scar commonly occurs running perpendicular to the RTSL as a result of wound closure under tension (Fig. 23-5). Hematoma formation, wound infection, and inverted wound closure are the common causes of a depressed scar. It may also result from initially deep injury with loss of subcutaneous tissue and contracted fibrous tissue adhering to underlying fascia and muscle. Meticulous layered closure of

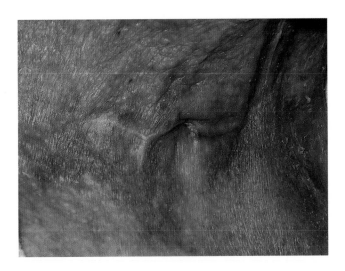

FIGURE 23-5 Depressed scar after previous tracheostomy.

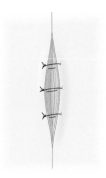

FIGURE 23-7 Improper alignment of wound edges resulting in step deformity.

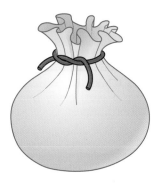

FIGURE 23-6 A circular wound contracts like a purse string.

the wound is important to prevent depressed scars. Tissue augmentation or dermabrasion or laser resurfacing can achieve recontouring of smaller depressed scars.

Z-plasty or W-plasty is used to correct the underlying tension problem, excising and elevating the scar in the same operation. Depression due to adherence of scar tissue to underlying structures requires excision of the scar, undermining of the subcutaneous tissue, and closure in layers to avoid recurrence.

Curved Scar

Healing of a curved scar produces contraction along the scar, resulting in a purse-string effect (Fig. 23-6). This produces a "trapdoor" appearance of the scar. Small trapdoor scars can be excised and primarily closed, but larger trapdoor scars are best revised with Z-plasty or multiple W-plasties to realign the scar to the RSTL. Wider undermining peripheral to the trapdoor flap may also help to oppose the trapdoor deformity. The possible mechanism of this effect is the outward pulling force that acts on the scar after the revision.

Pigmented Scar

Hyperpigmentation is not a common problem in whites but occurs more frequently in Asians and dark-skinned people. During the scar maturation process, exposure to sunshine and smoking are the risk factors associated with hyperpigmentation. Topical tretinoin is useful in the treatment of hyperpigmentation, but avoidance of sunshine until the scar matures is the best way to combat this condition. Laser treatment has been used for hyperpigmentation with limited success.

Stitch Marks

Tensionless suturing is the best way to avoid stitch marks. To minimize stitch marks, the use of skin hooks rather than forceps and a subcuticular method of suturing are desirable. If a simple interrupted suturing technique is adopted, fine sutures (i.e., 7-0) should be used and early removal (i.e., 3 days) is preferred.

Step-off Deformities

Step-off deformities are the result of inaccurate epidermal closure. Dermal abrasion and laser resurfacing with laser are commonly used techniques for this kind of scar. Generally, excision and resuturing are necessary if the step is greater than 1 mm (Fig. 23-7).

Painful Scar

Entrapment of a nerve ending in a healing wound results in a painful or tender scar. If conservative treatment with oral analgesic is not effective, the wound should be re-explored. The nerve should be cleancut and allowed to retract away from the wound and into muscle, if possible.

Patient's Tissue Response

The patient should be examined to detect the presence of other scars to determine whether there is a tendency to form keloid or hypertrophic scars. However, the presence of a well-healed scar can be misleading, because the formation of hypertrophic or keloidal scars depends heavily on other factors such as the degree of tissue crushing during trauma, orientation of the wound, and the site of the scar.

The mechanism of initial injury is the single most important factor in determining the formation of a scar. Blunt trauma injuries and crushed wound edges do badly compared to cleancut wounds. The presence of foreign bodies prolongs the inflammatory reaction and increases the likelihood of bad scar formation. Tissue loss and healing by secondary intention leads to an unsightly scar.

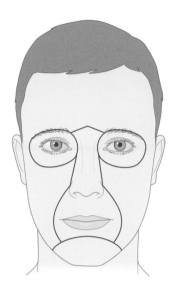

FIGURE 23-8   Cosmetic units consist of forehead, nose, periorbital area, perioral area, and chin.

Hypertrophic Scar or Keloid

A simple hypertrophic scar is limited to the tissue that constitutes the wound, whereas a keloid overgrows the wound and invades the surrounding tissue. Keloid grows slowly and may relapse for years before it becomes static. Hypertrophic scars become softer and paler as time passes. Histologically, both types of scar have the same appearance, and it is difficult to distinguish the two in the initial year after wound healing.

ESTHETIC UNITS

The face is divided into six esthetic units (Fig. 23-8): forehead, eye, nose, cheeks, mouth, and ears. Each can be further subdivided into smaller units.

Forehead

Scars in the forehead region can usually be improved with simple procedures. Forehead skin has a very rich blood supply, and so suction apparatus should be ready when operating in this area. During revision of forehead scars, special attention should be paid to the anatomical reconstitution of different layers such as frontalis muscle and skin. Preoperative documentation of the sensation status of the supratrochlear and supraorbital nerves should be made.

Eye
Eyebrows

It is important to recognize that injury to hair follicles will result in bald patches. Therefore, dissection in the eyebrow area should be carried out with extreme caution, and the incision should be made parallel to the direction of hair follicles to avoid damage. Small segments of alopecia should be removed, if feasible, and larger areas may require hair-bearing skin graft. The direction of the skin incision should be oblique to avoid transection injury to the hair follicles. Perfect alignment of the eyebrow is critical, because a step-off deformity is very obvious.

Eyelids

Scar contracture over the eyelids can cause ectropion or entropion and should not be tackled as a linear scar contracture. Addition of new tissue, by free skin grafting or local flaps, is necessary to achieve good results. Damage to the tarsal plate results in notching. The upper and lower eyelids consist of the thinnest skin of the body and should be grafted with paper-thin (<0.5 mm) skin for good results. The crow's feet at the lateral canthus provide a good area for disguise in scar revision. Multiple W-plasties to realign the scars along the crow's feet results in an inconspicuous scar. The degenerative laxity of the lower eyelid requires special attention, because this precipitates ectropion if the procedure creates downward tension.

Nose

The skin of the nose is strongly adherent to the underlying muscle and cartilage. Because of the underlying naris muscle pull, the skin has limited directions of movement. Excision of scars and closure of defects should always be undertaken with great care and may be helped by borrowing nearby tissue such as a bilobed flap.

Cheeks

The cheek is a flap with minimal wrinkles except in the older patient. Scars crossing this area are extremely difficult to hide. Laser resurfacing has a particularly important role in the treatment of scars over this area.

Mouth

The mucocutaneous vermilion border of the lip should be perfectly restored in the revision of scars crossing the lip. Other anatomical borders such as the red line and white line should be accurately restored. A three-layer closure of mucosa, muscle, and skin must be performed.

Ears

The ears themselves are not prone to any special scarring except keloid formation at the earlobe after earring puncture. The pinna provides a valuable composite skin-cartilage-skin graft for reconstruction of alar tissue loss (Figs. 23-9 and 23-10).

FACTORS AFFECTING SCAR QUALITY

Age

The older the patient, the better the scar and the results of revision. Younger people have a greater overall skin tension, which causes a scar to spread and become hypertrophic. Skin tension is one of the most important factors in the esthetic outcome of scar surgery.

Relaxed Skin Tension Lines

The skin is draped over the body in a fashion that permits mobility, retraction, extension, expansion, and flexion. Areas that allow greater movement, such as the perioral area, stretch and create excess skin to accommodate the movement of muscles. Over time, the excess skin, in conjunction with the loss of elastic tissue, creates wrinkles and age lines. These wrinkles often coincide with RSTLs (Fig. 23-11).

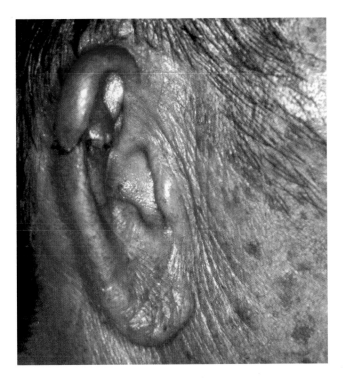

FIGURE 23-9 Composite graft harvested from the pinna consisting of skin and cartilage.

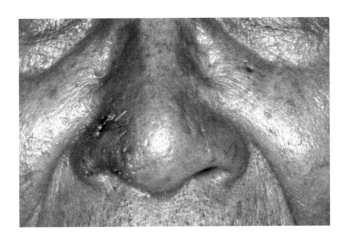

FIGURE 23-10 Application of composite graft to reconstruct an alar defect.

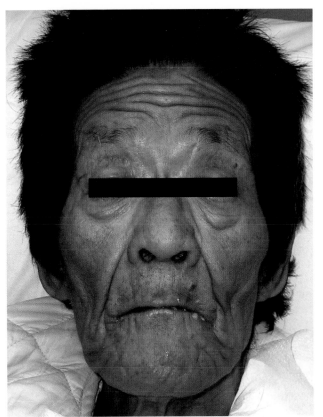

FIGURE 23-11 Wrinkles on the elderly face.

PRACTICAL MANAGEMENT OF FACIAL SCARS

EARLY SCAR MANAGEMENT

History of the Injury

The patient's history should be recorded clearly, including how, when, and where the injury occurred and the chance of foreign body presence in the wound. The history may indicate the possibility of injury to other vital organs and degree of tissue damage.

Psychological Support for the Patient

Every injury results in a more or less obvious scar. A scar may stigmatize a person and possibly affect social contacts, so psychological counseling should be started as soon as possible. Anticipation is the key to success in minimizing long-lasting emotional injury.

Communication

Good rapport and adequate explanation are necessary for the patient to understand the unavoidable scar formation. Reassurance should be given concerning the expected progress of the scar, the time sequence of the treatment, and possible future revision measures.

Documentation

After good communication and good surgical technique, documentation is the surgeon's best defense against legal claims. It is important to document the essence of all communications with the patient. Particular attention should be paid to the factors that affect wound healing. Host factors include ethnic group, extremes of age, diabetes mellitus, chronic renal failure, obesity, malnutrition, and the use of immunosuppressive therapy. The tendency of the patient to form keloid should be assessed, because it may predict the formation of a poor scar.

The site and degree of contamination and tissue trauma should be clearly documented. The size, depth of wound, and injury to deep structures such as tendons, nerves, and vessels should be accurately recorded for possible future legal purposes.

A history of drug allergy, especially to local anesthetic agents and antibiotics, should be determined, because these agents are likely to be administered in the acute stage of the injury.

Photographic Record

A photographic record for comparison of preoperative and postoperative comparison is necessary. A record of the initial wound and subsequent wound progress is mandatory for legal purposes. Although digital cameras are widely used, images are accepted as documentation for legal purposes only if they are produced as hard copies.

Patient Participation

The patient's contribution is important in producing a good scar. A motivated patient is necessary for good compliance with scar management during the first 6 to 9 months after injury. This starts in the immediate postoperative period. Keeping the head above the heart level to reduce wound edema is necessary for the initial 24 hours. The wound should be observed for any signs of infection such as erythema, warmth, swelling, and discharge. There should be a thorough discussion with the patient about the possible outcome, and the patient should be advised to seek prompt medical attention if infection sets in or doubt arises.

After the wound is healed, the patient needs to accept responsibility for sun avoidance and protection from ultraviolet light. Sunlight exposure increases the risk of scar hyperpigmentation. Sunscreens with a high sun-protective factor (SPF) must be used appropriately. Possible alterations in the patient's outdoor occupational and recreational activities may be necessary.

Surgical Options

The simplest method of primary wound closure should be used, unless there is substantial tissue loss that renders primary wound closure impossible. A local flap is the best choice in cases of significant tissue loss. Adjacent skin usually provides the best replacement in terms of color and texture. Full-thickness skin grafting should be the last option; a graft harvested from the postauricular and supraclavicular areas provides the best color match to facial skin.

Silicone Sheet

A silicone gel sheet may be used as a conservative treatment for hypertrophic scar or keloid[6,7] (Fig. 23-12). The sheet should be worn for as much as 24 hours per day. The mechanism is largely unknown but the silicone gel possibly increases the local temperature of the scar, enhancing the collagenase activity. Another postulated mechanism is a pressure effect that causes a lowering of oxygen tension and occlusion of the scar. A direct chemical effect of silicone on the scar is unlikely, because there is no evidence that silicone enters the scar tissue.

There are drawbacks. The sheet cannot be worn for long periods in hot and humid conditions. Sweat can cause skin excoriation and eczema, and scratching in response to the itchiness causes further damage. As a result, the keloid or hypertrophic scar can become more severe. The application of silicone gel on the face is much less acceptable cosmetically than on other parts of the body.

Corticosteroid Intralesional Injection

Intralesional injection of triamcinolone in combination with local anesthesia and other therapies has been used to control

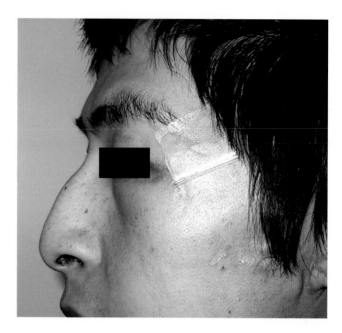

FIGURE 23-12   Application of silicone gel sheet on facial hypertrophic scar.

scars. It was reported to have a 50% response rate in keloid treatment over 5 years in terms of flattening the scar and decreasing discomfort. Various regimens with different concentrations (10, 20, 30, 40 mg/mL) at an interval of 4 weeks were used. The improvement is brought about by inhibition of the transcription of matrix protein genes such as α_1 type I and α_1 type III procollagen, fibronectin, TGF-β and other cytokines, and by inhibition of collagenase activity by α_2-macroglobulin synthesis.

Pain is substantial in intralesional steroid injection, so a local anesthetic should be infiltrated around the scar before treatment. Telangiectasia, infection, and necrosis of the skin are the possible complications of steroid injection. Incorrect injection of the steroid into the subcutaneous tissue leads to subcutaneous fat atrophy and formation of a depressed scar.

The systemic effects of steroids can be avoided by spacing the intervals between injections. Female patients should be asked about pregnancy, because this treatment should not be given to pregnant women. It is also important to mention possible irregularity of periods and the increased amount of flow after steroid injection. Other relative contraindications to the use of steroid include a previous history of breast or endometrial cancer.

Intralesional injection of a calcium channel blocker[8] (verapamil hydrochloride) is an effective alternative for treating hypertrophic scarring. The mechanism may be similar to that of trifluoperazine, a calmodulin inhibitor that causes cells to round up through an unknown intracellular, calcium-independent process involving alteration or rearrangement of the actin cytoskeleton. Surgical excision and intraoperative perilesional injection of verapamil is effective to prevent keloid recurrence.

Pressure Dressings

Constant compression (Fig. 23-13) of a hypertrophic scar has proved to be beneficial in preventing excessive growth of scar

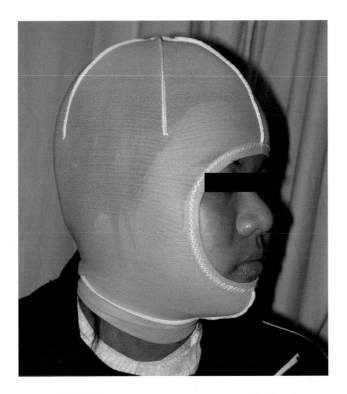

FIGURE 23-13   Tailor-made pressure garment for facial scar.

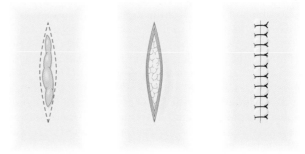

FIGURE 23-14   A linear scar was excised in a fusiform manner and closed primarily.

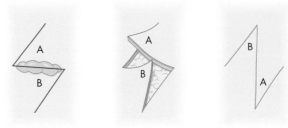

FIGURE 23-15   Z-plasty.

tissue. To be effective, a constant pressure of 15 to 40 mm Hg for at least 18 hours per day for 4 to 6 months is necessary.[9] This can be used in conjunction with silicone gel. It should be tailored to fit the involved parts of the body; examples are elasticized cervical collars, elastic ski masks, and spring-pressure earring devices for use after earlobe keloidectomy. This treatment modality should be explained carefully to the patient beforehand. Pressure sensors should be used to monitor the efficacy of the pressure garment at follow-up consultations.

DELAYED SCAR REVISION

Timing of Scar Revision

Complete scar maturation takes 2 to 3 years. There is a common consensus that scar revision should be delayed until the scar has reached full maturation. However, the appearance of the scar is worst during the 2 weeks to 4 months after injury. If the orientation of the scar crosses the RSTL, it will never heal in an optimal manner. Borges[10] therefore advocated that an interim scar revision and reorientation should be carried out at 2 months after injury to achieve the best result in the process of delayed scar revision. However, the average time to scar revision ranges from 6 months to 1 year.

Technical Aspects

The main objective of scar revision is to make the scar less conspicuous. This can be achieved by excision of scar tissue and rearrangement to maximize the length and reorient the scar along the RSTL.[11] This method enables the scar to heal with minimum tension and in the optimal direction.

Simple Excision

The oldest and simplest technique in scar revision is fusiform scar revision (FSR), which consists of excision of the scar followed by direct closure of the wound. This is possible if the scar is oriented approximately along the RSTL. FSR is very effective for treatment of a wide scar or a scar that is tethered to underlying structures. It may not be necessary to excise the whole scar; partial treatment (Fig. 23-14) can still achieve marked improvement.

The drawback of FSR is the formation of a deep furrow caused by the vertical contraction of scar tissue. Excision of all the underlying scar tissue and closure in layers can reduce the chance of this result.

Serial Excision

If the scar is too wide and a single FSR would result in undue tension for wound closure and unfavorable conditions for subsequent wound healing, serial intralesional excision of the scar can be used to provide time for the nearby skin and tissue to expand and allow a tensionless wound closure.

Z-Plasty

The main function of Z-plasty is to prevent thickening and contraction and to reorient the scar. This is achieved by lengthening and, more importantly, by changing the direction of scar to align it more closely to the RSTL. Z-plasty should be undertaken if the scar is slanted 60 degrees or less from the RSTL (Fig. 23-15). In multiple Z-plasties with limbs that follow the RSTLs, the direction of each postoperative oblique scar (diagonal) is the same as that of the original scar. The adjoining tissues must be elastic enough to make Z-plasty possible. Often after release of the scar contracture and undermining of the flaps of the Z-plasty, the flaps automatically realign to the final configuration.

It is convenient to wait until the scar has matured before performing the Z-plasties to avoid unnecessary sacrifice of tissue. Early Z-plasty is indicated in selected cases in which the wound could only be worsened as the scar contracts, such as a circular wound or malalignment of the vermilion border. Trapdoor deformity (Fig. 23-16) is inevitable. Therefore, multiple Z-plasties should be undertaken as soon as the wound has healed.

W-Plasty

W-plasty is used in the initial incision in elective surgery, to prevent later contracture, and in the conversion of an existing scar to a less apparent one. The latter is done by zigzag excision of scars, which produces a shortened, acutely angulated incision that can be closed by advancement without rotation of tissue to produce a scar that aligns along the RSTL (Figs. 23-17 through 23-19).

W-plasty is used to break up a long scar and realign it as much as possible along the RSTLs. A depressed scar can be eliminated by advancing V-shaped arms of tissue across the field of the scar.

Dermabrasion

Dermabrasion can be carried out with a high-speed dermabrader with a diamond fraise.[12] Fraises are stainless steel wheels with industrial-grade diamonds bonded to them. The scar should be pretreated with 0.05% tretinoin cream to shorten the re-epithelialization time and reduce the incidence of postoperative milia formation and hyperpigmentation. The procedure can be carried out with the use of local or regional blockade together with sedation.

Laser

Laser light is used in the treatment of scars because its precise cutting and welding properties cause less tissue damage than other methods. Its photochemical reaction may also provide a beneficial effect in altering metabolic function within the keloid. Superpulsed carbon dioxide laser[13] causes a significant increase of keloid dermal fibroblast growth factor-β (FGF-β) secretion and inhibits the secretion of TGF-β. These effects stabilize the cellular phenotype and inhibit excess collagen secretion. Laser therapy also causes thermal contraction of collagen, resulting in dermal tightening.

The neodymium:yttrium-aluminum-garnet (Nd:YAG) laser has a suppressive effect on collagen synthesis without changing DNA synthesis or causing loss of viability. Clinically, it is useful for moderate reduction of keloid size and consistency. The 585-nm flashlamp-pumped pulsed-dye laser is used for its specific hemoglobin absorption characteristic.

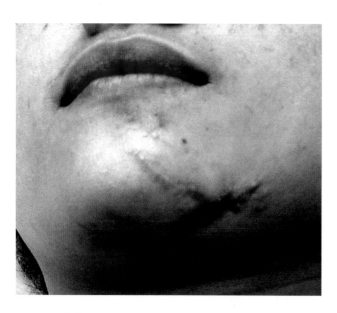

FIGURE 23-16   Trapdoor scar on the chin.

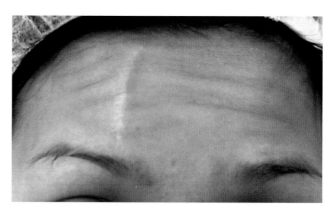

FIGURE 23-18   Forehead scar oriented across the relaxed skin tension lines.

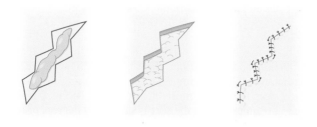

FIGURE 23-17   Realignment of scar to relaxed skin tension lines with W-plasty.

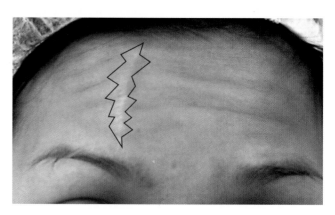

FIGURE 23-19   Design of W-plasty to realign the forehead scar.

Laser therapy is used for its ablative nature and to apply the specific wavelength for the vascular component of the hypertrophic scar. The 585-nm pulsed-dye laser has been shown to be effective in the treatment of microvascular lesions such as telangiectasia and port-wine stains. Studies have shown that it reduces the erythematous component and scar height and increases pliability. Posttreatment scar biopsy showed sclerotic collagen bundles and local mast cell proliferation.

The mechanism of laser action is selective photothermolysis. Selective absorption of light by hemoglobin leads to local heating of cutaneous blood vessels; the vessels are then thrombosed, and vasculitis follows. There is gradual local repair with neovascularization. Microvascular destruction leads to ischemia of the scar and affects collagen synthesis and the release of collagenase. The heat produced is conducted via the blood vessels to the surrounding dermis and alters the collagen composition of the scar. However, the 585-nm pulsed-dye laser is not useful in treating keloid, except for minimal improvement in erythema.[14] Combined therapy with intralesional injection of steroid does not give additional benefit except in the treatment of symptomatic hypertrophic scar.[15] In treating patients with Fitzpatrick skin type 4 through 6, one must lower the energy fluence and use multiple treatment sessions to minimize complications.[16,17]

Dermabrasion on raised scar with the carbon dioxide laser or erbium laser may cause hyperpigmentation, hypopigmentation, significant downtime, and prolonged erythema. This is especially common for Fitzpatrick skin type 4 or higher. Fractional laser resurfacing is a new concept that uses arrays of microscopic thermal damage in a pattern stimulating a wound healing response. It creates microscopic columns of thermal injury surrounded by uninjured tissue. Repair of epidermis occurs within a few hours, and the underneath dermis undergoes healing and reorganization and becomes flattened. Depth of penetration depends on the level of energy used. Fractional laser resurfacing avoids bulk heating of tissue and reduces the risk of irreversible nonspecific thermal injury. Ablative laser therapy with a wavelength of 2940 nm and nonablative laser therapy with a mid-infrared 1540-nm wavelength can be used. The latter method requires more treatment sessions but with less downtime and greater efficiency. Typically, ablative fractional laser resurfacing requires 5 to 10 sessions to achieve satisfactory results. It can be used to treat early or matured scars.

Another method for scar remodeling is the creation of microinjury that is deeper than that created with fractional laser. Orentreich and Fernandes independently described "subcision" or dermal needling.[18,19] Percutaneous collagen induction stimulates collagen production by triggering the normal chemical cascade for healing. Dermaroller therapy uses numerous small needles, ranging from 1 to 3 mm long, to produce injury at the epidermopapillary dermal level. Injury deeper than 6 mm will not cause additional improvement. Studies show that relatively intact epidermis has a lesser chance to cause hyperpigmentation.[20] During the treatment, platelets and neutrophils release growth factors such as TGF-α, TGF-β, PDGF, connective tissue activation protein III, and connective tissue growth factor to increase the production of intercellular matrix. Monocytes produce growth factors to increase collagen III, elastin, and glycosaminoglycans. Collagen III later converts to collagen I, resulting in tightening of skin, smoothing scars weeks and months after treatment.[21] The application of vitamin A in the form of retinyl palmitate or retinyl acetate and of vitamin C further induces collagen production during the treatment.

Platelet-Rich Plasma

Platelet-rich plasma has been used to improve wound healing.[22] Extra growth factors elicited by platelet-rich plasma and stem cells have been postulated to aid scar remodeling. Platelet-rich plasma has been used to improve wound healing for soft and bony tissue repair, and even in osseo-integration. Trials have been conducted on the use of platelet-rich plasma in the remodeling of new and matured scars. Platelet-rich plasma is obtained by collecting autologous blood, centrifuging the blood, and extracting the plasma portion. Injection of platelet-rich plasma to the intradermal or subdermal level has been shown to produce some improvement in scar quality. The mechanism is not clear, and it is not known whether it is the subcision done during the injection or the actual platelet-rich plasma that helps in scar remodeling.

Stem Cell

The use of stem cells in remodeling scar is still controversial. Stem cells have been isolated from bone marrow, adipose tissue, and blood serum. To date, many research studies have been carried out to test the efficacy of stem cell therapy in various types of tissue healing including tendon, cartilage, and heart muscle. The mechanism remains unknown.

Tissue Expander

Nearby tissue offers the best esthetic outcome in terms of color match and texture for facial skin reconstruction, but the supply is always limited. Tissue expansion is invaluable in the reconstruction of extensive scars with inadequate tissue nearby. Previously expanded skin flaps have an improved survival rate compared with similar flaps developed in nonexpanded skin.

Scar alopecia can be treated by expanding the remaining scalp. As much as half of a hair-bearing scalp defect can be reconstructed with tissue expansion (Fig. 23-20). Similarly, expansion of forehead skin for a forehead defect is feasible (Fig. 23-21). The innervation of the forehead frontalis muscle should be preserved to avoid later brow ptosis. Expansion of forehead skin can also provide extra good-quality, thin skin for reconstruction of the nasal area.

To reconstruct the cheek area, the tissue expander is best placed in the preauricular area, superficial to the superficial aponeurosis muscle. Further dissection superficial to the platysma muscle at the neck is necessary for placement of the tissue expander and expansion of the neck skin. Extra skin can then be acquired by a rotational flap. Neck skin is expanded for the reconstruction of cheek and perioral scars and defects.

Skin Grafting

Skin grafting usually cannot provide a satisfactory cosmetic result for facial scars and defects. However, it is invaluable for wound coverage in the acute stage so that later flap reconstruction (e.g., tissue expansion) may be planned. Split-thickness skin grafts can be harvested from the thigh or scalp. Full-thickness skin grafts can be harvested from the

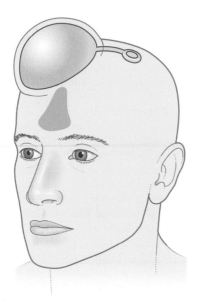

FIGURE 23-20   Placement of the forehead tissue expander for reconstruction of a forehead scar.

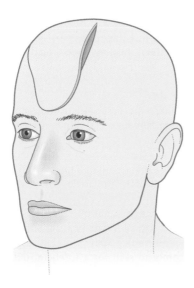

FIGURE 23-21   Reconstruction of forehead with the expanded skin.

preauricular, postauricular, neck, nasolabial, and supraclavicular regions.

Soft Tissue Augmentation

The ideal material for soft tissue augmentation should be safe, easy to apply, permanent, and nonallergenic.

Collagen Injection

Injectable bovine collagen has been used for treatment of depressed scars.[23] This xenogenic substance has the problem of allogenicity, which needs to be evaluated before treatment with a small test dose. In the 1980s, the U.S. Food and Drug Administration (FDA) approved Zyderm collagen implants (Collagen Corporation, Palo Alto, Calif) and the gelatin

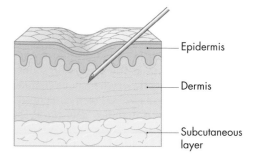

FIGURE 23-22   Depressed scar as a result of deficient dermis.

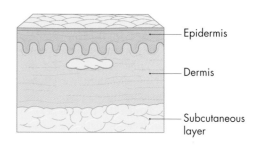

FIGURE 23-23   Leveling off of a depressed scar was achieved with the injection of augmentation material.

matrix implant Fibrel (Mentor Corp., Goleta, Calif) for clinical use. Zyderm I contains 35 mg/mL type I collagen, Zyderm II has 65 mg/mL type I collagen, and Zyplast is a glutaraldehyde cross-linked collagen. Each has different physical properties and different uses. Zyderm I is indicated for shallow scars or fine wrinkles, Zyderm II for intermediate deep depressed scars, and Zyplast for deep scars and deep dermal defects. However, intermittent swelling, vascular changes, and necrotic changes of the overlying skin are possible complications. This is caused by the heavy suspension of the Zyplast collagen, which results in infarction of larger subdermal vessels and local tissue necrosis.

The injection should be carried out with a 30-gauge needle using a multiple-puncture or fanning technique at a 35-degree angle to the skin. Care must be taken to avoid both implant extrusion through pores or around the needle orifice and injection deep to the subcutaneous tissue. In dealing with fibrotic scars, one has to undermine the scar with a needle to create a pocket for the injected collagen. Local anesthesia by regional blockade is necessary to avert possible pain caused by the undermining.

Injection treatment is contraindicated if there is history of keloid formation, sensitivity to gelatin, or a history of a bleeding disorder; cardiac, renal, or herpetic disease; or autoimmune disease.

With skillful injection, the depressed scar can be leveled off (Figs. 23-22 and 23-23). However, the difference in surface texture between the scar and the surrounding skin cannot be altered with this treatment. The best approach is to avoid development of the depressed scar in the first instance by layered closure of underlying muscle, which prevents the separation of muscle and adherence of scar to the underlying structure.

Silicone Injection

Silicone microdroplet technique is used for injection to stimulate an encapsulating ring of collagen that elevates a depressed scar. Silicone is a foreign, nonphysiological material, and there are serious concerns about its safety. After complications arose from the use of silicone breast implants, the FDA withheld approval for the use, distribution, and promotion of silicone injection for skin augmentation.

Fat Injection

Autologous adipose tissue acquired during liposuction is used to correct skin and soft tissue contour defects. It is a viable graft and should be harvested with care. A 14-gauge needle with limited negative pressure has been advocated for harvesting. The tissue is used for replacement of lost subcutaneous tissue but not as a dermal filler and not to rebuild dermal defects. The complications of lipoinjection are bruising, prolonged inflammation, induration, local infection, and hematoma formation. An unsolved problem with lipoinjection is gradual graft loss; it is estimated that only 30% to 40% of the graft remains after 1 year.

Tissue Transfer Flaps

Tissue transfer can be accomplished by local random flaps, local pedicled flaps, or distant free flaps. The choice of flap depends on the availability of local tissue and which flap offers the best texture and color match; distant free flaps depend on available surgical expertise and resources.

Radiotherapy

Radiotherapy is an efficient and time-honored method of treating resistant keloid. The mechanism of radiotherapy involves fibroblast destruction without replacement. A common concern is the potential risk of radiation-induced malignancy and immunosuppression in various degrees.[24] Several types of radiotherapy have been used in treatment, including kilovoltage irradiation (e.g., superficial x-rays), electron-beam irradiation, and interstitial radiotherapy. Sarcoma is the most likely radiation-induced tumor; it usually develops 8 to 10 years after treatment.

Isotretinoin

Isotretinoin is used in the treatment of keloid. There is a raised T-lymphocyte count in keloid tissue, and it has been postulated that sebum that leaks from the pilosebaceous structure acts as an antigenic stimulus, triggering T-lymphocyte migration, proliferation, and activation and the production of lymphokines, all of which influence fibroblasts to produce more collagen. Isotretinoin eliminates sebocytes and causes sebum suppression.

Wound Care

Although it is not surgically exciting and does not involve advanced technology, the role of wound care is extremely important. Good appropriate dressings certainly help wound healing. A moist environment speeds cell migration, and negative-pressure dressings speed up healing, especially in the presence of infection; silicone dressings may reduce hypertrophic scar formation, and adhesives may reduce tension across a wound. In a busy unit, great benefits can be obtained from fully involving wound care specialists, and the reader is directed to the appropriate literature.

INNOVATIONS

SKIN CLOSURE MATERIAL

Use of subcutaneous absorbable sutures to relieve the tension of the overlying skin is a standard procedure to minimize scar formation. Fine, nonabsorbable monofilament sutures are often used to minimize stitch marks. Stitches are usually removed early, on postoperative day 3.

Cyanoacrylate adhesives have been used as an alternative for skin closure in Canada and Europe for more than 20 years with no adverse effects reported. They are effective in closing superficial lacerations under low tension and can also be used for closure of surgical wounds (e.g., parotidectomy, thyroidectomy). Studies have shown that the results are comparable to those of monofilament sutures. However, the cyanoacrylate adhesives are superior in ease of application and cost-effectiveness and have obvious advantages in children. Major limitations of butylcyanoacrylates include low early breaking strength and a brittle consistency when dry. Therefore, their use should be avoided over skin creases. Proper application is necessary to achieve optimal results (Figs. 23-24 and 23-25).

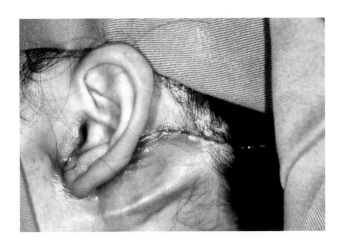

FIGURE 23-24 Facelift incision after parotidectomy closed with glue.

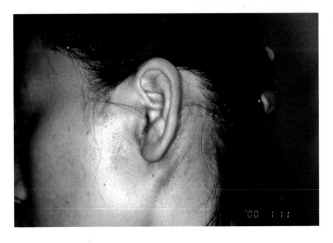

FIGURE 23-25 Postparotidectomy wound 2 weeks after the operation.

SCARLESS HEALING

Healing in the early-gestation fetus is by regeneration, whereas in adults it happens by fibrosis. This phenomenon has a profound impact in clinical practice and is being extensively investigated. The repair process requires turnover of extracellular matrix, and fetal skin has been found to have a higher matrix metalloproteinase level than adult skin. These proteinases are responsible for matrix degradation and are released by various cell types (e.g., zymogens) and activated by removal of amino-terminal propeptides. The TGF-β1 level is deficient in the fetus. TGF-β1 stimulates the deposition of collagen and other matrix components by fibroblasts, inhibits collagenase, blocks plasminogen inhibitor, enhances angiogenesis, and has a chemotactic effect on fibroblasts, monocytes, and macrophages. Administration of TGF-β1 to a fetus makes the fetal wound heal with scarring. The injection of TGF-β1–neutralizing antibodies into the wound may lead to antigenicity problems, limiting the clinical potential. The application of sugar mannose-6-phosphate blocks the IGF-2/mannose-6-phosphate receptor, which in turn decreases the activation of TGF-β1. Anti–TGF-β1 therapeutic strategies would be a way of reducing scarring during wound healing.[25-32]

REFERENCES

1. Bernstein EF, Mauviel A, Uitto J, et al: Wound healing. In Lask GP, Moy RL, editors: *Principles and techniques in cutaneous surgery*, New York, 1996, McGraw-Hill.
2. Muir IFK: On the nature of keloids and hypertropic scars. *Br J Plast Surg* 43:61-69, 1990.
3. Niessen FB, Spauwen PH, Schalkijk J, et al: On the nature of hypertropic scars and keloids: a review. *Plast Reconstr Surg* 104:1435-1458, 1999.
4. Seckel BR, Greene AB: *Facial danger zones: avoiding nerve injury in facial plastic surgery*, St. Louis, 1994, Quality Medical Publishing.
5. Haas AF, Grekin RC: Antibiotic prophylaxis in dermatologic surgery. *J Am Acad Dermatol* 32:155-176, 1995.
6. Fulton JE Jr: Silicon gel sheeting for prevention and management of evolving hypertrophic and keloid scars. *Dermatol Surg* 21:947-951, 1995.
7. Lindsey WH, Davis PT: Facial keloids: a 15-year experience. *Arch Otolaryngol Head Neck Surg* 123:397-400, 1997.
8. Lee RC, Doong H, Aileen F: The response of burn scars to intralesional verapamil. *Arch Surg* 129:107-111, 1994.
9. Carr-Collins JA: Pressure techniques for the prevention of hypertropic scar. *Clin Plast Surg* 19:733-743, 1992.
10. Borges AF: Timing of scar revision techniques. *Clin Plast Surg* 17:71-76, 1990.
11. Harahap M: *Surgical techniques for cutaneous scar revision*, New York, 2000, Marcel Dekker.
12. Coleman WP: Dermabrasion and hypertropic scars. *Int J Dermatol* 30:629, 1991.
13. Nowak KC, McCormack MB, Koch RJ: The effect of superpulsed carbon dioxide laser energy on keloid and normal dermal fibroblast secretion of growth factors: a serum-free study. *Plast Reconstr Surg* 105:2039-2048, 2000.
14. Paquet P, Hermanns J-F: Effect of the 585 nm Flashlamp-pumped pulsed dye laser for the treatment of keloids. *Dermatol Surg* 27:171-174, 2010.
15. Alster T: Laser scar revision: comparison study of 585-nm pulsed dye laser with and without intralesional corticosteroids. *Dermatol Surg* 29:25-29, 2003.
16. Kono T, Ercocen AR: Treatment of hypertrophic scars using a long-pulsed dye laser with cryogen-spray cooling. *Ann Plast Surg* 54:487-493, 2005.
17. Kono T, Ercocen AR: The flashlamp-pumped pulsed dye laser (585 nm) treatment of hypertrophic scars in Asians. *Ann Plast Surg* 51:366-371, 2003.
18. Orentreich DS: Subcutaneous incisionless (subcision) surgery for the correction of depressed scars and wrinkles. *Dermatol Surg* 6:543, 1995.
19. Fernandes D: Percutaneous collagen induction: an alternative to laser resurfacing. *Aesthetic Surg J* 22:315, 2002.
20. Aust MC, Reimers K: Percutaneous collagen induction: minimally invasive skin rejuvenation without risk of hyperpigmentation—fact or fiction? *Plast Reconstr Surg* 122:1553-1563, 2008.
21. Aust MC, Fernandes D, Kolokythas P, et al: Percutaneous collagen induction therapy: an alternative treatment for scars, wrinkles and skin laxity. *Plast Reconstr Surg* 121:1421-1429, 2008.
22. Eppley BL, Pietrzak WS: Platelet-rich plasma: a review of biology and applications in plastic surgery. *Plast Reconstr Surg* 118:147e-159e, 2006.
23. Coleman WP, Lawrence N, Sherman R, et al: Autologous collagen? Lipocytic dermal augmentation: a histologic study. *J Dermatol Surg Oncol* 19:1032-1040, 1993.
24. Darzi MA, Chowdri S, Kaul SK, et al: Evaluation of various methods of treating keloids and hypertropic scars: a 10-year follow-up study. *Br J Plast Surg* 45:375-379, 1992.
25. Adzick NS, Longaker MT: Scarless wound healing in the fetus: the role of the extracellular matrix. In Barbul A, Caldwell MD, Eaglstein WH, et al, editors: *Clinical and experimental approaches to dermal and epidermal repair: normal and chronic wounds.* New York, 1991, Wiley-Liss, pp 177-192.
26. Bullard KM, Cass DL, Banda MJ, et al: Transforming growth factor beta-1 decreases interstitial collagenase in healing human fetal skin. *J Pediatr Surg* 32:1023-1027, 1997.
27. Massague J: The transforming growth factor-beta family. *Ann Rev Cell Biol* 6:597-641, 1990.
28. Wikner NE, Persichitte KA, Baskin JB, et al: Transforming growth factor β stimulates the expression of fibronectin by human keratinocytes. *J Invest Dermatol* 91:207-212, 1988.
29. Vassalli P: The pathophysiology of tumour necrosis factors. *Ann Rev Immunol* 10:411-452, 1992.
30. Sullivan KM, Lorenz HP, Meuli M, et al: A model of scarless human fetal wound repair is deficient in transforming growth factor beta. *J Pediatr Surg* 30:198-203, 1995.
31. Singer AJ, Clark RAF: Mechanisms of disease: cutaneous wound healing. Review article. *N Engl J Med* 341:738-746, 1999.
32. Singer AJ, Hollander JE, Quinn JV: Current concepts: evalution and management of traumatic lacerations. *N Engl J Med* 337:1142-1148, 1997.

CHAPTER 24

Secondary Osteotomies and Bone Grafting

David Richardson, D. Carl Jones

M odern techniques of fracture management allow easy access to the whole craniofacial skeleton, accurate fracture reduction, internal fixation with miniplating and microplating systems, and primary bone grafting where necessary to replace missing bone. The goal of primary treatment is to restore normal anatomy and therefore normal form and function to the craniofacial complex. However, patients may present with posttraumatic deformity for a variety of reasons. They may fail to present in the acute phase, or injuries may go undiagnosed if specialist expertise is not available. Other serious injuries or medical conditions may preclude or compromise immediate treatment of facial injuries, and the results of primary treatment may be unsatisfactory if the extent of the injury is underestimated or in cases of severe comminuted panfacial fractures.[1]

CLASSIFICATION

There is no entirely satisfactory system for classification of posttraumatic facial deformity that incorporates the necessary mix of hard and soft tissue deficits or takes account of resultant esthetic or functional difficulties. Tessier[2] proposed a system based on the major esthetic aspects of the disfigurement and included an orbital syndrome with enophthalmos, a craniofacial syndrome including stigmata of residual frontal and nasoethmoidal fractures, a maxillary syndrome with occlusal abnormalities, and a nasal syndrome characterized by naso-orbital dislocation. Other workers such as Manson[3] and Gruss[4] devised systems related to the previous location of bone fractures comprising frontobasilar fractures; Le Fort I, II, and III fractures of the maxilla; and naso-orbitoethmoid, zygomatic, nasal, mandibular, complex, and panfacial deformities.

PRINCIPLES OF MANAGEMENT

The principles underlying management of secondary posttraumatic skeletal deformity include (1)accurate assessment by history, clinical examination, and special investigations; (2) treatment planning; and (3) surgery, using a variety of techniques for management of soft and hard tissue deficits or deformities, including osteotomies and bone grafting.

ASSESSMENT

Assessment of any deformity requires a detailed history, examination, and special investigations.

History

A full history is essential for diagnosis of secondary posttraumatic deformity. Of particular importance is documentation of the patient's complaints or concerns. A number of potentially correctable deformities may be present, and it is important to assess which of these require correction to address the concerns of the patient. A brief assessment of the psychosocial effect of the deformity may help to highlight important areas, because relatively minor physical abnormalities may give rise to significant psychological, social, or occupational problems. Understanding of the history of the original injury, whether any primary surgery was carried out, and, if so, what this involved are important to plan secondary surgery and anticipate potential difficulties or complications. For example, previous craniotomy with or without dural repair makes subsequent craniotomy more difficult due to dural adhesions, which predispose to increased risk of dural tear and subsequent cerebrospinal fluid (CSF) leak; eye injury or visual loss increases the significance of the risk to vision during operation on the contralateral orbit. The time that has elapsed between the original injury or its primary management and the presentation of secondary deformity may be significant in regard to the timing of secondary surgery. Some problems are better corrected early, whereas in others the timing is less critical (e.g., correction of enophthalmos, orbital and nasal reconstruction).

Examination

A comprehensive clinical examination of the craniofacial complex is mandatory and should include assessment of both hard and soft tissues.

Soft Tissues

Although soft tissues are not directly the subject of this chapter, they deserve mention. The presence of cutaneous scars, soft tissue deficiency, and distortions or subcutaneous fat atrophy may limit the extent of bony movement or the degree of soft tissue response to the underlying bony movement and may leave a persisting esthetic or functional deficit even if a perfect underlying skeletal position can be achieved.

This should be appreciated in the planning phase so that soft tissue adjustment can be carried out at the appropriate time, usually after the skeletal reconstruction.[1,4] In addition, what may seem to be a bony asymmetry may be solely a consequence of soft tissue problems, and surgical technique for correction is likely to be different from that chosen when the underlying problem is truly skeletal in nature. If complaints of orbitozygomatic deformity are being considered, soft tissues of the bony orbit are of paramount importance. Globe displacement in the vertical or anteroposterior (AP) plane needs to be accurately assessed, and the presence of characteristic stigmata of enophthalmos, such as pseudoptosis, implies a degree of displacement of the orbital tissues.

Examination of eye movement and the forced duction test allow assessment of tethering of the extraocular muscles (Fig. 24-1), and traction on the insertions of the medial and lateral recti (usually with the patient under general anesthesia before surgery) gives an indication of the potential for improvement in AP eye position after enophthalmos correction. On occasion, intraorbital fibrosis may preclude anterior eye repositioning despite good orbital volume correction. The position of the lateral and medial canthi should be assessed, intercanthal distances measured, and note made of any abnormality of eyelid position such as retraction or ectropion.

Hard Tissues

A thorough assessment of any bony distortion, deficiencies, or asymmetry must be carried out by inspection and palpation. Techniques used for assessing the bony (and cartilaginous) craniofacial skeleton are well documented in the craniofacial, rhinoplasty, and orthognathic literature. Assessment should be applied in a logical manner and must incorporate all areas of the craniofacial skeleton, including the calvaria and forehead, frontal sinus, orbits, zygomas, external and internal nose, temporomandibular joints (TMJs), mandible, upper and lower dental arches, and dental occlusion. Assessment should be made of displacements in each area examined in the three planes of space (AP, vertical, and transverse) and should include assessment of asymmetries in each of these planes.

Special Investigations

Special investigations may include plain films, dental study models, photographs, and computed tomography (CT) or magnetic resonance imaging (MRI), with three-dimensional (3-D) stereolithographic modeling or virtual planning if appropriate (see Chapter 33).

Plain Films

Plain films demonstrate the site and extent of the original injuries and the presence of bone plates and grafts used in primary treatment. Detailed measurements to assess malposition and asymmetries, including AP and lateral cephalometry, may be useful for delineating the underlying problem and for planning surgical correction. This particularly applies to fractures of the mandible, for which plain films can demonstrate a fibrous union or nonunion, the direction and extent of displacements, and major occlusal abnormalities such as an anterior open bite or mandibular asymmetry.

Dental Study Models

Dental study models are mandatory for assessment of posttraumatic deformity involving the tooth-bearing segments of the maxilla or the mandible. If a posttraumatic malocclusion exists, an assessment can be made of the achievable occlusion and whether any secondary dentoalveolar compensatory changes have occurred; the findings may result in a need for orthodontic or restorative correction or segmental surgery. Face bow recording and anatomical articulation may be useful, particularly in cases of bilateral condylar malunion, in which vertical face height changes are planned and mandibular autorotation is anticipated.

Computed Tomography

CT scanning in the axial and coronal planes yields very useful information, particularly in complex midface and orbitozygomatic deformities and calvarial defects. Two-dimensional imaging is useful to delineate areas of deformity or deficiency; as with plain films, accurate measurements taken from stable and unaffected portions of the craniofacial skeleton can provide an assessment of the degree of displacement or deformity. However, an additional benefit of CT scanning is its

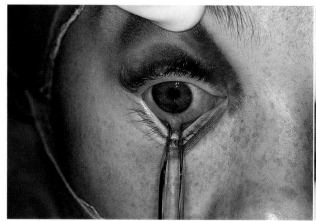
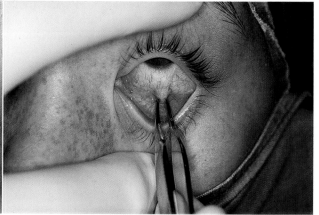

FIGURE 24-1   Forced duction test. **A,** Tethering of inferior rectus. **B,** Normal contralateral eye.

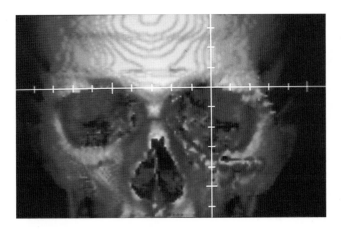

FIGURE 24-2 Three-dimensional computed tomographic scan of malunited fracture of the left zygoma with measurement of displacement.

ability to generate 3-D images that allow the surgeon to visualize all aspects of the deformity at the same time; 3-D images can sometimes reveal the underlying cause of a deformity or discrepancy that is difficult to assess by two-dimensional scans (Fig. 24-2).

In addition, the recent introduction of stereolithographic modeling and virtual planning allows direct visualization of the defect. Direct measurement of required bony movements or augmentation is possible, and surgical simulation, if necessary, may be carried out. It also facilitates the prefabrication of alloplastic implants and production of templates as a guide for size, shape, and positioning of bone grafts, as well as prebending of plates or mesh for graft fixation. Stereolithographic and virtual modeling has been a major advance in the management of complex posttraumatic bony deformities.

TREATMENT PLANNING

After the concerns of the patient have been identified, treatment goals established, and all areas of anatomical and functional abnormality documented, detailed operative planning is required. If a portion of a craniofacial skeleton is malpositioned or deficient and is giving rise to patient concerns or complaints, it should be restored to its normal anatomical position, shape, or volume. However, correction of one deformity may result in accentuation of another that was not previously noticed by the patient. For example, malar osteotomy may make a previously mild enophthalmos more obvious, or correction of mandibular asymmetry may exaggerate an ipsilateral mild nasal deviation. In this situation, the milder, unnoticed defects may require simultaneous or subsequent correction even if they are not of direct concern to the patient initially.

Detailed planning of surgical interventions and movements depends on the information gathered from the history and examination but in particular on the results of the special investigations. When planning bony surgery, it is essential that an accurate plan of surgery and movements is established before operation. This entails a detailed assessment of the extent of movement required in the three planes of space. If onlay grafts are to be used, the site and extent of augmentation should also be established preoperatively.

Intraoperative judgment of the extent of necessary bone movement or augmentation to achieve symmetry is extremely difficult because of distortion of overlying soft tissues due to the surgical access, edema, the presence of an endotracheal tube, and inaccessibility of normal reference points beneath sterile drapes. If 3-D or virtual modeling is available, prebending of plates, preforming of implants, or production of bone graft templates helps to facilitate accurate correction of the deformity and may reduce operating time.

It is important to ensure a coordinated approach to the correction of both bony and soft tissue abnormalities. This usually means correcting the bony abnormality first and then carrying out any necessary soft tissue revision subsequently.

It is essential to discuss with the patient the proposed correction and ensure a realistic expectation of outcome, including both the positive and negative effects of any proposed surgery.

TREATMENT TECHNIQUES

SURGICAL ACCESS

Surgical access to the entire craniofacial skeleton is afforded by bicoronal flap, lower eyelid, or transconjunctival and intraoral buccal sulcus incisions. In addition, a variety of intraoral and extraoral incisions are available for access to the mandible, particularly the vertical ramus and condyle.

Coronal Flap

A coronal flap provides excellent surgical exposure of the upper craniofacial skeleton. Preauricular extension of the incision and dissection in the temporal region immediately adjacent to the deep temporal fascia allow excellent exposure down to and including the zygomatic arches. The dissection in the subgaleal plane is kept on the surface of the deep temporal fascia and may pass deep to the superficial layer where it splits above the zygomatic arch, elevating the frontal branch of the facial nerve with the flap and leaving pericranium attached to the outer table of the skull. Once the flap is raised to within a centimeter of the supraorbital margins, the pericranium can be incised along the temporal crest on each side and across the vertex of the skull posteriorly. The pericranial flap pedicled anteriorly can be raised to expose the underlying skull and is available as vascularized tissue for isolation of the cranial cavity from the nose or for subfrontal dural repair if needed. Freeing of the supraorbital nerves from their foramina can be carried out by means of small osteotomies medial and lateral to the nerves. The calvaria, forehead, supraorbital rim, orbital roof, and lateral orbital rim are exposed, and after mobilization and reflection of the temporalis muscle, access is gained to the lateral wall of the orbit and the temporal fossa.

At the end of the operation, the temporalis muscle must be anchored to the lateral orbital rim with sutures (after anterior mobilization of the muscle, if necessary) to prevent postoperative retraction and temporal hollowing (Fig. 24-3). Access to the infraorbital margin and orbital floor is possible through a coronal flap but is limited, and fixation of osteotomy cuts or grafts can be difficult from this approach without a lower eyelid incision. In addition, if at the start of the

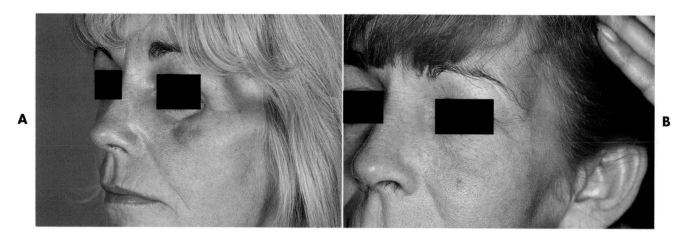

FIGURE 24-3   Postoperative retraction of temporalis muscle. **A,** Before treatment. **B,** After treatment by onlay augmentation of temporal fossa and correction of lower eyelid tethering.

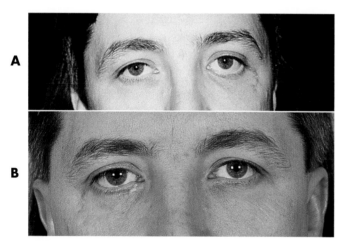

FIGURE 24-4   Postoperative lid retraction. **A,** Before treatment. **B,** After correction by placement of auricular cartilage graft.

operation the medial canthal ligament is intact and attached to the anterior lacrimal crest, it should never be detached during elevation of the flap, because this would require a transnasal canthopexy on closure, the results of which are often disappointing. The attachment of the medial canthal ligament can therefore limit access to the medial orbital wall. If full access to the medial orbital wall is necessary, a lower eyelid incision is required in addition to access gained via the orbital roof exposure of the bicoronal flap.

Lower Eyelid Incision

Transconjunctival, subciliary, or midtarsal incisions, with retro-orbicular preseptal dissection, all give excellent access to the infraorbital rim, orbital floor, infraorbital foramen, and anterior surface of the maxilla. We avoid the infraorbital incision for cosmetic reasons. Occasionally, postoperative lower eyelid retraction and increased scleral show may occur, but this is unusual and is amenable to correction if it fails to resolve spontaneously (Fig. 24-4).

Intraoral Buccal Sulcus Incisions

A horseshoe-shaped incision in the upper buccal sulcus provides excellent access to the lower half of the maxilla and zygomatic buttress and limited access to the infraorbital rim. It should be placed at the height of the sulcus, extending from first molar to first molar, and directed out into the cheek posteriorly to avoid tearing and ensure maintenance of a good vascular pedicle to the maxilla. Repair of the paranasal muscles at the end of the procedure may reduce the risk of alar flaring postoperatively.[5]

Extraoral Approach to the Mandible

Whereas lower buccal sulcus incisions give good intraoral access to the horizontal ramus and angle of the mandible, on rare occasions avoidance of the transoral route is necessary. In addition, intraoral access to the vertical ramus and mandibular condyle is poor, and surgical procedures on these areas of the lower jaw often require an extraoral approach. The introduction of endoscopically assisted surgery may on occasion preclude the need for extraoral access.

The submandibular approach provides good access to the horizontal ramus and angle and allows limited access to the vertical ramus of the mandible. The marginal mandibular branch of the facial nerve must be protected, either by dissection deeply on the cervical fascia or by dissection on the deep surface of platysma and formal identification of the nerve in the subplatysma fascial layer. Excessive traction may result in temporary paralysis of the lower lip due to stretching of the marginal mandibular branch of the facial nerve, but permanent weakness should be uncommon with this approach. However, nerve injury is more likely if the submandibular approach has been used previously, causing fibrosis, loss of surgical planes, and distortion of the local anatomy.

Retromandibular incision with blunt dissection between the buccal and marginal mandibular branches of the facial nerve can provide excellent access to the vertical ramus and condylar neck, and a preauricular incision with temporal extension allows access to the condylar head and TMJ. As with the bicoronal flap, dissection on the surface of the temporalis fascia avoids injury to the frontal branch of the facial nerve.

Other Incisions

Other local incisions such as the upper eyelid blepharoplasty incision, lateral eyebrow incision, Lynch incision, or use of existing scars may be indicated in selected cases in which more extensive exposure is not necessary.

CORRECTION OF DEFORMITY

Correction of bony deformity may be carried out by the use of osteotomy, onlay grafting, or a combination of these techniques. If an individual component of the facial skeleton is of normal morphology but in an abnormal position (displacement), osteotomy is usually the technique of choice. If the bulk of the bone is in a normal position but there is abnormal morphology such as a localized contour deficit (deficiency), onlay grafting may be appropriate.[4] If both displacement and deficiency exist, both techniques may be required. However, the choice of technique must take account of the concerns of the patient as well as the nature and degree of the deformity, the extent of surgery required, potential complications, and a realistic assessment of the likely outcome. These considerations may necessitate a departure from or modification of the basic principles outlined earlier.

Osteotomy

A variety of osteotomies are available and are well documented.[1-4] These effectively re-create the original fracture pattern in the area of concern. Secondary osteotomies for trauma patients are usually carried out by conventional surgical techniques with the use of interpositional bone grafting, if required, to fill gaps created by the bony movements and to ensure primary bone healing, stability of the bony movement, and support for overlying soft tissues. Osteogenic distraction of the craniofacial skeleton is becoming more widespread and may offer another treatment option in selected cases.[6] However, its role in the correction of posttraumatic deformity has yet to be established.

Onlay Grafting

Onlay grafting to correct bone deficiencies may be carried out using a number of materials. Autografts, homografts, heterografts, and alloplastic materials have been described, and each has its advantages and disadvantages. The ideal characteristics of onlay grafts have been outlined by a number of authors and include the following:

- Biocompatible
- No risk of disease transmission
- Resistant to infection
- Dimensionally stable
- Easy to shape or mold
- Amenable to skeletal fixation
- Long shelf life
- Cheap

Bone

Autogenous bone may be used as an interpositional graft or for onlay augmentation. It has several advantages over other materials, including its biocompatibility and lack of disease transmission. Resistance to infection is good, particularly if the bone is vascularized.[7] Dimensional stability is variable and depends on several factors:

- Vascularity: vascularized is better than nonvascularized bone[8,9]

- Embryological origin: membranous bone is better than cartilaginous bone[10]
- Fixation: rigid fixation is better than nonrigid fixation[10]
- Graft site: interpositional graft is better than onlay
- Functional loading: functional loading is better than no functional loading

A number of donor sites, including tibia, iliac crest, mandible, and calvaria, are available. We prefer iliac crest for cancellous or corticocancellous bone grafting to mandibular nonunion and calvarial bone grafting for almost all other situations, such as where osteotomy gaps or bony deficiency exist, masticatory loading is expected, or dimensional stability is important.

The use of nonvascularized grafts requires a healthy, well-vascularized graft bed. This is usually present in patients with secondary posttraumatic deformity, but occasionally the graft bed is of such poor quality that it requires vascularized bone grafts. Vascularized calvarial bone pedicled on temporalis muscle or on the superficial temporal vessels and temporoparietal fascia provides an excellent source of vascularized bone for midface and mandibular reconstruction.[11] A disadvantage in mandibular reconstruction is the possibility of postoperative restriction in mouth opening. If a large bulk of vascularized bone is required, microvascular free flap transfer is the treatment of choice. There are a variety of potential donor sites, including iliac crest (deep circumflex iliac artery) and fibula. In selected cases, bone regeneration by distraction osteogenesis may be an option,[6] but this has not been widely applied to treatment of posttraumatic deformity.

The disadvantages of autogenous bone grafting include prolongation of operating time and the creation of a graft donor site, with its potential associated morbidity. Variability of calvarial thickness may result in inadvertent cutting into the intracranial space during graft harvesting,[12] but complications are rare.

Cartilage

Autogenous cartilage is an excellent material for reconstruction in some situations.[13] It is biocompatible, maintains its viability, is dimensionally stable, and is easy to carve and shape. It can be fixed with wires or sutures. Although its resistance to infection is limited, it has proved to be a reliable material when implanted into a vascular bed, especially in the orbit and nose. It is an excellent space filler but is not rigid and therefore is unsuitable for load bearing. Potential donor sites are auricular concha and nasal septum, which yield a relatively thin sheet with limited area and volume, or costal cartilage, which has an abundant supply and can provide large volume. As with autogenous bone, prolongation of operating time and donor site morbidity, particularly if costal cartilage is used, are relative disadvantages.

Other Materials

A variety of homografts, heterografts, and alloplastic materials are available, and the reader is referred to Chapters 8 and 31 for discussion of these. In principle, we prefer to use autogenous materials in most situations to minimize the risk of disease transmission, peri-implant infection, or late extrusion. Exceptions are large calvarial defects, for which sufficient autogenous bone may not be available; temporal or forehead contour defects, for which bone graft substitutes (e.g., tricalcium phosphate) may be used; and minor malar deficiencies, for which alloplastic onlay grafts are an option.

FOLLOW-UP

Postoperative follow-up is essential to monitor the results of treatment and to assess the need for further procedures. It is not uncommon for several reconstructive procedures to be necessary to achieve the best possible result. Cohen and Kawamoto[1] presented a series of complex posttraumatic deformity cases in which an average of 3 to 4 procedures per patient (range, 1-15 procedures) was needed to obtain optimal correction. However, it is important to appreciate the limitations of corrective surgery and to accept that some patients cannot be restored to complete normality. There is a danger that unrealistic expectations of outcome on the part of the patient or the surgeon may result in an increasing number of surgical interventions yielding diminishing returns. If this point is reached, psychological counseling may be appropriate to help the patient accept and cope with any residual deformity.

In the remainder of this chapter, we discuss the application of the principles of secondary correction of posttraumatic deformity in the following areas: cranial vault deformity, orbitozygomatic injuries, nasoethmoidal injuries, posttraumatic malocclusion, and complex cases involving bone deficiency.

DEFECTS AND DEFORMITY OF THE SKULL

Cranial vault deformities are discussed under the headings of calvarial defects, frontal sinus fractures, and orbital roof fractures.

Full-Thickness Calvarial Defects
Background

Full-thickness calvarial defects may be seen in a number of situations such as after gunshot wounds, after loss of osteoplastic craniotomy flaps, or as a result of a growing skull fracture.

Growth of a linear or nonlinear skull fracture with time is a specific and unusual variant on the full-thickness calvarial defect. Ninety percent of the cases are seen in children younger than 3 years of age[14] (Fig. 24-5), although the process may also be observed in older children and adults.[15] This delayed complication of skull fracture is rare and occurred in only 0.6% of the cases in one large series.[16] Growing skull fractures manifest with soft swelling in the region of a previous skull fracture and clinical and radiographic evidence of increased width and length of the previous fracture. The predominant factor responsible for the increased size of the fracture seems to be a dural defect[17] with abnormal growth of the underlying cerebral tissues,[18] usually in the form of a leptomeningeal cyst but also from herniated cerebrum or dilated underlying ventricle with porencephalic cyst.

Full-thickness calvarial defects may require treatment for a number of reasons. There may be a risk of further trauma from blunt injury or a penetrating object, and a significant cosmetic defect may be apparent (see Fig. 24-5). In addition, infections of the scalp present a significant risk of intracranial spread due to loss of the natural barrier of the calvarial bone, with potentially serious consequences.[19]

Reconstruction using alloplastic prostheses has historically been the most commonly used method for correction of the larger full-thickness calvarial defect. In the early 20th century, active interest developed in autogenous cranioplasty from various donor sites such as tibia, ilium, ribs, or skull.

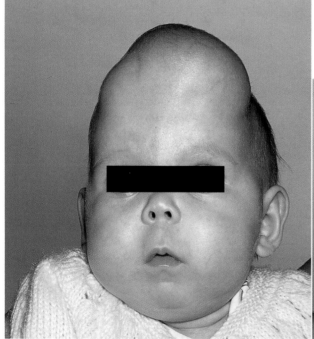
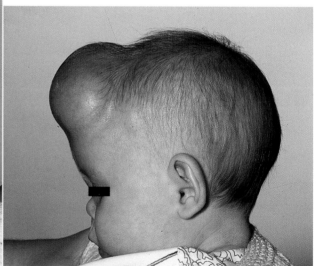

A, **B**

FIGURE 24-5   Clinical presentation of a growing skull fracture. **A,** Frontal view. **B,** Lateral view.

More recently, the trend has been to use split-thickness calvarial bone grafting. Calvarial bone grafts have become more popular because of their greater dimensional stability and lower donor site morbidity compared with other bone graft donor sites. However, harvesting of these grafts still involves small risks of dural tears, meningitis, brain abscess, encephalitis, and sagittal sinus tears. These risks depend on the size of the graft harvested, whether full-thickness or split-thickness grafts are used,[20] the location of the donor site, and the skill and experience of the surgeon.

Assessment

A full history of the cranial defect should be established together with previous surgical details, including any prior attempts at reconstruction, to anticipate potential surgical complications such as dural tears or the need to remove plates or other implants placed previously. As always, a thorough clinical examination is required. Special attention should be given to the site and size of the skull defect. The positions of previous surgical scars should be noted and the quality of the soft tissues overlying the bony defect assessed.

Plain radiographs show a characteristic irregular oval or elliptical skull defect. CT scanning provides more detailed images as well as useful information about the underlying brain. This is of special relevance when growing skull fractures are being managed. MRI is often used in addition because of its excellent soft tissue imaging characteristics. Reformatting of axial and coronal CT images can be performed to create 3-D images that give excellent visualization of the cranial defect. Modern software allows the milling of an exact model of the skull and defect. This is particularly useful for very large defects because it allows the fabrication of a custom-made alloplastic cranioplasty implant (Fig. 24-6).

Treatment Planning

The decision to reconstruct a full-thickness calvarial defect depends on a number of factors including age, risk of injury, the size of the defect, any underlying pathology, and the cosmetic consequences of the defect. The decision to operate is based on the merits of each individual case. Whether a calvarial bone graft or an alloplastic implant is used depends largely on the size of the defect and the availability of sufficient calvarial bone to cover it without leaving a deficiency in

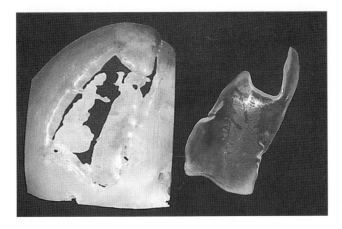

FIGURE 24-6   Three-dimensional model of skull defect and prefabricated implant.

the donor area. Large full-thickness calvarial defects are usually reconstructed with the use of alloplastic implants, whereas smaller defects are amenable to the use of split calvarial bone grafts.

Operative Technique

Surgery is performed with a standard coronal flap approach. Great care is needed when elevating the flap in the region of the bony defect to avoid producing a dural tear. The margins of the defect are exposed by subpericranial and extradural dissection, and any soft tissues within the fracture line or defect are excised or repositioned, including excision of nonviable cerebral tissue and dural repair where necessary.

If a calvarial bone graft is to be used, a template of the defect is cut out of sterile paper to aid in accurate harvesting of the graft. The exact form of the calvarial bone graft depends on the size of the defect being reconstructed. Shave grafts consist of fine strips of bone harvested from the outer table with osteotomes. Their advantage is that multiple grafts can be harvested from a wide area without leaving a significant donor defect. However, their small size means that they cannot be rigidly fixed in their new position, and therefore they are not recommended.

Sliding bone grafts are in many ways analogous to the advancement flaps used in skin surgery. An area of bone is exposed adjacent to the defect, and a bone graft somewhat larger than the defect is marked out with saws or burs. The outer table of the skull is harvested through the diploic layer, leaving the inner table intact. The bone graft is then slid across the defect in such a manner that it still partially lies across the inner table of the donor site. Such overlap allows increased primary stability and may possibly lead to earlier bony union.

Transposition calvarial bone grafts are now the most widely accepted method of reconstructing sizeable full-thickness skull defects.[20] After complete exposure of the edges of the bony defect, a template is fashioned, and a suitable area for the harvest of calvarial bone is identified. This is most often in the parietal region on the contralateral side from the preexisting defect. A full-thickness piece of calvarial bone slightly larger than the template is removed, with great care taken not to damage the underlying dura. The bone graft is then split with the use of fine osteotomes and saws along the diploic layer, producing two similarly sized pieces of bone consisting of the inner and outer table (Fig. 24-7). The outer table bone graft can be returned to the donor site, and the inner table graft can then be adapted to reconstruct the bony defect.

Fixation is achieved at the donor site and the grafted sites by microplates or miniplates (Fig. 24-8). For growing skull fractures in pediatric patients, consideration should be given to use of resorbable plates to avoid "drift" of the plate from the outer to the inner aspect of the calvaria with continued skull growth. The donor site should be covered with a layer of absorbable cellulose polymer (Surgicel). The pericranial layer is then closed and the scalp is repaired over a suction drain if necessary.

Outcome of Calvarial Defect Reconstruction

The outcome of reconstruction of simple calvarial defects using split calvarial bone grafts is excellent. In a follow-up study of 27 patients, Posnik et al.[21] found minimal complications with no infections, graft exposures, or intracranial injuries. However, a growing skull fracture is a different clinical entity. In a study of 41 patients with growing skull fractures, Gupta et al.[16] reported a death rate of 7%, postoperative CSF leaks in 7%, and local wound infection in 14%. In a review of 132 cases reported in the literature, Pezzota et al.[22] found a high incidence of seizures and focal neurological deficits; functional recovery was linked to the clinical presentation and early diagnosis. Reconstruction of simple calvarial defects is therefore associated with a better outcome than that of growing skull fractures, in which the postoperative morbidity is largely related to abnormalities of the underlying brain.

Frontal Sinus Fractures

Background

Frontal sinus fractures are most commonly managed in the acute setting, where open reduction and internal fixation (ORIF) of the disrupted bone is performed together with any necessary maxillofacial or neurological surgery.[23] If the

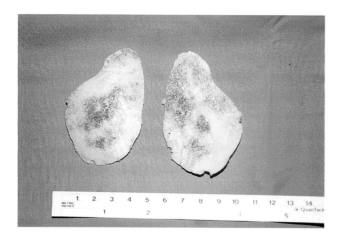

FIGURE 24-7 Split calvarial bone graft with outer and inner tables separated.

posterior wall of the frontal sinus is fractured, cranialization of the sinus and stripping of the lining mucosa, together with obliteration of the frontonasal duct with muscle, fat, or cancellous bone chips, are necessary to prevent late complications of CSF leakage, mucopyocele, osteomyelitis, and meningoencephalocele.[24] A dural repair is usually required if the posterior wall is fractured. On occasion, however, patients may present for late correction of a depressed fracture of the frontal bone, usually for reasons of cosmesis.

Assessment

A thorough history of the injury and its subsequent management should be taken. If the posterior table was involved in the original fracture, it is important to know whether a cranialization procedure was performed, because this has important consequences for the reconstruction of the bony defect. In this situation, fibrosis and adhesions increase the risk of further dural tear, and avoidance of extradural dissection is desirable. Onlay bone graft or use of an alloplastic filler material may be more appropriate than osteotomy to reduce risk of complications.

The frontal bone contour and the condition of the overlying skin are examined. The sensation subserved by the supraorbital and supratrochlear nerves should be assessed before the coronal flap is raised.

Plain radiographs can provide useful information especially with regard to the presence and location of metalwork from previous surgical procedures. CT scans are required to show greater detail of the anatomy of the anterior and posterior walls of the frontal sinus. The presence of active frontal sinus disease, if any, can be assessed and should be treated before reconstruction.

Treatment Planning

There are two principal methods of management, both of which usually involve a coronal approach. First, the bone may be re-osteotomized along the previous fracture lines and the bone fragments fixed in their original position with miniplates or microplates. If the posterior table has been involved, this is likely to entail a formal craniotomy. Alternatively, the defect can be masked with an onlay bone graft or an

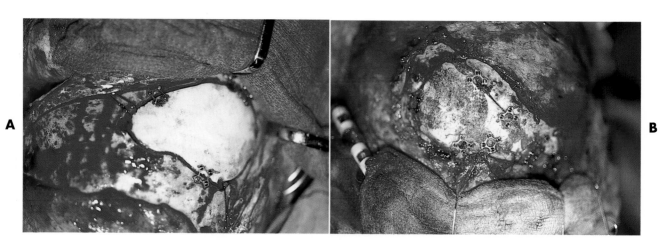

FIGURE 24-8 Split calvarial bone graft. **A,** Outer table replaced at donor site. **B,** Inner table reconstructing defect.

alloplastic implant. However, if the contour defect is minor, it may be corrected more simply by using calcium triphosphate bone replacement material keyed to the bone with microscrews or fine titanium mesh.

Operative Technique

Figure 24-9 illustrates the operative technique.

Outcome

The outcome after secondary osteotomy or bone grafting for displaced anterior wall fractures is excellent. Most complications are associated with the original injury and depend on whether the posterior wall is involved with dural tear, presence of CSF leaks, involvement of the nasofrontal duct, and whether adequate treatment (including, if necessary, dural repair, cranialization, or obliteration of the sinus and nasofrontal duct) was carried out. In a series of 33 patients with frontal sinus fracture,[25] long-term complications occurred in

4 patients, only 2 of which were cosmetic. The requirement for secondary surgery is therefore small in well-managed frontal sinus fractures.

Orbital Roof Fractures

Background

Orbital roof fractures are a consequence of severe trauma and are associated with a considerable likelihood of neurological and ophthalmological injury. In general, such injuries are managed in the acute phase, but if they were not treated or if treatment was inadequate, significant secondary deformity may occur. Before the age of 3 years, the orbital roof may be the site of a growing skull fracture.[15]

Assessment

A history of the original injury and previous treatment, together with the original notes, radiographs, and scans, is of great help in planning surgery.

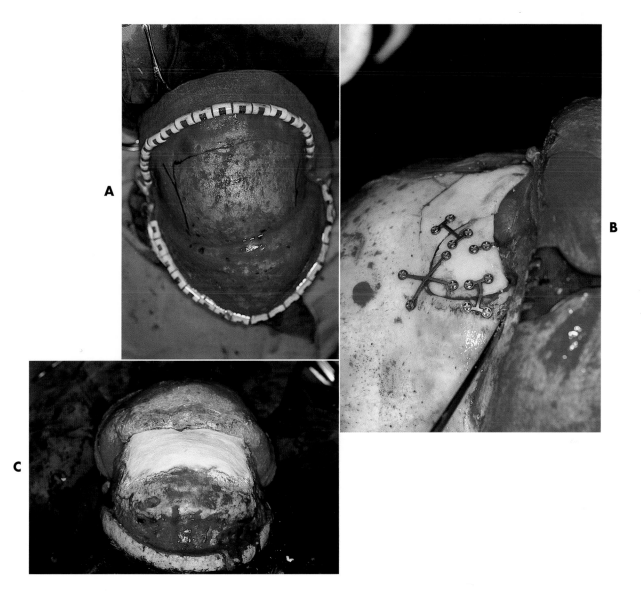

FIGURE 24-9 Frontal sinus fracture. **A,** Bicoronal flap. **B,** Osteotomy and fixation of fragments. **C,** Augmentation with tricalcium phosphate bone cement.

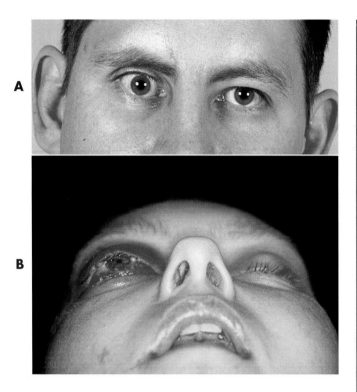

FIGURE 24-10   Orbital roof fracture. **A,** Inferior displacement of eye. **B,** Proptosis.

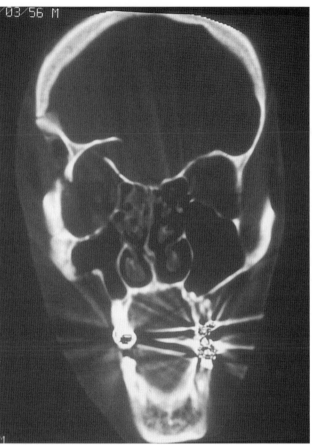

FIGURE 24-11   Computed tomographic scan of orbital roof fracture shows significant displacement of fracture segment.

A full assessment of the external bony contour should be made. Irregularity or asymmetry of the supraorbital rims should be noted. An assessment of enophthalmos or exophthalmos (including pulsating exophthalmos indicative of orbital roof defects) should be made. Sensory function of the supraorbital and supratrochlear nerves should be assessed. As with any orbital reconstruction, an ophthalmological opinion should be sought before any surgery is performed to document vision and ocular motility preoperatively, identify any problems, and act as a baseline for postoperative follow-up. If the orbital roof itself has been depressed, ocular dystopia with inferior displacement of the globe will occur (Fig. 24-10). Larger defects of the orbital roof put the patient at risk of dural herniation, which may result in pulsating exophthalmos and disturbance of ocular function.

Special Investigations
Fine-cut axial and coronal CT scans should be obtained to provide detailed images of the orbital roofs of both orbits (Fig. 24-11). This allows accurate surgical planning, and measurements can be made of bony displacement, deficiency, or asymmetry.

Operative Technique
In most cases, a coronal flap is the most appropriate approach. Occasionally, it is possible to access the surgical area via an existing scar or local incisions, and for small defects confined to the supraorbital rim, this approach may be adequate. However, larger deformities and any significant displacement or deficiency of the orbital roof will require a transcranial approach with unilateral frontal craniotomy, retraction of the frontal lobe, and, on occasion, removal of the supraorbital

bar. This requires joint management by neurosurgical and maxillofacial specialists.

Small depressions or contour irregularities may be masked by bony recontouring with burs and by the application of small onlay bone grafts or, alternatively, one of the proprietary bone cements. Large displacements or defects in the orbital roof require accurate reduction or reconstruction with split-thickness calvarial bone graft (after dural repair, if necessary). If a frontal craniotomy has been performed, the graft can be harvested from the inner table of the frontal bone flap, thereby avoiding any visible or palpable donor site defect.[26]

Outcome
There is very little in the literature regarding secondary correction of orbital roof fractures.[27] With accurate reconstitution of the anatomy, the outcome should be good in both pediatric and adult patients. However, some inaccuracy in vertical and AP globe repositioning, as well as postoperative diplopia, may occur.

DEFORMITY OF THE ORBITOZYGOMATIC REGION

Background
Fractures of the orbit and fractures of the zygoma are discussed together because of the great overlap of these topics. Injuries to this area can produce complex deformities, and

careful planning is required when secondary corrective surgery is contemplated. In general, deformity is caused by inadequate primary surgery[28]; it is related in part to the underlying bony skeletal abnormality and in part to the soft tissue component, including scarring, thickening, and incorrect draping of the soft tissue envelope on the facial bones. Deformities of upper and lower eyelids may be seen, often from the initial trauma but occasionally from a previous surgical approach.

Patient complaints may be related to cosmetic or functional deficit, or both. It is important to establish from the outset the specific concerns of the patient and expectations of the outcome of treatment. This will allow surgery to be tailored to the patient's concerns rather than the surgeon's view of the deformity and will provide the opportunity to dispel any unrealistic expectations.

Assessment

A full history should include the mechanism of the original injury, the treatment previously received, and the current concerns of the patient. A number of factors contribute to unsatisfactory appearance after orbitozygomatic injuries.

Enophthalmos is common because of increased orbital volume or herniation of orbital contents through defects in the orbital walls, usually the inferior or medial wall (Fig. 24-12). Ocular dystopia may occur with inferior displacement of the globe when Whitnall's tubercle is inferiorly displaced as a result of zygomatic malunion after an inferiorly displaced fracture. Loss of zygomatic prominence leading to cheekbone asymmetry is common, and increased facial width due to bowing of the zygomatic arch may occur secondary to an inadequately reduced, posteriorly displaced zygomatic fracture. Telecanthus may be present if the original fracture involved the portion of bone bearing the medial canthal ligament or if the ligament was detached during surgical access for primary treatment.

Esthetic concerns with regard to the periorbital soft tissues are frequently related to the position of the eyelids and canthi. Lid retraction or true ectropion (or both) may be seen, usually as a result of previous treatment (see Fig. 24-4).

Functional deficits after orbital trauma frequently relate to injury to the globe itself and are therefore within the preserve of the ophthalmological surgeon. Tethering and scarring of the periorbita and extraocular muscles may cause diplopia, which, if severe, can be disabling. Epiphora is a frequent complaint and may be related to damage to the bony or soft tissue component of the lacrimal drainage apparatus, including abnormalities of lower lid and lacrimal punctum position. If epiphora persists, corrective surgery may be necessary.

Clinical examination should include assessment of the degree of enophthalmos, which should be assessed subjectively by clinical examination and objectively by exophthalmometry. The classic signs of enophthalmos may be apparent, including obvious ocular retrusion, hypoglobus, deep supratarsal fold, pseudoptosis, and narrowing of the palpebral fissure (see Fig. 24-12). The normal anterior projection of the globe relative to the lateral orbital rim is between 12 and 16 mm. Although formal exophthalmometry would seem likely to give a more objective assessment than clinical examination, it is based on comparison between the position of the globe and that of the lateral orbital wall; if this bony landmark

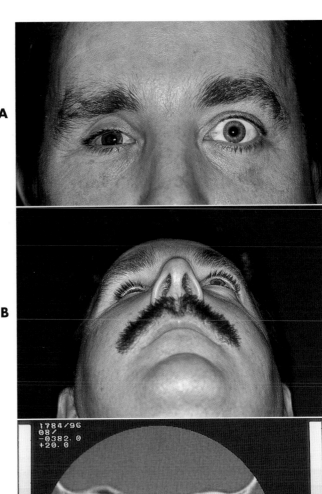

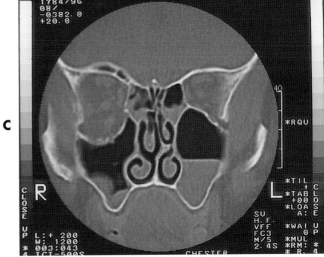

FIGURE 24-12 Enophthalmos. **A** and **B,** Clinical appearance. **C,** Computed tomogram shows large floor blowout.

was altered by the original trauma, the reading may be unreliable.

Any asymmetry of the malar prominences should be noted. The malar eminence on the injured side may be displaced medially, posteriorly, and inferiorly. Rarely, if previous surgery has overreduced the zygomatic complex, it may be lateral to its normal position and therefore overprominent (Fig. 24-13). Facial width should be assessed by comparing the relative prominence of the zygomatic arch on the injured and uninjured sides. If the zygoma is displaced posteriorly, there will be a "bowing out" of the zygomatic arch, increasing the facial width on the injured side.

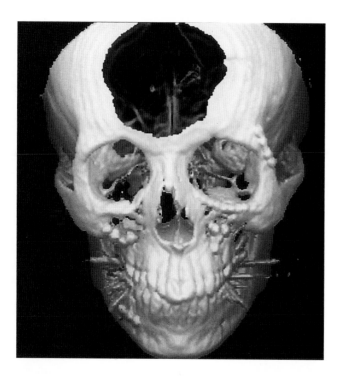

FIGURE 24-13 Three-dimensional computed tomogram shows overreduction of the fracture of the left zygoma.

An assessment of the overlying soft tissues should be made. The quality and thickness of the tissues should be noted. Scarred, contracted tissues may require correction at the time of osteotomy or later. Loss of sensation in the distribution of the infraorbital nerve is common after orbital trauma, whereas loss of supraorbital and supratrochlear nerve sensation is less frequently seen. There is no evidence to suggest that secondary surgery has a beneficial effect on compromised nerve function; indeed, the patient should be aware that surgery carries the risk of further nerve damage.

Special Investigations

Plain radiographs have a limited role in surgical planning for correction of midface deformity. They are useful in identifying the type and position of internal fixation used in previous operations, which will almost certainly need to be removed if further surgery is performed. A submentovertex radiograph will show the form of the zygomatic arches. Subtle variations in the shape of the arches can have a profound effect on facial width and overall facial balance.

CT scans are invaluable in surgical planning. Images should be obtained in the coronal and axial planes, and 3-D images can be particularly useful in orbitozygomatic injuries. Measurements from unaffected fixed points such as the pterygoid plates or contralateral uninjured orbit allow establishment of a quantitative measurement of the bony deformity with respect to the contralateral, uninjured side. These measurements should be established in three planes (vertical, mediolateral, and posteroanterior) so that the necessary movements or augmentations of the zygomatic-maxillary complex can be predicted. These movements should be accurately established before surgery is undertaken (Fig. 24-14).

MRI scans are little used in the planning of facial bone osteotomies, but they do have a role in assessing the nature and quality of the overlying soft tissues and may be useful in difficult cases. The degree of herniation of tissues through the medial, the inferior, and (to a lesser extent) the lateral orbital wall may be assessed with MRI. It may also be possible to image trapping or tethering of extraocular muscles.

Dental study casts have little role to play in the management of orbitozygomatic deformity unless a simultaneous osteotomy of the maxilla or mandible to correct a malocclusion is planned. The availability of computer-generated 3-D models of the bony facial skeleton derived from CT scans has been a major step forward in this regard. Exact measurements can be made on the models, and the surgery can be accurately preplanned. If alloplastic materials are to be used, they can be custom made on the 3-D models. Recent advances in computer software allowing detailed virtual planning and intraoperative image guidance are likely to facilitate much more accurate surgical planning and execution of bony surgery, but it must be borne in mind that variation or limitation in the soft tissue response to bony surgery may still yield imperfect results even if the bony symmetry is restored.

Sinus endoscopy is a relatively recent innovation and may be useful to assess the condition of the orbital floor. In the acute situation, some success with definitive fracture management has been achieved, but whether endoscopically assisted surgery will have any role in the management of the secondary deformity is unclear. One case has been reported of correction of enophthalmos secondary to a medial wall defect using alloplastic material inserted via an endoscopic approach medial to the lacrimal caruncle.[29]

If surgery is being considered, a full ophthalmic and orthoptic assessment is required to establish a baseline. This is especially important if the patient is experiencing diplopia.

Surgical Technique

For successful correction of the orbitozygomatic deformity, complete regional exposure is required,[28] although some authors advocate a more conservative approach.[30,31] Exposure is achieved through a bicoronal flap combined with a lower eyelid incision and an upper buccal sulcus incision. The bicoronal flap gives excellent access to the orbit and zygomatic arch and body and permits harvesting of calvarial bone graft. Stripping of the temporalis muscle facilitates exposure of the lateral orbital wall. The lower eyelid approach gives access to the infraorbital rim and orbital floor and allows visualization and protection of the infraorbital nerve. It may be done through a skin incision (blepharoplasty, midtarsal, or infraorbital) or a transconjunctival incision. The transconjunctival incision, which is usually combined with a lateral canthotomy, is technically more difficult to perform but has the advantage of leaving less facial scarring compared with the cutaneous approaches; it also may be associated with a lower incidence of lid retraction. The combination of the bicoronal flap and the lower lid approach allows circumferential subperiosteal dissection within the orbit. The lateral canthal ligament should be tagged and reattached at the end of the procedure. The medial canthal ligament, which is notoriously difficult to reattach, should have its origin carefully preserved.

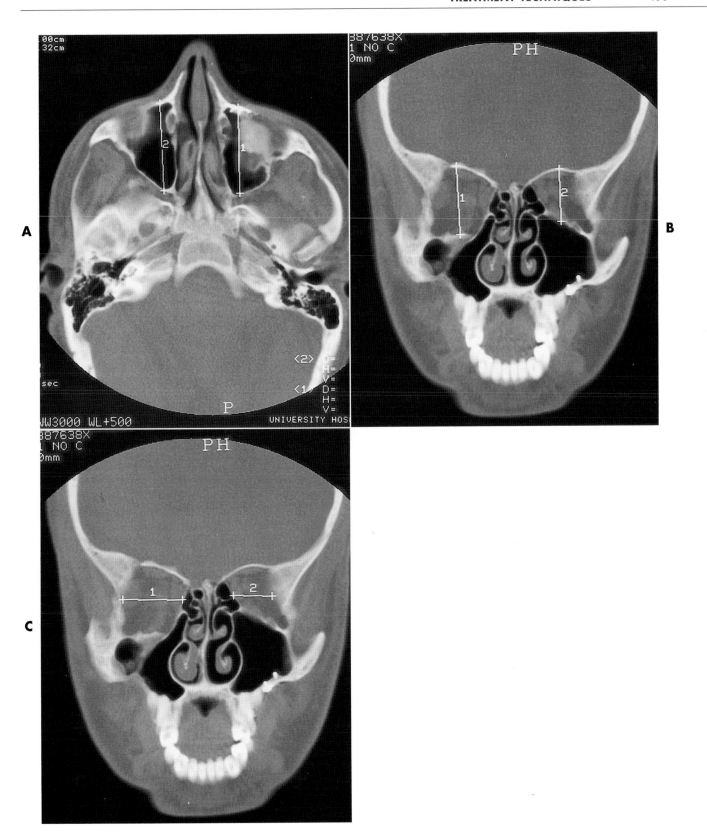

FIGURE 24-14 Surgical planning using computed tomographic scans. **A,** Anteroposterior measurement. **B,** Vertical measurement. **C,** Transverse measurement.

The orbital floor must be dissected with great care, because the infraorbital nerve is frequently embedded in dense scar tissue and may easily be damaged. A similar situation applies where gaps in the bony skeleton (e.g., in the lateral orbital wall) have led to fusion of the intraorbital and extraorbital soft tissues. The buccal sulcus incision gives access to the anterior surface of the maxilla, the zygomatic buttress, and, via the maxillary sinus, the inferior aspect of the orbital floor.

Correction of bony deformities in the orbitozygomatic area depends on the performance of several key maneuvers. Zygomatic osteotomy reproduces the fracture lines of the original injury. After exposure, bone cuts are made from the infraorbital rim just lateral to the nerve extending down the anterior maxillary wall, passing posteriorly, to the zygomatic buttress. The bone cut is continued around the lower extent of the buttress onto its posterior face. Within the orbit, the cut passes from the infraorbital rim posteriorly to the anterior end of the inferior orbital fissure. The cuts are then continued superiorly through or just anterior to the greater wing of the sphenoid and to the zygomatic-frontal suture. Completion of the osteotomy at the posterior aspect of the buttress is best performed with the use of a fine, curved osteotome, which is inserted via the coronal approach behind the lateral orbital rim within the temporal fossa; the incision extends from the anterior end of the inferior orbital fissure to join with the cut already made in the inferior part of the buttress. The root of the zygomatic arch is sectioned, resulting in complete freeing of the zygoma from its bony attachments. For the less experienced operator, appreciation of the exact 3-D anatomy is enhanced if a dry skull or a 3-D model is available in the operating theater.

Before the zygoma is mobilized, the bony movements should be marked at the infraorbital rim, the zygomatic-frontal suture, and the zygomatic arch. The most common posttraumatic displacement of the zygoma involves impaction posteriorly, inferiorly, and medially. Usually, bone removal is required at the zygomatic-frontal suture to permit superior repositioning of the zygoma, whereas advancement and lateral movement will create bony gaps. The zygoma is fixed into its new position with microplates. Repositioning of the body of the zygoma often produces contour deformities and steps in the zygomatic arch, and the arch itself may require local osteotomies to allow it to be recontoured.

Anterior, lateral, and superior movement of the osteotomized zygoma creates bony gaps and step deformities at several sites, and these require bone grafting to ensure bony union, stability, and soft tissue support and to avoid palpable irregularities and edges beneath the thin periorbital skin. Gaps occur at the infraorbital margin, orbital floor, the frontozygomatic cut, lateral orbital wall, zygomatic arch, and zygomatic buttress. In addition, the zygomatic repositioning may have created an orbit larger in volume than before, allowing herniation of periorbital tissues through bony defects of the orbital walls. Considerable widening of the inferior orbital fissure may occur as a result of repositioning. This increased orbital volume predisposes to the development of enophthalmos. The inferior orbital fissure should be exposed and the soft tissues divided (no significant structures pass through it); it should then be obliterated with a graft.

Bone grafting is essential to treat preexisting enophthalmos and to prevent its occurrence after osteotomy. Contoured calvarial bone is used for this purpose. Calvarial bone graft exhibits considerably less tendency for resorption than the previously used rib or iliac crest grafts, particularly if rigid fixation techniques are used.[10] Calvarial bone should now be considered the gold standard for grafting in and around the orbit. The bone is readily available and does not require a separate incision for its harvest. Enough bone is available in most cases, and the morbidity associated with its harvest is very low.[32] The technique has been described elsewhere, but the bone is usually obtained as thin rectangular strips, which are ideally suited for grafting orbital defects.

For the correction of enophthalmos, it is important that the bone graft be largely situated behind the equator of the globe so that the eye is displaced forward. Hypoglobus may be corrected if the bone graft is placed in the orbital floor beneath the globe, but care must be taken in placing orbital bone grafts not to produce unwanted elevation in globe position. Bone grafts placed posteriorly within the orbit do not usually require fixation, although a number of specifically designed plates are available for this purpose. For grafts that are more anteriorly placed, fixation is recommended to minimize the amount of resorption and prevent migration. If possible, the metalwork should be placed within the orbital margin so that it is not subsequently palpable through the thin infraorbital skin. A forced duction test is performed immediately before and again after placement of bone graft to ensure that ocular motility has not been jeopardized (see Fig. 24-1).

If a bone graft is being placed to correct a preexisting enophthalmos, overcorrection is advisable at the time of surgery to allow for swelling and a degree of bone graft resorption.[28] Some authors have recommended placing incisions within the scarred periorbital tissues to allow the globe to take up a more anterior position. However, it is likely that the scarring will recur, and this maneuver is not recommended. Advancement of the displaced zygoma and orbital rim depends on the ability to simultaneously correct the enophthalmos, because otherwise the appearance of the enophthalmos itself may be worsened (Fig. 24-15).

Onlay Grafting

Onlay grafting may be used in mild cases of malar asymmetry and can usually be carried out easily through a lower eyelid incision. Calvarial bone, bone substitutes, or alloplastic implants may be used (Fig. 24-16).

NASOETHMOID FRACTURES

Detachment of the medial canthal ligaments together with their bony insertion is relatively common after orbital and nasoethmoidal fractures. Inadequate primary management leads to telecanthus and blunting of the medial canthal angle. Osteotomy and repositioning of the nasoethmoidal segment may be required. Complete correction of the medial canthal position is notoriously difficult, and overcorrection should be the aim. If the medial canthal ligament is not attached to an identifiable bone fragment, a transnasal canthopexy is required (Fig. 24-17). If a nasoethmoidal fracture has been a significant part of the orbital injury, a graft will almost invariably be needed to the dorsum of the nose to re-create the degree of nasal projection present before the injury. Calvarial bone was widely used for this in the past. Although it gives a satisfactory appearance, its "feel," especially toward the nasal

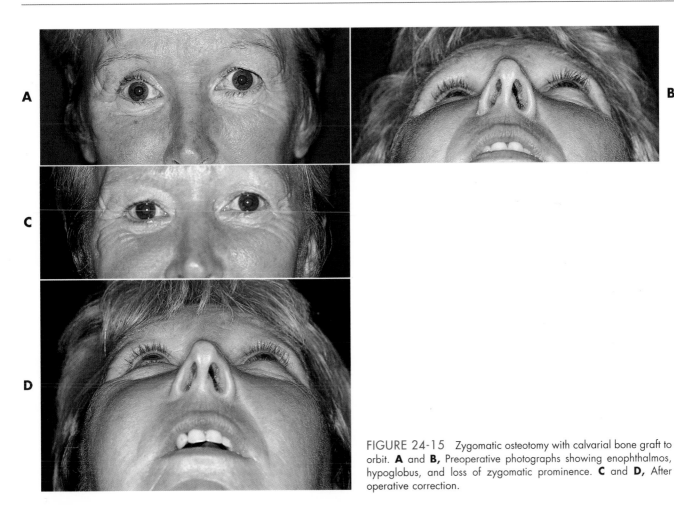

FIGURE 24-15 Zygomatic osteotomy with calvarial bone graft to orbit. **A** and **B**, Preoperative photographs showing enophthalmos, hypoglobus, and loss of zygomatic prominence. **C** and **D**, After operative correction.

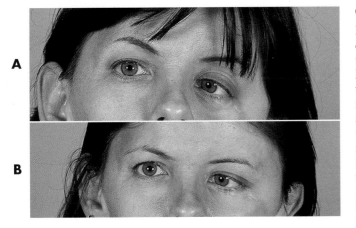

FIGURE 24-16 Onlay augmentation of left zygoma using vascularized calvarial bone pedicled on temporalis muscle. **A**, Preoperative view. **B**, Postoperative view.

tip, is too solid to be natural, and grafts that are cantilevered superiorly without support at the nasal tip may subsequently displace. A nasal dorsal graft of carved costal cartilage supported inferiorly by a columella strut gives a more natural feel and a stable augmentation (Fig. 24-18).

Outcome

Long-term outcome depends on the extent of the secondary deformity, detailed planning, choice of technique, and meticulous surgery. In a series published by Freihofer and Borstlap,[33] osteotomy was found to give superior results compared with onlay techniques. In 16 cases of posttraumatic nasoethmoid facture, 14 reconstructions were assessed as good or satisfactory, with only 2 being rated as unsatisfactory due to undercorrection, overcorrection, or persistence of enophthalmos. The authors found no decrease in visual acuity. Among five cases with associated posttraumatic enophthalmos, two were corrected fully and three were only partially corrected. Infraorbital nerve sensory loss occurred in approximately half of the group. In a series of four cases, Perino et al.[34] reported good results and a low complication rate. However, in both reports, there was a significant requirement for further procedures to ensure optimal outcome. In Cohen and Kawamoto's series[1] including 14 cases of orbitozygomatic deformity, the average number of operations required was 3.76. Further procedures may be required to reduce overcorrected malar position or to correct medial or lateral canthal dystopias, recurrence of enophthalmos, or abnormalities of eyelid position.

Hammer and Prein[28] reported good or satisfactory esthetic results after secondary orbitozygomatic reconstruction in 20 of 26 patients. Where diplopia was present before secondary correction, improvement occurred in just over half of the

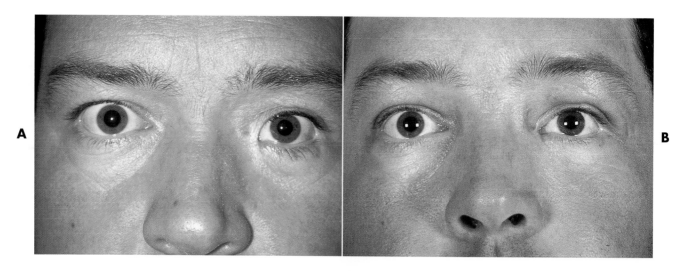

FIGURE 24-17 Secondary deformity after nasoethmoidal injury. **A,** Medial canthal detachment.
B, Appearance after transnasal canthopexy.

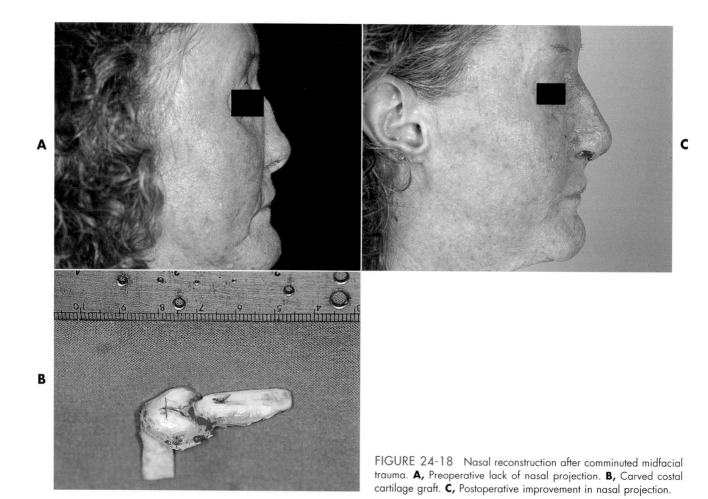

FIGURE 24-18 Nasal reconstruction after comminuted midfacial
trauma. **A,** Preoperative lack of nasal projection. **B,** Carved costal
cartilage graft. **C,** Postoperative improvement in nasal projection.

group. There was a complication rate of 15% including visual loss due to displacement of bone graft, endophthalmitis, orbital abscess, and exposure of a nasal bone graft.

Hans and Freihofer[35] reported a series of patients who underwent secondary correction of fractured zygomas with a good result obtained in 80%. Medial canthopexy was carried out in 19 patients; 3 required further procedures, but all 19 achieved a satisfactory or good final outcome.

POSTTRAUMATIC MALOCCLUSION

Background

Posttraumatic malocclusion may occur after malunion of any fracture that directly or indirectly involves the alveolar segments of the maxilla or mandible. These include isolated dentoalveolar fractures of the maxilla or mandible; maxillary fractures including Le Fort I, II, and III fractures with or without palatal split; and mandibular fractures.

Before the introduction of miniplating, stabilization of the occlusion by intermaxillary fixation (IMF) was the primary aim of treatment of facial fractures. The introduction of internal fixation makes direct anatomical segment reduction the primary aim. If this is achieved, a normal occlusion should automatically follow, and it does so in most cases. However, in some comminuted maxillary or mandibular fractures, a perfect occlusion is difficult to achieve, and most fractures of the mandibular condyle tend to be managed by closed techniques, with the potential for displacement after removal of the intermaxillary fixation. In addition, large muscle forces in the mandible may cause movement of the fracture site, resulting in fibrous union or nonunion. Infection of mandibular fractures, particularly those involving the tooth-bearing segment of the mandible or the angle, may result in nonunion and segment displacement with malocclusion.

Diagnosis

In the presence of small displacements of segments, patients usually complain of functional difficulties in biting and chewing and the inability to find a positive, comfortable intercuspal position. In large displacements, an effect on facial appearance may be added, particularly with increases in the mandibular angle that cause an anterior open bite and mandibular asymmetry, both usually due to malunion of mandibular condylar fracture. Complaints related to TMJ dysfunction may follow malunion of condylar fractures, and mechanical joint derangement may result in severe deviation or limitation of mouth opening.

Assessment of TMJ function is mandatory, because restriction of mouth opening or severe deviation may necessitate TMJ surgery in addition to osteotomies or bone grafting. It is important to check for mandibular displacement and ensure that the mandible is fully retruded when the malocclusion is assessed. Occasionally, a patient presents with occlusal complaints but shows an apparently good occlusion. This problem may be a minor mandibular displacement, indicating a discrepancy between the retruded condylar position of the mandible and the intercuspal position. In addition, fibrous union of a body fracture, which allows a very small degree of movement between segments, may lead to good intercuspation but only at the expense of bone movement at the site of the fibrous union. It may be difficult to see obvious

fracture mobility in this situation by standard clinical examination, but careful inspection of the fracture site while occluding and discluding the teeth may demonstrate movement. The use of articulating paper may help assessment if the discrepancy is small.

Investigation usually includes study models and plain radiographs. CT scans may occasionally help, particularly in the assessment of condylar injuries.

Dental study models are necessary to assess whether segmental surgery or whole-jaw surgery should be undertaken. If the pretraumatic occlusion is obtainable with the existing arch form, then one-piece jaw surgery is indicated. If an acceptable occlusion is not obtainable, there may be a malunited segmental fracture or a degree of dentoalveolar compensatory change secondary to the altered occlusion and jaw position. In this situation, one-piece jaw surgery alone will not establish the pretraumatic occlusion, and adjunctive treatment is necessary. If the occlusal discrepancy is slight, selective occlusal grinding may allow a reasonable seating of the occlusion. If this is considered undesirable or will not achieve a satisfactory occlusion, then orthodontic treatment may be considered. However, a number of cases are unsuitable for orthodontics due to lack of anchorage, poor oral hygiene or dental condition, or lack of sufficient motivation. If orthodontics is precluded for any of these reasons, occlusal rehabilitation by restorative techniques may be considered, but this may also be limited by existing dental condition, oral hygiene, or patient motivation. In this situation, segmental surgery may be the only viable option.

Face bow recording and anatomical articulation provide information that is useful in planning treatment for correction of an anterior open bite. They allow accurate assessment of the degree of posterior maxillary impaction required and an approximate assessment of the degree of mandibular autorotation. This is helpful in planning the need for mandibular osteotomy to correct AP jaw relationships.

Plain radiographs, particularly the orthopantomogram (OPG) and lateral cephalogram, demonstrate fibrous union, gross segment displacement, and the site of previously inserted metalwork; if orthognathic techniques are being used, they also provide a basis for orthognathic workup.

Treatment Planning

It is important to consider the need for multidisciplinary involvement before treatment is undertaken. This may involve an orthodontist and occasionally a restorative dental surgeon, because some occlusal discrepancies are amenable to occlusal adjustment, restorative treatment, or orthodontics. As mentioned previously, other patients may require a joint orthodontic and surgical approach using standard orthognathic techniques, particularly if a preexisting malocclusion or dental crowding existed or if sufficient time has elapsed since the injury to allow some compensatory dentoalveolar changes to occur. On occasions the amount of movement required at osteotomy is relatively small, resulting in only a small acceptable margin of error in jaw and segment positioning at surgery. If positioning errors occur, elastic traction may be adequate for correction in the early postoperative phase, but if this proves inadequate, an assessment of the feasibility of orthodontic or restorative solutions is useful.

The detailed surgical movements are dictated by the establishment of an acceptable dental occlusion. Intraoperative occlusal wafers to assist accurate jaw and segment positioning are essential. Preformed arch bars facilitate intraoperative intermaxillary fixation. If significant edentulous areas exist, especially posteriorly, acrylic saddles should be incorporated within the arch bars to facilitate jaw positioning, and they should be left in situ postoperatively to improve jaw stability and prevent loss of posterior ramus height in the early postoperative period.

Osteotomies

Maxilla

Indications To correct occlusal abnormalities caused by maxillary malunion, Le Fort I osteotomy is indicated. Osteotomy at the Le Fort II or III level, or variations of these procedures tailored to the individual needs of the patient, may be required in some instances if simultaneous correction of midface deformity is necessary. However, primary treatment by ORIF and primary bone grafting have substantially reduced the need for more extensive maxillary osteotomies in the treatment of secondary posttraumatic deformity. Le Fort I osteotomy is therefore indicated for most cases of maxillary occlusal abnormality when segmental or one-piece maxillary repositioning is necessary. In addition, maxillary osteotomy may be required to close an anterior open bite after bilateral condylar malunion.

Operative Technique A standard Le Fort I down-fracture is carried out via a horseshoe-shaped buccal sulcus incision. Bone cuts of the lateral maxillary wall, zygomatic buttress, lateral nasal walls, pterygomaxillary junction, and nasal septum are carried out in a manner similar to standard orthognathic surgery. After down-fracture, the maxilla is mobilized, and, if indicated, segmentation of the maxilla can be carried out from the nasal aspect by making a horseshoe-shaped cut in the bony palate and extending it radially between the roots of the teeth either side of the site of the desired segmental cut. After segmentation, an acrylic palate retained with Adams cribs helps to control the segments, and temporary intermaxillary fixation is applied with the use of a prefabricated occlusal wafer to establish the desired position of the maxilla relative to the mandible. Any areas that cause interference with establishment of the desired position of the maxilla are removed. This is particularly important in the nasal septum to avoid postoperative septal deviation and at the posterior maxilla in cases of maxillary impaction. The maxilla is then fixed with miniplates at the piriform apertures and zygomatic buttresses.

Once the maxilla is fixed, the intermaxillary fixation is removed to check the newly established dental occlusion. This must be exactly as planned and must be achievable by gentle upward pressure on the chin point, ensuring that no distraction of the mandibular condyles out of the glenoid fossae has occurred. If distraction happens, an anterior open bite will be detectable after removal of the intraoperative intermaxillary fixation, or certainly in the early postoperative period. If on careful checking of the occlusion, any discrepancy, in particular anterior open bite, is detected, then the occlusal wafer and intermaxillary fixation must be reapplied and the maxilla repositioned and replated, after removal of any persistent bony interferences, especially in the region of the maxillary tuberosity and pterygoid plates.

Once the correct maxillary position is established, any significant bony gaps or deficiencies are bone grafted. This is particularly important at the piriform and zygomatic buttresses and at the anterior maxillary wall. These ensure union, stability, and support for the overlying soft tissues of the cheek. However, the use of bone grafts in Le Fort I osteotomies to correct posttraumatic occlusion is uncommon because of the relatively small movements involved.

If segmental surgery is necessary to reposition a dentoalveolar segment only, it is best carried out by means of a full Le Fort I down-fracture in the manner described earlier. This approach facilitates access for bone cuts, particularly in the palate, and removal of bony interferences between segments. Care must be taken to avoid injury to the dental roots adjacent to the segmental bone cut, especially if preoperative orthodontic treatment has not been carried out. If palatal expansion is carried out, then bone graft may be placed in the palatal osteotomy gaps to improve transverse stability.[1] Previously described local segmental maxillary osteotomies have largely been superseded by the Le Fort I down-fracture technique.

Outcome There is very little literature devoted to the outcome of maxillary osteotomies, either one-piece or segmental procedures, for the correction of posttraumatic deformity. Stability after osteotomies for posttraumatic deformity depends to an extent on the nature of the original injury, its treatment and subsequent secondary procedures, and the presence of soft tissue scarring, which is likely to increase relapsing forces, a phenomenon well known in cleft osteotomy. Cohen and Kawamoto[1] reported the results of 25 patients with severe posttraumatic facial deformities, including 10 Le Fort I osteotomies. Although they presented no detailed analysis of long-term outcome, they took the view that malocclusion after secondary correction should be rare. However, any adult nonorthodontic, orthognathic surgery demands meticulous technique and accurate positioning of segments.

Mandible

Patients presenting with malocclusion after mandibular injuries have nonunion, fibrous union, or malunion.

Nonunion and Fibrous Union Nonunion and fibrous union may occur after fracture of any part of the mandible but most commonly affects fractures of the mandibular angle.[36] In a study of 1432 mandibular fractures, Mathog et al.[37] found a 2.8% incidence of nonunion. They reported an increased incidence in male patients, in fractures affecting the body of the mandible, and in patients with multiple fractures. Inadequate stabilization or reduction and osteomyelitis were found to be common. Other contributory factors included lack of prophylactic antibiotics, delay in treatment, presence of teeth in the line of the fracture, alcohol and drug abuse, an inexperienced surgeon, and lack of patient compliance.[37] Moreno et al[38] found that the rates of overall complications, postoperative infection, and postoperative malocclusion were significantly correlated with the severity of the original fracture. Similar risk factors were identified by Haug and Schwimmer.[39]

Treatment Treatment requires débridement of the fracture site and eradication of infection, with accurate reduction and fixation. In the absence of significant bone deficit, this treatment should result in successful union. Because infected nonunions manifest with a mandibular continuity gap, temporary fixation of fragments is desirable to allow resolution of infection before bone grafting. If there is intact overlying mucoperiosteum, this may be achieved by rigid internal fixation. However, in long-standing severe cases, the quality and availability of mucosal cover for the fracture may be poor. If internal fixation is used in these cases, dehiscence of the intraoral wound may occur with resultant plate exposure. In this situation, immobilization is best achieved by use of an external fixator (Fig. 24-19). Once infection is eradicated and mucosal healing has occurred, cancellous or corticocancellous bone graft and internal fixation in the form of mesh or plates is carried out, usually via an extraoral approach to avoid contamination of the bone graft by intraoral bacteria.

Operative Technique The fracture site is approached by a standard intraoral or extraoral incision. The fracture is mobilized, bone ends are cut back to healthy bleeding bone, and segments are repositioned with the aid of temporary intraoperative intermaxillary fixation and use of an occlusal wafer for accurate location of the teeth. If little or no bone gap is present, bone grafts may be unnecessary, but in most cases cancellous or corticocancellous bone harvested from the iliac crest restores mandibular continuity defects and ensures bony union.

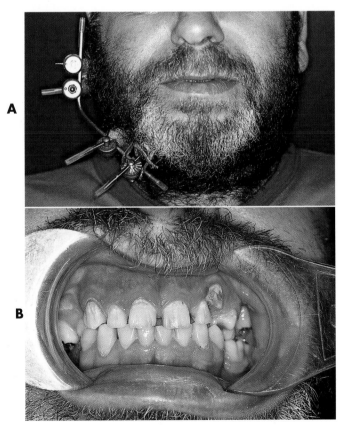

FIGURE 24-19 Infected nonunion of fractured mandible. **A,** External fixator in place. **B,** Maintenance of occlusion with fixator.

Outcome Outcome is usually good, although sensory loss in the region of the inferior dental nerve is common due to inevitable scarring and damage as a result of the original injury, primary treatment, and secondary bone grafting.

Malunion Malunion may occur in the horizontal or vertical ramus of the mandible.

Horizontal Ramus Malunion of a fracture of the horizontal ramus usually requires direct osteotomy to re-create the fracture, mobilization and repositioning of the segments, and placement of internal fixation. The expectation is for an excellent outcome.

Angle, Vertical Ramus, and Condylar Fractures
Background Malunion of fractures behind the tooth-bearing segment of the mandible results in displacement of the whole dentoalveolar arch. Uncomplicated angle and ramus fractures rarely result in malunion because they are amenable to ORIF. However, mandibular condyle fractures are often treated nonsurgically by closed methods of reduction, intermaxillary fixation, and elastic traction. Displacement of the mandible and resulting malocclusion may occur for a variety of reasons. Severe condylar malposition with dislocation allows vertical shortening of the ascending ramus, and this may be associated with restricted mouth opening or deviation on opening due to mechanical disruption of the TMJ.

The functional status of the TMJ is an important factor in the choice of technique adopted for correction of the occlusal deformity. If TMJ function is significantly compromised, reduction of the dislocation may be necessary, along with disc repositioning. If TMJ function is acceptable, ramus osteotomy is indicated to avoid joint surgery and the possibility of surgically induced limitation of mouth opening. Vertical ramus shortening may also occur after angular displacement of the condylar neck without dislocation if telescoping of the proximal and distal fragments occurs, particularly if the molar teeth are absent and there is lack of posterior occlusal support. It may also be seen after condylar resorption.[39]

In unilateral condylar fractures, malunion results in shortening of the ipsilateral ramus height, transverse cant of the lower occlusal plane, gagging of the occlusion on the ipsilateral posterior molars, and contralateral open bite. In addition, there may be posterior displacement of the ipsilateral mandible resulting in obvious chinpoint asymmetry, as well as crossbite or scissors bite. If bilateral malunion occurs, both ascending rami shorten; this causes an increase in the mandibular and lower occlusal plane angle, bilateral occlusal gagging on the posterior molars, anterior open bite with a class II jaw relationship, and, if severe, lip incompetence (Fig. 24-20).

Unilateral Treatment The aim of treatment in unilateral cases is to restore the pretraumatic ramus height and rectify any posterior mandibular displacement. This corrects the occlusal plane cant and restores a normal occlusion. These aims can be achieved by performing an osteotomy at the site of the original fracture, with repositioning and, if necessary, interpositional bone grafting to maintain the lengthening of the ramus, or by a ramus osteotomy distant from the fracture site, such as a vertical subsigmoid, inverted L, or sagittal split osteotomy. Direct fracture line osteotomy is appropriate if the

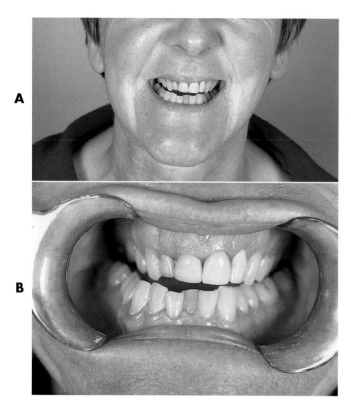

FIGURE 24-20 Bilateral condylar malunion. **A,** Obvious chinpoint asymmetry. **B,** Occlusal derangement with open bite.

fracture site involves the angle or ascending ramus. However, if the fracture involves the condylar neck, direct osteotomy and grafting can be difficult and carry significant risk of postoperative trismus or ankylosis. In this situation, vertical subsigmoid osteotomy, inverted L, or sagittal split osteotomy is indicated provided TMJ function is adequate. If TMJ function is compromised, reduction of the condylar fragment and disc repositioning may be necessary despite the surgical difficulty and risk of surgically induced restriction of mouth opening postoperatively.

If TMJ surgery or condylar reduction is not necessary, the particular type of osteotomy chosen is governed by the direction and extent of displacement. Rubens et al.[40] recommended that, when horizontal movement is the primary goal, sagittal split osteotomy is appropriate. If vertical correction is required, they recommended use of an intraoral or extraoral ramus osteotomy. However, they pointed out that other factors, such as facial scarring, ease of condylar segment manipulation, and available bone, also influence the approach selected.

Bilateral Treatment Bilateral condylar malunion usually results in an anterior open bite and class II jaw relationship. This is best treated in the same way as a developmental high-angle class II anterior open bite, using standard orthognathic and, if necessary, orthodontic techniques. This approach effectively accepts the reduced ramus height and therefore a reduced posterior face height. The correction is achieved by adjusting the maxilla to accommodate this reduced posterior face height by carrying out a posterior maxillary impaction. This results in an increase in the occlusal plane angle, but this

is of little significance and results in a stable correction of the anterior open bite component of the deformity as a consequence of mandibular autorotation. Mandibular autorotation also produces a degree of anterior mandibular projection, and this may be sufficient to correct the mild class II skeletal relationship. The degree of anterior projection resulting from autorotation may be assessed preoperatively by surgical simulation using an anatomical articulator. If autorotation is insufficient to correct the AP discrepancy, bilateral sagittal split mandibular advancement is indicated. As in orthognathic cases, the addition of advancement genioplasty in some patients may enhance the esthetic result and improve lip competence where needed.

Unilateral Operative Technique Access is gained via a posterior intraoral buccal sulcus incision or a submandibular, retromandibular (Fig. 24-21B), or preauricular extraoral incisions. Depending on the technique chosen, the old fracture line is osteotomized or a ramus osteotomy is carried out distant from the fracture site (see Fig. 24-21C). Once this has been done, temporary, intraoperative intermaxillary fixation with an occlusal wafer is applied (see Fig. 24-21D).

Next, posterior and upward traction is applied to the proximal fragment to keep the condyle in its retruded position. The condyle may be located outside the confines of the glenoid fossa if it is dislocated. In this situation, intraoperative judgment of the correct condylar position is a little more difficult, but the surgeon should err on the side of overcorrection if doubt exists. Seating of the condyle reveals the extent of the ramus height deficit. If direct fracture osteotomy or an inverted L osteotomy has been carried out, a suitably sized bone graft is inserted into the osteotomy gap and internal fixation is applied. If a vertical ramus osteotomy or sagittal split has been carried out, no bone graft is necessary and fixation is applied after repositioning of the proximal segment (see Fig. 24-21E).

In some cases of unilateral injury, a contralateral sagittal split osteotomy may be required to achieve the preplanned occlusion. This can be assessed preoperatively with the use of an anatomical articulator and intraoperatively when the occlusion can be assessed after osteotomy on the injured side. If a satisfactory occlusion is achieved, contralateral osteotomy may be unnecessary. If satisfactory occlusion cannot be achieved, contralateral osteotomy must be carried out (Fig. 24-22).

Bilateral Operative Technique Posterior maxillary impaction, mandibular autorotation, and advancement are well described in the orthognathic literature. The use of these techniques in a posttraumatic situation usually demands little or no modification (Fig. 24-23).

Outcome The techniques described are effective in correcting the esthetic and functional problems associated with posttraumatic malocclusion. In a study of 21 patients, Becking et al.[41] reported stable dental and cephalometric results in 20 patients. Similarly, Spitzer et al.[42] reported occlusal correction and normal mandibular movement in a group of 14 patients. Rubens et al.[40] presented four cases with successful outcome, including correction of occlusion and resolution of TMJ and muscle pain.

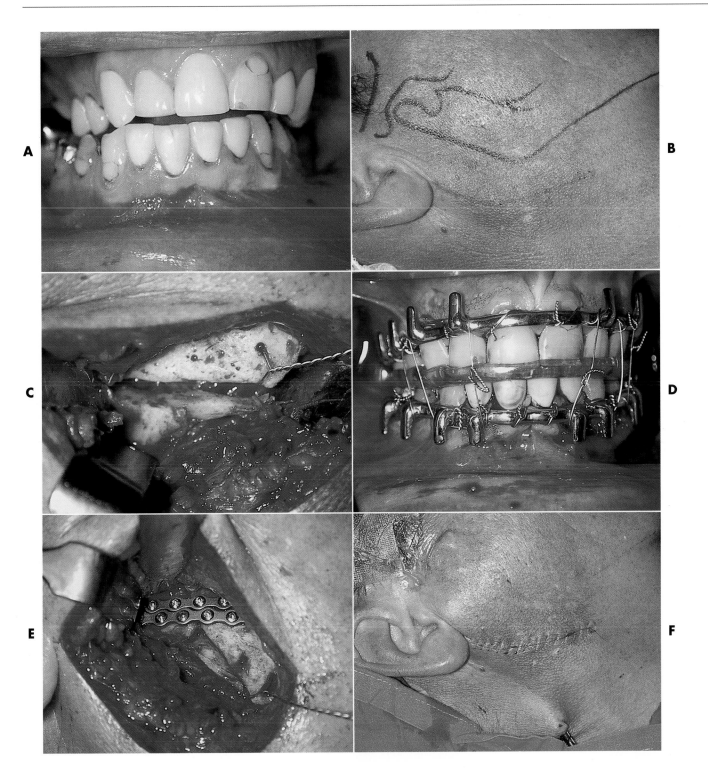

FIGURE 24-21 Vertical ramus osteotomy to correct posttraumatic malocclusion. **A,** Preoperative malocclusion. **B,** Retromandibular incision marked. **C,** Vertical ramus osteotomy performed. **D,** Temporary intermaxillary fixation with occlusal wafer. **E,** Fixation of osteotomy. **F,** Wound closure.

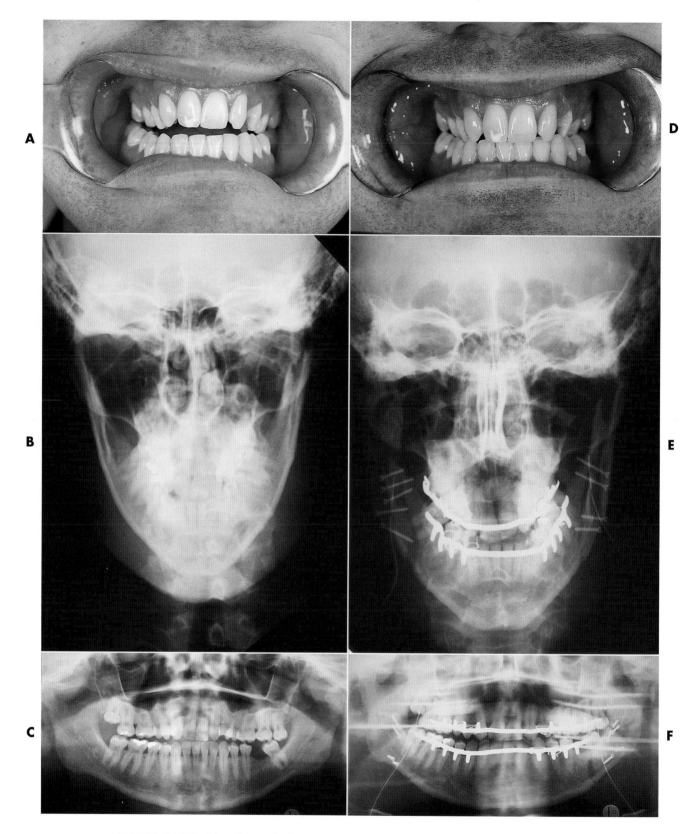

FIGURE 24-22   Bilateral sagittal split osteotomy to correct postoperative malocclusion. **A,** Preoperative malocclusion due to unilateral condylar fracture. **B,** Preoperative cephalogram. **C,** Preoperative orthopantomogram (OPG). **D,** Postoperative occlusion after osteotomy. **E,** Postoperative posteroanterior cephalogram. **F,** Postoperative OPG.

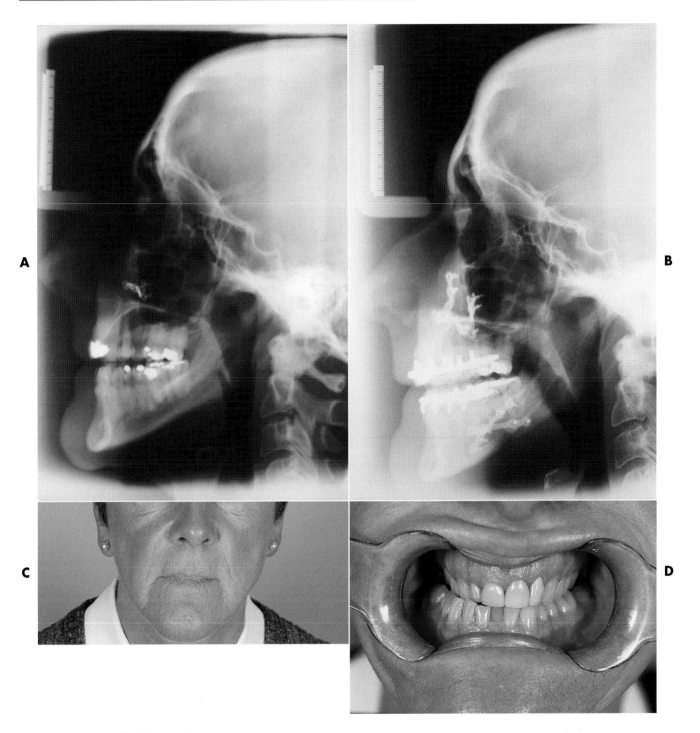

FIGURE 24-23 Bimaxillary osteotomy to treat anterior open bite and mandibular asymmetry after bilateral condylar fracture. See Figure 24-20 for the preoperative clinical appearance. **A** and **B,** Preoperative and postoperative lateral cephalograms. **C** and **D,** Postoperative facial appearance and occlusion.

TRAUMATIC TISSUE LOSS

Severe posttraumatic tissue loss is uncommon in civilian practice. It may occasionally be encountered after gunshot wounds, high-speed road traffic accidents, or industrial accidents. Often, there is a combination of hard and soft tissue loss demanding a variety of primary and secondary reconstructive techniques with multiple operations to restore lost form and function. Initial management usually follows the traditional principles of trauma management, and subsequent correction may involve pedicle or free tissue transfer to replace hard and soft tissue. The recent development of osteogenic distraction in the craniofacial skeleton provides another option for replacement of bony deficits along with their closely associated soft tissues. Each case is different and must be planned and treated on its own merits, but Figure 24-24 shows a case that illustrates many of the principles and problems involved.

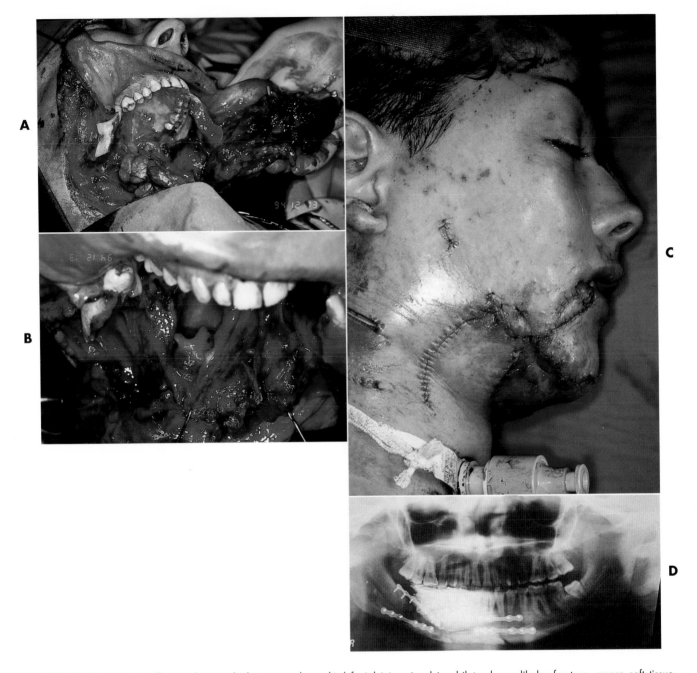

FIGURE 24-24   Road traffic accident resulted in severe lower-third facial injury involving bilateral mandibular fracture, severe soft tissue disruption, and complete traumatic glossectomy. **A** and **B,** Appearance on presentation. **C,** Tracheotomy, plating of fracture, and soft tissue repair; the defect in the floor of the mouth is dressed with Whitehead varnish pack. **D,** Orthopantomogram (OPG) shows mandibular fixation.

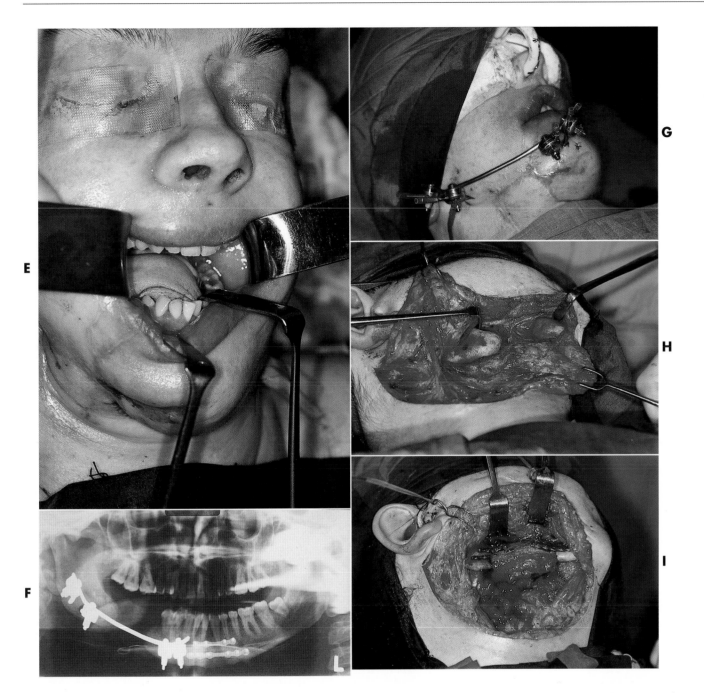

FIGURE 24-24, cont'd **E,** Radial forearm free flap to repair the floor of the mouth and the tongue defect. **F** and **G,** Avascular necrosis of right mandibular body treated by removal of fixation, débridement, and application of external fixator. **H,** Mandibular defect after nonunion. **I,** Reconstruction with deep circumflex iliac artery (DCIA) free vascularized bone flap.

Continued

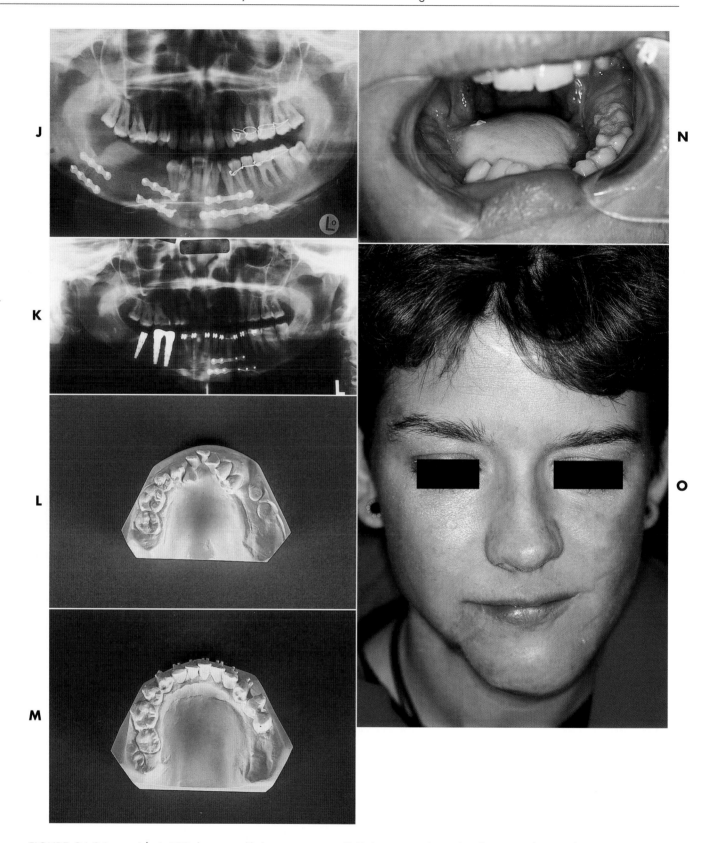

FIGURE 24-24, cont'd   **J,** OPG shows mandibular reconstruction. **K,** Endosseous implants placed into DCIA bone graft. **L,** Lingual movement of lower incisors due to lip pressure after loss of tongue. **M,** Appearance after orthodontic treatment using implants as anchorage. **N,** Intraoral appearance of radial forearm flap. **O,** Facial appearance at commencement of orthodontic treatment.

REFERENCES

1. Cohen SR, Kawamoto HK: Analysis and results of treatment of established post traumatic facial deformities. *Plast Reconstr Surg* 90:574-584, 1992.

2. Tessier P: Total osteotomy of the middle third of the face for faciostenosis or for sequelae of Le Fort III fractures. *Plast Reconstr Surg* 48:533-541, 1971.

3. Manson PN: Facial injuries. In McCarthy JG, editor: *Plastic surgery*, Philadelphia, 1990, Saunders, pp 867-1141.

4. Gruss JS: Fronto-naso-orbital trauma. *Clin Plast Surg* 9:557-589, 1982.

5. Schendel SA, Lewis W, Williamson DDS: Muscle reorientation following superior repositioning of the maxilla. *J Oral Maxillofac Surg* 41:235-240, 1983.

6. Shvykov MB, Shamsudinov AK, Sunarckov DD, et al: Non-free osteoplasty of the mandible in maxillofacial gunshot wounds: reconstruction by compression-osteodistraction. *Br J Oral Maxillofac Surg* 37:261-267, 1999.

7. McCarthy J, Zide BM: The spectrum of calvarial bone grafting: introduction of the vascularised calvarial bone flap. *Plast Reconstr Surg* 74:10-18, 1984.

8. Berggren A, Weiland AJ, Dorfman M: Free vascularized bone grafts: factors affecting their survival and ability to lead recipient bone defects. *Plast Reconstr Surg* 69:19-29, 1982.

9. Paskest JP, Yaremchuk MJ, Randolph MA, et al: Prolonging survival in vascularised bone allograft transplantation: developing specific immune unresponsiveness. *J Reconstr Microsurg* 3:254, 1987.

10. Zins JE, Whitaker LA: Membranous versus endochondral bone autografts: implications for craniofacial reconstruction. *Plast Reconstr Surg* 72:778-785, 1983.

11. Yaremchuk MJ: Vascularised bone grafts for maxillofacial reconstruction. *Clin Plast Surg* 16:29-39, 1989.

12. McCarthy JG, Cutting CC, Shaw WW: Vascularised calvarial flap. *Clin Plast Surg* 14:37-47, 1987.

13. Zalzal GH, Cotton RT, McAdams AJ: Cartilage grafts: present status. *Head Neck Surg* 8:363-374, 1986.

14. Yen CP, Cheung CM, Loh JK, et al: Growing skull fracture. *Kaohsiung J Med Sci* 15:175-181, 1999.

15. Colak A, Akbasak A, Biliciler B, et al: An unusual variant of a growing skull fracture in an adolescent. *Paediatr Neurosurg* 29:36-39, 1998.

16. Gupta SK, Reddy NM, Khosla VK, et al: Growing skull fractures: a clinical study of 41 patients. *Acta Neurochir* 139:928-932, 1997.

17. Sener RN: Growing skull fracture in a patient with cerebral hemiatrophy. *Paediatr Radiol* 25:64-65, 1995.

18. Scarfo GB, Mariottini A, Tomaccini D, et al: Growing skull fractures. *Childs Nerv Syst* 5:163-167, 1989.

19. Hunter PD, Pelofsky S: Classification of autogenous skull grafts in cranial reconstruction. *J Craniomaxillofac Trauma* 1:8-15, 1995.

20. Hunter D, Baker S, Sobol SM: Split calvarial grafts in maxillofacial reconstruction. *Otolaryngol Head Neck Surg* 102:345-350, 1990.

21. Posnick JC, Goldstein JA, Armstong D, et al: Reconstruction of skull defects in children and adolescents by the use of fixed cranial bone grafts: long-term results. *Neurosurgery* 32:785-791, discussion 791, 1993.

22. Pezzota S, Silvani V, Gaetani P, et al: Growing skull fractures of childhood. *J Neurosurg Sci* 29:129-135, 1985.

23. Ionnides CH, Freihofer HP, Friens J: Fractures of the frontal sinus: a rationale of treatment. *Br J Plast Surg* 46:208-214, 1993.

24. Luce EA: Frontal sinus fractures: guidelines to management. *Plast Reconstr Surg* 80:500-510, 1987.

25. Gonty AA, Marciani RD, Adornato DC: Management of frontal sinus fractures: a review of 33 cases. *J Oral Maxillofac Surg* 57:372-379, discussion 380-381, 1999.

26. Penfold CN, Lang DD, Evans B: The management of orbital roof fractures. *Br J Oral Maxillofac Surg* 30:97-103, 1992.

27. Horowitz JH, Persing JA, Winn HR, et al: The late treatment of vertical orbital dystopia resulting from an orbital roof fracture. *Ann Plast Surg* 13:519-524, 1984.

28. Hammer B, Prein J: Correction of post traumatic orbital deformities: operative techniques and review of 26 patients. *J Craniomaxillofac Surg* 23:81-90, 1995.

29. Barone CM, Gigantelli JW: Endoscopic repair of posttraumatic enophthalmos using medial transconjunctival approach: a case report. *J Craniomaxillofac Trauma* 4:22-26, 1998.

30. Watzinger F, Wanschitz F, Wagner A, et al: Computer-aided navigation in secondary reconstruction of post traumatic deformities of the zygoma. *J Craniomaxillofac Surg* 25:198-202, 1997.

31. Jones RH, Ching M: Intraoral zygomatic osteotomy for correction of malar deficiency. *J Oral Maxillofac Surg* 53:483-485, 1995.

32. Frodel JL, Marentette LJ, Quatela VC, et al: Calvarial bone graft harvest: techniques, considerations and morbidity. *Arch Otolaryngol Head Neck Surg* 119:17-23, 1993.

33. Freihofer PM, Borstlap WA: Reconstruction of zygomatic area: a comparison between osteotomy and onlay techniques. *J Craniomaxillofac Surg* 17:243-248, 1989.

34. Perino KE, Zide MF, Kinnebrew MC: Late treatment of malunited malar fractures. *J Oral Maxillofac Surg* 42:20-34, 1984.

35. Hans PM, Freihofer P: Effectiveness of secondary post-traumatic periorbital reconstruction. *J Oral Maxillofac Surg* 23:143-150, 1995.

36. Ellis E 3rd: Treatment methods for fractures of the mandibular angle. *Int J Oral Maxillofac Surg* 28:243-252, 1999.

37. Mathog RH, Toma V, Clayman L, et al: Nonunion of the mandible: an analysis of contributing factors. *J Oral Maxillofac Surg* 58:746-752, discussion 752-753, 2000.

38. Moreno JC, Fernadez A, Ortiz JA, et al: Complication rates associated with different treatment for mandibular fractures. *J Oral Maxillofac Surg* 58:273-280, discussion 280-281, 2000.

39. Haug RH, Schwimmer A: Fibrous union of the mandible: a review of 27 patients. *J Oral Maxillofac Surg* 52:832-839, 1994.

40. Rubens BC, Stoelinga PJW, Weaver TJ, et al: Management of malunited mandibular condylar fractures. *Int J Oral Maxillofac Surg* 19:22-25, 1990.

41. Becking AG, Zijerveld SA, Tuinzing DB: Management of post traumatic malocclusion caused by condylar process source. *J Oral Maxillofac Surg* 56:1370-1374, discussion 1374-1375, 1998.

42. Spitzer WJ, Vanderborght G, Dumbach J: Surgical management of mandibular malposition after malunited condylar fractures in adults. *J Craniomaxillofac Surg* 25:91-96, 1997.

CHAPTER 25

Facial Distraction Techniques

Alexander C. Kübler, Joachim E. Zöller

HISTORY OF DISTRACTION

The first clinical application of bone distraction was described in 1905 by Codivilla, who performed a bone distraction of the lower leg.[1] The distractor was fixed with plaster at the upper and lower leg, providing only minor stability, and severe soft tissue problems such as necrosis occurred. Various experimental studies followed regarding the rate and distance of distraction and the effects of the periosteum and soft tissue on the distraction process. In 1927, Rosenthal reported the first distraction of the mandible.[2] He treated a patient with a mandibular retrognathism by bone distraction and fixation of the distractor along the teeth. In 1952, Anderson used cortical bone pins for the fixation of the distractor, as described by Coleman et al. in 1967.[3] This was a milestone in the technique of bone distraction because it enabled rigid fixation of the bone fragments.

The real father of bone distraction was a Russian orthopedic surgeon named Ilizarov, who popularized the technique more than 30 years before it became recognized in the West. In the late 1980s, he published in the United States for the first time his research and clinical results on bone distraction, prompting a wave of developments in bone distraction techniques worldwide.[4]

PRINCIPLE OF BONE DISTRACTION

The aim of bone distraction is to obtain new bone tissue and gain bone length by slow distraction of the callus. The basic principle of bone distraction is the process of bone fracture healing. Osteotomy can be performed by two methods. In the original method, as described by Ilizarov, a corticotomy is performed in which only the cortex of the bone is separated and the cancellus stays untouched. Another method, which is more often used in head and neck surgery, is to split the cortex and the cancellus of the bone to facilitate the process of distraction. With this technique, the forces needed to distract the bone are significantly lower, allowing use of smaller distractors that can be placed under the skin or the mucosa.

After the osteotomy and a latent period of 5 to 7 days, the bones on both sides of the osteotomy line are slowly pulled apart to stretch the fracture cleft and the newly formed callus.[5,6] A latent period between the osteotomy and the start of the distraction process allows callus formation and soft tissue healing. Higher activity of the osteoblasts and blood vessel growth within the osteotomy line and the callus can be achieved.[7] Various experimental and clinical studies have reported a latent period ranging from 0 to 14 days between the osteotomy and the start of the distraction, depending on the individual situation.[7] In the field of head and neck surgery, an average waiting period of 5 to 7 days is advisable. However, patient age, bone size, and soft tissue coverage may influence the latent period.

Distraction must take place slowly to achieve new bone formation within the callus. An average distraction rate of 1 to 1.5 mm/day provides the best clinical results.[6] At a lower rate of 0.5 mm/day or less, early ossification takes place, whereas at a higher rate of 2 mm/day or more, no bone formation occurs.[8] Another important fact is the frequency of distraction. The ideal situation is a continuous distraction of callus,[6] but because this is difficult, repeated distraction once or twice each day (1-1.5 mm/day total) seems to be useful.

Numerous experimental and clinical studies have investigated the effects of bone distraction and the progress of bone formation during distraction. It has been shown that the gap between the distracted bone edges is first occupied by fibrous tissue.[9] As distraction proceeds, the fibrous tissue becomes longitudinally oriented in the direction of distraction. Early bone formation starts from the cut bone edges and advances along the fibrous tissue. Bone is formed predominantly by intermembranous ossification.[10,11] Histological observations showed a gradual change from an amorphous matrix to a fibrous matrix and then to an osseous-like tissue.[10] Bone columns crystallize along longitudinally oriented collagen bundles, expanding circumferentially to surrounding bundles.[11] While the distraction gap increases, the bone columns increase in length and diameter, whereas the fibrous interzone remains constant at a few millimeters.[6] Clinical and animal experimental data have shown that distraction osteogenesis provides unlimited new bone formation that remodels at a daily rate ranging from 200 to 400 μm.[8,11] Most of the experimental data were obtained from orthopedic studies, and only limited information about the indications for maxillofacial surgery is available.

Various methods have been described for fixation of the distractor.[12] The easiest method of fixation is to use bone pins that are placed in the bone near the osteotomy line and through the skin. The pins are fixed externally to the distractor, which can be slowly expanded. The external distractors are easy to fix and very stable, but most of them are rather bulky, and the transcutaneous pins can cause scars.[11] These factors encouraged the development of smaller devices that can be placed intraorally. Today, minidistractors and microdistractors are currently used; they are small enough to be placed completely subcutaneously or under the mucosa. Only the screw for the activator of the distractor is visible.

Another distractor for the midface is the halo frame.[13] The frame is fixed at the skull by screws and attached to the midface.

An important aspect of all distractors is their stability and stiffness. Experimental studies have shown that mobility during the process of distraction can cause micromovements, resulting in impaired bone formation.[8] Distractor size is therefore limited by physical stability and rigidity.

After reaching the intended bone length, the distractor (or plate fixation) must stay in place for many weeks until mineralization and ossification of the newly formed callus has been completed and sufficient bone strength has been attained.[14] The length of this period depends on individual factors such as the location of the osteotomy, the bone length gained, and the age of the patient.[15,16] A retention period of 8 to 12 weeks seems to be sufficient for the facial skeleton. Some surgeons remove the distractor and use plates to provide stabilization for the consolidation period.

followed by bone distraction until the intended occlusion is reached.[18,19] With osteotomies of the cortex alone, the risk of nerve injury is less likely. This approach also may have a role in cases of severe trauma.

Other indications include congenital, traumatic, or infection-induced hypoplasia of the mandible in young children (Figs. 25-1 through 25-3) if functional orthopedics does not work and the airway is impaired. With distraction of the mandible, the space for soft tissues such as the tongue and the floor of the mouth increases, improving airflow.[20] This application can avoid a permanent tracheotomy, and it can be used from the age of 6 months, when ossification of the mandible allows fixation of the distractor.

The part of the mandible that must be distracted depends on the location of the bone growth deficit.[21] Because some distractors have only one vector of distraction, the bone must be advanced in one direction, and the position of the distractor is critical for the final clinical result. The placement of the distractor parallel to the occlusal plane results in horizontal mandibular advancement. If the distractor is placed at an angle to the occlusion plane, the results are mandibular advancement and a tendency for an open bite. A distractor set vertically in relation to the occlusion plane produces malocclusion of the molars. The position and angle between the distractor and the occlusal plane must be determined carefully preoperatively by a cephalometric analysis or model surgery, or both. In some cases, bilateral osteotomy and distraction may be necessary.

Timetable for Bone Distraction

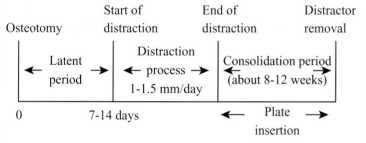

INDICATIONS AND TECHNIQUES FOR BONE DISTRACTION

Congenital malformations of the mandible originally were the most common indications for distraction. McCarthy et al. first described the use of a miniaturized distractor as an extraoral device to lengthen the malformed mandible.[17] Soon, smaller distractors were developed that were placed completely intraorally to avoid scars and hide the distractors. Currently, distraction of the mandible can be classified as distraction of the horizontal mandible ramus, the vertical mandible ramus, the mandible symphysis, or the alveolus.

HORIZONTAL OR VERTICAL DISTRACTION OF THE RAMUS OR ANGLE OF THE MANDIBLE

Malformations of ramus growth horizontally or vertically are the most common indications for distraction in the field of head and neck surgery. In less severe orthognathic surgery cases, a unilateral or bilateral sagittal split can be performed,

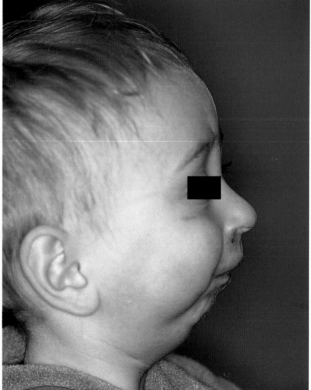

FIGURE 25-1 A 2-year-old boy with infection-induced hypoplasia (osteomyelitis) of the mandible and severe breathing problems before distraction of the mandible.

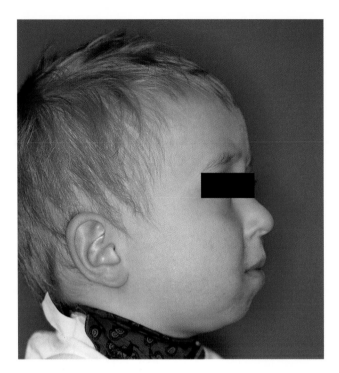

FIGURE 25-2   Same patient as in Figure 25-1. Three months after distraction of the mandible on both sides near the mandibular angle for about 15 mm, the breathing problems had disappeared completely.

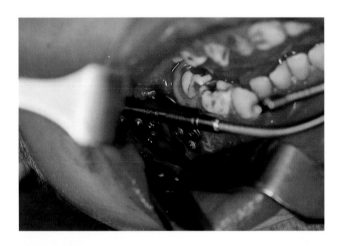

FIGURE 25-3   Same patient as in Figure 25-1. Intraoperative view at the osteotomy line and placement of the distractor near the mandibular angle on one side.

The operation is usually performed with the patient under general anesthesia. After local disinfection and injection of a vasoconstrictor, the mucosa is opened, and the mandible is exposed subperiosteally. The distractor is placed at the intended position and fixed temporarily with two monocortical screws. The osteotomy line is marked on the buccal side of the mandible using a drill. The distractor and the screws are removed, and the osteotomy is performed. The lingual side of the osteotomy is performed carefully to prevent exposure of the lingual periosteum, which is important for the blood supply. The bone is mobilized, and the distractor is fixed using the holes drilled earlier and the remaining screws.

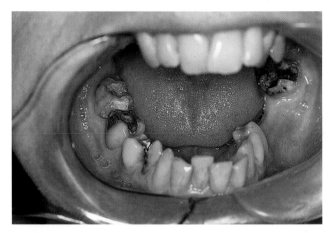

FIGURE 25-4   A 40-year-old patient with a narrow mandible before distraction.

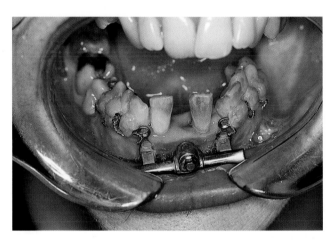

FIGURE 25-5   Same patient as in Figure 25-4. One week after initiation of the distraction process, separation of the incisors becomes obvious.

The soft tissue is closed so that the thread of the distractor is visible and can easily be reached by the patient. After a waiting period of about 5 to 7 days, distraction can be started at a rate of 0.5 mm twice daily until the intended mandible length is obtained.

The retention period lasts about 12 weeks before the distractor can be removed under local or general anesthesia. Some surgeons replace the distractor with plates to complement the consolidation period.

DISTRACTION OF THE MANDIBULAR SYMPHYSIS

In patients with a congenital or trauma-induced narrow mandible (e.g., after mandible fracture), surgical widening may be necessary (Figs. 25-4 through 25-6). Vertical osteotomy of the mandible between the incisors followed by horizontal distraction results in a significant increase in width. Because of the principle of distraction, the condyles are rotated, but this causes no permanent problems.

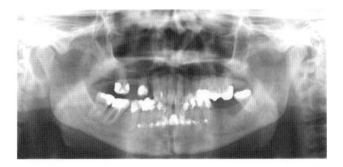

FIGURE 25-6 Same patient as in Figure 25-4. Radiograph obtained during distraction.

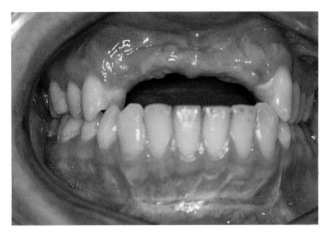

FIGURE 25-7 A 25-year-old patient with traumatic loss of the upper incisors and a significant lack of vertical height of the alveolar ridge before therapy.

With the patient under general anesthesia, the vestibular mucosa between the canines is opened and the mandible is exposed. The distractor is temporarily placed using two monocortical screws. The upper arms of the distractor must be placed anterior to the teeth. Only the lower arms of the distractor are fixed at the bone with monocortical screws. The osteotomy line is marked with the use of a drill, and the distractor is removed. Thereafter, the mandible is separated between the two first incisors. The lingual periosteum is not exposed because the depth of the cut can be felt with the finger. After mobilization of the fragments, the distractor is fixed with the use of screws for the lower arms. The upper arms of the distractor are fixed at the teeth with wires or dental composite.

Dental anchorage of the upper arms of the distractor is important to avoid twisting of the segments; if both arms of the distractor are fixed at the bone, an uncontrolled rotation of both sides of the mandible may occur. The mucosa is closed, and the distraction can start at a rate of 0.5 mm twice daily after a waiting period of about 1 week. A retention period of 12 weeks for mineralization and ossification of the newly formed callus must be observed.

VERTICAL DISTRACTION OF THE ALVEOLAR RIDGE

Since the development of minidistractors and microdistractors, vertical distraction of the alveolar ridge of the mandible and maxilla has become very popular[22] (Figs. 25-7 through 25-16). There are many indications[23] for this technique, which can be used in edentulous parts of the mandible after segmental resection in tumor surgery or after trauma instead of bone transplantation. Patients who lose their teeth as a result of periodontal disease and those with badly fitting dentures often suffer from reduced bone volume. In these cases, vertical distraction of the alveolar ridge can improve the bone volume to enable placement of dental implants or to provide a prosthesis. A residual mandible height of at least 7 mm is necessary to enable horizontal splitting and rigid fixation of the distractor.

The osteotomy and placement of the distractor can be done with the patient under general anesthesia and mobilization of smaller segments with local anesthesia. The mucosa is opened on the buccal side, and the alveolar ridge is exposed. The distractor is placed and fixed temporarily using two monocortical screws. The osteotomy line is marked with a

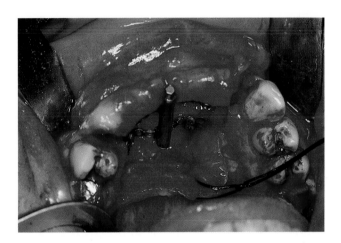

FIGURE 25-8 Same patient as in Figure 25-7. Intraoperative view at the placement of the distractor for vertical distraction of the alveolar ridge.

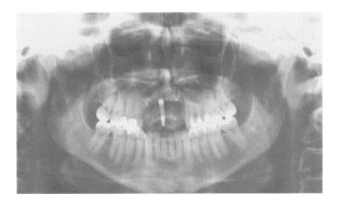

FIGURE 25-9 Same patient as in Figure 25-7. Radiograph obtained during distraction.

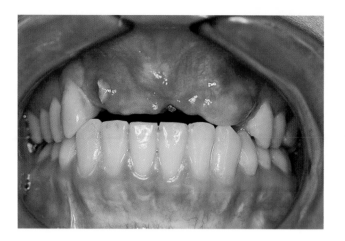

FIGURE 25-10   Same patient as in Figure 25-7. Clinical result of newly gained height of the alveolar ridge after vertical distraction during the process of retention.

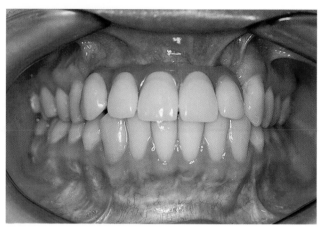

FIGURE 25-11   Same patient as in Figure 25-7. Clinical result after insertion of dental implants and prosthetic rehabilitation.

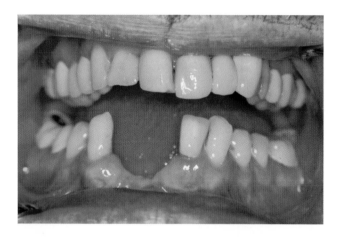

FIGURE 25-12   A 32-year-old man with traumatic loss of the lower front teeth. (Courtesy of the University Clinic, Freiburg, Germany).

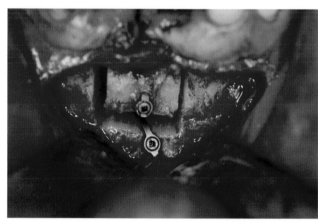

FIGURE 25-13   Same patient as in Figure 25-12. Intraoperative view during placement of the distractor (i.e., implant distractor).

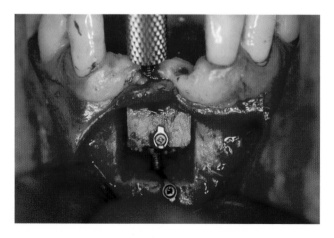

FIGURE 25-14   Same patient as in Figure 25-12. In this intraoperative view, the bone segment is temporarily distracted for testing.

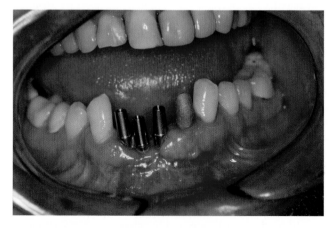

FIGURE 25-15   Same patient as in Figure 25-12. After distraction and after the placement of three implants.

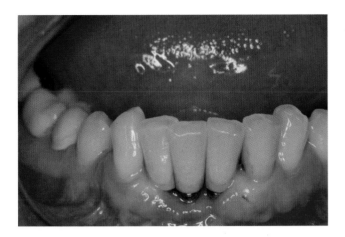

FIGURE 25-16 Same patient as in Figure 25-12. Clinical result after distraction and prosthetic rehabilitation with implantation of single crowns.

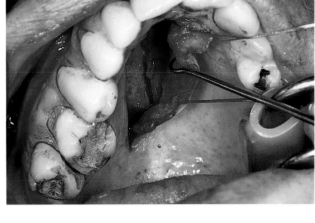

FIGURE 25-17 A 22-year-old patient with a narrow maxillary arch. An intraoperative view shows that the maxillary suture is exposed and separated.

drill, and the distractor is removed. The osteotomy is carried out with the use of a drill or a small saw, ensuring that the lingual mucosa and periosteum are not injured. After osteotomy, the segmented cranial part of the bone segment of the mandible is mobilized. Survival of this segment depends on preservation of the lingual mucoperiosteal flap. The distractor can then be attached by screws, and the bony segment is stabilized for 7 days. Distraction is performed at a rate 0.5 mm twice daily. Within 15 days, a vertical increase of 15 mm can be obtained. After the required bone height is reached, the thread of the distractor can be removed for the patient's comfort. The distractor stays in place for another 10 to 12 weeks. Four weeks after the end of the distraction process, there is mineralization of the new bone and reunion of the transported bone in the alveolar ridge. Mineralization studies suggest that insertion of dental implants is possible after 3 months, at the time of removal of the distractor under local anesthesia.

In tooth-bearing areas of the mandible or maxilla, vertical distraction of the alveolar ridge can transport tooth-bearing segments. This approach may be indicated in patients with an open bite, in those who have vertical deficiencies of the alveolar ridge caused by ankylosed teeth, or for orthopedic reasons. The principle of distraction is similar for edentulous regions of the alveolar ridge, and the procedure can be performed with the patient under local or general anesthesia.

A vestibular approach is used; the distractor is placed, and the osteotomy lines are marked. After removal of the distractor, the segment is osteotomized using a small saw or a Lindemann bur. Preservaton of the lingual mucoperiosteum ensures vitalization of the tooth-bearing segment and wound healing. The lingual cortex must be separated with the use of a small chisel. After mobilization of the tooth-bearing segment, the distractor is fixed and the wounds are closed. The schedule for distraction is the same as for edentulous segments. If necessary, the distractor can be removed after 4 weeks. To prevent a relapse of the segment, a bracket stabilization of the distracted segment to the neighboring teeth with an orthopedic wire is advisable for another 4 to 8 weeks. During distraction, the vitality of the mobilized teeth remains intact, and neighboring teeth are not damaged. There are few

limitations to the size of the distracted segment. If necessary, several teeth can be distracted simultaneously within one segment.

BONE TRANSPORTATION DISTRACTION TECHNIQUE OF THE MANDIBLE

The technique of bone distraction of the mandible was first described by Ilizarov in 1988.[3] In patients with a traumatic or operative defect of the continuity of the mandible, this horizontal distraction technique can be used to regain bone contact. The principle of this technique is based on bone distraction, but due to technical problems, it remains experimental.[24,25]

With the patient under general anesthesia, both ends of the mandible near the continuity defect are exposed. A distractor is placed between the two ends, and a 1.5- to 2-cm-wide section of the mandible is split off near the defect using a saw. This piece of bone is slowly moved from one end of the mandible defect to the other end until bone contact is obtained. Both ends of the mandible and the separated piece of mandibular bone must be fixed by a distractor that enables movement of this part. Movement of this separated segment of bone according to the principles of bone distraction with regard to waiting periods and distraction speed results in a gain of new mandible bone, and the defect can be closed by obtaining a new mandibular continuity. This technique also has been successful after radiotherapy of the mandible. It also transports good-quality mucosa attached to bone.

DISTRACTION OF THE MAXILLA ARCH

The principle of opening of the palatal suture by surgery followed by orthopedic expansion of the maxilla was described in 1961 by Haas.[26] Various surgical techniques have been described that focus on surgical weakening of the maxillary suture.[27]

The procedure should be performed with the patient under general anesthesia, but local anesthesia is possible. The maxillary suture is separated with a small chisel beginning at a small vestibular incision above the incisors (Fig. 25-17).

Weakening of the zygomatic buttress by use of a drill or a saw is advisable (Fig. 25-18). The pterygoid process usually does not have to be fractured, and a complete Le Fort I osteotomy is unnecessary. For expansion of the suture, a bone-anchored distraction device is fixed with miniscrews (Fig. 25-19). The distraction rate is 0.5 mm twice daily (Fig. 25-20). Retention of about 10 weeks is needed to prevent a relapse. Orthopedic treatment can be continued 4 weeks later (see Fig. 25-19).

DISTRACTION OF THE MIDFACE

The main reasons for distraction of the midface are congenital growth disorders, but indications also include posttraumatic situations with insufficient primary osteosynthesis or wrong bone or midface placement. Midface distraction is undertaken for cosmetic motives and for functional reasons such as restricted airflow, malocclusion, and visual problems.

Distraction of the midface can be classified by the lines of osteotomy and can be performed at the Le Fort I, II, or III

level, depending on the indications. The zygoma can be distracted separately.

For distraction at the Le Fort I level, an external distraction device (i.e., halo frame) or an internal distractor can be used[28,29] (Fig. 25-21). A conventional Le Fort I osteotomy is performed with the patient under general anesthesia using a vestibular approach. After the osteotomy, the maxilla is distracted by a dental-anchored device that is fixed to the skull by means of the halo frame; alternatively, two internal distractors are placed at both sides of the sinus walls (see Fig. 25-21). With the use of internal distractors, determination of the distraction vector is more difficult, and it cannot be altered after the operation. With a halo frame, the direction and the vector of distraction can be altered during the process of distraction to obtain a perfect occlusion. An average distraction speed of 1 to 2 mm/day is advisable.

After completion of the distraction process, a retention period of about 8 weeks must be observed, after which the distractors (external or internal) can be removed with the use of local anesthesia. However, in patients with clefts, longer stabilization is needed. This period is followed by treatment with an orthodontic device that maintains the occlusion for another 2 months.

For the Le Fort II and III levels, external distraction using the halo frame seems to be the most effective modality[28,29] (Figs. 25-22 and 25-23). Internal distractors for the LeFort III level distraction also are available (Fig. 25-24). Osteotomy of the midface is carried out with the patient under general anesthesia using a bicoronal approach and standardized operation techniques. After osteotomy and mobilization of the midface within the Le Fort II or III level, two wires are fixed at the anterior nasal aperture toward the center of the midface. The wires can also be fixed at the teeth by means of a dental splint. The wires are directed through the skin by a small incision or directed through the oral opening and fixed to the halo frame, which is located in front of the face.

After a waiting period of about 5 days, distraction starts by pulling the wires at a rate of 1 to 2 mm/day. During the process of distraction, the direction of advancement and the

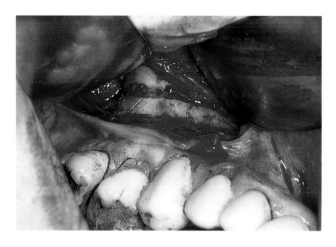

FIGURE 25-18 Same patient as in Figure 25-17. Intraoperative view of the crista zygomaticus. The crista is exposed and separated for distraction of the maxillary arch.

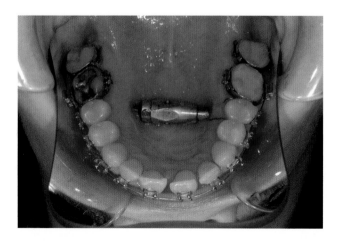

FIGURE 25-19 Same patient as in Figure 25-17. Clinical result after separation of the suture with the distraction device in place but before the start of the distraction.

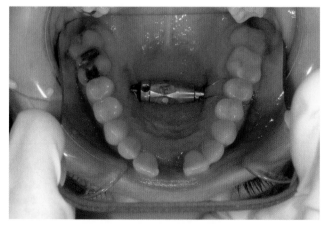

FIGURE 25-20 Same patient as in Figure 25-17. Clinical result after distraction of the maxillary arch. The incisors are separated.

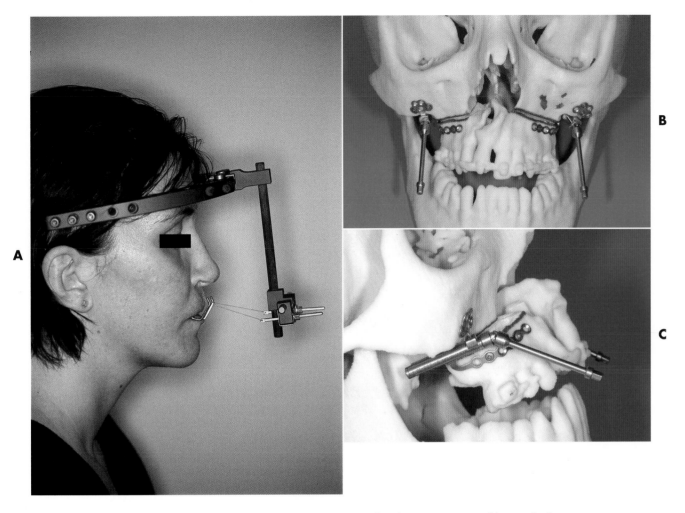

FIGURE 25-21 **A,** A 28-year-old patient with trauma-induced posterior position of the maxilla during the process of distraction on the Le Fort I level. The halo frame is fixed to the skull, and the dental-anchored device is attached to the maxillary teeth. **B,** Front view of the internal distractor for LeFort I distraction. **C,** Lateral view of the internal distractor for LeFort I distraction.

distraction vector can be adjusted according to the intended position of the midface and dental occlusion.

For distraction at the Le Fort III level, subcutaneous distractors fixed at the zygoma do not offer the possibility of changing the direction of advancement and the distraction vector[30,31] (see Fig. 25-24). General anesthesia must be used for removal of these distractors.

By following the rules of distraction, a midface advancement of up to 3 cm can be obtained if necessary. After achieving the final position of the midface, a retention period of 8 weeks must be observed, after which the halo frame can be removed with the patient under local anesthesia. This operation is followed by treatment with an orthopedic device that maintains the obtained occlusion for another 2 to 3 months.

DISTRACTION OF THE SKULL SUTURES

Techniques have been described for distraction of the skull sutures,[32,33] but they are mainly experimental and are seldom used in clinical practice. Currently, surgical widening remains the technique of choice.

PREOPERATIVE PLANNING

Each distraction treatment requires careful preoperative planning. In addition to clinical examination, two-dimensional radiography is required. If feasible, computed tomography (CT) with three-dimensional reconstruction offers the best option for successful planning and distraction treatment. The osteotomy lines and placement of the distractor can be planned and simulated. Software programs enable the surgeon to plan and simulate the movement of the bone under distraction. The location of the osteotomy lines and the direction of distractor placement determine the direction of the distraction vector and bone movement. With the exception of the halo frame, the direction of distraction cannot be changed after placement of the distractor and completion of the operation. Care must be taken to avoid compound fractures, nerve damage, and ischemic necrosis. Vertical distraction of the mandible must take into account the placement of implants into the new bone.

In some cases, such as distraction of the hypoplastic mandible in younger children, the placement of the distractor is

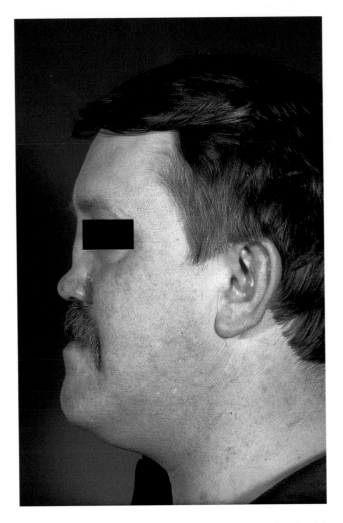

FIGURE 25-22 A 48-year-old man with trauma-induced "dish face."

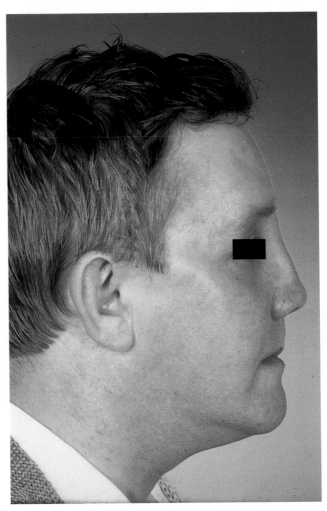

FIGURE 25-23 Clinical result after distraction of the midface on the Le Fort III level using a halo frame.

difficult because of small size and reduced space. It may be useful to manufacture a lithography model based on the CT data, followed by a simulated operation on the model and experimental placement of the distractor. With this technique, placement of the distractor can be planned, and the distraction procedure and the clinical result after the distraction can be simulated.

An important aspect in planning the procedure is the location of the distractor's thread. It must be placed so that it does not harm the soft tissues, and it must be easily reached by the patient, who has to activate it once or twice every day.

COMPLICATIONS

One of the most frequent mistakes is incorrect placement of the distractor and an incorrect distraction vector. Only when the halo frame is used can the distraction vector be altered during the process of distraction. If an error becomes obvious, the complication can be managed by applying the floating bone principle. The distractor must be removed as soon as the complete distance of distraction is reached. At this stage, the callus is still soft and malleable because the process of

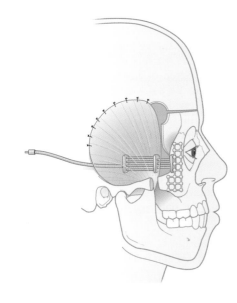

FIGURE 25-24 Principle of distraction at the Le Fort III level with the use of subcutaneously implanted distractors on both sides.

mineralization and ossification is not complete. The direction of the newly formed bone can easily be corrected. For intraoral devices, special orthognathic components such as plates or activators can be used. For extraoral devices, the forces of the soft tissue often may be responsible for a partial relapse or reshaping of the new bone.

Soft tissue problems include exposure of the new bone or the distractor. In cases with intraorally placed distractors, this is not a problem. The process of distraction usually can be continued, and the soft tissue will heal.

Fractures of the distractor or the distractor thread seldom occur and mainly indicate an inadequate osteotomy, wrong selection of distractor, or very strong soft tissue forces. In these cases, only an exchange of distractor can help.

A lack of ossification occurs if the distraction process is performed too fast. If the distraction speed of 1.5 mm/day is exceeded, the gap between the bone ends will be remodeled by fibrous tissue, not by newly formed bone. Sometimes, callus compression can be tried, but usually surgical removal of the soft tissue and a new, slower redistraction must be performed.

A relapse of the newly formed bone to the preoperative position can occur after midface distraction and premature removal of the distractor. Frequent clinical examinations must be performed after removal of the midface distractor, and the clinical results must be checked carefully. Therapeutically, orthognathic devices such as the Delaire mask must be used, or the distractor must be replaced.

REFERENCES

1. Codivilla A: On the means of lengthening in the lower limbs, the muscles and tissues which are shortened through deformity. *Am J Orthop Surg* 2:353-369, 1905.
2. Rosenthal W: Kiefergelenksankylose und Mikrogenie. *Dtsch Zahnarztl Z* 4:786-793, 1949.
3. Coleman SS, Noonan TD: Anderson's method of tibia lengthening by percutaneous osteotomy and gradual distraction. *J Bone Joint Surg* 49:263-279, 1967.
4. Ilizarov GA: The principle of the Ilizarov method. *Bull Hosp Joint Dis* 48:1-11, 1988.
5. Ilizarov GA: The tension-stress on the genesis and growth of tissues. Part I. The influence of stability of fixation and soft-tissue preservation. *Clin Orthop* 238:249-281, 1989.
6. Ilizarov GA: The tension-stress on the genesis and growth of tissues. Part II. The influence of the rate and frequency of distraction. *Clin Orthop* 239:263-285, 1989.
7. White SH, Kenwright J: The importance of delay in distraction of osteotomies. *Orthop Clin North Am* 22:569-579, 1991.
8. Aronson J: Experimental and clinical experience with distraction osteogenesis. *Cleft Palate Craniofac J* 31:473-481, 1994.
9. Karp NS, McCarthy JG, Schreiber JS, et al: Membraneous bone lengthening: a serial histological study. *Ann Plast Surg* 29:2-7, 1992.
10. Califano L, Cortese A, Zupi A, et al: Mandibular lengthening by external distraction: an experimental study in the rabbit. *J Oral Maxillofac Surg* 52:1179-1183, 1994.
11. Aronson J, Good B, Stewart C, et al: Preliminary studies of mineralization during distraction osteogenesis. *Clin Orthop* 250:43-49, 1990.
12. Sproul JT, Price CT: Recent advances in limb lengthening. Part I. Clinical advances. *Orthop Rev* 21:307-314, 1992.
13. Polley JW, Figueroa AA: Management of severe maxillary deficiency in childhood and adolescence through distraction osteogenesis with an external, adjustable, rigid distraction device. *J Craniofac Surg* 8:181-185, 1997.
14. DeBastini G, Aldegheri R, Renzi-Brivio L, et al: Limb lengthening by callous distraction (callostasis). *J Pediatr Orthop* 7:129-134, 1987.
15. Paley D: Problems, obstacles and complications of limb lengthening by the Ilizarov technique. *Clin Orthop* 250:81-104, 1990.
16. Fischgrund J, Paley D, Suter D: Variables affecting time to bone healing during limb lengthening. *Clin Orthop* 301:31, 1994.
17. McCarthy JG, Schreiber J, Karp N, et al: Lengthening the human mandible by gradual distraction. *Plast Reconstr Surg* 89:1-8, 1992.
18. Wangerin K, Gropp H: Multidimensional intraoral distraction osteogenesis of the mandible—4 years of clinical experience. *Int J Oral Maxillofac Surg* 26(suppl 1):14, 1997.
19. Gropp H, Wangerin K, Paello F, et al: Skeletal stability following distraction osteogenesis of the mandible with transorally applied devices. *J Craniomaxillofac Surg* 26(suppl 1):64, 1998.
20. Janette AJ, Vicari FA, Bauer BS, et al: Treatment of upper airway obstruction secondary to mandibular deficiency by distraction osteogenesis. *J Oral Maxillofac Surg* 53(suppl 4):96, 1995.
21. Wangerin K, Gropp H: Mandibular distraction osteogenesis using intraorally applied devices. In Härle H, Champy M, Terry B, editors: *Atlas of craniomaxillofacial osteosynthesis*, Stuttgart, 1999, Thieme, pp 148-152.
22. Block MS, Chang A, Crawford D: Mandibular alveolar ridge augmentation in the dog using distraction osteogenesis. *J Oral Maxillofac Surg* 54:309-314, 1996.
23. Hidding J, Zöller JE: Alveolar bone distraction. In Härle H, Champy M, Terry B, editors: *Atlas of craniomaxillofacial osteosynthesis*, Stuttgart, 1999, Thieme, pp 139-140.
24. Costantino PD, Friedman CD, Shindo ML, et al: Experimental mandibular regrowth by distraction osteogenesis: long term results. *Arch Otolaryngol Head Neck Surg* 119:511-516, 1993.
25. Annino DJ, Goguen LA, Karmody CS: Distraction osteogenesis for reconstruction of mandibular symphyseal defects. *Arch Otolaryngol Head Neck Surg* 120:911-916, 1994.
26. Haas AJ: Rapid palatal expansion of the maxillary dental arch and nasal cavity by opening the midpalatal suture. *Angle Orthod* 31:73-76, 1961.
27. Hidding J, Breier M: Distraction-osteogenesis of the maxilla. *Int J Oral Maxillofac Surg* 26(suppl 1):76, 1997.
28. Molina F, Ortiz Monasterio F, Paz A, et al: Maxillary distraction: aesthetic and functional benefits in cleft lip-palate and prognathic patients during mixed dentition. *Plast Reconstr Surg* 101:951-963, 1998.
29. Polley JW, Figueroa AA: Rigid external distraction: its application in cleft maxillary deformities. *Plast Reconstr Surg* 102:1360-1372, 1998.
30. Chin M, Toth BA: Le Fort III advancement with gradual distraction using internal devices. *Plast Reconstr Surg* 100:819-830, 1997.
31. Cohen SR: Craniofacial distraction with a modular internal distraction system: evolution of design and surgical techniques. *Plast Reconstr Surg* 103:1592-1607, 1999.
32. Persing JA, Babler WJ, Nagorsky MJ, et al: Skull expansion in experimental craniosynostosis. *Plast Reconstr Surg* 78:594-603, 1986.
33. Tschakaloff A, Losken HW, Mooney MD, et al: Internal calvarial bone distraction in rabbits with experimental coronal suture immobilization. *J Craniofac Surg* 5:318-326, 1994.

26
Secondary Rhinoplasty for Traumatic Nasal Deformities

Barry L. Eppley

The nose is the most frequently traumatized structure on the face due to its prominent central location and its elevation from the relatively flat frontal facial plane. The composite osteocartilaginous structure and its complex interconnections make the nose easily deformed when exposed to blunt trauma. Primary treatment of traumatic nasal deformities is presented in Chapter 13. Secondary nasal reconstruction is not rare because of the high incidence of persistent deformities after primary treatment. Some authors have reported a very high failure rate, up to 80%,[1] mainly due to failure to correct the septum, not just in the immediate postoperative period but over a longer time.

There are numerous reasons for the high incidence of secondary deformities of the nose after trauma. These include inadequate initial treatment due to a failure to appreciate the deranged anatomy, unstable bony and cartilaginous anatomy due to fracture lines and dislocations, insufficient postoperative stabilization, delayed presentation for treatment, and recurrent trauma in the early postoperative period. Regardless of the reason, patients need to be informed of the potential need for secondary rhinoplastic surgery after any nasal injury.[2]

Secondary nasal deformities are associated with a variety of cosmetic and functional issues. Typically, the nose is deviated or depressed or both. Nasal breathing is often impaired, usually by being unilateral on the side of the deviation. Surgical correction of such nasal deformities can present some of the most difficult challenges in rhinoplasty. This chapter discusses the various deformities that may be found and some common techniques for their correction.

ANATOMICAL DEFORMITIES AND EVALUATION

The effects of trauma to the nose and central face have been well described.[2,3] With initial low-velocity trauma, the nasal tip alone can become malpositioned. Typically, the lower portion of the fracture rotates inward and the upper portion is pushed upward and outward. This action causes a supratip depression with a small, more cephalic hump (Fig. 26-1). With increasing force, the cartilaginous and bony dorsum becomes fractured. Often, however, there is an incomplete fracture, which leads to a late deviation. This is frequently confused with a dislocation of the septum from the groove in the palatal shelf.

CLINICAL EXAMINATION

With experience and careful examination, it is possible to evaluate the external deformity and understand the underlying structural deformity. However, it is important to have a logical approach to the clinical examination of the nose. The variables are

- symmetry
- depression of the nasal dorsum
- tip deformity
- nasal skin scars
- condition of the internal septal and inferior turbinate

SYMMETRY

Asymmetry of the face is very common, and examination of the nose for asymmetry must be undertaken in context with the whole face. Pre-injury photographs are important to exclude long-standing asymmetry. Nasal symmetry is best assessed by looking from above the patient, with the head tilted back. This allows the nasal form to be examined afresh, with the eyebrows and chin point as reference points. Once these key landmarks have been evaluated, the cupid's bow of the upper lip can be brought into the visual field by further tilting and related to the nasal tip. In many cases, the symmetry varies along the length of the nose, and this should be noted. Deviation of the upper third of the nose most likely reflects nasal bone deformation, deviation in the lower two thirds reflects the symmetry of the septum. This should give a clear understanding about the extent and position of any asymmetry. The columella should be examined from below to confirm any tip deviation and symmetry of the nares and domes. Finally, the nasal spine should be palpated. Traumatic displacement of the nasal spine can make true central alignment of the nose impossible.

DEPRESSION OF THE NASAL DORSUM

To appreciate the position of the nasal bridge or dorsum, both lateral and anterior views must be evaluated. Laterally, the nose should come off the nasion and frontal bone at an angle of about 135 degrees. This line should continue until the slight rise at the nasal tip, to give the characteristic tip break.

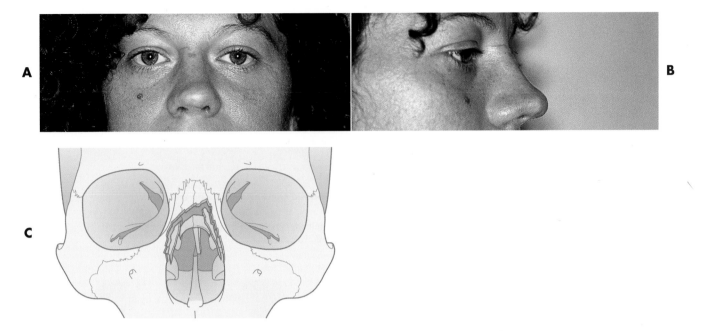

FIGURE 26-1   Secondary nasal deformity from old fracture with depression of the end of the right nasal bone and middle vault displacement. **A,** Frontal view. **B,** Right lateral view. **C,** Diagrammatic representation of fracture pattern.

The columella should make an angle with the upper lip of 90 to 110 degrees. From these normal values, an appreciation of the defect should be possible, allowing appropriate planning, such as how much nasal augmentation is needed.

In the anterior or full face examination, any broadening of the nasal bridge or the alar base should be evaluated. The alar width should fall on a vertical line from the inner canthi. In trauma cases, it is important to be sure the injury did not extend into the nasoethmoid complex, as this can produce a traumatic telecanthus. The normal width in a Caucasian adult is about 34 mm.

Any pseudoelevation of the tip, caused by a saddle deformity, should be distinguished from a true traumatic elevation caused by upward displacement of the nasal spine (which is rare).

NASAL SKIN SCARS

Any lacerations or abrasions should be carefully noted, because they must not be confused with planned surgical incisions (e.g., for an open rhinoplasty). If any scars by chance are in the correct position they should be used. Any scarred areas may represent a potential weakness and could reopen at secondary surgery, especially early after trauma. There may also be an opportunity to revise any scar.

INTERNAL EXAMINATION

The internal examination is probably the most important part of the examination. For it to be useful, one needs a good head light and a speculum of appropriate length to examine the whole nose or a fiberoptic endoscope. The clinical examination should first test function (i.e., the nasal airway), ideally obtaining and documenting the ease of nasal airflow. The effect of opening the internal nasal airway by

pulling the soft tissue on the lateral nose laterally and the effect of vasoconstrictors, which reduce posttraumatic edema, may help to identify and focus on the cause of any obstruction. Specifically, any collapse of the middle vault should be noted.

Observation of the internal nose aims to identify:

- Deviated septum
- Resolving septal hematomas
- Mucosal hyperemia and/or edema
- Inferior turbinate hyperplasia
- Displacement of lateral nasal bones
- Evidence of nasal valve trauma

Septal hematomas are common with nasal trauma, because the nose is distorted on impact and the palatal shelf is a solid, fixed point. In children, a missed septal hematoma leads to a late delayed deviation and impaired symmetry of growth in addition to the distortion caused by the organizing hematoma.

Septal fracture and dislocation may accompany hematomas. Initially, the dorsum may be merely deflected to one side, but with increased force comes a more retro-displacement of both cartilage and bone (Fig. 26-2). The septum is central to correcting the symmetry and prominence of the nasal bridge. Guyuron et al. described six typical variations of septal position observed in more than 1000 revision procedures[4]; 40% had a simple tilt of the septum, which probably indicates no fracture. Other common presentations included a C-shaped deformity, either horizontally or vertically, and an S-shaped deformity, usually horizontally. These more extensive deformities reflect severe distortion with likely fracture or partial fracturing of the septum. It is the healing of these fractures that generates tensions leading to late deformation of the septum, which is reflected in a distorted nose.

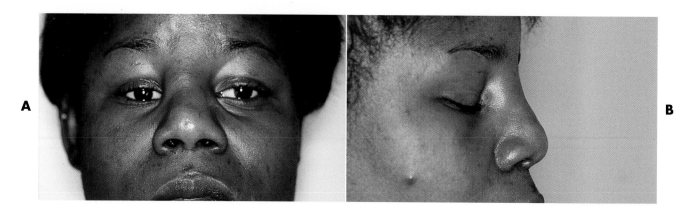

FIGURE 26-2 Secondary nasal deformity with more significant impaction of nasal bones, shortening of the septum, and superior tip rotation. **A,** Frontal view. **B,** Lateral view.

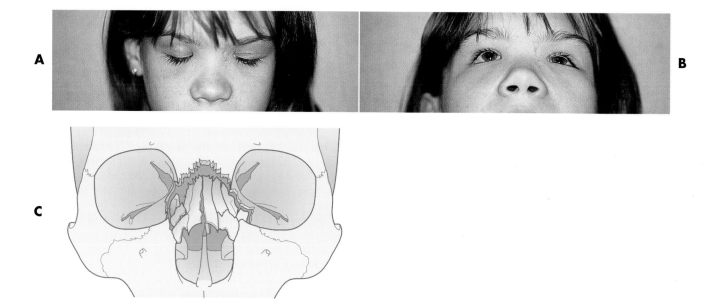

FIGURE 26-3 Secondary deformity showing naso-orbitoethmoid (NOE) fracture pattern with nasal impaction and telecanthus. **A,** Frontal view. **B,** Submental view. **C,** Diagrammatic representation of fracture pattern.

Initial fracture of the nasal bones may extend to involve the nasal process of the frontal bone, the nasal process of the maxilla, the lacrimal bone, and the lamina papyracea. With larger blunt forces that occur directly over the bridge of the nose or from an inferior direction, naso-orbitoethmoid (NOE) fractures occur with telecanthus. This results in a flat, wide nasal dorsum with decreased nasal length, decreased nasal projection and support, and columellar retraction (Fig. 26-3). NOE fractures are frequently part of more extended midfacial fractures. An understanding of these common fracture patterns aids in the assessment of the secondarily deformed nose, but the need for a thorough preoperative evaluation is not obviated.

In contrast to cases of primary esthetic rhinoplasty, those involving a deformed traumatized nose more often are associated with some degree of nasal obstruction, reflecting damage to the septum or, less commonly, damage to the intranasal valve. This is more commonly seen in cases involving lacerations or penetrating injuries. Its correction requires identification of both fixed and dynamic components of the obstruction. A thorough examination of the nasal passages must be performed before and after the topical application of a vasoconstrictive agent. The shrinkage of the mucosa aids in identifying surgically reversible causes of nasal obstruction. With a nasal speculum, the position of the septum, size of the turbinates, and internal and external valves should be assessed.[3] The fractured septum is often displaced off the maxillary crest to one side or telescoped on itself. Nasal valve obstruction is frequently found with either upper lateral cartilage displacement medially or collapse. This may be confirmed by performing the Cottle maneuver, which should improve with lateral displacement of the cheek on the obstructed side. Enlarged turbinates, especially with lateral wall displacement medially, can also contribute to further nasal obstruction.

ESTHETICS

A trauma patient seeking revision is no different from a patient seeking a cosmetic rhinoplasty. Clearly, some trauma patients fit into the "warrior class" and have little regard for appearance or social behavior, but they are unlikely to seek revision surgery. Some patients who have been injured in a domestic dispute may be more demanding than a patient seeking a cosmetic rhinoplasty, because their deformity carries much more emotional impact, such as anger associated with the injury.

As with any cosmetic aspect, the patient's wishes not only guide the surgical process but can inform the surgeon about the patient's psychological makeup (see Chapter 30). Trauma patients are just as likely to be dysmorphic as any other group. The two important warning signs are vague, nonspecific comments about appearance and concerns about appearance that seem inappropriate to the clinical findings.

It is also important to determine just how the nose looked before the injury and exactly how the fractured nose compares. Old pictures may be beneficial in determining which deformities have always been present and which are secondary to the nasal trauma.

INVESTIGATIONS

After a history and thorough examination, radiographic assessment is often helpful to exclude other facial fractures and to aid in planning any bony surgery. However, plain radiographs are even less useful than they are in primary nasal fracture repair (Fig. 26-4A,B). They simply do not provide an anatomic assessment of the internal nasal airway, which is often the ambiguous issue. Computed tomographic (CT) scans are the most helpful in this regard, and their axial and coronal slices provide the most complete view of the internal nasal airway (see Fig. 26-4C,D). They are not particularly helpful for evaluation of external nasal morphology.

Some controversy exists, because it is often believed that a thorough intranasal examination makes CT scanning superfluous. In certain cases, this is probably true, but the traumatized nose superimposes variable anatomical derangements on top of the patient's native nose, which may or may not have been normal before the injury. If the intranasal examination is not clear, a paranasal CT scan is warranted. In rare cases, usually those involving untreated or undertreated NOE fracture patterns, a three-dimensional CT reconstruction may be useful to assess surrounding facial skeletal morphology as well the fracture (see Fig. 26-4E); however, because of the thin, fine bones in this area, the computer reconstruction may create artifacts.

SUMMARY OF PREOPERATIVE EXAMINATION

The aspects of the preoperative examination are as follows:

- Identifying the patient's concerns
- Careful external examination of the nose and face for symmetry and deformity, both lateral and full face;

examination of the whole face and nose from above is the most reliable method of determining symmetry of the face and nose
- Careful internal examination with speculum and endoscope
- Airway examination
- Radiological examination in some cases

COMMON TRAUMATIC NASAL DEFORMITIES

Whereas traumatic nasal rearrangement can produce a wide variation of deformities, a pattern of nasal dysmorphologies can be identified. These include the expected alterations that can occur with any projected tripod structure: loss of height, deviation, and asymmetries. Most traumatized noses have all of these components, and the anatomical contribution of each component must be understood if an ideal correction is to be achieved.

SADDLE NOSE

A saddle nose deformity leaves the patient with a lack of structure (of bone, cartilage, or both) in the nasal dorsum.[1,2] This defect leads to a scooped-out appearance from the lateral view and an appearance of a flattened nasal bridge from the frontal view. An illusion of tip rotation accompanies the depression; in some cases in which significant middle vault collapse has occurred, this rotation may be real. Also, there is an apparent widening of the nasal vault on frontal view without displacement of the nasal bones or cartilage. Loss of height and lack of a light reflex lead to this illusion.

SHORT NOSE

The short nose deformity is characterized by a decreased distance from the nasion to the tip defining point, a low ratio of tip projection to nasal length, and a more obtuse than normal nasolabial angle.[1] Overall the nose appears overrotated and deprojected. This nasal deformity can have many causes, including weakening of the lower lateral cartilages, shortening of the septum, and destabilization or detachment of the upper lateral cartilages from the nasal bones. This is the characteristic appearance of a depressed nasoethmoid fracture, which should be excluded. In well-pneumatized frontal sinuses, a minimal injury is needed to depress the whole complex.

NASAL DEVIATION

Blunt trauma from a lateral direction can cause the nasal dorsum or tip to become deviated. A portion or all of the nose is deviated off a straight line drawn from the glabella down through the central aspect of the cupid's bow. This is most often caused by displacement of one or both nasal bones, but the injury may extend down through the structures of the middle vault as well. Illusions of deviation of the nose may also be seen with collapse of an ipsilateral upper lateral cartilage and bone, leading to shadowing along one side.

There is no doubt that deviation of or damage to the cartilaginous septum is extremely important as a cause of nasal

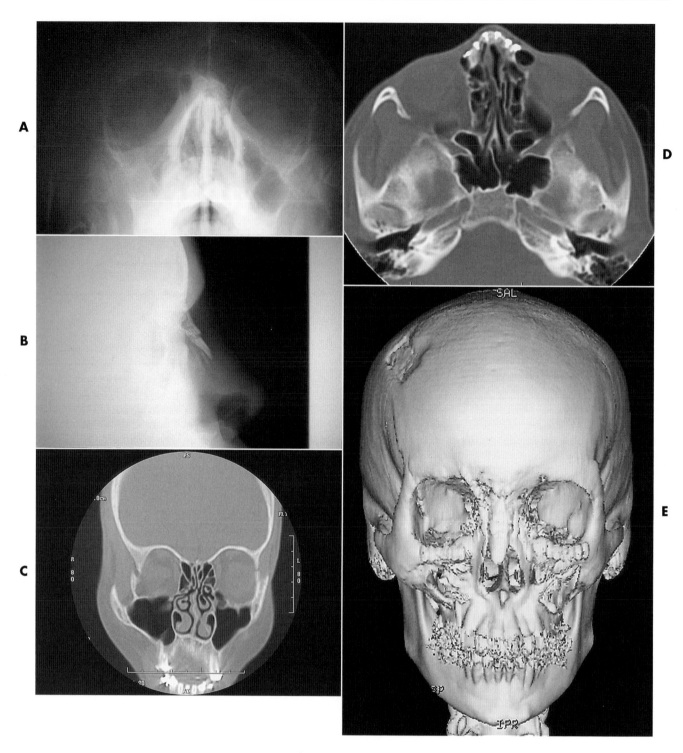

FIGURE 26-4 Plain radiographic assessment of secondary nasal deformities is even less useful than that of primary nasal fractures. **A,** Submental view of an old nasal fracture in a patient who presented with a secondary depressed nasal deformity. **B,** Lateral view. The bony pattern of an old nasal fracture can be appreciated in these plain radiographs, but they do not add to what a good physical examination would show. Computed tomographic (CT) scans are more useful, particularly axial and coronal paranasal views, and occasionally a three-dimensional (3-D) reconstruction can be appreciated. **C,** Coronal view in an older teenager with severe nasal depression and airway obstruction after primary treatment of a naso-orbitoethmoid (NOE) injury. **D,** Axial CT view. **E,** 3-D reconstruction. The internal nasal derangement as well as the surrounding facial bone treatments can be visualized.

deviation. Its importance is as much about the difficulty in correcting the damage as it is about making the diagnosis.

It has long been recognized a resolving hematoma on the septum in a child produces deviation that deteriorates as the nose grows. The resultant deviation and nasal obstruction are extremely significant. However, diagnosis and drainage of the hematoma largely prevents the problem.

In adults, the problem is controversial not because of the well-recognized effects of a deviated septum but because of the etiology. At one time, it was suggested that nasal deviation was entirely due to displacement of the septum from the palatal groove or from its position between the crura anteriorly. It has now been shown experimentally and clinically that the deviation develops from small linear fractures of the cartilage just superior to the palatal groove. This healing fracture then produces the deviation. Localized submucous resections are advocated acutely to prevent long-term deviations.

Because the nasal bones are so frequently fractured (being the most common type of nasal fracture), bridge and sidewall deformities are common. Because of the fractures, the location of the nasal bones is asymmetrical, possibly because of their attachments to the maxilla and orbit up to the apex of the dorsum.

COLUMELLAR RETRACTION

The normal distance from the nasal ala to the base of the columella is 2 mm on lateral view. With nasal trauma, the amount of columellar show can change depending on the direction of the displacing force and the nasal structures disrupted. It can be decreased or become nonexistent due to retro-displacement of the caudal septum that pulls the columellar skin posteriorly. This usually occurs from a direct blow impacting the base of the nose. With upper and middle vault collapse, the tip may rotate superiorly, which can result in increased columellar show.

STATE-OF-THE-ART MANAGEMENT

TIMING

The timing of a secondary corrective rhinoplasty is not critical in most patients. The deformities encountered, although distressing to the patient and often restrictive of some nasal airflow, are not life-threatening, and good healing of the nasal structures should have occurred before manipulation is attempted. For some patients, timing is not an issue because their injury had occurred months to years previously and the present surgeon was not involved in the management of the original problem.

If the secondary deformity is an extension of the original treatment or the patient is presenting late (months) after a primary nasal injury, the decision as to when to operate can be more difficult. Ideally, nasal mucosal swelling and inflammation should have resolved and the deformities of the osteocartilaginous structures should have become completely apparent with resolution of the cutaneous edema. The surgical axiom of waiting 6 to 12 months after the injury is often quoted, but operating earlier may be indicated based on the patient's desires, a full appreciation of the aberrant anatomy, and the type of surgical approach.

APPROACHES

The choice of an open versus a closed approach depends on the surgeon and the defect. It is reasonable to use the open approach for all secondary rhinoplasties unless the surgeon has complete confidence in both the diagnosis of the nasal deformities and his or her ability to correct them through the more limited exposure of the closed approach. Usually, an endonasal approach in secondary surgery requires either a more limited nasal problem or an extensive experience in rhinoplastic surgery on the part of the surgeon. Nevertheless, many secondary nasal deformities can be adequately treated through a closed approach involving the use of traditional and intercartilaginous incisions, as has been well described in the past (Fig. 26-5). In cases requiring more extensive correction, which almost always involves the placement of cartilage grafts, the open approach provides superior visualization of the nasal structures and better facilitates graft placement onto the upper and middle vaults as well as the nasal tip (see Fig. 26-5).

SURGICAL TECHNIQUES

Grafting of the Nasal Dorsum

Nasal dorsal grafting is a common technique used for repair of the saddle nose deformity. Which material is best for augmentation in this area has been a source of great controversy over the years. The materials available for nasal augmentation are similar to those used elsewhere in the face and can be divided into autografts, homografts, and alloplastic biomaterials.

Both bone and cartilage autograft materials may be appropriate, offering the advantage of incorporation into the recipient site and a lack of any risk of rejection. They do have to be harvested, which takes time and, in certain donor sites, carries some limited morbidity. Many surgeons make the choice of bone versus cartilage based on the amount of augmentation needed. For small to moderate-sized dorsal grafts, cartilage is usually chosen because it is fairly easy to harvest and shape.

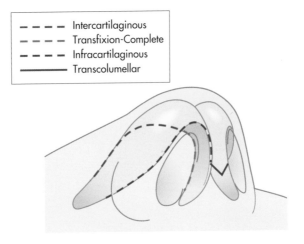

FIGURE 26-5 Diagrammatic representation of incisional options in nasal approaches: 1, intercartilaginous; 2, complete transfixion; 3, infracartilaginous (marginal rim); 4, transcolumellar.

The most common donor sites are the underlying septum, ear, and rib.

Septal cartilage has the advantage of being in the same operative field and can offer a large amount of graft material, because only a centimeter of dorsal and caudal cartilage must be retained for adequate dorsal support in a traditional septal harvest (Fig. 26-6). With a previous nasal injury, however, this cartilage is usually less than optimal, and straight pieces of sufficient length may not be harvestable due to previous fractures and potential shortening of vertical septal height. This cartilage, when relatively undamaged, is easy to sculpt, often matches the deficient structure, and is usually the first choice of most surgeons.[5] With increasing graft thickness, septal cartilage must be stacked and sutured together, which requires some skillful crafting. In the thin-skinned patient, this may result in some palpable edges.

Auricular cartilage is also in the same operative field, and harvest of the concha through a postauricular incision is rapid and causes little morbidity. The curved shape of this cartilage may or may not be beneficial depending on the defect. With smaller dorsal defects for which a long length is not required, conchal cartilage may be adequate (Fig. 26-7). For nasal tip work, its inherent curved shape is often useful. For long, straight-line grafts of the dorsum, conchal cartilage is problematic in both shape and length.

Costal cartilage offers the advantage of a large amount of donor tissue, but it has some inherent drawbacks that may be difficult to overcome. Of all the cartilage donor sites, rib is the most likely to warp or curl. This is because the eighth and ninth rib harvest sites are curved and cannot provide a long, straight graft. Bending the graft by scoring the perichondrium or removing it completely may make it straight intraoperatively, but postoperative memory or recoil often occurs.

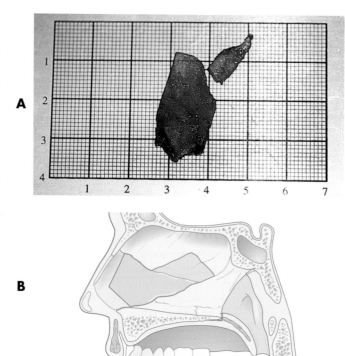

A

B

FIGURE 26-6 When the septum is relatively undamaged, septal harvest can provide a large amount of graft tissue. **A,** It is very important to maintain enough dorsal and caudal septum to ensure external support of the dorsal line, tip, and columella. **B,** The lined area indicates the maximum amount of septum that should be harvested.

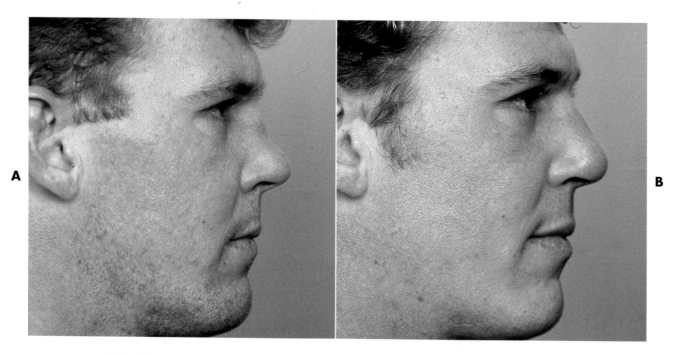

A

B

FIGURE 26-7 Dorsal reconstruction with a combination of conchal cartilage and acellular human dermis (Alloderm) in a depression of the upper and middle vaults. **A,** Preoperative appearance. **B,** Appearance 6 months after operation.

Some surgeons have attempted to overcome this tendency by placing a K-wire through the center of the graft before dorsal placement, and this appears to be effective.

Besides warping, the other concern with all types of cartilage grafts is resorption. Most cartilage grafts do undergo some resorption with an unpredictable change in graft volume. Whether this is significant for the dorsal profile depends on the size of the graft, its source, and the amount of augmentation needed. One technique that I have found particularly useful for nasal rib cartilage is that of *dicing*. It virtually eliminates all of the problems of the solid one-piece rib graft. Placed inside a fascial sleeve, it is moldable, does not warp, and is associated with little to no resorption. Its only downside is the time required to put together the fascial-cartilage ensemble.

Another collagen-based nasal augmentation option is that of dermal grafting. Processed human dermis, which comes in a variety of sizes and thicknesses, is almost ideal for augmentation of only 1 or 2 mm. It is soft, has no sharp edges, and does not undergo resorption. If greater thickness is needed, stacking and suturing several layers can be done to get dorsal augmentations of up to 3 or 4 mm.

Autogenous bone grafts provide greater support and augmentation, which may be required in larger defects. The most common donor sites are rib, iliac crest, and calvaria. The advantages of calvarial bone include being close to the operative field and greater maintenance of volume over time. Adequate length and size as a single piece can usually be obtained from the occipital area or anywhere along a hemicoronal or scalp incision in the hair-bearing scalp.[6] The outer cortex is taken, and reconstruction of the resultant defect is not usually necessary, because the defect is minimal. Some skill and experience are required in harvesting the graft to avoid the potential for inner cortex disruption and dural violation. Grafts are never harvested across suture lines because of the attachment of the underlying dura, and in particular they are never taken across the midline of the skull because of the presence of the underlying sagittal venous sinus. Sculpting of the graft requires a powered bur and irrigation to obtain a desirable, boat-like shape for dorsal augmentation. Many cranial bone grafts, because of their size and length, benefit from some form of fixation. When the graft is placed through an open approach, securing of the distal graft end to the upper or lower alar cartilages may be adequate (Fig. 26-8). Screw fixation to the frontonasal junction is most easily done through a coronal incision and is most commonly performed in reconstruction of more severely impacted or NOE-type injuries (Figs. 26-9 and 26-10). The main drawbacks of autogenous bone are the time required for harvest and sculpting, the need for fixation of some grafts, and potential donor site morbidity, including a scalp scar.

Homograft cartilage or bone can also be used for dorsal augmentation. Use of banked cartilage and bone is limited by concerns about processing and potential disease transmission as well as the numerous available autogenous options. Improving methods of allogeneic tissue processing promise that this option may some day rival autogenous grafts. Irradiated cartilage is also available; it provides a sterile and nonantigenic source of homograft cartilage, but the resorption potential is high.[1]

A variety of alloplastic materials have been used over the years to augment the nasal dorsum, including silicone rubber,

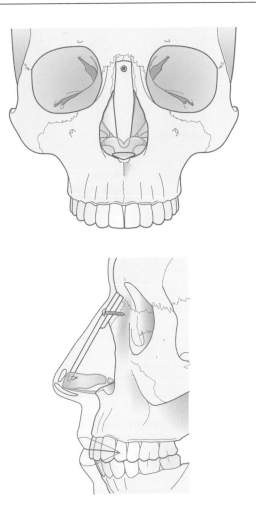

FIGURE 26-8 Augmentation of the nasal dorsum with a cranial bone graft placed deep to the cartilage domes, lag screw fixation, and cartilage grafts to the columella and tip.

Supramid (polyamide), Mersilene mesh (polyethylene terephthalate), and Gore-Tex (polytetrafluoroethylene). Alloplasts offer the advantage of an unlimited supply and the avoidance of any donor site morbidity. Silicone rubber has been associated with an unreasonably high extrusion rate and is not widely used today. Although Supramid and Mersilene mesh have been reasonably well tolerated in the nasal dorsum, they have both been found to have a significant resorption rate over time, and the occurrence of infection poses a potentially difficult problem. Gore-Tex is by the far the most commonly used alloplast placed in the nasal dorsum today (Fig. 26-11). There is considerable controversy about its use, with strong voices on both sides of the issue.[7,8] Its ease of use and effectiveness in dorsal augmentation are undeniable, but the presence of an alloplast under only a cutaneous cover brings up long-term concerns about infection, thinning of the nasal skin, and potential extrusion.

In most cases, alloplasts are chosen because of their availability off the shelf and their favorable handling properties, but lack of autogenous donor tissue is not a legitimate reason, given the many potential sites for harvest of fascia, cartilage, and bone in any individual. No patient lacks adequate autogenous tissue, only the surgeon's desire and experience to harvest it. The introduction of processed dermal grafts has

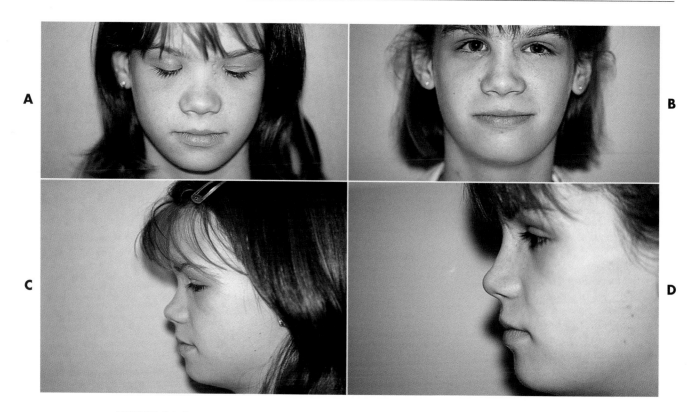

FIGURE 26-9 This 14-year-old girl sustained a naso-orbitoethmoid (NOE)-type facial fracture and was referred for treatment of secondary deformities after primary facial fracture repair. She was treated with cranial bone graft augmentation and lag screw fixation, medial canthoplasties with transnasal wiring, removal of indwelling metal hardware, and dacryocystorhinostomies (external incisions) through her previous coronal incision. **A,** Preoperative frontal view. **B,** Frontal view 1 year after operation. **C,** Preoperative lateral view. **D,** Lateral view 1 year after operation.

quelled this controversy somewhat; they offer a biologically safe and well-tolerated alternative without the need for autogenous harvest. They are very pliable, easy to cut and shape, and have utility in rhinoplastic surgery as a dorsal camouflage of either underlying grafts or osteocartilaginous irregularities[9] (Fig. 26-12). The processed dermal graft is almost ideal for augmentations that require need 1 or 2 mm. It is soft and will have no sharp edges or resorption. If greater thickness is needed, stacking and suturing of several layers can be done for dorsal augmentations of up to 3 or 4 mm.

Osteotomies

Correction of deformities of the bony nasal vault is typically done with osteotomies. Nasal osteotomies can achieve closure of an open roof deformity, straightening of a deviated nasal dorsum, and narrowing of the nasal side walls. All osteotomy techniques essentially infracture one or both of the nasal bones. Widening of the nasal dorsum via outfracturing of a nasal bone, although useful, is an inherently more unstable procedure.

Commonly used osteotomy techniques include lateral osteotomy, intermediate osteotomy, medial osteotomy, and superior osteotomy (Fig. 26-13). Lateral osteotomies are typically performed in a high-low-high fashion in a linear direction from an intranasal incision at the superior edge of the inferior turbinate. Starting the osteotomy from this position

ensures preservation of the lateral and nasal suspensory ligament attachments to the piriform aperture. Elevation of the inner lining of the nose is carried out with a Freer elevator. The actual bony cuts are then made with a small (3-mm) unguarded osteotome. The intermediate osteotomy is used when there is a marked height difference between the two nasal bones or when a marked convexity of one of the nasal bones exists. The position between the medial and the lateral osteotomy depends on the clinical situation. When used for correction of height, it should be placed close to the nasal facial groove. For correction of nasal convexity, a path through the area of convexity should be used. Medial osteotomies are required for correction of the markedly deviated nose. The path of the medial osteotomy begins at the junction of the septum and the nasal bone and proceeds in an angulated fashion to meet either the back fracture site or the superior osteotomy site. If a saddle nose deformity or an open book deformity exists, a medial osteotomy should not be required.

The nose that is severely deviated to one side should be approached with osteotomies in a sequential fashion, in the same way as opening a book (Fig. 26-14). The medialized nasal bone is first approached with a lateral osteotomy and then a medial osteotomy, allowing lateralization of the bone. Next, a medial osteotomy is performed on the laterally deviated side, allowing return of the septum to the midline.

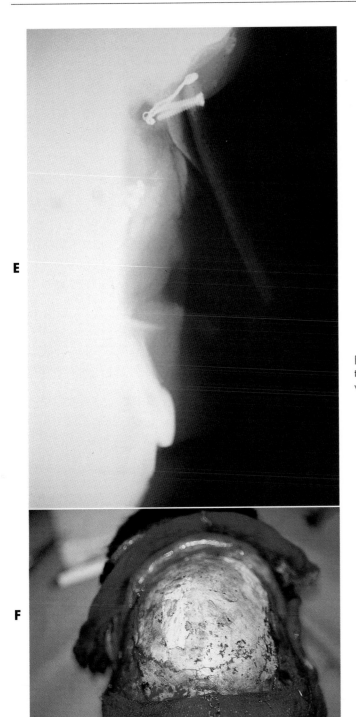

FIGURE 26-9, cont'd E, Lateral radiograph 1 year after operation. **F,** Cranial bone graft donor site (upper frontal) was recontoured with hydroxyapatite bone substitute.

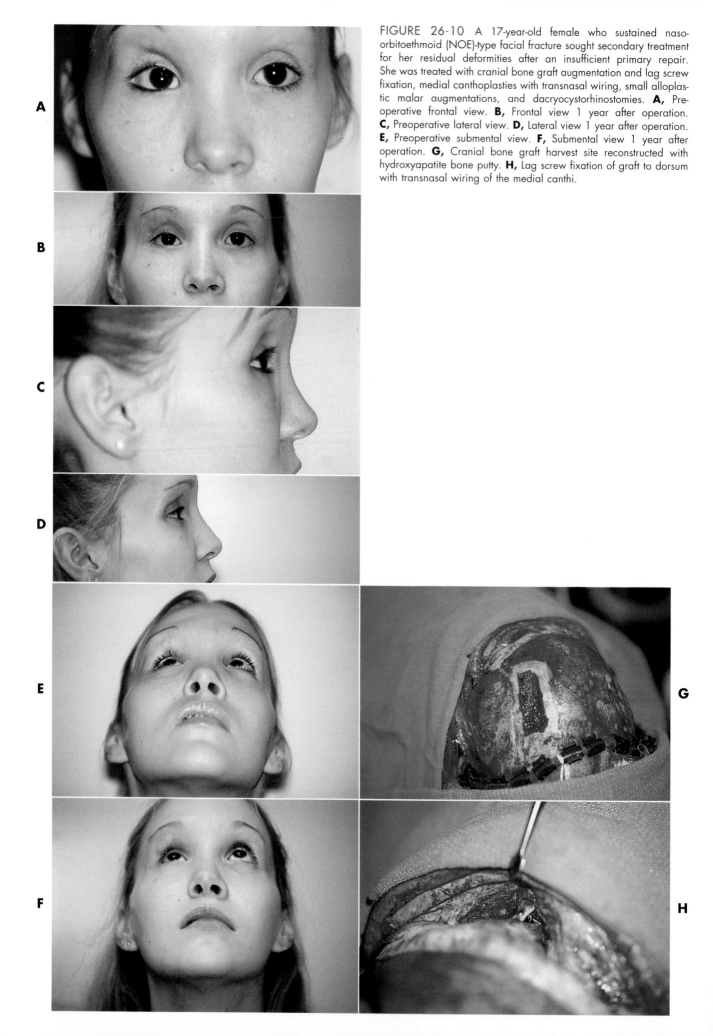

FIGURE 26-10 A 17-year-old female who sustained naso-orbitoethmoid (NOE)-type facial fracture sought secondary treatment for her residual deformities after an insufficient primary repair. She was treated with cranial bone graft augmentation and lag screw fixation, medial canthoplasties with transnasal wiring, small alloplastic malar augmentations, and dacryocystorhinostomies. **A,** Preoperative frontal view. **B,** Frontal view 1 year after operation. **C,** Preoperative lateral view. **D,** Lateral view 1 year after operation. **E,** Preoperative submental view. **F,** Submental view 1 year after operation. **G,** Cranial bone graft harvest site reconstructed with hydroxyapatite bone putty. **H,** Lag screw fixation of graft to dorsum with transnasal wiring of the medial canthi.

Finally, the laterally displaced bone is brought back toward the midline with a lateral osteotomy.

Spreader Grafts

Deformity of the middle nasal vault can lead to both nasal obstruction and airway obstruction due to collapse of the internal nasal valve (angle of <15 degrees). Spreader grafts provide a solution to both of these problems and are one of the most important contributions to corrective rhinoplastic surgery introduced in the past two decades[10] (Fig. 26-15). With significant dorsal septal deflections for which scoring of the septum would be inadequate, spreader grafts can be used unilaterally to create the illusion of a straight middle nasal vault (Fig. 26-16). Bilateral middle nasal vault narrowing (i.e., inverted-V deformity) may be corrected with bilateral spreader graft placement.

The placement of spreader grafts can be done through either a closed or an open approach, but it is inherently easier for most surgeons to properly position and secure them through an external approach. After elevation of the skin envelope, a submucosal pocket is developed between the upper lateral cartilage and the septum. The pocket should span the entire length of the upper lateral cartilage. Spreader grafts can be fashioned from septal cartilage, conchal cartilage, or resected vomer. Some surgeons have used grafts fashioned from resorbable polymers with good success, believing that the residual scar is sufficient as a volumetric expander.[11] Length should allow extension from just under the nasal bones to the caudal edge of the upper lateral cartilage. Width is determined by the defect being repaired but typically varies between 1 and 3 mm. Grafts are secured in position with 5-0 resorbable monofilament sutures in a horizontal mattress

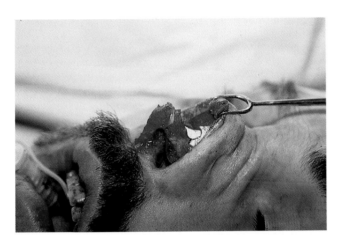

FIGURE 26-11 Gore-Tex (polytetrafluoroethylene) graft placed over the dorsum in reconstruction of a traumatic saddle nose deformity through an open approach.

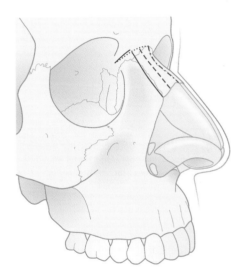

FIGURE 26-13 Nasal osteotomy options: lateral (solid line), intermediate or midlevel (dashed line), medial (dotted line), superior (dot-dash line).

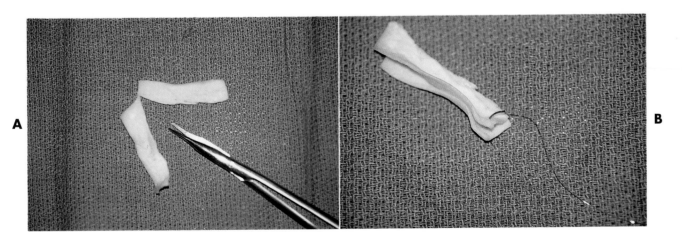

FIGURE 26-12 Processed human dermis (acellular dermis) provides a soft and reasonably thick (0.75-1.5 mm) graft material for the nasal dorsum that can be easily cut (**A**) and securely sutured. **B,** Its revascularization is rapid and assured and its volume is well preserved.

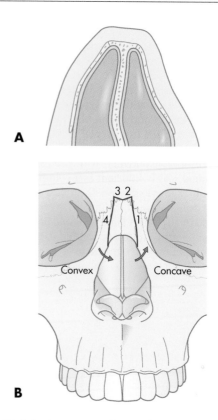

FIGURE 26-14 Osteotomy technique for severe nasal pyramid deviation. **A,** Typical deviated nose caused by trauma with convex and concave deformities of the bones and septal angulation. **B,** Pattern and sequence of osteotomies for straightening of nasal bone asymmetry.

fashion through the upper lateral cartilage, the graft, the septum, and the opposite side graft if used (see Fig. 26-15).

Septoplasty

The nasal septum functions as the backbone of the nose and has an enormous effect on the appearance of the dorsum. Deflections of the septum can make both the middle third and the lower third of the nose appear deviated. Although septal deviation and deflections can exist in a wide variety of anatomical forms, the traumatized nose most frequently develops an S-shaped or reverse S-shaped anteroposterior deformity due to buckling and fracture of the septum from oblique forces.[4] The orientation of the S-shape depends on the initial direction of the traumatizing blow (Fig. 26-17A). With more severe superior or direct displacing forces on the nasal tip or dorsum, the septum fractures, telescopes, and shortens onto itself.

Correction of the deviated septum is usually done through a hemitransfixion incision. Deviated portions of the septum are removed, preserving at least a 1-cm strut both dorsally and caudally (see Fig. 26-6B). Whenever possible, removed cartilage is morselized and returned to the septum if it is not used as grafts. If minor deviations exist in this important preserved strut area, light vertical scoring may be used on the concave side of the septal deformity. For maximal septal cartilage preservation, the S-shaped deformity is corrected by removal of the posterior portion of the bone and cartilage,

bilateral cephalocaudal scoring on the concave areas, and osteotomy and repositioning of the nasal spine and vomer bone (Figs. 26-18 and 26-19; see Fig. 26-17B). For more major deflections in which the caudal septum remains deviated, spreader grafts should be used, with the upper lateral cartilage opposite the deviated side sewn differentially to the spreader graft–septal composite to pull it to the midline.[4] Intranasal extramucosal splints may also be used to improve cartilage memory if spreader grafts are not used.

Illusion of Nasal Lengthening

Traumatized noses that have only minimal shortening may be amenable to illusion techniques by which a small amount of lengthening can be achieved. One such technique involves inferior rotation of the nasal tip.[12] The lower lateral cartilages are freed from their surrounding attachments, and the tip is rotated downward (Fig. 26-20). The net achievement is deprojection of the tip along with inferior rotation, but no real net increase in length is actually obtained. Radix grafts also provide the illusion of increased nasal length.[13]

Septal grafts are harvested and sculpted in a beveled fashion. They are placed through an intercartilaginous incision and laid over the area of the radix. A mattress suture of 5-0 plain gut placed through the overlying skin can be used to secure the graft in position. Simply stuffing the grafts into a dorsal subcutaneous pocket should be avoided, because they are prone to potential migration. This technique is most beneficial for those patients who had a preexisting deep radix before their injury. A gain of 1 to 2 mm in radix height can usually be achieved. A need for greater augmentation in this area suggests an overall lowering of the dorsum, which is best addressed by other techniques.

Nasal Lengthening

A variety of surgical maneuvers may be used to create an actual increase in nasal length. In most nasal fracture deformities, both increased nasal length and increased tip projection are needed. All techniques involve cartilage grafting and include tip grafts, columellar struts, and septal extension grafts.

A very versatile method is the dynamic adjustable rotational tip tensioning (DARTT) technique, which aims to achieve all of these maneuvers in a single procedure.[14] It is performed through an open rhinoplasty approach; multiple septal cartilage grafts are placed as a single columellar strut with two other grafts serving as septocolumellar interpositional grafts (Fig. 26-21). These three grafts are used to create a new tip complex that provides columellar support, allows repositioning of the nasal tip in an inferior direction, and opens the internal nasal valve. A wide arc of rotation is possible, and the appropriate tip projection and rotation can easily be selected. This technique offers adaptability as well as maximal stability.

Another grafting technique is that of a two- or three-tiered graft that is sutured to the caudal edge of the medial crura.[15] With the use of septal or conchal cartilage, the graft is buttressed against the very stable medial crura and distal septum through an open approach (Fig. 26-22). The redraping of the skin over the graft creates an increased dorsal length, although it is not as significant as that obtained by the DARTT technique.

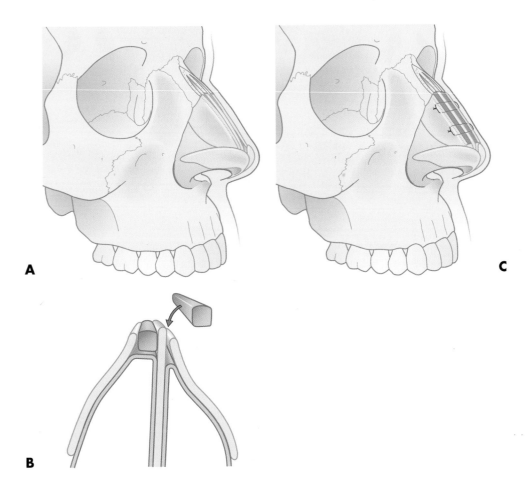

A

B

C

FIGURE 26-15 Spreader graft placement technique. The middle vault is narrowed due to medial collapse of the upper lateral cartilages. **A,** Spreader grafts often extend from the osseous-cartilaginous junction to beneath the domes to open up the internal nasal valves. **B,** Spreader grafts (usually from septum) are placed into position between the upper lateral cartilage and the nasal septum. **C,** The grafts are best secured by 5-0 resorbable horizontal mattress sutures.

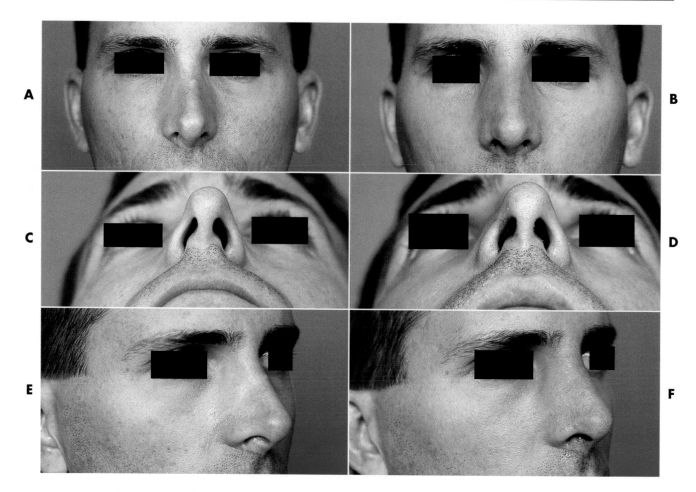

FIGURE 26-16   Male patient with 2-year-old nasal fracture initially treated with closed reduction technique at an outside institution with airway obstructive symptoms and nasal asymmetry. The patient was treated through an endonasal approach with unilateral spreader graft and nasal side wall graft of septal cartilage. **A,** Preoperative frontal view. **B,** Frontal view 2 weeks after operation. **C,** Preoperative submental view. **D,** Submental view 2 weeks after operation. **E,** Preoperative right oblique view. **F,** Right oblique view 2 weeks after operation. The patient's airway obstructive symptoms are completely resolved, and the right upper and middle vaults have been restored. The spreader graft has done a good job of opening the internal nasal valve and correcting the collapse of the right lower alar cartilage.

FIGURE 26-17   **A,** Correction of S-shaped anteroposterior deformity with removal of posterior bone and cartilage *(dark area)* and bilateral anteroposterior scoring on the concave side of the cartilage *(straight and hatched lines)*. **B,** Repositioning of the caudal end of the septum is almost always needed with removal of the overlapping portions of the septal cartilage and maxillary crest bone *(lined areas)* and fixation of the freed cartilage end to the bony anterior nasal spine area.

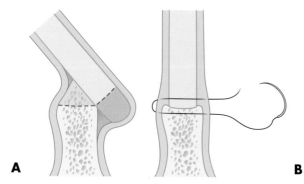

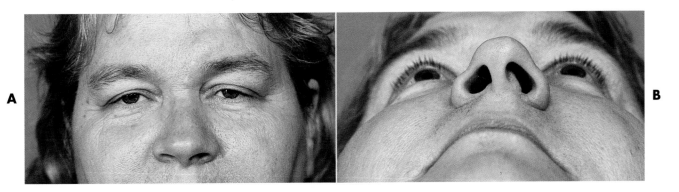

FIGURE 26-18   Female patient with 1-year-old nasal fracture inadequately treated by closed reduction techniques with resultant left-sided septal deviation, right middle and upper vault collapse, and left nasal airway obstruction. She was treated through an endonasal approach with septoplasty and caudal septal fixation, left inferior turbinate reduction, septal spreader graft to the right middle vault, and septal graft to the right nasal side wall. **A,** Preoperative frontal view. **B,** Preoperative submental view.

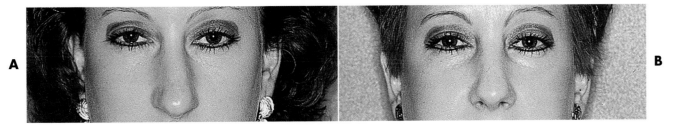

FIGURE 26-19   Female patient with 12-year-old nasal deformity secondary to an untreated fracture she sustained as an adolescent. The resultant septal deformity is superimposed on a preexisting dorsal hump and drooping tip deformity. She was treated with a simultaneous correction of the deviated septum through anteroposterior scoring, limited septal resection, dorsal hump reduction, and superior tip rotation techniques. **A,** Preoperative frontal view. **B,** Frontal view 6 months after operation.

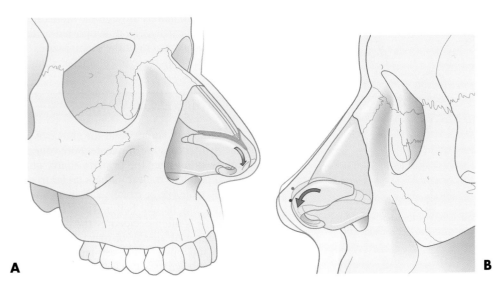

FIGURE 26-20   Inferior tip rotation technique for lengthening an esthetically short nose. **A,** Release of the lower lateral cartilages from their attachments to the upper lateral cartilages, suspensory ligaments, and septum. **B,** Direction of rotation of lower lateral cartilages and their effect on nasal length and tip position.

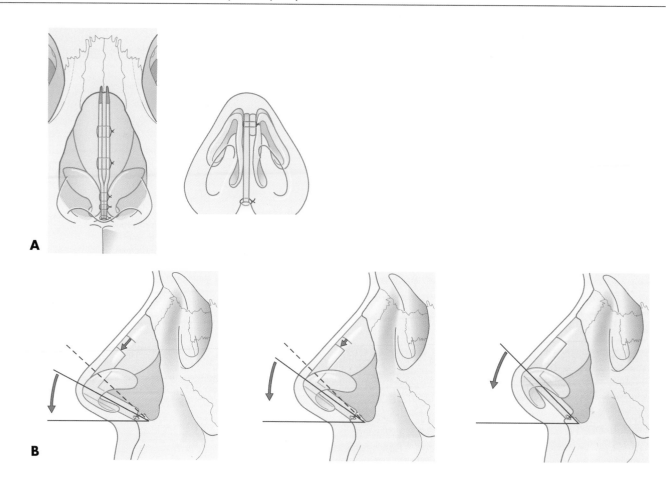

FIGURE 26-21   Dynamic adjustable rotational tip tensioning (DARTT) technique. **A,** Frontal and basal views. **B,** Lateral view demonstrates the degree of tip rotation that can be achieved by adjusting the placement of the septocolumellar interpositional grafts.

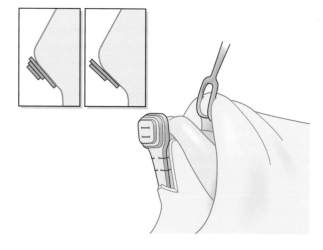

FIGURE 26-22   Lengthening the foreshortened nose through tiered cartilage grafts placed on a primary columellar strut. A stack of two or three grafts can be used.

Columellar Extension

Isolated retraction (impaction) of the columella can be corrected in a variety of ways. Composite auricular grafts added to the caudal end of the septum have been traditionally described as a method of creating columellar extension.[16] A

more effective technique also employs a small auricular cartilage graft, but staggered septal-columellar incisions are made, completely releasing the septal-columellar unit. The graft is then placed through the more caudal incision with the composite cartilage graft supported by the opposite mucosal flap. This extension of the membranous septum provides for a noticeable increase in columellar show.

CONTROVERSIES

The timing of surgery and the choice of grafting material are the primary issues of debate. Some surgeons advocate early intervention after the primary injury once the extent of the nasal problem is clear. Others prefer to wait until the nose is more stable (i.e., cartilage and bone have healed), when the tissues may handle better. There is no clearcut answer, and the issue is often decided by the magnitude of the deformity, the degree of airway obstruction, and the patient's desires. Since the open approach has achieved wide acceptance, earlier intervention can be more easily performed with higher assurance of postoperative stability due to the visibility provided and the ability to more securely fix grafts into the desired positions.

Graft materials are more hotly debated, and there are advocates of both autogenous and alloplastic implants. As elsewhere on the face, both can work successfully if good technique is used and the skin and mucosal cover are of good quality. Autogenous materials clearly require more work to harvest, shape, and place but their long-term benefits almost always justify the effort. This is particularly true for secondary reconstruction of the traumatized nose, where significant restructuring and grafting may be needed and the mucosal coverage may be scarred and less plentiful.

CONCLUSION

The posttraumatic nose can be a difficult problem to correct secondarily, and successful treatment involves an appreciation of the contributions of the nasal bones, septum, and upper and lateral cartilages to both the esthetic and f unctional problems that the patient is experiencing. Optimal correction of the architectural deformities of the traumatized nasal framework, such as saddle nose and short nose problems, requires accurate diagnosis and reconstruction, which is best done through an open approach given the complexity of the anatomical changes. Stable long-term results depend on the surgeon's ability to restore a balance between the tensile and compressive forces of the nasal superstructure.

A wide variety of deformities may be encountered during the secondary treatment of these difficult nasal injuries. A thorough knowledge of the plethora of available techniques is required to achieve optimal results. Onlay and interpositional cartilage grafts, osteotomies, septal repositioning, use of dermal grafts, and occasionally the judicious use of alloplastic materials are the mainstays of treatment. Most patients require a combination of these techniques to either correct or camouflage the nasal problem. These techniques are applied to achieve nasal symmetry, elevation and straightening of the dorsal line, and opening of the internal nasal valve. Improvements in breathing and appearance are almost always achieved, but complete return of the nasal morphology to its pre-injury state may not be attainable in all patients.

ACKNOWLEDGMENT

The authors wish to thank Mark M. Hamilton for his contribution to this chapter in the first edition.

REFERENCES

1. Frodel JL Jr: Primary and secondary nasal bone grafting after major facial trauma. *Facial Plast Surg* 8:194, 1992.
2. Stuzin JM, Kawamoto HK: Saddle nasal deformity. *Clin Plast Surg* 15:83, 1988.
3. Rohrich RJ, Krueger JK, Adams WP Jr, et al: Rationale for submucous resection of hypertrophied inferior turbinates in rhinoplasty: an evaluation. *Plast Reconstr Surg* 108:536-544, 2001.
4. Guyuron B, Uzzo CD, Scull H: A practical classification of septonasal deviation and an effective guide to septal surgery. *Plast Reconstr Surg* 104:2202, 1999.
5. Collawn SS, Fix J, Moore JR, et al: Nasal cartilage grafts: more than a decade of experience. *Plast Reconstr Surg* 100:1547, 1997.
6. Posnick JC, Seagle MB, Armstrong D: Nasal reconstruction with full-thickness cranial bone grafts and rigid internal skeletal fixation through a coronal incision. *Plast Reconstr Surg* 86:894, 1990.
7. Owsley TG, Taylor CO: The use of Gore-Tex for nasal augmentation: a retrospective analysis of 106 patients. *Plast Reconstr Surg* 94:241, 1994.
8. Daniel R: Gore-Tex for nasal augmentation (reply). *Plast Reconstr Surg* 96:229, 1996.
9. Gryskiewicz JM, Rohrich RJ, Reagan BJ: The use of Alloderm for the correction of nasal contour deformities. *Plast Reconstr Surg* 107:561, 2001.
10. Sheen JH: Spreader graft: a method of reconstructing the middle vault following rhinoplasty. *Plast Reconstr Surg* 106:922, 2000.
11. Stal S, Hollier L: The use of resorbable spacers for nasal spreader grafts. *Plast Reconstr Surg* 106:922, 2000.
12. Gunter JP, Rohrich RJ: Lengthening the aesthetically short nose. *Plast Reconstr Surg* 83:793, 1989.
13. Naficy S, Baker SR: Lengthening the short nose. *Arch Otolaryngol Head Neck Surg* 124:809, 1998.
14. Dyer WK II, Yune ME: Structural grafting in rhinoplasty. *Facial Plast Surg* 13:269, 1997.
15. Hamra ST: Lengthening the foreshortened nose. *Plast Reconstr Surg* 108:547, 2001.
16. Dingman RO, Walter C: Use of composite ear grafts in correction of the short nose. *Plast Reconstr Surg* 43:117, 1969.

CHAPTER 27

Secondary Orbital Surgery

Kenneth J. Sneddon, Jeremy Collyer

Residual deformities in the orbital region have several causes: extent and severity of the original injury, tissue loss, associated injuries, inadequate initial diagnosis, compromised initial management, and complications of initial treatment. The severity of the facial injury may make it impossible to achieve a good result after the initial surgical repair, especially if there is extensive tissue loss resulting from the traumatic injury. The extent and severity of associated injuries may preclude optimal management of the facial injuries in the immediate and early posttraumatic periods, leading to delayed or compromised primary surgery. Neurological damage associated with a head injury or direct nerve damage can result in deformities such as ptosis. The damage usually is not repaired at the time of initial management and requires secondary correction. Inadequate diagnosis of the true nature of the injury or poor initial management may lead to poor outcomes. These patients present with residual deformities with cosmetic and functional implications (Fig. 27-1).

ASSESSMENT OF ORBITAL DEFORMITY

An essential step in managing secondary orbital deformity is to list and prioritize problems based on what is causing the patient concern. The typical secondary deformities can be categorized as deformities affecting the external appearance of the orbit or deformities affecting the function of the orbit. Some secondary deformities affect the patient's appearance:

- Defects of the cheek and orbital rim
- Scars: tethering of skin, pigmentary changes
- Changes in position of the globe
  - Anteroposterior position: enophthalmos or exophthalmos (rare)
  - Vertical position: orbital dystopia
  - Lateral position: hypertelorism (rare)
- Lid changes
  - Upper lid: ptosis
  - Lower lid: lid lag, ectropion, entropion
  - Canthal changes: telecanthus

Other types of deformity cause functional problems:

- Visual loss
- Diplopia
- Sensory nerve problems: infraorbital, supraorbital
- Epiphora: lacrimal drainage, abnormal lid contact with the eye
- Dry eyes, corneal exposure
- Obstruction of the coronoid process
- Obstruction of sinus drainage

Patients seek treatment for secondary deformities for many reasons. These injuries can result in obvious and sometimes severe cosmetic defects. Patients can suffer enormous psychological trauma as a result. They may lose self-confidence, and people with previously outgoing personalities can become shy and retiring. In extreme cases, they may withdraw from society and find themselves unable to cope with their work or mix socially with friends. Patients vary enormously in their perception of problems, and the most serious psychological reactions are not necessarily seen in those with the most serious injuries. The patient and the clinician may perceive a deformity very differently. Patients have increasingly high expectations and think that an injury should be corrected and that they should be returned to their pre-injury state. This is not always possible, and one of the clinician's tasks is to combine encouragement and support with realistic expectations of what can be achieved. Injuries causing secondary deformities also are important from a medicolegal standpoint.

The zygomatic complex is the key to the orbital skeleton, and many deformities result from inadequate or misplaced reduction of zygomatic fractures. Inadequately reduced zygomatic fractures and fractures of the orbital walls (i.e., blowout fractures) cause changes in orbital volume and shape, producing enophthalmos and orbital dystopia.

Scarring around the orbital region can have profound effects on facial appearance. Even well-healed scars in this area are obvious and difficult to camouflage. Scar contracture can have serious consequences leading to distortion of anatomical landmarks, particularly in the lower eyelid, where it may result in unsightly ectropion (Fig. 27-2). Tethering of the relatively thin skin of the eyelid and the periorbital area to the underlying bone results in loss of the animation required for normal facial expression.

It is difficult and somewhat artificial to separate the bony and soft tissue elements of these injuries. Inadequate support of the soft tissues due to insufficiet bony reduction further complicates the issue, and difficulties in dealing with scarred,

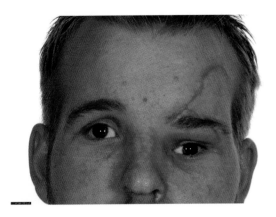

FIGURE 27-1   The combined effects of skeletal and soft tissue elements produced scarring, orbital dystopia, enophthalmos, and loss of cheek contour. Because of the severity of the head injury, management of the facial injuries was not possible in the immediate posttraumatic period.

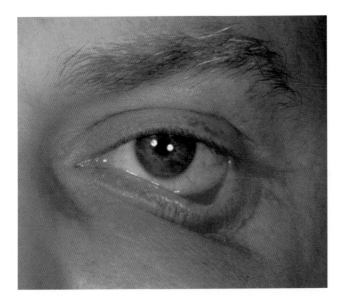

FIGURE 27-2   Infection around an orbital rim plate led to tethering of the overlying skin and an unsightly ectropion.

thickened, and fibrosed soft tissues may lead to poor cosmetic results despite a perfect bony reconstruction. Combinations of skeletal and soft tissue problems produce deformities such as telecanthus and canthal malpositions.

HISTORY AND CLINICAL EXAMINATION

Much information can be gained from a thorough history and clinical examination. The time that has elapsed since the initial injury is relevant; orbital fractures are healed at 3 weeks, but nerve recovery takes months. Some nerve injuries, including superior orbital fissure syndrome and neurapraxia of the infraorbital nerve, have a relatively good prognosis for recovery. Injuries involving the optic nerve have a worse prognosis.

Careful clinical assessment leading to an accurate diagnosis of the deformity is essential for successful management.

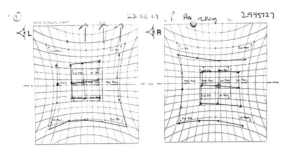

FIGURE 27-3   The Hess chart shows tethering of the inferior rectus.

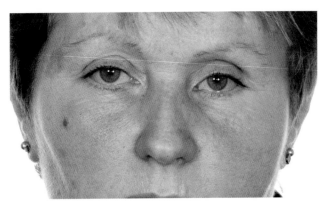

FIGURE 27-4   Supratarsal hooding and obvious shadowing above the left eye are clinical signs of enophthalmos.

Examination must assess facial shape and symmetry as well as the position of the globe in three dimensions and compared with the contralateral side. The eyelids, the brows, and the position of the medial and lateral canthi must also be assessed. The distance from the medial canthus to the facial midline and from the pupil to the lateral orbital rim should be measured and compared bilaterally for symmetry. The position of the malar fat pad over the cheek is crucial to the cosmetic appearance. As a result of trauma or previous subperiosteal dissections, it may migrate inferomedially, accentuating the effect of posterior displacement of the zygomatic complex. Evaluation may identify functional problems, the most common of which is diplopia. Evaluation of diplopia is best achieved by means of Hess charts (Fig. 27-3), fields of binocular vision, or prism bars, which allow objective assessment of ocular movements and estimation of the degree of diplopia.

Enophthalmos is commonly associated with orbital trauma. An eye that sinks into the orbital cavity generates the characteristic clinical appearance of supratarsal hooding, or a supratarsal sulcus deformity, which produces shadowing above the eye (Fig. 27-4). This clinical sign indicates loss of inferoposterior support of the globe. True orbital dystopia may be an associated finding. Clinically, enophthalmos is best assessed by examining the patient from above and behind, looking down on the eyes, and gently retracting the upper eyelids to reveal the globes. This means of clinical examination is surprisingly sensitive, and enophthalmos of 2 to 3 mm can be detected by this method. More formal measurement of enophthalmos is carried out by use of a Keeler frame or

Hertel exophthalmometry; however, both devices use the orbital rim as a reference point and are potentially inaccurate for patients in whom the orbital rim is not intact or is displaced.

IMAGING

Orbital defects are typically assessed with computed tomography (CT). Other choices include conebeam tomography and magnetic resonance imaging (MRI). Conventional helical CT has the advantage of a rapid acquisition time and good detail of hard and soft tissues. The downside of conventional CT is the radiation dose, which increases in proportion to the resolution of the scan. The eye is one of the most radiosensitive tissues, and the threshold for inducing cataracts in adults can be as low as 500 to 2000 mGy. In children, this threshold is even lower, and development of cataracts has been documented at less than one half of the adult dose of radiation. Typically, the dose to the eye is about 50 mGy, depending on the instrument and protocol.

Conebeam tomography scanners are becoming increasingly available to maxillofacial surgeons. They have the advantage of lower radiation dosage, typically about 10% that of conventional tomography. The disadvantage is a lack of soft tissue definition and limitation of scanning volume dictated by the size of the cone.

The least commonly used modality for examination of the orbit is MRI. Standard MRI protocols have long acquisition times and render relatively poor images of the bony anatomy. Soft tissue imaging with MRI is superior to that with CT, and in some circumstances, such as extraocular muscle assessment, MRI is helpful.

DIGITAL PLANNING WITH IMAGING DATA

Rapid expansion in the availability and affordability of computer power in the past 20 years has had a profound impact on every aspect of clinical practice. Imaging has been greatly affected by the underlying digital processes used to acquire data.

Early CT scanners acquired data in a single plane—usually axial because of the patient's position in the scanner. Acquisition of coronal images involved extending the patient's neck so that the coronal plane of the orbits was coincident with the axial plane of the rest of the body. Any restriction of neck extension resulted in an oblique plane of cut through the orbit, making image interpretation difficult. These problems disappeared with the advent of multislice spiral CT scanning. The patient is scanned in the axial plane, and image acquisition is easy, even when the patient is unconscious. The acquired data are used to immediately reconstruct images in axial, sagittal, and coronal planes, making interpretation easier (Fig. 27-5).

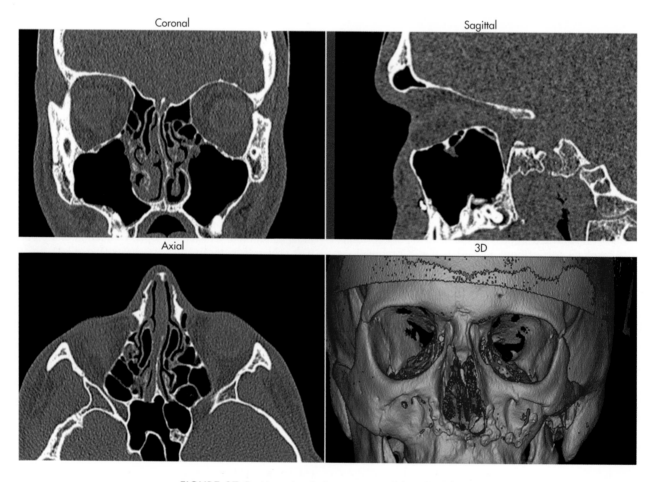

FIGURE 27-5 Normal multiplanar images of the orbital floor.

Orientation of the slices is not fixed with respect to the original acquired slices, which allows for rotation to correct for imprecise alignment of the patient in the scanner. It is therefore feasible to obtain bilateral comparisons that are useful for orbital reconstruction. Accurate orbital volume measurements can be made, arbitrarily shaped pieces can be isolated and moved around, and operations can be simulated. Portions of the normal orbital anatomy can be isolated, duplicated, mirrored, and transposed to the affected side to facilitate planned reconstruction. Even without further application of technology, the detail that can be gained from images of this quality greatly facilitates an accurate diagnosis and formulation of a treatment plan. For example, accurate measurement of the posterior limit of orbital floor defects from the inferior orbital rim gives the surgeon greater confidence in continuing with a posterior dissection without fear of coming across the optic foramen.

Computer-aided manufacture of scanners has greatly extended the scope of this technology. In the early days, modeling was achieved by means of a removal process using models manufactured of expanded polyurethane with a computer-guided milling machine. Reproduction of undercuts was limited with the more widely available machines, which had only three degrees of freedom, but more expensive, five-axis machines were capable of more accurate reproduction. The cost of such machinery was a serious limiting factor. The other main form of model construction under development was stereolithography. In contrast to milling, this was a constructive process in which layer-by-layer polymerization of a curable resin is achieved by a computer-driven laser. This technology was capable of producing models of stunning accuracy but was a lengthy and expensive process. Newer manufacturing processes, including surface deposition modeling, have reduced the costs significantly (Fig. 27-6).

USE OF MIRROR-IMAGE SOFTWARE

A key reason to use software for craniofacial planning is the ability to select portions of the craniofacial skeleton and create mirror copies of the data, resulting in a digital copy of the missing or misplaced hard tissue. This allows the surgeon to visualize the displacement of the orbital fragments and assess the missing tissue. The mirror template can be used in implant manufacture and for intraoperative guidance (Fig. 27-7).

Mirror-image reconstruction was first used for construction of mirror-image milled models of the orbital floor to allow manufacture of custom titanium implants. The small implants are reasonably successful, and they are rigid and accurate[1] (Fig. 27-8). However, this type of reconstruction method relies on a surface anatomical fit for correct positioning of the implant; the contour is not always obvious and can lead to error. The titanium sheet must be produced carefully, taking into account the likely surgical path of insertion. Large titanium implants may exceed the size of the available surgical access in orbital floor reconstruction. This situation can be complicated by the rigidity and hardness of the material; it may not be possible to trim the material in an operating room environment. The final disadvantage is one of cost. Custom materials are always more expensive than off-the-shelf equivalents.

Polyetheretherketone (PEEK) implants are produced based on principles similar to those used for titanium implants. However, the design process is purely digital; no physical models are made during production of the implant. PEEK originally was used as a material in engineering applications. The polymer is highly resistant to degradation in in vivo settings. It is nonporous and easy to sterilize. PEEK is easier to use than titanium for manufacture of complex, three-dimensional shapes such as the bone of the outer orbital frame (Fig. 27-9), and it can be adjusted and drilled using operating room instrumentation. The disadvantage remains the high manufacturing cost.

INTRAOPERATIVE GUIDANCE WITH STEREOTACTIC IMAGING

Frameless stereotactic imaging systems have been used in neurological surgery since the early 1990s. The arrangement consists of a three-dimensional camera system attached to a computer terminal displaying the patient's preoperative imaging (CT or MRI) (Fig. 27-10). The surgical instrumentation is marked with optical markers to allow the camera

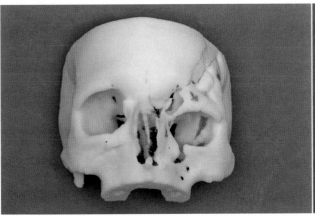
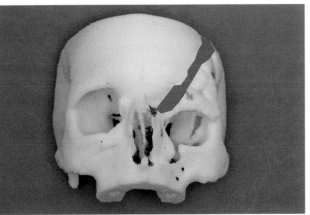

A   **B**

FIGURE 27-6   Stereolithic model of an orbital roof injury (**A**) and outline of a plan for an orbital roof osteotomy (**B**).

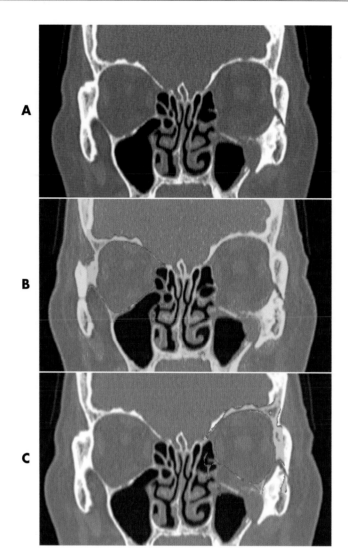

FIGURE 27-7   Computed tomography shows an orbital floor and zygoma fracture (**A**), the normal orbit marked in *blue* (**B**), and a normal orbit mirrored to the injured side to demonstrate fracture displacement (**C**).

system to identify and display their real time position on preoperative imaging. Because these systems can see the anatomical position of instruments in areas of limited surgical access close to vital structures, they have valuable applications in neurosurgery. The same anatomical conditions exist around the orbital apex. However, it is rarely necessary to dissect posterior to the orbital plate of the palatine bone in secondary orbital repair. Navigation offers a significant advantage in orbital dissection when the orbital anatomy is grossly distorted and scarred, but the real advantage is intraoperative verification of the position of reconstructions (Fig. 27-11).

Mirror software can create a virtual position of the ideal reconstruction and then use navigation to confirm that the actual reconstruction is an accurate copy. An advantage of this technique is that it does not depend on a particular reconstructive material. Any graft or alloplastic material can be positioned in the same way. Avoiding custom materials reduces consumable costs, although the capital cost of navigation systems is very high.

Another criticism of navigation systems is the steep learning curve required because of their complexity. A technically simpler approach is to use intraoperative C-arm scanning (combined with mirror-image technology) to confirm the position of reconstructions. However, there are numerous disadvantages, including radiation dosage, the lack of real-time verification, and restriction to radiopaque materials during orbital reconstruction.

ENOPHTHALMOS

Treatment of enophthalmos depends on a thorough understanding of the underlying pathophysiology. Several mechanisms are postulated for the development of posttraumatic enophthalmos:

- Herniation of orbital fat
- Loss of ligamentous globe support
- Increase in orbital volume
- Fat atrophy
- Herniation of extraocular muscles
- Soft tissue contraction

The relative contributions of these factors are controversial. However, it is known that posttraumatic enophthalmos represents an imbalance between orbital contents and orbital volume.

FAT HERNIATION AND LIGAMENTOUS SUPPORT

Manson et al.[2] investigated the relationship between fat and ligaments in the provision of globe support. Orbital fat is traditionally separated into extramuscular and intramuscular compartments, with fine ligaments dividing these compartments.[3] Most of the extramuscular fat compartment exists in the anterior portion of the orbit, whereas posteriorly, almost all of the fat is intraconal. Investigations showed that removal of intraconal fat produced globe displacement similar to clinical enophthalmos. Removal of the extramuscular fat, although it produced globe displacement, was of less significance than loss of the posterior intraconal fat. The average change in globe position in patients undergoing cosmetic blepharoplasty was less than 1 mm, suggesting that anterior extramuscular fat plays little part in globe position. The ligamentous system alone was incapable of maintaining the full forward projection of the globe, for which intramuscular conal fat was required. The importance of the ligamentous sling system of the orbit is evidenced by the observation that removal of the orbital floor as part of a maxillectomy procedure does not lead to a change in globe position as long as the periosteum and sling system remain undisturbed. Removal of bone from multiple orbital walls, by changing the mechanics of the sling system, does alter globe position and is part of the rationale behind orbital decompression for thyroid eye disease.

ORBITAL VOLUME AND FAT ATROPHY

CT allows detailed investigation of the relationship between orbital volume changes and enophthalmos. Several investigators have described the changes in orbital volume and soft

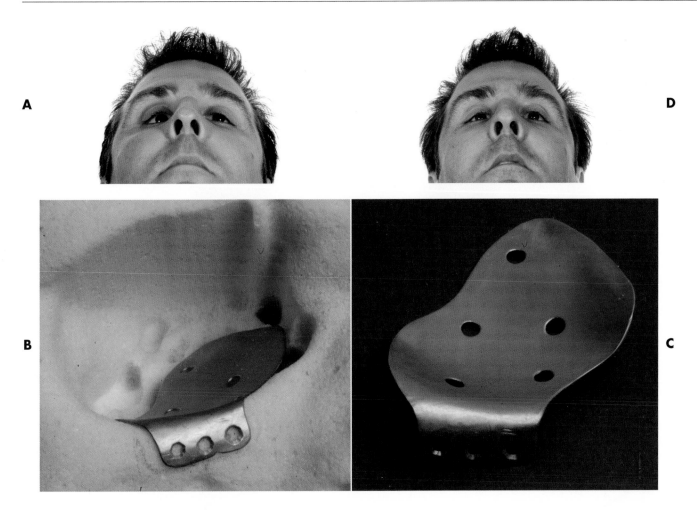

FIGURE 27-8   **A,** Preoperative view of a patient with enophthalmos. **B** and **C,** Custom-made titanium implant used to reconstruct the orbital floor. **D,** Postoperative result.

tissue orbital volumes after injury.[4-6] Thin-slice CT scans can be used to assess orbital volume accurately. They show a linear relationship between increased orbital volume and enophthalmos, with each 1 cm^3 increase in orbital volume leading to 0.47 mm of enophthalmos. Whitehouse et al.[7] demonstrated 0.8 mm of enophthalmos for each 1 cm^3 of orbital expansion. These relationships are valid for fractures more than 4 weeks old when initial posttraumatic edema has settled. Manson et al.[6] investigated bony orbital volume changes and soft tissue volumes within the orbit. Their study revealed a slight (5%) increase in total soft tissue volume and retrobulbar volume (5%), whereas bony orbital volume was increased by up to 18%. Fat and globe volume changes were not significant. Fat atrophy was not a predominant feature in most patients. They also demonstrated that reconstruction of the bony orbit reversed these volume changes and restored globe position. Manson et al.[6] drew the following conclusions:

- The principal mechanism of posttraumatic enophthalmos involves displacement of a relatively constant volume of orbital tissue in the enlarged bony orbit.

- Changes in the shape of the orbital soft tissue to a more spherical configuration allow posterior, inferior, and medial globe displacement.

Although in this chapter we are discussing only the management of secondary deformities, it is clear that early correction of enophthalmos gives superior results. From the data, investigators determined criteria that accurately predicted the likelihood of enophthalmos developing, and they identified cases in which early surgical intervention would be beneficial. Raskin et al.[8] described group 1 fractures (<13% orbital expansion), which failed to demonstrate enophthalmos on follow-up examination, and group 2 fractures (>13% orbital expansion), which frequently demonstrated enophthalmos when managed conservatively.

Manson et al.[6] believed that they can predict the development of enophthalmos in cases in which the orbital floor disruption exceeds a total area of 2 cm^2, the bony orbital volume increase exceeds 1.5 cc or 5%, and significant fat and soft tissue displacement occurs.

Orbital volume is the most relevant factor in posttraumatic enophthalmos. The converse is also true for the rare

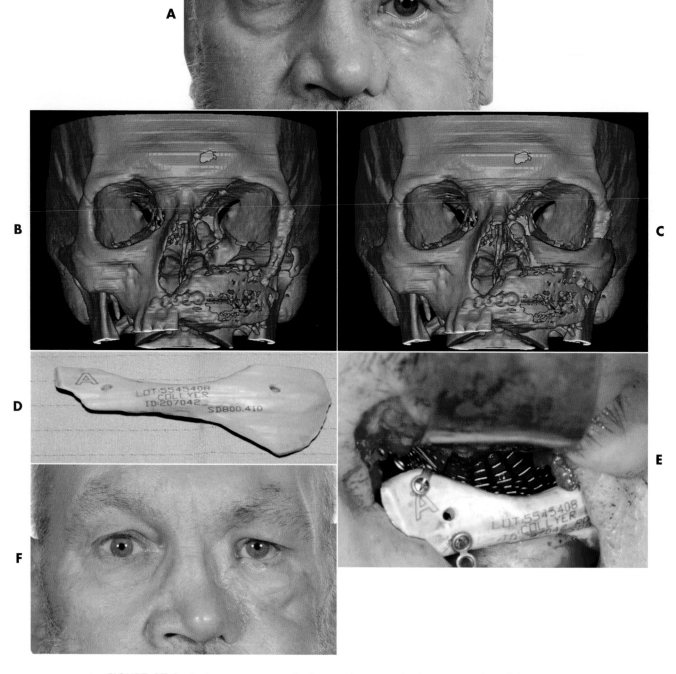

FIGURE 27-9   **A,** Preoperative view. **B,** Computed tomography demonstrates loss of the zygoma and orbital floor and reconstruction of the maxilla with a free flap. **C,** Mirror image of the zygoma in *green* and the orbital floor in *magenta*. **D,** Missing zygoma manufactured in polyetheretherketone (PEEK). **E,** PEEK component in situ with the orbital floor reconstructed in titanium. **F,** Postoperative result.

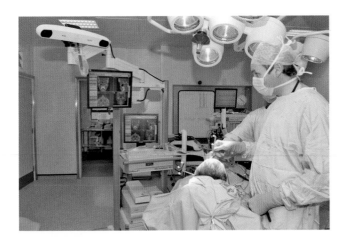

FIGURE 27-10 Navigational setup in the operating room showing an optical camera, optical markers on the patient, and an instrument in the surgeon's right hand.

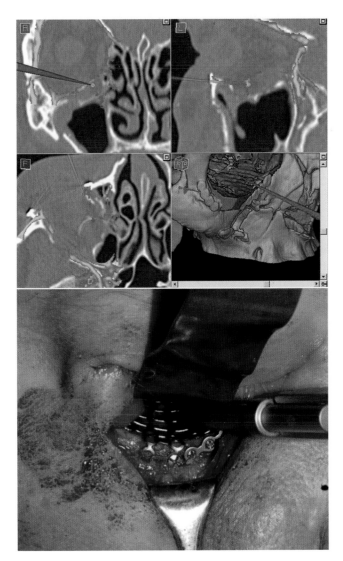

FIGURE 27-11 Intraoperative verification of the position of the orbital floor mesh using navigation.

condition of posttraumatic exophthalmos, in which the orbital volume is reduced as a result of brain herniation through the orbital roof. The curious condition of pulsatile exophthalmos results from high blood flow to the brain.

MATERIALS FOR ORBITAL RECONSTRUCTION

Many materials have been used in the repair of bony orbital wall defects. Each has advantages and disadvantages, and none fulfills all the requirements of the ideal graft material:

- The material should be strong enough to support the orbital contents without herniation into the defect.
- It should be available in thin sheets to bridge defects or to provide bulk for volume expansion.
- It should be easily shaped and molded to the complex anatomical shape required and should retain that shape without memory.
- It should remain dimensionally stable in the long term.
- It should be biocompatible.
- It should be resistant to infection.
- It should be radiopaque but not produce scatter artifact, which impairs future radiological investigations.

Autologous materials include bone (multiple donor sites), septal cartilage, periosteum, and fascia lata. Alloplastic materials can be used and include Silastic, hydroxyapatite, polytetrafluoroethylene (PTFE), coral, titanium, polydioxanone (PDS) sheet, poly-L-lactide (PLLA), and PEEK.

Working on the principle of replacing like with like, autogenous bone is the obvious choice. Bone can be harvested from several sites; for small floor defects, the contralateral antral wall[9] provides a suitably shaped and thin piece of bone. The morbidity associated with the harvest of this graft is the least of the available donor sites. For larger grafts, calvaria and iliac crest are most commonly used.

The calvaria has much to recommend it as a donor site for orbital reconstruction. If a coronal flap has been raised as part of the access for the reconstruction, the graft can be harvested without the need for further incisions and with negligible added morbidity. Even if the orbital floor is approached through a lid incision, only a small hemicoronal flap is required to harvest a suitable piece of bone. The calvaria produces sheets of graft about 2 to 3 mm thick. After repair of the overlying scalp, there is a barely noticeable defect in the skull. If for any reason a craniotomy is required as part of the reconstructive process, the calvaria can be split and the inner table used as graft before the craniotomy is replaced. However, calvarial bone is very dense, and there is a limit to the extent to which it can be shaped. Leaving the periosteum attached to the outer surface allows the bone to be sectioned through its full thickness to give a flexible sheet of bone and periosteum. The very dense nature of this bone is thought to be the reason why it is the most dimensionally stable of the available grafts, particularly when rigidly fixed.

Iliac crest is a useful source of bone grafting material, and it can provide large quantities of bone. The bone is somewhat easier to shape than calvarial bone, but it does exhibit greater resorption. The donor site morbidity is higher and requires a second distant operative site.

Despite the problems of donor site morbidity and lack of dimensional stability due to resorption, autogenous bone remains the material of choice for the reconstruction of large defects. It is less susceptible to infection and more tolerant of it should it develop. Septal cartilage offers a useful autologous alternative to bone.[10] It is easily accessible, is relatively abundant, and provides adequate support to the orbital floor. Donor site morbidity is negligible.

To avoid a donor site and overcome some of the problems associated with the use of autogenous bone, many alloplastic materials have been used in orbital reconstruction. Silastic (i.e., medical-grade silicone polymer) was available in a range of thicknesses and in reinforced and plain forms. It became popular because it was easy to cut to size and shape, and it had sufficient strength to support the orbital contents, particularly in small and medium-sized defects. As with all alloplastic materials, it was susceptible to infection, and rates between 0.4% and 7% were cited. Silastic promotes a foreign-body reaction around it, taking the form of encapsulation of the implant in a dense, nonadherent, fibrous capsule. This fibrous capsule accounts for problems of extrusion of the implants and chronic sinus formation reported up to 20 years after surgery.[11] As a result, Silastic has fallen out of favor and can no longer be recommended as a material for orbital reconstruction.

Titanium has been widely used in orbital reconstruction and has several advantages. It usually is in the form of a mesh and is available in sheets of various thicknesses. It is malleable and therefore easily adapted to the shape of the orbital defect, but it has sufficient strength to support the orbital contents when bridging relatively large defects. It is the most biocompatible of all the available materials. Because of the mesh structure, connective tissue can grow around and through the implant, preventing migration. However, this has the potential disadvantage of making the implant very difficult to remove if required. Titanium produces relatively little artifact on CT and does not therefore preclude subsequent radiological assessment. The mesh structure enables relatively straightforward fixation by placing screws through the mesh. Titanium can be used in solid sheets and perhaps has its greatest potential when used in conjunction with computer-aided design and computer-aided manufacturing (CAD/CAM), of custom-fabricated implants.

Of the nonmetallic alloplastic materials, Gore-Tex (high-density polyurethane) is the most commonly used. As with titanium, it is available in a number of thicknesses to offer various degrees of support to the orbital contents. The thicker sheets have more strength but are more difficult to shape, and the material has a degree of memory, tending to return to its original shape after placement. Medpor can be used in sheet form with channels incorporated in the material, into which can be inserted plates to anchor and secure the material. This is achieved by cantilevering the sheet off the inferior orbital rim. Medpor has a rough surface into which connective tissue can grow to stabilize the implant. However, several cases of infection and displacement have been reported, and as with titanium mesh, removal can be difficult.

A resorbable material that can provide sufficient rigidity and support until bony healing is followed by total resorption is appealing. The advent of PDS sheets generated much excitement, because it initially appeared to offer these desired properties. As research results were published, however, some complications became apparent. Common postoperative sequelae included sensory disturbance, restriction of globe motility, and enophthalmos developing after orbital repair. PDS is resorbed by a process of hydrolytic dissolution. Early loss of support after only 4 weeks has been demonstrated; this is not sufficient time to allow adequate bony healing of the orbital defect. Moreover, cyst-like lakes and so-called sterile sinus formation were associated with the implant material. This material is not considered suitable for the repair of large defects.

Poly-L-lactic acid/polyglycolic acid copolymer (Lacto-Sorb) has been investigated.[12] It has potential for orbital floor repair.

TREATMENT

When dealing with secondary corrections, it is useful to differentiate cases in which the initial injury is confined to the internal orbit (often referred to as orbital blowout injuries, although more accurately identified as orbital wall and floor defects) from those in which there is disruption of the orbital framework. The latter cases result from previously untreated or inadequately treated zygomatic or nasoethmoidal injuries. Treatment in these cases always involves initially correcting the orbital framework before moving on to correct internal orbital damage.

INTERNAL ORBITAL INJURIES

For internal orbital injuries, the aim of treatment is to restore globe position and release any mechanical entrapment that may be contributing to diplopia. Because the orbital framework is intact, there is no change in facial contour. The classic pure blowout fracture typically produces an orbital floor defect of less than 2 cm^2 that occurs in the anterior or middle part of the orbit.

Small Defects

Repair of small defects (<2 cm^2) usually is straightforward. A cutaneous or transconjunctival approach to the orbital floor is used,[6-9] and the defect is reached by subperiosteal dissection of the orbital contents, proceeding from the orbital rim backward. After the defect is outlined, the herniated orbital contents are freed from the maxillary sinus and gently returned to the confines of the orbital cavity. The choice of material for orbital repair in these fractures is not critical. A thin sheet of the chosen repair material is shaped to cover the defect, and if it can be made to overlap the margins of the defect onto sound bone all around, it usually does not require fixation (Fig. 27-12). The weight of the orbital contents resting on it serves to stabilize the repair.

Large Defects

Correction of some orbital floor defects is not straightforward. This is especially the case with secondary reconstructions.

In complex orbital wall defects, the defect extends to involve more than one of the orbital walls (most often the floor and medial wall, but any combination is possible) and backward into the posterior third of the orbit (Fig. 27-13). For these large defects (>2 cm^2), the orbital volume must be

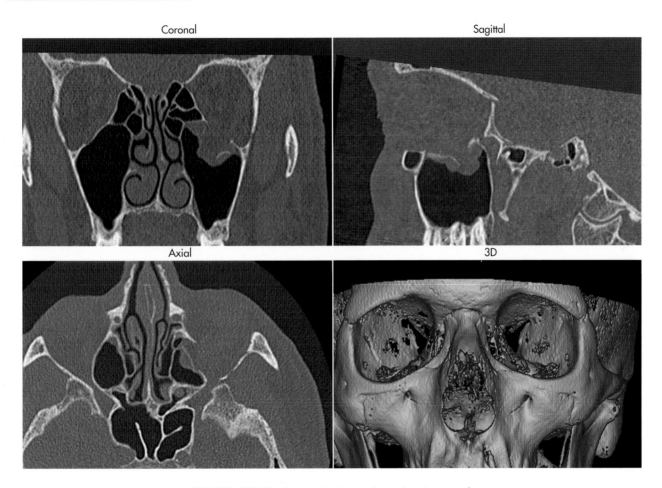

Coronal

Sagittal

Axial

3D

FIGURE 27-12 The small orbital defect is less than 2 cm².

restored, and to achieve satisfactory results, the precise shape of the orbit must also be reconstructed.

The orbit is classically described as an open pyramid with its apex posteriorly; however, the walls of the pyramid are not flat. The orbital floor behind the orbital rim is concave until a point just behind the equator of the globe, where it becomes convex, inclining upward at about 30 degrees and creating a retrobulbar constriction in the orbit. This arrangement combines with a roughly 45-degree inclination of the floor from the lateral to the medial wall to produce a prominent posteromedial and inferomedial bulge. This bulge behind the globe and adjacent to and on the medial side of the posterior extent of the inferior orbital fissure is a critical area in orbital reconstruction. This posterior medial wall area is the region Hammer[13] described as the *key area* (Fig. 27-14), and its reconstruction is essential in gaining anterior projection of the globe.

Reconstruction of these complicated, multiwall orbital defects is difficult. Essential to a satisfactory repair is adequate exposure and dissection around the entire defect. Exposure in these cases is rarely sufficient through a lower lid approach alone. A transconjunctival incision with the addition of a lateral canthotomy allows far greater exposure of the orbital cavity, and a transcaruncular extension medially gives even greater exposure of the medial wall. These two extensions of the standard transconjunctival incision still give access to only about two thirds of the circumference of the

orbit. To allow full 360-degree dissection of the orbit as advocated by Hammer,[13] a lower lid incision must be combined with a coronal approach. This gives the best exposure of the medial wall and is the only incision to provide adequate exposure of the nasoethmoidal complex. To maximize the nasoethmoidal exposure, it is necessary to incise the periosteum on the deep side of the flap in the region of the nasal bridge.

ORBITAL DISSECTION

Subperiosteal orbital dissection can be more difficult in secondary corrections because of dense scarring and adherence of orbital tissue to periorbital structures. The correct plane of dissection is most easily established by starting from an uninjured part of the orbit and approaching the defect from all sides. To gain complete exposure of the orbital cavity, a number of structures must be divided, including several small vessels that run from the infraorbital bundle to the periorbita. Dissecting back along the orbital floor, using the infraorbital nerve as a guide, the surgeon comes across the contents of the inferior orbital fissure, which prevent further dissection in a posterior direction. There are no anatomical structures of importance running through the inferior orbital fissure, and its contents should be divided after careful coagulation with bipolar diathermy.

The orbital fissure can be followed posteromedially toward the apex of the orbit. At the anterior margin of the orbital

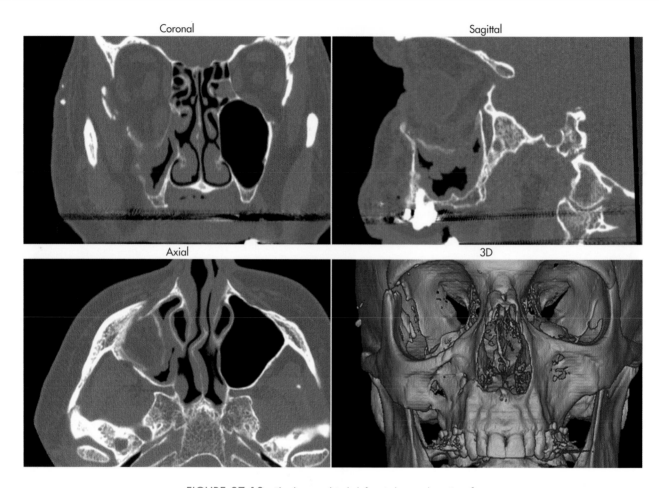

FIGURE 27-13   The large orbital defect is larger than 2 cm².

apex lies the orbital plate of the palatine bone. This structure is a key landmark[14] in orbital reconstruction because it is frequently preserved after orbital trauma, and it represents a sound posterior bony ledge on which to rest a reconstruction (Fig. 27-15). After the anterior and posterior limits of the floor are established, dissection of the medial wall can take place. Division of the anterior ethmoidal artery high on the medial wall significantly improves access in this area.

If the periorbita has been perforated, orbital fat herniates through and bulges over the retractors on the medial and lateral sides, further hampering visibility. Two retractors are often more useful than one large malleable strip. The most useful retractor is fashioned by cutting a sheet of Silastic to the approximate dimensions of the orbit. This instrument is placed underneath normal malleable strips, preventing herniation of fat over the edge of the retractor.

After the defect has been identified, the herniated orbital contents must be freed and returned to the confines of the orbital cavity. In the acute setting, this can usually be achieved with little difficulty, but this task is much less readily accomplished in a secondary reconstruction. The surgeon often must resort to careful sharp dissection to release the orbital contents from the margins of the defect and adjacent periorbital tissues. This tissue can be surprisingly vascular, and thorough bipolar coagulation is required during dissection.

After the displaced orbital contents have been released, the true nature and extent of the orbital wall defects become apparent. If difficulty is experienced in freeing the defect, extra access can be gained by orbitotomies. Removal of a portion of the orbital rim improves visualization of the defect and access to it (Fig. 27-16), especially for posteriorly placed defects. A suitable plate is first shaped and temporarily fixed to the orbital rim to allow accurate repositioning of the segment at the end of the procedure. A portion of the orbital rim is removed with a fine saw or bur. In effect, an orbitotomy—a zygomatic fracture—may already have taken place. In cases of a combined fractured zygoma and orbital floor reconstruction, it is wise to complete the orbital floor dissection before reducing the zygomatic fracture.

BONE VERSUS ALLOPLAST IN RECONSTRUCTION

Once identified and fully exposed, the defect is often extensive and has a complicated, three-dimensional shape. For these large and complex defects, the reconstructive material is rigid and dimensionally stable. The shape and contour of the material must be controlled to reconstruct the depression in the orbital floor immediately under the globe and the inferomedial bulge posterior to the globe's equator. Reconstruction of these areas with a flat material overcorrects the area under the globe and undercorrects the area behind the globe. The result is a globe that is elevated and enophthalmic (Fig. 27-17).

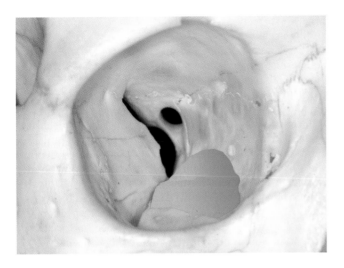

FIGURE 27-14   The inferomedial bulge, which Hammer[13] describes as a key area, is shown in *orange*.

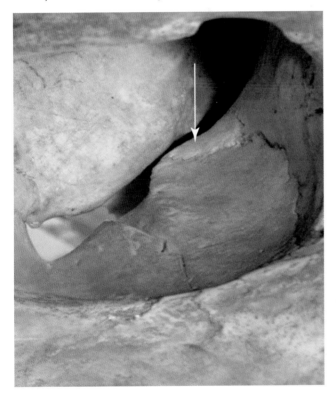

FIGURE 27-15 The *arrow* indicates the orbital plate of the palatine bone.

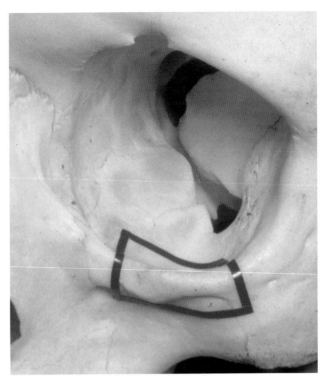

FIGURE 27-16   Inferior orbitotomy. Removing a section of rim from the inferior, lateral, or superior aspect affords greater access to and visibility of posterior defects.

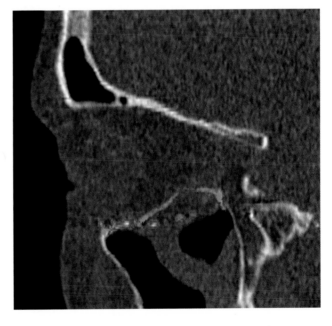

FIGURE 27-17   The error of using a flat plate. The plate position is marked in *blue*, and the ideal position of the orbital floor is marked in *green*.

One solution is to reconstruct the orbit with multiple layers of flat material. This can be achieved by starting with a flat bone graft that lies along the orbital floor and is held in place at the infraorbital margin. Additional layers of bone grafting can be added posterior to the globe to restore the inferior medial bulge. This method of using bone as graft was advocated by Hammer.[13]. In the correction of enophthalmos, overcorrection is considered to be the key to long-term success. Globe position changes after reconstruction. It is assumed that this reversion is related to resorption of bone graft material (about 30%), although some minor reduction in soft tissue volume is also likely after reconstruction.

Perioperative edema at the time of reconstruction can be misleading and can result in an underestimate of the degree of enophthalmos correction that has been achieved.

The other solution is to use a single piece of material that is correctly contoured to the shape of the orbital floor.

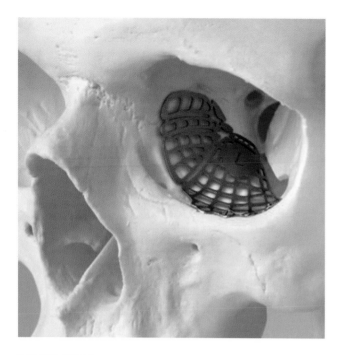

FIGURE 27-18 The orbital floor plate is prebent to the average shape of the orbital floor. (© by Synthes)

Re-creation of the complex curves and bulges of the orbital floor is impossible with a single piece of calvarial bone, but it can be done with titanium mesh. The mesh must be malleable enough to contour to the correct shape but rigid enough to allow insertion of the plate without distortion of the carefully contoured shape. A refinement is to construct the plate on the basis of the average shape of the orbital floor and medial wall (Fig. 27-18). These plates represent a significant advance because the inferior medial bulge is an inherent part of the plate design. The challenge that remains is positioning the plate correctly. This is difficult when substantial amounts of the medial orbital wall are missing, because there is no medial bony ledge on which to rest the reconstruction plate. In these cases, innovations such as intraoperative navigation can help to verify the plate's position.

ORBITAL FRAME INJURIES: ZYGOMATIC FRACTURES

In all cases of orbital trauma repair, the first stage of treatment is reconstruction of the orbital skeleton. This concept applies equally to secondary repair, although there are significant added difficulties compared with the early management of these injuries. For example, the fractures have healed, and bony continuity has been reestablished. Osteotomies of the zygomatic complex are therefore required to mobilize the bony fragments and allow repositioning. The situation varies slightly between cases in which there has been no previous surgery and those in which there has been inadequate reduction in the past. In cases of no previous surgery, there may be gross dislocations of large fragments resulting in significant deformities of the zygomatic complex. There may be bony union or areas of fibrous union with soft tissues interspersed between bone fragments. In cases of previous attempts at

surgical correction, better bony contact and good bone healing usually exist.

The principal problem in these cases is inaccurate reduction of the original bony injury, usually with rotation around the vertical axis of the zygomatic complex. Very small rotational discrepancies can lead to significant changes in the orbital volume. This problem can best be visualized by looking at the lateral orbital wall behind the lateral rim. This substantial piece of bone usually reduces well. Steps seen in this area indicate rotational discrepancies and an inaccurate reduction. The other common problem is fixation of the zygomatic arch. This is an area where mistakes are often made. It often is assumed that the arch is indeed an arch form and is therefore fixed with a gentle curve. However, on closer inspection, this is not the case. The zygomatic arch projects in a relatively straight line and is often fixed with too much of a curve. This shortening and overbending of the arch lead to outward rotation of the zygoma, creating a defect in the lateral orbital wall, lack of anterior projection of the maxilla, and an increase in facial width.

In fracture repair, the reconstruction is essentially a jigsaw puzzle with all bony fragments present. After the fragments have been adequately reduced, they tend to fit nicely together and can be fixed in position to give a true anatomical reduction. This typically is not the case with secondary or delayed reconstructions. Soon after injury, the bone ends round off and change shape slightly. Small fragments may devitalize and subsequently resorb. The net effect of these changes is that simple reduction of the fragments (as in early fracture repair) does not lead to restoration of the original pre-injury state, and indeed, this may not be possible. The best orbital framework that can be achieved is produced by realignment of the fragments. This often results in small gaps, which can be spanned by plates or filled with bone graft to restore continuity (Fig. 27-19).

Exposure

In secondary corrections, wide exposure is essential to allow accurate three-dimensional reconstruction. Although a zygomatic osteotomy can be successfully achieved through local incisions alone in some simpler cases, a coronal flap usually is required to gain adequate exposure. This flap must be brought down sufficiently to expose subperiosteally the whole area involved in the original injury, exposing the entire zygomatic arch and the body of the zygoma. Some argue that to achieve the greatest accuracy in reconstruction and to gauge symmetry, the coronal flap should be reflected sufficiently to expose the contralateral zygoma for comparison. This extra exposure is not necessary if intraoperative navigation is used to verify the position of the fragments. In addition to the coronal flap, access is required to the area of the zygomatic buttress through an incision intraorally in the buccal sulcus and an incision to expose the infraorbital rim.

Careful planning of the approach to the orbital rim is required in secondary corrections. The choice of incision may be predicated by incisions used in previous operations, or there may be scars resulting from the original injury that can be used and revised at the same time. There may be existing problems of lower eyelid position as a result of the original injury, and some degree of shortening of the lower eyelid may exist. The incision used must take these factors into account and must not risk worsening the situation. For these reasons,

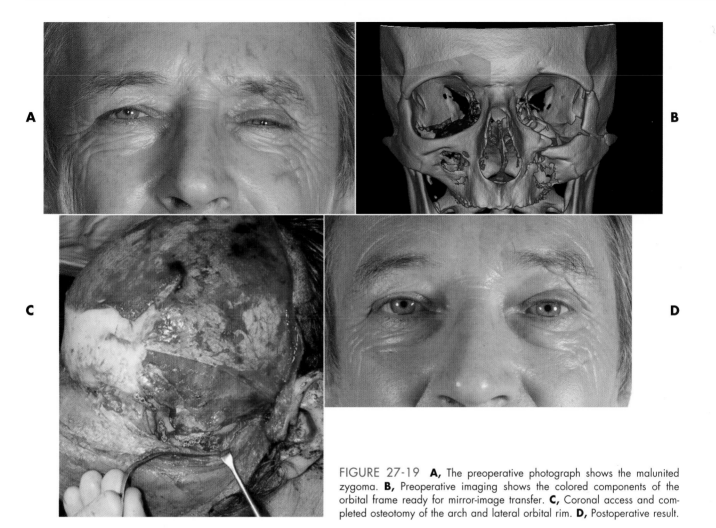

FIGURE 27-19 **A,** The preoperative photograph shows the malunited zygoma. **B,** Preoperative imaging shows the colored components of the orbital frame ready for mirror-image transfer. **C,** Coronal access and completed osteotomy of the arch and lateral orbital rim. **D,** Postoperative result.

very high subciliary or blepharoplasty incisions often are best avoided in secondary corrections. The choice of incision often rests between an infraorbital incision made transcutaneous close to the infraorbital rim and a lid swing approach. The lid swing approach starts with a lateral canthotomy and inferior cantholysis, releasing the lower eyelid. The lower eyelid is then retracted, allowing dissection posterior to the orbital septum. The aim of both approaches is to avoid scarring in the orbital septum, which causes middle lamellar shortening and lid lag. It is often better to complete the approach to the infraorbital rim before raising the coronal flap. Subperiosteal exposure of the zygomatic complex is required, and it may be more difficult in areas where there is tethering of the overlying soft tissue to underlying fracture lines or plates. Areas where the overlying soft tissues have been damaged by the original injury may make elevation difficult.

Reduction

After full exposure of the injured area, the site and extent of the deformity are usually obvious. Even if there has been good bony healing, the original fracture lines are usually apparent. The fractures have to be re-created to allow repositioning of the fragments. Bony repair often is not fully consolidated, making it possible to open these fracture lines by prising them apart with an osteotome. If this is not the case, a combination

of chisels or a surgical saw may be used. Separation is achieved at the frontozygomatic (FZ) suture, the zygomatic arch, and the infraorbital rim. The cut at the infraorbital rim is extended downward to pass through the area of the zygomatic buttress being accessed at this point through the intraoral incision. The next step is to join the cuts at the infraorbital rim and the FZ suture. This is best achieved about 4 to 5 mm inside the orbital margin by means of a fine bur or osteotome.

It is often necessary to remove bone to allow correct realignment of the fragments, and this is particularly the case at the FZ suture. The amount of bone that needs to be removed can be calculated by measuring the degree of orbital dystopia against the uninjured side. With the FZ suture temporarily wired at the correct height, the zygoma is repositioned using the lateral orbital wall as a guide to avoid rotation. Straightening the zygomatic arch and comparing it with the contralateral side helps to achieve a good position. The fragments are rigidly fixed with plates. Microplates usually are sufficient across the infraorbital rim, where there is considerable advantage in their small size, but heavier plates are placed at the FZ suture, the zygomatic buttress, and across the zygomatic arch. To achieve stable fixation in three dimensions, fixation is placed at least at three points.

Because of the nature of these injuries, there are often gaps between the bone ends; although they can be bridged by plates, they should be filled with bone graft to ensure a smooth postoperative contour. Small, negative-contour deformities often remain after repositioning the zygoma, and they can be filled with bone chips or small onlays. Positive deformities can be smoothed with a bur.

NASOETHMOIDAL FRACTURES

The nasoethmoidal area poses some of the biggest challenges in secondary reconstruction. Small degrees of deformity, if symmetrical, may be acceptable, but any degree of asymmetry is usually disfiguring and unacceptable to the patient. Although many patterns of fracture may present, they are traditionally classified according to the size of the central canthal-bearing fragment[15]:

- Type I fractures exhibit a large central fragment consisting of the entire medial portion of the orbital rim with the medial canthal ligament attached to it.
- Type II fractures show disruption of the inner orbital frame into several pieces, but with the ligament attached to a piece of bone of sufficient dimensions to allow direct fixation.
- In type III fractures, the central fragment is severely comminuted. There may be complete avulsion of the canthal ligament, or more commonly, it remains attached to a very small fragment of bone that is, however, too small to allow direct fixation.

There is some doubt about the correlation of this classification with clinical outcomes, and it is not frequently used. For secondary corrections, the classification is less clinically relevant because the fractures often have united.

Secondary deformity of the nasoethmoidal region manifests as flattening and foreshortening of the nose, resulting in an upturned appearance of the nostrils. Traumatic telecanthus (Fig. 27-20) is cosmetically unacceptable because of increased spacing of the eyes and blunting of the canthal angle at the medial end of the palpebral fissure. There may be associated injuries to the frontal sinus or the lacrimal drainage system. A dacryocystogram is useful in the assessment of these injuries.[16]

In principle, the approach to secondary correction is straightforward: One mobilizes or refractures the fragments and fixes them in the correct position after reduction. However, practice is much more complicated than theory.

The first step is to mobilize the bony nasal skeleton, including the lacrimal crest and the canthal attachment. If it remains attached, the canthal insertion must not be stripped during the subperiosteal exposure, because a perfect re-creation of the normal anatomical configuration is rare. The nasal complex tends to telescope inside the frontonasal region, and reduction requires that the central nasal fragment be pulled out to full length. Fixation of the nasal root to the frontal bone can be achieved by means of miniplates; an inverted Y-plate often works well in this region (Fig. 27-21). Associated fractures of the frontal sinus must be repaired first.

The nasal bones at the time of secondary repair often appear to have healed well but are splayed. Simple fixation of the central fragment would result in increased nasal width, militating against complete correction of the telecanthus. Nasal widening is accentuated by the often significantly increased soft tissue thickness in this area as a result of previous injury. To combat these problems, it is important to obtain as much skeletal narrowing as possible. If there has been extensive comminution, healing can result in the production of considerable callus, which widens the nasal bridge. This callus must be reduced with a bur. A small plate can be placed horizontally across the bridge of the nose to compress the two sides into an acceptable shape. Surgeons claim that it is almost impossible to overcorrect traumatic telecanthus. If there is no large, central nasal fragment, bone grafting may be required to recontour the nasal bridge or to re-create the nasofrontal angle. Bone grafting may also be required to reconstruct the medial orbital wall and to provide a site to which the medial canthal ligament may be reattached. Calvarial bone grafts harvested from the outer or inner table of the parietal skull are ideal for these purposes and can be obtained through a surgical approach.

If there has been extensive comminution or loss of bone from the nasal area, it is reconstructed with the use of a strut graft cantilevered off the frontal bone. In cases of secondary

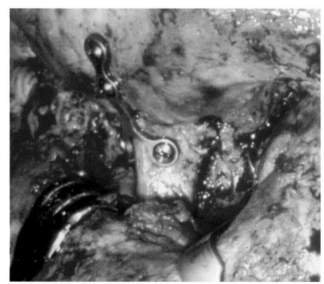

FIGURE 27-21 A Y-plate is used to stabilize the nasal bridge. The inferior limbs of the Y can be compressed to narrow the nasal bone, and if sufficiently posterior, the screw hole can anchor a suture passed through the medial canthus.

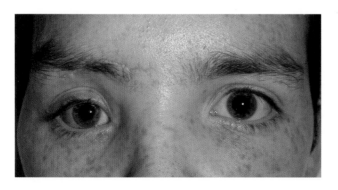

FIGURE 27-20 Traumatic telecanthus.

reconstruction, scarring and contraction of the overlying skin may render placement of a sufficiently large graft to provide the required contour difficult. There is always a danger of too large a graft perforating through the overlying skin, and care must be taken to avoid this complication.

MEDIAL CANTHUS DETACHMENT

Reattachment of the medial canthus is one of the most demanding aspects of secondary reconstruction. Proper reduction of telecanthus depends on accurate repositioning of the medial canthal ligament, and an understanding of the anatomy is crucial.[17] The medial canthal ligament is a complex, three-dimensional structure, not a simple single ligament as is often imagined. The key to optimal canthal reattachment is appreciation of the fact that the true anatomical attachment is more posteriorly placed than is often realized. If the reattachment is placed too anteriorly, a disappointing cosmetic result is obtained, with the medial palpebral angle distracted from the globe. This produces an unsightly asymmetry even though the true intercanthal distance may be correct.

The nature of the canthal detachment determines the technique used for reattachment. The canthus usually remains attached to a small fragment of bone, and with available microplates, it is possible to obtain fixation of this canthus-bearing fragment to its anatomical position.[18] If this can be achieved with a good degree of solidity, a stable result can be expected. Rarely, the canthus is avulsed from the bone and has no bony fragment attached to it, making identification and reattachment of the canthus difficult. To aid in the identification of the canthal ligament, the deep aspect of the inner canthal angle can be picked up with a fine dissecting forceps. When traction is placed on the forceps in a medial direction, the canthal angle is seen to move freely if the canthus has been correctly identified. If the medial end of the detached canthus remains elusive, it can be located near the lacrimal sac by passing a needle through the canthal angle and identifying it on the deep surface posterior to the lacrimal sac. A fine wire suture is passed through the canthus, and if the site is properly identified, pulling on this wire should pull the canthal angle in the desired direction and reduce the telecanthus.

If this test result is satisfactory, some form of canthopexy must be performed. It may be possible to perform a direct canthopexy, attaching the canthus to plates placed in the region of the anterior and posterior lacrimal crests. If there is a sufficiently substantial piece of bone in the correct position, tendon anchors may be used to attach the canthus.[19] Both means of direct canthopexy have an advantage over the more traditional transnasal canthopexy in that it is somewhat easier to obtain posterior positioning of the canthal attachment. If there is insufficient bone, a transnasal canthopexy must be performed. The wire suture attached to the canthus is passed across the nasal skeleton, and fixation achieved on the contralateral side.

The holes are positioned to allow passage of the wires through the nose to obtain the desired direction of pull on the medial canthus. Placement of the holes is aided by identifying any portion of the lacrimal crest or by referencing the contralateral side. The holes are made with a drill bur or nasal awl. The holes must be placed farther posteriorly than is often imagined. This can be technically challenging because it is often difficult to obtain the correct angulation of the drill without interference from the globe.

After being passed through the nose, the canthopexy wires are fixed to a small plate or screw on the opposite nasal bone. If bilateral canthopexy is required, wires are passed from either side of the nose. Fixation in these patients was always difficult, and it used to be the practice to pass the wires back over the nasal bridge and twist the right and left wires together, producing a circumferential wire. With modern microplates, this is rarely required, and adequate fixation usually can be achieved. Tightening of the canthopexy wires is continued while the intercanthal distance is measured to achieve a correct reduction. It is wise to overcorrect somewhat to allow for some relapse. Final tightening of the canthopexy is the last step in a secondary correction, because after the canthal attachment has been reestablished, access to the medial orbital wall and lacrimal system is impeded.

It is often prudent to support the canthopexy from the cutaneous surface. This can be achieved by the use of clear acrylic buttons. It is important not to overtighten the button, because there is a risk of skin necrosis. The clear acrylic makes surveillance for necrosis easier.

LACRIMAL SYSTEM DAMAGE

The lacrimal system is often damaged by midfacial and especially by nasoethmoidal trauma. Damage is best repaired early because the lacrimal system can become encased in dense scar tissue, making secondary repair very difficult. Lacrimal drainage may be problematic despite a patent system. This occurs when the medial eyelid is not in proper alignment with the lacus. Eyelid contraction and canthal malposition can be responsible for this problem. The lacrimal system is investigated with a dacryocystogram.[13] Secondary repair by dacryocystorhinostomy is indicated, but it is technically challenging in the presence of often considerable scar tissue. The use of Lester Jones tubes is an alternative.

SOFT TISSUES

RECONSTRUCTION CONSIDERATIONS

Accurate repositioning of the bony elements of the zygoma and orbital rim does not lead to uniformly successful results, largely because of the overlying soft tissue drape. The soft tissue changes associated with severe bony injuries are often underestimated and militate against good results in secondary reconstruction. Soft tissue injury may be evident, with extensive lacerations or degloving-type injuries. These injuries leave scars, but the more subtle soft tissue injuries often contribute to secondary deformity. Tethering of the overlying soft tissue to areas of underlying bony injury may produce an obvious deformity. Displacement of the cheek fat pad produces obvious sagging of the face, with accentuation of the nasolabial fold and apparent flattening in the infraorbital area.

For esthetic reconstruction the soft tissue, all elements must be fully considered, and after completion of the bony skeletal reconstruction, the soft tissues must be redraped across the cheek. For the soft tissues to be mobilized sufficiently to allow redraping, extensive subperiosteal dissection is required to release any tethering. Deep-plane face-lift techniques are used to resuspend the soft tissues in their correct position. Subperiosteal sutures are used anteriorly to anchor the cheek fat pads to the inferior orbital rim, and laterally, a superficial musculo-aponeurotic system (SMAS) plication gives support to the tissue over the lateral cheek. If a coronal flap has been raised to gain access, excess skin can be excised to tighten the soft tissues when final suturing takes place, as is done in a standard face-lift procedure.

Attention must be paid to the correct canthal position. The medial canthal position was previously discussed in terms of nasoethmoidal injuries, but the lateral canthal position is also important. Unlike the medial canthal ligament, whose attachment is preserved if possible, the lateral canthal ligament is routinely detached when raising a coronal flap. This is done because it significantly increases exposure while being relatively straightforward to reattach. The lateral canthal ligament should be reattached to the lateral orbital rim in a slightly overcorrected position. This is best achieved by drilling a small hole at an appropriate point in the lateral orbital wall and suturing the ligament to it with a non-resorbable suture.

Minor contour irregularities often remain after bony reconstruction. They are best managed by small onlay grafts.

EYELIDS

After orbital trauma, asymmetry of the eyes is one of the most obvious deformities. Changes in the width of the palpebral fissure, canthal malpositions, and lid abnormalities are immediately noticeable.

Ectropion is a common lid problem. There are several possible causes of ectropion, but in the posttraumatic scenario, cicatricial ectropion is the most likely. In addition to the esthetic deformity, several functional problems may arise, including drying of the eyes with corneal irritation and epiphora if the punctum is no longer in contact with the tear pool. Six elements of pathology may manifest in an ectropic eyelid: horizontal lid laxity, medial canthal tendon laxity, punctal malposition, vertical tightness of the skin, orbicularis paresis, and disinsertion of the lower eyelid retractors. One or more of these features may be present in any one lid. Accurate identification of the underlying anatomical abnormality allows selection of the appropriate procedure for surgical correction.

Other than trauma, the most common cause of ectropion is vertical shortening of the anterior lamella, which pulls the eyelid away from the globe. Vertical shortening may arise from a single vertical scar crossing the lid margin. Scar contraction leads to ectropion, and there is often associated notching of the lower lid. Vertical tightness may result from contraction of surgical approaches to the lower lid. Infraorbital incisions are more prone to late ectropion than transconjunctival approaches. Overenthusiastic suturing of the deeper layers is often responsible. It is recommended that only the periosteum over the orbital rim should be closed and then the overlying skin. Vertical shortening is best treated by Z-plasty or skin grafting.

Z-Plasty

A Z-plasty is used to release the tension in a scar and reorient the limbs of the scar in a more appropriate direction. The Z-plasty works by the principle of transferring tissue to reduce pull in one direction at the expense of a line perpendicular to it. In the case of a vertical scar running across the lower eyelid, this releases the downward pull leading to ectropion and converts the scar to run parallel to the lid margin.

The linear margins of the scar are outlined. A line is drawn from the superior and inferior ends of the scar at 60 degrees and in opposite directions. These lines should be equal to the vertical length of the scar. The old scar is excised by cutting round the markings, and the lines drawn are incised. The resultant skin flaps, when raised, produce two equal triangles. They are undermined widely until they can be transposed with ease and without undue tension. The delicate skin flaps must be handled with care to avoid damage to the skin margin. The flaps are sutured in position with 6-0 nylon sutures. The lower lid should be supported and placed under some tension by a temporary tarsorrhaphy or, more comfortably, by using a Frost suture taped to the brow. For longer vertical scars, two or more Zs can be placed along the vertical limb.

Skin Grafting

When the vertical shortening extends over a more diffuse area, skin grafting is the treatment of choice. In terms of functional and esthetic results, full-thickness grafts are preferable to split-thickness skin in the lower lid area. The skin can be harvested with relative ease from the postauricular area. A horizontal incision is made parallel to and about 2 to 4 mm below the lid margin. The incision is carried down to the depth necessary to release all scar bands and allow the eyelid to return to its normal position. A Frost suture is used to place gentle upward traction on the lower lid. A template is fashioned from a suture packet, and a full-thickness graft is harvested from the postauricular region. The graft must be thoroughly defatted before application. Meticulous hemostasis is required before placing the graft, because hematoma formation beneath it will jeopardize survival.

The graft is best secured using 6-0 silk sutures spaced evenly around the margins of the defect. Alternate sutures are left long to secure a proflavine-soaked bolus tie-over dressing, which should remain in situ for 1 week. It is prudent to support the lower lid with a Frost suture for the first postoperative week.

Horizontal Laxity

Horizontal laxity of the lower lid may manifest medially or laterally (Fig. 27-22). It is the result of stretching of the medial or lateral canthal ligaments rather than elongation of the tarsal plate. Several procedures are available for correction of this problem, including a full-thickness wedge excision of the lower lid with primary closure. Rather than excision of a simple wedge, resection of a pentagon of tissue gives better results. A criticism of this procedure is that it can lead to blunting of the lateral canthal angle and does not address the underlying pathology of stretching of the lateral canthal tendon. The lateral canthal sling or tarsal strip procedure is most appropriate for these cases.

The procedure begins by making a lateral canthotomy with sharp scissors. It is deepened through the orbicularis until the lateral orbital rim is reached. The tip of a Freer elevator is placed just inside the lateral orbital rim, and the periosteum is exposed but not incised. By pulling the lower lid in a medial direction, the lower limb of the lateral canthal ligament can be felt as a tight band. The ligament is exposed and then

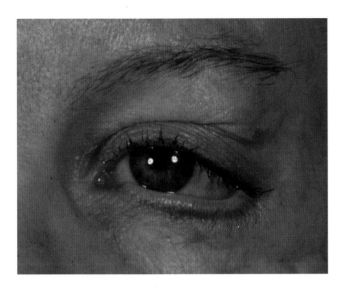

FIGURE 27-22 Lateral ectropion and inferior displacement of the lateral canthus.

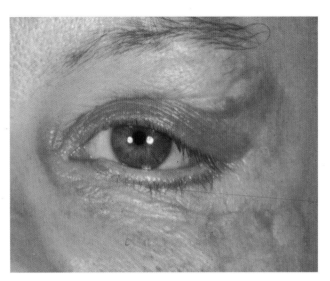

FIGURE 27-23 Postoperative view shows tightening of the lower lid and elevation of the lateral canthus.

divided. After cantholysis is performed, the whole lower lid becomes mobile. The ligament is grasped and put under tension while pulling laterally. Scissors are passed subconjunctivally, and the lower lid is divided along the gray line into anterior and posterior lamellae. The length of this incision in the gray line is determined by the amount of horizontal laxity that requires correction. Skin, orbicularis, and conjunctiva are excised to the point where the new lateral canthus is to be fashioned. The newly fashioned lateral canthus is passed deep to the upper limb of the lateral canthus and reattached to the periosteum of the lateral orbital rim with a non-resorbable suture. There should be sufficient tension to slightly overcorrect the horizontal laxity. The ligament should also be placed in a slightly more superior position than normal to allow for some minor degree of stretching. The lateral canthotomy is closed with 6-0 nylon sutures (Fig. 27-23).

CONCLUSIONS

Secondary orbital deformities present some of the greatest challenges in the management of facial trauma. Advances in imaging and modeling have increased our understanding of the anatomy of these injuries and, together with developments in plating technology and materials, have helped to produce accurate skeletal reconstructions. However, results often are disappointing for the patient and surgeon. Limitations mainly arise because of problems with the overlying soft tissues, which can shrink or become fibrosed and tethered. The challenge remains better management of the skin integument to reflect the accurate underlying reconstruction.

REFERENCES

1. Perry M, Banks P, Richards R, Friedman EP, Shaw P: The use of computer-generated three-dimensional models in orbital reconstruction. *Br J Oral Maxillofac Surg* 36(4):275-284, 1998.

2. Manson PN, Clifford CM, Su CT, Iliff NT, Morgan R: Mechanisms of global support and posttraumatic enophthalmos: I. The anatomy of the ligament sling and its relation to intramuscular cone orbital fat. *Plast Reconstr Surg* 77(2):193-202, 1986.

3. Koorneef L: *Spatial aspects of the orbital fibro-muscular tissue in man.* Amsterdam, 1977, Swets and Zeitlinger.

4. Bite U, Jackson IT, Forbes GS, Gehring DG: Orbital volume measurements in enophthalmos using three-dimensional CT imaging. *Plast Reconstr Surg* 75(4):502-508, 1985.

5. Kreipke DL, Moss JJ, Franco JM, Maves MD, Smith DJ: Computed tomography and thin-section tomography in facial trauma. *AJR Am J Roentgenol* 142(5):1041-1045, 1984.

6. Manson PN, Grivas A, Rosenbaum A, Vannier M, Zinreich J, Iliff N: Studies on enophthalmos: II. The measurement of orbital injuries and their treatment by quantitative computed tomography. *Plast Reconstr Surg* 77(2):203-214, 1986.

7. Whitehouse RW, Batterbury M, Jackson A, Noble JL: Prediction of enophthalmos by computed tomography after "blow out" orbital fracture. *Br J Ophthalmol* 78(8):618-620, 1994.

8. Raskin EM, Millman AL, Lubkin V, della Rocca RC, Lisman RD, Maher EA: Prediction of late enophthalmos by volumetric analysis of orbital fractures. *Ophthal Plast Reconstr Surg* 14(1):19-26, 1998.

9. Lee HH, Alcaraz N, Reino A, Lawson W: Reconstruction of orbital floor fractures with maxillary bone. *Arch Otolaryngol Head Neck Surg* 124(1):56-59, 1998.

10. Lai A, Gliklich RE, Rubin PA: Repair of orbital blow-out fractures with nasoseptal cartilage. *Laryngoscope* 108(5):645-650, 1998.

11. Sewall SR, Pernoud FG, Pernoud MJ: Late reaction to silicone following reconstruction of an orbital floor fracture. *J Oral Maxillofac Surg* 44(10):821-825, 1986.

12. Cordewener FW, Bos RR, Rozema FR, Houtman WA: Poly(L-lactide) implants for repair of human orbital floor defects: clinical and magnetic resonance imaging evaluation of long-term results. *J Oral Maxillofac Surg* 54(1):9-13; discussion 13-14, 1996.

13. Hammer B: *Orbital Fractures: diagnosis, operative treatment, secondary corrections.* Seattle, 1995, Hogrefe and Huber.

14. Evans BT, Webb AA: Post-traumatic orbital reconstruction: anatomical landmarks and the concept of the deep orbit. *Br J Oral Maxillofac Surg* 45(3):183-189, 2007.

15. Markowitz BL, Manson PN, Sargent L, Vander Kolk CA, Yaremchuk M, Glassman D, et al: Management of the medial canthal tendon in nasoethmoid orbital fractures: the importance of the central fragment in classification and treatment. *Plast Reconstr Surg* 87(5):843-853, 1991.

16. Gruss JS, Hurwitz JJ, Nik NA, Kassel EE: The pattern and incidence of nasolacrimal injury in naso-orbital-ethmoid fractures: the role of delayed assessment and dacryocystorhinostomy. *Br J Plast Surg* 38(1):116-121, 1985.

17. Zide BM, McCarthy JG: The medial canthus revisited—an anatomical basis for canthopexy. *Ann Plast Surg* 11(1):1-9, 1983.

18. Shore JW, Rubin PA, Bilyk JR: Repair of telecanthus by anterior fixation of cantilevered miniplates. *Ophthalmology* 99(7):1133-1138, 1992.

19. Okazaki M, Akizuki T, Ohmori K: Medical canthoplasty with the Mitek Anchor System. *Ann Plast Surg* 38(2):124-128, 1997.

CHAPTER 28

Facial Nerve Injuries: Reconstruction, Reanimation, and Masking Procedures

Rainer Schmelzeisen, Ralf Schön, Pit J. Voss

Facial nerve paralysis is one of the most devastating peripheral nerve injuries, and patients with facial palsy suffer from massive functional and esthetic problems.

AIMS

For every patient, an individualized solution has to be made considering the underlying disease, the patient's desire, age, and life expectancy. The aim must be to provide the patient with the best possible esthetic appearance of the face at rest and during motion. Usually, combinations of procedures have to be used. Static procedures alone aim at an improved appearance of the face at rest but fail to rehabilitate the patient when expressing emotions and for swallowing and speaking. Some static procedures improve the patient's situation for a defined time period only.

ANATOMY OF THE FACIAL NERVE

Injuries of the facial nerve not only cause a paresis of the target muscles. Because the facial nerve is responsible for the range of facial expressions, injuries to the nerve cause serious disturbances in social life due to impairment in the translation of emotions to others.

The facial nerve is a mixed motor and sensory nerve with the main function of innervation of the muscles of voluntary facial expression. It originates from the homolateral facial nucleus in the caudal pons. Cortical projections to the facial nuclei pass through the internal capsule into the pons, where they diverge, innervating both the contralateral and the homolateral nucleus.

Autonomic fibers from the greater petrosal nerve reach the sphenopalatine ganglion and supply the lacrimal and nasal minor salivary glands. Next within the facial canal, the nerve to the stapedius muscle exits, followed by the chorda tympani nerve, which provides taste efference from the anterior tongue and secretor motor efference to the submandibular gland approximately 5 mm proximal to the stylomastoid foramen.

Because the facial nerve travels through the labyrinthine segment of the facial canal and the greater petrosal nerve (exiting anteriorly) and the geniculate ganglion resides anterior to the somatic motor fibers, turning at the first genoposteriorly into the tympanic or horizontal segment, the facial canal is smallest in diameter in this segment (Fig. 28-1). More than 90% of facial nerve injuries from blunt temporal bone trauma occur in this region as a result of the traction forces exerted by its three branches.[1-3]

Lesions proximal to the meatus and within segments of the fallopian canal cause disturbances of tear and saliva production and taste sensation, impairment of the stapedius muscle, and various patterns of facial paralysis. Lesions distal to the stylomastoid foramen result in selective dysfunction of the facial muscles.

At the exit from the stylomastoid foramen, the facial nerve divides into the temporofacial and the cervicofacial branches (see Fig. 28-1). At the pes anserinus, five classic distal branches: temporal, zygomatic, buccal, mandibular, and cervical. The temporofacial branch anastomoses with the auriculotemporal nerve (cranial nerve V3) and divides into branches destined for the cutaneous muscles of the skull and face. It leaves as the:

- superior buccal branches (buccinator, upper part of the orbicularis oris muscles).
- infraorbital branches (greater and lesser zygomatic muscles, levators of the upper lip and nasal alae, transverse and dilator nasal muscles).
- frontal and palpebral branches (palpebral part of the orbicularis oculi, frontal part of the epicranius muscles).
- temporal branches (muscles of the outer aspect of the external ear).

After the anastomosis of the cervicofacial branch with the auricular branch of the cervical plexus, the branch divides into several others in the region of the mandibular angle:

- Inferior buccal branches (lower half of the orbicularis oris muscle)
- Cervical branch (platysma)

FUNCTIONAL PROBLEMS

CAUSES OF INJURIES

Unilateral palsy or paralysis of the face can be divided into damage above the upper motor neuron and damage involving the lower motor neuron and its distal termination on the

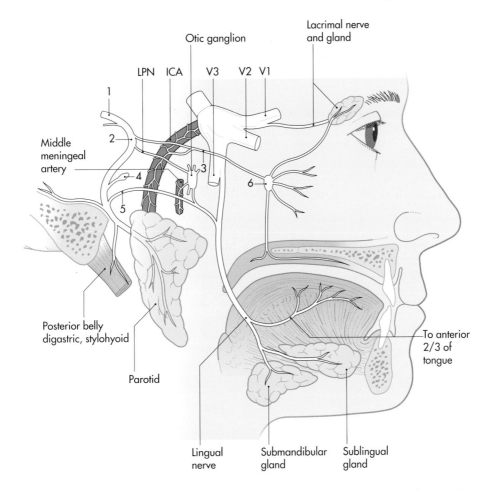

FIGURE 28-1   Schematic drawing of the facial nerve. 1, Facial nerve. 2, Geniculate ganglion. 3, Greater petrosal nerve. 4, Stapedius branch. 5, Chorda tympani. 6, Sphenopalatine ganglion. ICA, internal carotid artery; LPN, lesser petrosal nerve.

facial musculature. Supranuclear palsy spares the frontalis muscle because of the bilateral innervation of the nucleus from both cerebral hemispheres. In these supranuclear palsies, the facial involvement is often the most minor part of the patient's problems.

Lesions of the lower motor neuron usually involve the entire face. Nuclear lesions usually involve adjacent brainstem structures (abducens, trigeminal nerve). The part of the nerve most commonly damaged appears to lie within the facial canal and at each end of the canal.

The largest etiological category of facial palsy is idiopathic facial palsy (Bell's palsy), which is often diagnosed by exclusion of other etiologies.[3] It is characterized by a rapid onset of unilateral facial palsy including movements of the forehead, orbicularis oculi, perioral muscles, and platysma. Defective taste sense (anterior two thirds of the tongue) and hyperacusis may additionally be present. The etiology of Bell's palsy is unknown. There are a number of other causes of facial nerve palsies, which are listed in Box 28-1.

Central upper facial nerve injuries may occur as a result of tumor surgery at the cerebellopontine angle or from skull base fractures or trauma.[4,5] In its extracranial course, the facial nerve is most often injured by sharp lacerations. However, the most frequent cause of injury is iatrogenic, occurring during resection of tumors in the parotid gland.

Under these conditions, immediate microsurgical repair, including the use of grafts, is indicated. Resection of malignant parotid gland or skull base tumors may necessitate resection of branches of the facial nerve or the nerve itself. It must be decided on an individual basis whether a primary reconstruction of the facial nerve using nerve grafts is indicated. In trauma situations with obvious separation of the facial nerve or its branches, an immediate coaptation must be performed. If during primary trauma care, injury is only suspected or not proved, an expectant attitude should be preferred.

INVESTIGATION OF FACIAL NERVE FUNCTIONS

In the clinical investigation of a patient with a facial palsy, determination of onset characteristics is very important. In patients with Bell's palsy, an acute onset (e.g., on waking in the morning after normal facial motion the night before) is typical. Sudden onset may also be present in infectious or inflammatory conditions affecting the facial nerve (e.g., herpes zoster oticus, multiple sclerosis). Patients with tumors usually demonstrate progressive paresis over long periods with initially mild symptoms (e.g., weakness of the labial depressor muscle).

In trauma patients, a delayed onset of facial palsy carries a significantly better prognosis than immediate onset.[2]

BOX 28-1	Causes of Facial Nerve Palsy

Congenital
Moebius syndrome (congenital nuclear aplasia) (possibly + palsy of external rectus muscles)
Myotonic dystrophy
Melkersson-Rosenthal syndrome + lingua plicata, swelling of the face/upper lip
Congenital cholesteatoma/congenital facial nerve palsy

Neurological
Myasthenia gravis
Multiple sclerosis
Guillain-Barré syndrome

Neoplastic
Facial nerve tumors (schwannoma, neurofibroma, neurogenic sarcoma)
Glomus tumors (glomus jugulare/tympanicum)
Others (meningioma, acoustic neuroma)
Parotid tumors
Temporal bone/external auditory canal tumors

Infectious
Otitis media
Bacterial causes (diphtheria, tuberculosis)
Viral causes (herpes zoster oticus, mumps, infectious mononucleosis)

Other Causes
Toxic
Metabolic
Idiopathic

Iatrogenic
Parotidectomy
Rhytidectomy
Lateral skull base surgery

Traumatic
Temporal bone fractures (longitudinal, transverse)
Penetrating trauma (gunshot)
Facial lacerations
High altitude palsy

Associated symptoms may also indicate certain diseases. Oral pain, respiratory infections, and hearing loss may accompany acute otitis media, whereas initial fever, arthritis, and neuropathies may be indicative of Lyme disease. Herpes zoster oticus shows typical additional symptoms (i.e., vesicular eruptions, severe pain).

Temporal bone neoplasms may cause other cranial nerve involvements (cochlear/vestibular nerves and cranial nerves IX, X, and XI → jugular foramen; cranial nerves V, VI, and VII → temporal bone). Lesions of the second, third, fourth, and sixth cranial nerves may suggest multiple sclerosis.[2]

First, a careful observation of voluntary facial movements is undertaken. The symmetry of forehead wrinkling is investigated when the patient is asked to raise the brows. A functioning orbicularis oculi muscle allows for complete closure of the eyelids and absence of visible upward rotation and exposure of the sclera (Bell's phenomenon).

A forced wide smile distinguishes symmetries of the perioral muscles depending on the buccal and marginal mandibular branches. Comparison of the depth of the nasolabial folds and the symmetrical contraction of the platysma muscle is also important. The Schirmer test measures tear production over a 5-minute period.

Objective methods of determining the secretory function of the parotid and submandibular glands exist. Pure taste sensation may be investigated by using samples of sweet, bitter, acid, and salty substances on the anterior tongue. An audiological investigation may reveal the dysacusis caused by a nonfunctional stapedius muscle, which usually moves the tympanic membrane inward for sound absorption. Laboratory tests of sedimentation rate, treponemal antibody titer, and Lyme disease titer are scheduled. High-resolution computed tomography (CT) is indicated for patients with suspected temporal bone disease (e.g., skull base fracture). Magnetic resonance imaging (MRI) is indicated to detect lesions at the cerebellopontine angle. The typical symptoms of facial nerve injuries are listed in Box 28-2.

The House-Brackmann classification is often used for rating facial palsy. Grade I refers to normal function without weakness; slight facial asymmetry with a minor degree of synkinesis is classified as grade II. Obvious but not disfiguring asymmetry (e.g., with contracture or hemifacial spasm but residual forehead movement) is judged as grade III. Grade IV represents obvious, disfiguring asymmetry with lack of forehead motion and incomplete eye closure. Asymmetry at rest and only slight facial movement is rated as grade V. Complete absence of tone or motion is grade VI.[6]

Electromyography (EMG) and electroneurography are routinely employed. In cases of acute injury, nerve excitability tests are used, but normal results are less reliable than abnormal results, because functional deficits may occur at a later time. EMG analyzes the function of the muscles during needle insertion and gives information on the existence of spontaneous activity (action potentials) arising from voluntary muscle contraction. Spontaneous activity indicates a pathological process within the nerve, whereas fibrillation potentials may be a sign of nerve disruption.

During evoked EMG, a supramaximal stimulus is applied at the skin surface near the stylomastoid foramen. Intact axons will provide action potentials that can be recorded distally. In facial nerve injury, the amplitude of the action potential is defined as a percentage of the amplitude on the normal side. Magnetic transcranial and electrical stylomastoid stimulation procedures allow for differentiation of lesions and distinction between central and peripheral facial nerve palsies.[7,8]

PRINCIPLES

SURGICAL MANAGEMENT

If the distal facial nerve branches and musculature are intact, reinnervation from the proximal facial nerve is ideal. Reinnervation using another motor nerve may be indicated if the proximal facial nerve cannot be identified. Cases with partial return of nerve function are always problematical. The risk of destruction of functional nerve branches during surgery must be weighed against the possible advantages of reconstructive procedures.

BOX 28-2 Typical Symptoms of Different Facial Nerve Injuries

Complete peripheral facial paralysis:
- Ipsilateral forehead: absence of frontalis function
- Brow ptosis
- No closure of upper eyelid
- Drooping of lower eyelid
- In closing the eyelids, the globe rotates upward, resulting in a visible sclera (Bell's phenomenon)
- Absence of nasolabial fold; corner of mouth droops downward
- Generalized flattening of the face

Central facial paralysis (cerebral vascular accident; tumor above the level of the facial nucleus):
- Function of frontalis muscles and orbicularis oculi preserved (uncrossed fibers maintain innervation to the upper face)
- Bell's phenomenon not present
- Involuntary expression of emotion often preserved

Lesion of the facial nucleus in the pons:
- Symptoms like those of peripheral paralysis
- Tear and saliva production preserved
- Taste sensation of the anterior two thirds of the tongue preserved (intermedial nerve enters the facial nerve caudally)

Facial nerve lesions at the cerebellopontine angle cephalad to internal auditory meatus (i.e., acoustic neuroma):
- Complete peripheral facial paralysis
- Tearing, salivation, and taste often abnormal (intermedial nerve approaches the internal auditory meatus)
- Stapedius muscle function impaired

Facial nerve lesion caudal to the geniculate ganglion, cephalad to the nerve stapedial branch:
- Complete peripheral facial paralysis (e.g., lesion at the internal auditory meatus)
- Exception: lacrimal gland production preserved (greater petrosal and sphenopalatine ganglion)
- Lesions between the stapedial nerve and the chorda tympani: normal tear production, normal stapedial muscle function with complete peripheral facial paralysis
- Lesions caudal to the chorda tympani: peripheral extracranial paralysis

Facial nerve lesion at the stylomastoid foramen:
- Complete peripheral nerve paralysis (no disturbance of tear/saliva production, taste, stapedius muscle function)

Lesions occurring within the confines of the parotid gland:
- Selective paralysis of voluntary motor functions
- Paralysis of temporal branch: asymmetrical motion of the forehead, some dysfunction of the upper and possibly the lower eyelid
- Paralysis of zygomatic branch: paralysis of the muscles zygomaticus major, zygomaticus minor, levator anguli oris, levator superioris—impairment of smile
- Paralysis of buccal branch: buccinator muscle, orbicularis oris muscle distortion—buccozygomatic connections make complete branch dysfunction rare
- Paralysis of mandibular branch: innervates muscles triangularis, risorius, quadratus labii inferioris, mentalis, orbicularis oris—asymmetry of smile, affected commissure pulled upward and internally rotated
- Paralysis of cervical branch: innervation of platysma, little functional loss in cases of injury

The following basic strategies are applied most frequently for surgical correction of facial paralysis and its sequelae.

In light of the types of nerve injury and the general chance of a spontaneous regeneration in neurapraxia and axonotmesis, exact information about the mechanism of the facial nerve injury is mandatory. In cases of a sharp transection in the absence of significant adjacent soft tissue trauma or infection, immediate primary management by a well-trained operating team may be indicated.

Often, it is not known what type of nerve injury is present. Although peripheral dissected facial nerve branches may be identified under magnification or with electrical stimulation, the clinical consequences of these injuries often cannot be judged immediately. Therefore, during primary wound closure, suspected branches of the facial nerve are marked with non-resorbable sutures. The suture material is positioned at the external wound surface to help identify the nerve fibers at a later stage. This allows assessment of the clinical consequences of a nerve injury and performance of micronerve anastomosis under sterile conditions. Primary nerve grafting procedures are avoided.

Nerve reconstruction is performed immediately or within 2 months after the injury through the use of direct nerve coaptation or placement of a nerve graft.

Reconstructions of the facial nerve are limited by the atrophy of the musculature that occurs 6 to 12 months after the injury. Reanimation procedures such as faciofacial and 7th-to-12th nerve (VII-XII) anastomosis are performed not earlier than 6 to 12 months after the trauma. In long-standing facial nerve palsy, muscle grafts are often necessary due to the increasing atrophy of the facial muscles. A suggested algorithm of a staged facial reanimation is shown in Box 28-3 (modified after Volk et al.[9]).

Microsurgical Techniques

In all microsurgical techniques for facial nerve reconstruction, attempts should be made to get impulses from the

BOX 28-3 Steps in Staged Facial Reanimation

1. **Early Reconstruction:**
   Direct nerve suture
   Interpositional graft
   Lid loading
   (Additional soft tissue procedures)

2. **Early/Delayed Reconstruction (Eventual Impossibility of Performing Step 1):**
   Hypoglossal/facial jump anastomosis
   Lid loading
   Cross-face nerve suture
   Masticatory muscle transfer
   (Eyebrow lift/nasolabial fold creation/eyebrow lift)

3. **Late Reconstruction:**
   Mimic musculature existing
   Hypoglossal/facial jump anastomosis
   Lid loading
   Cross-face nerve suture
   Mimic musculature not existing
   Microvascular muscle transfer
   Temporalis muscle transfer (nasolabial fold creation/eyebrow lift/face-lift)

ipsilateral facial nerve, such as by a surgical preparation of the nerve out of the tumor or by the use of nerve grafts. If these possibilities do not exist, other procedures (e.g., VII-XII procedures) may be considered.

In cases of primary or early secondary nerve reconstruction after a defined injury, direct identification and preparation of the nerve stumps is usually possible. Coaptation or grafting techniques can then be performed easily.

In secondary microsurgical nerve repair, exploration of the site of the lesion and the stumps of the facial nerve always follows a certain order, especially in cases of peripheral facial nerve palsies in which the extent of the injury is uncertain.

It is easy to identify the facial nerve stumps that have been marked with sutures beforehand. In older secondary lesions, this is not possible, and in these cases, the first step is the systematic preparation of the extratemporal course of the central facial nerve.[9-13] The identification of the nerve at the stylomastoid foramen is the approach of choice, and tracing the nerve back from the periphery should be attempted only if the central approach is not possible.

The preauricular skin incision runs in an anteriorly curved fashion into the submandibular neck fold. The skin can then be dissected away from the fascia of the parotid gland. The cartilaginous auditory canal and the pointer, anterior to the tragus cartilage, are identified. The main trunk of the facial nerve lies approximately 1 cm caudal to that pointer at the transition level between the cartilaginous and the osseous auditory canal. If the origin of the sternocleidomastoid muscle at the mastoid and the biventer muscle are additionally prepared, the facial nerve trunk will be found to lie cranial to the angle created by these two muscles (Fig. 28-2).

For further preparation, the fibrous tissue fibers between the parotid gland and the osseous auditory canal are separated step by step, and crossing vessels are carefully coagulated. Fatty tissue cranial to the facial nerve is mobilized

anteriorly. Then, the approximately 2-mm-thick facial nerve stump is identified with the help of a nerve stimulator. The division into its main branches usually occurs after 1 cm. With a small trunk scissors, the tissue overlying the nerve is dissected away from the nerve and elevated. With a second scissors, this tissue is transected. In this manner, the branches are traced into the periphery of the gland. Among the peripheral branches, the marginal branch may be identified most easily. It lies lateral to the superficial neck fascia and crosses the facial artery and vein. Via the submandibular skin incision, it can be identified at the lateral surface of the submandibular gland and then traced dorsally.

At the superior border of the parotid gland, the temporal and zygomatic branches leave the parotid gland and are identified below the zygomatic arch in the subcutaneous tissue. The buccal branches are found cranial to Stensen's duct.

After identification of the nerve branches, the first procedure in surgical intervention is external neurolysis with preparation of the tissue surrounding the nerve and resection of the scarred perineurium. If the nerve itself is scarred, intraneural neurolysis is performed to remove cicatricial compression of the nerve fiber bundles caused by an epineural or paraneural scar. Healthy perineurium is left intact so as not to interrupt the blood supply to the individual nerve bundles and the exchange of fibers among the various fascicles.

After neurolysis, the nerve is moved away from the scar tissue bed and placed into healthy tissue to avoid further scar formation.

Direct Nerve Suture Nerve Grafts

If the nerve is interrupted, direct suturing of the nerve stumps may be performed without tension. Because the facial nerve is monofascicular or oligofascicular at its central aspect, with polyfascicular branches, we do not perform an interfascicular preparation and suture. The main trunk of the facial nerve and the small distal branches are repaired by placement of epineural sutures, which are technically easier and provide less surgical trauma to the inner nerve structures. Depending on the nerve diameter, two, four, or six 10-0 nylon sutures are applied.

In nerve coaptation, fibrous tissue proliferation at the sutured area may endanger axons arising from the central nerve stump and may impair penetration of the axons into the distal stump. Axons that have already regenerated may be compromised by scar formation. Fibrous tissue formation may be initiated by traumatization of the nerve ends, interpositioning of blood clots between the nerve stumps, or application of tension.

Because the epineural fibroblasts proliferate faster than the fibroblasts in the Schwann cells of the endoneural space, the epineurium at the central nerve stump may be carefully diminished. The protruding axons are cut to prepare a smooth nerve surface and facilitate adaptation of the stumps.

With a saw-type scissors, the nerve is cut in a definitively uninjured area, and an eventually existing neuroma is resected. The epineurium is shortened, and after further trimming of the axons, the needle is passed superficially through the fibrous tissue sheath (epineurium/perineurium). The knots are cut short to avoid foreign material reactions in the vicinity of the sutures. Torsion of the nerve stumps must be avoided (Fig. 28-3).

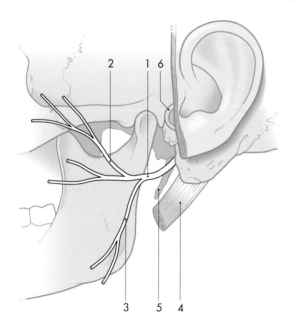

FIGURE 28-2 Identification of the facial nerve. 1, Facial nerve. 2, Temporofacial branch. 3, Cervicofacial branch. 4, Digastric muscle. 5, Styloid process. 6, Cartilaginous pointer.

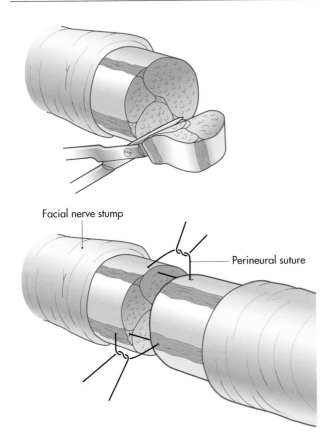

Facial nerve stump

Perineural suture

FIGURE 28-3 Perineural suture technique. If an epineural suture technique is chosen, the epineurium is not stripped back. The fascicles are trimmed before the anastomosis is performed.

Nerve Grafts

End-to-end coaptation can be performed only after sharp injury of the facial nerve. After tumor resection of malignant parotid tumors, larger nerve defects necessitate nerve grafting; this is also required in cases of secondary posttraumatic defects after resection of neuromas. Appropriate donor sites must be easily accessible and must cause minimal donor site morbidity.

The great auricular nerve can easily be found below the auricle on the external surface of the sternocleidomastoid muscle.

The sural nerve can be exposed by an oblique incision behind the lateral malleolus. After exposure of the sural nerve, its further course is identified by pulling the nerve and palpating in the proximal direction. Through additional horizontal incisions at intervals of 6 to 8 cm, the nerve can be followed to the area below the knee. The proximal end is cut, and the nerve is mobilized at its distal side. In this way, long grafts that are suitable for cross-face grafting can be harvested (Figs. 28-4 and 28-5).

The technique of aligning the stump of the recipient nerve with that of the transplanted nerve is similar to end-to-end suturing. If the cross-sections of the stumps of the recipient and transplanted nerves are of different size, it is possible to use two or even more grafts for bridging. Particularly in reconstruction of the branches of the facial nerve, the distal diversions of the sural and great auricular nerves allow for one central nerve anastomosis and several anastomoses in the periphery to the distal branches of the facial nerve (Fig. 28-6).

From the main trunk, three grafts may be placed to the main distal branches. Also, two grafts may be coapted to the upper and lower branches, bypassing the central branches to prevent mass movements of the midface. In cases with potential malignant neural invasion, the contralateral greater auricular nerve may be used.

Immediate nerve grafting gives the best functional results.[10] The postoperative results after facial nerve reconstruction correlate with the delay between trauma and reconstruction (Tables 28-1 and 28-2).

Hypoglossal/Facial Jump Anastomosis

If a direct nerve suture is not indicated, another motor nerve may be chosen as a donor motor nerve. In most cases, the hypoglossal nerve is selected; it can easily be detected underneath the intermediate tendon of the biventer muscle. The nerve is traced dorsally onto the surface of the carotid artery. Classic techniques recommend a total resection of the nerve distal to the descending branch. The complete hypoglossal nerve stump is then coapted to the peripheral facial nerve stump (Fig. 28-7).

The hypoglossal/facial nerve anastomosis may cause additional functional problems for the patient. Tongue atrophy with functional disturbance of swallowing, speech, and mastication may occur after complete interruption of the hypoglossal nerve. Therefore, tongue-sparing techniques involving modified coaptation using the descending branch or splitting of the hypoglossal nerve are favored.[11] The hypoglossal nerve may be only partially severed so that only one third or one half of the nerve is coapted with the nerve graft.[12,14-17]

Cross-face Grafts

Reinnervation of the paralyzed side with a cross-face nerve graft requires division of facial nerve branches on the undisturbed side to serve as axon donors. The donor branches are chosen from the buccozygomatic region, which has extensive crossbranching, rather than the single temporal or marginal mandibular branches. Careful selection of redundant buccozygomatic branches of the facial nerve on the normal side avoids impairment of the motions of eye closure, smile, and pucker.

Between 30% and 40% of the healthy facial nerve branches are severed and coapted to corresponding peripheral branches of the paralyzed side with sural nerve grafts of adequate length. The advantage of the procedure is the emotional correlation of both sides of the face.

The cross-face procedure may be performed along with the grafting procedure on the healthy side, with a coaptation to the paralyzed facial nerve branches performed 4 months later. More often, however, the procedure is performed as a single stage.

After cross-face nerve grafting, transient weakness of the risorius and zygomatic muscles on the healthy side is observed, but movement of the normal hemiface does not appear to be permanently affected.[18] Particularly in cross-face grafts, the degree of recovery is critically dependent on the time elapsed since onset of the facial palsy.[19] However, clinical experience shows that not all expectations about ideal symmetrical function coordinated with the healthy side are

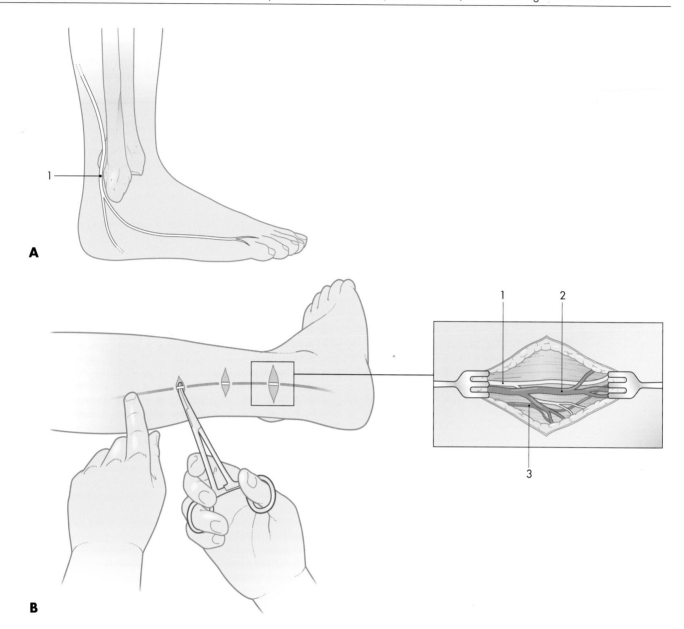

FIGURE 28-4 **A** and **B,** Harvesting of a sural nerve graft. Incision of the skin at the external surface of the lower leg 1 cm dorsal to the lateral malleolus. After identification of the sural nerve medial to the peroneal artery, the nerve is traced cranially. According to the length of the graft required, several additional horizontal incisions are performed. 1, Sural nerve. 2, Short saphenous vein. 3, Peroneal artery.

fulfilled, probably also related to a progressive atrophy of the mimic musculature.

After cross-face nerve grafting performed before transplantation of a pectoralis minor muscle graft, the number of regenerating axons was not correlated with age, nor with regeneration time. Lack of a distal connection did not appear to lead to secondary degeneration of the regenerated myelinated fibers, which remained in an immature state for months.[13,20,21]

Transposition of Masticatory Muscles
Transposition of masticatory muscles may be considered as a single step or in combination with other procedures. This procedure may become necessary if microvascular muscle

grafts are contraindicated or not indicated in patients with limited life expectancy. Disadvantages of muscle transposition are the limited direction of movements and the requirement for exercise and self-control.[22]

The masseter muscle is approached by a preauricular face-lift incision. The anterior part of the muscle, pedicled cranially and with preservation of the trigeminal nerve fibers entering the muscle posteriorly, is sharply dissected from the lower border of the mandible to provide an adequate length of the muscle to be transferred. A tunnel is dissected, the muscle is divided and inserted near the modiolus. The masseter muscle parts may be coupled to the healthy half of the orbicularis oris muscles by means of a tendon graft.[22] Eventually, an additional nasolabial fold can be created. Bleeding

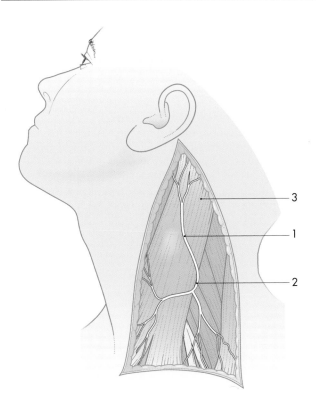

FIGURE 28-5   Harvesting of a great auricular nerve graft. A vertical incision is made lateral to the sternocleidomastoid muscle. 1, Great auricular nerve. 2, Transverse cervical nerve. 3, Sternocleidomastoid muscle.

TABLE 28-1   Functional Results after Microneurosurgical Reconstruction of the Facial Nerve*

Patient No.	Int. T/R	t (months)	Technique	Outcome (Points)†
1	2 mo	77	Graft	75
2	—	58	Graft	100
3	48 mo	66	Graft	60
4	5 days	105	Graft	72
5	5 days	24	End-to-end	83
6	—	48	Graft	75
7	36 mo	104	Graft	30
8	12 mo	18	VII–XIIn	72
9	7 mo	51	VII-XIIn	30

Int. T/R, interval between trauma and reconstruction; t, time from reconstruction to follow-up investigation; T, technique; VII-XIIn, 7th-to-12th nerve anastomosis.
*Results were evaluated according to the modified method of Fisch and Rouleau.[44]
†Outcome: 30-50 points = poor result; 51-70 points = moderate result; 71-90 points = good result; 91-100 points = normal facial nerve function.

TABLE 28-2   Photographic Evaluation after Reconstruction of the Facial Nerve ($N = 9$)

Score	Rating	No. of Patients	%
91-100	Excellent (normal)	1	11.1
71-90	Very good	5	55.6
51-70	Good	1	11.1
30-50	Moderate	2	22.2
≤29	Bad	0	0
TOTAL		9	100

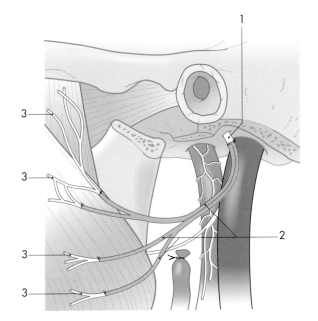

FIGURE 28-6   Coaptation of two sural nerve grafts at the central stump of the facial nerve with peripheral splitting of the grafts for anastomosis with the facial nerve branches. 1, Central stump of the facial nerve. 2, Grafts. 3, Peripheral branches of the facial nerve.

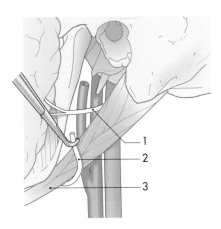

FIGURE 28-7   Schematic drawing of hypoglossal/facial nerve anastomosis. First the anterior border of the sternocleidomastoid muscle is identified. The hypoglossal nerve is identified underneath the biventer muscle; its proximal segment crosses the carotid artery. The hypoglossal nerve is sectioned after the parotidectomy incision is extended into the submandibular fold. 1, Facial nerve. 2, Hypoglossal nerve. 3, Biventer muscle.

must be controlled carefully. An overcorrection should be intended. This fold and its incisions may be used for perioral fixation of the muscle slips (Fig. 28-8).

The temporalis muscle transposition is performed via a preauricular incision that extends superiorly into the temporal area of the scalp. The incision is carried down to the temporal muscle fascia. The middle or central portion of the muscle is used. Fascia, muscle, and periosteum with a cranial extension of the periosteal incision are used. Additional mattress sutures may reinforce muscle, periosteum, and fascia. The attached fascia-periosteum is divided into two slips. They are inserted through a tunnel according to the preoperative measurements and the smile pattern. The muscle sling is

folded over the zygomatic arch, and in selected cases the arch must be trimmed or resected. Again, an overcorrection should be considered. An external splint for support of the angle of the mouth may be applied[23] (Fig. 28-9).

Free Vascularized Muscle Grafts
The main indication for microneurovascular free muscle transplantation is in cases of facial paralysis in which primary or secondary nerve repair is not likely to produce a successful result (e.g., if the facial muscles have severely degenerated). Other indications are mainly unsuccessful procedures with nerve grafting or local muscle transposition.

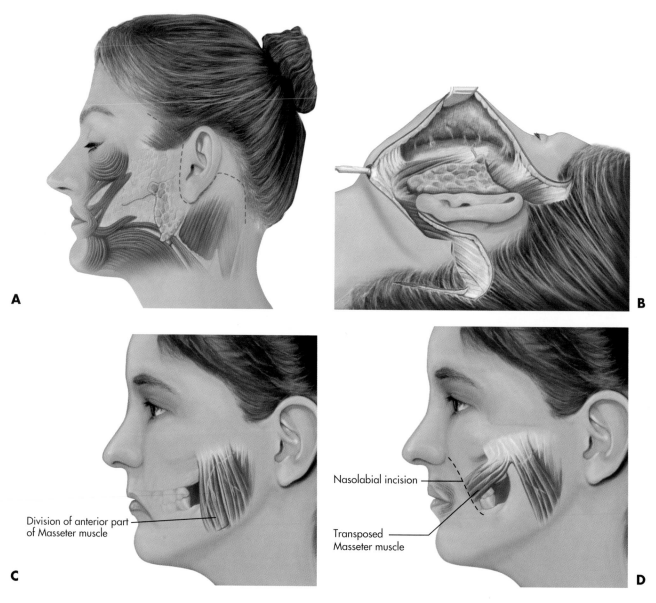

A

B

C Division of anterior part of Masseter muscle

D Nasolabial incision — Transposed — Masseter muscle

FIGURE 28-8   **A,** Face-lift incision for soft tissue suspension. A preauricular incision is led around the earlobe and retroauricularly continued under or into the hairline. **B,** After elevation of the skin, the masseter muscle can be identified for transposition of the anterior part of the muscle. Also, the temporal muscle can be approached and transposed via a cranial extension of that incision. **C,** Schematic drawing of the masseter muscle. The anterior part of the muscle is divided. **D,** The anterior part is elevated and fixed into the newly created nasolabial fold. It also can be extended with the fascia lata strip into the perioral region.

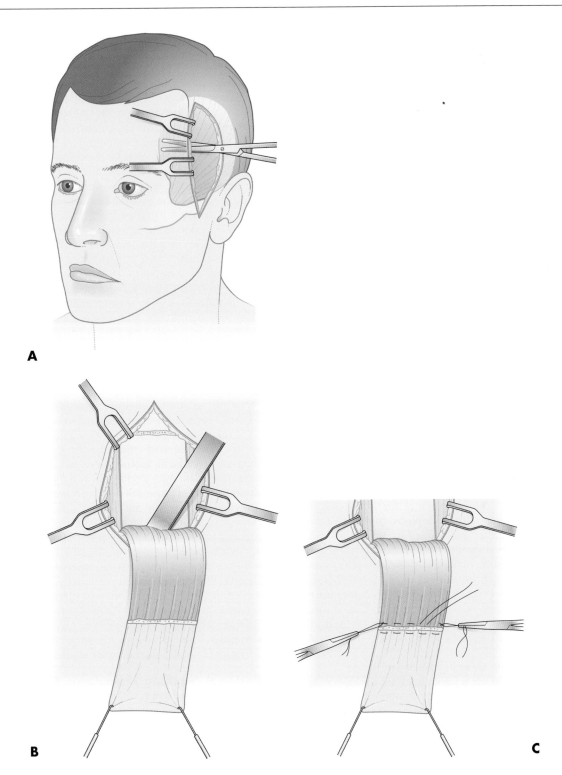

FIGURE 28-9 **A,** Transfer of the temporalis muscle via a preauricular/coronoid incision. **B,** The muscle is raised with the fascia and the periosteum. **C,** The muscle and fascia transition may be reinforced with mattress sutures.

The first clinical application of vascularized gracilis muscle grafts was described by Harii et al. in 1976.[24] A great variety of muscle grafts, including pectoralis minor, latissimus dorsi, rectus abdominis, extensor digitorum brevis, and abductor hallucis longis, have been described for reconstruction in long-standing facial palsies. These muscle grafts also allow for complex reanimation procedures of the face. The latissimus dorsi muscle is used for substitution of the zygomatic and levator labii muscles, whereas the serratus anterior segment is used for substitution of the depressor labii muscles.

Today, the gracilis muscle is regarded as the graft of choice because it is relatively easy to harvest, has great versatility, and leaves no donor site problems. Most often, the gracilis muscle is used in the standard two-stage procedure, with cross-face nerve grafting performed 6 to 12 months before muscle transplantation. The main indication for (gracilis) muscle transplantation is for recovery of the smile, which requires relatively strong muscle power and good excursion.[24-28]

The gracilis muscle originates from the inferior ramus of the pubic bone and inserts at the medial aspect of the tuberosity of the tibia (pes anserinus). Proximally, the muscle is located superficial to the adductor longus and magnus muscles; distally, it is located in the vicinity of the sartorius and the semimembranosus and semitendinosus muscles. The vascular supply is from the medial circumflex femoris artery, which originates from the deep femoral artery. The average diameter of the artery is 1.5 mm, and it is usually accompanied by two veins. The muscle is innervated by the obturatorius branch, which lies proximal to the vascular pedicle (Fig. 28-10A).

Before the operation, the position of the nasolabial fold on the healthy side and the direction and amount of excursion of the corner of the mouth are transferred and marked on the paralyzed cheek. With these permanent markings, the patient enters the operating room.

The paralyzed cheek is widely undermined through a pre-auricular face-lift incision that extends into the submandibular fold, where suitable recipient vessels are identified. Because the temporal vessels and especially the superficial temporal vein are often very fragile, they are not typically used for vascular anastomosis.

The undermining starts just above the superficial parotid fascia and extends slightly into the upper and lower lip, where the lateral portion of the remnants of the orbicularis oris muscles is exposed. Stay sutures are placed in the orbicularis oris muscle in the upper and lower lips as well as in the modiolus. Additional sutures are then placed in these three positions for later fixation of the distal portion of the muscle. The effect of the fixation sutures has to be repeatedly tested by pulling the sutures cranially. These sutures determine the effect of the muscle pull that is later applied. Care must be taken not to fix the sutures too superficially underneath the skin to avoid creating unnatural folds.

Harvesting of the Gracilis Muscle

Usually, the gracilis muscle is harvested from the side contralateral to the palsy. The surgeon stands opposite to that leg. The patient is placed in a supine position with the knee flexed and the hip abducted. A line is drawn between the pubic tubercle and the medial condyle of the tibia, the gracilis muscle being positioned posterior to that line. At the proximal upper leg, a 10-cm incision is made along the posterior border of the adductor longus muscle. After separation of the fascia overlying the adductor longus and gracilis muscles, which can be identified by the straight orientation of the muscle fibers, the vascular pedicle is approached beneath the adductor longus muscle. The vascular pedicle enters the muscle approximately 8 to 10 cm distal to the pubic tubercle and runs on the surface of the adductor brevis muscle. As the pedicle is traced to its origin at the deep femoral vessels, several small vascular branches that enter the adductor longus muscle have to be clipped carefully. The motor nerve originating from the obturator nerve enters the muscle in the vicinity

of the vascular pedicle but then runs more proximally in an oblique fashion toward the hip.

With a nerve stimulator, a muscle segment of adequate length and contractility can be identified. To avoid too much muscle bulk, the anterior segment of the muscle can be separated from the residual gracilis muscle. The epimysium should be left intact on the muscle surface to allow the muscle later to glide within that epimysium (see Fig. 28-10B,C).

After harvest of the muscle, the distal portion is split to insert muscle parts into the lateral aspects of the upper and lower lip. Before the muscle is secured with the stay sutures previously placed, the proximal and distal muscle ends are reinforced with resorbable mattress sutures to prevent rupture of the stay sutures within the muscle. Then the cranial fixation of the muscle to the zygoma is performed (see Fig. 28-10D). The neurovascular repair is performed with the use of the operating microscope.

Harii favors cross-face nerve grafts for neural anastomosis of the gracilis muscle to give an emotional link with the healthy side. Cross-face grafts have a tendency to recover even over long periods. There is no correlation between the number and diameter of the nerve fibers in the distal end of the cross-face nerve graft and the functional recovery of the transplanted muscle, but the quality of the healthy nerve used for crossover innervation is important. If a facial nerve branch innervating the slow buccinator muscle is used, the originally fast gracilis muscle is transformed into a slow muscle by this kind of reinnervation.[29,30]

It is recommended that the hypoglossal nerve be chosen as a recipient motor nerve in patients for whom muscle transplantation combined with a cross-face nerve graft cannot be performed because of bilateral facial paralysis or previous surgery on the healthy side. As with VII-XII anastomosis, we prefer the technique of hypoglossal nerve sectioning rather than separation of the whole nerve. Ueda et al. recommended use of the bundle of the hypoglossal nerve that diverges inferiorly to innervate the suprahyoid muscles as the recipient motor nerve to permit natural movements of the grafted muscle without functional disability of the tongue.[31]

The masseteric branch may also be used for neurosurgical anastomosis of the gracilis muscle nerve. It can be identified at the sigmoid notch penetrating the medial pterygoid muscle.

Additional Masking Procedures and Skin Surgery Procedures

Creation of a Nasolabial Fold

One esthetic problem of the paralyzed side of the face is the absence of a nasolabial fold, especially in contrast to the unparalyzed side. A new nasolabial fold improves the symmetry and also helps to elevate the upper lip, creating more symmetry by provision of a better visible upper lip mucosa. In muscle transposition or grafting procedures, the incision can be used for fixation in the perioral area.

The symmetry of the nasolabial fold is marked with the patient in a sitting position before surgery. The incision runs from the lateral aspect of the nasal base to the desired position above and lateral to the oral commissure. Necessary procedures for fixation of tendon or muscle slips are performed.

A small strip of skin is de-epithelialized from the inferior skin area and inserted into a subdermal pocket of the superior

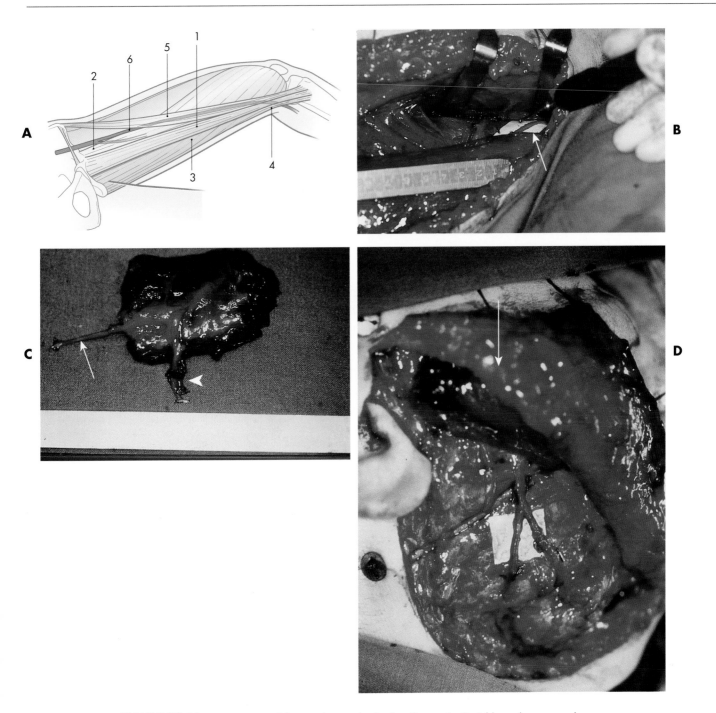

FIGURE 28-10   **A,** Anatomy of the gracilis muscle. 1, Gracilis muscle. 2, Adductor longus muscle. 3, Adductor magnus muscle. 4, Semitendinosus muscle. 5, Sartorius muscle. 6, Deep femoral artery and veins and entrance of the neurovascular bundle. **B,** Harvesting procedure for a gracilis muscle graft. Intraoperative situation after identification of the motor branch of the gracilis muscle *(arrow)*. The corresponding contractile region is identified with a nerve stimulator. **C,** Anterior segment of the gracilis muscle with vascular pedicle *(arrowhead)* and motor branch *(arrow)*. **D,** Intraoperative aspect after neurovascular anastomosis and fixation of the muscle at the zygoma *(arrow)*.

cheek portion by deepening sutures. In this way, an impression of depth can be created (Fig. 28-11A).

The nasolabial fold is marked on the unaffected side with the patient in a sitting position. On the paralyzed side, the incision line is chosen slightly below the line of the unaffected side so as to elevate the red of the lip. Then a corresponding area of upper lip is de-epithelialized starting from the incision

line. In the cheek area, a corresponding pocket is undermined for insertion of the de-epithelialized upper lip part (see Fig. 28-11B-E).

Brow Lift
The drooping of the brow is not only an esthetic problem; it also interferes with the upper lid and limits the upward gaze.

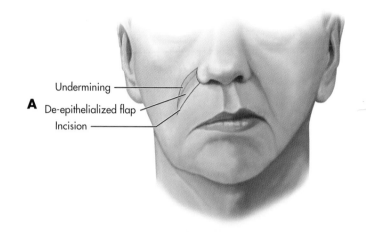

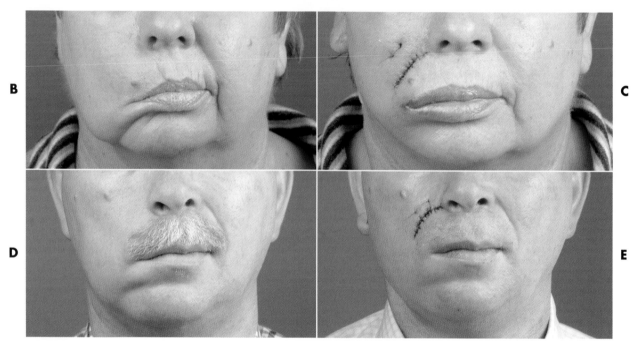

FIGURE 28-11 **A,** Schematic drawing of the new creation of a nasolabial fold. **B,** Patient with facial nerve palsy on the right side. **C,** Situation immediately after creation of a new nasolabial fold, with stay sutures for the de-epithelialized upper lip skin. **D,** Patient with facial palsy lid excision. **E,** Newly created nasolabial fold with stay sutures still in place.

By means of a brow lift, the eye can be opened more fully. If lid loading is to be done, the brow lift procedure should be performed first.

Before surgery, the brow position is marked with the patient sitting. The new position should match that of the unaffected side. The amount of skin to be removed is marked directly above the brow. After excision, the new position is secured by attaching the orbicularis muscle to the periosteum above. Alternatively, skin in the temporal/forehead region can be excised close to the hairline.

For isolated marginal branch lesions and other selected indications, a partial lip resection with transposition of the orbicularis oris may provide a local orbicularis transposition with a satisfying result.[32]

Face-lift

Patients with Facial Nerve Palsy on One Side As an isolated procedure but more often in combination with other surgical techniques, a unilateral or bilateral face-lift may be indicated for patients with facial paralysis, especially if sagging of facial skin and loss of skin tone are exaggerated by long-standing facial paralysis. Tightening of the skin and the superficial musculo-aponeurotic system with removal of excess skin improves the overall result (Fig. 28-12).

Before surgery, the desired amount of skin to be resected and the direction of cranioposterior pull must be marked with the patient in a sitting position. In particular, the projection to the lower border of the mandible and the amount of soft tissue to be elevated must be identified. The typical

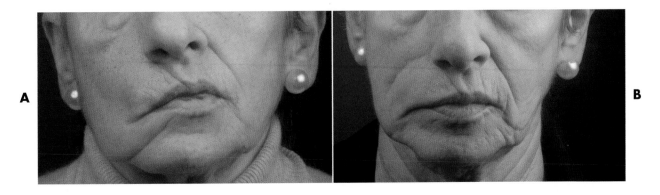

FIGURE 28-12 **A,** Patient with mild facial nerve palsy on the right side: preoperative aspect. **B,** Situation after bilateral face-lift with elevation of soft tissue and creation of a new nasolabial fold.

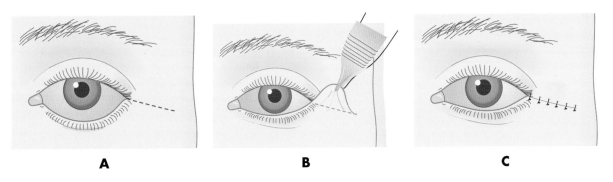

FIGURE 28-13 **A** and **B,** Determination of skin excess before full-thickness skin excision of the lid. **C,** Reconstruction of the muscle with absorbable sutures followed by skin closure.

face-lift incision is marked in the preauricular fold extending into the hairline posterior to the earlobe. The face-lift incision also allows for transfer of parts of the masseter muscle and, with the cranial extension, transposition of the temporalis muscle.

Surgical Correction of the Eyelid

Our experience with lid loading techniques accords with that reported in the literature, providing good esthetic and functional results with high predictability.[33-36]

Ueda et al.[34] observed superior functional results with temporalis muscle transfer for closure of the eye compared to lid loading with gold implants. However, cornea protection was also provided in the lid loading procedures used in combination with other procedures. Muscle transposition for ocular protection may impose an increased strain on the patient and need for reeducation.

In lid loading, the weight is usually first temporarily fixed to the skin of the eyelid before surgery. The weight should not impair opening of the eyelid but should provide complete closure at rest. The weight is usually about 1 to 1.4 g.

An upper eyelid incision is used, and the curved weight is fixed to the tarsal plate. Additionally, the levator aponeurosis may be advanced over the implant and the final eyelid height may be adjusted with levator myotomies.

A circumscribed procedure such as isolated correction of the upper or lower eyelid may also improve the patient's situation. More often, lower eyelid techniques are employed, using wedge resections combined with rotations of the lower

lid skin. During that procedure, the lateral canthal tendon may also be repositioned (Fig. 28-13).

In some patients, a composite skin and cartilage graft may be useful to support the lower lid.

POSTOPERATIVE TREATMENT

All patients must undergo physical therapy and mimic therapy. At best, this should start when the first signs of reinnervation are visible clinically or by EMG after micronerve surgery or muscle graft transposition and grafting. In patients with hypoglossal/facial jump nerve anastomosis, the training should first focus on tongue movements; the patient will then learn which kinds of tongue movements generate facial movements.[9]

OUTCOMES

In micronerve surgery, results obtained by end-to-end coaptation and cable nerve grafting are superior to those achieved by hypoglossal/facial jump grafts.[37] In central lesions, no statistical correlation was found between the length of the graft and the degree or timing of clinical recovery.[38] Facial nerve reconstruction in cases of nerve discontinuity, or in reanimation procedures with the contralateral facial or ipsilateral hypoglossal nerve as the donor nerve, gives overall satisfactory results with symmetry at rest and complete eye closure equivalent to a House-Brackmann grade III in 69% of cases.

Green et al.[21] reported that no patient with a neural repair (direct anastomosis or cable graft) had better results than House-Brackmann grade III. Patients undergoing direct anastomosis of the nerve obtained House-Brackmann grade III. Most often in patients undergoing cable nerve grafting, grade IV was obtained. Patients with normal or almost normal facial nerve function (grade I or II) had undergone only decompression of the facial nerve.[13,21] Hypoglossal/facial nerve anastomosis gave excellent results in 56% of the patients ($n = 32$), and 66% would have repeated the operation. The procedure is most effective when it is used as soon as possible after the palsy has developed.

The results of crossover techniques depend on the grade of atrophy of the facial nerve: Results are better if the atrophy is less than 50% that of the normal nerve. Even 2 to 7 years after nerve injury, good results may be obtainable. Combinations of hypoglossal/facial anastomosis with transposition of temporal or masseter muscles are also possible.[15] Video analysis demonstrates that rehabilitation with hypoglossal/facial jump grafts may give better results than bioplasties with temporalis muscle.[39]

We have performed 20 gracilis muscle grafts. All patients showed significant improvements of face symmetry at rest and with emotion after the operation (Figs. 28-14 and 28-15). The simplified semiquantitative evaluation of our long-term results in six patients is shown in Table 28-3. In addition to the functional results demonstrated by photography, we regard the subjective estimation of the patient as very important. All of these patients reported that they would have the surgical procedure again and that the muscle transfer was a significant contribution to better self-esteem and an important basis for improved social contacts. One patient had expected a normal function of the mimic muscles postoperatively and rated the results inferior to his expectations.[40,41]

CONTROVERSIES

Increasing age at the time of injury may be associated with generally poorer reconstruction outcomes.[37] In contrast to other authors' descriptions, micronerve reconstruction with end-to-end coaptation, cable grafting, and hypoglossal/facial anastomosis can have good results after time periods longer than 2 years from onset of the facial palsy.[2] Also, so-called babysitter procedures before free muscle grafting may improve the patient's situation during the longer period of the two-stage cross-face and free muscle graft procedure.[23,42,43]

In some patients with selected indications, static procedures may be beneficial for an esthetic improvement. Fascia lata or foreign materials can be used to correct the static position of the angle of the mouth. Various techniques have been described for elevation of the angle of the mouth. Most often, the soft tissue is suspended with fascia lata toward the zygomatic arch. Most static procedures produce only a temporary effect (Fig. 28-16).

As an alternative to microvascular procedures and in patients whose general status or previous operations do not allow microvascular surgery, regional muscle transpositions with the temporal muscle, the masseter, or the platysma may be considered.[38,39]

In addition to muscle bulk lateral to the zygomatic arch, a visible volume defect in the region of the temporal muscle often occurs postoperatively.

Masseter muscle transfer can be performed extraorally as transfer of the whole muscle belly or as transposition of the anterior half of the muscle via an intraoral approach. The blood and nerve supplies to the muscle enter from the infratemporal fossa through the coronoid notch. The muscle is removed sharply with its tendinous insertion and bluntly elevated from the periosteum to the coronoid process. The

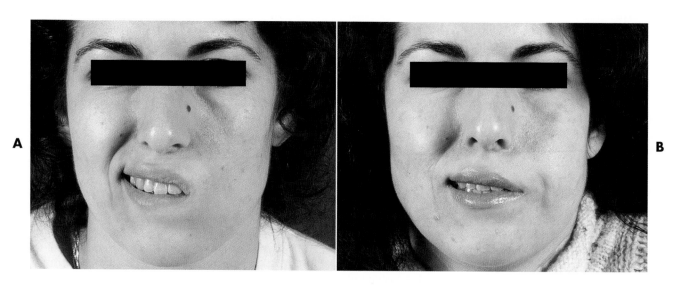

FIGURE 28-14 **A,** Twenty-year-old female patient with facial nerve paralysis on the left side. **B,** Postoperative result 3 years after surgery with improved balance of the mouth and lateral pull of the gracilis muscle (anastomosis to hypoglossal nerve).

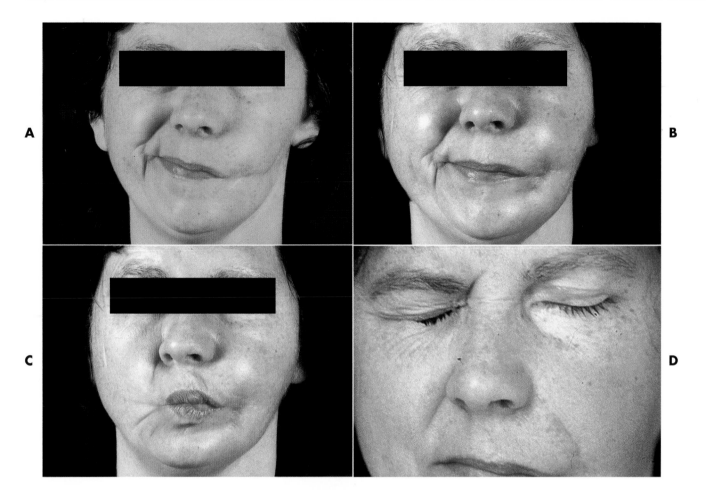

FIGURE 28-15 **A,** Left facial nerve palsy after surgery for an acoustic neuroma: preoperative aspect. **B,** Postoperative result 1 year after gracilis muscle transplantation with nerve coaptation to a cross-face graft performed 9 months earlier. **C,** Gold weight implantation. A weight of 1.5 g has been inserted into the upper eyelid. **D,** Postoperative result with complete eye closure.

TABLE 28-3	Postoperative Results of Vascularized Muscle Grafts							
				OBJECTIVE (INVESTIGATOR)		SUBJECTIVE (SELF-ESTIMATION)		
Patient No.	Age at Surgery (yr)	Months from Surgery to Follow-up	Nerve	Stat.	Smile	Stat.	Smile	Acceptance*
1	16	67	X	+++	++	++	++	Yes
2	53	65	X	++	++	+	+	Yes
3	47	59	Cross-face	+++	++	++	+	Yes
4	40	55	Cross-face	++	++	++	+	Yes
5	36	29	Right masticatorius	++	+	+	+	No
6	60	24	XII	++	++	++	+	Yes

+++ = results correlate with healthy side; ++ = significant improvement; + = minor improvement.
*Situation improved, patient would have procedure again.

inferior tendon is used for anterior fixation of the muscle. As with the temporalis, the muscle is split at the anterior portion to preserve the nerve supply to both muscle slips. These muscle slips are fixed with nonabsorbable sutures to the underlying dermis. Overcorrection is performed. Disadvantages of the procedure are the volume deficit in the angle of the mandible and the lateralized direction of pull.

Often, the success of the transfer of masticatory muscles is limited by a complex reeducation process for the patient and a failure of these muscles to reach sufficiently large areas. In these cases, procedures such as extending the temporal

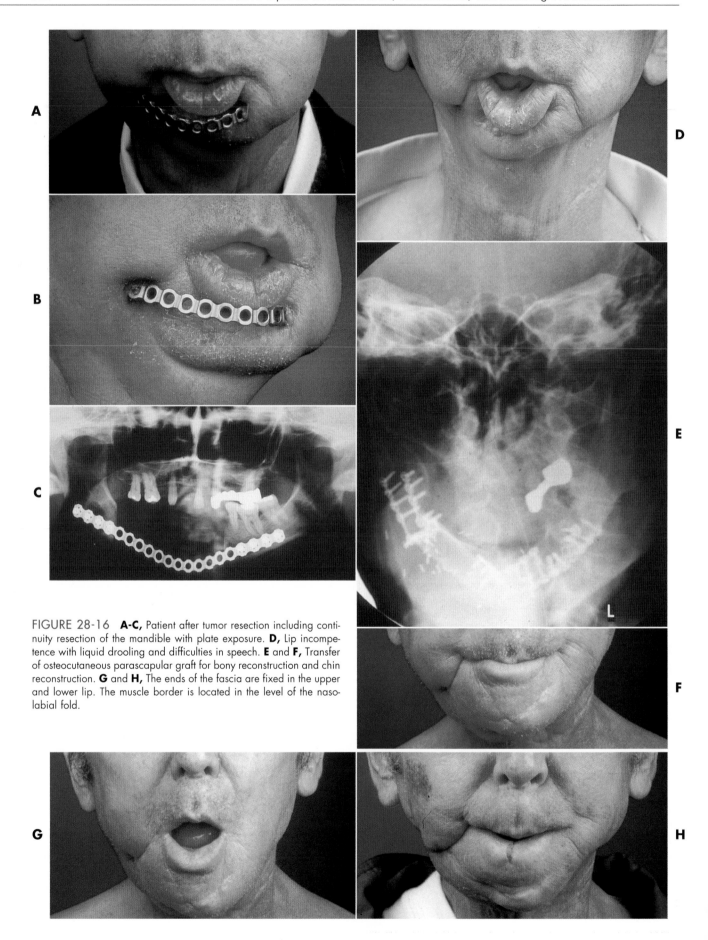

FIGURE 28-16   **A-C,** Patient after tumor resection including continuity resection of the mandible with plate exposure. **D,** Lip incompetence with liquid drooling and difficulties in speech. **E** and **F,** Transfer of osteocutaneous parascapular graft for bony reconstruction and chin reconstruction. **G** and **H,** The ends of the fascia are fixed in the upper and lower lip. The muscle border is located in the level of the nasolabial fold.

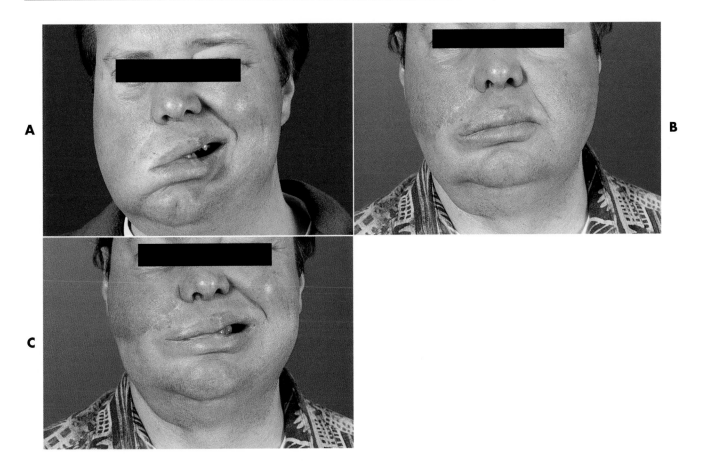

FIGURE 28-17 **A,** Preoperative aspect of a patient with facial nerve palsy on the right side.
B, Static result 2 years after masseter muscle transfer. **C,** Dynamic result 2 years postoperatively.

muscle flap with galea allows more extended rotation (Fig. 28-17).

Temporalis muscle transposition may also be used for early, temporary treatment of complete facial palsy when recovery of the nerve function is predicted to be extended and incomplete, because the procedure does not interfere with neural regeneration.

An alternative reanimation procedure using a vascularized muscle graft involves transfer of the free rectus femoris muscle. The long motor nerve is led through the upper lip and sutured to the contralateral facial nerve without the need for a two-stage procedure.

KEY POINTS

- Exact knowledge of the anatomy of the facial nerve is necessary.
- There must be precise clinical and electrophysiological investigation of facial nerve functions.
- A treatment plan is established according to:
  - the patient's expectations
  - the general conditions of the patient
  - the best possibility for individual outcome
- The procedure is planned with regard to the type of lesion and the interval between trauma and repair.
- Hypoglossal/facial nerve anastomosis is probably the most reliable procedure for micronerve reconstruction.
- For long-standing facial palsies, neurovascular anastomosed muscle grafts are the method of choice.

REFERENCES

1. Wang RC, Barrow H, Weiss MH, et al: Diagnosis of disorders within the temporal bone causing facial paralysis. In Rubin LR, editor: *The paralyzed face,* St. Louis, 1991, Mosby–Year Book, pp 91-100.
2. Leblanc A: *Anatomy and imaging of the cranial nerves: facial nerve,* Berlin, 1992, Springer Verlag, pp 171-210.
3. Louis SM, McKnight P: Medical causes of facial paralysis, including Bell's palsy. In Rubin LR, editor: *The paralyzed face,* St. Louis, 1991, Mosby–Year Book, pp 87-90.
4. Roland JT Jr, Hammerschlag PE, Lewis WS, et al: Management of traumatic facial nerve paralysis with carotid artery cavernous sinus fistula. *Eur Arch Otorhinolaryngol* 251:57-60, 1994.
5. Tatagiba M, Matthies C, Samii M: Facial nerve reconstruction in neurofibromatosis 2. *Acta Neurochir* 126:72-75, 1994.
6. House J: Facial nerve grading systems. *Laryngoscope* 93:1056-1069, 1983.
7. Glocker FX, Magistris MR, Rösler KM, et al: Magnetic transcranial and electrical stylomastoidal stimulation of the facial motor pathways in Bell's palsy: time course and relevance of electrophysiological parameters. *Electroencephalogr Clin Neurophysiol* 93:113-120, 1994.
8. Rösler KM, Magistris MR, Glocker FX, et al: Electrophysiological characteristics of lesions in facial palsies of different etiologies: a study using electrical and magnetic stimulation techniques. *Electroencephalogr Clin Neurophysiol* 97:355-368, 1995.
9. Volk GF, Pantel M, Guntinas-Lichius O: Modern concepts in facial nerve reconstruction. *Head Face Med* 6:25, 2010.
10. Vaughan ED, Richardson D: Facial nerve reconstruction following ablative parotid surgery. *Br J Oral Maxillofac Surg* 31:274-280, 1993.
11. Meltzer NE, Alam D:Facial paralysis rehabilitation: state of the art. *Curr Opin Otolaryngol Head Neck Surg* 18:232-237, 2010.
12. Cusimano MD, Sekhar L: Partial hypoglossal to facial nerve anastomosis for reinnervation of the paralyzed face in patients with lower cranial nerve palsies: technical note. *Neurosurgery* 35:532-533, 1994.
13. Samii M, Matthies C: Indication, technique and results of facial nerve reconstruction. *Acta Neurochir* 130:125-139, 1994.

14. Linnet J, Madsen FF: Hypoglosso-facial nerve anastomosis. *Acta Neurochir* 133:112-115, 1995.

15. Kunihiro T, Kanzaki J, Yoshihara S, et al: Analysis of the prognosis and the recovery process of profound facial nerve paralysis secondary to acoustic neuroma resection. *Otorhinolaryngology* 56:331-333, 1994.

16. Arai H, Sato K, Yanai A: Hemihypoglossal-facial nerve anastomosis in treating unilateral facial palsy after acoustic neurinoma resection. *J Neurosurg* 82:51-54, 1995.

17. Kukwa A, Marchel A, Pietniczka M, et al: Reanimation of the face after facial nerve palsy resulting from resection of a cerebellopontine angle tumour. *Br J Neurosurg* 8:327-332, 1994.

18. Cooper TM, McMahon B, Lex C, et al: Cross-facial nerve grafting for facial reanimation: effect on normal hemiface motion. *J Reconstr Microsurg* 12:99-103, 1996.

19. Inigo F, Ysunza A, Rojo P, et al: Recovery of facial palsy after crossed facial nerve grafts. *Br J Plast Surg* 47:312-317, 1994.

20. Jacobs JM, Laing JH, Harrison DH: Regeneration through a long nerve graft used in the correction of facial palsy: a qualitative and quantitative study. *Brain* 119:271-279, 1996.

21. Green JD Jr, Shelton C, Brackmann DE: Surgical management of iatrogenic facial nerve injuries. *Otolaryngol Head Neck Surg* 111:606-610, 1994.

22. Michaelidou M, Tzou C-HJ, Gerber H, et al: The combination of muscle transpositions and static procedures for reconstruction in the paralyzed face of the patient with limited life expectancy or who is not a candidate for free muscle transfer. *Plast Reconstr Surg* 123:121-128, 2009.

23. Terzis JK, Olivares FS: Mini-temporalis transfer as an adjunct procedure for smile restoration. *Plast Reconstr Surg* 123:533-542, 2009.

24. Harii K: Microneurovascular free muscle transplantation. In Rubin LR, editor: *The paralyzed face*, St. Louis, 1991, Mosby–Year Book, pp 178-200.

25. O'Brien B, Kumar V: Cross-face nerve grafting with free vascularized muscle grafts. In Rubin LR, editor: *The paralyzed face*, St. Louis, 1991, Mosby–Year Book, pp 201-212.

26. Jiang H, Guo ET, Ji ZL, et al: One-stage microneurovascular free abductor hallucis muscle transplantation for reanimation of facial paralysis. *Plast Reconstr Surg* 96:78-85, 1995.

27. Zhao L, Miao H, Wang W, et al: The anatomy of the segmental latissimus dorsi flap for reconstruction of facial paralysis. *Surg Radiol Anat* 16:239-243, 1994.

28. Ueda K, Harii K, Yamada A: Free vascularized double muscle transplantation for the treatment of facial paralysis. *Plast Reconstr Surg* 95:1288-1296, 1995.

29. Ueda K, Harii K, Yamada A: Long-term follow-up of nerve conduction velocity in cross-face nerve grafting for the treatment of facial paralysis. *Plast Reconstr Surg* 93:1146-1149, 1994.

30. Frey M, Happak W, Girsch W, et al: Histomorphometric studies in patients with facial palsy treated by functional muscle transplantation: new aspects for the surgical concept. *Ann Plast Surg* 26:370-379, 1991.

31. Ueda K, Harii K, Yamada A: Free neurovascular muscle transplantation for the treatment of facial paralysis using the hypoglossal nerve as a recipient motor source. *Plast Reconstr Surg* 94:808-817, 1994.

32. Yavuzer R, Jackson T: Partial lip resection with orbicularis oris transposition for lower lip correction in unilateral facial paralysis. *Plast Reconstr Surg* 108:1874, 2001.

33. De Min G, Babighian S, Babighian G, et al: Early management of the paralyzed upper eyelid using a gold implant. *Acta Otorhinolaryngol Belg* 49:269-274, 1995.

34. Ueda K, Harii K, Yamada A: A comparison of temporal muscle transfer and lid loading in the treatment of paralytic lagophthalmos. *Scand J Plast Reconstr Surg Hand Surg* 29:45-49, 1995.

35. Catalano PJ, Bergstein MJ, Sen C, et al: Management of the eye after iatrogenic facial paralysis. *Neurosurgery* 35:259-262, 1994.

36. Gladstone GJ, Nesi FA: Management of paralytic lagophthalmos with a modified gold-weight implantation technique. *Ophthal Plast Reconstr Surg* 12:38-44, 1996.

37. Malik TH, Kelly G, Ahmed A, et al: A comparison of surgical techniques used in dynamic reanimation of the paralyzed face. *Otol Neurotol* 26:284-291, 2005.

38. Stephanian E, Sekhar LN, Janecka IP, et al: Facial nerve repair by interposition nerve graft: results in 22 patients. *Neurosurgery* 31:73-76, 1992.

39. Kecskes G, Herman P, Kania R, et al: Lengthening temporalis myoplasty versus hypoglossal-facial nerve coaptation in the surgical rehabilitation of facial palsy: evaluation by medical and nonmedical juries and patient-assessed quality of life. *Otol Neurotol* 30:217-222, 2009.

40. Schliephake H, Schmelzeisen R, Tröger M: Revascularized muscle transfer for facial reanimation after long standing facial paralysis. *Int J Oral Maxillofac Surg* 29:243-249, 2000.

41. Schmelzeisen R, Neukam FW, Reich RH, et al: Neurovaskulär reanastomosierte Muskeltransplantate bei der Behandlung langbestehender N.-facialis-Paresen. [Neurovascular reanastomosed muscle grafts for the treatment of long-standing facial nerve palsy]. *Dtsch Z Mund Kiefer Gesichtschir* 18:145-149, 1993.

42. Terzis JK: "Babysitters": an exciting new concept in facial reanimation. The facial nerve. In Castro D, editor: *Proceedings of the Sixth International Symposium on the Facial Nerve*, Rio de Janeiro, Brazil, October 2-5, 1988. Amsterdam, 1990, Kugler & Ghendini, pp 525.

43. Mersa B, Tiangco DA, Terzis JK: Efficacy of the "baby-sitter" pocedure after prolonged denervation. *J Reconstr Microsurg* 16:27-35, 2000.

44. Fisch U, Rouleau M: Facial nerve reconstruction. *J Otolaryngol* 966:437-492, 1980.

CHAPTER 29

Psychological Support and Intervention in Facial Injuries

Alexandra Clarke

As biomedical techniques become increasingly sophisticated, patients who might in the past have had a poor prognosis are successfully completing treatment. However, those who undergo treatment are often left with impaired function or appearance, and the process of treatment may last months or years with no clear guarantees about outcome. This situation applies to maxillofacial conditions from head and neck cancers to severe burn injuries. Pioneering treatments such as facial transplantation[1] have added to the potential reconstructive options for patients with significant facial injury, but these approaches require a considerable investment in terms of patient selection, preparation, and management, including a commitment to a multiprofessional approach to care.

Although the importance of psychological rehabilitation has been acknowledged since the pioneering work of McIndoe and his team at East Grinstead during the 1940s, there is increasing interest in the psychological problems that patients experience and the psychological predictors of good long-term outcome. This area of research has produced a much better understanding of the factors and processes that predict psychological adjustment and a corresponding focus on evidence-based psychological interventions with clear and measurable goals. The National Institute for Clinical Excellence (NICE) guidelines,[2] National Service Frameworks,[3] and the National Burn Care Review[4] in the United Kingdom have emphasized rehabilitation and psychological processes that often are delivered by a stepped-care approach.

SOCIAL PSYCHOLOGY AND THE FACE

The neurological basis of face perception and recognition is a fascinating area of research whose complexity highlights the importance of the face in the social context. Each of us is unique, although the transfer of facial characteristics to our offspring ensures the family and racial characteristics that underpin the cohesiveness of social groups. The face is an important determinant of our internalized sense of who we are. Just as we are instantly recognized by friends and family, we have an internalized body image that is highly resistant to change. Accepting a change in appearance is not the same thing as habituating to it, and patients often describe shock at catching sight of themselves in a shop window or in a photograph many years after the initial trauma. Adapting to

any disfiguring condition, even when the change is minor, can be a very long process, which often is described as one of bereavement with a clear focus on grieving for lost looks.[5,6]

Physical attractiveness is judged to a significant extent on facial characteristics such as skin texture, size and shape of eyes, and facial symmetry, with vast amounts spent each year on cosmetics that enhance these features. Disfiguring conditions have a huge personal impact in terms of perceived attractiveness, with interesting sex differences. Whereas facial scarring, for example, can exaggerate the sexual stereotype for men (e.g., more macho, aggressive, willing to take risks), for a woman, the stereotype is weakened, and she may appear less feminine and less attractive. This does not mean that disfigurement is less of an issue for men. The largest study[7] of concern about appearance dispelled several myths about which patients are disturbed about appearance. In a sample of 1265 participants recruited from community and clinical settings, gender and age were not powerful predictors of distress, and there was a large amount of variation in the responses. Young men in particular may struggle and may behave in a hostile or aggressive way in social encounters as a result of negative responses from their peer group.

Barriers to sexual activity, such as altered facial sensation and the ability to kiss a partner, can cause enormous distress. Withdrawal from intimacy is a major problem for people with anxiety about their bodily appearance, and gradual avoidance of social activity occurs as the prospect of an intimate relationship is perceived as more remote.

The head, neck, and face provide us with the basis of communication. Laryngectomy and removal of the vocal cords permanently abolishes the ability to speak, with future "speech" achieved through a variety of alternative mechanical means. Cancer and the treatment for invasive disease or significant trauma can have a major impact on appearance, speech, swallowing, and shoulder function after neck dissection.[8]

In addition to providing the neural and muscular basis of speech production, nonverbal signaling, such as eye contact, facial gesture, and blushing, depend on facial structure. These nonverbal behaviors support verbal exchanges, helping to pace and structure conversation and allowing us to express emotion and to indicate personal attitudes.[9] Interruption of these mechanisms, often because patients try to avoid eye contact or smiling when there is a facial palsy, can add to the awkwardness of social encounters. Problems may also occur with swallowing. Ingestion of food, chewing, swallowing, and salivation are frequently affected after maxillofacial trauma, with profound implications for ensuring optimal nutrition and impacting dramatically on the social aspects of eating. Patients can be embarrassed about the difficulties of drooling, spilling food, or using special utensils or straws. Interruption of what is an important social activity may be expected to impact self-esteem. The inability to express personality through speech and social exclusion from activities such as having a drink or a meal with friends can affect self-image as much as an objective change in physical appearance.[10] For patients who experience major surgery or accidental trauma to the face, the psychological impact of facial dysfunction may affect any or all of these areas.

PSYCHOSOCIAL IMPACT OF FACIAL DISFIGUREMENT

Research studies are remarkably consistent in describing the problems that people with a disfigurement encounter. The predominant difficulties lie within the area of social interaction, with people being subjected to unwanted intrusions such as staring or comments. Macgregor's classic study[11] has not been bettered in terms of summarizing patients' self-reported data. "In their attempts to go about their daily lives, people are subjected to visual and verbal assaults and a level of familiarity from strangers, including naked stares, startled reactions, double takes, whispering, remarks, furtive looks, curiosity, personal questions, advice, manifestations of pity or aversion, laughter, ridicule, and outright avoidance".[11]

First impressions are important in our image-conscious society, and adapting to disfigurement, even when minor, can be profoundly difficult.[12] First encounters are particularly stressful, staring and intrusions are common, and social avoidance can rapidly develop as the simplest means of survival. As in other anxiety disorders, avoidance of the feared situation provides only temporary relief and removes the opportunity to learn by experience or build up a repertoire of coping strategies. Confronting social situations becomes increasingly difficult, and one of the components of psychological intervention is graded exposure to eliminate the anxiety response, reframe beliefs about the social environment, and develop positive coping strategies.

Not surprisingly, this group of people may have very low self-esteem and expectations about life chances. For example, many believe that they need to make compromises in terms of relationships (e.g., take what you can get) or think that they have diminished employment prospects.[13] For children, all the problems of chronic illness, such as repeated hospitalizations, time off from school, and disruption of peer relationships and education, may be compounded by bullying at school and the lowered expectations of teachers and parents. Studies have demonstrated that even in normal classroom situations, sensitivity about appearance can impact behavior, with children unwilling to put up their hands to answer questions if they feel uncomfortable about what they look like.[14]

Although the perceived hostility from other people has led to the description of facial disfigurement as the last bastion of discrimination in the United Kingdom,[15] the situation is not completely one sided. The increased uncertainty, embarrassment, and self-consciousness that people experience when their appearance changes can often prompt changes in behavior that elicit a negative response from other people. Altered posture, avoidance of eye contact, hiding the face with the hand and hair, and overzealous use of cosmetic camouflage and clothing, especially hats, can elicit the very responses that the individual is trying to avoid.

It is easy to see how repeated exposure to negative events can lead to a behavioral change, particularly increasing avoidance of social situations, but the role of individual beliefs is also important. People behave differently in response to someone who is visibly different, and the expectation of a negative response is enough for the visibly different person to perceive and report events differently. Social psychologists have examined the impact of these beliefs about disfigurement. Actors were made up to look disfigured, but under the guise of having fixative added and unknown to them, the experimental group had that make-up removed before being exposed to the experimental situation.[16] Subjects who believed themselves to be scarred reported stronger reactions from other people than the control group. This finding might have resulted from heightened sensitivity leading to the misinterpretation of events or to subtle alterations in the subject's behavior, such as poor posture or eye contact, producing genuinely stronger reactions from the onlooker. However, sensitivity to the disfigurement and the tendency to attribute all negative experiences to facial appearance, even when unrelated, is a commonly reported problem and a possible explanation for the significance to the individual of apparently only minor disfigurement.

From the clinical perspective, these findings are important because the modification of inappropriate cognitions (i.e., beliefs) and the introduction of more appropriate cognitions and behavior form the basis of effective psychological intervention in this group. Social anxiety and avoidance can be effectively targeted using this well-established approach.[17,18]

Relatively few studies have attempted to look beyond the description of psychosocial problems in the target population to the factors associated with good adjustment in the long term. There is a strong, erroneous presumption that psychological distress is proportionate to the severity of the disfigurement, a finding that has no basis in research findings but nevertheless drives referral patterns and services. It is instead the individual factors driven by cognitive processes that predict long-term adjustment.[19,20] Macgregor[11] illustrated this idea many years ago, identifying coping style as important. Those who cope well and report fewer problems tend to use the positive coping strategies summarized in Box 29-1, all of which allow them to manage social situations. Negative coping strategies are those that facilitate the avoidance response.

Findings of the Appearance Research Collaboration further clarified the factors and processes that are associated with positive adjustment in the long term. They demonstrated that biomedical factors such as the cause, timeline, and severity of the condition do not predict adjustment, although visibility to others is important. The psychological characteristics of those who were positively adjusted included higher levels of optimism, greater feelings of social acceptance and satisfaction with social support, a lack of concern about negative evaluations by others, and a self-system with lower levels of salience and valance afforded to appearance-related information.[7]

BOX 29-1 **Coping Style as a Predictor of Good Long-term Adjustment after Facial Disfigurement**

Positive Coping Strategies
- Good social skills
- Assertiveness
- Taking the initiative in new situations

Negative Coping Strategies
- Poor social skills
- Aggressiveness
- Avoidance or withdrawal from new situations
- Use of alcohol
- Unrealistic pursuit of surgical solutions

Data from Macgregor F: *Transformation and identity: the face and plastic surgery.* New York, 1974, Quadrangle/New York Times Book Company.

This research is important to those working in the maxillofacial trauma field, primarily because it identifies individual behavior, rather than the condition or appearance, as a determinant of successful long-term outcomes. This is encouraging because behavior is learned and can be modified. These ideas provide the basis for psychological management of patients with altered appearance, who do not have to rely solely on biomedical solutions aimed at restoring appearance.

PSYCHOLOGICAL ASPECTS OF MAXILLOFACIAL TRAUMA

ANXIETY, DEPRESSION, AND POSTTRAUMATIC STRESS DISORDER

Disfigurement exposes individuals to a range of social stressors and psychological stresses that are predisposing factors for a trio of disorders. The relevant literature in this area indicates that depression, anxiety, and posttraumatic stress disorder (PTSD) are the most commonly reported psychological sequelae of burn injury or other types of trauma. The three often exist together, and high levels of comorbidity are expected. Many individuals who suffer burn injury or trauma already show a range of behaviors that place them at risk for mental illness, substance abuse, social problems, or previously existing psychiatric problems. The challenges of dealing with facial injury and disfigurement add to the psychological difficulties that may already be present. The degree to which an individual feels responsible for the injury may affect his or her attitude about asking for help. Shame is an important construct in this context, and survivors of trauma often are preoccupied with the idea that they have survived while others have not.[4,21]

PSYCHIATRIC ASSESSMENT AND MANAGEMENT

Studies based on psychiatric models measure symptoms of mental distress, such as depression, anxiety, and PTSD, which are clearly defined within the fourth edition of the *Diagnostic and Statistical Manual of Mental Disorders* (DSM-IV) crite-

ria[22] and measured using standardized scales such as the Hospital Anxiety and Depression Scale.[23]

Depression

Depression can be understood in many ways. Depressed mood often is explained in terms of a subjective feeling of unhappiness, encompassing feelings of guilt, worthlessness, listlessness, apathy, and self-loathing. Depression can be associated with other medical problems and develop as a secondary reaction. Depressed mood can be seen as a reaction to circumstances that an individual can work through with assistance from others and that will dissipate over time. Clinical depression is more serious and more pervasive, and it often requires formal intervention to be resolved.

To obtain a diagnosis of clinical depression, an individual must display a cluster of symptoms that usually comprise depressed mood, loss of interest, anxiety, sleep disturbance, loss of appetite, lack of energy, and suicidal thoughts.[22] Additional symptoms may include weeping, slowness of speech and action, extreme withdrawal, hallucinations (often of ridiculing voices), and delusions that the person has been responsible for a horrific catastrophe. Thoughts of death, self-harm, or suicide can occur.

It is more difficult to recognize depression in someone who is physically unwell or who has been injured. Many of the physical symptoms typically described for depression can overlap with symptoms of physical illness. For example, appetite loss is to be expected if an individual has difficulties eating. An instrument such as the Hospital Anxiety and Depression Scale,[23] which was designed to detect depression and anxiety while disregarding ambiguous physical symptoms, can help to screen patients at risk for anxiety or depression, or both.

Anxiety Disorders

Fear is a natural response to anything perceived as threatening. Patients are often anxious about their diagnosis and treatment, and the heightened arousal can cause difficulties in attending to information in the consultation or following instructions for rehabilitation. Medical treatment is often associated with pervasive anxiety. An anxious patient is particularly tuned into threatening stimuli and is more likely to interpret information as threatening and find it difficult to assess risk objectively. The process of repeat scanning as part of follow-up can produce a cycle of dread in anxious patients, who become more and more preoccupied as the target date approaches, gaining only temporary relief afterward as the build-up to the next scan begins.

Responses occur on a number of levels: behavioral, cognitive (thoughts), affective (emotions), and physiological. Social fears and anxiety related to disfigurement are common. Much of this chapter discusses approaches that can be used to help individuals to overcome these fears and anxieties.

Adjustment Disorder

Adjustment disorder is a somewhat vague term used by psychiatrists to describe the cluster of symptoms, including depressed mood, anxiety, and physical complaints such as pain, that are common in people who struggle to engage in rehabilitation, including physiotherapy and resuming a normal diet. Although it is not abnormal to find a change in circumstances challenging, some may require additional support and reassurance. People also vary in their acceptance of prostheses, including walking and hearing aids. Managing chemotherapy with the associated changes in energy levels, appearance, and general well-being may be exceptionally difficult for some people, and psychological intervention can assist them to set realistic goals, pace activities, and focus their attention appropriately.

TREATMENT

Effective treatment may be delivered by a combination of approaches. Psychological treatment (particularly cognitive-behavioral approaches, which produce the best outcomes) has become much more widely understood, and access to these techniques has been improved by the Increasing Access to Psychological Treatment (IAPT) protocols in primary care in the United Kingdom for people with mild or moderate depression and anxiety.[24]

Depression can result from negative thinking styles and biases in perception and cognitive functioning. The therapist and patient work together to change this worldview using cognitive approaches and behavioral experiments in the context of a warm, empathic, and genuine relationship. Evaluation of these approaches demonstrates improvement of longer duration and generalizability. So-called third-wave approaches include mindfulness, which combines Western psychotherapy and Eastern meditation to focus the individual in the present rather than on thoughts about the past and future. This is a particularly effective approach to preventing relapse. Medication is used for people with severe symptoms, but it should be combined with psychological therapy as set out in the NICE guidelines for the treatment of depression.[25] Anxiety disorders typically respond well to a combination of psychological therapy (e.g., cognitive-behavioral approaches) and medication. These approaches are clearly defined in the NICE guidelines for the treatment of anxiety.[26]

POSTTRAUMATIC STRESS DISORDER

Most patients being treated for maxillofacial injuries sustained the damage in a traumatic incident. This section considers the possible consequences of exposure to trauma, effects on psychological functioning, and treatment approaches. This is not a comprehensive review of this vast area, and further information can be found in other textbooks.[27]

Humans exist in a continuous state of homeostasis. As the environment changes, we try to adapt to the shifting demands. This applies to everyday occurrences and to extraordinary experiences. As we age, we learn to make sense of what has been encountered and to place it in context. When an event occurs that is far outside ordinary expectations, a major process of adjustment may have to take place, and feelings may be unique, powerful, and unfamiliar. When we are threatened or frightened, the body and brain are programmed to ensure our survival (i.e., fight, freeze, or flight reactions).

If exposed to threat, the individual usually tries to deal effectively with the event by thinking about it and attempts to learn how to cope better with the threat if it occurs again in the future. However, traumatic events may be processed very differently from the way in which other events and memories are processed. Brewin[28] offers a clear explanation of the dual processing theory, which proposes that highly emotionally charged images are processed and stored without access to the perceptual processing pathways that confer meaning. Flashbacks occur when sensory triggers (i.e., sights, sounds, or scents) stimulate the re-emergence of images without the ability to place them in context, with the result that they become relived or re-experienced. Considerable research supports this explanation, including the recommended treatment approaches set out for adults and children in the NICE guidelines.[29]

Maxillofacial trauma implies exposure to some type of trauma that results in injury to the face. Interpersonal violence is becoming the most common cause of maxillofacial trauma for adults in Western society. Being exposed to violence from another individual can be seriously challenging to our beliefs regarding the world as a safe, benevolent place to be. The response to violence may be to view everyone as malevolent. Other causes of injury, such as car crashes and accidents in the home or at work, also can challenge the view of the world as a predictable and safe place. It is understandable that the immediate response is often one of avoidance and reluctance to leave the safety of a familiar environment; however, the sooner people can get back to their familiar, everyday lives, the earlier their recovery.

Definition of Posttraumatic Stress Disorder

The syndrome of PTSD was officially recognized in 1983 by the American Psychiatric Association. After several updates and revisions, the current definitions in the DSM-IV[22] are those in common circulation. They are outlined in Box 29-2.

Facial disfigurement can compound many of the symptoms shown in Box 29-2 by giving constant reminders of the trauma and increasing feelings of social isolation. Many individuals with maxillofacial trauma have experienced events that can predispose them to PTSD.

BOX 29-2   Definitions of Posttraumatic Stress Disorder

The diagnosis of posttraumatic stress disorder (PTSD) requires a person to have been exposed to a traumatic event of exceptional severity and to be re-experiencing distressing symptoms. People with PTSD usually show emotional detachment from people, places, or activities previously enjoyed; numbing; hyperarousal; and avoidance of stimuli associated with the trauma. Either of the following factors, which usually arise within 6 months of the trauma, must also be present:

1. Partial or complete impaired recall for some aspects of the period of exposure to the stressor
2. Persistent symptoms of increased psychological arousal that were not present before the trauma
   - Sleep disturbance (falling or staying asleep)
   - Anger or irritability
   - Concentration difficulties
   - Hypervigilance
   - Exaggerated startle response

Adapted from National Institute for Health and Clinical Excellence (NICE): *NICE guidelines for the treatment of post-traumatic stress disorder, 2005:* http://www.nice.org.uk/CG26. Accessed May 1, 2011.

Incidence and Prevalence of Posttraumatic Stress Disorder

Epidemiological research suggests that most people experience at least one traumatic event during their lifetimes. Intentional acts of violence are more likely to lead to PTSD than accidents. Men tend to experience more trauma than women, but women tend to experience higher-impact events. Women are more likely to develop PTSD in response to a traumatic event than men.

Posttraumatic Stress Disorder in Children and Adolescents

There has been little systematic research about children with PTSD. Children affected by trauma demonstrate symptoms of re-experiencing, avoidance, numbing, and increased arousal, and younger children show more obvious aggression. Parental behavior is very influential, and children often choose not to talk about trauma or their reactions to it with their parents. This means that the condition is underdiagnosed and that a parental report alone does not constitute an adequate assessment.

Identification of Posttraumatic Stress Disorder

Normal Reactions and Symptoms

It is common for those who have been exposed to trauma to experience, at least briefly, some of the previously described symptoms. They typically pass quickly without treatment. Those who have been traumatically injured often thought that they were going to die. Re-experiencing the traumatic event in flashbacks or nightmares is common, but this reaction usually passes with time. Reminders of the accident, including seeing the disfiguring injury itself, can cause a recurrence of symptoms. This can lead to avoidance of the feared stimulus that can bring back the disturbing images.

NICE Guidelines for Treatment

Most people have a period of sleeplessness, preoccupation, and distress related to trauma. This is not PTSD according to the NICE guidelines, and it is important not to intervene too early.

Watchful Waiting in the First Month

Input from involved professionals involves support and education. Through reassurance, explanation, and normalization, individuals and their families can learn about their reactions. Simple anxiety management strategies focused on controlled breathing and distraction can help during this time. If this approach is followed, an assessment should be offered at the end of this period.

Treatment of Posttraumatic Stress Disorder

If an individual appears to be suffering from the symptoms described previously and they persist for longer than 1 month after injury, assistance from other sources should be sought. The NICE guidelines recommend psychological intervention as the first-line treatment before medication is considered. Psychological treatments take the form of trauma-focused cognitive-behavioral therapy (CBT) and eye movement desensitization and reprocessing (EMDR). Trauma-focused CBT usually requires 8 to 12 sessions. By retelling the experience in detail over repeated sessions, the highly sensory images are organized and reprocessed so that they become experienced as memories rather than as reliving the event. Avoidance behaviors are managed by gradual exposure and anxiety reduction.

EMDR involves the use of rapid side-to-side eye movements while revisualizing the trauma. This appears to help the processing of flashbacks in a way similar to trauma-focused CBT. It is a recognized treatment with good outcomes.

Medication can be considered for adults. The NICE guidelines recommend selective serotonin reuptake inhibitors (SSRIs) or the tetracyclic antidepressant mirtazapine. When medication is used, it usually is continued for at least 12 months. However, these medications should be offered only in certain circumstances:

- The person chooses not to have psychological treatment.
- The person has not benefited from psychological treatment.
- The person cannot start treatment because of the risk of further trauma.
- The person has a comorbid depression that reduces the effectiveness of psychological treatment.

Treatment of Posttraumatic Stress Disorder in Children

The NICE guidelines recommend a course of trauma-focused CBT for older children with severe symptoms within the first month after trauma. There is no evidence for the benefit of single-session debriefing at any age. After 3 months, advice for children is as follows:

- CBT should be offered and adapted to the developmental level, age, and circumstances.
- CBT should be a course of 8 to 12 sessions for children or young people who have chronic PTSD.
- When appropriate, parents and child should be involved in the treatment plan.
- Psychological treatment should be continuous (one session per week) and delivered by the same person.
- Parents or guardians should be informed that trauma-focused CBT is the recommended treatment and that there is no evidence for play therapy or family therapy.

Treatment for PTSD is highly effective, and outcomes are good even when there has been a long gap between the trauma and the start of treatment. Support for the family of an injured individual is often essential at the time of early treatment. Family reactions can have a huge impact on longer-term functioning, and preparing relatives for the appearance of their injured loved one so that they do not appear shocked or horrified can have a positive effect on self-acceptance. Those close to the individual also might have been exposed to the traumatic event, and they may be suffering from PTSD. If their functioning is compromised, it can influence the psychological recovery of the injured party.

FACTORS CONTRIBUTING TO EXPOSURE TO TRAUMA

The epidemiology of maxillofacial trauma is reviewed Chapter 1), which points out that assaults and road traffic accidents provide most cases of this type of trauma worldwide. Severe facial injuries increased among military casualties after development of body armor that protects the vital organs but leaves the face and extremities vulnerable, resulting in multiple amputations and facial disfigurements.[30]

The misuse of alcohol also plays a role in facial injuries, particularly among the young. Programs have been developed to provide early intervention to manage problem drinking, with patients targeted in accident and emergency settings. Successful nurse-led programs include those set up in Glasgow, Scotland, where the incidence of problem drinking is the highest in the United Kingdom.[31] A review of actions designed to prevent injuries in problem drinkers[32] concluded that there is some evidence for a variety of medical and psychological interventions reducing injuries, including falls, drinking-related injuries, domestic violence, and suicide. Interventions included education, medication, cue exposure, brief interventions, and motivational interviewing. By offering support, education, and referral to specialist services, it seems likely that professionals working in the trauma field can assist their patients in reducing their risk behaviors and the likelihood of repeat injury. Patients who are identified as drinking in a dependent or problem fashion should be counseled appropriately and offered the chance to be referred to local alcohol services for specialized help.

Patients who have been burned have been studied extensively. Most patients admitted to the hospital due to burn injuries are categorized as sensory impaired because of drug or alcohol use, age (very young or very old), or psychiatric illness. Premorbid psychopathology in those who sustain burn injuries severe enough to warrant hospitalization includes depression, personality disorders, and alcohol and drug abuse.[4] Dementia and other neurological disorders are commonly reported, and individuals from lower socioeconomic groups are disproportionately represented. Estimates of previous psychiatric illness range from 28% to 75%. Individuals who have suffered burn injury also seem to have a high frequency of risk-taking behavior, and those with psychiatric illness may be careless, actively self-harming, and disturbed or have reduced levels of competence.

COURSE OF UNTREATED PSYCHOLOGICAL PROBLEMS OVER TIME

The popular idea that "time is the best healer" is not supported by the evidence in the maxillofacial injury setting. An early study looking at the change in outcomes for the head and neck cancer population reported that psychosocial problems increase and medical problems decrease with time after surgery.[33] Semple et al.[8] reviewed the quality of life issues for these patients and stressed the ongoing challenges that patients experience with regard to appearance, speech, and eating. Patients often lack the appropriate coping skills to manage the profound change that they have experienced, and the study suggests that this pattern can be prevented with better clinical input using cognitive-behavioral approaches that teach an active approach to management. Although studies suffer from small sample sizes and other methodological weaknesses, a growing literature supports the use of active rehabilitation programs in this area.[34,35] This has also been found in the long-term follow-up of patients who have had severe burns.[36]

The finding that psychosocial problems remain and may become worse with time while medical problems may resolve is significant. It stimulates the ethical arguments about moderation of procedures that have a devastating impact and supports a more comprehensive approach to the study of outcomes, such as the quality of life model. It also provides support to researchers working in a coping skills framework who are attempting to discover factors that predict successful coping and who are beginning to develop models for clinical intervention.

QUALITY OF LIFE RESEARCH

The value of using a quality of life framework for investigating the long-term impact of medical conditions lies in the intrinsic acknowledgment of the patient as a person with life roles beyond those of a sick patient. The model includes the basic premise that the value of a procedure is determined by the impact on the course and progress of the disease and by its effect on the individual. Medical issues such as side effects of drugs and measurement of anxiety and depression are important, but social issues such as the ability to continue with employment also are key indicators of the value of a procedure. It is not difficult to see that this model provides a comprehensive picture of outcome within conditions and has the potential for comparing across conditions and treatment modalities.

The definition of quality of life has proved challenging. A widely adopted definition is that *quality of life* refers to patients' appraisal of and satisfaction with their current level of functioning compared with what they perceive to be possible or ideal.[37] The World Health Organization (WHO) Quality of Life group defined quality of life as patients' perceptions of their position in life in the context of culture and value systems in which they live and in relation to their goals, expectations, standards, and concerns. The group developed the World Health Organization Quality of Life Assessment-BREF (WHOQOL-BREF), which is widely used in European studies.[38] As the model has been developed, issues such as religious beliefs have been added to it, and a large number of researchers have been involved in devising, validating, and measuring quality of life scales. Self-report has become a contentious issue, with some suggestion that a large part of the literature on quality of life is redundant because it is based on health professionals' assessment of what is essentially an individual issue. Self-report is considered vital if the measure is to have any meaning. As scales have become more and more precisely validated for specific populations, other researchers have stressed the artificiality of imposing set categories on questionnaires, and the need for people to generate their own categories has been stressed.[39]

Despite all these difficulties, the quality of life literature has grown enormously, and within many medical settings, it has produced the most useful approach to measuring outcome. According to Talmi,[40] a MEDLINE search in 1970 produced only 6 reports that included quality of life as a major outcome measure, but by 2000, a similar search produced 4797 reports. However, Semple et al.[8] noted that most of the work has been in the development and validation of scales and that proliferation of measures leads to problems in collating the results from different studies. Despite these problems, Llewellyn et al.[41] published a systematic review of psychosocial and behavioral factors related to health-related quality of life and concluded that several psychosocial factors were potentially modifiable and offered possibilities for intervention to improve patients' quality of life in the long term.

In an important paper published in 1995, Bjordal et al.[42] compared patient-rated quality of life scores with physicians' ratings. Patients consistently rated their quality of life as lower than that rated by the clinicians. This study stresses the importance of self-report and the need for interventions that attempt to improve patients' coping strategies and meet their rehabilitation needs. Semple et al.[8] used a qualitative approach to explore the changes and challenges to lifestyle after treatment for head and neck cancer. Their sample of patients described the impact of their condition across many different aspects of everyday living rather than problems in one domain. This finding supports the need to manage patients holistically.

Although there have been some attempts to develop psychosocial interventions rather than report that they are needed, studies have been criticized for methodological weaknesses, including small sample sizes and lack of control groups. There has been little practical development of these approaches in the clinical setting.

COPING THEORIES AND INTERVENTIONS

Coping theories have generated much work in clinical and health psychology, particularly about cancer patients. These studies have an a priori model within which they attempt to describe psychological issues and how patients manage them. Some studies go on to suggest or investigate potential intervention strategies within this coping framework. For example, in a study investigating the effects of nursing care guided by self-regulation theory on coping with radiation therapy, by preparing patients carefully before treatment, less disruption to life activities was found during and after treatment.[43] Although this older study is of breast and prostate cancer patients, it is well designed and controlled, and it has a clear practical application for the way in which nurses can prepare patients with other conditions for invasive procedures.

Another approach to rehabilitation after head and neck cancer surgery uses Lazarus' cognitive-transactional theory of stress.[44] It proposes that a patient will respond to the stress of surgery by trying to identify and develop an appropriate coping response. From this approach developed the stress-coping model, also known as the Dropkin model (named after its author), which allowed exploration of the process of rehabilitation and prediction of aspects of behavior that facilitate good outcome. This model has been developed and applied to many groups of patients whose disfigurements may place them at a social disadvantage, including patients with head and neck cancer, traumatic disfigurement after surgery, and facial transplanation.[45]

The Dropkin model has been translated into a practical care plan with specific objectives defined for each postoperative day (Box 29-3). For example, early socialization is identified as a predictor of good long-term outcome, and patients are encouraged to leave their rooms and use the whole ward during early ambulation. Immediate postoperative care includes early confrontation of the facial disfigurement by looking in the mirror. Although attempted avoidance may be common, this is vigorously challenged, and patients are

---

BOX 29-3 | Behavioral Observation and Action Plan for Maxillofacial Patients

Postoperative Days*

	1	2	3	4	5	6	7
Motor Activities							
Lying in bed					A		A
Sitting in chair in room					S		S
Ambulation in room					S		S
Ambulation out of room					E		E
Ambulation beyond ward					S		S
					S		S
Self-Care Behaviors					M		M
Wash face (mirror)					E		E
Brush hair					N		N
Dress unaided					T		T
Assist with dressings							
Social Interaction							
Ambulation out of room					P		P
Eye contact?					O		O
Posture?					I		I
Interaction with staff					N		N
Eye contact?					T		T
Posture?							
Verbal?							
Interaction with other patients							
Eye contact?					O		T
Posture?					N		W
Verbal?					E		O

Action Plan

Days 1-7:	Monitor and assist the patient.
Day 5:	Review and prompt ambulation attempt if the patient is not out of the room.
Day 7:	All items should have been achieved. Discuss targets with the patient, reviewing particular concerns. Consider referral to a specialist.

*The protocol and postoperative dates are based on Dropkin's plan for head and neck cancer patients.[44] Target dates for other conditions should be determined by reference to the relevant cohort.

---

encouraged to take part in self-care, such as helping with dressings, from the earliest possible stage. Postoperative day 5 is an important watershed, with patients who are still having difficulty in taking part in their care more likely to have long-term problems. By day 7, very active clinical intervention from an experienced nurse is indicated for patients who still have problems in the area of socialization and early ambulation. This intervention takes the form of challenging unhelpful beliefs and emphasizing the importance of surgery; it is a cognitive intervention aimed at encouraging the patient to develop a behavioral response. This is one of the first studies to introduce the idea of coping into the literature, and it is an extremely effective piece of applied research, using psychological theory to generate and test very practical outcomes. However, there is room to develop more creative and innovative forms of intervention.

The goals of rehabilitation can be summarized in terms of reintegration into social and work settings. The importance of a rehabilitation program that starts early, preferably preoperatively, should be stressed, and it includes strategies such as those outlined earlier to ensure that the potential for healthy psychosocial recovery is maximized. Together with the research on quality of life in head and neck cancer, studies using a coping model to underpin the work consistently stress the need for patients to be offered some kind of support after surgery. Given the evidence of need and the promise of early studies' results, it is surprising that work is just beginning to develop and evaluate psychosocial intervention. Group interventions in particular offer the benefits of increasing social support while maximizing cost-effectiveness. Fiegenbaum first described the benefits of this approach in 1981, and Clarke drew on this approach 20 years later to design an intervention that developed the training needs of clinical nurse specialists in head and neck cancer and in burns.[35] This approach is based on a model for understanding much of the dysfunction after treatment of head and neck cancer in terms of social embarrassment. Patients may look and sound differently, and they may report problems with eating in public. Using a coping skills approach, patients can learn different strategies for managing these difficulties in the same way as they manage social interaction problems associated with disfigurement, with positive impact on social functioning and quality of life. Clarke demonstrated that nurses could deliver effective intervention that had a positive impact on quality of life for patients, but the work suffers from small sample sizes.

Bessell et al.[46] built on the CBT approaches used in clinical practice to develop a computerized intervention for people with disfiguring conditions. This was effective, with benefits evident at the 6-month follow-up, and it proved to be very acceptable to patients of all ages. It offers a highly innovative approach to managing patients remotely. This field remains an area in which the evidence for the benefits of psychological rehabilitation is beginning to accrue[47] and one that awaits robust, long-term evaluation.

PSYCHOLOGICAL IMPACT OF MAXILLOFACIAL TRAUMA

Cumulative research confirms that maxillofacial trauma may have a major impact on the individual. Patients represent a high-risk group for severe psychiatric illness, especially given the high incidence of premorbid conditions such as alcoholism and substance abuse, which increase the probability of severe depression, anxiety, and suicide postoperatively.

Psychosocial problems may persist and get worse over time, even after medical problems resolve. Measurable psychiatric symptoms may persist months or years after the traumatic event, with a resulting breakdown in lifestyle. When avoidant coping strategies are used, individuals do not have the opportunity to develop a repertoire of positive coping responses, and social avoidance may develop into complete social isolation. Length of time since trauma is not a useful predictor of outcome without considering the patient's coping style.

For many maxillofacial patients, separating the relative impact of disfigurement and dysfunction is difficult to do, but it is intriguing that studies of other conditions in which there is no associated dysfunction (e.g., dermatological conditions) find no relationship between severity (usually size or noticeability) of the lesion and psychological distress. This apparently counterintuitive finding has been repeatedly reported.[19,20] Similarly, Cordeiro et al.[48] compared patients presenting with purely esthetic facial concerns with those whose altered facial appearance was caused by an underlying medical condition and a third group with both functional and esthetic changes (i.e., scleroderma). Psychological distress was highest among those with purely esthetic conditions and lowest among those with additional functional impairment. Given this evidence, it is important to consider the psychological impact of any change of appearance after trauma; there is no basis for assuming that patients with minor scarring are at less risk for psychological distress than those with severe scarring. Similarly, after surgery for head and neck cancer, patients with severe disfigurement may adapt as well as patients with a much less obvious defect. Adjustment involves psychological processes, including dispositional optimism, cognitive appraisal of the outcome in light of other issues, level of social support, and a nonavoidant approach to management. The ways in which these factors combine can be understood in terms of the impact of the disease on the individual.[49] In other words, how well can this person adapt to changes caused by trauma or treatment given his or her lifestyle and the extent of social support available?

The importance of social interaction is highlighted in the literature on disfigurement across conditions and re-emerges in the quality of life literature as a major determinant of long-term outcome after maxillofacial trauma. The use of prostheses, pressure garments for burn injury, and exposure of the individual to situations that are perceived as socially embarrassing are emphasized. Speech and eating difficulties can affect the individual because of their social effects rather than because of the day-to-day management in practical terms. Interventions aimed at facilitating a patient's ability to maintain social function within the family, at school, and at work are a logical development from these findings, and a few successful studies have been reported.

Social support, as in many studies of adaptation after major surgery or disease, is important in predicting good outcome. This is a challenging finding given the premorbid characteristics of patients who experience burns, trauma, and head or neck cancer, with the very factors that increase risk of injury or disease also predicting poor social support. Maximizing support is nevertheless an important goal for rehabilitation, with relatives involved in planning long-term care when possible and, if support is not necessarily evident in close family attachments, introduction to lay support groups.

Impact of age, gender, and ethnicity must be considered. Research studies on disfigurement across conditions find no effect for these variables, but this may be because there has been relatively little research on large populations, particularly ethnic populations. Given the importance of the face in reinforcing feminine stereotypes, however, there remains an assumption that facial injuries for girls and women are linked with poorer outcomes,[50] but later research has stressed the importance of appearance for men and older populations.[7]

PLANNING AND MANAGING PSYCHOLOGICAL SUPPORT AFTER MAXILLOFACIAL TRAUMA

BUILDING PSYCHOSOCIAL SUPPORT INTO ROUTINE PATIENT CARE

Patient Advocacy

Increasingly in specialist services, a multidisciplinary team with representation from many disciplines manages patients. From the patient's perspective, this translates into many people to see, often at one visit and frequently in one room (i.e., goldfish bowl effect). This is a daunting prospect for anybody, and the efficiency with which information exchange takes place is reduced by the patient's anxiety. For children, there may be concerns that have not been shared with parents or caregivers.

One way of overcoming these problems is through advocacy. An initial interview with the patient by one member of the team can explain procedures and elicit questions and concerns. This member of the team takes responsibility for ensuring that everything that is of importance to the patient is discussed with the relevant team member. A second review session in a one-to-one setting can ensure that all advice is clearly understood and that outstanding issues are dealt with. In practice, this role can be filled by a designated nurse, clinical nurse specialist, or member of the medical team. This is a particularly helpful model for managing rounds in large wards.

Information about Patient Satisfaction

The request for information is a consistent finding in research into patient satisfaction with diagnosis and treatment in studies of quality of life during rehabilitation and throughout the health psychology literature. Most patients want to be adequately and honestly informed at each stage of treatment, although it is important to respect the subgroup of patients who prefer to leave all decision making in the hands of their medical team.

Balanced against the desire for information, patients sometimes complain of being bombarded with information at certain points in the treatment course, such as at diagnosis, and of feeling bewildered and unable to take it all in. Information given verbally at any stage may not be remembered accurately. The patient may lack the appropriate framework for asking questions, and information may be poorly understood. The same problems are reported by relatives and caregivers, even if present during consultation, who may remain uninformed or misinformed and therefore unable to offer the optimal level of appropriate support during treatment and after the patient goes home. Given the evidence of the importance of social support in health outcomes, caregivers can be seen as a huge untapped or wasted resource.

Although health professionals recognize that patients need information to manage their working and social lives, they have been slower to recognize the role of the individual in actively managing the condition. Despite the evidence that an informed and knowledgeable patient can expect a better outcome, patients may still be viewed with suspicion if they ask for a second opinion, want to read professional literature, or take notes in the consultation. Access to information on the Internet, which has no efficient quality control, is becoming a problem in medical settings. It remains difficult to provide the kind of information patients are asking for, which facilitates rather than challenges the working arrangement between health professional and patient. Clarke et al.[51] reviewed the information needs of patients contacting the charity Changing Faces and reported that most patients were seeking advice about their own role in the management of the condition. Newell et al.,[52] similarly reviewed the information needs of patients with head and neck cancer.

In some units, patients are routinely offered a folder of information about various aspects of their care or invited to hold their own care plans, compiling information on each aspect of their care as it becomes relevant. An example is the Teamwork Project for cancer patients in the United Kingdom, which is run in association with the National Cancer Alliance. Patient-led organizations such as CancerBackup and Changing Faces produce a variety of publications that can be made available routinely. A more patient-centered and less-expensive approach is to provide details of what is available, when the patient is most likely to find it helpful, and which member of the team is the appropriate person to ask. This allows the individual to pace the process of information gathering and reduces the chances of misinformation gathered from the least-experienced member of the team. It also allows the patient to take the lead in eliciting information. All written material offered to patients should have the source attributed and be dated to ensure quality control standards. A small ward or outpatient library can be easily assembled and accessed, and it makes good use of time spent waiting for appointments. Web resources are available, but high-quality information and ease of navigation are important criteria for patients accessing the Internet.[53]

PSYCHOSOCIAL SUPPORT

Patients seeking psychological adjustment require psychosocial support from family members or other sources. Quality of support appears to be more important than the number of sources, but the supporters often need some assistance to enable them to continue to help a family member. Many patients express a desire for ongoing support, and charities such as Changing Faces are highly regarded in terms of the information and activities they can provide for anyone experiencing or caring for someone who is experiencing a disfiguring condition. Support groups for specific conditions, such as acoustic neuroma and laryngectomy, are well organized and highly regarded in the United Kingdom. Specialized psychological support is becoming more prevalent and often is provided by clinical nurse specialists and psychology services specializing in patients with altered appearance.

STEPPED-CARE APPROACH TO PSYCHOSOCIAL MANAGEMENT

The stepped-care approach is fully embedded in cancer services, but it has utility in all multidisciplinary settings. Patient care includes a psychosocial component in the same way that all patients are offered analgesia, routine physiotherapy, and wound care management. This care may be designed and managed by one designated person, but it is delivered by all members of the multidisciplinary team. The aim is to ensure that treatment outcomes are maximized by providing information in a way that promotes understanding, reduces anxiety, promotes self-care, and develops appropriate coping strategies in the short and long term. This approach provides a patient-centered environment that looks beyond the condition to the individual's needs and the needs of the family. This is psychological support as patients commonly refer to it in self-report studies. Their experience is characterized by staff attitudes, time available to talk through issues that concern them, and information available when they need it. This support may be experienced as relative informality, but it depends on careful management to ensure that protocols of care are in place. Inclusion of the term *psychological support* as part of the nursing process is not enough without ensuring that all staff members are appropriately trained and that psychological issues are not dismissed as secondary to the physical aspects of care.

In some medical units, psychologists may be central in organizing support, but in others, mental health professionals may not be involved at all. It can be difficult for ward team members who offer this standard of care to understand what a consulting psychiatrist or clinical psychologist can add. "We do all of our own psychological support" is a common view.

PLISSIT MODEL

The PLISSIT model[54] has four levels of intervention: permission, limited information, specific suggestions, and intensive treatment. It has been used to provide psychosocial screening and intervention for persons with sexual dysfunction, and Rumsey et al.[7] adapted it for use in treating patients with disfiguring conditions.

Level One: Permission

A direct approach is encouraged. Permission applies to both sides of the interaction, with all patients and all health professionals encouraged to ask questions about psychosocial issues.

We recommend that all patients develop a response to answering questions about their appearance that manages curiosity by providing a minimal amount of information.[21,55] In practice, this means that all practitioners are responsible for raising questions about appearance (Box 29-4).

A good answer is one that demonstrates that the person has anticipated the situation and has a plan or is clearly not distressed about the likelihood of this kind of intrusion. A response that suggests the patient is hoping no one will notice or is putting life on hold until he or she looks normal again should prompt an offer of more information.

Level Two: Limited Information

Health professionals must manage the responses that they get directly or by referral. No one is likely to ask if he or she has no idea about how to manage the answer or believes this approach will be time consuming.

Resources such as details of support organizations or website addresses provide a limited information response. At a minimum, anyone who has an unusual facial appearance

---

BOX 29-4 **Psychological Screening Process for Identifying Patients' Appearance-Related Concerns**

Step One
Question 1: How do you think the change in your appearance will affect your life, if at all (record response)?
- If the patient indicates no impact, confirm with a query: "Is there nothing that you will feel uncomfortable about when you first go home?"
- If yes, go to step 2. If no, go to step 3.

Step Two
Question 2: What specific things do you feel less comfortable about (list three examples)?
1.
2.
3.

Step Three
Patients sometimes ask what to do when other people ask questions about their condition. The patient may ask, "What kind of thing would you do in my position?" Use the patient's condition as the example, and record your response.

Step Four
The patient's behavior is observed during the assessment.
- Did the patient avoid making eye contact with you?   Y/N
- Did the patient try to conceal his face by turning to one side or covering his face with his hand?   Y/N

Step Five
Action planning is based on analysis of the situation.
1. Based on the patient's verbal and nonverbal responses to your questions, do you think there are any social or emotional consequences of the change in his appearance due to maxillofacial trauma?   Yes   No   Maybe   (circle one)
2. If your answer is Yes or Maybe, will you:
   - Suggest that he speaks to the psychologist
   - Ask the psychologist to speak to him
   - Offer him relevant information
   - Suggest a coping strategy yourself

Data from a personal communication from G.M. Coughlan, 2000.

---

should be encouraged to have an answer to questions about his or her face.

Level Three: Specific Suggestions

At the third level of intervention, the health professional provides help guided toward a specific problem. This has been called the *target stressors approach*, which builds strategies for managing commonly reported problems. This approach is used by Changing Faces in their direct work with patients and through their information resources.

Nurses in a counseling role, clinical nurse specialists, occupational therapists, and maxillofacial technicians are well placed to deliver a psychosocial intervention at this third level of the PLISSIT model (Table 29-1). Computer-based interventions such as FaceIT, developed by Bessell et al.,[46] are a recent addition to psychological treatment, and evaluation of this approach indicates that it is extremely effective.

TABLE 29-1	Stepped-Care Framework for Interventions to Promote Psychosocial Adjustment in Appearance Concern		
Level of Intervention	Description	Example of Intervention	Health Professional Background
Level 1	Permission	Sensitive exploration of psychosocial concerns	All health practitioners including general practitioners, practice nurses, National Health Service (NHS) Direct
Level 2	Limited information	Written information, recommended websites and contact details for support groups; answers basic questions about visible differences	All health practitioners working with target groups, including doctors and nurses in relevant specialties
Level 3	Specific suggestions	Social skills training, dealing with staring, comments, and questions; managing social situations proactively	Nurses in a counseling role, clinical nurse specialists, occupational therapists, maxillofacial technicians, support groups
Level 4	Intensive treatments	Cognitive-behavioral therapy aimed at identifying and modifying maladaptive appearance schemes	Specialist training in cognitive-behavioral therapy

From Rumsey N, Clarke A, Harcourt D, for the Appearance Research Collaboration (ARC): *Factors and processes associated with positive adjustment to disfiguring conditions. Report to the Healing Foundation, 2009*: www.thehealingfoundation.org. Accessed April 28, 2011.

Level Four: Intensive Treatment

Psychologists use higher intensity evidence-based approaches to manage behavior. Intervention may occur before surgery to deliver appropriate smoking or alcohol cessation programs, to assess information needs and expectations of surgery, or to manage other problems identified by the multidisciplinary team. Problems may be identified postoperatively in terms of poor coping or socialization in line with a Dropkin-style protocol, or patients may have increased anxiety or depression, flashbacks, or other symptoms requiring treatment. Long-term follow-up can disclose failure to re-engage in day-to-day activities, social avoidance and isolation, poor adherence with treatment (e.g., use of pressure garments), or for children, school refusal or failure.

Any psychological approach is only as good as the screening process that identifies the patient's problems. At the inpatient stage, progress with early socialization, monitoring of mood and self-care behaviors, and an apparent lack of social support can be important indicators for identifying who needs further help. Standardized measures such as screening instruments for anxiety and depression and quality of life measures can be useful in assessing long-term outcome, but

a good clinical interview can be equally important. Many psychological issues, particularly problems such as poor sexual function, rarely are volunteered by the patient and are not identified unless there is a commitment to discussing psychosocial issues by all members of the care team.

Children are particularly difficult to assess, because they may deny their problems completely or rate them as much worse than the ratings given by their parents. A specialist's assessment is indicated when there are signs of problems, which may first be evident as a breakdown in behavior routines or concern about bullying.

In practice, a stepped-care approach works effectively only in settings in which psychological support is a routine part of the treatment package, appropriate assessment procedures are in place, and pathways to appropriate referral are available and properly understood.

PLANNING FOR ELECTIVE SURGERY

MODIFICATION OF RISK BEHAVIORS

The nature of maxillofacial trauma means that many patients are treated on an emergency basis. However, for patients with conditions for which a series of surgical procedures is planned as part of reconstructive surgery, psychological assessment can be beneficial. In addition to screening for PTSD or other psychiatric symptoms that require treatment, psychological support may target risk behaviors. A smoking cessation program can provide real benefits in terms of lung function and wound healing, even if the patient stops smoking a few days or weeks before surgery. Alcohol intake should be carefully assessed because detoxification over a few days can prevent problems of acute confusional states postoperatively. Protocols for managing substance abuse range from early admission of patients (by a few days), so that alcohol can be withdrawn and appropriate medication substituted, to individual sessions supporting smoking withdrawal.[49]

LOOKING IN THE MIRROR AND EARLY SOCIALIZATION

Most specialist units remove mirrors so that the introduction to a new appearance can be planned; in practice, most patients catch sight of themselves in reflective surfaces anyway. It makes sense to ensure that appearance is optimized as much as possible (e.g., wait until the edema is reduced). However, it is important that protocols do not unwittingly promote a policy of avoidance. The key to successful rehabilitation is confrontation and management of change, and this approach should begin as soon as possible.

The first step is education. In this phase, the patient needs to understand that appearance will continue to change dramatically and that the current status is not the end of the process. Questions should be answered frankly, and uncertainty about the outcome should be framed as much as possible in terms of the control that the individual can exert. For example, the long-term presence of disfigurement or scars can be discussed in terms of the use of pressure garments.

However well prepared, patients do experience shock and need time to talk about their feelings. They may choose to talk about how they feel, they may wish to have time before talking, or they may choose not to disclose their feelings. Managing this process at a time when the patient is assured of the opportunity for contemplation, rather than just before visitors are due, is important. This process has been likened to bereavement or grieving for the lost self, and the emphasis is on the chance for someone to talk about his or her feelings rather than offering management strategies at this stage.

Beliefs about the future are likely to be confused. People may feel that their plans and hopes about the future have vanished. Catastrophizing or magnifying negative events may lead to a situation in which the patient thinks that he will never work again, never have friends, or never form relationships. Acknowledging this pattern of thinking without necessarily probing too far is a helpful intervention at this stage. Talking in general terms about these patterns of thinking, particularly when changing dressings or helping patients with self-care activities, helps to acknowledge these thoughts as a normal part of the response to trauma. This is also a chance for extreme reactions or altered mood to be identified.

As the initial shock of the trauma becomes less extreme, focusing on behavior becomes a key intervention. Involving patients in their own self-care, such as dressings, and encouraging relatives to ask whether cutting up food or doing up buttons is helpful before assuming the care role help to promote independence from the outset. Early mobilization around the unit provides the earliest opportunities for social interaction and the basis for building key nonverbal strategies. Encouraging patients to stand up with a good posture, to maintain eye contact, to nod, and to stop and talk to other patients and discouraging behaviors such as covering the face with the hand or trying to let hair fall forward over the face are important strategies.

Gradually building on this behavior each day provides the foundations of effective coping and influences patients' beliefs and feelings about themselves and their opportunities for the future. Verbal coping strategies can be supported by written information, but learning to answer simple questions about appearance is a useful skill. Anyone who has sustained a facial injury will be questioned (What happened to your face?). Giving a simple answer to the question is something that everyone should be prepared for and should feel confident about.

Early socialization can be implemented as a protocol with assessment at key stages and planned intervention when problems arise. In practice, this is the same process as wound management, in which stitches are inspected for signs of infection, they are removed on a set day, and antibiotic therapy (i.e., remedial process) is triggered when problems arise. For example, the patient who is particularly tearful or reluctant to leave his room by the end of the first week may be referred for help from the psychologist. A three-point standard for all patients who have altered appearance at the point of discharge is provided in Box 29-5.

BOX 29-5	Three-Point Standard for Patients with Altered Appearance at Discharge

- Patients should have the name of the appropriate support group.
- Patients should have access to relevant information about their condition and its management.
- Patients should be able to answer simple questions about their condition.

Data from Rumsey N, Clarke A, White P, Hooper E: Exploring the psychosocial concerns of outpatients with disfiguring conditions, *J Wound Care* 12:247-252, 2003.

PLANNING FUTURE CARE

After the immediate life-threatening phase is over, the patient's concerns are about the uncertainty of the future and what can be done in terms of medical and surgical input. The uncertainty of outcome after maxillofacial trauma is compounded by the length of time involved in waiting to see how well reconstructive techniques have worked before planning the next phase. Understanding that the medical team does not yet know precisely what further surgery will be needed can be difficult. It is frustrating to the medical team too to word responses in a way that can come across as evasive.

Putting a time frame on decisions, preferably within a written care plan, is of great value to the patient. A clear indication of how frequently appointments will be planned and the kinds of decisions that will be made at each one is very reassuring. Structuring the time between decisions in terms of patients' and relatives' roles turns what is effectively a wait-and-see process into one of active management and control. For example, diary keeping of significant personal events and treatment compliance (e.g., wearing of pressure garments, taking medication) and the use of photographs pasted in to record change are ways the family can measure progress. These kinds of approaches are especially helpful with children who have less understanding of time. It is also important to stress that physical and psychological recovery may proceed at different rates. Patients have not necessarily recovered because the wound has healed. Relatives can find this very difficult to absorb and lay organizations or support groups can help people through this stage.

PSYCHOLOGICAL ASPECTS OF FACIAL TRANSPLANTATION

Facial transplantation was proposed as a reconstructive option after severe trauma in 2002,[56] and it became a clinical reality with the first partial facial transplantation carried out in France in 2005.[57] Several successful procedures have been reported.[1] Initial concerns centered on the technical challenges of the procedure, the necessity of long-term immunosuppression, and the psychological issues associated with transplantation of facial tissue, particularly altered appearance.[58] The initial response to the concept of facial transplantation from both the general public and The Royal College of Surgeons (RCS) was very cautious with a strong recommendation that the potential unknown consequences of the procedure outweighed any clinical benefit. Concern about the likelihood of transferring identify from donor to recipient was very prevalent with considerable doubt about whether people would be prepared to donate facial tissue. The justification for immunosuppression for an essentially quality of life procedure also generated much debate. These issues have been gradually resolved by the steady publication of research studies examining the evidence and the use of computer generated images to illustrate the proposed procedures. Ultimately, it was the successful undertaking of the first partial face transplantation and its meticulous documentation that paved the way for this procedure to enter the clinical field.[57]

The prediction of major psychological problems for patients after transplantation has not been substantiated, with recipients positive about the procedure and re-engaged in social activity. Quality of life is improved, and the lifestyle goals of the patients have been achieved. Acute rejection has been managed by a temporary increase in the dosage of immunosuppressive medication, although long-term outcomes are not yet available. The incidence of chronic rejection has not yet been reported.

There have been major changes in the regulation of the procedure. The Royal College of Surgeons[58] and American Society of Plastic Surgery guidelines[59] stress the importance of highly skilled teams with surgeons, psychologists, transplantation clinicians, and therapists. This multidisciplinary approach characterizes the successful programs underway. The biggest threat to facial transplantation would be an unethical procedure or one carried out without appropriate assessment or team support for the patient over the long term.

PSYCHOLOGICAL ISSUES IN RECONSTRUCTIVE SURGERY

Although there is a clear and logical imperative for surgery that aims to restore function, techniques used for restoring appearance stimulate a wider debate. The medical team and the patient can find psychological support useful in the process of decision making. Reconstructive surgery can continue forever in the sense that there is always the opportunity to revise a scar and to make minor improvements to appearance. Sometimes, the patient seeks additional surgery, and sometimes, surgeons feel a responsibility to suggest further revision if improvement is possible. Both groups may find it difficult to work out the cost-benefit analysis, which focuses on the individual and the likely improvement in his or her lifestyle and self-esteem rather than on the surgical result. Perceived noticeability (the subjective view of the patient) is very important, although patient expectations of what is possible may exceed what the surgeon can achieve. Psychological assessment can help patients to understand the benefits of surgery in this context, to examine their motivations and to decide the point at which they feel comfortable about stopping the search for surgical solutions. Intervention can be useful when there are unrealistic expectations about what surgery can achieve, and when the motivation for surgery is principally about self-confidence, psychologists can help to clarify the relationship between objective physical appearance and self-esteem.

This is a field in which reliable instruments for measuring change are invaluable. Development and publication of the Derriford Appearance Scale[60] has enabled much better evaluation of long-term outcomes. It has helped us to learn more about the factors and processes that underpin adjustment of patients with disfiguring conditions.

PROVIDERS OF PSYCHOSOCIAL SUPPORT

One of the difficulties for the medical team working in this area is to understand the differences between the many disciplines offering psychological support. Referral to a clinical psychologist, a psychiatrist, a psychotherapist, or a counselor may result in quite different goals for the patients and different approaches to their management. Even within these disciplines, different therapists have preferred models for understanding behavior. What works for whom is an important topic, and a brief outline of these approaches and their appropriateness in various situations is given to facilitate effective clinical referral, service planning, and therapy delivery.

PSYCHIATRISTS

Physicians who work within a medical model understand psychiatric symptoms, such as depression, in terms of illness. Psychologists understand depression more in terms of a response to a set of maladaptive thoughts, beliefs, and behaviors. Some psychiatrists offer psychotherapy. Others refer to other health professionals if they think that psychotherapy may be helpful, but only psychiatrists are qualified to treat patients using medication.

CLINICAL PSYCHOLOGISTS

Qualified psychologists have undergone postgraduate training. They are essentially problem solvers, drawing heavily on their knowledge of research to help their clients understand the nature of their difficulties and designing and testing effective solutions. Clinical psychologists may use a number of approaches in their work, but they usually set clear targets and measure outcomes.

COUNSELORS

Counselors may have only 1 or many years of training. They use their relationships with their clients to provide an environment in which clients can work on living more resourcefully and successfully. The counselor's role is to listen and to help the client to clarify and organize his or her thoughts. A counselor does not give advice in the sense of suggesting solutions. Counselors may not have a degree in psychology or use the scientific understanding of behavior in their work, but they often have expertise in working in a specific area, such as cancer, bereavement, and disfigurement.

PSYCHOTHERAPISTS

Psychotherapists are most easily defined by comparing what they do with the work of counselors. There is much overlap between counseling and psychotherapy, with many counselors arguing that what they do is psychotherapy. In practical terms, counseling may address what is happening here and now, whereas psychotherapy may evaluate repetitious patterns of behavior. This means that counselors usually are working with their clients on a specific problem, and psychotherapists are working on a more general approach to managing a problem in a different way.

CHOOSING A SPECIALIST

All of the specialists described may have a role in treating patients with maxillofacial trauma. There is a clear role for a consultant psychiatrist in managing PTSD, anxiety, and depression with appropriate medication. Clinical psychologists often work with psychiatrists in the management of anxiety and depression; they use a cognitive-behavioral approach to help patients to challenge unhelpful beliefs and develop more appropriate behaviors. Clinical psychologists may also employ a coping framework to help patients develop more positive coping strategies through anxiety management and graded exposure aimed to overcome social avoidance. Psychologists may work with schools to ensure that a child's needs are fully understood and that there are recognized procedures in place to manage discrimination.

Psychiatrists and clinical psychologists offer forms of therapy that are highly structured and directive. Patients are prescribed a course of treatment or consent to a series of therapeutic sessions in which the focus of intervention is behavioral change. Targets are set, and outcomes are measured. In contrast, psychotherapy and (usually) counseling are nondirective, with the therapist following the lead of the patient.

Although there has been little research into what works for this population, there is evidence for the directive approach to management. Coping skills training has been demonstrated to be effective in individual and group settings. Counselors employed in health settings often take a more solution-focused approach to treatment than in other settings, but long-term individual psychotherapy is probably indicated only when there are long-standing emotional difficulties. Long-term psychotherapeutic groups have not been evaluated for this population.

The distinction between directive and nondirective approaches is important in considering lay support groups. The stereotypical support group, a collection of people sympathizing with each other about their problems, is not helpful. However, good patient-led support groups adhere much more closely to a coping model, promoting self-management, inviting speakers to talk about specialized aspects of their condition, and providing focused and informed support to their members. They are an increasingly important resource in the long-term management of all chronic medical conditions.

CONCLUSIONS

Patients who have undergone maxillofacial trauma require psychological support, with particular emphasis given to the management of appearance-related concerns. A stepped-care approach is used to manage psychological issues.[61]

Providing a supportive environment for patients is important for preventing long-term problems and for identifying issues that require more focused input. Effective support is delivered by the whole multidisciplinary team rather than exclusively by mental health professionals. Changing Faces is an organization that can provide support in the form of training courses and study days and through access to relevant resources.

Access to mental health specialists varies in different units. Psychiatry consultations may be more easily accessed than help from psychologists, although this direct help is also available through lay routes. The important message is that psychological support is more than simply providing a listening ear, and clinical intervention using the kind of directive approaches that have been outlined provides patients with psychological alternatives for managing the impact of maxillofacial trauma.

ACKNOWLEDGMENT

We respectfully remember Lisa Alexander and acknowledge her contribution as co-author in the first edition of this chapter in 2003.

REFERENCES

1. Clarke A, Butler PEM: Psychological management of facial transplantation. *Expert Rev Neurother* 9:1087-1100, 2009.
2. National Institute for Health and Clinical Excellence: NICE: www.nice.org.uk. Accessed May 1, 2011.
3. National Health Service: *National service frameworks and strategies*: www.nhs.uk/nhsengland/NSF/pages/Nationalserviceframeworks.aspx. Accessed May 1, 2011.
4. National Health Service: *National burn care review, 2001*: www.nbcg.nhs.co.uk/national-burn-care-review. Accessed May 1, 2011.
5. Changing Faces: *Changing faces*: www.changingfaces.co.uk. Accessed May 1, 2011.
6. Rumsey N, Harcourt D: Body image and disfigurement: issues and interventions. *Body Image* 1:83-97, 2004.
7. Rumsey N, Clarke A, Harcourt D, for of the Appearance Research Collaboration (ARC): *Factors and processes associated with positive adjustment to disfiguring conditions. Report to the Healing Foundation, 2009*: www.thehealingfoundation.org. Accessed April 28, 2011.
8. Semple CJ, Dunwoody L, Kernohan WG, et al: Changes and challenges to patients' lifestyle patterns following treatment for head and neck cancer. *J Adv Nurs* 52:85-93, 2008.
9. Argyle M: *The psychology of interpersonal behavior*, New York, 1994, Penguin.
10. Diamond J: *C—because cowards get cancer too*, London, 1999, Vermillion.
11. Macgregor F: *Transformation and identity: the face and plastic surgery*, New York, 1974, Quadrangle/New York Times Book Company.
12. Rumsey N, Harcourt D: *The psychology of appearance*, Berkshire, UK, 2005, Open University Press.
13. Rumsey N, Clarke A, White P, et al: Altered body image: appearance-related concerns of people with visible disfigurement. *J Adv Nurs* 48:443-453, 2004.
14. Lovegrove E, Rumsey N: Ignoring it doesn't make it stop: adolescents, appearance and anti-bullying strategies. *Cleft Palate Craniofac J* 42:33-44, 2005.
15. McGrouther DA: Facial disfigurement: the last bastion of discrimination. *Br Med J* 314:991, 1997.
16. Strenta F, Kleck R: Physical disability and the attribution dilemma: perceiving the causes of social behaviour. *J Soc Clin Psychol* 3:129-142, 1985.
17. Robinson E, Rumsey N, Partridge J: An evaluation of the impact of social interaction skills training for facially disfigured people. *Br J Plast Surg* 49:281-289, 1996.
18. Kleve L, Rumsey N, Wyn-Williams M, White P: The effectiveness of cognitive behavioural interventions at Outlook: a disfigurement support unit. *J Eval Clin Pract* 8:387-395, 2002.
19. Moss T: The relationship between objective and subjective ratings of disfigurement severity, and psychological adjustment. *Body Image* 2:151-159, 2005.
20. Ong JL, Clarke A, Johnson M, et al: Does severity predict distress? The relationship between subjective and objective measures of severity in patients treated for facial lipoatrophy. *Body Image* 4:239-248, 2007.
21. Coughlan G, Clarke A: Shame and burns. In Gilbert P, Miles J, editors: *Body shame: conceptualisation, research and treatment*, London, 2002, Routledge.
22. American Psychiatric Association: *Diagnostic and statistical manual of mental disorders*, ed 4, Washington, DC, 1994. American Psychiatric Association.
23. Zigmond A, Snaith R: The hospital anxiety and depression scale. *Acta Psychiatr Scand* 67:361-370, 1983.
24. UK Department of Health: *Increasing access to psychological therapies*: www.dh.gov.uk. Accessed May 1, 2011.
25. National Institute for Clinical Excellence: *NICE guidelines for depression, 2009*: http://guidance.nice.org.uk/CG/WaveR/24. Accessed May 1, 2011.
26. National Institute for Clinical Excellence: *NICE guidelines for anxiety, 2007*: http://guidance.nice.org.uk/CG22/NICEGuidance/pdf/English. Accessed May 1, 2011.
27. Yule W, editor: *Posttraumatic stress disorders: concepts and therapy*, Chichester, UK, 1999, John Wiley.
28. Brewin CR: *Post-traumatic stress disorder: malady or myth?* London, 2007, Yale University Press.
29. National Institute for Health and Clinical Excellence: *NICE guidelines for the treatment of post-traumatic stress disorder, 2005*: http://www.nice.org.uk/CG26.Accessed April 28, 2011.
30. Butler PEM, Clarke A, Hettiaratchy SL: Facial transplantation: a new option in reconstruction of severe facial injury. *BMJ* 331:1349-1350, 2005.
31. Goodall C, Oakey F, Ayoub A, et al: Effect of motivational interviewing in reducing alcohol consumption in patients with alcohol related facial injury. *Br J Oral Maxillofac Surg* 43:356-361, 2005.

32. Dinh-Zarr T, DiGuiseppi C, Heitman E, Roberts I: Interventions for preventing injuries in problem drinkers. *Cochrane Database Syst Rev* (2):CD00157, 2000.

33. Rapaport Y, Kreitler S, Chaiklick S, et al: Psychosocial problems in head and neck cancer patients and their change with time since diagnosis. *Ann Oncol* 4:69-73, 1993.

34. Semple C, Sullivan K, Dunwoody L, Kernohan WG: Psychosocial interventions for patients with head and neck cancer. *Cancer Nurs* 27:434-441, 2004.

35. Clarke A: *Resourcing and training head and neck cancer nurse specialists to deliver a social rehabilitation programme to patients. Unpublished doctorate thesis*, London, 2000, University of London.

36. Kleve L, Robinson E: A survey of psychological need amongst adult burn-injured patients. *Burns* 25:575-579, 1999.

37. Cella DF, Tulsky DS: Measuring quality of life today: methodological aspects. *Oncology* 4:29-38, 1990.

38. WHO: *Measuring quality of life*, Geneva, 1997, World Health Organization.

39. O'Boyle CA, McGee H, Hickey A, et al: The schedule for the evaluation of individual quality of life. Administration manual of the Department of Psychology, Dublin, 1993, Royal College of Surgeons.

40. Talmi YP: Quality of life issues in cancer of the oral cavity. *J Laryngol Otol* 116:785-790, 2002.

41. Llewellyn CD, McGurk M, Weinman J: Are psychosocial and behavioural factors related to health quality of life in patients with head and neck cancer? A systematic review. *Oral Oncol* 41:440-454, 2005.

42. Bjordal K, Freng A, Thorvik J, Kaasa S: Patient reported and clinician rated quality of life in head and neck patients: a cross-sectional study. *Eur J Cancer B Oral Oncol* 31B:235-241, 1995.

43. Johnson JE, Fieler VK, Wlasowicz GS, et al: The effects of nursing care guided by self-regulation theory on coping with radiation therapy. *Oncol Nurs Forum* 24:1041-1050, 1997.

44. Dropkin MJ: Coping with disfigurement and dysfunction after head and neck cancer surgery: a conceptual framework. *Semin Oncol Nurs* 5:213-219, 1989.

45. Brill SE, Clarke A, Veale DM, Butler PEM: Psychological management and body image issues in facial transplantation. *Body Image* 3:1-15, 2006.

46. Bessell A, Clarke A, Harcourt D, et al: Incorporating user perspectives in the design of an online intervention tool for people with visible differences: Face IT. *Behav Cogn Psychother* 38:577-596, 2010.

47. Bessell A, Moss TP: Evaluating the effectiveness of psychosocial interventions for individuals with visible differences: a systematic review of the empirical literature. *Body Image* 4:227-238, 2007.

48. Cordeiro CN, Clarke A, White P, et al: A quantitative analysis of psychological and emotional health measures in 360 plastic surgery candidates: is there a difference between aesthetic and reconstructive surgery? *Ann Plast Surg* 65:349-353, 2010.

49. Feber T, editor: *Head and neck oncology nursing*, London, 2000, Whurr.

50. Gardiner MD, Topps A, Richardson G, et al: Differential judgments about disfigurement: the role of location, age and gender in decisions made by observers. *J Plast Reconstr Aesthet Surg* 63:73-77, 2010.

51. Clarke A, Psychol C: Managing the psychological effects of altered appearance: the development of an information resource for people with disfiguring conditions. *Patient Educ Couns* 43:305-309, 2001.

52. Newell R, Zielger l, Stafford N, Lewin R: The information needs of head and neck cancer patients before surgery. *Ann R Coll Surgeons Engl* 86:407-410, 2004.

53. Parikh A, Lloyd M, Clarke A, et al: How to design a website. *Health Serv J* Nov:26, 2005.

54. Annon J: *The behavioural treatment of sexual problems*, vol 1, Honolulu, 1974, Enabling Systems.

55. Rumsey N, Clarke A, Musa M: Altered body image: the psychosocial needs of patients. *Br J Commun Nurs* 7:563-566, 2002.

56. Hettiaratchy S, Butler PEM: Face transplantation—fantasy or the future. *Lancet* 360:5-6, 2002.

57. Devauchelle B, Bodet L, Lengete B, et al: First human face allograft: early report. *Lancet* 368:203-209, 2006.

58. Morris PJ, Bradley JA, Doyal L, et al: Facial transplantation: a Working Party report from the Royal College of Surgeons of England. *Transplantation* 77:330-338, 2004.

59. American Society for Reconstructive Microsurgery (ASRM) and American Society of Plastic Surgeons: *Facial transplantation: ASMS/ASPS guiding principles*: www.microsurg.org/ftGuidelines.pdf. Accessed May 1, 2011.

60. Moss TP, Harris D, Carr T: *Manual for the Derriford appearance scale 24 (DAS24)*, Bradford on Avon, UK, 2004, Musketeer Press.

61. Rumsey N, Clarke A, White P, Hooper E: Exploring the psychosocial concerns of outpatients with disfiguring conditions. *J Wound Care* 12:247-252, 2003.

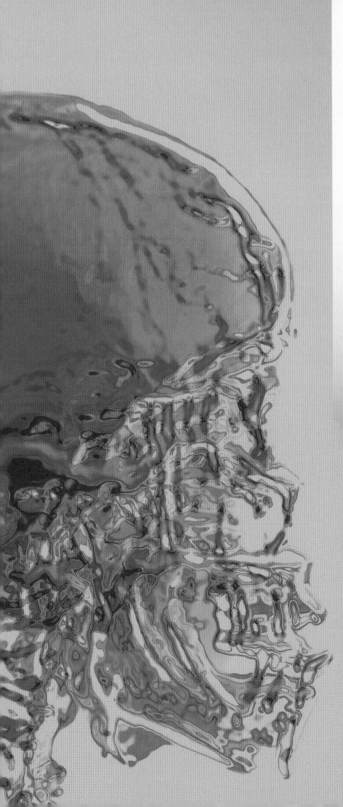

Innovations

CHAPTER 30

Biomaterials in Craniomaxillofacial Surgery

Rudolf R.M. Bos, Henk J. Busscher

aterials used to support or replace diseased tissues, collectively called *biomaterials*, play an important role in craniomaxillofacial surgery. Collaboration among material scientists, biomaterial engineers, clinicians, and clinical investigators has accelerated understanding of the requirements and potentials of various implant materials. Alloplastic materials play an essential part in the reconstruction of function and contour in craniomaxillofacial surgery. Many different polymers, metals, ceramics, and composites are used as biomaterials. Some, such as osteosynthesis materials, are used to achieve a temporary goal; others, such as artificial joints, need to function for sometimes a lifetime. There are many requirements that biomaterials must meet if they are to form either a temporary or a lasting union with the part of the body being treated. Adequate strength or, more probably, suitable mechanical characteristics, is a necessary but not the only feature; chemical and electrical factors and biological responses all contribute to success or failure.[1]

Very often, the primary requirement is mechanical strength. Biocompatibility is considered a secondary requirement, despite the fact that many biomaterials applications in the human eventually fail due to infection. In his *Science* paper, the famous biomaterial scientist, Antony G. Cristina, went as far as to call biomaterials in the human body a "microbial time bomb," because they seem to have an almost "magnetic" action on infectious microorganisms. Whether a biomaterial becomes infected depends in part on what is described as a "race for the surface" between tissue cells and microorganisms.[2] The so-called wetability of a biomaterial's surface determines the outcome of this race, either full integration of an implant (when the race is won by tissue cells) or infection (when it is won by microorganisms) (Fig. 30-1).

This chapter reviews the biomaterials most commonly used in craniomaxillofacial surgery.

BONE SUBSTITUTES

Bone grafts are increasingly used in cases of trauma, tumor surgery, and congenital absence or hypoplasia and for strictly esthetic purposes. Many surgeons prefer the use of autogenous bone grafts to reconstruct bony defects. Autogenous bone grafts have disadvantages including shortage of donor sites, donor site morbidity, growth deformity, and unpredictable resorption. The favorite donor sites for craniomaxillofacial reconstruction are calvaria, rib, and iliac bone. It seems that there is less resorption or at least slower with cranial bone than with rib or iliac bone.[3] Over the past 20 years, many kinds of biomaterials have been developed that can be used as bone graft substitutes. They have demonstrated their usefulness in craniomaxillofacial reconstruction with their ability to augment and replace portions of the craniofacial skeleton.

DEMINERALIZED BONE

Demineralized bone can be used for reconstruction of craniomaxillofacial defects.[4] The advantages of using demineralized bone are that it is pliable, easy to shape and to fit, available in limitless supply, and free from donor morbidity, which is particularly useful in children. Implantation of demineralized bone hardly affects tissue reaction and osteoclastic activity; 8 to 12 weeks after the implantation of demineralized bone, new bone formation was noticed in histological evaluations. Fragmentation of the implanted demineralized bone was observed 12 weeks postoperatively but in combination with new bone formation and without multinuclear cell activity. Hydrolytic enzymes may be the cause of this fragmentation. At 4 years after implantation, there were still large areas of nonvital bone without osteocytes in the bone lacunae and osteoblasts on the surface. Several areas showed fragmentation of the autogenous bone matrix. Several areas contiguous with nonvital bone showed evidence of transformation into living bone and remodeling. Active resorption, osteoclasts, and inflammation of fibrous changes were not observed in the long term.

Demineralized bone pastes[5] are composed of living osteoblasts derived from homograft materials. Theoretically, they provide osteogenic cells capable of inducing osteogenesis. Demineralized bone pastes can be used alone or in combination with other materials such as hydroxyapatites. The advantage of such a combination is that it provides a structural supporting matrix with cells that have osteogenic ability.

HYDROXYAPATITE

Hydroxyapatite (HA) is the principal mineral component of bone and determines 60% of the calcified human skeleton. It has been manufactured synthetically for more than 30 years and has been in clinical use for at least 20 years.[6] Certain

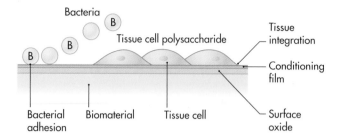

FIGURE 30-1   The "race for the surface." If the race is won by tissue cells, a stable implant is achieved. If infecting organisms are able to colonize an implant before the arrival of the first tissue cells, failure is imminent.

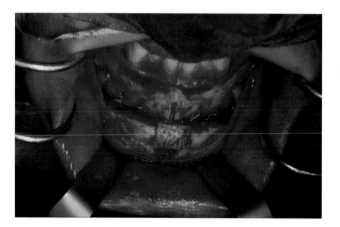

FIGURE 30-2   A block of porous hydroxyapatite used for widening of the chin.

marine corals consist of HA and have a structure that is similar to that of human bone. There are two forms of HA: ceramic and nonceramic. Nonceramic HA is not sintered after the HA crystals have been formed and therefore is more absorbable in vivo than the ceramic form. Ceramic forms of HA have excellent biocompatibility and show osteoconduction and osseointegration when placed in direct contact with viable bone. Osteoinduction is not evident because of the absence of inductive growth factors.[7] Nonceramic HA can also be formed into cements, whereas ceramic HA cannot.

Ceramic Hydroxyapatite

Ceramic HA is synthesized in crystal form at low pH and then heated (sintered) at 700° C to 1300° C to form a solid mass of HA. Ceramic HA is available in two forms: dense and porous. The dense form is completely synthetic, it has no pores and can be fabricated into blocks or granules, which are difficult to shape and do not permit tissue ingrowth. Granules have greater contour adaptability than the solid blocks but have no intrinsic structural integrity and do not become mechanically stable until surrounded by fibro-osseous tissue. Dense HA granules are difficult to contain within the desired site of implantation, and there is a possibility of migration to unwanted areas after several months or years.[8]

Porous HA can be produced synthetically, or it can be based on the skeletons of marine coral. The calcium carbonate skeleton of the coral is chemically converted to HA, with the original porous structure of the coral retained.[9] Porous ceramic granules appear to be less prone to migration over

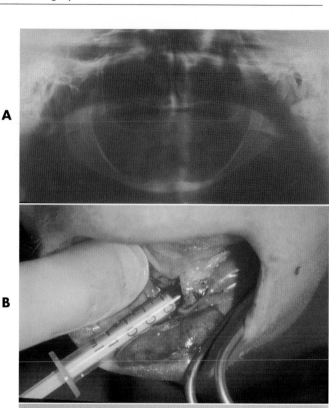

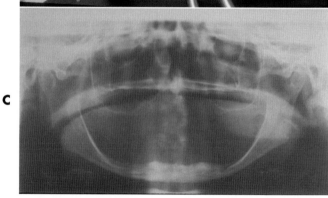

FIGURE 30-3   **A,** Orthopantomogram of a patient with an extremely resorbed mandible. **B,** Subperiosteal injection of hydroxyapatite granules for augmentation of the mandible. **C,** Orthopantomogram 12 weeks after augmentation with hydroxyapatite granules.

time. Another means of preventing migration is to combine HA granules with resorbable carrier compounds. The very important advantage of porous HA is the ingrowth of fibro-osseous tissue: the implant becomes fixed to the surrounding bone within a few weeks. After completion of fibro-osseous tissue ingrowth, the implant consists of approximately 40% residual HA implant and 60% fibro-osseous tissue. Porous HA in block form is rather fragile and very difficult to contour (Fig. 30-2). Therefore, its application has been limited in craniomaxillofacial surgery. Use of porous HA for alveolar ridge augmentation (Fig. 30-3) has demonstrated that the implant is resistant to infection after fibro-osseous tissue ingrowth is finished, but it easily becomes exposed, especially if the overlying soft tissue is thin or compromised.[10]

Porous ceramic HA can be chemically combined with various biomaterials to improve its physical properties. It can also be used as a carrier of bioactive substances such as bone morphogenetic proteins, which increase the ingrowth of bone into the pores.[11]

Nonceramic Hydroxyapatite

Tetracalcium phosphate cement (HA cement) is a form of nonceramic HA. It is the only calcium phosphate cement that sets into a stable shape and is converted in vivo to pure HA. It can be produced by direct crystallization of HA at physiological pH and temperature and does not require heating to form a structurally stable implant. The dry cement is composed of tetracalcium phosphate and dicalcium phosphate. It sets in approximately 15 minutes and converts to HA within 4 hours.[12] After conversion to HA it is no longer water soluble and is slowly replaced by bone over time. Its contour is stable. Animal studies[13] proved that 35% of implanted HA was replaced by fibro-osseous tissue; after 12 months, bone replaced 75% of this fibro-osseous tissue. Even in human clinical trials, the cement was found to be functionally nonresorbable over 42 months on the basis of computed tomographic scans and incidentally by direct intraoperative inspections during secondary surgery.

These biologically active forms of HA cement are especially useful in situations where contour is not an important factor or where bone replacement of the implant material is necessary, such as reconstruction of skull base defects, orthopedic applications, and pediatric craniomaxillofacial surgery. HA cement may be used in the growing skull because it has been observed to have no adverse effects on development.[13] HA has no toxic reactions, and it has a low rate of infection (about 4%) even when the HA implant is in contact with the paranasal sinuses or oral cavity.[14] An important disadvantage of HA cement is that it is very difficult to give it the desired contour because it tends to settle with gravity during the setting process. HA granules may also be mixed with fibrocollagen and autogenous blood to form a paste that can be injected into subperiosteal pockets. It becomes firmly fixed by fibrous tissue ingrowth from the surrounding tissues. It has been used to augment the malar bone, premaxilla, nasal dorsum, and glabella area. Large volumes of this paste have been used to fill cranial defects in children. The infection rate was about 3%.[14]

A mixture is on the market consisting of type I bovine dermal fibrillar collagen (PFC) and a mixture of 65% ceramic HA and 35% β-tricalcium phosphate (TCP) granules. The HA-TCP granules and the PFC are separately packed; they are mixed in the operating room to form a granular, nonsetting paste. Autogenous bone marrow can be added to the mixture to give it more osteoinductive and osteogenic properties. This mixture allows bony ingrowth and rapid vascularization. However, it is nonsetting and can easily become deformed before fibro-osseous tissue ingrowth has occurred. Contour change and volume loss occur because of resorption of both the collagen and the TCP component, amounting to about 40% of the total mixture. The addition of autogenous bone marrow to the mixture decreases the infection rate from 5% to 2.5%.[15]

POLYMERS

In general, polymers are thought of as plastics, relatively weak solid materials that soften as temperature increases. Polymers are ubiquitous in the human environment and have begun to displace metals and ceramics from traditional applications. Polymers and polymer-based composites represent one of the most exciting areas of modern materials science. They combine moderate strength, low cost, and easy raw material availability with the ability to regulate physical properties by design of composition, internal structural arrangement, and processing. Nowhere has the impact of modern polymeric materials been greater than in medicine, with the resulting wide use of polymeric disposable supplies, dressings, and sutures and the incorporation of polymers into medical devices, surgical instruments, and implants.[1] The most widely used applications are discussed in this chapter.[16,17]

POLYDIMETHYLSILOXANE

Polydimethylsiloxane, better known as silicone, has been widely used in craniomaxillofacial surgery. It has proved to be highly compatible with soft tissues. It is easy to shape, is resistant to the physiological environment, and can be produced with a wide range of mechanical properties. Its surface is hydrophobic (Table 30-1). Depending on the number and nature of side chains and crosslinks and the average molecular weight, the resulting materials may be liquid or solid, rubbery or brittle. They may be produced as thermoplastics or as two-part thermoset materials. The latter are used to manufacture a custom mold either before implantation or in situ. The natural host response to the smooth surface of silicone is a fibrous encapsulation. To prevent extrusion of silicone implants, the overlying soft tissues should not be thin, unstable, or under tension (Fig. 30-4). Injections of large amounts of liquid silicone for purposes such as breast augmentation may induce systemic toxicity.

The poor abrasion resistance of silicone rubbers prevents their use in weight-bearing applications. Abrasion of silicone causes a granulomatous inflammatory reaction, both locally and in regional lymph nodes. Because of an ongoing controversy regarding the charge that silicone breast implants can cause connective tissue disease,[18] silicone as a craniomaxillofacial implant material has disappeared from the market almost completely. Silicone blocks have been widely used for craniofacial augmentation purposes, such as malar

TABLE 30-1	Chemical Structure of Various Polymeric Biomaterials and Metals	
Polymer Name	Chemical Functionality	Water Contact Angle (degrees)
Silicone rubber	-(O-Si-CH$_3$)-	111
Polyethylene	=CH$_2$'-CH$_3$	95-100
Polypropylene		94
Polytetrafluoroethylene (PTFE)	=CF$_2$'-CF$_3$	104
Polymethylmethacrylate (PMMA)		70-80
Polylactide (PLA)		
Titanium (oxide)		35-45
Stainless steel		65-75

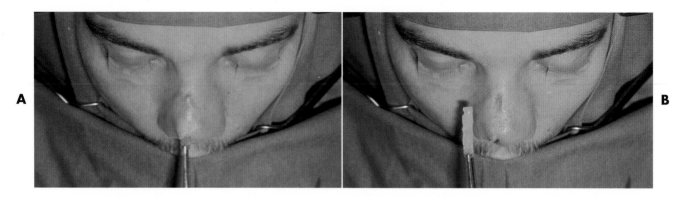

FIGURE 30-4 **A,** Dehiscence of a silicone implant used for cosmetic reconstruction of the nasal dorsum. **B,** The silicone implant after removal from the nose.

bones, chin, and nasal dorsum. Care should be taken to prevent migration of the blocks and erosion of the underlying bones as well as perforation of the compromised overlying skin.[16]

POLYETHYLENE

Polyethylene is one of the most commonly used biomaterials.[1] It is the base polymer for other materials such as polypropylene and polytetrafluoroethylene (PTFE). It elicits a minimal tissue reaction, especially when manufactured in a high-density, high-molecular-weight form. In this form, it serves as a reference standard for other materials because of its minimal tissue reaction. Ultra-high-molecular-weight polyethylene (UHMWPE) has proved to date to be the best polymer for load-bearing applications in metal-polymer wear pairs such as artificial joints. Artificial temporomandibular joints have been developed in which UHMWPE serves as an artificial disc placed between a metal fossa part and a ceramic condylar head[19] (Fig. 30-5).

Polyethylene is also available in a porous form. The porous structure of this implant material allows ingrowth of soft tissues 1 week after implantation and bony ingrowth by 3 weeks. The porous polyethylene is easy to shape but difficult to remove after ingrowth.[20] A porous polyethylene reinforced with titanium is available to reconstruct bony defects of the skull after tumor ablation or trauma. Excellent craniofacial symmetry and stability are achievable. Many implant forms are commercially available, including malar, chin, mandible, nasal bone, and orbital floor implants. Flexible porous polyethylene blocks can be ideally suited to repair small to medium-sized cranial defects. Host response to polyethylene is mild, and complications are rare. Porous polyethylene has an advantage over autogenous bone in that it is not susceptible to contour change. It has proved to be a safe and effective bone substitute for contouring of the facial skeleton.

POLYMETHYLMETHACRYLATE

Polymethylmethacrylate (PMMA) has been used as bone cement for 40 years. It is an acceptable space filler that is not resorbed.[1] Its mechanical properties are excellent to serve as a bone replacement in the craniofacial area, and its surface is moderately hydrophobic (see Table 30-1).

Methyl methacrylate has two different components, a mixing powder polymer and a liquid monomer. The chemical reaction is exothermic, and the associated toxicity is related to the free monomer component. Cardiovascular collapse and even death have been described in patients undergoing a total hip replacement with freshly mixed methyl methacrylate but not with its use in craniofacial surgery. The free methyl methacrylate monomer can cause asthmatic reactions.

PMMA has been used for reconstruction of skull defects for many years, in cement form and in a presurgically shaped and polymerized solid implant form (Fig. 30-6). Patients with isolated cranioplasty rarely experience infections, but the infection rate increases considerably (to about 23%) in patients undergoing a cranioplasty simultaneously with reconstruction of the orbital wall or nose. If the facial contour requirement is important, especially preshaped PMMA delivers a predictable contour without any resorption.[21] PMMA may be used in adult patients with healthy overlying soft tissues and no infection. It is not an adequate implant material for reconstruction of craniofacial bones in the growing child.

POLYTETRAFLUOROETHYLENE

Polytetrafluoroethylene (PTFE) is used as a base material for various implants.[1] It is frequently used for so-called guided tissue regeneration of dental alveolar bone in dental implantology (Fig. 30-7) and periodontology. PTFE sheets, sold under the trade name Gore-Tex, prevent fibrous tissue ingrowth and allow bony regeneration of a blood clot covered by the Gore-Tex fabric.

A composite of PTFE reinforced with carbon fibers or with aluminum oxide (Proplast) has been widely used for malar (Fig. 30-8) and chin augmentation. Proplast is a microporous material that does not allow fibrous or bony ingrowth. It was initially reported that Proplast did not give rise to many complications. It seemed to have a low infection rate of about 4%, displacement was rare (3.5%), and implant removal was required in about 8%. However, this implant material is no longer manufactured, perhaps because of a high incidence of infection and displacement in the long run.[22] We used Proplast for bilateral malar augmentation in a series of 10 patients operated on at the beginning of the 1980s; 19 of the 20

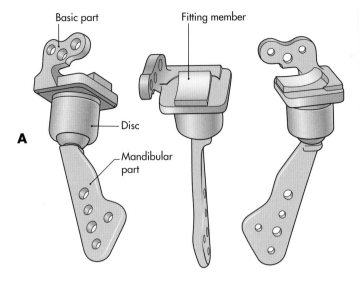

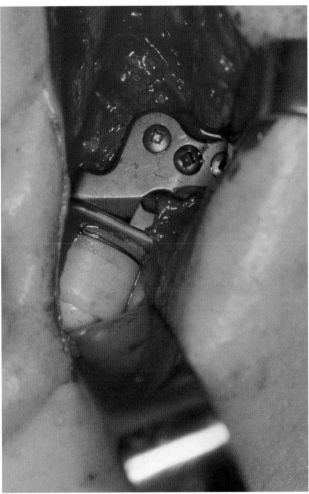

FIGURE 30-5 **A,** Schematic drawing of the Groningen temporomandibular joint prosthesis with its polyethylene disc. **B,** Intraoperative view of the polyethylene disc during insertion of the prosthesis.

implants had to be removed because of chronic fistulae or even chronic sinusitis due to migration of the Proplast implant into the maxillary sinus. Proplast has also been used as a lining for the fossa part of the Vitek temporomandibular joint prosthesis. However, rapid wear and, more importantly, an aggressive foreign body response to the wear debris have rendered this material unusable for implant applications in which wear phenomena are possible.[23]

POLYETHERETHERKETONE

Polyetheretherketone (PEEK) is a relatively new biomaterial with very good mechanical properties; it is substantially stiffer and stronger than for example PMMA (polymethylmethacrylate). An advantage over most other polymers is that PEEK is autoclavable. It originally was used in knee and hip prostheses and artificial vertebrae[24] and later as a biomaterial for craniomaxillofacial reconstruction. Computer-designed customized PEEK implants are available for skull defect reconstruction[25] and for reconstruction of maxillofacial defects.[26] No prospective or long-term longitudinal studies of PEEK implants are available.

RESORBABLE POLYMERS

The polymers discussed so far are intended to retain their shape and their essential properties after implantation. However, there are a number of applications for which it would be desirable to have properties change or even to have the material completely disappear with time. This principle has been long recognized in the use of resorbable subcutaneous sutures. One of the most challenging of these potential applications is in internal fixation of fractures and osteotomies (Fig. 30-9).[9] It would be ideal to have a device that slowly weakens and eventually disappears, transferring load to the healing bone and encouraging maximal Wolff's Law remodeling.

In the past 3 decades, much progress has been made in the development of biodegradable materials for osteosynthesis. Most bioresorbable osteosynthesis materials used today are produced from synthetic semicrystalline poly(α-hydroxy acid) polymers (PHAs).[27] Polylactide (PLA) is most often used, because it is most suitable for producing implants with acceptable mechanical properties (Fig. 30-10). Polyglycolide (PGA) is often used; it degrades faster and is used primarily

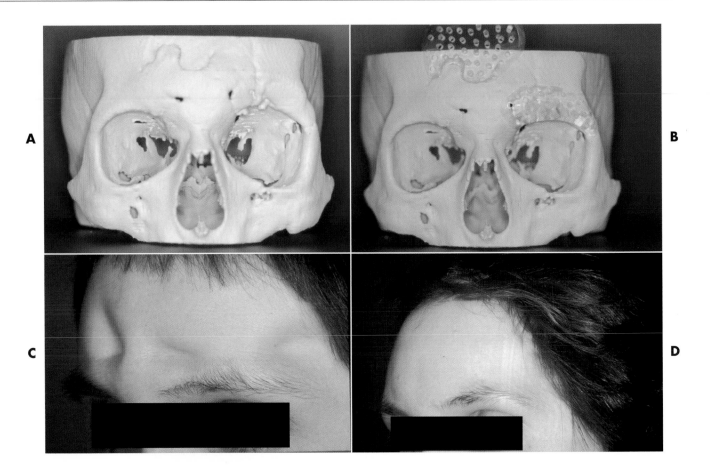

FIGURE 30-6 **A,** Stereolithographic model of a patient with frontal deformities after a fireworks accident. **B,** Polymethylmethacrylate (PMMA) implants on the stereolithographic model. **C,** Preoperative view of a patient with frontal defects after a car accident. **D,** Postoperative view after implantation of PMMA implants through a coronal incision.

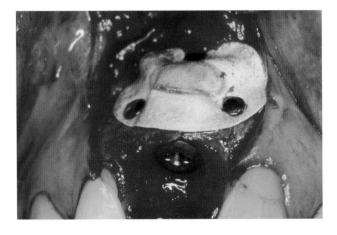

FIGURE 30-7 A Teflon sheet used for guided tissue regeneration of a bony dehiscence along a dental implant.

in applications in which high strength is not the most important factor. Polymer blends of PLA and PGA are also often used to tailor the properties of a polymer to a specific application. In addition to PLA, PGA, and PLA/PLG copolymers, a number of other aliphatic polyesters such as poly(*p*-dioxanone) (PDS) and poly(ε-caprolactone) (PCL) have been

investigated for these uses. PDS is used to make pins (Orthosorb) and orbital floor implants. However, PDS and PCL are primarily used for the production of bioresorbable sutures such as Monocryl, a PCL/PGA monofilament suture, and PDS monofilament suture.

Biodegradable osteosynthesis materials perform satisfactorily in many aspects. However, considerable problems are encountered that stand in the way of their general clinical use. First, the mechanical properties of the resorbable materials are still not as good as those of metallic ones. Moreover, the perioperative handling of resorbable devices is far more critical and difficult. The mechanical properties of resorbable plates and screws or pins are easily destroyed during bending or by torsional forces during insertion.

Another main issue is biocompatibility. For a long time, the biocompatibility of bioresorbable PLA and PGA polymers has been considered to be beyond reproach. This, however, seems to be an over simplification. Degradation of these polymers occurs primarily by hydrolysis; enzymatic activity is thought to contribute in the later stages of degradation. Free radicals, in particular hydroxy radicals, also appear to play a role in the degradation process. The end products of degradation of PLA and PGA, lactic acid and glycolic acid, are hypothesized to be eliminated from the body mainly as carbon dioxide and water, with a small portion excreted in the urine and feces. Homopolymers of PLA and PGA give

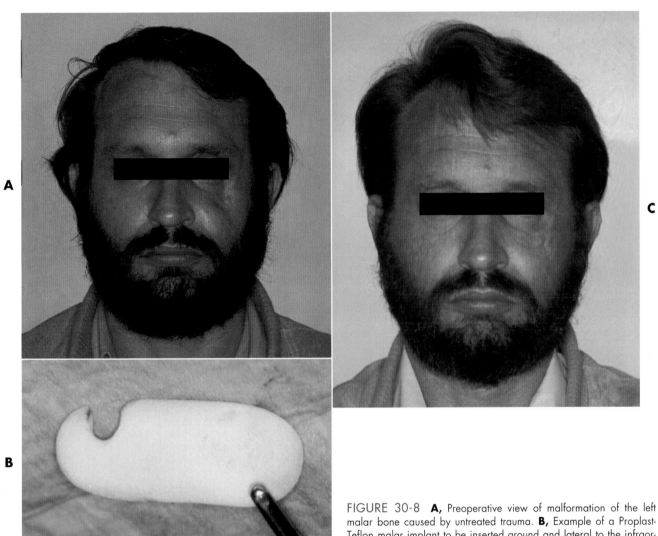

FIGURE 30-8 **A,** Preoperative view of malformation of the left malar bone caused by untreated trauma. **B,** Example of a Proplast-Teflon malar implant to be inserted around and lateral to the infraorbital nerve. **C,** Postoperative view 3 months after transcutaneous implantation of the Proplast-Teflon malar implant.

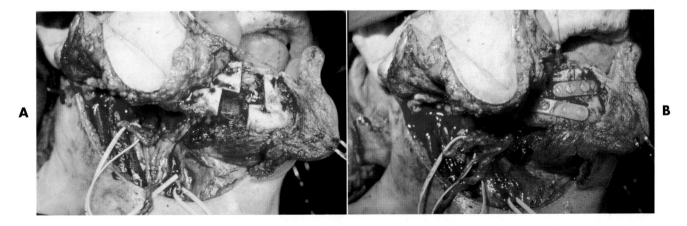

FIGURE 30-9 **A,** Lateral swing osteotomy of the mandible in a patient with a planocellular carcinoma of the oropharynx. **B,** Fixation of the osteotomy with two resorbable polylactic acid (PLA) plates and screws.

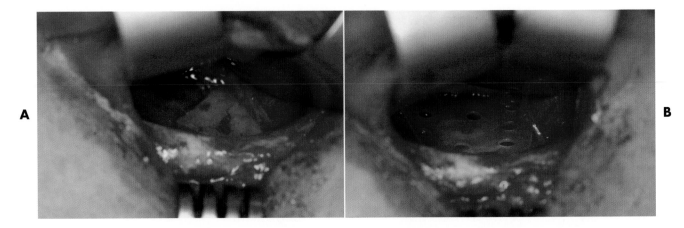

FIGURE 30-10 **A,** Intraoperative view of a blowout fracture of the orbital floor. **B,** Reconstruction of the orbital floor with a resorbable polylactic acid (PLA) sheet (0.4 mm thickness).

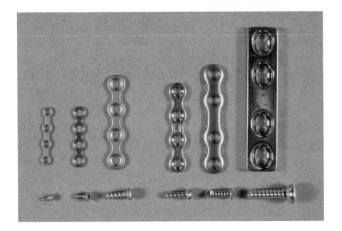

FIGURE 30-11 A variety of osteosynthesis plates and screws used in craniomaxillofacial surgery.

rise to a clinically detectable foreign body reaction. Blending copolymerization or crosslinking seem to be a solution to limit or avoid foreign body reactions during degradation. However, a 2000 study documented the presence of very persistent nanoparticles and microparticles in the degradation pathway of a PLA/PGA copolymer in use as a so-called bioresorbable implant material.[28] This study indicated that PHA implants may not completely degrade within 15 to 20 years. At present, it seems prudent to assume that crystalline debris from PHA implants will remain present in the recipient indefinitely with the potential for the development of unforeseen complications. Especially if use of multiple or large implants is being considered, such remnants may pose a long-term health risk. These problems need to be solved so that bioresorbable osteosynthesis implants can perform to their full potential and, eventually, come into general clinical application.

Another routine application of biodegradable materials could be as a scaffold for bone reconstruction. An ideal bone substitute would be a biomaterial that has osteoconductive and inductive properties and will be replaced by regenerating host bone. Biodegradable meshes have been produced that can be filled with particulate bone marrow or mixtures of bone marrow and HA. These have been used in experimental studies for mandibular reconstruction.

Biodegradable foams have also been used in experimental studies. They are loaded with bone morphogenetic proteins, platelet-derived growth factor, or transforming growth factor or with osteoblasts or chondroblasts. All these studies have been experimental.[29] Only some meshes are available for clinical use.

METALS

Metals enjoy wide application in craniomaxillofacial surgery as structural, load-bearing materials in devices for fracture fixation, for partial or total joint replacement (see Fig. 30-5), in instruments, and as external splints. The principal reasons for this broad popularity are excellent mechanical properties and biocompatibility. Today, one principally uses metals such as stainless steel, chromium-molybdenum alloys, or commercially pure titanium.[1] Until 1986, the metal of choice in craniomaxillofacial surgery was stainless steel. However, titanium is now the material of choice for the maxillofacial field. The superior biocompatibility of titanium is conveyed by its oxide skin, which forms spontaneously on exposure to an oxygen-containing environment (e.g., room air).

Internal fixation with various systems of plates and screws is a widely accepted method in craniomaxillofacial trauma (Fig. 30-11), orthopedic surgery, and reconstruction after tumor surgery. Many surgeons prefer not to remove metallic plates and screws used for fixation, because it requires an additional surgical intervention with all of the attendant risks and socioeconomic and psychological disadvantages. In regard to biocompatibility, commercially pure titanium is thought to be superior to stainless steel products because of its completely inert oxide skin. Although titanium is more expensive than steel, it may be cost-effective in the long run because of its favorable characteristics. Because it is thought to be nonallergenic and completely inert, a second intervention to remove titanium plates and screws is not necessary.[30] For internal fixation in the maxillofacial area, titanium is now almost exclusively the material of choice. Because of the coincidental finding that titanium has a more or less exclusive property of osseo-integration, it is used worldwide as a dental implant material and as an osseous implant to fix maxillofacial prosthetics. Computer-designed titanium implants can also be used for cranial reconstruction after trauma or tumor surgery. The infection rate of titanium implants is extremely low.

BIOFILM FORMATION

The formation of a biofilm on the surface of biomaterials in the human body results from adsorption of macromolecular components such as salivary proteins and the adhesion of infectious microorganisms. The biofilm mode of growth protects the organisms against host defenses and environmental attacks (e.g., antibiotic treatment). Consequently, their formation very often necessitates removal of a biomaterial implant.[21,31]

Interactions of biomaterials with bacteria and tissue cells are directed not only by specific receptors and outer membrane molecules on the cell surface but also by the atomic geometry and electronic state of the biomaterial surface. Understanding these mechanisms is important to all fields of medicine and is derived from and relevant to studies in microbiology, biochemistry, and physics. Modifications to biomaterial surfaces at an atomic level allow programming of cell-to-substratum events, thereby diminishing infection by enhancing tissue compatibility or integration or by directly inhibiting bacterial adhesion.

The Bränemark implant system, consisting of an endosteal titanium screw and a transmucosal abutment, is prone to biofilm formation. The abutment surface properties dictate the amount of biofilm formed. Roughened abutment surfaces have been found to harbor 25 times more bacteria than smooth abutment surfaces after 3 months.[32] Influences of surface hydrophobicity on biofilm formation are generally more evident in situations of fluctuating shear conditions than in a pocket. In vivo studies over a 9-day period demonstrated far less biofilm formation on hydrophobic Teflon strips glued on the front incisors of human volunteers than on native, more hydrophilic tooth surfaces[32] (Fig. 30-12).

CONCLUSION

Biomaterials are being used with increasing frequency for tissue substitution. The major barriers to their use are the possibility of bacterial adhesion, which causes biomaterial-centered infection, and the lack of successful tissue integration or biocompatibility with biomaterial surfaces.

When the literature over the past decade is reviewed,[33] it is striking that really new biomaterials have not been developed. Well-designed comparative studies with statistical analyses on differences in success rates between different biomaterials or bone grafts for specific indications are not available.

When looking for suitable biomaterials, one should critically examine scientific papers on that material. The fact that bony ingrowth in HA granules occurs in young rabbits does not automatically mean that bony ingrowth also occurs in elderly people who need filling out of bony defects or augmentations before insertion of dental implants. When looking

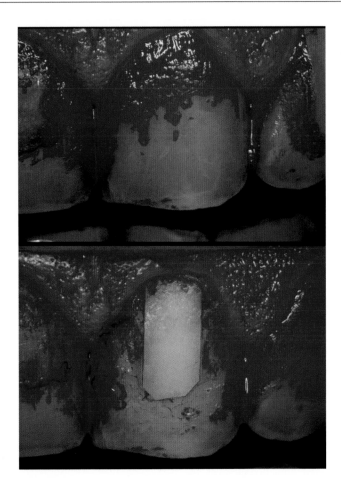

FIGURE 30-12 The amount of biofilm formed on a hydrophobic material glued to the front incisor of a human volunteer was considerably less than that formed on a more hydrophilic tooth surface in the absence of tooth brushing over a period of 9 days.[32]

for so-called resorbable materials, one should carefully assess how intensively investigators have looked for remnants of material to discriminate between real resorption or degradation and disintegration only.

Many articles report higher complication rates with some biomaterials compared to autogenous tissue. It is often difficult to attribute these rates solely to the implant material itself. Many factors, such as surgical techniques, host response, and potential toxicity of the implant, influence complication rates. For example, variations in the antibiotic regimen, attention to aseptic techniques, the normal flora, susceptibility to antibiotics, and the method of mechanical fixation can influence infection rates for a given material. Modern biomaterials produce a very low level of acute local or systemic host response in patients. However, mechanisms have been identified for a variety of immunological responses, including neoplastic transformation. Increasing periods of implantation, resulting from earlier surgical intervention, and increased surface areas of implants, as required for fixation by biological ingrowth, may be placing patients at increasing risk. As material researchers and clinicians become more sensitive to the biological response implications of the biomaterials that they use, patient analyses will clarify the situation and provide upper boundaries on the prevalence of such effects.

BIOMATERIALS FOR TISSUE ENGINEERING

Although advances in surgical techniques and bone grafting have significantly improved the functional and cosmetic restoration of craniofacial structures lost due to trauma or disease, there are still limitations in the ability to regenerate these tissues. Tissue engineering is an interdisciplinary field of research that combines the principles of engineering with those of biology and medicine toward the development of biological substitutes that restore, maintain, and improve normal function.

No current technology has led to complete solutions, but progress in the preclinical field gives confidence that clinically applicable methods will become achievable. Tissue engineering, gene therapy, and stem cell biology combine cells, biomaterial scaffolds, and cell signaling factors to anatomically and functionally reconstruct bony defects, avoiding donor site morbidity.

Natural, synthetic, and composite materials have been investigated to serve as scaffolds. Natural scaffolds such as collagen, chitosan, calcium alginate, hyaluronic acid, and composites have proved to be osteoconductive in vitro and in vivo but are lacking in mechanical stability. Alternatives with better mechanical properties, such as synthetic polymers and copolymers including PLA, PGA, poly(lactic-co-glycolic acid) (PLGA), PMMA, PCL, and poly(trimethylene carbonate) (PTMC) have been developed. Polymer/ceramic composites such as PLLA/HA, PTMC/HA, and PCL/HA have been used successfully to reconstruct osteochondral defects.

Craniomaxillofacial tissue engineering research has developed enormously over the past 2 decades. Although the results of this research are promising, general application in craniomaxillofacial surgery still lies in the future.[34-38]

REFERENCES

1. Black J: *Orthopedic biomaterials in research and practice*, Edinburgh, 1988, Churchill Livingstone.
2. Cristina AG: Biomaterials-centered infection: microbial adhesion versus tissue integration. *Science* 237:1588-1595, 1987.
3. Zins JE, Whitaker LA: Membranous versus enchondral bone: implications for craniofacial reconstruction. *Plast Reconstr Surg* 72:778-785, 1983.
4. Neigel JM, Ruzicka PO: Use of demineralized bone implant in orbital and craniofacial reconstruction and a review of the literature. *Ophthal Plast Reconstr Surg* 12:108-120, 1996.
5. Glowacki J, Kaban CB, Murray JE: Application of the biological principle of induced osteogenesis for craniofacial defect. *Lancet* 1:959-962, 1981.
6. Jarcho M: Calcium phosphate ceramics as hard tissue prosthesis. *Clin Orthop Rel Res* 157:259-278, 1981.
7. Ono I, Takheiko O, Murata M: A study on bone induction in hydroxyapatite combined with bone morphogenic protein. *Plast Reconstr Surg* 90:870-879, 1992.
8. Harvey WK, Pincock JL, Matukas VJ, et al: Evaluation of subcutaneous implanted hydroxyapatite-Avitene mixture in rabbits. *J Oral Maxillofac Surg* 43:277-280, 1985.
9. Cottrell DA, Wolford LM: Long-term evaluation of the use of coralline hydroxyapatite in orthognathic surgery. *J Oral Maxillofac Surg* 56:935-941, 1998.
10. Salyer KE, Hall CD: Porous hydroxyapatite as an onlay graft substitute for maxillofacial surgery. *Plast Reconstr Surg* 84:236-244, 1989.
11. Ripamonti U, Ramoshebi LN, Matsaba T, et al: Bone induction by BMPs/OPs and related family members in primates. *J Bone Joint Surg Am* 83(suppl 1, pt 12):116-127, 2001.
12. Jackson IT, Yavuzer R: Hydroxyapatite cement: an alternative for craniofacial skeletal contour refinements. *Br J Plast Surg* 53:24-29, 2000.
13. Lykins CL, Friedman CD, Costanino PD, et al: Hydroxyapatite cement in craniofacial skeletal reconstruction and its effects on the developing craniofacial skeleton. *Arch Otolaryngol Head Neck Surg* 124:153-159, 1998.
14. Costantino PD, Chaplin JM, Wolpoe ME, et al: Application of fast setting hydroxyapatite cement: cranioplasty. *Otolaryngol Head Neck Surg* 123:409-512, 2000.
15. Cornell CN: Initial clinical experience with use of Collagraft as bone graft substitute. *Tech Orthop* 7:55-63, 1992.
16. Rubin JP, Yaremchuk MJ: Complications and toxicities of implantable biomaterials used in facial reconstructive and aesthetic surgery: a comprehensive review of literature. *Plast Reconstr Surg* 100:1336-1353, 1997.
17. Homsy CA: Complications and toxicities of implantable biomaterials for facial aesthetic and reconstructive surgery. *Plast Reconstr Surg* 102:1766-1768, 1998.
18. Sanchez-Guerrero J, Colditz GA, Karlson E, et al: Silicone breast implants and the risk of connective tissue disease and symptoms. *N Engl J Med* 332:1666-1670, 1995.
19. Van Loon JP, Bont LGM, Stegenga B, et al: Groningen temporomandibular joint prosthesis: development and first clinical application. *Int J Oral Maxillofac Surg* 31:44-52, 2002.
20. Odum BC, Bussard GM, Lewis RP, et al: High-density porous polyethylene for facial bone augmentation. *J Long Term Eff Med Implants* 8:3-17, 1998.
21. Gosain AK, Persing JA: Biomaterials in the face: benefits and risks. *J Craniofac Surg* 10:404-414, 1999.
22. Moos KF, Jackson IT, Henderson D, et al: The use of Proplast in oral and maxillofacial surgery. *Br J Oral Surg* 16:187-197, 1979.
23. Mercuri LG: Considering total temporomandibular joint replacement. *Cranio* 17:44-48, 1999.
24. Kurtz SM, Devine JN: PEEK biomaterials in trauma, orthopedic, and spinal implants. *Biomaterials* 28:4845-4869, 2007.
25. Scolozzi P, Martinez A, Jaques B: Complex orbito-fronto-temporal reconstruction using computer-designed PEEK implant. *J Craniofac Surg* 18:224-228, 2007.
26. Kim MM, Boahene KD, Byrne PJ: Use of customized polyetheretherketone (PEEK) implants in the reconstruction of complex maxillofacial defects. *Arch Facial Plast Surg* 11:53-57, 2009.
27. Suuronen R, Haers PE, Lindqvist C, et al: Update on bioresorbable plates in maxillofacial surgery. *Facial Plast Surg* 15:61-72, 1999.
28. Cordewener FW, Schmitz JP: The future of biodegradable osteosyntheses. *Tissue Eng* 6:413-424, 2000.
29. Stock UA, Vacanti JP: Tissue engineering: current state and prospects. *Annu Rev Med* 52:443-451, 2001.
30. Meningaud JP, Poupon J, Bertrand JC, et al: Dynamic study about metal release from titanium miniplates in maxillofacial surgery. *Int J Oral Maxillofac Surg* 30:185-188, 2001.
31. Donlan RM, Costerton JW: Biofilms: survival mechanisms of clinically relevant microorganisms. *Clin Microbiol Rev* 15:167-193, 2002.
32. Quirijnen M, Marechal M, Busscher HJ, et al: The influence of surface free energy on planimetric plaque growth in man. *J Dent Res* 68:796-799, 1989.
33. Neovius E, Engstrand T: Craniofacial reconstruction with bone and biomaterials: review over the last 11 years. *J Plast Reconstr Aesthet Surg* 63:1615-1623, 2010.
34. Ward BB, Brown SE, Krebsbach PH: Bioengineering strategies for regeneration of craniofacial bone: a review of emerging technologies. *Oral Dis* 16:709-716, 2010.
35. Shanti RM, Li WJ, Nesti LJ, et al: Adult mesenchymal stem cells: biological properties, characteristics, and applications in maxillofacial surgery. *J Oral Maxillofac Surg* 65:1640-1647, 2007.
36. Srouji S, Kizhner T, Livne E: 3D scaffolds for bone marrow stem cell support in bone repair. *Regen Med* 1:519-528, 2006.
37. Handschel J, Wiesmann HP, Depprich R, et al: Cell-based bone reconstruction therapies: cell sources. *Int J Oral Maxillofac Implants* 21:890-898, 2006.
38. Marx RE: Platelet-rich plasma: evidence to support its use. *J Oral Maxillofac Surg* 62:489-496, 2004.

CHAPTER 31

Minimally Invasive Surgery

Ralf Schön, Rainer Schmelzeisen

Experience with arthroscopy of the temporomandibular joint (TMJ) and with endoscopic sinus and skull base surgery equips the oral and maxillofacial surgeon for the endoscopic-assisted treatment of maxillofacial trauma. Endoscopic-assisted management of maxillofacial trauma has been described for treatment of fractures of the mandibular condyle, the zygomatic complex, the orbit, and the frontal sinus.[1-4] The reduction and fixation strategy of open fracture treatment with osteosynthesis has not changed. However, with the use of endoscopic-assisted techniques, extraoral incisions can be limited or avoided in favor of intraoral approaches. Intraoperative fixation after fracture reduction in areas of limited exposure and visibility can be obtained with these techniques.[5] However, the choice to use endoscopic techniques has no influence on the indication for surgical treatment. It is a relatively new surgical field, which continues to expand, yet its long-term benefit in many scenarios, still awaits confirmation.

STATE-OF-THE-ART MANAGEMENT

MANDIBLE

Mandibular Condyle Fractures

Fractures of the mandibular condyle are common and account for 9% to 45% of all mandibular fractures.[6,7] Closed reduction is the method most widely employed for the treatment of displaced condylar fractures.[7] Anatomical reduction is rarely achieved, and rehabilitation and TMJ function depend on adaptation of the altered condylar morphology or formation of a new joint. With precise fracture reduction by preauricular, retromandibular/transparotid, or submandibular approaches, damage to the facial nerve and the creation of visible scars have been described.[8] Because of these possible complications, the indications for open reduction versus closed treatment are still in debate.[9,10]

The risks of facial nerve damage and extensive visible scars can be minimized by minimally invasive endoscopic techniques using a transoral approach.[1,5,11-13] However, in cases of severely displaced or comminuted fractures, the extraoral approach seems to be advantageous over endoscopic-assisted reduction of mandibular condyle fractures.[5]

Other Mandibular Fractures

For mandibular fractures in other locations, such as the mandibular angle and the ramus, the transoral approach is less time-consuming and is preferable to avoid visible scars and possible facial nerve damage. The transoral approach is indicated if there is no comminution. However, with a transoral approach, the inferior and posterior aspects of the fracture and possible lingual gaps cannot be visualized. Endoscopic examination of the fracture site after transoral reduction and fixation of fractures provides further information about the accuracy of the fracture reduction. The alignment of the posterior and inferior aspects of angle fractures and the presence of a lingual gap in ramus fractures can be detected endoscopically and corrected intraoperatively if necessary.

Midfacial and Frontal Sinus Fractures

Endoscopic-assisted techniques for treatment of fractures of the zygoma, the midface, and the orbit have been reported.[2,3,14-16] In patients with fractures of the zygomatic complex, the orbital floor and infraorbital rim are often inspected by transconjunctival or mid–lower eyelid incisions. Nondisplaced fractures of the orbital floor that do not need to be treated yet are often noted. Inadequate results after repositioning may occur due to rotation of the fragment if the repositioning at the sphenozygomatic buttress is not fixed.

Inspection of the lateral orbital wall in cases of displaced fractures of the zygomatic complex can be performed endoscopically by means of a limited blepharoplasty incision.[2] In zygoma fractures, the orbital floor can be endoscopically inspected transorally via the maxillary sinus. The result after fracture reduction can also be evaluated at the infraorbital rim and the lateral orbital wall. Additional transconjunctival or infraorbital incisions can be avoided if there is no displaced fracture of the orbital floor and no displacement of the fragments at the infraorbital rim after repositioning. When indicated, osteosynthesis of the infraorbital rim can be performed endoscopically by the transoral approach.

The endoscopic treatment of comminuted fractures of the zygomatic arch is reported to avoid open reduction via coronal incisions, in the rare cases when an open approach is needed.[3]

Frontal sinus fractures of the anterior wall may be reduced with the use of minimally invasive techniques.[4] At least two incisions posterior to the hairline are needed for insertion of the endoscope and instruments for repositioning of fractures. Stab incisions may be needed for direct manipulation and fixation of the fragments. The indications for minimally invasive endoscopic surgery of the frontal sinus may be limited to single-fragment fractures of the anterior table of the frontal sinus.

SURGICAL TECHNIQUE

Endoscopic Equipment

The results of our experience are presented below, as this is rapidly developing field of surgery, clear clinical outcomes are not yet available for many procedures.

Initially, a prototype of an endoscopic plate application device (Synthes, Paoli, Penn) with a 30-degree angle, 4-mm diameter endoscope (Karl Storz, Tuttlingen, Germany) was used via an extraoral approach, because of the limited vision with this angulation during plate insertion using the plate application device there was a need for transbuccal incisions. The device was successfully only used in selected cases if the submandibular approach was performed.

In selected cases, 45- and 70-degree angle endoscopes, when used by experienced endoscopic surgeons, can be successful. These endoscopes are more difficult to employ, because there is limited forward vision when inserting the endoscope. A suction and irrigation device allows irrigation of the endoscope tip in limited optical cavities if vision through the lens is blurred by blood.

The monitor and the endoscopic equipment should be placed in the operating room facing the surgeon and assistant. Intraoperatively, it is important to watch the endoscopic picture on the monitor while sitting in a comfortable position. The light source and the camera should be close to the patient's head to avoid limiting the movement of the endoscope. A second suction device is recommended, even if an endoscope equipped with a suction and irrigation instrument is used.

Mandibular Condyle Fractures

The type of fracture, degree of displacement, and result of reduction were evaluated intraoperatively using the endoscope. Of course, conventional preoperatively and postoperatively Towne's and panoramic radiographs or computed tomographic (CT) and conebeam computed tomographic (CBCT) scanning are required (Figs. 31-1 to 31-3).

Transoral Approach

The transoral incision is similar to the surgical approach for sagittal split osteotomies of the mandible in orthognathic surgery. Local anesthetic is injected 8 to 10 minutes before incision to control bleeding. To create the optical cavity, the periosteal tissue on the ascending mandibular ramus is elevated, freeing the posterior aspect of the ascending ramus and the mandibular angle. The inferior inserting fibers of the temporalis muscle are stripped from the lower aspect of the muscular process. The endoscope is inserted subperiosteally and advanced cranially toward the fracture without dissection of the masseter muscle to avoid bleeding and damage to the facial nerve (see Fig. 31-7).

Repositioning and Fixation

Distraction of the TMJ region by pressure on the mandibular molars via the transoral approach is performed to facilitate repositioning of the condylar fragment. The periosteum and the soft tissues in the vicinity of the proximal fragment are removed carefully to allow the miniplates to be placed without detaching the lateral pterygoid muscle or impairing the blood supply to the condylar head.

Special instruments are inserted for the reduction of the condylar fragment. Stab incisions in the condylar region are made for transbuccal insertion of the screws. Transbuccal incisions are avoided when angulated drills and screw drivers

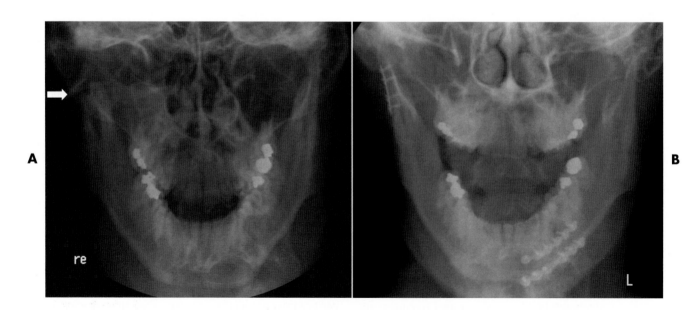

FIGURE 31-1   Panoramic and Towne's radiographs taken preoperatively (**A**) and postoperatively (**B**) after endoscopic-assisted transoral reduction and fixation of a displaced condyle fracture with lateral override *(arrow)*.

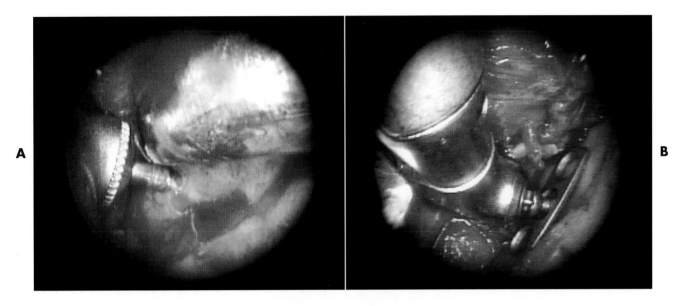

FIGURE 31-2 Intraoperative view of angulated drill (**A**) and screwdriver (**B**) during transoral fixation of a displaced condylar fracture without transbuccal step incision.

TABLE 31-1	Indications for Endoscopic-Assisted Trauma Procedures in 66 Patients between April 1997 and May 2002
Indication	No. of Patients
Condylar fractures	45
Investigation and treatment of midface fractures with additional orbital injury (e.g., orbital floor)	49
Decompression of optic nerve	3
Fixation of distraction devices in the mandible	2
Treatment of mandibular fractures or plate removals	21
Revisions of frontal sinus	7
Other (e.g., exploration of skull base; treatment of lesions in combination with conventional surgical procedures)	14

are used endoscopically via a transoral approach (see Fig. 31-2).

After insertion of the first screw in the condylar fragment, the fracture reduction is facilitated by pulling the miniplate with modified nerve hooks. The second screw is then inserted next to the fracture in the mandibular fragment. Osteosynthesis is performed with a 2.0-mm miniplate with at least two screws on each side of the fracture. After fracture reduction and fixation using two screws, the alignment at the posterior border of the ascending ramus is controlled endoscopically before osteosynthesis is completed (see Figs. 31-3 and 31-8).

Mandibular Fractures in Other Locations

In patients with mandibular fractures, endoscopic-assisted control after transoral fracture reduction is performed in areas of limited vision such as the inferior and posterior aspects of the ascending ramus in mandibular angle fractures (Table 31-1). The result after fracture reduction was controlled endoscopically in areas of limited visibility during the transoral approach to avoid displacement at the inferior and posterior aspect of the fracture and prevent lingual gaps before osteosynthesis is completed.

Midfacial and Frontal Sinus Fractures

In patients with fractures of the zygomatic complex and the orbit, endoscopic-assisted treatment can be undertaken. Limited incisions were performed, and because of the superior visibility with endoscopic techniques, further incisions (e.g., a transconjunctival approach) could be avoided in selected cases. However, the advantage of endoscopic-assisted techniques in the treatment of midfacial trauma remains controversial.[16]

Zygomatic Fractures

Because of possible rotation of the zygomatic bone, the result after repositioning can be evaluated intraoperatively before osteosynthesis is performed. The repositioning cannot be determined precisely from the lateral orbital wall with an intraoral approach. An additional extraoral approach for exploration of the orbital floor and the infraorbital rim is recommended if displaced zygoma fractures are suspected. Using these additional incisions, one can often identify non-displaced fractures that do not need treatment at the orbital floor and infraorbital rim.

In case of zygoma fractures, the endoscope is inserted via a limited blepharoplasty incision to control the fracture-dislocation at the sphenozygomatic buttress at the lateral orbital wall (Figs. 31-4 and 31-5). In displaced zygoma fractures, defects of the outer wall of the maxillary sinus often exist and can be used to insert the endoscope for transoral inspection of the orbital floor (Fig. 31-6). Mobility of the orbital floor is noted endoscopically when pressure is applied to the orbital content. Fractures of the infraorbital rim can also be investigated transorally with the use of a head lamp. After fracture reduction, evaluation of the alignment of the infraorbital rim, the sphenozygomatic buttress, and the

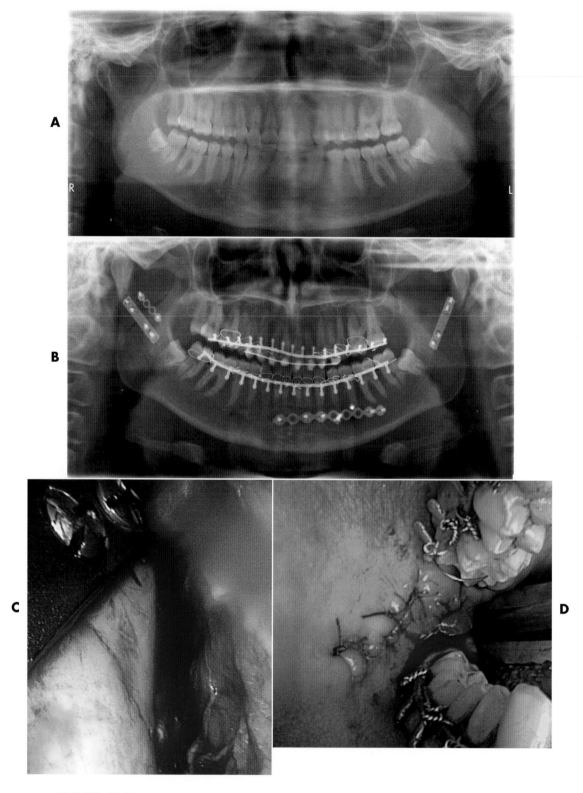

FIGURE 31-3 Preoperative (**A**) and postoperative (**B**) panoramic radiographs show a bilateral condyle fracture with an additional mandibular fracture and dental trauma in the anterior upper jaw. The intraoperative endoscopic view shows the quality of the reduction at the posterior aspect of the left condyle fracture after osteosynthesis (**C** and **D**) and the extent of the intraoral incision.

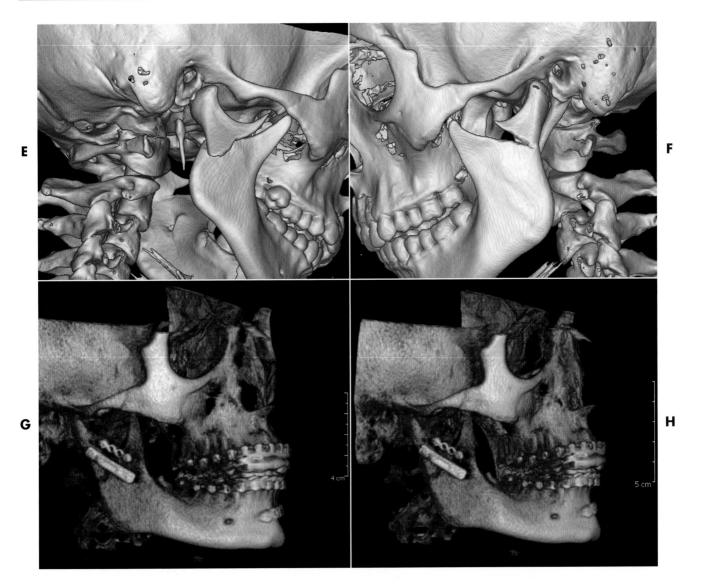

FIGURE 31-3, con't Preoperative three-dimensional computed tomograms (**E** and **F**) and a postoperative conebeam computed tomographic scan (**G** and **H**) demonstrate the amount of dislocation and shortening of the ascending ramus and the result after anatomical reduction and fixation of the displaced bilateral condyle fracture. Pre-injury function of the temporomandibular joint without malocclusion was achieved postoperatively.

zygomaticomaxillary buttress is performed. After temporary osteosynthesis at the lateral orbital aspect and the zygomaticomaxillary buttress with two screws for each plate, the result of repositioning and fixation is evaluated before osteosynthesis is completed. Moderate displacement of the infraorbital rim can be treated transorally. In selected cases, osteosynthesis at the infraorbital rim can be performed endoscopically via the transoral approach. If there is no displacement of the orbital floor, further investigation via transconjunctival or infraorbital incisions can be avoided.

If displaced orbital floor fractures are present, the endoscopic-assisted repositioning of orbital soft tissues into the maxillary sinus and orbital floor fractures can be performed transorally (see Fig. 31-6). In comminuted fractures of the orbital floor and infraorbital rim, open reduction and insertion of resorbable foils, bone grafts, or titanium mesh may be indicated to reconstruct the orbital floor and

infraorbital rim. In these cases, exposure of the fracture site by means of a transconjunctival incision is indicated (Fig. 31-7). The result of repositioning of the orbital soft tissue and reconstruction of the orbital floor can be checked endoscopically via the maxillary sinus (see Figs. 31-6 and 31-7).

Fractures of the anterior wall of the frontal sinus may be reduced by minimally invasive techniques if the fracture is not comminuted. Two or three limited incisions in the scalp for insertion of the endoscope, suction, and instruments (e.g., an elevator) can be used for reduction of the fracture, similar to the procedure used in endoscopic brow lift surgery. Fixation without further stab incisions is difficult. Depressed fragments may be elevated using single screws inserted via stab incision under endoscopic control. However, because of the difficulty in fracture reduction, this approach is not established as a routine procedure, and superior results may be obtained with open reduction and fixation via a laceration or

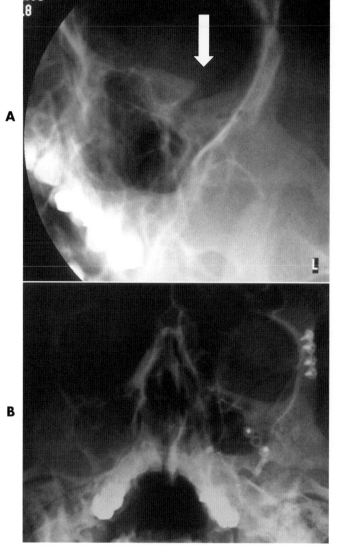

FIGURE 31-4 Towne's radiographs obtained preoperatively (**A**) and postoperatively (**B**) after endoscopic-assisted reduction and fixation of a dislocated zygoma fracture *(arrow)* carried out via a laceration in the upper left eyelid (see Fig. 31-5).

coronal approach. If displaced fractures of the posterior table are present, open treatment via a coronal incision is indicated.

Other authors have described the endoscopic-assisted injection of bone substitute to fill contour defects of the forehead secondarily after frontal sinus fractures without impairment of frontal sinus function.[16a]

OUTCOME

MANDIBLE

Mandibular Condyle

Plate fixation and control of reduction was facilitated endoscopically (see Figs. 31-3 and 31-8). Transbuccal stab incisions for insertion of the screws were performed in all patients for whom the submandibular approach was used. In those patients with a transoral approach, angulated drills and screwdrivers facilitated fixation of the fractures without the need for transbuccal incisions (see Fig. 31-2). The transoral approach therefore has become the standard approach for open reduction of condyle fractures.

Temporary weakness or permanent damage of the mandibular branch of the facial nerve was observed more often in patients with the submandibular approach compared to the minimally invasive endoscopic-assisted transoral approach. Six months after open reduction of displaced condyle fractures, the mouth opening in all patients exceeded 40 mm interincisal distance without significant deviation and with good TMJ function. There were no signs of TMJ dysfunction, and none of the patients had pain in the TMJ area. The average length of the submandibular scar was 4 to 5 cm. The scars were esthetically acceptable in all patients. The transoral endoscopic approach proved to be more time-consuming. However, because of a steep learning curve, the time for transoral endoscopic treatment was reduced to less than 1 hour on average.

Mandibular Fractures in Other Locations

Precise fracture repositioning was achieved by transoral endoscopic control in patients with fractures of the mandibular angle and ramus. Checking the fracture reduction was obtained endoscopically in areas of limited vision. Initially, only two screws were fixed temporarily and evaluated before the osteosynthesis was completed. In selected patients, the fixation had to be corrected because of inadequate positioning that could not have been discerned without the endoscopic control. Postoperatively, all patients had a good result of repositioning and fixation without signs of malocclusion.

MIDFACE AND FRONTAL SINUS FRACTURES

Intraoperatively, the degree of dislocation of zygoma fractures and the results after reduction were checked endoscopically via limited incisions. Fractures of the lateral orbital wall were endoscopically inspected via blepharoplasty incisions (see Figs. 31-4 and 31-5). The orbital floor and the infraorbital rim were visualized via the transoral approach (see Figs. 31-6 and 31-7). For treatment of nondisplaced orbital floor fractures, endoscopic-assisted techniques were used to avoid additional eyelid incisions. Postoperative images demonstrated good results. None of the patients presented with diplopia.

Displacement of orbital soft tissues into the maxillary sinus was detected in patients with comminuted fractures of the orbital floor (see Figs. 31-6 and 31-7). Transconjunctival incisions are indicated in comminuted fractures of the orbital floor to allow for adequate fracture reduction, stabilization, or reconstruction of the orbital floor using resorbable foils, bone grafts, or titanium mesh under complete visual control. The use of a head lamp is advantageous in reconstructive orbital surgery.

Fractures of the anterior wall of the frontal sinus were reduced with the use of minimally invasive techniques in selected cases when there were no signs of a comminuted fracture. However, because of the limited bone thickness of the frontal sinus, the injury was underestimated on

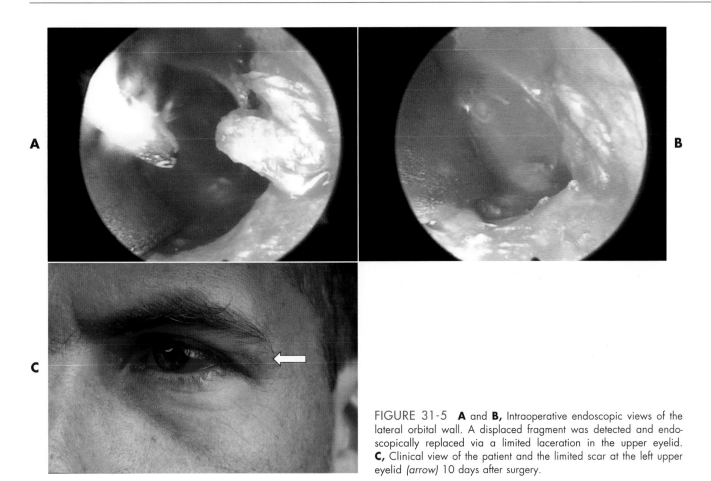

FIGURE 31-5 **A** and **B,** Intraoperative endoscopic views of the lateral orbital wall. A displaced fragment was detected and endoscopically replaced via a limited laceration in the upper eyelid. **C,** Clinical view of the patient and the limited scar at the left upper eyelid *(arrow)* 10 days after surgery.

high-resolution CT scans before surgery. After elevation of the periosteal tissue, multiple fragments were noticed and the treatment strategy had to be changed to an open reduction via coronal incision. Open reduction and fixation via the coronal approach proved to be advantageous compared to endoscopic-assisted techniques for the treatment of frontal sinus fractures.

CONTROVERSIES

Minimally invasive endoscopic procedures have been described for various indications in the craniomaxillofacial area.[2,3,4,14,16] To minimize the risks of damage to the facial nerve and visible scars, endoscopic-assisted techniques via limited or transoral incisions have been confirmed.[1,5,9-13,17-20]

In cases of oral and maxillofacial trauma, adequate exposure for comminuted fractures is mandatory to allow for precise three-dimensional fracture reduction. The indication for endoscopic-assisted treatment is limited to fractures that can be treated without wide exposure. Creation of an optical cavity is required to obtain endoscopic vision of the fracture site through limited incisions. The extent of the incision depends also on the type of fracture and the treatment planned. However, the volume of the optical cavity has to allow for the handling of instruments. Special instruments designed for endoscopic repositioning and fixation have been developed. Because the work is done in an optical cavity, incisions in inconspicuous areas can be used as surgical ports.

Minimally invasive techniques and limited incisions facilitate reduction and the insertion of screws and plates in oral and maxillofacial trauma surgery, especially in fractures of the mandibular condyle. Good vision of fracture sites in areas with limited visibility is obtained with the use of endoscopic techniques. After endoscopic-assisted treatment of the condylar fractures by an intraoral approach, precise anatomical reduction, good postoperative function, and restoration of occlusion were achieved.[16-21] Good function after endoscopic-assisted treatment compared with treatment via extraoral incisions was also demonstrated in a prospective randomized trial.[21] Different approaches for the treatment of displaced condylar fractures have been demonstrated. The surgical approach is chosen according to the type and location of the fracture. The extraoral approach was preferably selected for displaced fractures with medial override and for comminuted or condylar neck fractures in cases managed from April 1998 to December 1999. Since 1999, all subcondylar fractures with indication for open reduction and fixation have been treated successfully by a transoral approach,

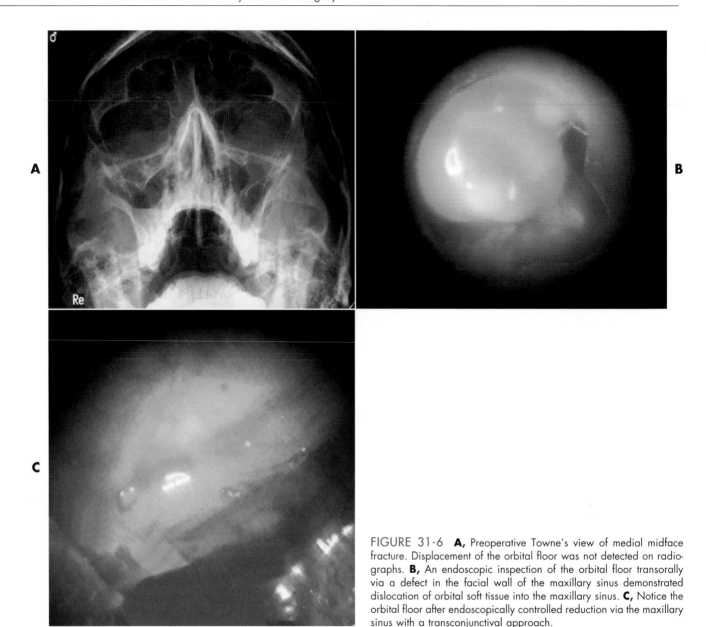

FIGURE 31-6 **A,** Preoperative Towne's view of medial midface fracture. Displacement of the orbital floor was not detected on radiographs. **B,** An endoscopic inspection of the orbital floor transorally via a defect in the facial wall of the maxillary sinus demonstrated dislocation of orbital soft tissue into the maxillary sinus. **C,** Notice the orbital floor after endoscopically controlled reduction via the maxillary sinus with a transconjunctival approach.

even when a medial dislocation of the proximal fragment was present.[1,5,11]

Angled drills and screwdrivers facilitated the transoral management of condylar fractures without the need for transfacial stab incisions in both adult and pediatric patients.[5,17-20]

Compared with the submandibular approach, the endoscopic-assisted transoral approach is less time-consuming, the intraoral scars are invisible, and the risk of facial nerve damage is minimal.

The transoral use of endoscopes for checking fracture reduction in areas of limited vision, such as the posterior aspect of the ascending ramus and the inferior aspect of the mandible, provided further information about the quality of fracture reduction. In addition, a load-sharing situation could be achieved to improve surgical results and to reduce complications such as screw loosening and plate fractures.[16] Therefore, the transoral endoscopic approach for condyle fractures became routine procedure in our clinic. Since 1999,

we have used the transoral endoscopic approach for all condyle fractures for which an open procedure was indicated, even when severe displacement was present. However, careful patient selection is mandatory.

The aim of minimally invasive management of midfacial trauma is to minimize the operative trauma. However, as in mandibular fractures, the indication may be limited in the midfacial area, where comminution and multiple displaced fragments may require wide exposure.[16] Fractures of the zygomatic complex are often inspected by means of transconjunctival and infraorbital incisions to check fractures of the orbital floor and infraorbital rim. The endoscopic inspection of the lateral orbital wall and sphenozygomatic buttress by means of a limited blepharoplasty incision has proved to be helpful for the evaluation of suspected displaced zygoma fractures before and after repositioning and fracture reduction. Often, nondisplaced fractures are seen that do not need further treatment. To avoid incisions that serve a diagnostic

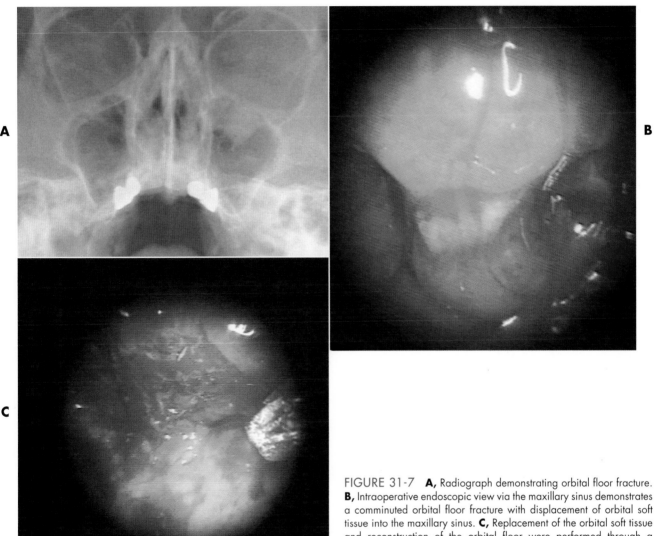

FIGURE 31-7 **A,** Radiograph demonstrating orbital floor fracture. **B,** Intraoperative endoscopic view via the maxillary sinus demonstrates a comminuted orbital floor fracture with displacement of orbital soft tissue into the maxillary sinus. **C,** Replacement of the orbital soft tissue and reconstruction of the orbital floor were performed through a transconjunctival approach with transoral endoscopic control after repositioning of the orbital soft tissue via the maxillary sinus.

purpose only, endoscopic control of the orbital floor can be performed transorally via the maxillary sinus.

However, because of the increased availability of CBCT and CT, a precise preoperative diagnostic examination can be performed without the need for intraoperative inspection. If exposure of the fracture is performed, good visibility can be obtained with the use of a head light.

Endoscopic-assisted reduction of comminuted zygomatic arch fractures using preauricular and transconjunctival incisions with lateral canthotomy has been reported.[3] Because of the presence of multiple fragments, wide exposure is often required, and extracorporeal realignment of the arch fragments may be indicated. For fixation with a long 2.0-mm osteosynthesis plate in the anterior aspect, incisions in the visible area by lateral canthotomy have been used. These incisions leave visible scars in an exposed area of the face.[3] In severely comminuted fractures of the zygomatic complex, open reduction via coronal incision provides better exposure for a safer reduction without visible scars.

The endoscopic nasal approach for reduction of medial orbital wall fractures has been described.[15] In fractures of the medial orbital wall with orbital soft tissue displaced into the ethmoid area, placement of bone grafts or resorbable foils may be indicated for reconstruction of the orbital volume to prevent enophthalmos. Bone grafts or resorbable foils that are indicated for the reconstruction of the medial orbital wall in extended fractures cannot be inserted transnasally. Medial orbital wall fractures without displacement of orbital soft tissue into the ethmoid area and without signs of double vision do not need to be treated. For frontal sinus fractures, minimally invasive techniques can be applied in selected cases.[4] However, more predictable and precise results are obtained by an open approach via coronal incision.

If comminuted fractures or involvement of the posterior table of the frontal sinus or the anterior skull base is present with suspected leakage of cerebrospinal fluid, open treatment via a coronal incision with wide exposure of the fracture site in collaboration with the neurosurgeon is indicated, and

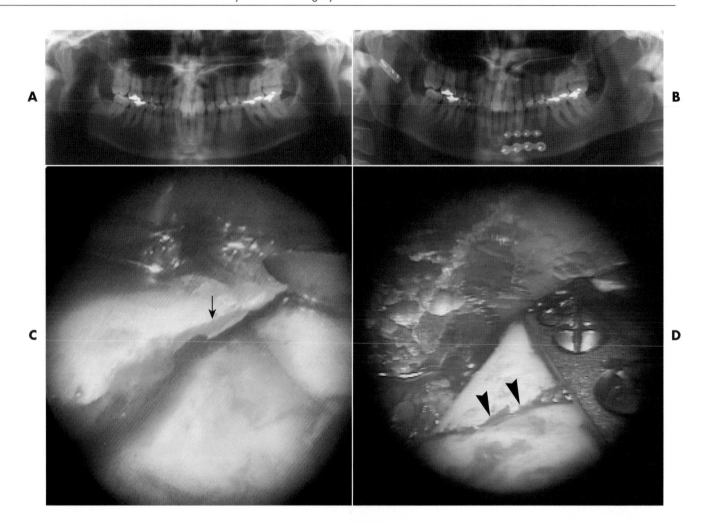

FIGURE 31-8 Displaced mandibular condyle fracture and paramedian fracture of the mandible resulting from a football accident. **A** and **B,** Preoperative and postoperative panoramic radiographs. **C** and **D,** Intraoperative transoral views of the mandibular condyle fracture with lateral override using a 30-degree angle endoscope, before *(arrow)* and after *(arrowheads)* osteosynthesis.

endoscopic techniques should not be performed. Because of the limited thickness of the bone involved in frontal sinus fractures, the degree of comminution is often misjudged on CT scans. This may cause difficulties in reduction through limited incisions, because the degree of comminution and displacement can often be appreciated only after elevation of the periosteal tissue and exposure of the fragments. Therefore, the indications for endoscopic-assisted fracture reduction of the frontal sinus area may be limited.

Contour defects of the forehead can be treated by minimally invasive techniques using bone substitutes injected under endoscopic control after a frontal sinus wall has healed in dislocation. Esthetically compromising contour defects manifesting after craniotomy for neurosurgical treatment also can be evened out by this approach.

CONCLUSION

Future perspectives for increasing the indications for minimally invasive surgery are planned using the combination of endoscopic techniques and computer-assisted surgery. The endoscope position can be monitored with the use of computer-assisted techniques that allow endoscopic-assisted surgery of the anterior skull base or next to anatomical structures such as the optic nerve and the internal carotid artery. Further developments of bone cements or bone glues may lead to other indications and new treatment strategies for endoscopic surgery in craniofacial trauma. The repair of contour defects and fixation of nondisplaced fractures may be carried out using bone cements and glues.

Intraoperative imaging with CT and CBCT allows for immediate quality control after minimally invasive procedures for the repositioning of craniomaxillofacial fractures.

Intensive training in endoscopic techniques and the handling of special instruments is mandatory before endoscopic-assisted treatment of oral and maxillofacial fractures is performed. Because of the steep learning curve, the operation time required for the initially time-consuming endoscopic-assisted procedures can be reduced significantly.

REFERENCES

1. Lauer G, Schmelzeisen R: Endoscope-assisted fixation of mandibular condylar process fractures. *J Oral Maxillofac Surg* 57:36-39, 1999.

2. Schön R, Gellrich N-C, Schramm A, et al: Endoskopische Chirurgie im Mund-, Kiefer- und Gesichtsbereich: Video demonstration einer endoskopisch assistierten Versorgung einer dislozierten Jochbeinfraktur [Endoscopic oral and maxillofacial surgery: video demonstration of the endoscopic assisted treatment of a displaced zygoma fracture]. *J DGPW* 12:21, 2000.

3. Lee CH, Lee C, Trabulsy PP: Endoscopic-assisted repair of a malar fracture. *Ann Plast Surg* 37:178, 1996.

4. Graham HD, Spring P: Endoscopic repair of frontal sinus fracture: case report. *J Craniomaxillofac Trauma* 2:52-55, 1996.

5. Schön R, Gutwald R, Schramm A, et al: Endoscopic assisted treatment of condylar fractures: extraoral vs. intraoral approach. *Int J Oral Maxillofac Surg* 31:237-243, 2002.

6. Schön R, Roveda SIL, Carter B: Mandibular fractures in Townsville, Australia: incidence, etiology and treatment using the 2.0 AO/ASIF miniplate system. *Br J Oral Maxillofac Surg* 39:145-148, 2001.

7. Walker RV: Condylar fractures: nonsurgical management. *J Oral Maxillofac Surg* 52:1185, 1994.

8. Weinberg MJ, Merx P, Antonynshyn O, et al: Facial nerve palsy after mandibular fractures. *Ann Plast Surg* 34:546, 1995.

9. Ellis E III, Dean J: Rigid fixation of mandibular condyle fractures. *Oral Surg Oral Med Oral Pathol* 76:6, 1993.

10. Hall MB: Condylar fractures: surgical management. *J Oral Maxillofac Surg* 52:1189, 1994.

11. Lauer G, Schmelzeisen R, Wichmann U: Endoskopgestützte: Fixation von Gelenkfortsatzfrakturen des Unterkiefers [Endoscopic assisted fixation of condylar fractures of the mandible]. *Mund Kiefer Gesichtschir* 2(suppl 1):S168-S170, 1998.

12. Chen C-T, Lai J-P, Tung T-C, et al: Endoscopically assisted mandibular subcondylar fracture repair. *Plast Reconstr Surg* 103:160-165, 1998.

13. Jacobovicz J, Lee C, Trabulsky PP: Endoscopic repair of mandibular subcondylar fracture. *Plast Reconstr Surg* 101:160-165, 1998.

14. Vasconez LO, Core GB, Oslin B: Endoscopy in plastic surgery: an overview. *Clin Plast Surg* 22:585, 1995.

15. Michel O: Isolierte mediale Orbitawandfrakturen: Ergebnisse einer minimalen invasiven endoskopisch-kontrollierten endonasalen Operationstechnik [Isolated fractures of medial orbital wall: results using a minimal invasive endoscopic controlled endonasal operation technique]. *Laryngorhinootologie* 72:450-454, 1993.

16. Forrest CR: Application of endoscope-assisted minimal-access techniques in orbitozygomatic complex, orbital floor, and frontal sinus fractures. *J Craniomaxillofac Trauma* 5:7-12, 1999.

16a. Picetti GD III, Ertl JP, Bueff HU: Endoscopic instrumentation, correction, and fusion of idiopathic scoliosis. *Spine J* 1:190-197, 2001.

17. Schön R, Schramm A, Gellrich N-C, et al: Follow up of condylar fractures of the mandible in 8 patients at 18 months after transoral endoscopic-assisted open treatment. *J Maxillofac Surg* 61:49-54, 2003.

18. Schön R, Fakler O, Gellrich N-C, et al: Five year experience with the transoral endoscopic-assisted treatment of displaced condylar mandible fractures. *Plast Reconstr Surg* 116:44-50, 2005.

19. Schön R, Gellrich N-C, Schmelzeisen R: Minimal invasive open reduction of dislocated pedriatric condylar fracture. *Br J Oral Maxillofac Surg* 43:258-260, 2005.

20. Schön R, Fakler O, Metzger M, et al: Preliminary functional results of endoscope-assisted transoral treatment of displaced bilateral condylar mandible fractures. *Int J Oral Maxillofac Surg* 37:111-116, 2008. Epub September 5, 2007.

21. Schmelzeisen R, Cienfuegos-Monroy R, Schön R, et al: Patient benefit from endoscopically assisted fixation of condylar neck fractures: a randomized controlled trial. *J Oral Maxillofac Surg* 67:147-158, 2009.

CHAPTER 32

Computer-Assisted Oral and Maxillofacial Surgery: Technology and Clinical Developments

Stefan Hassfeld, Joachim Mühling, Marc C. Metzger, Georg Eggers

Computers are used increasingly as a supportive tool for diagnosis, operative planning, and treatment in medicine and dentistry. They are used in combination with ultrasound and digital imaging techniques such as computed tomography (CT) and magnetic resonance imaging (MRI) to improve the visualization of anatomical and physiological conditions. Almost every medical specialty shows a tendency toward less invasive procedures, and good imaging is essential for diagnosis and surgery, particularly for minimally invasive procedures. Within our own surgical specialty, this extends into all areas, from dental implantology to the treatment of craniofacial malformations and advanced tumors. It is particularly important in this complex anatomical maxillofacial region.

Whereas in diagnostic imaging enormous progress has been made, the intraoperative use of imaging techniques has been relatively restricted. Intraoperative three-dimensional (3-D) imaging with ultrasound, CT, and MRI is still costly and is available only at an experimental level and for exceptionally complex cases. Computer-assisted surgery will be a help in this field in the future, and techniques of virtual reality will become increasingly important in relation to medical devices.

The goal of the interactive, intraoperative application of 3-D imaging has been used in part through instrument navigation systems. These systems enable the surgeon, for the first time, to show the actual instrument position in the surgical site on the 3-D reconstructed image dataset of the patient. It is also possible to focus on the position of a pathological or anatomical structure within the operative field. "Mirroring" of the non effected side is invaluable in trauma reconstruction.

DIAGNOSTIC IMAGING

3-D imaging techniques such as CT, conebeam computed tomography (CBCT), MRI, and ultrasound can present almost every anatomical and pathological structure with high resolution and quality. Present developments concentrate on artifact reduction and on techniques for automatic fusion of the various imaging modalities.

SEGMENTATION PROCEDURES

The segmentation procedure is necessary to mark anatomical structures for further data manipulation and planning.[1] Hounsfield-specific units (e.g., delineating bone, soft tissue, muscles, tumors) on a 3-D dataset can be selected in each slice of the dataset or by defining the area of interest.[2,3] Performing the segmentation slice by slice is very time-consuming, whereas defining the area of interest and performing a threshold segmentation by selecting specific Hounsfield units often is not sufficiently precise (Fig. 32-1). In craniomaxillofacial surgery, the midface area with its thin anatomical bone structures often leads to the presence of virtual "pseudoforamina" or artifact holes after the segmentation procedure.

Because of these complications, modern software offers so-called automatic atlas segmentation procedures. After the data is imported into the planning software, a menu is available from which the surgeon can select the area of interest. A deformation algorithm transfers the information of a standarized and segmented skull atlas into the patient-specific dataset. After this procedure, the adapted parts can be used for further planning in the patient dataset (Figs. 32-2 and 32-3).

PLANNING AND SIMULATION

Automated generation of the proposed operation with simulation of surgical procedures and outcome is nearly possible within the framework of virtual surgery. For the simulation of operative results (i.e., virtual 3-D graphic simulation of various treatment alternatives on the computer), software must be developed to allow for interactive manipulation. This should be in real time within the 3-D visualization, including viewing from various angles, cutting, palpation, and insertion of implants. Here, the user's interaction has to be conform with the usual surgical actions. In the future, input media with power feedback (haptic interfaces from the field of virtual reality technologies) will offer options for intuitive control of complex 3-D simulation environments.

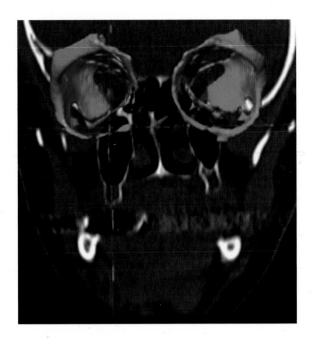

FIGURE 32-1   Threshhold-segmentation of the orbital cavity. Due to areas with thin bone, pseudoforamina often result after the segmentation procedure.

INTRAOPERATIVE SUPPORT

The imaging data acquired preoperatively during diagnosis should be available for interactive use by the surgeons at all times. In this way, modern techniques of computer-assisted surgery can help to decrease the operative risks and postoperative morbidity rates. Future interactive support for the surgeon can be characterized within three areas:

- *Passive tools for support of the intraoperative orientation* will allow for routine transfer of the preoperative plan onto the patient. These tools include projection techniques, head-mounted displays, and instrument navigation systems.
- *Guiding systems (semiactive manipulator systems)* will show the surgeon a risk-free path for the surgical instruments to achieve the operative plan. By this means, operative strategies can be transferred to the surgical site precisely and safely.
- *Surgical robots will execute specific operative steps* In this case, the surgeon will leave control to the robot for certain parts of the operation. The best-known example is the highly precise milling of the femur shaft for adaptation of

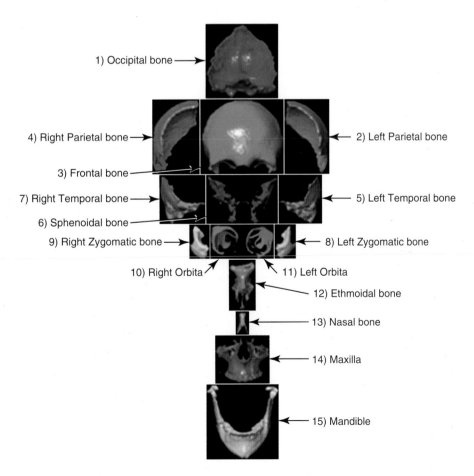

FIGURE 32-2   A standarized and segmented skull is used for the automatic atlas segmentation procedure.

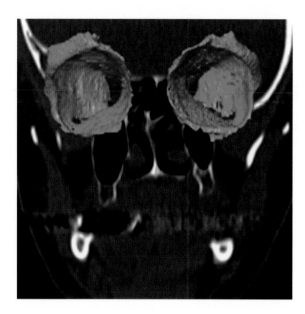

FIGURE 32-3   Atlas segmentation of the orbital cavity. Deforming the atlas leads to patient-specific parts without any pseudoforamina.

a hip joint endoprosthesis, which is already in routine clinical use.

INTRAOPERATIVE IMAGING

Intraoperative imaging is most helpful for maxillofacial procedures that require precise postoperative symmetry with limited intraoperative visualization. If the surgeon would consider obtaining a postoperative CT to check implant placement or symmetry, then intraoperative imaging could also be considered. It will provide the surgeon with the required anatomical information in the operating room and allow for a revision if necessary.

There are two modalities for intraoperative CT scanning: fan beam scanners (CT) and conebeam scanners (CBCT). Both are rapid (requiring <2 minutes per scan) and give adequate bone resolution. Due to better handling, lower costs, and less x-ray exposure, intraoperative imaging by CBCT (C-arm machine) has won recognition.

The C-arm provides 3-D reconstructions that are acquired by rotation around an isocentric point. With panning of the C-arm over the surgical field, no reposition of the patient is necessary. The acquired 3-D data can easily be imported into the existing planning software of the navigation device. With the use of image fusion, the preoperative plan can be compared with the intraoperative imaging data (Fig. 32-4). This shifts the postoperative control into the operating room, decreasing complications, and costs.

POSTOPERATIVE EVALUATION

Postoperatively, a comparison between the control imaging data and the original imaging data for evaluation of the real surgical result will permit scientific studies using the follow-up

controls. The resulting data can be used for optimization of operative strategies using the software tools to improve prediction of the surgical outcome.

DIAGNOSTIC IMAGING APPLICATIONS

The existence of suitable imaging data in the form of 2-D and 3-D datasets is critical for successful preoperative planning and intraoperative navigation. In many cases, we use several, partly complementary imaging devices in the same anatomical area to obtain detailed, supplementary clinical information.

CT offers the advantages of a precise, reproducible and high-contrast presentation of osseous structures. The image quality of CT is diminished by patient movement, as well as the presence of metal artifacts, and if there is limited soft tissue contrast. Advantages of MRI are its excellent soft tissue imaging choice of image planes, and the possibility of functional imaging (diffusion- and perfusion-weighted acquisitions, magnetic resonance angiography). In addition, the patient is not subjected to radiation exposure. Disadvantages are the various artifacts (e.g., distortion), both appliance specific and patient induced, including the chemical shift, susceptibility artifacts, movement, and metal artifacts.

Sonography (ultrasound) offers the advantages of quick access, high resolution, the choice of image planes, and especially the possibility of tracking anatomical structures and determining function (e.g., blood flow, and vascularity). Disadvantages are the dependence on the examiner's skill and the geometrical distortions and associated "noise". The use of 3-D sonography creates more indications, with the possibility of reconstruction of the image layers parallel to the CT or MRI images. In addition it may be aligned to give the view for the surgeon, resulting in improved orientation.

The possibility of intraoperative use offers an additional advantage of sonography and, to a lesser extent, of CT and MRI.[5] Imaging must be considered not only with respect to diagnosis but also in connection with operative planning and other methods based on these data. Especially important are the imaging parameters chosen by the surgeon in cooperation with the radiologist, such as the plane of the cuts, layer spacing and thickness, and use of contrast media.

Because of the increasing need to include all imaging information in treatment planning, it is desirable sometimes to combine the data from various sources to achieve a fused imaging dataset (Fig. 32-5). For this purpose, an automated fusion of the various image modalities and automated segmentation of the anatomical and pathological structures should be available but is not yet possible with the present state of the art. So far, only bones and skin surfaces can be segmented automatically using CT data. However, knowledge of the exact positions of "at-risk" structures such as vessels and nerves is especially important—for example, to avoid damage during the planning phase of the operative steps to be performed by a robot.

Many implantologists wish to have a 3-D visualization of the bone status for planning of complex cases. So far, CT has been used infrequently as a diagnostic aid, not least because of the associated radiation exposure. However, dental implantologists are interested primarily in bony

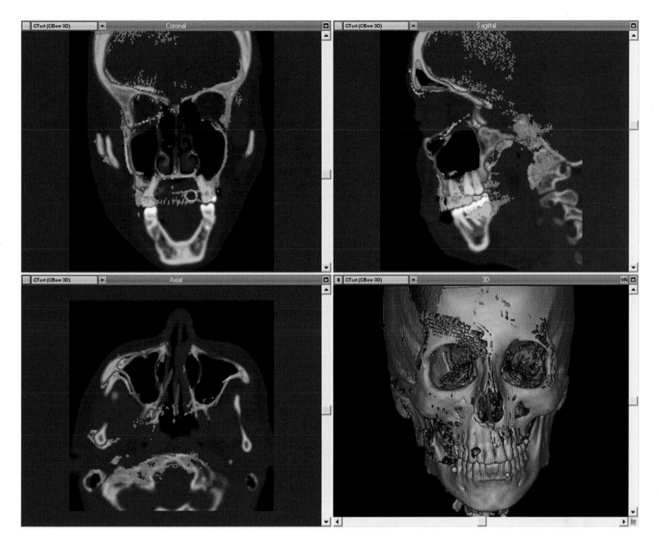

FIGURE 32-4 Multiplanar view of a patient with secondary zygomatic bone reconstruction of the right side shows the preoperative planning by mirroring the left to the right side *(red)* and the image fusion including the actual surgical situation of the surgery in the operating room *(blue)*.

structures, and high soft tissue resolution is not necessary. Dose reduction seems promising. Dose-reduced CT allows exact metric measurements in the range of 1 mm or less as well as 3-D representation of the jawbone, facilitating a precise 3-D implantation plan with justifiable radiation exposure. Therefore, we consider CT-assisted planning to be indicated before dental implantations in patients with limited bone volume, for example near the maxillary antrum or the mandibular canal, and when multiple implants are planned.

Following technical developments, 3-D radiographic techniques are expected to become increasingly important in oral surgery. CBCT scanners produce a 3-D imaging data record without the need to move the patient table. With the cone-beam technique, dedicated devices can be built especially for dentistry; in design, these could be similar to conventional devices (Fig. 32-6). It seems realistic to expect the development of further devices with costs comparable to those of current orthopantomography devices.

PLANNING AND SIMULATION APPLICATIONS

In contrast to the rapid progress in diagnostic imaging, development and clinical use of new technologies for planning and performing therapy are lagging behind. This can clearly be seen from the fact that 3-D CT imaging data are still exposed as 2-D images on X-ray film. Analysis is mostly restricted to general statements or a few measurements. Planning is carried out mentally by the treating physicians and depends very much on their experience and powers of imagination.

The aim of operative planning in oral and maxillofacial surgery is optimization of the surgical result in terms of function and esthetics. The prerequisite for successful operative planning is preparation of preoperative patient imaging data. For segmentation of the original imaging data, individual pixels or voxels are assigned to certain classifications such as skin, bones, at-risk structures, and tumors. Powerful graphic workstations are necessary for interactive manipulation in great detail.

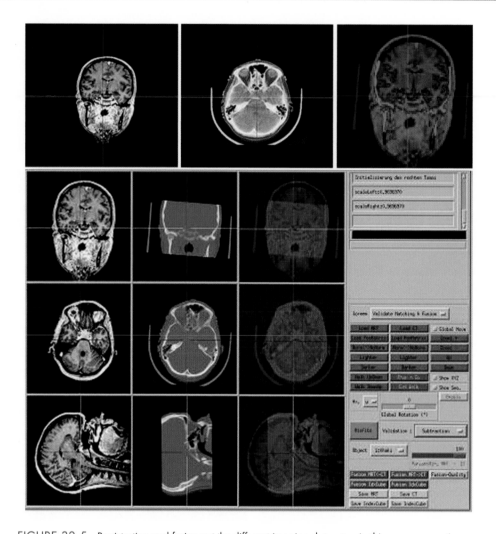

FIGURE 32-5 Registration and fusion put the different imaging datasets—in this case, magnetic resonance tomography (MRT, *above left*) and computed tomography (CT, *above middle*)—into a common geometrical context (fused imaging dataset with MRT in *red* and CT in *green, above right*). The software makes it possible to represent the individual datasets and the fused dataset in different frames on the monitor.

With the aid of the patient model generated from the original imaging data, the operative goal can be defined and the operation planned. However, the model is only an approximation of the patient. Certain information, such as that contained between the layers or "slices" of the imaging data, is missing, so precision is limited by layer thickness.

At the present time, there is a serious discrepancy between the scientific development of tools with highly complex software systems and the simple handling requirements the surgeon uses. This problem prevents the conversion of a theoretical process into practical application, because the interactive planning of a complex bone-shifting operation requires more than 1 hour.

Optimal use of new technologies to safely plan and carry out surgical interventions requires an operative planning system that can be consulted by the surgeon during preoperative planning, intraoperative intervention, and postoperative evaluation. During preoperative planning, the first task is to define the operative aim. For example, the bone segments to

be moved must be specified and virtually cut, moved, and positioned.

Two application areas are described here to highlight the clinical importance of preoperative planning and simulation.

Computer-Assisted Planning in Dental Implantology

Conventional preimplantation planning is usually conducted with a 2-D panoramic radiograph. This method cannot supply an assessment of the actual bone volume in a buccolingual dimension. Often, it becomes apparent during surgery that the bone is too narrow or is not suitable for an implant due to concave cortical surfaces. When the third dimension is unknown, large distances must be left between implants and neighboring structures for safety reasons, and the use of all the available bone cannot be optimized. CT-based planning systems for dental implantology have been introduced with the goal of overcoming these limitations. To choose the

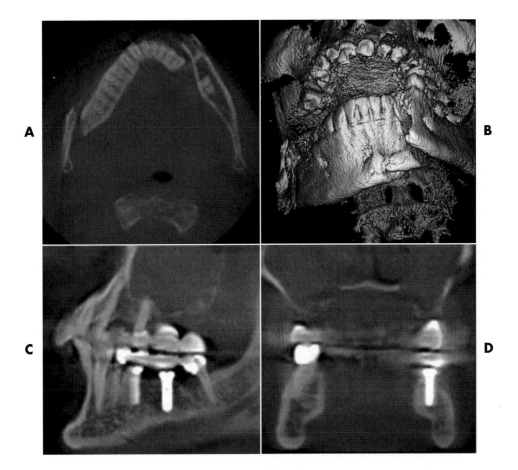

FIGURE 32-6   Image examples produced with conebeam computed tomography (NewTom QR-DVT 9000). Axial (**A**) and three-dimensional (**B**) representations of a mandibular angle and a paramedian fracture with a free basal fragment. Sagittal (**C**) and coronal (**D**) reformats demonstrate bone volume in the vicinity of the implant.

most suitable implant insertion site, it is possible to move through an almost unlimited succession of finely graduated cross-sectional and panoramic sections. At any time, the treating physician can reconstruct the exact information required for treatment planning without having to reexamine the patient. These software-generated secondary sections from the CT dataset of a jaw allow, for the first time, the mucosal surfaces and evaluation of the vestibulo-oral dimension of the alveolar process and immediate metric registration directly on the screen. However, most software systems commercially available today have one serious disadvantage: real time 3-D visualization is not possible.[6]

Software programs for interactive 3-D planning of dental implantations have only recently become available. This data provides high resolution, and corresponding detailed visualization of the patient's bone volume data. Therapy planning additionally requires the representation of virtual surgical equipment such as implants, drills, and saws which can more precisely utilized. For operator convenience, frame rates of several images per second are necessary; only then will intuitive and interactive positioning of the implants possible.

A system for interactive 3-D planning for dental implantology, developed at our hospital (Fig. 32-7), allows the 3-D positioning of implants with high image quality. The position of the mandibular canal requires only identification of the

mandibular foramen and the mental foramen; from that, the software automatically performs an analysis of the most probable course of the mandibular canal within the CT image. Based on bone availability, the distance to critical structures, and the planned prosthetic superstructures, the surgeon decides on the position of the implants.[7]

From a prosthetic view, to prevent interferences between the optimal number, position, angulation, and type of implants and the existing anatomy, it is necessary to match the preoperatively obtained data (bone quality and bone quantity) with prosthetic demands (statics, dynamics, and esthetics) during the planning. The successful result of an implant superstructure can be optimized and guaranteed for the long term. Future developments in this area will also encompass the integration of 3-D simulation of prosthetic superstructures and their esthetic effects into the planning software environment. In this way, the virtual implantation procedure, from a prosthetic and surgical viewpoint, will be achieved for the first time.

The advantages of CT-based implantation planning do have to be considered in relation to the disadvantages of availability of scanners, higher costs, and higher radiation exposure for the patient. Many authors consider it better to apply standard orthopantomography techniques for routine examinations and to reserve CT-based implantation planning for

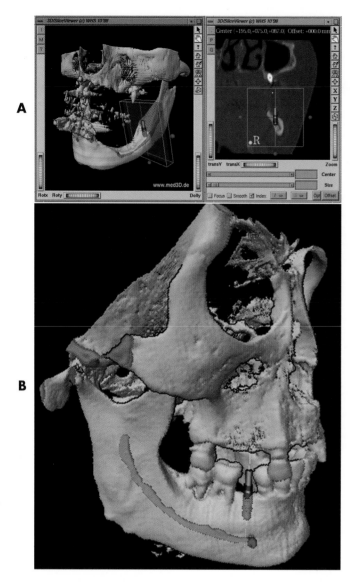

A

B

FIGURE 32-7   **A,** Positioning of an implant on the monitor. The implant's position and orientation can be interactively changed in the two-dimensional layer or on three-dimensional (3-D) visualization. In the semitransparent representation on the *left,* the 3-D relation of the implant to the mandibular canal is obvious. **B,** Semiautomatic segmentation of the mandibular canal. For user interaction, it is merely necessary to click on the mandibular foramen and the mental foramen. (**A,** *Courtesy of Dr. W. Stein, Heidelberg, Germany; www.med3D.de [accessed May 2, 2011].*)

particularly complex cases, such as those with reduced bone volume, especially near the maxillary sinus and mandibular canal, and for planning the insertion of multiple implants.

The decisive step to an exact implant insertion has not yet been achieved. In the simplest case, 3-D planning data can be used to produce individual drill guides made with titanium tubes. Also, combination with intraoperative navigation systems for implant insertion is possible. From a technical viewpoint, medical robotics could also be used for implant insertion. Many things are still at the developmental or prototype stage, but significant effects on surgical routine are expected soon.

Computer-Assisted Planning for the Correction of Malformations

New software and hardware technologies have led to successful use of surgical navigation systems in many disciplines (e.g., removal of foreign bodies and tumors). To use these new technologies optimally and safely to plan and carry out a surgery, planning systems are needed that support the surgeon during preoperative planning as well as intraoperatively.

Software developments for the virtual cutting and shifting of bone parts now allow a patient-specific simulation of complex osteotomies.[3-11] Through contact detection, it becomes apparent which bone parts must be remodeled further. For a better graphic quality, the individual bone segments are differentiated through the use of different colors. After determination of the optimal movement on the computer screen, the calculated data can be applied precisely to the operative site (i.e., to the patient), for example with the aid of a navigation system, to ensure optimal precision of the surgery (Figs. 32-8 and 32-9).

The simulation of the surgical outcome (i.e., 3-D graphic representation of the various osteotomies on the computer) supports the surgeon in the planning and choice of the best operation. The 3-D visualization facilitates assessment of the planned operation and permits discussion with colleagues and patient. Conventional limits with regard to the surgeons, planning are overcome, and this method also allows the patient to be involved in the the operation planning. Another goal is to achieve simulation of soft tissue changes in the 3-D presentation of the results of a planned intervention.[12] The patient would then be able to decide on the surgical method together with the physician, strengthening the relationship between physician and patient.

The use of the term *operative planning* varies in the literature. With most operative planning systems, only a simulation of the postoperative image can be carried out; only a few systems also support intraoperative visualization of the preoperative planning. The individual planning systems can be classified into three categories:

1. *Systems without technical support*: These carry out, above all, a visualization of the postoperative state.
2. *Systems with passive support for intraoperative navigation*: These systems allow the surgeon to run through a preoperatively planned access path using visual control. Apart from the access path, many systems also show objects such as tumors, foreign bodies, and tissues at risk that must be avoided.
3. *Systems with active support*: This may be provided, for example, by a surgical robot.

In complex surgical interventions, such as preoperative planning of a fronto-orbital advancement, the increase in intracranial volume achieved by the bone shift can be visualized. To simulate interventions of this kind, computer-based geometric models have to be produced from the CT images; these models clearly represent the anatomical structures and simulating the interventions that are relevant for the operation, such as drilling, sawing, or deformation. Methods for interaction that guarantee an exact and intuitive input of the surgical actions must be seen on the computer.

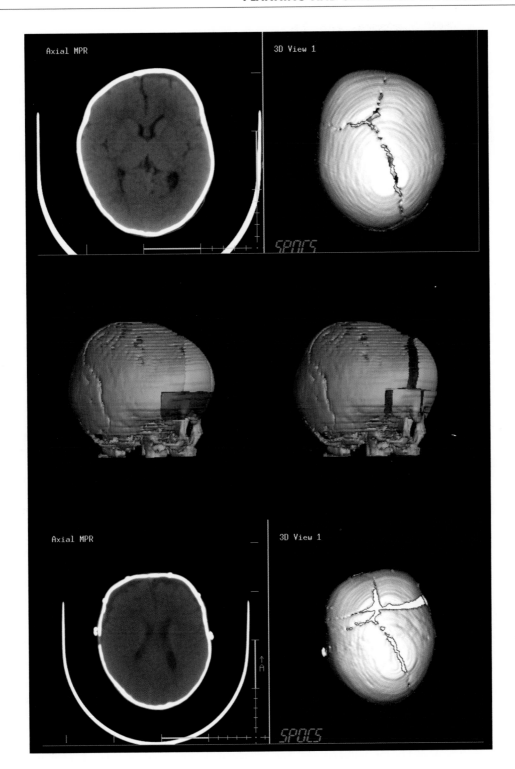

FIGURE 32-8 Simulation of correction of a plagiocephaly through fronto-orbital bone advancement. A postoperative comparison of the control computed tomographic (CT) imaging data with the basic CT imaging data for evaluation of the operative real result is shown. *Top,* preoperative status; *bottom,* postoperative status; *middle left,* simulation before operation; *middle right,* simulation after operation.

FUTURE OF SURGERY SIMULATION

Tools for 3-D interaction with the imaging data (human-machine interface) require the selection of points or partial volumes in the 3-D scene. Usually, a 2-D mouse is used for this task, but 3-D input devices can accelerate the processing and increase the precision of the whole procedure. Another improvement can be achieved by giving a "feel" or sense of touch in this interaction. For this reason force-feedback devices are becoming increasingly integrated as part of the human-machine interface. Surgeons performing the planning "feel" as if they have actually made an incision into the skin or bone surface[9,13] (Fig. 32-10).

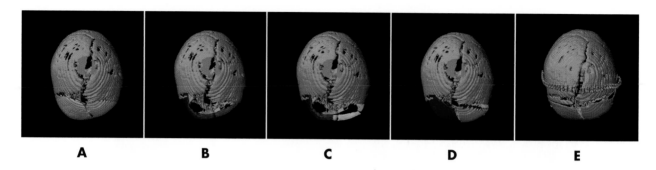

A   **B**   **C**   **D**   **E**

FIGURE 32-9   Simulation of correction of a plagiocephaly, showing detailed planning of segments: **A,** Segmentation of the bone segments; **B,** temporary removal of the frontal bone; **C,** shaping and foreshifting of the orbital segment; **D,** reorientation of the frontal bone; **E,** postoperative situation.

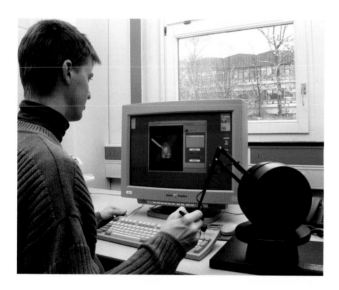

FIGURE 32-10   Input of incision planning via a haptic interface.

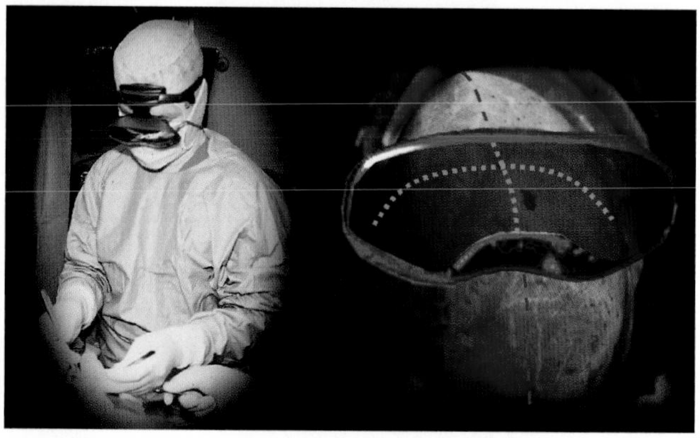

FIGURE 32-11   Semitransparent glasses to overlap the computer simulation with the real operative area.

COMPUTER-ASSISTED INTRAOPERATIVE SUPPORT APPLICATIONS

PROJECTION OF THE OPERATIVE PLAN ONTO THE PATIENT

Anatomically and pathologically relevant structures or planning data such as the incision line can be directly projected onto the patient or virtually mirrored into 3-D glasses (Fig. 32-11). Such see-through devices or head-mounted displays (HMD) are already available for military use. For medical uses, they have to be modified. Apart from simple handling problems (e.g., the surgeon standing at the table cannot put on and take off the glasses and may have to refocus them or look above or below them to see well), there are technical problems regarding the resolution and frequency of the image representation.

The alternative is direct projection of the desired information onto the patient. This requires exact planning and a coordination of the patient's head, the eyes of the observer, and the projector. Because deeper anatomical structures cannot be projected correctly with respect to their position, their interface with the surface has to be visualized, and the

surface position must therefore be known at all times. Technically, this is already possible, but it requires a great deal of effort.[14] The aforementioned augmented reality techniques will facilitate a much easier interactive use of diagnostic images and planning data intraoperatively in the future.

INTRAOPERATIVE SUPPORT BY INSTRUMENT NAVIGATION

In the areas of neurosurgery; ear, nose, and throat surgery; orthopedics; and oral and maxillofacial surgery, intraoperative instrument navigation is already routinely used in many hospitals and clinics. The navigation system records the spatial position and orientation of a probe or a surgical instrument. After the registration has been completed, the preoperatively acquired imaging data of the patient is merged into the actual position of the instrument through 2-D and 3-D visualization. During intraoperative navigation (Fig. 32-12C), the spatial position data for the navigation instrument are permanently presented on the CT or MRI dataset of the patient. Simultaneously, the instrument tip position is shown as a crosshair in the original layers and in two vertical, secondary computed levels on the screen; for example, with axial original layers, additional sagittal and frontal views may be shown. The 3-D reconstruction of the CT data is shown in a fourth screen window that displays the

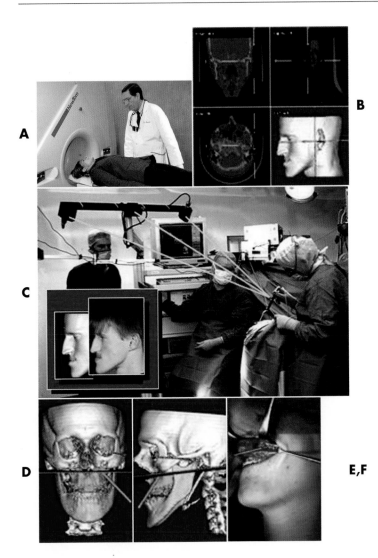

FIGURE 32-12   Principles of intraoperative instrument navigation. **A,** Computed tomographic or magnetic resonance imaging data. **B,** Three-dimensional (3-D) visualization. **C,** Optoelectronic navigation system for registration of imaging data to patient position. **D** through **F,** 3-D visualization of imaging data and instruments corresponding to the actual clinical position. (*A, From Dawson P:* Functional occlusion, *St. Louis, 2007, Mosby.)*

position and orientation of the whole instrument (e.g., a probe) and a projected virtual extension of the instrument axis (see Fig. 32-12B).

Assessment of Navigation Technology and Accuracy

The intraoperative use of operative planning data on the basis of radiographic images was first performed in neurosurgery with stereotactic systems firmly attached to the skull. These systems allow for localization of deep-seated intracranial structures and are used today for neurosurgical operations because of their good precision and it is a well-proven procedure.[15]

By transition from the computer-assisted plan to the operative phase based on frameless navigation and localization techniques, surgeons can see their actual instrument position for the first time on the 3-D reconstructed imaging dataset of the patient. Conversely, it is also possible to determine the position of a pathological or anatomical structure shown on the images of the individual patient's anatomy. The precision of such navigation systems is usually reported to be in the range of 2 to 5 mm.[15-19] The accuracy is substantially higher in rigid structures such as bones and osseous areas than in soft tissue areas.

From a technical point of view, instrument navigation in medical surroundings is possible *mechanically,* through position calculation with a gear of movable angles. Also it can be done *electromagnetically,* through detection of field changes with coils; using *ultrasound,* through real-time measurements of the sound signals; and *video-optically,* through position calculation with infrared diodes or recognition of patterns with charge-coupled device (CCD) cameras.

The *mechanical systems* offer the advantages of good technical precision (about 1 mm), low susceptibility to failure, and are easy to sterilize with covers. The disadvantages are the unwieldy handling, restricted range and mobility, and space requirement at the operating table.[17]

Electromagnetic systems offer the advantages that very small detector coils can be used, no visual contact between the instrument and the sensor system is required, a rapid computation of the signals can be made, and sterilization is easy. Their disadvantages are susceptibility to interference through magnetic fields and metal objects and, consequently, possible limited accuracy. Incorrect position sensing of up to 4 mm may occur.[8,19-21]

The *ultrasound-based systems* offer the advantages of a technically acceptable precision in the range of 1 to 5 mm, convenient handling, and easy sterilization. However, because these systems are subject to interference through reflection, the Doppler effect, air movement, background noise, and obstructions in the sound path, they are rarely used today.

Systems with *optical coupling* are used increasingly in intraoperative navigation.[18-22] Optical navigation systems offer the advantages of a high technical precision in the range of 0.1 to 0.4 mm, convenient handling, and easy sterilization. The disadvantages lie in the necessity for constant visual contact between cameras and instruments and the susceptibility to interference through light reflections on metallic surfaces in the operating environment.

The resolution of CT data is very high. Our team, for example, experimentally determined the precision to be between 0.3 mm and 0.5 mm.[23] This resolution is so small that we can safely assume, with regard to the interactive use of the imaging data, that the limiting factor is the precision of the intraoperative realization, not the image generation. Radiation remains an important consideration for some elective procedures.

The resolution of MRI data achieves similar results, but problems may occur in some cases due to massive irregular geometrical deviations in the examination volume. The combination of CT data and MRI data on a geometrical basis offers a viable solution.

Possible errors exist with the segmentation and 3-D reconstruction of the datasets. Flaws in the respective calculation algorithms may lead to inaccuracies of the 3-D object (e.g., enlargement, reduction, distortion). Another possibility is the incorporation of image parts that were not supposed to be part of the structure to be reconstructed; conversely, necessary parts might also possibly be excluded.

Registration

The basic requirement of any navigation technique is the registration of the patient's position in relation to the imaging dataset, which can be performed according to various principles.

In the case of frame-based stereotaxy, this is accomplished by attaching the frame to the patient's head before taking the required images. For frameless navigation techniques in general, anatomical landmarks or artificial markers are used. Subsequently, they are marked with the computer mouse (or automatically) on the imaging dataset in the operating room and traced onto the patient with the navigation system. The workstation then computes the correlation between the actual patient position and the imaging dataset. This procedure requires absolute fixation of the patient or continuous high-precision measurements of the patient's movements,.

The choice of registration procedure itself has a direct influence on navigation accuracy. Registration with anatomical landmarks is not precise enough, with divergences of 2 to 5 mm being described. Adhesive markers are described as being sufficiently exact. The markers should be attached to skin portions that do not tend to shift too much and are not expected to experience a change due to swelling, distortion through draping, or other causes during the time between CT scanning and the operation. Problems with lost or, more critically, slightly displaced skin markers can occur because of the time lapse between tomography and surgery (often >24 hours). Miniscrews inserted preoperatively into the bone are substantially more precise.

Surface-based scans for automatic registration of the patient's position are increasingly mentioned. With these systems, the patient surface is traced by laser scanners or illuminated by a structured light, and the resulting dataset is matched with the preoperatively obtained diagnostic imaging data of the patient.

Additional *reference frames* using infrared diodes such as the operating instruments make it possible to move the operating table together with the fixated patient without having to repeat the registration.[17] However, these reference frames are often blocked by or hidden behind the surgeon. Referencing systems fixated directly on the patient are supposed to permit patient movements and to recognize and adjust to unnoticed shifts automatically. The patient does not necessarily need to be immobilized. Such systems supply a firm mechanical fixation but should also be removable, not too invasive, and resilient (Fig. 32-13). Noninvasive devices using the auditory canals and a nasion support can cause an error of approximately 1 mm between the frame's position during preoperative image production and its attachment in the operating room. Hauser et al.[24] described the intraoperative accuracy of this kind of system when combining a facial bow with an optical navigation system of 2 mm or less.

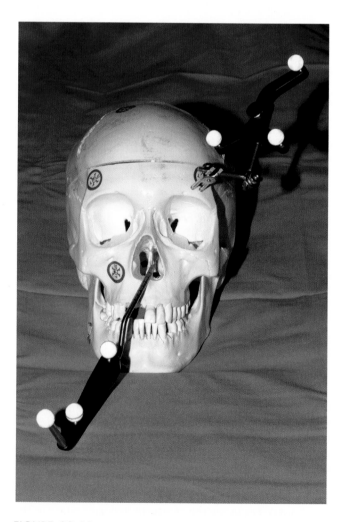

FIGURE 32-13   Instrument set for passive optical navigation. The pointer and reference frame are rigidly fixed to the supraorbital rim for registration of the patient's movements.

We currently prefer the use of intraosseous screws,[17] because this method eliminates a number of problems associated with adhesive markers or surface scan registration. The quality of registration is independent of the application pressure of the probe, the positioning of the probe tip on the marker is unmistakable, and the danger of a shift of markers between the scan and the operation is eliminated. The temporary insertion of screws into the cranial bones of the patient can certainly be justified in cases of tumor resection, but this procedure seems to be somewhat excessive for elective surgery. In such cases, the fixation of adequately formed markers to the remaining teeth of the patient through an acid-etching technique or by positioning of a plastic dental splint would be a possible alternative. This method also provides absolute stability, is noninvasive, and is associated with easy postoperative removal.

Only a few comparable studies regarding the precision of navigation and measurement of intraoperative navigational systems can be found in the literature. They describe experiences gained through clinical applications and test series on various phantoms, reporting navigation accuracy values in the range of 1 to 5 mm (1-3 mm in bony structures).[23] This shows that an error, defined as divergence of the imaged position from reality, is always possible in computer-aided surgery. An accumulation of errors ranging from image reproduction to actual surgery with navigation is unavoidable. Today, the intraoperative accuracy of the navigation systems in bones and in soft tissues in the vicinity of bone is usually less than 3 mm.

Clinical Application of Navigation Systems

Between the autumn of 1993 and mid-2001, more than 200 clinical applications of navigation technology took place at the Department of Maxillofacial and Craniofacial Surgery, University of Heidelberg, using mainly CT data (layer thickness, ≤2 mm). Some of the surgical episodes were performed in interdisciplinary cooperation with the Heidelberg University Clinic Department of Neurosurgery, ENT Department, and Department of Ophthalmology.

According to our own experience, CT-based navigation can achieve an accuracy of 3 mm or less in bones and in soft tissue areas in the vicinity of bones. Registration of the patient's position with preoperatively inserted screw markers, which eliminates skin shifts, achieved accuracy values of 2 mm or less.[17,23] With the use of MRI scans as a navigation basis, application accuracy values of 4 mm or less were achieved in soft tissue regions surrounding the skull base. In pure soft tissue surgery, the flexibility of the tissue can render the preoperatively obtained data obsolete.

Two clinical cases are presented here to demonstrate the advantages of intraoperative instrument navigation technology.

Use in Complex Surgical Situations

A 10-year-old patient suffering from a left temporomandibular ankylosis with severely restricted mouth opening after trauma in early childhood underwent surgery. During the operative planning, the system facilitated a precise 3-D analysis of the changes in the temporomandibular joint (Fig. 32-14A). In the operative revision, the navigation system contributed to precise and safe orientation near the severely altered lateral cranial base (see Fig. 32-14B and C).

Localization of Foreign Bodies

The second patient had been shot in the face, and bullet fragments were scattered in the maxillary and mandibular regions. After use of the system for detailed visualization and analysis of the positions of the fragments and the bony fractures, the navigation technique was used intraoperatively to precisely locate and remove the bullet fragments in the left pterygopalatinel and submandibular regions (Fig. 32-15).

Clinical Evaluation of Navigation Technology

Based on literature review and our own experience, instrument navigation techniques have proved to be very advantageous for:

- localization of anatomical and pathological structures (e.g., foreign bodies, tumors) in the operative field.
- planning surgical access.
- precise intraoperative planning of the individual 3-D plan in jaw asymmetries and craniofacial malformations.
- protection of essential structures.
- control of resection borders in tumor surgery.
- planning and insertion of implants.
- teaching and postgraduate medical education.

With the use of these techniques, the spatial orientation for surgeons operating in complex anatomical regions may be improved considerably. The possibility of checking resection borders opens up new perspectives in tumor surgery and osteotomies. Tumor resections may be carried out faster and more precisely, but due to the time-consuming registration of the patient's position, the total operative time cannot as yet be reduced.

In our extensive clinical evaluation of the instrumental navigation technique we have also found the following deficiencies:

- At the moment, there are no navigation systems with an intraoperative accuracy of less than 2 mm, as desired by surgeons.
- There are no reliable details referring to the actual accuracy during the surgical intervention.
- The systems are time-consuming due to fault-prone registration procedures when correlating the system's coordinates and the patient's location. Software operation is not particularly well integrated ergonomically into the operative procedure, and visualization on the monitor is not adapted to the surgeon's view of the operative site.
- The connection of motor-driven instruments (e.g., drills, milling cutters, saws) is not yet possible due to lack of real-time visualization.
- With increasing operative time, the preoperative imaging data no longer correspond to the actual operative status.

Intraoperative Imaging

Fundamental problems of intraoperative instrument navigation techniques can arise from the potential for deviation of the preoperatively obtained imaging data from the actual operative situation. This can be caused, for example, by changes due to swelling or by distortions resulting from the removal of bone or other tissues. Inaccuracies during the phases of data acquisition, data preparation, or registration of

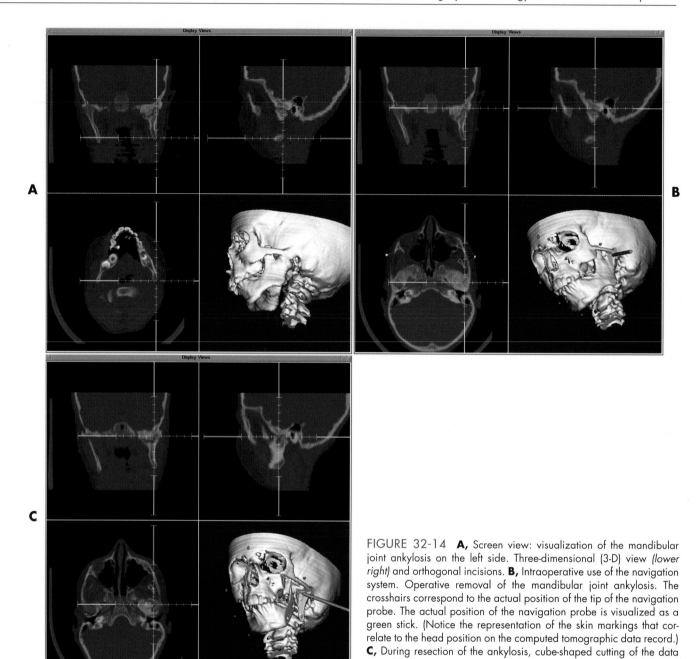

FIGURE 32-14   **A,** Screen view: visualization of the mandibular joint ankylosis on the left side. Three-dimensional (3-D) view *(lower right)* and orthogonal incisions. **B,** Intraoperative use of the navigation system. Operative removal of the mandibular joint ankylosis. The crosshairs correspond to the actual position of the tip of the navigation probe. The actual position of the navigation probe is visualized as a green stick. (Notice the representation of the skin markings that correlate to the head position on the computed tomographic data record.) **C,** During resection of the ankylosis, cube-shaped cutting of the data record in the 3-D view corresponds to the actual position of the tip of the navigation probe.

the patient's position and the navigation technique itself may also produce problems. Because of the stability of the structures, deviations during surgery involving osseous structures are considerably less than during operations involving soft tissues alone. A possible solution for these deviations is the use of intraoperatively applicable imaging procedures such as ultrasound, CT, and open MRI.[5]

Further concepts aim at applying ultrasound, CT, and MRI techniques in the operating room to validate the preoperatively obtained patient data, update them if necessary, and then visually pass them on to the operating surgeon in their updated form.

Finally, we also have to think of an intraoperative 4-D technique (i.e., moving 3-D images). For example, this technology would allow inclusion of functional aspects in joint areas as part of the planning, simulation, and operation.

INTRAOPERATIVE USE OF MEDICAL ROBOTS

Rapid technological progress in hardware, falling prices, and the rapid development of planning and controller software increasingly allow the use of robots in the operating room. Medical robotic systems are being tested or are already in commercial use in stereotactic neurosurgical interventions, in orthopedic surgery of the hip or knee, and in active endoscopic systems for minimally invasive surgery. Robots in the operating room are the last link in

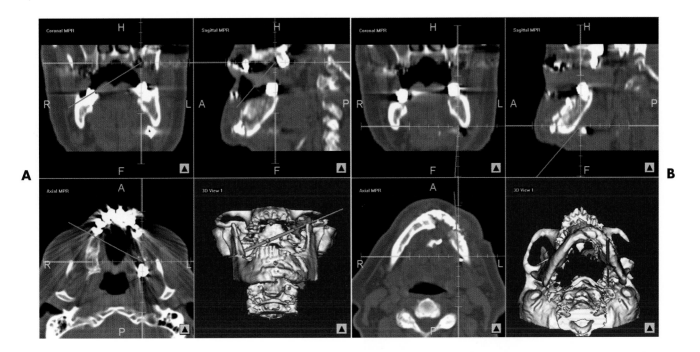

FIGURE 32-15   Visualization of a gunshot wound with multiple bullet fragments scattered in maxillary and mandibular regions. The navigation system was used intraoperatively to localize and remove bullet fragments in the left submandibular region. **A,** Three-dimensional view *(lower right)* and orthogonal images. The crosshairs correspond to the actual position of the tip of the navigation probe. The actual position of the navigation probe is visualized as a green stick. **B,** Intraoperative use of the navigation system for localizing and removing bullet fragments in the left retromaxillary region.

the chain of efforts to give the surgeon comprehensive technical support. They make it possible to carry out precise incisions in large bony structures after preoperative planning, including optimal application of implants and transplants.[25]

With the autonomous use of robots, the surgeon permits the robot to perform certain parts of the operation completely. After finishing the procedure, the robot arm goes back to its base and remains away from the operating table as the surgeon continues the operation. Therefore, the robot should be considered as a tool that relieves the surgeon of certain tasks requiring high precision. The development of such systems is a challenge, because the precision and safe handling requirements are extremely important in surgery.

The development of semiactive systems, in which the operative plan supplies the surgeon with a guide for direction of the surgical instrumentation, seems promising. This could be used, for example, by a manipulative computer-controlled arm that guides the surgeon's instrument on the calculated osteotomy cut, serving as a remote-controlled guide for the surgeon. The surgeon controls the instrument while it is connected to the manipulative arm. Each deviation from the planned operative procedure can be announced or even avoided by the system, using active power feedback systems to protect at-risk areas such as nerves and vessels. A robot of this kind could, for instance, support an inexperienced surgeon by preventing penetration into high-risk areas. We have already tested a prototype system of this kind with phantom and animal experiments, and further clinical use is planned (Fig. 32-16).

Present surgical interventions with robotic assistance exhibit the following characteristics:

- The robot-assisted intervention itself is relatively simple, and no surgeon is capable of manually working with the same high precision as the robot.
- Complex interventions, such as cardiac surgery or laparoscopic operations, can be performed only under the direct control of the surgeon, such as by telemanipulation.

In contrast to robots previously used in orthopedics and neurosurgery, a robotic system for craniomaxillofacial surgery makes higher conceptual demands on the system. The bone structures involved are more complex, and there are more vital structures such as nerves and vessels in the operative area.

The central precondition for successful intervention with a robotic system is an adapted patient model that contains all relevant information. This relies on data obtained from the imaging techniques that are used to define the patient's individual anatomical and pathological characteristics.

The Maxillofacial and Craniofacial Surgery Unit of the University of Heidelberg, in cooperation with the Institute of Real-Time Computer Systems and Robotics at the Faculty of Computer Science, University of Karlsruhe, is working on a robotic system to be used in maxillofacial and craniofacial surgery (Fig. 32-17). The robot is a modified industrial model with six degrees of freedom and a load of 6 kg. The robot is installed on the rotating foot of an operating table. During the operation, the foot is lowered onto the floor to keep the surgical robot's base in a firm position. The following system components are included:

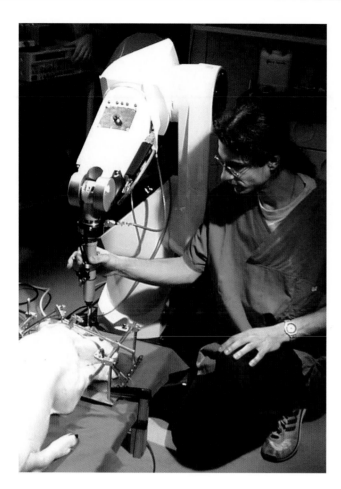

FIGURE 32-16   Test of the interaction between surgeon and robot in the semiactive mode with a pig preparation.

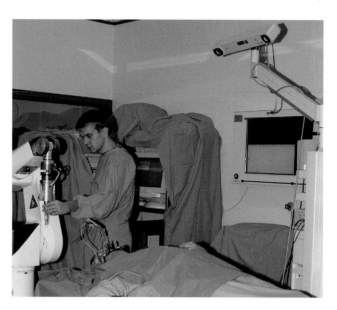

FIGURE 32-17   Preclinical tests with a surgical robot painting incision lines on a volunteer's skin.

- Robot Unimation RX90 with control software
- End effector, consisting of bone milling machine and bone drill, force/torque sensor (which facilitates power-controlled manual guidance of the robot), and overload protection
- Infrared navigation system for positional determination, registration, and control of the patient, the robot, and other tools
- Coordination processor for the sensory data
- Planning and simulation data processor

The precision of this prototype robotic system has been tested by an extensive accuracy analysis with phantoms and animal cadavers. Clinical use of this system is planned soon.

We are also testing the use of preoperative 3-D planning for dental implantology through a smaller robot. In this case, the robot positions an instrument for guidance of the surgical handpiece (Fig. 32-18). The initial drilling is carried out manually by the physician, with the position, drilling direction, and depth specified by the robot-assisted guide. As a result, the surgeon can transfer the implant's position, which has been optimally defined previously on the computer, exactly onto the patient.

Future robotic techniques in oral and maxillofacial surgery could include the following:

- Drilling holes with an automatic stop after penetration of the bone to protect the tissue lying deep to the bone
- Milling bone surfaces in plastic surgery according to a 3-D operative plan
- Performing deep saw cuts for osteotomies and allowing for the precise 3-D transposition of the subsequent bone segments
- Defined drilling of the implant bed for positioning of dental or surgical implants
- Preoperative automatic selection of the necessary osteosynthesis plates, their bending by a special machine, and their intraoperative positioning in defined positions

INTEGRATION OF COMPUTER-ASSISTED DESIGN

Applications of the computer-aided design and computer-aided manufacturing (CAD/CAM) technique are also used in surgery, with the main focus being the computer-assisted construction and manufacture of bespoke three-dimensional implants. Titanium implants for precise replacement of osseous defects of the skull,[26] for example, may now be produced directly rather than by use of physical models or templates, as has previously been necessary. Figure 32-19 demonstrates a skull reconstruction with CAD/CAM technology-based direct fabrication of a titanium implant.

EVALUATION OF SURGICAL OUTCOME

Rapid progress in the field of Internet technology means that the routine use of teleradiology and telemedicine will become a reality in oral and maxillofacial surgery. Clinical and imaging data from all stages of treatment will be available to all referring physicians associated with the patient's management. Smart cards will enable patients to carry their relevant medical data with them. Multicenter and multidisciplinary

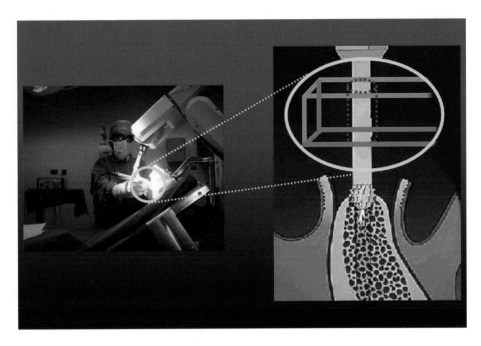

FIGURE 32-18 Interaction between surgeon and robot during tests on a phantom. The robot is serving as a three-dimensional interactive drill guide for the precise insertion of dental implants. *(Courtesy of Dr. R. Boesecke, Medical Robotics, Schwabmünchen, Germany.)*

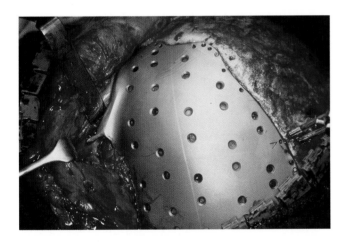

FIGURE 32-19 Secondary skull reconstruction after extensive trauma with CAD/CAM technology-based direct fabrication of a titanium implant. *(Implant planning and fabrication by Prof. Dr. H. Eufinger, Maxillofacial Surgery Unit, University of Bochum, Germany. Information at www.cranioconstructe.de/2001 [accessed May 2, 2011].)*

databases will enable new research options. These developments, however, do raise questions of data safety and security that will have to be discussed thoroughly by the medical community.

Postoperative computer-assisted assessment of 3-D morphology can be achieved by surface scanning technologies. The operation's success may be checked, and the data obtained may be used in planning and operative simulation for future procedures, thus improving the likely operative outcome. Further work should be aimed at developing tools for the semiautomatic generation of operative plans in a virtual surgical environment. In craniofacial surgery, for example, a proposal with individually optimized bone cuts and 3-D repositioning of bone segments could be presented by the computer to the surgeon, who would then be able to accept or change the plan before performing the surgery.

CONCLUSION

Computer and robotic technologies can optimize operative planning and improve the precision and quality of the operative performance. Through improved control of operative risks, preexisting limits may be disregarded and completely new operations may be performed. The following prerequisites are required from any future integrated system for computer-assisted oral and maxillofacial surgery.

All phases of the treatment—preoperative diagnostic procedures, operative planning, performance of the operation, and evaluation of the results—must be integrated. The system should be capable of supporting the surgeon in performing conventional operations performed without technical aids, technically supported operations involving passive navigation, and, ultimately, operations performed with active robotic assistance.

Today, the instrument navigation technique, with its interactive use of patient imaging data, already supports surgeons precisely and reliably. It has provided a substantial improvement in the areas of orientation and safety in complex anatomical regions, localization of pathological changes or foreign objects, and surgical correction of distinct malformations. Osteotomies and resections in the areas of tumor surgery, especially at the skull base, and reconstructive surgery may now be performed faster and more precisely.

From a surgical perspective, a system accuracy of less than 2 mm would be highly desirable. However, despite the described deficiencies, these prototype navigation systems are already being successfully used for the benefit of the patient and the support of the surgeon. In the near future, as a result of the techniques of computer-assisted surgery and their associated quality improvements and reduced operative risks, there may well be a considerable decline in patient-related stress. Nonetheless, the total operative time cannot yet be reduced because of the required set-up time and complex registration procedures. The economic consequences of such high-technology surgical applications should always be discussed, but there are already reports of decreased hospitalization time as a result of the use of navigation systems in neurosurgery.

Many authors believe that the use of instrument navigation systems will become the standard for complex operations.[1,14,17,18] In some fields, especially osseous surgical interventions with high demands on precision, operative robots have already proved their worth in routine clinical practice.[21] General limitations on the intraoperative use of navigation and robotic systems emerge from the fact that the preoperative imaging data become increasingly inexact due to changes caused by the operative procedure itself. It is here that we must work on the integration of intraoperative imaging data (from ultrasonography, MRI, CT, and conventional radiography) into the planning, simulation, and navigation systems.[1] Considerable limitations in the field of image generation, computer hardware, and software have as yet prevented the routine use of such intraoperative imaging updates.

Now that the initial feasibility has been proven, it is our aim to produce an economical operative system with handling as simple and intuitive as possible. This will encourage a broad clinical use of computer-assisted oral and maxillofacial surgery.

ACKNOWLEDGMENTS

Figures 32-5, 32-10, 32-16, and 32-17 are based on a collaboration with the Institute for Process Control and Robotics, Prof. Dr. H. Woern, Faculty of Computer Science, University of Karlsruhe, Germany. Figure 32-11 is based on a collaboration with the Institute for Process Control and Robotics, Prof. Dr. R. Dillmann, Faculty of Computer Science, University of Karlsruhe, Germany. Both projects are funded by the Sonderforschungsbereich 414 "Information Technology in Medicine—Computer and Sensor Supported Surgery" of the Deutsche Forschungsgemeinschaft.

Finally we would like to acknowledge the important work of Prof. Joachim Mühling, who has sadly died since the first edition was published.

REFERENCES

1. Altobelli DE, Kikinis R, Mulliken JB, et al: Computer-assisted three-dimensional planning in craniofacial surgery. *Plast Reconstr Surg* 92:576-585; discussion 586-577, 1993.
2. Deufelhard P, Dossel O, Louis AK, et al: Mehr Mathematik wagen in der Medizin. *ZIB Report* 25:26, 2008.
3. Stalling D, Zockler M, Sander O, et al: Weighted labels for 3D image segmentation. *Preprint SC* 98-39, 1998.
4. Zachow S, Zilske M, Hege HC: 3D reconstruction of individual anatomy from medical image data: segmentation and geometry processing. *ZIB Report* 07-41, 2007.
5. Wirtz CR, Knauth M, Staubert A, et al: Clinical evaluation and follow-up results for intraoperative magnetic resonance imaging in neurosurgery. *Neurosurgery* 46:1112-1120, 2000.
6. Verstreken K, van Cleynenbreugel J, Martens K, et al: An image-guided planning system for endosseous oral implants. *IEEE Trans Med Imaging* 17:842-852, 1998.
7. Hassfeld S, Stein W: Dreidimensionale Planung für die dentale Implantologie anhand computertomographischer Daten. [3D-planning in dental implantology based on CT data]. *Dtsch Zahnärztl Z* 55:313-325, 2000.
8. Kikinis R, Gleason PL, Moriarty TM, et al: Computer-assisted interactive three-dimensional planning for neurosurgical procedures. *Neurosurgery* 38:640-649, 1996.
9. Neumann P, Siebert D, Faulkner G, et al: Virtual 3D cutting for bone segment extraction in maxillofacial surgery planning. *Stud Health Technol Inform* 62:235-241, 1999.
10. Robb RA, Aharon S, Cameron BM, et al: Patient-specific anatomic models from three dimensional medical image data for clinical applications in surgery and endoscopy. *J Digit Imaging* 10(suppl 1):31-35, 1997.
11. Vannier MW, Marsh JL: Three-dimensional imaging, surgical planning, and image-guided therapy. *Radiol Clin North Am* 34: 545-563, 1996.
12. Keeve E, Girod S, Kikinis R, et al: Deformable modeling of facial tissue for craniofacial surgery simulation. *Comput Aided Surg* 3:228-238, 1998.
13. Munchenberg J, Woern H, Brief J, et al: Intuitive operation planning based on force feedback. *Stud Health Technol Inform* 70:220-226, 2000.
14. Xia J, Ip HH, Samman N, et al: Computer-assisted three-dimensional surgical planning and simulation: 3D virtual osteotomy. *Int J Oral Maxillofac Surg* 29:11-17, 2000.
15. Zamorano L, Jiang Z, Kadi AM: Computer-assisted neurosurgery system: Wayne State University hardware and software configuration. *Comput Med Imaging Graph* 18:257-271, 1994.
16. Birkfellner W, Watzinger F, Wanschitz F, et al: Systematic distortions in magnetic position digitizers. *Med Physics* 25:2242-2248, 1998.
17. Hassfeld S, Zoeller J, Albert FK, et al: Preoperative planning and intraoperative navigation in skull base surgery. *J Craniomaxillofac Surg* 26:220-225, 1998.
18. Hauser R, Westermann B: Optical tracking of a microscope for image-guided intranasal sinus surgery. *Ann Otol Rhinol Laryngol* 108:54-62, 1999.
19. Marmulla R, Hilbert M, Niederdellmann H: Inherent precision of mechanical, infrared and laser-guided navigation systems for computer-assisted surgery. *J Craniomaxillofac Surg* 25:192-197, 1997.
20. Gunkel AR, Freysinger W, Thumfart WF: Experience with various 3-dimensional navigation systems in head and neck surgery. *Arch Otolaryngol Head Neck Surg* 126:390-395, 2000.
21. Watzinger F, Birkfellner W, Wanschitz F, et al: Positioning of dental implants using computer-aided navigation and an optical tracking system: case report and presentation of a new method. *J Craniomaxillofac Surg* 27:77-81, 1999.
22. Reinhardt HF, Trippel M, Westermann B, et al: Computer assisted brain surgery for small lesions in the central sensorimotor region. *Acta Neurochir Wien* 138:200-205, 1996.
23. Hassfeld S, Mühling J: Comparative examination of the accuracy of a mechanical and an optical system in CT and MRT based instrument navigation. *Int J Oral Maxillofac Surg* 29:400-407, 2000.
24. Hauser R, Westermann B, Probst R: Noninvasive tracking of patient's head movements during computer-assisted intranasal microscopic surgery [published erratum in *Laryngoscope* 107:1000-1001, 1997]. *Laryngoscope* 107:491-499, 1997.
25. Taylor RH, Joskowicz L, Williamson B, et al: Computer-integrated revision total hip replacement surgery: concept and preliminary results. *Med Image Anal* 3:301-319, 1999.
26. Eufinger H, Wehmoeller M: Individual prefabricated titanium implants in reconstructive craniofacial surgery: clinical and technical aspects of the first 22 cases. *Plast Reconstr Surg* 102:300-308, 1998.

CHAPTER 33

Clinical Application of Computer-Assisted Reconstruction in Complex Traumatic Deformities

Nils-Claudius Gellrich, Alexander Schramm, Rainer Schmelzeisen

Correction of complex traumatic deformities remains a challenge; in the diagnostic evaluation of the deformity, in setting up the therapeutic schedule, and in the surgical correction itself. Until now, computer-assisted preoperative planning (CAPP) and computer-assisted surgery (CAS) have not been practiced as part of the surgical routine in the field of traumatic deformities.[1-5] The aim of this chapter is to demonstrate the value of modern computer-assisted analysis, simulation, and especially intraoperative navigation through the use of optical navigation systems in the field of traumatic reconstructive craniomaxillofacial surgery. In our experience, the direction of development of conventional navigation systems toward a multifunctional planning-navigation-control unit sets new standards in craniofacial plastic and reconstructive surgery.

Primary diagnostics are indispensable in assessing the mostly combined bony and soft tissue deformities in major craniofacial traumatic disorders. Advances in imaging techniques such as spiral computed tomography (CT) with multiplanar reconstruction and three-dimensional (3-D) imaging and associated technologies such as stereolithographic (STL) models, have led to improved preoperative planning for the craniomaxillofacial surgeon.[6-11] STL models create the 3-D situation only of hard tissue defects. They permit, to some degree, the preoperative or intraoperative manufacturing of individual implants, but they do not fulfill further requirements of reconstructive surgery. STL models, reflect just one segment within the gray scale of the acquired spiral CT dataset. Their use carries the risk of producing pseudoforamina artefacts instead of thin bony structures, which are widely present, especially in the midfacial skeleton (Fig. 33-1).

A spiral CT dataset provides information on a variety of both soft and hard tissues, limited only in the communication between radiologist and surgeon.[10] To obtain sufficient information about the preoperative situation, surgeons must familiarize themselves with the patient's individual anatomy. Today, modern navigation systems make it possible to increase the amount of CT/MRI information and to handle it easily. The surgeon can adjust the gray scale and reconstructions to current demands.[12-15] This is particularly important

in traumatic enophthalmos for precise assessment of the displacement of orbital contents before surgery (Fig. 33-2). The features of CAS/CAPP are listed in Box 33-1.

Proper assessment of asymmetry is the first and most important step before the reconstructive plan is designed. The correct measurement of distances between anatomical structures helps to determine the severity of displacement, for example, if bony prominences are displaced or deviations from the original midline or occlusal plane are concerned. Sometimes even well-established clinical measurements such as Hertel's index are limited and must be regarded with great skepticism. They do not take into account the amount of bony dislocation at the lateral orbital rim, which is often present in severe midface fractures. In this case, objective computer-based measurement technique is advantageous: the CT-based corrected Hertel's index (the perpendicular distance between projection of the corneal surface and the lateral orbital rim) allows for quantification of globe projection, including the additive effect of bony displacement (see Fig. 33-2).[16] Further transverse, craniocaudal, and posterior-anterior measurements within the orbit suggest where the problem is situated and how much bone grafting or reconfiguration of periorbital bone is necessary.[17] Using this planning procedure, the surgeon becomes familiar with the individual deformity in a three-dimensional manner.

Among a total of 125 patients with midface fractures and skull base deformities, severe ankyloses of the temporomandibular joint (TMJ), optic nerve decompression, complex craniosynostosis, midface skull base tumor resections, primary and secondary reconstructions and complex dental implant insertion were being treated with CAPP and CAS. Six fields of computer-based craniofacial reconstruction were evaluated.

1. Secondary correction of panfacial fractures
2. Traumatic enophthalmos with or without re-osteotomy and advancement of the malar bone
3. Optic nerve decompression in the treatment of traumatic optic neuropathy
4. Navigated endoscopic frontal sinus revision after severe skull base comminution

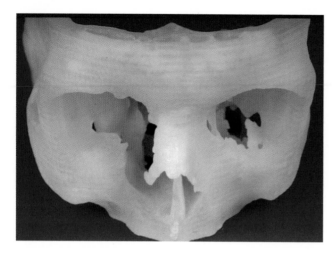

FIGURE 33-1 Stereolithographic model with a right midfacial defect. Pseudoforamina are widely present in the normal left orbit.

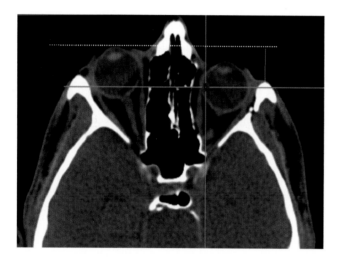

FIGURE 33-2 Axial computed tomographic (CT) view of a unilateral enophthalmos with a retruded left malar bone. The *interrupted horizontal white line* shows the intended projection for the left globe; the *perpendicular yellow line* demonstrates the CT-based Hertel's index.

BOX 33-1   Advantages of CAPP and CAS in Posttraumatic Reconstruction

- Measurement of distances
- Volume measurements (e.g., orbital contents)
- Mirroring parts of the dataset to an individually created plane with virtual reconstruction of form in definable ranges
- Virtual insertion and positioning of autologous bone grafts, realizing preoperative simulation of augmented deficient body contours
- Identifying structures at risk such as the optic nerve
- Intraoperative navigation that allows checking of the individual anatomy online and preoperative comparison of planned contour changes
- Assessment of changes between the preceding measurements and the actual CT/MRI dataset when postoperative spiral CT/MRI is performed for control

---

CAPP, computer-assisted preoperative planning; CAS, computer-assisted surgery; CT, computed tomography; MRI, magnetic resonance imaging.

5. Combined periorbital recontouring with computer-aided design and computer-aided manufacturing (CAD/CAM) of titanium implants and autologous bone grafts
6. Recontouring of severe bone and soft tissue deformities by augmentation of the contours with alloplasts (e.g., calcium phosphate cement, titanium mesh)

Starting with CAPP and CAS in 1997, the protocol for CT data acquisition was to acquire spiral CT datasets (Somatom Plus 4 scanner, Siemens, Erlangen, Germany; 1-mm collimation slice thickness, 2-mm table feed, 1-mm increment) to serve for CAPP and CAS on the STN navigation system (Surgical Tool Navigator, Stryker-Leibinger, Aalen, Germany) with STP 4.0 software (Zeiss, Oberkochen, Germany). By 2010, CT data acquisition had significantly improved, and conebeam computed tomography (CBCT) was being used for planning of even more complex craniofacial deformity and navigated surgery. Modern CBCT machines such as the Zenith (Orangedental, Biberach, Germany) allows for scanning of a field of view of 24 × 19 × 19 cm. The number of patients with craniofacial deformities we have treated using CAPP and CAS exceeds 700. Planning software nowadays is independent of the navigation system itself (i-Plan 3.0, Brainlab, Feldkirchen, Germany; Voxim 6.0, IVS-Solutions, Chemnitz, Germany); it is network-based and allows for direct combination with the navigation workstations. Furthermore, STL import and export have become standard. Virtual world (.wrl) files (including color and texture of 3-D photography) can be implemented in the DICOM data format.

Because of the insufficient accuracy of commercially available noninvasive registration systems, the combination of CAPP with virtual correction, intraoperative navigation, and postoperative control has not yet become a routine procedure in the treatment of orbital deformities. We overcame this problem by using an individual noninvasive registration system that we developed (Fig. 33-3).[18,19] Thermoplastic splints are fabricated individually by a dental technician, permitting reuse in the same patient. Occlusal splints are routinely used in the upper jaw with four markers in different XYZ axes. All four markers are kept out of artifact zones such

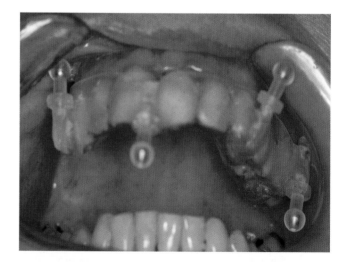

FIGURE 33-3 Noninvasive system: upper occlusal splint with four markers.

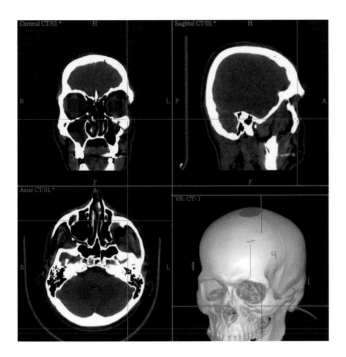

FIGURE 33-4 Multiplanar and three-dimensional view of a patient with severe left midface trauma.

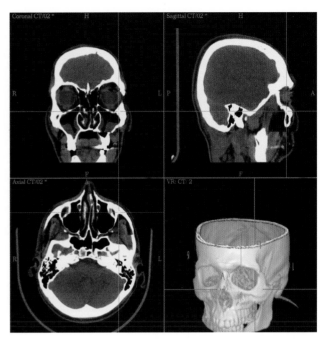

FIGURE 33-5 Same patient as in Figure 33-4. Simulation of an ideal virtual correction by mirroring of a subvolume from the unaffected right side onto the left side.

as prosthodontic restorations (see Fig. 33-3). The markers can be alternated according to the demands of the selected imaging modality (MRI, CT) and intraoperative use. The major advantage of this registration system is its easy reproduction, but it is limited in emergency cases in which quick assessment of a spiral CT dataset is mandatory (e.g., traumatic optic neuropathy) and in edentulous patients. In such cases, either temporary inserted bone markers or surface matching are used.

At the workstation itself, the full dataset can be adapted to the surgeon's requirements regarding gray scale (i.e., whether hard or soft tissues are to be weighed). On the workstation, the patient's individual anatomy is assessed in multiplanar (axial, coronal, sagittal) and 3-D views (Fig. 33-4). Virtual corrections can be made by drawing new contours or by designing virtual implants at the workstation (see Fig. 33-2). For unilateral deformities (that do not cross the midline), the mirror tool that we developed in cooperation with the Stryker-Leibinger company in 1998, permits an ideal reconstruction by superimposing the normal side over the affected or deformed side, thereby creating a new dataset (Fig. 33-5).[20] Most traumatic and tumor-related orbital deformities are unilateral, so many cases can be approached with a side-to-side comparison. In reconstructive surgery, the surgeon must define the individual plane to which the selected range of the dataset should be mirrored from the unaffected to the deformed side. The software guides the surgeon exactly through this procedure. Intraoperatively, either the native CT dataset or the modified CT dataset can be referred to, so that navigation of the intraoperatively achieved reconstruction in comparison with the preoperative virtual correction is possible at any step of the operation. The time required for setting up and using intraoperative navigation, once mastered, is an extra 30 minutes, whereas the preoperative planning takes about 1 hour.

The limit of precision of intraoperative navigation between the virtual patient on the workstation and the actual patient on the operating table is approximately 1 mm. This can be achieved by use of the aforementioned, individually fabricated occlusal thermoplastic splints with four reference markers in different XYZ positions. Experimental and clinical evaluation of this system proved this overall accuracy of 1 mm.[18]

Intraoperative navigation was performed using frameless stereotaxy (Fig. 33-6). Three infrared cameras controlled the pointer (P) via integrated light-emitting diodes (LEDs), and the patient's position was controlled by a dynamic reference frame (DRF) fixed rigidly to the Mayfield clamp.

Intraoperative pointer-based navigation with the STN workstation was used not only to navigate the present bony contours but also to check on new contours, such as surfaces augmented with autologous bone grafts, bone substitutes, or advanced facial bones (Fig. 33-7). The augmentation procedure was finished when the intraoperative situation matched the preoperatively planned virtual contours on the workstation.

CLINICAL APPLICATIONS OF CAPP AND CAS

CORRECTION OF A PANFACIAL FRACTURE

After trauma resulting in a panfacial fractures that was treated at another institution, the patient in Figure 33-8A underwent, as a first step, bilateral orbital reconstruction with autologous calvarial split-bone grafting and telecanthus correction according to the Hammer method.[1] The second step in secondary reconstruction was to perform correction of the displaced mandibulomaxillary complex by bimaxillary

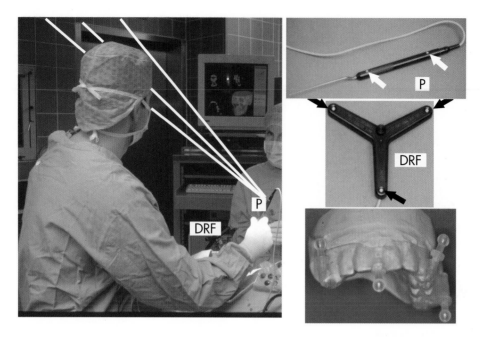

FIGURE 33-6 Setup for intraoperative navigation. The dynamic reference frame (DRF) is firmly attached to the Mayfield clamp by which the patient's position is controlled. Instrument and pointer (P) positions are monitored by integrated light-emitting diodes (LEDs). The maxillary occlusal splint with four markers in different XYZ axes allows for noninvasive referencing.

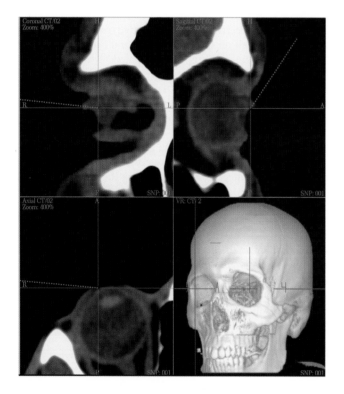

FIGURE 33-7 Same patient as in Figure 33-4. Screen capture during navigated surgery with the virtually reconstructed computed tomography (CT) dataset in multiplanar (coronal, sagittal, axial) and three-dimensional views. The pointer (dotted lines) monitors the virtually reconstructed CT dataset to determine whether the advanced left globe matches the computer-assisted preplanned contour.

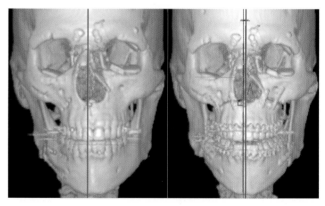

FIGURE 33-8 Three-dimensional view of a patient injured in a traffic accident who underwent correction of secondary enophthalmos and telecanthus, before (**A**) and after (**B**) repositioning of the bimaxillary complex.

re-osteotomy. CAPP was used to define the repositioning in regard to the overall asymmetry. Vectors for the ideal correction of the maxilla were defined (Fig. 33-9) and were followed during later surgery with navigational control. The bony result of the bimaxillary correction is demonstrated in Figure 33-10B. Figure 33-11 demonstrates a clinical frontal view before orbital correction and after bimaxillary surgery.

TRAUMATIC ENOPHTHALMOS WITH AND WITHOUT RE-OSTEOTOMY AND ADVANCEMENT OF THE MALAR BONE

Symmetry in orbital reconstruction is important for functional and esthetic reasons.[21] Orbital asymmetry mostly results from combined soft and hard tissue deformities

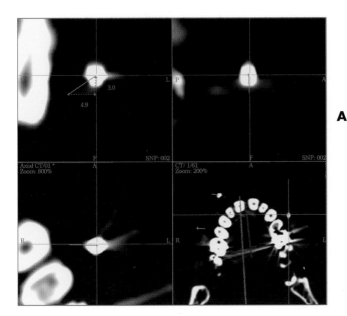

FIGURE 33-9   Same patient as in Figure 33-8. Planning of the vectors for ideal maxillary shifting. The *light blue lines* in the multiplanar view resemble the amount of movement of defined points (center of referencing points).

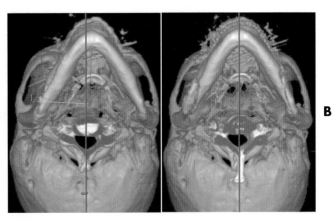

FIGURE 33-10   Same patient as in Figure 33-8. Preoperative (**A**) and postoperative (**B**) view from below showing the corrected left shift of the maxillomandibular complex.

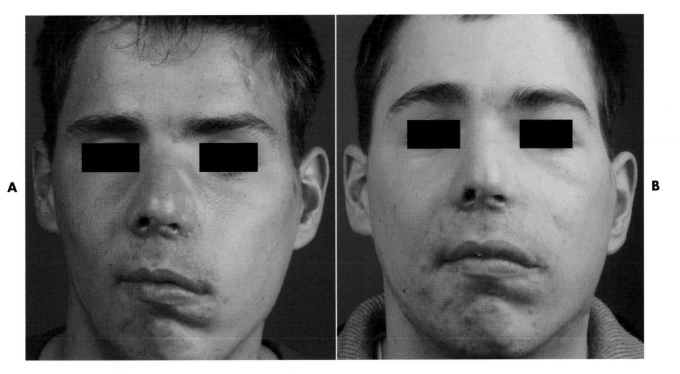

FIGURE 33-11   Same patient as in Figure 33-8. Clinical view before orbital correction (**A**) and after bimaxillary surgery (**B**).

including the orbital contents, the bony orbit, and the periorbital soft tissues including the canthal ligaments.

Enophthalmos due to the enlargement of orbital volume is a severe complication in traumatic orbital deformities if primary reconstruction cannot be correctly achieved.[22]

Particularly in traumatic orbital deformities, measurement of sagittal globe projection can be done in the same position at the workstation as if the patient were on the operating table.[23] The sagittal projection of the globe can be virtually marked and corrected (see Fig. 33-2). The globe projection changes

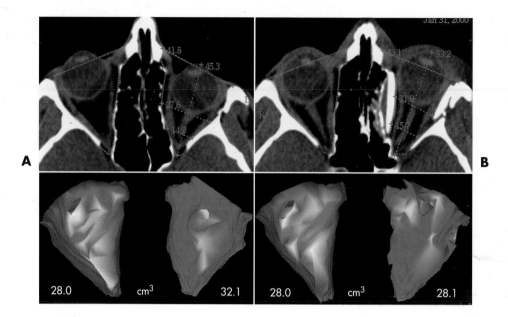

FIGURE 33-12   Axial computed tomographic images from a patient with left enophthalmos before (**A**) and after (**B**) correction with corresponding bilateral orbital volumes. The figures show a 4.0 cm³ reduction in orbital enlargement on the left side.

can be measured in reference to the corneal surface and the optic canal entrance; the latter is the most reliable landmark in traumatic patients as far as quantifying sagittal changes in orbital contents is concerned (Fig. 33-12). In addition to measuring functions, the software permits 3-D evaluation of orbital contents with individual figures (see Fig. 33-12). With this method, the orbits can be directly compared to each other and the postoperative outcome can be objectively quantified.

The average decrease after single orbital reconstruction in a group of 18 secondary traumatic enophthalmos corrections was 4.0 ± 1.9 cm³, or 65% of an average adult eye-globe volume; the average overcorrection of sagittal globe projection was 2.7 mm.[16] However, the clinical outcome, which was achieved in all patients by only one operation, seems to justify this temporary excess in sagittal globe projection, because there is always a certain relapse in globe projection after enophthalmos correction.

Figure 33-13A shows a patient with right enophthalmos caused by midface trauma sustained 2 years earlier. The right malar bone and orbital frame were retruded. In addition, the patient showed right temporal hollowing, eyebrow displacement, telecanthus, and a displaced lateral canthal ligament. The right malar bone with the superior-lateral periorbital frame was advanced via a coronal approach. Hollowing caused by temporalis muscle atrophy was reconstructed by augmentation of the right temporal region with a calvarial split-bone graft. The orbit was recontoured using calvarial split-bone grafts. The right medial and lateral canthal ligaments were repositioned. Figure 33-13B shows the postoperative result after reconstruction of the enlarged orbit with autologous split-bone grafts. During the operation, the bone graft position can be checked by navigation at any moment, as can the distance to highly vulnerable structures such as the optic nerve (Fig. 33-14).[23] For intraoperative navigation, the mirrored dataset was used as a virtual model for the intended

ideal reconstruction. The individually mirrored plane and the extension of vertical, sagittal, and transverse ranges to be mirrored have to be selected at the workstation. This method of superimposing a contour by mirroring results in a virtual template that can serve directly for intraoperative navigation and postoperative control is an easy way to achieve symmetry. The postoperative evaluation of the orbital volumes showed a clear improvement on the corrected side; the decrease in orbital volume in this patient was 80% that of an average adult globe volume (Fig. 33-15).

All patients with secondary enophthalmos corrections were operated on using a coronal combined with a transconjunctival approach. In patients with additional malar bone advancement, an intraoral incision was added.

Figure 33-16 shows a screen capture obtained during navigational control for reconstruction of the left medial orbital wall in which the mirrored dataset from the patient in Figures 33-4, 33-5, and 33-7 was used intraoperatively. The surgical plan included advancement of the retruded left malar bone and augmentation of the left orbit. Figures 33-17 and 33-18 show different 3-D views for preoperative planning and simulation and postoperative control.

In primary unilateral orbital reconstructions with severe destruction of the bony frame and orbital cone, navigated surgery can be performed based on an online side-to-side comparison. Figure 33-19 shows a screen capture during reconstruction of the left orbital floor in a comminuted midface fracture. The tip of the dotted line equals the tip of the pointer checking on the orbital floor that was primarily reconstructed with the use of autologous calvarial split-bone grafts. During the operation the bone graft position can be checked by navigation at any moment, as can the distance to highly vulnerable structures such as the optic nerve (Fig. 33-20). Figure 33-21 demonstrates multiple 3-D and multiplanar views to control the preoperative and postoperative CT scans (Figs. 33-21A and 33-21B, respectively). In addition

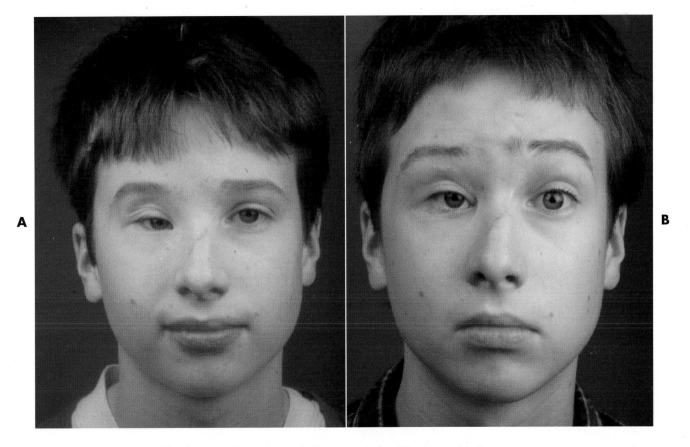

FIGURE 33-13   Clinical frontal views before (**A**) and after (**B**) right enophthalmos correction.

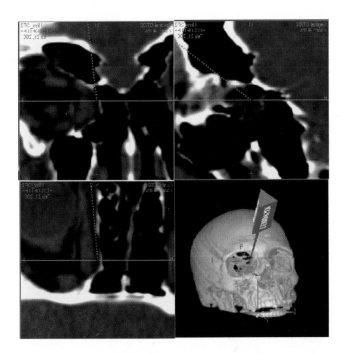

FIGURE 33-14   Same patient as in Figure 33-13. Intraoperative screen capture during navigated orbital reconstruction. With the pointer-based navigated surgery *(dotted line)*, the virtually reconstructed computed tomographic dataset can be used, for example, to determine whether the intraoperatively augmented medial orbital wall matches the computer-assisted preplanned contour.

to the craniomaxillofacial reconstruction, neurosurgical colleagues performed a left anterior skull base revision via a frontal osteoplastic approach.

OPTIC NERVE DECOMPRESSION FOR TREATMENT OF TRAUMATIC OPTIC NEUROPATHY

Among the various therapeutic options in the treatment of traumatic optic neuropathy, surgical optic nerve decompression is an important choice, especially if there is evidence of fractures in the posterior third of the orbit or the optic canal. In addition to clinical ophthalmological findings, the decision of whether to decompress can be based on electrophysiological evidence (i.e., flash visual-evoked potentials).[23]

The operation is performed with the use of a surgical microscope. Preoperative planning of the surgical approach can be transferred to the visual field of the microscope to guide the surgeon to the optic canal (Fig. 33-22). The focus of the microscope is correlated to the CT dataset so that the surgeon is able to identify the anatomical structures visualized through the microscope by watching the CT scan at any time (Fig. 33-23). With the use of frameless stereotaxy, the decompression of the optic nerve in trauma or tumor cases becomes a safe and minimally invasive procedure. The multiplanar CT shows a fracture in the bony optic canal as the radiological correlate for a bony lesion representing the pathophysiological mechanism for the optic nerve injury. The same CT dataset that was scanned for the primary

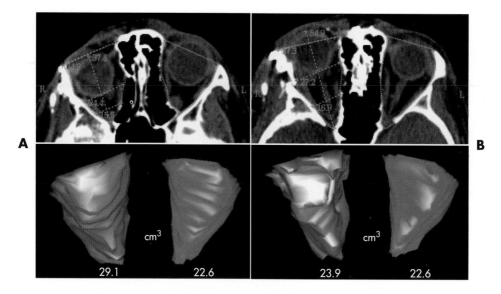

FIGURE 33-15 Axial computed tomographic images from the patient in Figure 33-13 showing the orbital region with corresponding bilateral orbital volumes before (**A**) and after (**B**) operation. Right orbital volume was decreased by 5.2 cm³.

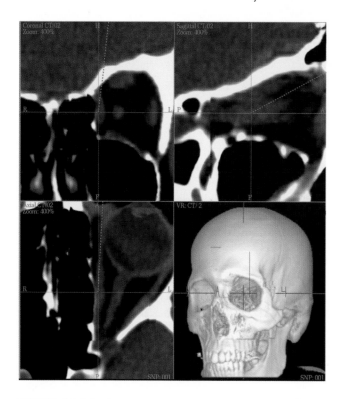

FIGURE 33-16 Same patient as in Figures 33-4, 33-5, and 33-7. Multiplanar and three-dimensional screen capture during navigated control of medial orbital wall augmentation. The tip of the pointer *(dotted line)* shows the correct reconstructed contour of the medial orbital wall compared with the mirrored dataset, resembling the ideal reconstruction. New position on top of the augmented calvarial grafts.

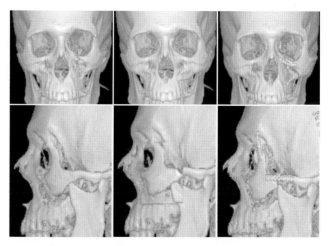

FIGURE 33-17 Frontal and lateral three-dimensional computed tomographic views from the patient in Figures 33-4, 33-5, 33-7, and 33-16 preoperatively, after simulation, and postoperatively.

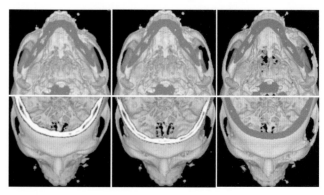

FIGURE 33-18 Bird's-eye and worm's-eye three-dimensional computed tomographic views from the patient in Figures 33-4, 33-5, 33-7, 33-16, and 33-17 preoperatively, after simulation, and postoperatively.

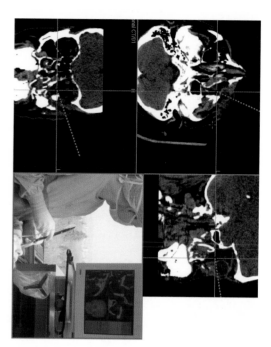

FIGURE 33-19 Screen capture from a patient with a comminuted left orbital fracture undergoing navigation-controlled primary orbital reconstruction. The pointer (dotted line) marks the intended position of the orbital floor to be reconstructed (i.e., side-by-side split grafts or titanium mesh can be contoured).

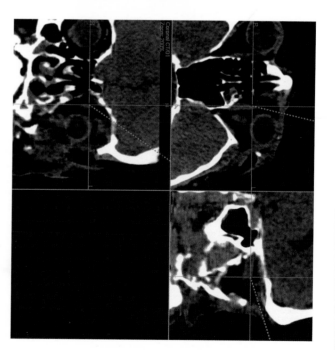

FIGURE 33-20 Same patient as in Figure 33-19. Screen capture during reconstruction of the left medial orbital wall. The dotted line represents the pointer; the tip of the pointer checks for the contour of the inserted calvarial split-bone grafts.

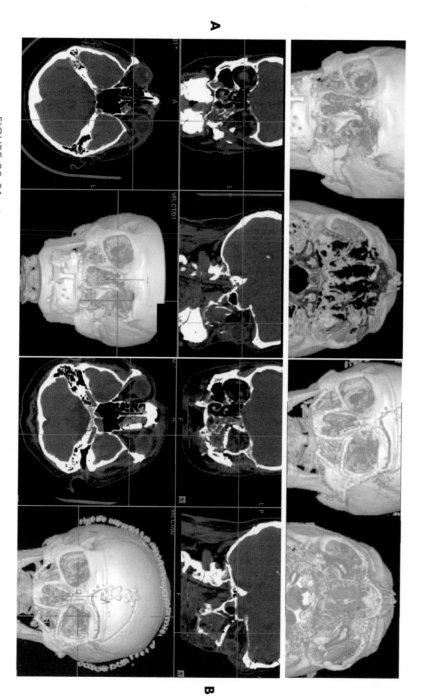

A

B

FIGURE 33-21 Same patient as in Figure 33-19. Control of preoperative (A) and postoperative (B) three-dimensional and multiplanar views.

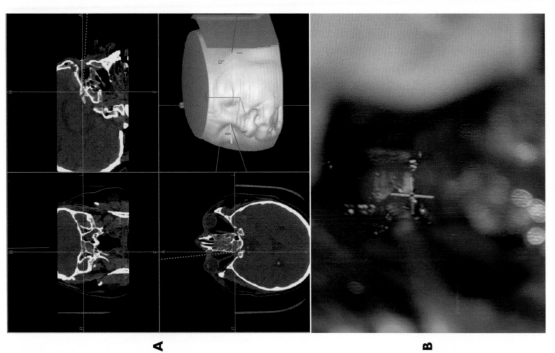

A

B

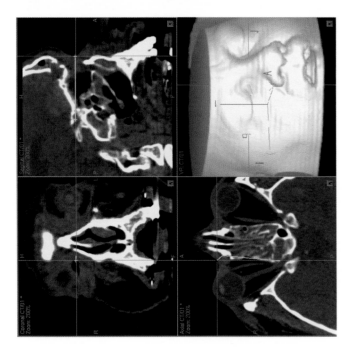

FIGURE 33-22 Computer-assisted preoperative planning of the approach for optic nerve decompression in multiplanar and three-dimensional views of a patient with a right traumatic optic nerve lesion.

craniofacial diagnostic workup can also be used for intraoperative navigation. The only prerequisite is that during the CT scanning process a registration system has to be applied to the patient. In this emergency situation, we used a prefabricated upper occlusal splint, mounted with the aforementioned four markers and filled with a silicone-based impression material. Intraoperatively, the CT dataset and the patient on the operating table could easily be matched by using the scanned four reference points.

Figure 33-23 shows an intraoperative screen capture in a multiplanar view during the transnasal/transethmoidal optic nerve decompression. Figures 33-24A and 33-24B compare the matched preoperative and postoperative views in the coronal and axial planes.

NAVIGATED ENDOSCOPIC FRONTAL SINUS REVISION AFTER SEVERE SKULL BASE COMMINUTION

After a car accident, a male adult patient lost his frontal bones due to major infection in the comminuted frontal sinus and ethmoidal area (Fig. 33-25A). Before reconstruction of the neurocranium, the severely deformed frontoethmoidal region was operated on with tracked endoscopic minimally invasive surgery (Figs. 33-26 and 33-27). The axis and the tip of the endoscope are indicated by a dotted line (see Fig. 33-27, inset). Figures 33-26 and 33-27 show the clinical view and Figure 33-27, inset, demonstrates a screen capture during tracked endoscopic surgery. Secondarily, a CAD/CAM-titanium implant (Cranio Construct Bochum, Bochum, Germany) was inserted to reconstruct the major frontal defect. Figure 33-28 shows the intraoperative lateral view, Figure 33-25B demonstrates the clinical view 10 days after reconstruction. Today,

FIGURE 33-23 Same patient as in Figure 33-22. **A,** Intraoperative multiplanar and three-dimensional views (screen capture) during navigated optic nerve decompression. **B,** The tip of the dotted line in **A** is correlated with the focus of the microscope, in which the optic nerve (cross-marked in the microscopic view) can be seen.

even in such cases, CBCT might be regarded as appropriate for acquiring 3-D data.[24]

COMBINED MALAR BONE ADVANCEMENT WITH CUSTOM-MADE TITANIUM IMPLANT

After a close gunshot injury, the subject of the CT scan in Figure 33-29 suffered from gross middle and upper facial deformity and was admitted for secondary reconstruction to our department. Figure 33-29 shows the eye prosthesis in place in the left deformed orbit. Before surgery, a titanium implant was custom-fabricated by computer numerical control (CNC) milling on the basis of a virtually ideally reconstructed subvolume of the CT dataset (Cranio Construct Bochum).

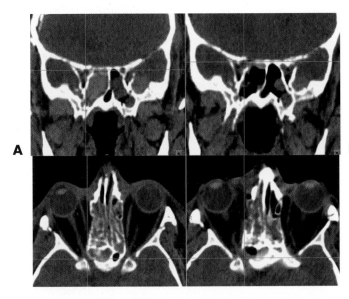

FIGURE 33-24 Same patient as in Figure 33-22. Matched preoperative (**A**) and postoperative (**B**) axial and coronal views. After transethmoidal optic nerve decompression, the bony ring of the optic canal has been opened.

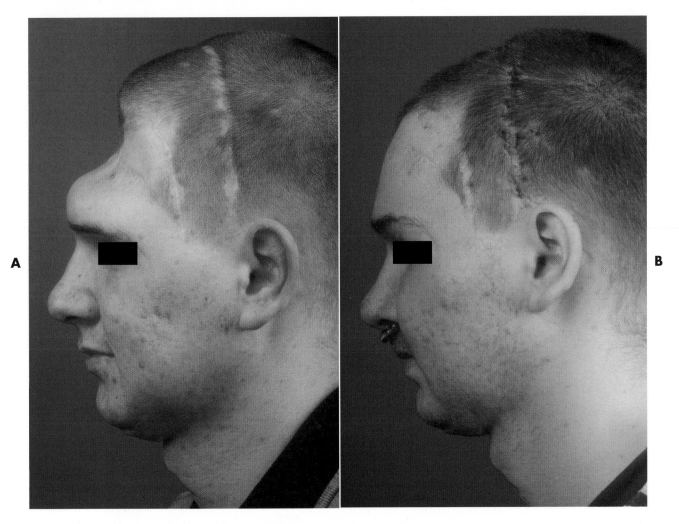

FIGURE 33-25 Preoperative (**A**) and 10 days postoperative (**B**) lateral views of a patient with an extended bifrontal defect sustained in a car accident.

The first step was to position the individual titanium implant in the left bifrontotemporal region, and the second step was re-osteotomy of the left malar bone and navigationally controlled advancement and fixation of the bone segment. For better control, the mirror tool was preoperatively applied again to achieve an ideal reconstructed virtual model.[16] This

served intraoperatively for navigated control of the advancement of the left malar bone segment before rigid fixation (Fig. 33-30). In a third step, an additional autologous calvarial split-bone graft was used to augment the left temporal hollowing, which was caused by severe muscle loss. The mirrored dataset was used again to check on the preplanned contours in the temporal region. Figures 33-31 and 33-32 show postoperative multiplanar and 3-D views, and Figure 33-32 demonstrates the correct reconstruction of the deficient left temporal region.

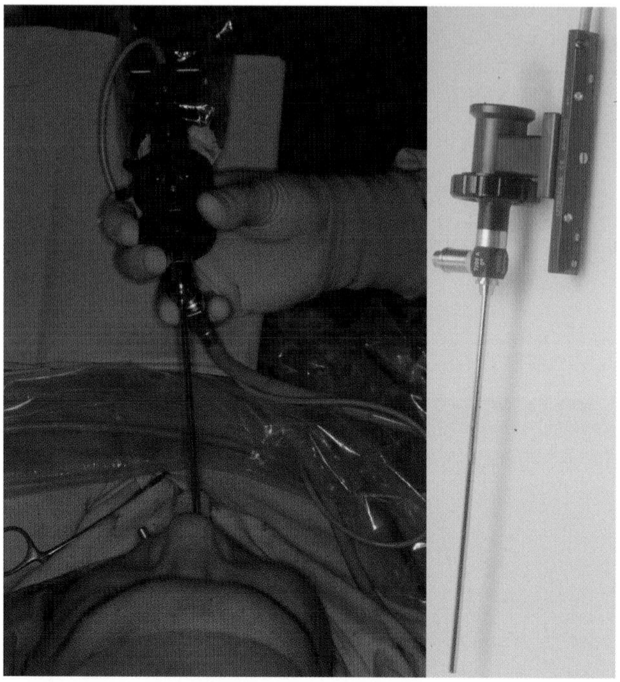

FIGURE 33-26 Same patient as in Figure 33-25. Bird's-eye view during navigated endoscopic surgery with a tracked endoscope *(right)*.

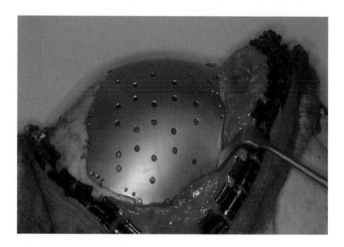

FIGURE 33-28 Same patient as in Figure 33-25. Intraoperative lateral view during secondary bifrontal reconstruction with a commercially available custom-made titanium implant (Cranio Construct Bochum, Bochum, Germany).

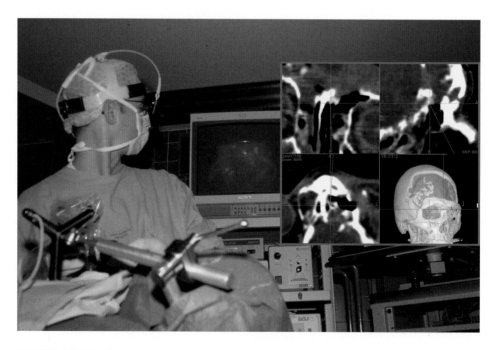

FIGURE 33-27 Same patient as in Figure 33-25. Intraoperative overview during computer-assisted endoscopic surgery. A multiplanar and three-dimensional view of the same patient *(inset)* is available to the surgeon in real time. The tip of the *dotted green line* marks the tip of the tracked endoscope.

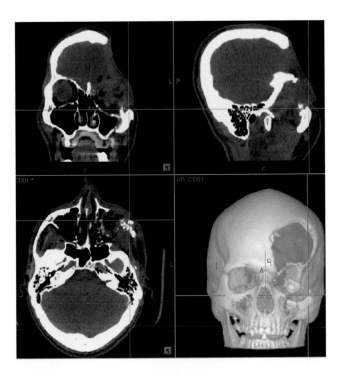

FIGURE 33-29 Multiplanar and three-dimensional view of a patient's computed tomographic dataset after a closely fired gunshot wound shows extended left soft and hard tissue loss.

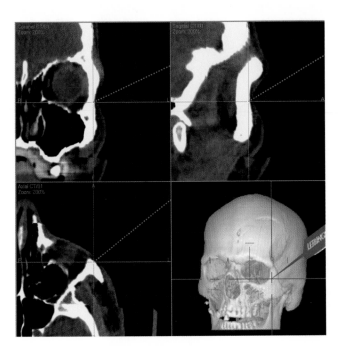

FIGURE 33-30 Same patient as in Figure 33-29. Intraoperative screen capture during navigated control of repositioning of the advanced left malar bone complex. The tip of the *dotted line* indicates the pointer tip. The correct position for the lateral orbital rim is achieved according to the virtually reconstructed dataset demonstrated here.

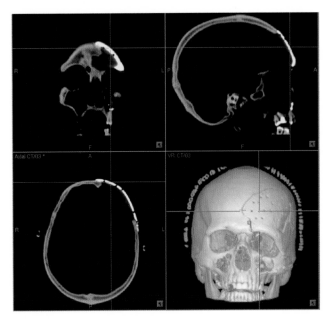

FIGURE 33-31 Same patient as in Figure 33-29. Postoperative multiplanar and three-dimensional view.

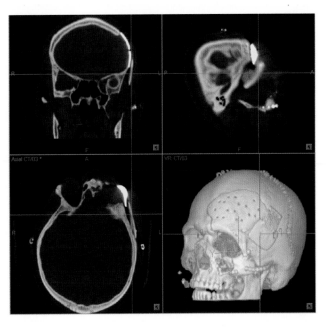

FIGURE 33-32 Same patient as in Figure 33-29. Postoperative multiplanar and three-dimensional view shows additional bone grafting to overcome the temporal hollowing.

RECONTOURING OF SEVERE BONE AND SOFT TISSUE DEFORMITIES BY AUGMENTATION OF THE CONTOURS WITH CALCIUM PHOSPHATE CEMENT

The preoperative CT scan in a multiplanar view (Fig. 33-33) shows a left periorbital and temporal bony and soft tissue defect after an osteoplastic trepanation without osseous reintegration of the temporal bone. The first step was to virtually ideally reconstruct the patient before operation by mirroring

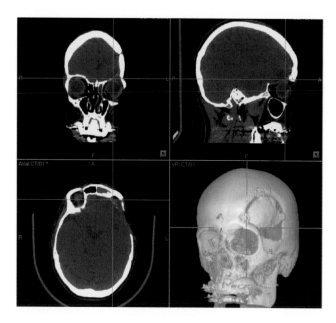

FIGURE 33-33 Preoperative multiplanar and three-dimensional view from a patient with left temporo-orbital soft and hard tissue loss.

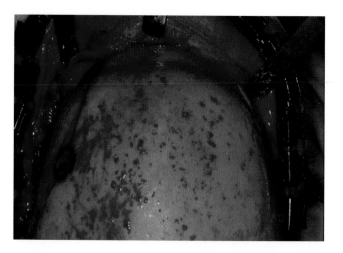

FIGURE 33-35 Same patient as in Figure 33-33. Clinical view from above after exposure of the deficient left temporo-orbital region via a bicoronal approach.

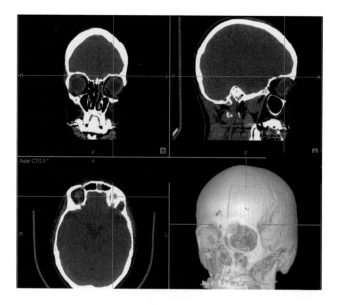

FIGURE 33-34 Same patient as in Figure 33-33. Corresponding views after virtual reconstruction with application of the mirror tool.

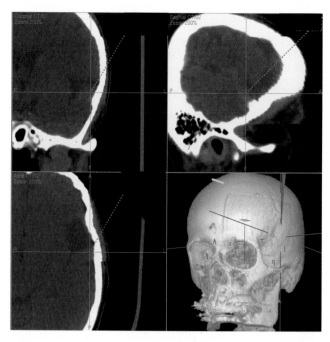

FIGURE 33-36 Same patient as in Figure 33-33. Intraoperative screen capture pointing at the surface of the deficient temporal region (tip of dotted line) in the virtually ideally reconstructed computed tomographic dataset.

a subvolume of the CT dataset from the unaffected right side onto the left side (Fig. 33-34). Intraoperatively (Fig. 33-35), autologous calvarial split-bone grafts were used to recontour the left orbit, and calcium phosphate cement served for recontouring of the severe left temporal hollowing. Figure 33-36 shows a screen capture obtained during navigation with the mirrored dataset; the pointer is checking the contour during reconstruction. To reduce the amount of calcium phosphate cement, a calvarial split-bone graft was used as an onlay graft to the forehead.

The intraoperatively achieved augmentation was stopped when it matched the preplanned contours (Fig. 33-37). Figure 33-38 shows postoperative CT multiplanar and 3-D views after recontouring of the periorbital and temporal left defect. Figure 33-39 shows matching of lateral 3-D views (preoperative, ideally virtually reconstructed, and postoperative CT datasets) of the same patient on the workstation of the STN navigation system.

The noninvasive registration system marked by radio-opaque spheres has been patented by the authors.

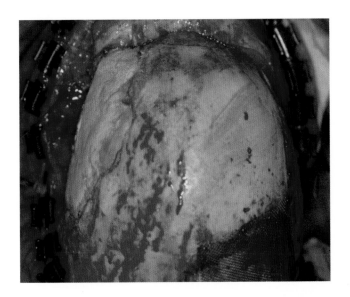

FIGURE 33-37   Same patient as in Figure 33-33. Clinical view corresponding to Figure 33-35 after augmentation of the left frontotemporo-orbital region with calcium phosphate cement.

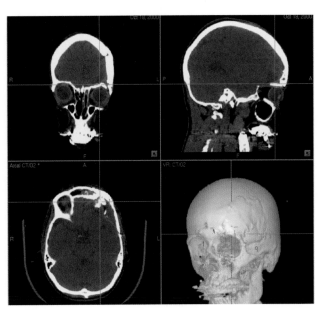

FIGURE 33-38   Same patient as in Figure 33-33. Postoperative multiplanar and three-dimensional view corresponding to Figures 33-33 (preoperative) and 33-34 (virtually reconstructed).

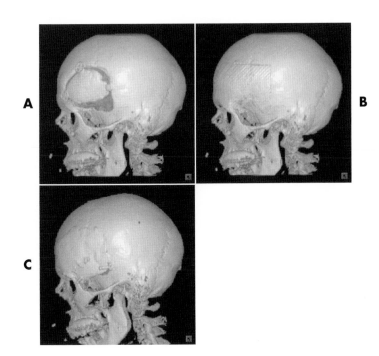

FIGURE 33-39   Same patient as in Figure 33-3. Matched lateral preoperative (**A**), simulated (**B**), and postoperative (**C**) three-dimensional computed tomographic views.

PRIMARY TRAUMATIC ORBITAL RECONSTRUCTION: STL MODELING AND PATIENT-SPECIFIC PREOPERATIVE IMPLANT MANUFACTURING VERSUS STANDARDIZED PREFORMED ORBITAL PLATES

A patient suffered a two-wall fracture of the right medial orbital wall and orbital floor as the result of an assault. Figure 33-40 shows the preoperative sagittal and coronal conebeam data acquired with the Zenith machine (Orange-dental). Preoperatively, an STL model was virtually manufactured using Brainlab software i-Plan 3.0 (Feldkirchen, Germany) (Fig. 33-41); after the STL file was exported, a custom-made, laser-sintered model was fabricated (Fig. 33-42), which allowed prefabrication of a patient-specific two-wall orbital implant (Fig. 33-43). This implant was compared with a standardized preformed orbital wall plate (Synthes, West Chester, Penn).

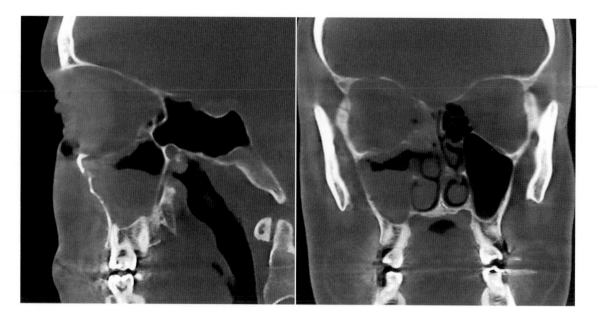

FIGURE 33-40 Preoperative sagittal and coronal conebeam data from a patient with a two-wall fracture of the right medial orbital wall and orbital floor.

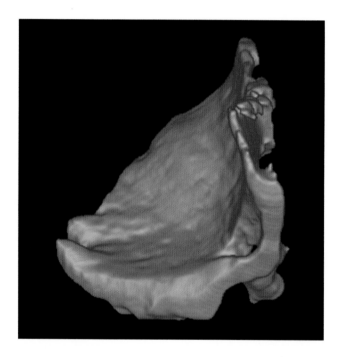

FIGURE 33-41 Same patient as in Figure 33-40. Stereolithographic (STL) model preoperatively manufactured virtually.

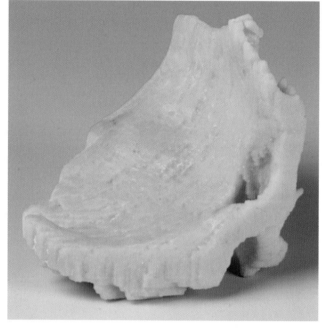

FIGURE 33-42 Same patient as in Figure 33-40. Custom-made laser-sintered model fabricated after exporting of the stereolithography (STL) file.

Figure 33-44 shows a frontal view of the two implants, with the standardized preformed plate on top of the patient-specific two-wall orbital implant (based on a Synthes fanplate orbital implant). The decision to use a patient-specific implant was made because of the vertical discrepancy in this specific case, although the overall precision of the standardized preformed plates is very satisfying in many cases. The implant was inserted via a retroseptal transconjunctival approach with a retrocaruncular extension to the medial orbital wall

(Fig. 33-45). Positioning of a perfect lid on the corresponding pot resp. of a perfectly shaped orbital implant in the injured orbit was checked by intraoperative navigation with the Brainlab navigation system (Colibri); the postoperative conebeam scan shows the orbital implant in its appropriate position (Fig. 33-46). Figure 33-47 shows the preoperative and 4 weeks postoperative view from below.

The future of computer-assisted planning and surgery is more and more directed towards an effective use of

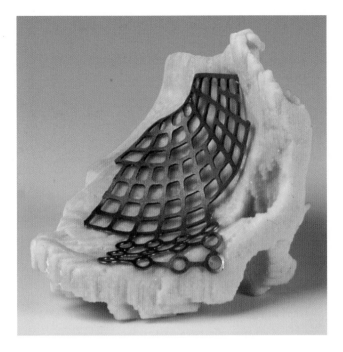

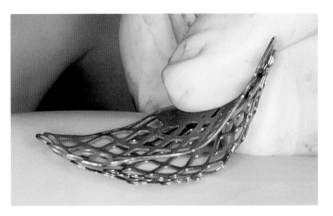

FIGURE 33-44 Same patient as in Figure 33-40. Frontal view of the implant from Figure 33-43 compared with a standardized preformed orbital wall plate (on top).

FIGURE 33-43 Same patient as in Figure 33-40. Prefabricated patient-specific two-wall orbital implant.

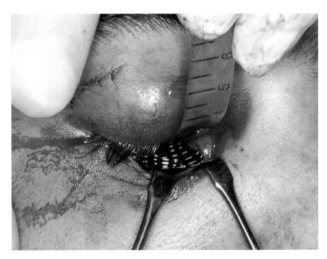

FIGURE 33-45 Same patient as in Figure 33-40. Insertion of the patient-specific two-wall orbital implant via a retroseptal transconjunctival approach with a retrocaruncular extension to the medial orbital wall.

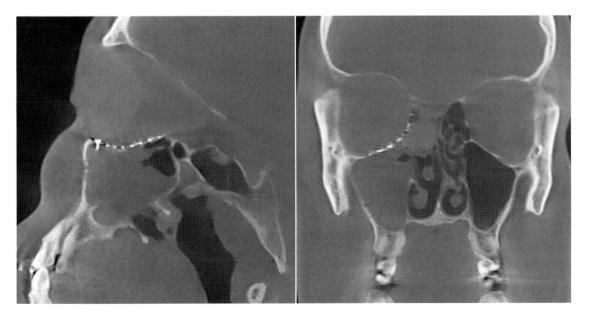

FIGURE 33-46 Same patient as in Figure 33-40. Postoperative conebeam scan shows appropriate position of the orbital implant.

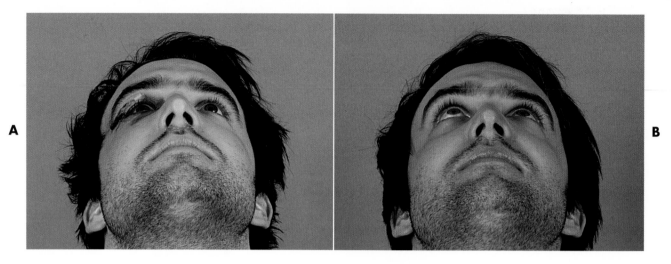

FIGURE 33-47 Same patient as in Figure 33-40. Preoperative (**A**) and 4 weeks postoperative (**B**) views from below.

preoperative, intraoperative, and postoperative phases, to improve the quality of the surgical outcomes. This must be integrated with rigorous audit of those outcomes.[25-30]

REFERENCES

1. Hammer B, Prein J: Correction of post-traumatic orbital deformities: operative techniques and review of 26 patients. *J Craniomaxillofac Surg* 23:81-90, 1995.

2. Howard G, Osguthorpe JD: Concepts in orbital reconstruction. *Otolaryngol Clin North Am* 30:541-562, 1997.

3. Kawamoto HK Jr: Late posttraumatic enophthalmos: a correctable deformity? *Plast Reconstr Surg* 69:423-432, 1982.

4. Manson PN, Grivas A, Rosenbaum A, et al: Studies on enophthalmos. II. The measurement of orbital injuries and their treatment by quantitative computed tomography. *Plast Reconstr Surg* 77:203-214, 1985.

5. Schmelzeisen R, Husstedt H, Zumkeller M, et al: Profilerhalt und Verbesserung bei primärer und sekundärer Orbitarekonstruktion. *Mund Kiefer Gesichtschir* 1(suppl 1):87-89, 1997.

6. Eufinger H, Wittkampf AR, Wehmoller M, et al: Single-step fronto-orbital resection and reconstruction with individual resection template and corresponding titanium implant: a new method of computer-aided surgery. *J Craniomaxillofac Surg* 26:373-378, 1998.

7. Heissler E, Fischer FS, Bolouri S, et al: Custom-made cast titanium implants produced with CAD/CAM for the reconstruction of cranium defects. *Int J Oral Maxillofac Surg* 27:334-338, 1998.

8. Hoffmann J, Cornelius CP, Groten M, et al: Orbital reconstruction with individually copy-milled ceramic implants. *Plast Reconstr Surg* 101:604-612, 1998.

9. Holck DE, Boyd EM Jr, Mauffray RO: Benefits of stereolithography in orbital reconstruction. *Ophthalmology* 106:1214-1218, 1999.

10. Luka B, Brechtelsbauer D, Gellrich NC, et al: 2-D and 3-D reconstructions of the facial skeleton: an unnecessary option or a diagnostic pearl? *Int J Oral Maxillofac Surg* 21:99-103, 1995.

11. Perry M, Banks P, Richards R, et al: The use of computer-generated three-dimensional models in orbital reconstruction. *Br J Oral Maxillofac Surg* 36:275-284, 1998.

12. Haßfeld S, Mühling J, Zöller J: Intraoperative navigation in oral and maxillofacial surgery. *Int J Oral Maxillofac Surg* 24:111-119, 1995.

13. Marmulla R, Niederdellmann H: Computer-aided navigation in secondary reconstruction of post-traumatic deformities of the zygoma. *J Craniomaxillofac Surg* 26:68-69, 1998.

14. Watzinger F, Wanschitz F, Wagner A, et al: Computer-aided navigation in secondary reconstruction of post-traumatic deformities of the zygoma. *J Craniomaxillofac Surg* 25:198-202, 1997.

15. Wirtz CR, Knauth M, Hassfeld S, et al: Neuronavigation: first experiences with three different commercially available systems. *Zentralbl Neurochir* 59:14-22, 1998.

16. Gellrich NC, Schramm A, Hammer B, et al: Computer-assisted secondary reconstructions of unilateral posttraumatic orbital deformities. *Plast Reconstr Surg* 110:1417-1429, 2002.

17. Ilankovan V, Jackson IT: Experience in the use of calvarial bone grafts in orbital reconstruction. *Br J Oral Maxillofac Surg* 30:92-96, 1992.

18. Schramm A, Gellrich NC, Naumann S, et al: Non-invasive referencing in computer assisted surgery. *Med Biol Eng Comput* 37(suppl):644i5, 1999.

19. Schramm A, Gellrich NC, Schimming R, et al: Rechnergestützte Insertion von Zygomaticus-Implantaten (Brånemark System(r)) nach ablativer Tumorchirurgie. *Mund Kiefer Gesichtschir* 4:292-295, 2000.

20. Gellrich NC, Schramm A, Hammer B, et al: The value of computer-aided planning and intraoperative navigation in orbital reconstruction. *Int J Oral Maxillofac Surg* 28(suppl 1):52-53, 1999.

21. Gruss JS: Naso-ethmoid-orbital fractures: classification and role of primary bone-grafting. *Plast Reconstr Surg* 75:303-317, 1985.

22. Manson PN, Ruas EJ, Iliff NT: Deep orbital reconstruction for correction of post-traumatic enophthalmos. *Clin Plast Surg* 14:113-121, 1987.

23. Gellrich NC: Controversies and state of the art in therapy of optic nerve lesions in craniofacial traumatology and surgery. *Mund Kiefer Gesichtschir* 3:176-194, 1999.

24. von See C, Bormann KH, Schumann P, et al: Forensic imaging of projectiles using cone-beam computed tomography. *Forensic Sci Int* 190:38-41, 2009.

25. Stuehmer C, Essig H, Bormann KH, et al: Cone beam CT imaging of airgun injuries to the craniomaxillofacial region. *Int J Oral Maxillofac Surg* 37:903-906, 2008.

26. Schramm A, Suarez-Cunqueiro MM, Rücker M, et al: Computer-assisted therapy in orbital and mid-facial reconstructions. *Int J Med Robot Comput Assist Surg* 5:111-124, 2009.

27. Kokemueller H, Zizelmann C, Tavassol F, et al: A comprehensive approach to objective quantification of orbital dimensions. *J Oral Maxillofac Surg* 66:401-407, 2008.

28. Metzger MC, Schön R, Tetzlaf R, et al: Topographical CT-data analysis of the human orbital floor. *Int J Oral Maxillofac Surg* 36:45-53, 2007.

29. Metzger MC, Schön R, Tetzlaf R, et al: Anatomical 3-dimensional pre-bent titanium implant for orbital floor fractures. *Ophthalmology* 113:1863-1868, 2006.

30. Metzger MC, Hohlweg-Majert B, Schön R, et al: Verification of clinical precision after computer-aided reconstruction in craniomaxillofacial surgery. *Oral Surg Oral Med Oral Pathol Oral Radiol Endod* 104:1-10, 2007.

Index

Note: Page numbers followed by f refer to figures; page numbers followed by t refer to tables; page numbers followed by b refer to boxes.